HODGKIN'S DISEASE

HODGKIN'S DISEASE

Editors

Peter M. Mauch, M.D.
Professor of Radiation Oncology
Harvard Medical School
Associate Chief
Department of Radiation Oncology
Brigham and Women's Hospital
Dana-Farber Cancer Institute
Boston, Massachusetts

James O. Armitage, M.D.
Professor and Chairman
Department of Internal Medicine
Section of Oncology and Hematology
University of Nebraska Medical Center
Omaha, Nebraska

Volker Diehl, M.D.
Professor and Chairman
Department of Internal Medicine
Klinik I für Innere Medizin
der Universität zu Köln
Köln, Germany

Richard T. Hoppe, M.D., F.A.C.R.
Henry S. Kaplan-Harry Lebeson Professor
of Cancer Biology and Chairman
Department of Radiation Oncology
Stanford University
Stanford, California

Lawrence M. Weiss, M.D.
Chairman
Department of Pathology
City of Hope National Medical Center
Duarte, California

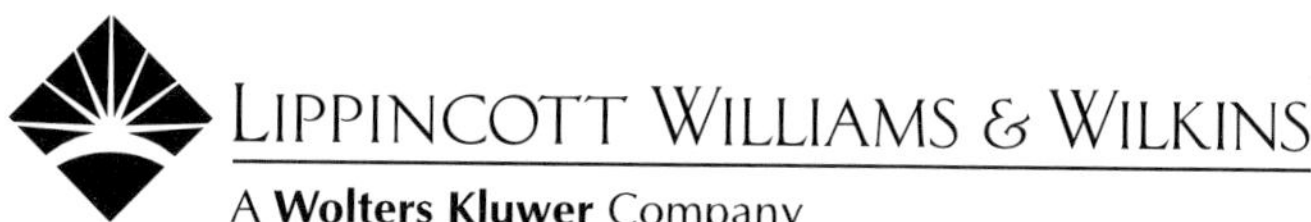

Philadelphia • Baltimore • New York • London
Buenos Aires • Hong Kong • Sydney • Tokyo

Acquisitions Editor: Stuart Freeman
Developmental Editor: Joyce A. Murphy
Manufacturing Manager: Tim Reynolds
Production Manager: Liane Carita
Production Editor: Tony DeGeorge
Cover Designer: Mark Lerner
Indexer: Robert Elwood
Compositor: Lippincott Williams & Wilkins Desktop Division
Printer: Edwards Brothers

Printed in the United States of America

9 8 7 6 5 4 3 2 1

Library of Congress Cataloging-in-Publication Data
Hodgkin's disease/Peter M. Mauch ... [et al.].
p. cm.
Includes bibliographical references and index.
ISBN 0-7817-1502-4 (alk. paper)
1. Hodgkin's disease. I. Mauch, Peter M.
[DNLM: 1. Hodgkin Disease. WH 500 H689231 1999]
RC644.H622 1999
616.99'446—dc21
DNLM/DLC
for Library of Congress 98-55677
CIP

Care has been taken to confirm the accuracy of the information presented and to describe generally accepted practices. However, the authors, editors, and publisher are not responsible for errors or omissions or for any consequences from application of the information in this book and make no warranty, expressed or implied, with respect to the contents of the publication.

The authors, editors, and publisher have exerted every effort to ensure that drug selection and dosage set forth in this text are in accordance with current recommendations and practice at the time of publication. However, in view of ongoing research, changes in government regulations, and the constant flow of information relating to drug therapy and drug reactions, the reader is urged to check the package insert for each drug for any change in indications and dosage and for added warnings and precautions. This is particularly important when the recommended agent is a new or infrequently employed drug.

Some drugs and medical devices presented in this publication have Food and Drug Administration (FDA) clearance for limited use in restricted research settings. It is the responsibility of the health care provider to ascertain the FDA status of each drug or device planned for use in their clinical practice.

To the memory of Henry S. Kaplan, clinician, teacher, and scientist, who was responsible for major contributions to our understanding of the natural history and treatment of Hodgkin's disease.

Contents

Contributors

Richard F. Ambinder, M.D.
Department of Oncology, Pharmacology, and Pathology
Johns Hopkins University School of Medicine
Baltimore, Maryland

James O. Armitage, M.D.
Professor and Chairman
Department of Internal Medicine
Section of Oncology and Hematology
University of Nebraska
Omaha, Nebraska

Michael Barton, M.D.
Associate Professor
Department of Medicine
University of New South Wales
Roadwick, New South Wales, Australia;
Research Director
Collaboration for Cancer Outcomes Research and Evaluation
Liverpool Hospital
Elizabeth Street
Liverpool, New South Wales, New Australia

Werner Bezwoda, M.D.
Department of Medicine
University of the Witatersrand
Parktown, South Africa

Philip J. Bierman, M.D.
Associate Professor
Department of Internal Medicine
Section of Oncology and Hematology
University of Nebraska
Omaha, Nebraska

Johan M. Björkholm, M.D., Ph.D.
Professor of Medicine
Department of Medicine
Karolinska Institute and Hospital
Stockholm, Sweden

Gianni Bonadonna, M.D., F.R.C.P.
Director, Division of Medical Oncology
Chief, Department of Medicine
Istituto Nazionale Tumori
Milan, Italy

Jürgen H. Bramswig, M.D.
Professor
Department of Pediatrics
University of Münster;
Department of Pediatrics
University Children's Hospital
Münster, Germany

Fernando Cabanillas, M.D.
Professor of Medicine and Chairman
Department of Lymphoma-Myeloma
M.D. Anderson Cancer Center
University of Texas
Houston, Texas

George P. Canellos, M.D., F.R.C.P., Sc.D. (Hon.)
William Rosenberg Professor of Medicine
Department of Medicine
Harvard Medical School;
Senior Physician
Department of Adult Oncology
Dana-Farber Cancer Institute
Boston, Massachusetts

Antonino Carbone, M.D.
Associate Professor
Department of Pathology
University of Padua
Padua, Italy;
Chief
Department of Pathology
Centro di Riferimento Oncologico,
Instituto Nazionale Tumori
Aviano, Italy

Patrice Carde, M.D.
Professor, Chief of Service
Department of Medicine Oncology/Hematology
Institute Gustave-Roussy
Villejuif, France

Angelo M. Carella, M.D., Ph.D.
Coordinator
Department of Hematology
Azienda Ospedale/Università
Genova, Italy

Ronald A. Castellino, M.D.
Professor of Radiology
Department of Radiology
Cornell University Medical College;
Chairman
Department of Radiology
Memorial Sloan-Kettering Cancer Center
New York, New York

Franco Cavalli, M.D.
Division of Oncology
Ospedale San Giovanni
Bellinzona, Switzerland

John K.C. Chan, M.D.
Consultant Pathologist
Department of Pathology
Queen Elizabeth Hospital
Kowloon, Hong Kong

Joseph M. Connors, M.D.
Clinical Professor of Medicine
Division of Medical Oncology
University of British Columbia
Vancouver, British Columbia

Louis S. Constine, M.D.
Professor
Department of Radiation Oncology and Pediatrics
University of Rochester Medical Center
Rochester, New York

Jean-Marc Cosset, M.D.
Professor and Chairman
Department of Radiation Oncology
Institut Curie
Paris, France

Vincent T. DeVita, M.D.
Yale Cancer Center
Yale University School of Medicine
New Haven, Connecticut

Volker Diehl, M.D.
Professor and Chairman
Department of Internal Medicine
Klinik I für Innere Medizin
der Universität zu Köln
Köln, Germany

Ketayun A. Dinshaw, D.M.R.T., F.R.C.R.
Professor and Head
Department of Radiation Oncology
Tata Memorial Hospital;
Director
Tata Memorial Center
Parel, Mumbai, India

Sarah S. Donaldson, M.D., F.A.C.R.
Catharine and Howard Avery Professor
Department of Radiation Oncology
Stanford University School of Medicine;
Associate Chair
Department of Radiation Oncology
Stanford Medical Center
Stanford, California

Eckhart Dühmke, M.D.
Professor and Chairman
Department of Radiotherapy and Radiation Oncology
Ludwig-Maximilians-Universität München;
Director
Department of Radiotherapy and Radiation Oncology
Klinikum Grasshadern u. Zumenstadt
München, Germany

Andreas Engert, M.D.
Klinik I für Innere Medizin
der Universität zu Köln
Köln, Germany

Geoffrey Falkson, M.D.
Emeritus Professor
Department of Medical Oncology
University of Pretoria
Pretoria, South Africa

Richard I. Fisher, M.D.
Dorothy W. and J. D. Stetson Coleman Professor of Oncology
Director, Cardinal Bernardin Cancer Center
Loyola University Stritch School of Medicine;
Director
Division of Hematology/Oncology
Foster G. MacGaw Hospital
Maywood, Illinois

Henning Flechtner, M.D.
Lecturer
Department of Child and Adolescent Psychiatry
Universität zu Köln;
Deputy Chief
Clinic of Child and Adolescent Psychiatry
University Hospital
Köln, Germany

Patricia Fobair, M.P.H.
Clinical Social Worker
Department of Radiation Oncology
Stanford University Medical School
Stanford, California

Christa Fonatsch, M.D.
Institut für Medizinische Biologie
der Universitat Wien
Wien, Austria

Jeremy Franklin, M.Sc.
Statistician
Klinik I für Innere Medizin
der Universität zu Köln
Köln, Germany

Eli Glatstein, M.D.
Department of Radiation Oncology
Hospital of the University of Pennsylvania
Philadelphia, Pennsylvania

Anthony H. Goldstone, F.R.C.P.
Honorary Senior Lecturer
Department of Hematology
University College London Hospital
Medical School;
Medical Director and
Director of Cancer Service
University College London Hospital
London, United Kingdom

Mary K. Gospodarowicz, M.D., F.R.C.P.C.
Professor
Department of Radiation Oncology
University of Toronto;
Director of Clinical Programs
Department of Radiation Oncology
Princess Margaret Hospital
Toronto, Canada

Seymour Grufferman, M.D., Dr.P.H.
Professor of Family Medicine
and Clinical Epidemiology
University of Pittsburg School of Medicine
Pittsburgh, Pennsylvania

Vincent F. Guinee, M.D., M.P.H.
Professor
Department of Internal Medicine
The University of Texas—
Houston Medical School;
Chairman (Retired)
Department of Patient Studies
M. D. Anderson Cancer Center
University of Texas
Houston, Texas

Rajnish K. Gupta, M.B., Ph.D., F.R.C.P.
Senior Lecturer
Department of Medical Oncology
St. Bartholomew's and The Royal London
School of Medicine and Dentistry;
Consultant
Department of Medical Oncology
St. Bartholomew's Hospital
London, United Kingdom

Barry W. Hancock, M.D., F.R.C.P., F.R.C.R.
Director
Division of Oncology and
Cellular Pathology
University of Sheffield;
Professor
Department of Medical Oncology
Weston Park Hospital
Sheffield, United Kingdom

Steven L. Hancock, M.D.
Professor
Department of Radiation Oncology
Stanford University
School of Medicine
Stanford, California

Martin-Leo Hansmann, M.D.
Head
Department of Pathology
University of Frankfurt
Frankfurt, Germany

Nancy Lee Harris, M.D.
Professor of Pathology
Harvard Medical School;
Director of Anatomic Pathology
Massachusetts General Hospital
Boston, Massachusetts

Dirk Hasenclever, M.D.
Senior Biometrician
Institut für Medizinische Informatik, Statistik und Epidemiologie
Universität Leipzig
Leipzig, Germany

Samuel Hellman, M.D., F.A.C.R.
A. N. Pritzker Distinguished Service Professor
Department of Radiation and Cellular Oncology
University of Chicago
Chicago, Illinois

Michel Henry-Amar, M.Sc., M.D.
Senior Scientist
Department of Clinical Research
Centre François Baclesse
Caen, France

Richard T. Hoppe, M.D., F.A.C.R.
Henry S. Kaplan—Harry Lebeson Professor of Cancer Biology
Chairman
Department of Radiation Oncology
Stanford University
Stanford, California

Sandra J. Horning, M.D.
Professor
Department of Medicine
Stanford University
Stanford, California

Alan Horwich, Ph.D., F.R.C.R., M.R.C.P.
Professor
Department of Radiotherapy and Oncology
The Royal Marsden Hospital and Institute of Cancer Research
Surrey, United Kingdom

Rachel E. Hough, B.M.B.S., M.R.C.P.
Clinical Research Fellow
Division of Oncology and Cellular Pathology
University of Sheffield;
Clinical Research Fellow
Department of Clinical Oncology
Weston Park Hospital
Sheffield, United Kingdom

Melissa Hudson, M.D.
Associate Member
Department of Hematology and Oncology
St. Jude Children's Research Hospital
Memphis, Tennessee

Michael Hummel, Ph.D.
Institute of Pathology
Universitätsklinikum Freien Universität Berlin
Berlin, Germany

Peter Jacobs, M.D., Ph.D.
Department of Hematology and Bone Marrow Transplant Unit
Constantiaberg Medi-Clinic
Plumstead, South Africa

Elaine S. Jaffe, M.D.
Chief, Hematopathology Section
Department of Pathology
National Cancer Institute
National Institutes of Health
Bethesda, Maryland

Suresh C. Jhanwar, Ph.D.
The Cytogenetics Service
Memorial Sloan-Kettering Cancer Center
New York, New York

Florence Joly, M.D.
Medical Oncologist
Department of Medicine
Centre François Baclesse
Caen, France

Andrea Jox, M.D.
Department of Internal Medicine
Klinik I für Innere Medizin der Universität zu Köln
Köln, Germany

Marshall E. Kadin, M.D.
Associate Professor
Department of Pathology
Harvard Medical School;
Senior Pathologist
Director of Hematopathology
Department of Pathology
Beth Israel Deaconess Medical Center
Boston, Massachusetts

Raymond H. S. Liang, M.D., F.R.C.P.
Professor
Department of Medicine
University of Hong Kong;
Chief
Department of Medicine
Division of Haematology/Oncology
Queen Mary Hospital
Hong Kong

David N. Liebowitz, M.D., Ph.D.
Associate Professor
Department of Medicine
University of Pennsylvania;
Director of Immunotherapy Programs
Leonard and Madlyn Abramson Family Cancer Research Institute
University of Pennsylvania Cancer Center
Philadelphia, Pennsylvania

T. Andrew Lister, M.D.
Professor and Head
Department of Medical Oncology
St. Bartholomew's Hospital
West Smithfield
London, United Kingdom

Markus Loeffler, M.D., Ph.D.
Professor
Institute of Medical Statistics and Epidemiology
University of Leipzig
Leipzig, Germany

Kenneth MacLennan, M.D.
Reader in Tumor Pathology
I.C.R.F. Cancer Medicine Research Unit
Saint James University Hospital
Leeds, United Kingdom

Theresa Marafioti, M.D.
Institute of Pathology
Universitätsklinikum Freien Universität Berlin
Berlin, Germany

Peter M. Mauch, M.D.
Professor of Radiation Oncology
Harvard Medical School
Associate Chief
Department of Radiation Oncology
Brigham and Women's Hospital
Dana-Farber Cancer Institute
Boston, Massachusetts

Nancy P. Mendenhall, M.D.
Professor and Chairman
Department of Radiation Oncology
University of Florida College of Medicine;
Shands HealthCare at the University of Florida
Gainesville, Florida

Silvio Monfardini, M.D.
Chief of the Division of Medical Oncology
Azienda University Hospital
Padova, Italy

Mary Ann Muckaden, M.D.
Professor
Department of Radiation Oncology
Tata Memorial Center;
Assistant Radiation Oncologist
Department of Radiation Oncology
Tata Memorial Hospital and Centre
Mumbai, India

Nancy E. Mueller, M.D.
Professor of Epidemiology
Harvard University School of Public Health
Boston, Massachusetts

Hans Konrad Mueller-Hermelink, M.D.
Professor of Pathology
Institute for Pathology
University of Wurzburg
Wurzburg, Germany

Andrea K. Ng, M.D., M.P.H.
Instructor
Department of Radiation Oncology
Brigham and Women's Hospital;
Harvard Medical School
Boston, Massachusetts

Evert M. Noordijk, M.D., Ph.D.
Professor in Clinical Radiotherapy
Head, Department of Clinical Oncology
Leiden University Medical Center
Leiden, The Netherlands

Peter O'Brien, M.D.
Department of Radiation Oncology
Newcastle Mater Hospital
Waratah, New South Wales, Australia

Odile Oberlin, M.D.
Department of Pediatrics
Institut Gustave-Roussy
Villejuif, France

Robert T. Osteen, M.D.
Associate Professor
Division of Surgical Oncology
Harvard Medical School;
Surgeon
Brigham and Women's Hospital
Boston, Massachusetts

Santiago Pavlovsky, M.D.
Medical Director
Angelica Ocampo Hospital and Research Center-Fundaleu
Buenos Aires, Argentina

Gordon L. Phillips, M.D.
Professor
Department of Blood and Marrow Transplant
University of Kentucky;
Director, Blood and Marrow Transplant Program
Department of Internal Medicine
Markey Cancer Center
University of Kentucky Medical Center
Lexington, Kentucky

Donald A. Podoloff, M.D.
Professor and Chairman
Department of Nuclear Medicine
Division of Diagnostic Imaging
M. D. Anderson Cancer Center
University of Texas
Houston, Texas

Sibrand Poppema, M.D., Ph.D.
Chairman
Department of Pathology and Laboratory Medicine
University of Groningen;
Chief
Department of Pathology and Laboratory Medicine
University Hospital Groningen
Groningen, The Netherlands

Carol S. Portlock, M.D.
Associate Professor
Department of Clinical Medicine
Cornell University Medical Center;
Department of Medical Oncology
Memorial Sloan-Kettering Cancer Center
New York, New York

Marc Potters, M.D.
Department of Pathology and Laboratory Medicine
University Hospital Groningen
Groningen, The Netherlands

Leonard R. Prosnitz, M.D., F.A.C.R.
Professor and Attending Physician
Department of Radiation Oncology
Duke University Medical Center
Durham, North Carolina

John Raemaekers, M.D., Ph.D.
Associate Professor
Department of Medicine
Division of Hematology
University Hospital of Nijmegan
Nymegen, The Netherlands

Saul A. Rosenberg, M.D.
Professor Emeritus
Department of Medicine and Radiation Oncology
Stanford University School of Medicine
Stanford, California

Ulrich Ruffer, M.D.
Department of Hematology/Oncology
Klinik I für Innere Medizin
der Universität zu Köln
Köln, Germany

Armando Santoro, M.D.
Director
Medical Oncology and Hematology
Istituto Clinico Humanitas
Milano, Italy

Andreas H. Sarris, M.D., Ph.D.
Associate Professor and Associate Internist
Department of Lymphoma-Myeloma
University of Texas
M.D. Anderson Cancer Center
Houston, Texas

Gunther Schellong, M.D.
Emeritus Professor
Department of Hematology and Oncology
University Children's Hospital
Münster, Germany

Norbert Schmitz, M.D.
Associate Professor
Head, BMT Unit
Department of Internal Medicine II
Christian-Albrechts-University;
Kiel, Germany

Dalila Sellami, M.D.
Radiotherapie
Institut Salah Azaiz
Tunis, Tunisia

Michael Sextro, M.D.
Klinik I für Innere Medizin
der Universität zu Köln
Köln, Germany

Samuel Singer, M.D.
Assistant Professor
Division of Surgical Oncology
Harvard Medical School;
Associate in Surgery
Brigham and Women's Hospital
Boston, Massachusetts

Reinier Somers (retired)
Valeriusstraat 42 II
1071 MK
Amsterdam, The Netherlands

Lena K. Specht, M.D., Ph.D.
Chief
Department of Oncology
Herlev Hospital
University of Copenhagen
Herlev, Denmark

Harald Stein, M.D.
Professor and Head
Institute of Pathology
Universitätsklinikum Freien Universität Berlin
Berlin, Germany

David J. Straus, M.D.
Professor
Department of Medicine
Weill Medical College of Cornell University;
Attending Physician
Department of Medicine, Lymphoma Service
Memorial Sloan-Kettering Cancer Center
New York, New York

Berthold Streubel, M.D.
Institut für Medizinische Biologie der Universität Wien
Wien, Austria

Simon B. Sutcliffe, Bsc, M.D.
Vancouver Cancer Center
Vancouver, British Columbia
Canada

Anthony J. Swerdlow, M.D., Ph.D.
Professor
Department of Epidemiology and Population Health
London School of Hygiene and Tropical Medicine
London, United Kingdom

Hans Tesch, M.D.
Professor
Klinik I für Innere Medizin
der Universität zu Köln
Köln, Germany

Umberto Tirelli, M.D.
Associate Professor
Department of Oncology
University of Udine
Udine, Italy;
Chief
Division of Medical Oncology and AIDS
Instituto Nazionale Tumori
Aviano, Italy

David Todd, M.D., F.A.C.P.
Professor
Department of Medicine
University of Hong Kong
Queen Mary Hospital
Hong Kong

Maurice Tubiana, M.D., Ph.D.
Emeritus Professor
Centre Antoine Béclère
Faculté de Medecine
Paris, France;
Honorary Director
Institut Gustave-Roussy
Villejuif, France

Margaret A. Tucker, M.D.
Chief
Genetic Epidemiology Branch
National Cancer Institute
Rockville, Maryland

Pinuccia Valagussa, M.D.
Head
Department of Biostatistics
Istituto Nazionale Tumori
Milan, Italy

Flora E. van Leeuwen, M.D.
Department of Epidemiology
The Netherlands Cancer Institute
Amsterdam, The Netherlands

Julie M. Vose, M.D.
Professor and Vice Chair
Department of Internal Medicine
University of Nebraska Medical Center
Omaha, Nebraska

Roger A. Warnke, M.D.
Professor
Department of Pathology
Stanford University Medical Center
Stanford, California

Lawrence M. Weiss, M.D.
Chairman
Department of Pathology
City of Hope National Medical Center
Duarte, California

Ute Winkler, M.D.
Post-Doctoral Fellow
Universität zu Köln;
Chief Resident
Klinik I für Innere Medizin
der Universität zu Köln
Köln, Germany

Jürgen Wolf, M.D.
Department of Internal Medicine
Klinik I für Innere Medizin
der Universität zu Köln
Köln, Germany

Joachim Yahalom, M.D.
Professor of Radiation Oncology
Cornell University Medical College;
Member and Attending
Department of Radiation Oncology
Memorial Sloan-Kettering Cancer Center
New York, New York

C. C. Yau, M.B., F.R.C.R.
Senior Medical Officer
Department of Radiotherapy and Oncology
Queen Mary Hospital
Hong Kong

Foreword

Hodgkin's disease has attracted the attention of physicians and researchers for more than a century, and to a degree out of proportion to its relative incidence. It is far less common than its cousins, the non-Hodgkin's lymphomas, and compared to many cancers it is a relatively rare disease. Yet a distinguished group of over 100 authors have contributed to this significant book of over 40 chapters describing our current knowledge about this unique human malady. Previous monographs, chapters, and sections of books have also been devoted to Hodgkin's disease, but only the two editions of the late Henry S. Kaplan's books are as comprehensive as this text, organized and edited by Peter Mauch and his four coeditors.

The reasons why Hodgkin's disease has attracted so much scientific and clinical attention during this century are well described throughout the book. The very nature of Hodgkin's disease, a true neoplasm, an inflammatory, even infectious disease, an unusual immunologic reaction, or a combination of these pathogeneses has long been and continues to be controversial. It remains a question whether Hodgkin's disease is a single human disease or several variations of an etiologic theme. The unique epidemiology of Hodgkin's disease, its familial and genetic features, needs explanation and understanding. These questions are complicated by the probable heterogeneity of what is called Hodgkin's disease by pathologists, by the absence of a true animal model of the disease, and the great difficulty, perhaps impossibility, of propagating Hodgkin's cell-lines for *in vitro* study. These problems and questions are described and reviewed in the book with our current state of knowledge carefully detailed by international experts in their disciplines.

There are other factors which have lead to the special interest in Hodgkin's disease, justifying the need and value of a comprehensive text. Hodgkin's disease frequently affects individuals in young adulthood, often at the prime of their life. If untreated, it is uniformly fatal in a matter of a few years. However, dramatic success has been achieved in the management of the disease, so that a cure is now accepted as the goal of treatment and is achieved in the great majority of patients worldwide. The concepts of the nature of the disease, its clinical behavior, and its response to therapies have evolved gradually this century, and rapidly since the 1960s continuing through today. Many of those responsible for these advances describe them fully in the text, providing an invaluable resource for clinicians, investigators, and students of the disease.

It can be predicted, however, that as valuable and current as this text is, major changes and discoveries will make it outdated in the near future. Just as the Kaplan texts are now of predominately historic interest, so will be this excellent book, and probably within a decade.

But that is why Hodgkin's disease remains a fascinating disorder and object of scientific inquiry. This comprehensive volume, written by the world's experts, brings us up-to-date for the moment and sets the stage for the developments of the future. For this, we congratulate the five editors and their over 100 contributing colleagues.

Saul A. Rosenberg, M.D.

Preface

Hodgkin's disease and childhood leukemia, both uniformly fatal prior to 1960, were the first cancers discovered to be highly curable with the development of multi-agent chemotherapy and modern radiation therapy. The outgrowth of the successful treatment of these diseases has provided a prototype for strategies for the curative treatment of other cancers over the past 30 years.

The last definitive text on Hodgkin's disease was published in 1980 by Harvard University Press. Dr. Henry S. Kaplan, a clinician and researcher whose many seminal contributions greatly improved our understanding and treatment of Hodgkin's disease, wrote editions of his book in 1972 and 1980. The text had no co-authors or co-editors, an amazing feat by today's standards. We have retained the original title of his book to credit and honor his work.

In designing the current text, we choose to be as inclusive as possible. We wanted a broad representation of the knowledge and treatment of Hodgkin's disease, and we wished to credit those who have made important contributions to our understanding of the disease. As a result the editors represent the disciplines of radiation oncology, medical oncology, molecular biology, and pathology. There are over 100 contributors from all parts of the world. In trying to be as representative as possible we apologize to those we may have inadvertently omitted in the process.

Hodgkin's Disease is divided into eight sections to represent the many advances in this disease that have occurred since 1980. Each chapter has been designed to stand alone and to comprehensively cover a topic. By intent a topic may be covered in several different chapters. Hodgkin's disease was felt to be an incurable illness by most physicians until the mid 1960s. Many of the physicians whose work was instrumental in developing a curative approach to this disease have generously contributed their perspectives to Section I.

Advances in the etiology and epidemiology of Hodgkin's disease, especially for the emerging role of the Epstein-Barr virus, are covered in Section II. Section III, composed of eight chapters on biology and pathology, presents the many new and exciting advances in our knowledge of the pathogenesis of Hodgkin's disease.

Sections IV (Staging and Initial Evaluation), V (Treatment Principles and Techniques), and VI (Selection of Treatment) outline the current treatment options and ongoing trials for patients with Hodgkin's disease. These chapters should prove to be a valuable resource to physicians, nurses, medical students, and patients.

The late effects of treatment are covered in Section VII. Increasing knowledge of these effects has dramatically changed our approach to the treatment of patients with Hodgkin's disease. Finally, special topics are covered in Section VIII.

We had several goals in designing this book. We wanted to provide a reference text for training programs and researchers. We wanted to provide information and guidance for practicing physicians. Finally we hoped to provide a foundation for new ideas in laboratory and clinical investigation.

The treatment of Hodgkin's disease is sufficiently effective that now we have the luxury of reducing treatment intensity to avoid late complications. We look forward to advances that will enable us to better understand the pathophysiology and etiology of Hodgkin's disease. These advances should aid in its prevention and in the development of safer treatment approaches.

Peter Mauch
James Armitage
Volker Diehl
Richard Hoppe
Lawrence Weiss

Acknowledgments

We are deeply indebted and most appreciative of the efforts of all the contributors whose expertise and promptness has eased the preparation of this text. Particularly, we would like to thank our families who endured our efforts in the preparation of this work, and our colleagues who provided support and supplied valuable suggestions.

We also want to thank J. Stuart Freeman, Jr., Senior Editor of the oncology program at Lippincott Williams & Wilkins, whose guidance helped shape the book, and Marge Keskin (Stanford, California), Elaine Ryan (Omaha, Nebraska), and Tara Sheridan and Barbara Silver (both of Boston, Massachusetts) who assisted in the preparation of materials for the book.

Color Plates

Plates 1 through 38 fall between pages 168 and 169.

Plate 26. *A nodule of nodular lymphocyte predominance Hodgkin's disease.*
Plate 27. *High magnification, showing characteristic L&H or "popcorn" cells (Giemsa stain).*
Plate 28. *Follicular dendritic cells form large networks in nodular lymphocyte predominance Hodgkin's disease (immuno–alkaline phosphatase, CD21).*
Plate 29. *Several L&H cells show a membrane-bound immunoreaction for CD20 (immuno–alkaline phosphatase).*
Plate 30. *A large progressively transformed germinal center surrounded by several small germinal centers (Giemsa stain).*
Plate 31. *The progressively transformed germinal centers are composed mainly of B cells.*
Plate 32. *Nodular infiltrate of lymphocyte-rich classical Hodgkin's disease.*
Plate 33. *Fluorescence in situ hybridization (FISH) with painting probes for chromosomes 7 (red) and 11 (green). L-428.*
Plate 34. *Fluorescence in situ hybridization (FISH) with painting probes for chromosomes 7 (red) and 11 (green). L-1236.*
Plate 35. *FISH with painting probes for chromosomes 2 (green) and 12 (red). L-428.*
Plate 36. *FISH with painting probes for chromosomes 2 (green) and 12 (red). L-1236.*
Plate 37. *FISH with painting probes for chromosomes 2 (red) and 8 (green). L-428.*
Plate 38. *FISH with painting probes for chromosomes 2 (red) and 8 (green). L-540.*

SECTION I

Historical Aspects

Hodgkin's Disease, edited by P. M. Mauch,
J. O. Armitage, V. Diehl, R. T. Hoppe, and L. M. Weiss.
Lippincott Williams & Wilkins, Philadephia ©1999.

CHAPTER 1

A Brief Consideration of Thomas Hodgkin and His Times

Samuel Hellman

It is difficult to describe this complicated man and the world in which he lived in a brief chapter. To those readers who are interested in a more detailed account, I recommend *Perfecting the World,* by Amalie and Edward Kass, and *Curator of the Dead,* by Michael Rose. The latter book title is an amalgamation of Hodgkin's official position at Guy's Hospital, where he served as "Inspector of the Dead" and "Curator of the Museum," and, while brief, the monograph gives the flavor of the man, which is more fully explicated in the Kasses book.

This is an especially propitious time to consider Thomas Hodgkin, as 1998 was the centenary year of his birth. Born August 17, 1798, to a family of staunch Quakers, Hodgkin was educated in and fully embraced the Quaker religion and worldview as a guide for his activities. This religious man was a major academic force despite spending most of his time in meliorist activities. A true Victorian, he was committed to the superiority of his civilization but also to the obligations required by noblesse oblige and his strong religious convictions. These missions informed much of his life. This chapter begins with a brief biographical sketch followed by a recitation of his medical accomplishments and then those reflecting his social conscience.

Following a brief period as an apothecary's apprentice, he chose a career in medicine and enrolled as a pupil able to walk the wards at Guy's Hospital. Since at that time Guy's and St. Thomas's had a close relationship, he was allowed to observe the clinical activity at both institutions. St. Thomas's is a venerable institution begun in the 12th century and named for Thomas à Becket. Much later, Thomas Guy, Jr., a wealthy benefactor, provided funds to build a new hospital related to St. Thomas's but devoted to investigation of new treatments for serious and incurable disease. Guy's Hospital opened in 1726 directly across from St. Thomas's. Essential to the development of that hospital into a leading world medical center was the extremely long tenure of Benjamin Harrison, Jr., who at age 26, succeeding his father in 1797, became the treasurer of Guy's Hospital. He lived at the hospital and served for over 50 years. While he was a despot who affected Thomas Hodgkin's life in important and unfortunate ways, he was strongly evangelical and a member of the Clapham set, which encouraged religious piety by the poor and extensive evangelical missionary works abroad. We shall return to Hodgkin's encounter with this man later.

Because Hodgkin was a Quaker, he was unable to enter the English universities of Oxford and Cambridge. Since a physician was required to complete a university course of study, about one-quarter of the physicians in Britain went to those venerable institutions, while the remaining three-quarters studied in Edinburgh, Scotland, or on the continent. Hodgkin went to Edinburgh, accepted largely on the basis of the recommendation of the distinguished surgeon Astley Cooper, whose acquaintance he had made while walking the wards at Guy's Hospital. It was at Edinburgh while still a medical student that he wrote his first paper, "On the Uses of the Spleen." This subject presages the description of the disease that bears his name. The Greeks believed the spleen to be a seat of laughter, and there was still a significant influence of Aristotelian and Hippocratic medicine on British physicians of the day. Hodgkin believed that the spleen's purpose was to regulate fluid volume within the body, to clean impurities from the body, to be a reservoir for excess nutrients coming from the gastrointestinal tract to the liver, and to store and dispose of black bile (melancholy). He suggested that the spleen supplied expandability to the portal system. He

S. Hellman: Department of Radiation and Cellular Oncology, University of Chicago, Chicago, Illinois.

noted that it was enlarged in many diseases but decreased in size with hemorrhage.

He interrupted his studies at Edinburgh to spend a year in Paris, then the center of medicine and intellectual life. In the 18th century medicine was primarily an intellectual exercise based on logic and studies of the Greek scholars, but gradually in the beginning of the 19th century it began to be based more on extensive observation and, later in the century, on experimentation. Medicine was considered to be a part of a broader intellectual universe, and British physicians were expected to have had a general education. While in Paris Hodgkin met with Laennec, who greatly influenced his approach to medicine. Laennec was among the most astute clinicians of the time, a careful observer who, among his many contributions, developed the stethoscope. But perhaps the most influential of the people Hodgkin met during that year was Baron von Humboldt, whom Hodgkin describes as the "hero of my youth," because of his interests in anthropology, particularly ethnography, a field for which Hodgkin had a great affinity. He also met Baron Cuvier, the distinguished anatomist and paleontologist whose Saturday soirees on both scientific and broadly intellectual subjects were often attended by the young medical student. A close contemporary was Thomas A. Bowditch, whose expeditions to Africa, concerned primarily with the ethnography of the natives, also greatly influenced Hodgkin's future activities. After this formative year in Paris, Hodgkin returned to Edinburgh to complete his studies. Following graduation from medical school he returned to Paris to be the companion and traveling physician to Abraham Montefiore, a distinguished Jewish philanthropist who at that time was suffering from tuberculosis. While Montefiore was dissatisfied with Hodgkin as a physician, they remained very good friends and Thomas Hodgkin developed a lifelong friendship with Moses Montefiore, Abraham's older brother.

He returned to London in 1825 to join the staff at Guy's Hospital, which had recently separated from St. Thomas's, to form a new medical school. In 1826 he was made "Inspector of the Dead" and "Curator of the Museum." He also worked as a physician to the London Dispensary, a medical facility dealing with the medical problems of the indigent, for which he received no fee but left after 2 years under acrimonious circumstances. During those years at Guy's Hospital, some of the leading doctors of the time were in active medical practice, including not only the surgeon Astley Cooper but the great physicians Richard Bright and Thomas Addison. And so, by his late 20s Hodgkin had met many of the intellectual and medical giants of the time: Laennec, Humboldt, Cuvier, Bright, Cooper, and Addison. In addition, he became interested in the microscope and had a close association with Joseph Jackson Lister, who developed the achromatic microscope and was the father of the more famous Joseph Lister, who was responsible for aseptic surgery. This role of morbid anatomist provided the opportunity for the clinicopathologic correlations central to his career. In addition to this activity he greatly desired appointment as physician to Guy's Hospital.

In 1837 disaster struck Hodgkin; he ran afoul of Benjamin Harrison. The number of appointed physicians at Guy's Hospital was limited, and so his appointment required the death or retirement of an incumbent. With the retirement of James Cholmeley, Addison, an assistant physician, was expected to succeed Cholmeley, thereby providing a vacant assistant physician position. Hodgkin was felt to be next in line for such a position, and he was quite optimistic that he would be appointed. Unfortunately, his nonmedical activities had caused him to have some differences with Harrison. Hodgkin was distressed by the way the Hudson Bay Company was treating natives of western Canada. It was trading guns and alcohol for furs, and thus the traditional way of life was being destroyed but not replaced by that of a Western society. Harrison was one of seven members of the Grand Committee of the Hudson Bay Company, and Hodgkin was convinced that Harrison was sympathetic to his own values concerning the treatment of native populations. He wrote to Harrison, "I cannot believe that Benjamin Harrison, whose life is almost entirely devoted to institutions which have for their object the relief and amelioration of his fellow creatures, will either regard the subject with indifference, or have his attention fixed upon it without conceiving the means which may correct and retrieve the evil, or that he would advocate the cause in vain, were he to undertake it." Harrison was affronted by this letter, while Hodgkin, largely naive and unaware of how he was viewed, expected his support. When the opportunity to appoint an assistant physician occurred, Harrison effectively prevented the appointment, resulting in Hodgkin resigning from all positions at Guy's Hospital.

His activities in medicine, including a small and largely unsuccessful private practice as well as involvement in a number of medical and public health activities, continued until his death in 1866. In 1842, he briefly joined St. Thomas's Hospital, which had fallen considerably as a medical school when Guy's Hospital separated. Hodgkin was asked to design a new medical curriculum and to revive the museum. Again his naiveté caused him to be shocked and disappointed when he was not reappointed, largely because it was felt he had spent excessive funds on the museum. The remainder of his medical activities were limited to his small practice and to lecturing and writing on issues of public health, while his major efforts were with the betterment of aboriginal populations abroad as well as the poor of England.

From 1857 through 1866, with his friend Moses Montefiore, Hodgkin was involved in five journeys primarily concerned with helping Jews and Christians in Moslem lands. The relationship between the two friends was interesting; Montefiore, an observant Sephardic Jew, and

Hodgkin, a religious Quaker, respected each other's religious views and were attracted to each other by their common adherence to religion and their actions on behalf of their fellow man consistent with their religious beliefs. On April 4, 1866, during the last of these trips, Hodgkin died of an unknown but lengthy illness and was buried in Jaffa. His brother John had inscribed upon the gravestone "Nothing of humanity was foreign to him." This was used earlier by Hodgkin when he dedicated his medical thesis to Humboldt. The quotation comes from the Roman slave Torrence: "He always thought that among all things nothing belonging to man was foreign to him."

MEDICAL ACCOMPLISHMENTS

Hodgkin played an important role in bringing the stethoscope to Great Britain while he was still a medical student. After spending a year as a medical student in Paris, he delivered a major lecture on the uses of the stethoscope devised by Laennec. This lecture at Guy's Hospital was considered to have been of major importance in the acceptance of the stethoscope in England, although there remained a significant number of practitioners who failed to appreciate its importance. As the Inspector of the Dead and Curator of the Museum of Morbid Anatomy, Thomas Hodgkin was in the vanguard of medical science. The correlation of clinical disease to pathologic material was quite new, and Hodgkin was the leading morbid anatomist of his day. Clinicopathologic correlation owes a great deal to Hodgkin who, in developing the museum at Guy's Hospital, had by 1829 over 1,600 specimens demonstrating the effects of disease. He taught the first core course in pathologic anatomy in Great Britain. He was critical of the vitalism of the time and emphasized the importance of the chemical nature of the body. From analyses of pathologic specimens he described appendicitis with perforation and peritonitis. He described the local spread of cancer to draining lymph nodes, noting that the tumor at both sites had similar characteristics. All this was accomplished well before the microscope was used in pathology.

Hodgkin was also quite interested in microscopy and recognized the importance of the achromatic microscope devised by Joseph Jackson Lister. With Lister, the senior, he described the biconcave nature of the erythrocyte and the fibrillar and striated nature of muscle. They provided detailed descriptions of nerves and the three layers of arterial walls. They demonstrated that the globular theory of disease was false because the globules, due to aberrations in microscopy, were not present with the achromatic microscope. While Dominic Corrigan is usually credited with first describing aortic insufficiency, it was Hodgkin who described the disease fully 20 years earlier. Using clinicopathologic correlation he identified the valvular insufficiency and the bruit and murmur associated with this abnormality. Well before the separation of public health from clinical medicine in universities, physicians made contributions to both. These two areas of physician responsibility epitomized by the daughters of Aesculapius—Panacea and Hygeia—are both realized in Hodgkin; Panacea in the clinicopathologic descriptions of disease and Hygeia in his concerns for public health. He emphasized the dangers of lead pipes and proposed coating them with tin. He suggested that excessive cream and butter were harmful, and that wheat, to be fully nutritious, required the hulk to be present. He recognized, I believe for the first time, the importance of fiber in the diet, since he indicated that the consumption of the husk avoided the constipation associated with eating refined wheat. He recommended a decrease of sugar and meats in the diet and an increase in vegetables. He cautioned against both tobacco and alcohol.

Perhaps Hodgkin's major influences on public health were through his lectures on sanitation and adequate food and housing for the poor. As Asiatic cholera began creeping across Europe toward England, Hodgkin suggested that its effects could be limited by improving the conditions of the poor. He also recognized the contagious nature of the disease. Despite these efforts, there were about 80,000 cases of cholera in Britain during that epidemic, with an approximately 40% mortality. Both of these important clinical and public health contributions were central to the contemporary reputation of Hodgkin. They represent the essence of the man much more than that for which he is remembered in posterity.

He described in 1832 the eponymous disease for which he is known, in a paper entitled, "On Some Morbid Appearances of the Absorbent Glands and Spleen" that was presented and subsequently published in the *Medical-Chirurgical Society Transactions.* It was known at that time that cancer, inflammation, tuberculosis, and syphilis could cause lymph node enlargement. He separated six cases from the experience at Guy's Hospital as different and added one sent to him in a detailed drawing by his friend Carswell. It is of interest that two of the six cases were patients of Bright and one of Addison. Subsequent histopathologic examination revealed that three of the cases, in fact, were Hodgkin's disease, which Hodgkin described from the gross anatomy since microscopic anatomy was not used until three decades later. He considered this lymph node enlargement different because it was not associated with pain or heat nor was it due to metastases from adjacent malignant tumors. This 1832 article was not widely recognized, although Bright in 1838 reported on the disease, emphasizing Hodgkin's original contributions. Samuel Wilks in 1856 described the disease, quoting Bright and indicating he had thought that the observation was original until Bright had directed him to Hodgkin's original paper. In 1865 Wilks described the disease in further detail and attached the name Hodgkin's disease to this lymph node and splenic enlargement. It was also Wilks who published in 1877

"Historical Notes on Bright's Disease, Addison's Disease and Hodgkin's Disease," referring to these physicians as the three great men of Guy's, an appellation that has continued to this time. While Wilks did not know of Hodgkin's priority until it was pointed out to him by Bright, Hodgkin mentions that the first reference that he could find to this or a similar disease was in fact by Malpighi in 1666. Hodgkin recognized that the disease spread primarily by contiguity of adjacent lymph nodes and that splenic involvement occurred late in the course of the disease. Nuland, in an interesting paper, has suggested that perhaps Wilks's generosity toward Hodgkin was not completely without pressure from Bright, although later, Wilks and Betany in *A Biological History of Guy's Hospital* wrote "It must be said that in Hodgkin, Guy's Hospital lost one of its greatest ornaments and the profession in England one who was destined to add luster to its ranks." Before leaving the medical contributions of Hodgkin, I must cite his efforts in creating the University of London and its medical schools, the first in Britain requiring no affiliation with the Church of England. Both University College and King's College are a part of this university.

In June 1840, the 18-year-old Edward Oxford attempted to assassinate Queen Victoria and Prince Albert. Hodgkin appeared at the trial as an expert witness in his defense, supporting the view of moral insanity, which he explained as the inability to understand the significance of one's deeds or to refrain from criminal acts, despite appearing normal under many other circumstances. This carried the day, augmented by Oxford's seeming nonchalance and eagerness to accept responsibility as well as a strong family history of mental illness. It was the first successful use of this concept in English law.

NONMEDICAL INTERESTS

Hodgkin's involvement in the Quaker movement is central to understanding him and his activities. Not only was he born to a devout family, but he remained a devout member of the Society of Friends throughout his life. Deeply in love with his first cousin, he petitioned the society to allow the marriage of first cousins. Because of its refusal the cousins did not marry, and he remained a bachelor until 1850.

He was a strong and committed abolitionist whose animus toward slavery was a defining part of his life. This stemmed from his religion, but added to that, I believe, were the general meliorist views of some Victorian English. The dislocations produced by colonialism and the Industrial Revolution produced a great sense of responsibility to native peoples and the poor. This sense of noblesse oblige had a certain condescending tone based on the implicitly felt superiority of the English and of evangelical Protestant Christianity. The meliorist aspect of these goals also was consistent with Hodgkin's longstanding interest in ethnography, the latter enlarged by his association with Humboldt. Antislavery, concern for native people throughout the world including Africa, North America, New Zealand, and Australia, as well as a strong sense of responsibility defined his life following his separation from Guy's Hospital. This was the time of extensive publicity and civic pride in the great English explorers, including Livingstone, Speck, Grant, and Burton in Africa; Palliser in the Canadian Rockies; as well as others in Australia. Livingstone, a medical missionary, embodied the many goals and responsibilities of mid–19th century Britain: civilizing, converting to Christianity, eliminating slavery, and exploring the world by the then dominant country. All those engaged in these explorations enjoyed wide publicity and public approbation, bringing to the British an awareness of indigenous civilizations. Many Victorians felt a responsibility to improving the plight of the natives, which included bettering their health as a justification for their imperialist goals. Hodgkin, while not particularly evangelical, was concerned with the well-being of the indigenous people. He founded and was the long-time president of the Aborigines Protection Society as well as a founder and long-term supporter of the Ethnological Society of London. The combination of his ethnologic interests and concerns for the welfare of indigenous civilizations was infused with his strong public health interests. Traveling with Moses Montefiore provided him opportunities for advocating public health measures not only in Britain but in North Africa, southern Europe, and the Middle East. Unfortunately, it was these very views that did not allow his advancement at Guy's Hospital.

SOME LESSONS FROM HODGKIN AND HIS TIMES

We cannot help but be awed by the prodigious accomplishments of this man. His medical accomplishments were primarily during the brief period (1825–1837) he served at Guy's Hospital. While these accomplishments continued after 1837, he more and more became enamored of his meliorist interests. The very breadth of his interests was grounded in an underlying worldview that many in the Victorian Age shared. This was still a time when medicine was considered a part of general intellectual activity, and physicians were expected to be broadly educated. Hodgkin is a paradigm of the best of Victorians and of physicians. Hodgkin's success and his disappointment were due to his focus, drive, and naiveté as well as his prickly personality. Cameron in his book *My Guy's Hospital* of 1954 states that there was in Hodgkin's nature that which made it hard for him to obtain ultimate success in life, some perverse spirit that seemed always to place him in opposition. While I believe that this characterization is neither accurate nor charitable, it does emphasize the way in which reformers and those that deviate from common practice are regarded.

Review of his scientific accomplishments reveals a mix of the prescient and what appears today to be ridiculous. His views must be considered in light of the then contemporary state of medicine with the continuing influence of the classic scholars and with the scientific method in its infancy. Systematic observation was just being appreciated as a requirement for acquiring new medical information and the experimental method not widely used until later in the 19th century. Also remarkable is his close contact with the medical and intellectual leaders of the time. Hodgkin's acquaintance with Addison, Bright, Cooper, Humboldt, Laennec, Lister, and Montefiore is truly remarkable. All of these figures have had their names attached to diseases or entities that make them familiar well beyond their years. Addison's disease—adrenal insufficiency; Bright's disease—those several renal diseases associated with albuminurea; Cooper's ligament; Cuvier's duct; Humboldt's current; Laennec's cirrhosis. Even Lister and Montefiore have eponymous representations today—Lister, through his son of aseptic surgery fame and for whom the genus *Listeria* is named, and Montefiore, for the many monuments recognizing his philanthropic efforts, including the Montefiore hospitals. One lesson from Hodgkin's eponymous recognition is that it often does not represent the discoverer's major accomplishment. Hodgkin, were he alive today, would be surprised, I believe, that it is for Hodgkin's disease that he is remembered. Few recognize Laennec for the breadth of his clinical contributions or for the stethoscope; rather it is by the liver disease that his name continues to be familiar to physicians. Hodgkin's disease also teaches us something about the accuracy of medical attribution. While the disease is associated with Hodgkin, he fully appreciated Malpighi's priority. Rene Gilbert, Vera Peters, and Henry Kaplan are associated with the notion of lymph node contiguity, but this was clearly described in Hodgkin's original article. The Reed-Sternberg cell was first described by Greenfield. While Hodgkin described aortic insufficiency, Corrigan gets the credit.

From Hodgkin we also learn of the breadth of contribution possible and of the extent to which a physician can extend his or her influence. He was concerned with individual patient care, medical research, and public health. But his commitments and contribution extended far beyond that to his obligations as a civilized human being. These latter were based on a particular and strongly felt worldview. This estimable person should serve as an exemplar for us all.

SUGGESTED READINGS

Bright R. Observations on abdominal tumors and intumescence, illustrated by cases of disease of the spleen. *Guy's Hosp Rep* 1838;3:401–409.

Cameron HC. *My Guy's Hospital.* London: Longman, 1954:154.

Hellman S. Thomas Hodgkin and Hodgkin's disease. Two paradigms appropriate to medicine today. *JAMA* 1991;265:1007–1010.

Hodgkin T. *A catalogue of the preparations of the anatomical museum of Guy's Hospital.* London: R. Watts, 1829.

Hodgkin T. On the object of post-mortem examinations. *Lond Med Gaz* 1828;2:423–431.

Hodgkin T. On the retroversion of the valves of the aorta. *Lond Med Gaz* 1829;3:433–442.

Hodgkin T. On some morbid experiences of the absorbent glands and spleen. *Med Chir Trans* 1832;17:69–97.

Hodgkin T. *Promoting and preserving health.* London: Cornhill Darton & Harvey Highley Fry, 1835.

Kass A, Kass E. *Perfecting the world: the life and times of Thomas Hodgkin (1798–1866).* New York: Harcourt Brace Jovanovich, 1988.

Kass EH, Carey AB, Kass AM. Thomas Hodgkin and Benjamin Harrison: crises and promotion in academia. *Med Hist* 1980;24:197–208.

Malpighi M. De viscerum structura exexcitato anatomica bononiae. *J Montij* 125–156. (Translated in *Ann Med Hist* 1925;7:245–263.)

Nuland SB. The lymphatic contiguity of Hodgkin's disease: a historical study. *Bull NY Acad Med* 1981;57:766–786.

Rose M. *Curator of the dead: Thomas Hodgkin (1798–1866).* London: Peter Owen, 1981.

Rosenblum J. An interesting friendship—Thomas Hodgkin, M.D., and Sir Moses Montefiore Bart. *Ann Med Hist* 1921;3:381–386.

Sakula S. Dr. Thomas Hodgkin and Sir Moses Montefiore Bart—the friendship of two remarkable men. *J R Soc Med* 1979;72:382–387.

Wilks S. Cases of enlargement of the lymphatic glands and spleen (or Hodgkin's disease), with remarks. *Guy's Hosp Rep* 1865;11:56–67.

Wilks S. Cases of lardaceous disease and some allied affections with remarks. *Guy's Hosp Rep* 1856;2:103–132.

Wilks S. Historical notes on Bright's disease, Addison's disease and Hodgkin's disease. *Guy's Hosp Rep* 1877;22:259–261,270–274.

Hodgkin's Disease, edited by P.M. Mauch,
J.O. Armitage, V. Diehl, R.T. Hoppe, and L.M. Weiss.
Lippincott Williams & Wilkins, Philadephia ©1999.

CHAPTER 2

The History of the Chemotherapy of Hodgkin's Disease

Vincent T. DeVita and Gianni Bonadonna

THE ROOTS OF CHEMOTHERAPY

The idea that chemicals might be useful in treating cancer received great impetus from the successful use of synthetic chemicals and natural products used to cure parasitic, common bacterial infections, and tuberculosis in rodents and humans. In each case, the possible success of drug therapy was greeted with great pessimism, but none more so than the possibility that chemotherapy could cure cancer.

At the turn of the 20th century, Paul Erlich, an optimist by all other accounts and considered the father of chemotherapy, was paid to work on the problem of cancer. This time he was not at all optimistic about the possible outcome. The part of the laboratory at that time that was devoted to cancer research is reported to have had a sign over it stating "Abandon all hope all ye who enter here." In 1898, Erlich discovered the first alkylating agent, but it was nearly 50 years before this observation was applied to the treatment of neoplastic diseases in humans at Yale University, specifically in the lymphomas. However, physicians knew of lymphomas and treated them as early as the late 19th century. Mention of the chemotherapy of lymphomas was made in 1894 in the first edition of Osler's textbook of medicine (1). In this case it was Fowler's solution, an arsenic-containing medicinal, that was considered the standard of the day and used for a number of cancers. Osler was an astute clinician, however, and recognized that waxing and waning adenopathy seemed to occur in Hodgkin's disease, and wondered out loud as to the true impact of this arsenic-containing material on the natural history of the disease. There was no way to test compounds in a model system prior to their use in humans until George Clowes, at Roswell Park Institute in Buffalo, New York, developed the first transplantable animal tumor models for this purpose in 1912 (2).

The first use of alkylating agents in humans actually resulted not from a discovery in Erlich's laboratory, or from animal screening studies, but from the development of the United States war gas program. An explosion in the harbor in Bari, Italy, during World War II exposed servicemen to the lethal toxic effects of mustard gases. Profound marrow and lymphoid aplasia were noted, and, as a consequence, a derivative of mustard gas, nitrogen mustard, was submitted for testing in humans to Goodman and Gilman at Yale in 1943 (2–4). Without the benefit of a Food and Drug Administration (FDA) review process, a group of six patients with Hodgkin's disease and lymphosarcoma were treated in the same year the compounds were submitted, 1943, in what has to be considered the first phase I/II cancer clinical trial on record. Because of the secrecy surrounding the war gas program, the results were not published until 1946 (5). Striking dissolution of tumor masses occurred in these patients with both Hodgkin's disease and lymphosarcoma following intermittent dosing with nitrogen mustard. Subsequent studies by Alpert and Petersen (6) and Dameshek and colleagues (7) confirmed these effects. These early studies, however, were the source of both great excitement and great disappointment. Excitement arose because never before had such marked regression of tumor masses occurred in humans as a result of drug treatment, and the possibility of curing cancer with drugs was first theoretically entertained; and disappointment followed because, with the rapid regrowth of the tumor masses and eventual death of these patients, a generation of pessimists was born and

V.T. DeVita: Yale Cancer Center, Yale University School of Medicine, New Haven, Connecticut.

G. Bonadonna: Division of Medical Oncology, Department of Medicine, Istituto Nazionale Tumori, Milan, Italy.

the long debate began—and persisted and permeated academic circles—as to whether anticancer drugs provided any significant palliative benefit, let alone cure, for patients with these diseases. In general, in these early times, even the use of the word *cure* was considered wild speculation and evidence of lack of critical judgment.

As a consequence, the 1950s was a decade of gloom about the utility of chemotherapy. The antitumor activity of the antifols was discovered in the 1950s, but they had no immediate bearing on the treatment of lymphomas. Their effectiveness in leukemia did, however, lead to a commitment by the U.S. government to set up the Cancer Chemotherapy National Service Center (CCNSC), a cancer drug development program under the auspices of the U.S. National Cancer Institute (NCI) that would ultimately add other agents to the therapeutic armamentarium (8,9). The controversial use of random screening of thousands of chemical compounds by the CCNSC, using a single transplantable mouse leukemia, Leukemia 1210 (L1210), was decried by many as a waste of money. However, there were features of this screening program that made it attractive and safe for the pharmaceutical industry to submit compounds for screening and low-cost development under a "commercial discreet agreement" with the NCI that gave impetus to a number of companies to begin searching for drugs against cancer, which in turn gave birth to the highly successful cancer drug discovery programs of today (9).

In the 1950s, the discovery of the corticosteroids also provided an additional therapeutic tool for physicians to use with alkylating agents, but even in combination, these agents did not seem to provide durable benefit for patients with lymphomas. Thus, during the 1950s, investigators were limited to comparing the effects of a variety of alkylating agents, evaluating various routes and schedules of administration, and debating their palliative benefits and arguing as to their effects on survival.

THE EARLY CLINICAL TRIALS IN HODGKIN'S DISEASE

The first study to have an impact on the management of patients with Hodgkin's disease was published by Scott (10) in 1963. Eighty-nine patients with advanced Hodgkin's disease received a conventional induction course of nitrogen mustard (0.4 mg/kg), of which 40 patients with satisfactory response were randomized to receive either no further treatment or continuous treatment with the newly developed oral alkylating agent chlorambucil. In the 16 patients who received chlorambucil, time to relapse averaged 35 weeks (range 4 to 84 weeks) compared to 11.7 weeks (range 4 to 51 weeks) without further treatment. This highly significant difference in the duration of a satisfactory remission provided the first useful information on alternatives in the management of patients with Hodgkin's disease. No mention was made in this study, however, as to whether any survival benefit accrued to the patients maintained on chlorambucil. Subsequent studies comparing remission induction with nitrogen mustard and maintenance with chlorambucil to induction and maintenance with another new alkylating agent, cyclophosphamide, which had both an oral and intravenous formulation, revealed no significant differences in either the response rate or remission duration between the two alternatives.

Jacobs and colleagues (11) presented one of the first survival curves published in the modern chemotherapy era. Drug treatment in patients with advanced Hodgkin's disease was associated with a median survival of less than 2 years, with only 5% living beyond 4 years, all with evidence of disease. These results were only slightly superior to a series of patients with all stages of Hodgkin's disease left untreated for the entire course of their disease, reported by Craft (12) in 1940; this report did not provide support for the position that chemotherapy was improving survival.

The next major advance in the chemotherapy of the lymphomas came with the identification of the plant-derived natural products called the vinca alkaloids (13). The availability of two apparently non–cross-resistant classes of antitumor agents and the conceptual separation of induction and maintenance therapy gave impetus to a large study initiated through the combined effort of two clinical cooperative groups supported by the NCI (Acute Leukemia Group B and the Eastern Solid Tumor Group) (14). In this important early study, which provided the foundation for the future studies on combination chemotherapy that were to prove so effective, 342 patients were randomized by disease and prior therapy to remission induction with cyclophosphamide or one of the vinca alkaloids. Vinblastine was used in Hodgkin's disease and vincristine in non-Hodgkin's lymphomas, known then as lymphosarcoma and reticulum cell sarcoma. The objectives of this study were to compare the effectiveness of the vinca alkaloids to an alkylating agent, in this case cyclophosphamide, in remission induction in lymphomas. These investigators also studied the duration of response. Patients received either cyclophosphamide or placebo to maintain the remission, and the investigators also compared the effectiveness of continuous therapy versus intermittent with regard to induction with cyclophosphamide. The results established the superiority of vinblastine over cyclophosphamide for remission induction in patients with advanced Hodgkin's disease. In all disease categories, the average duration of placebo-maintained remission was a remarkably short 4 to 6 weeks, irrespective of the drug used to induce the remission. Daily oral cyclophosphamide significantly prolonged remission duration when compared to placebo, confirming the observation of Scott (10). Remission duration with drug maintenance treatment was, however, only 32 weeks for Hodgkin's disease.

There were two other features of this study that were not initially emphasized but that had a profound influence on the studies later designed with curative intent by NCI investigators. First, patients were separated by whether they had partial or complete remissions, a practice used to evaluate treatments in leukemias but not generally employed at that time in solid tumors. Response duration was always significantly longer for patients who achieved complete remission, emphasizing the importance of this subset of responders, which remains true today. Second, regardless of the approach to treatment, overall survival in the various subgroups in each disease category was almost identical. These data indicated that, while maintenance drug treatment did prolong remission duration and provided a smooth way to manage patients in the normal practice of medicine, survival was not compromised by a decision to induce remissions and leave patients untreated until relapse. The value of obtaining a complete remission and the failure of the maintenance treatment to prolong survival allowed the investigators at the NCI, using combination chemotherapy, to set as their major initial goal achieving a high complete remission rate and to leave complete responding patients off all future therapy to evaluate the capacity of their new treatment program to eradicate the tumor (cure the disease, if you will).

The appearance of vinca alkaloids was followed shortly by the discovery of the antitumor activity of the methylhydrazine derivative procarbazine, then called ibenzmenthyzin, in Hodgkin's disease by Bollag and Grunberg (15), Mathe and colleagues (16), Martz and colleagues (17) in Europe, and by DeVita and colleagues (18) in the United States. These studies and others indicated that procarbazine was almost exclusively useful in Hodgkin's disease, a curious and unexplained observation even today.

THE BASIC PRINCIPLES OF CHEMOTHERAPY

With the two exceptions of choriocarcinoma and Burkitt's lymphoma, treatment with single agents, unlike the treatment of bacterial infections, is unable to cure patients with cancer (19,20). Therefore, there was interest very early in combining drugs, although as in the treatment of bacterial infections at the time the practice was frowned upon. Early attempts to design drug combinations were based on the principle of sequential biochemical blockage. Using known or suspected mechanisms of action of anticancer drugs, combinations were constructed that would theoretically strangle cancer cells biochemically (21–23). These attempts were ineffective due to the fact that most of the drugs selected by mechanism only were individually inactive against the cancers treated with the combinations. Another principle important to the design of successful combination chemotherapy was born from this observation. For a drug to be beneficial in combination with other agents, it had to demonstrate clinical activity by itself in the disease in question.

In the 1950s and 1960s, most drugs were given by routes and schedules empirically derived and administered in a fixed dose, without regard to body weight or surface area. It was standard practice for clinical protocols to call for therapy administered for a continuous 6-week period but not longer, regardless of response. In short, little scientific thinking went into protocol design. The basic underpinnings of the principles of cancer chemotherapy are owed to Howard Skipper and colleagues at the Southern Research Institute (SRI). The SRI had major contracts for screening compounds with the NCI's drug development program, the CCNSC, and its investigators were prompted to study the model used for screening, L1210, which at that time was an incurable transplantable rodent leukemia. By 1964, Skipper and colleagues had worked out the doubling time of L1210 using crude ascites cell counts and, by back extrapolating from the extensions of survival produced by anticancer drugs, were able to show that a given dose of a drug killed a constant fraction of cells, not a fixed number (the "fractional cell kill" hypothesis) (24,25). The implications were that by increasing the dose the fractional kill could be maximized. It also became obvious that cell number at the start of treatment was of overriding importance. Coupled with clinical testing in human leukemias, these principles suggested that leukemia was more treatable than previously supposed. From these data they also developed the inverse rule, the invariable inverse relationship between cell number and curability by chemotherapy, a rule that has stood the test of experimentation in rodents for decades. Although rarely testable in the clinic, the inverse rule was to be tested using nitrogen mustard, Oncovin (vincristine), procarbazine, and prednisone (MOPP) in early-stage Hodgkin's disease and in other lymphomas using combination chemotherapy.

Tolerable doses of single agents prolonged survival in L1210 but did not cure it. To cure this rodent leukemia, combinations of drugs were needed and they had to be individually effective and used in schedules actually optimized in this rodent model. In 1964 Skipper reported the first cure of a rodent tumor, the L1210 model, using these principles. These studies had an important impact on the thinking of clinical investigators developing new treatments that were to prove curative for childhood leukemia (reviewed in ref. 26). The concept that human malignancies could be cured by chemotherapy was bolstered by the early studies in the childhood leukemia model. These studies also had a profound stimulating effect on the early trials of the treatment of Hodgkin's disease, carried out in the same institution.

Applying these principles to the drug treatment of human cancers in patients with intact bone marrow function, however, required additional data on the differences between growth characteristics of rodent leukemia and those of human cancers, and the differences in growth rates of the main normal target tissue in mice and human, the bone marrow.

More precise data on the cell kinetics of the L1210 leukemia model and the kinetics of both mouse and human bone marrow were made possible by the availability of the then new tool tritiated thymidine for labeling of cells progressing through DNA synthesis. The cell kinetic data led to the development of the now-standard cyclical chemotherapy given for 2 weeks with 2-week rest intervals (25–31). A guiding principle was the scheduling of cycles of chemotherapy around the kinetics of bone marrow recovery after exposure to cytotoxic agents, which was about twice as long in humans as in the mouse. *In vivo* cell kinetic studies in humans with other solid tumors using tritiated thymidine also showed that cycle times of cancer cells were the same as normal cells, but the growth fraction was small, indicating that exposure to cytotoxic drugs over many cycle times would be necessary to expose all malignant cells to drugs during vulnerable periods of their cell cycle. These data suggested that the standard 6-week exposure to cancer drugs used in protocols of the day, including human leukemia studies, was likely to be too short.

THE BIRTH OF COMBINATION CHEMOTHERAPY FOR HODGKIN'S DISEASE

The first intensive drug combination program designed to exploit the new principles of chemotherapy in Hodgkin's disease began in 1963 and utilized the combination of cyclophosphamide, vincristine, methotrexate, and prednisone (MOMP) given for only 2½ months (32–34). The goal of this pilot protocol was to test the safety of combination chemotherapy in advanced Hodgkin's disease. Only 14 patients were studied, and all were hospitalized and kept in reverse isolation. Ultimately the approach was shown to be safe, and a high complete remission rate (80%) was attained. One other combination drug program was reported at that time. In 1964, Lacher and Durant (35) reported that the administration of low-dose vinblastine and chlorambucil in combination achieved a remission rate of approximately 30%. However, these remissions were not well documented and this was not a significant improvement over the response rate achieved with vinblastine alone. No further reports were ever published on the patients in this study. As experience accrued with procarbazine, the MOMP program was modified in several ways in 1964. Because of the data on the low growth fractions for human tumors, duration of treatment was increased to 6 months and procarbazine, by now an agent known to be active in Hodgkin's disease, was substituted for the antifol methotrexate for which there was less evidence of clinical utility. This new program was the above-defined MOPP (36,37).

Several of the principles previously outlined guided the selection of drugs in the MOPP program:

1. Only drugs known to be partially effective when used alone in Hodgkin's disease were selected for use in the MOPP combination. Drugs that produced some fraction of complete remissions were preferred to those that produced only partial responses.
2. Drugs were selected for toxicity that did not overlap with other drugs used in the combination. While vinblastine was thought to be more effective than vincristine in Hodgkin's disease at that time, there were sufficient data to suggest equal efficacy, and the absence of marrow toxicity from vincristine made it an attractive drug to partner the marrow-cytotoxic alkylating agent and procarbazine. This type of logic in the selection led to a wider range of side effects and greater general discomfort to the patient, but it minimized the risk of a lethal effect to a single target organ and allowed for maximizing dosage despite combining cytotoxic drugs, in an era when methods of supportive care were still quite primitive.
3. Drugs were used in their optimal dose and schedule, and doses were not routinely adjusted downward because a combination of drugs was to be used.
4. The drugs in MOPP were to be given at consistent intervals. This led to the development of the now-standard sliding scale for dose adjustment to preserve the integrity of the combination of drugs while adhering to schedules and minimizing toxicity.

In principle, it was also felt that the use of effective drugs in combination would cover more resistant cell lines present in a heterogeneous tumor mass, and prevent or slow the development of resistance.

The interval selected between cycles was the narrowest possible to allow for recovery of the most sensitive normal target tissue, the bone marrow. Cell kinetic studies had shown that the bone marrow had a storage compartment that could supply mature cells to the peripheral blood for 8 to 10 days after the stem cell pool had been exposed to a cytotoxic agent and temporarily ceased to function. The actual clinical data derived from these early studies showed that events measured in the peripheral blood were usually a week behind the events in the bone marrow. Therefore, even after a cytotoxic event in previously untreated patients, leukopenia and thrombocytopenia were discernible only after the 9th or 10th day after initial dosing. The nadir of these blood counts was reached by the 14th to 18th day, with some recovery apparent by the 21st and usually complete recovery by the 28th day. Prior treatment with drugs or x-ray altered the sequence by shortening the time to the appearance of leukopenia and thrombocytopenia and prolonging the recovery time. Curiously, the habit of giving the second half of the drug combination in the clinic 1 week later (day 8), just preceding the usual onset of leukopenia and thrombocytopenia, proved safe even though peripheral blood count suppression appeared even if the second dose was omitted. The most important cytotoxic dose-response effect turned out to be the duration of nadir white cell and platelet counts, not the absolute level of cytopenia. This was fortunate since the most dangerous depression of blood counts (a granulocyte count of less than 500/dL, and a platelet count less than 20,000/dL) lasted only 4 to 7 days and was tolerated by most patients even without supplemental support.

In 1967, the results of the use of MOPP in the first 43 patients were reported, and an 81% (35 patients) complete remission rate was noted. This was a fourfold increase over results achieved with the best use of single agents, and those remissions proved durable and influenced survival (36). Other controlled and uncontrolled studies confirmed the results of the MOPP program (38–44). Hugeley and associates (44) compared the use of MOPP chemotherapy to intensive use of the single agent, nitrogen mustard. Although the complete remission rate for the MOPP program (48%) in this study was less than that reported by the NCI, there was a statistically significant difference between the ability of MOPP and nitrogen mustard to induce complete remissions; nitrogen mustard induced complete remissions in only 13% of patients (40,44).

British investigators modified the MOPP program to alter the toxic profile. Sutliffe and colleagues reported on a modification of the MOPP program that substituted vinblastine for vincristine and was able to achieve a 42% complete remission rate (45). A complete remission rate comparable to that of the NCI was reported by the group from Stanford (41) and Frei and colleagues (39) in a large study from the Southwest Oncology Group, with remission rates ranging from 66% to 74%. While the Stanford group confirmed the NCI results, its concern with the neurotoxicity of vincristine led it to recommend capping the dose at 2 mg total dose in future studies, an approach that significantly altered the dose intensity of this drug, affected future studies of MOPP, and is unfortunately still widely practiced even though no evidence supports the practice. Patients previously treated with chemotherapy responded less well to MOPP chemotherapy than previously untreated patients, as reported by Lowenbraun and colleagues (46). Exposure to prior radiotherapy did not, however, seem to compromise the patient's ability to respond to chemotherapy (38,47–49).

NCI investigators reported in a 20-year follow-up study the results of treatment of the first 198 Hodgkin's disease patients with the MOPP program as their primary treatment (48,49); 159 of the 198 patients (80%) achieved a complete remission. These patients required a median number of three cycles to attain remission. The only characteristics significantly associated with a greater probability of attaining a complete remission in this population were the absence of fever, night sweats, and weight loss (B symptoms) and the rate of delivery of vincristine. For example, all 23 patients without symptoms attained complete remission, compared to 78% of the symptomatic patients. This difference was highly significant and only one asymptomatic patient has relapsed in subsequent years. Of the 32 patients who had received local radiotherapy, before MOPP treatment, all but two (94%) attained complete remission, compared to 78% of the unirradiated patients. While this difference was not significant, the p value was .065, and for the most part this trend has been consistent in most subsequent studies.

NCI investigators reported survival results in terms of tumor mortality since different treatments were not compared in the original MOPP studies. Sixty-three percent of patients achieving complete remission, who were at risk for longer than 10 years, remained disease free. The proportion of all treated patients who remained free of relapse at 10 years and beyond was 54.6%. Although most relapses tended to occur within 42 months after cessation of the therapy, three relapses occurred at 77, 82, and 92 months. The NCI authors further reported that three factors had a significant influence on the durability of the remissions. The first was, again, the absence of systemic symptoms. Only one of the 23 asymptomatic patients relapsed. The second was the histologic subtype of the disease. A significantly worse prognosis was noted in patients with nodular sclerosing Hodgkin's disease. When this group was further analyzed, the poor prognosis was related to patients with the lymphocyte depleted, nodular sclerosing disease subtype. The third factor was, again, the rate of delivery of vincristine, once again confirming that altering doses of this vinca alkaloid could affect outcome.

There were 98 recorded deaths, 23 (24%) of which represented patients who died without evidence of Hodgkin's disease. Autopsies were done in 15 of these 23 patients and no Hodgkin's disease was detected in 14, further supporting the contention that in patients who appear to be in clinical remission, the disease was eradicated by chemotherapy.

While 80% of patients treated with MOPP, or variants of MOPP, entered complete remission, approximately 35% of patients relapsed by the fifth year of follow-up. The next question posed by the NCI group was whether maintenance drug therapy would be beneficial after achieving a complete remission, as had been the case in human leukemias. The first such study in Hodgkin's disease was also conducted at the NCI. After achieving complete remission patients were randomly allocated to intermittent cycles of carmustine [bischloroethylnitrosourea (BCNU)] or no therapy or intermittent cycles of MOPP. Maintenance treatment was given for 15 months. When the results of this study were reported in 1973, and when reanalyzed in 1980 and since, no significant advantage was found for either continued intermittent MOPP or intermittent carmustine therapy (48,50). The toxicity in the two chemotherapeutic arms was significantly greater than in the no-maintenance-treatment arm. The Southwest Oncology Group did a comparison study between the use of intermittent MOPP as maintenance therapy, given as two cycles every 3 months, and no further therapy after the initial six cycles of MOPP. While these authors initially reported a prolongation of remission duration with MOPP maintenance, this difference was lost by the seventh year of follow-up. Eight other studies have addressed the same question using a variety of maintenance treatments, and none of these programs have shown a positive effect (39,40,45,50–56). These data made an impressive case for discontinuation of therapy after it has been carefully documented that a complete remission has been achieved. These data also provide further indirect evidence that a substantial number of patients who achieve a complete remission are indeed cured of their disease, since it might be expected that continuation of therapy, in the form of maintenance, would have no benefit in cured patients. The initial advantage in the relapse-free survival curve reported by Frei and colleagues (39) could be explained by the effect of drug maintenance on patients who failed to have a documented true complete remission and, therefore, profited by temporary suppression of tumor regrowth.

An important biologic principle related to the issue of de novo resistance to chemotherapy emerged from the study of patients who relapsed after achieving complete remission after MOPP treatment and were retreated with the same regimen; 59% of 32 patients who relapsed after treatment achieved a second complete remission (57). However, only 5 out of 17 patients (29%) whose initial complete remission was less than 1 year in duration achieved a second complete remission compared to 14 out of 15 (93%) patients whose initial complete remission was a year or longer, a statistically significant difference ($p = .001$), and once again remissions in this latter group were durable. The duration of the second remission was significantly longer in patients whose initial complete remission exceeded 1 year than in those whose initial remission was less than 1 year. Overall survival was significantly improved in those patients who achieved second remissions over those who did not achieve a second remission ($p = .005$). Long-term follow-up of this study group confirmed these results in terms of tumor mortality, but the overall survival of the group retreated after long initial remissions was compromised, and reduced by half, due to complications of repeated and prolonged chemotherapy, not by Hodgkin's disease (58).

Data on the importance of the initial remission duration and data that demonstrated that maintenance therapy in complete responders does not improve relapse-free survival have led to several conclusions. Patients who are truly cured during remission induction cannot experience beneficial effects from maintenance therapy. Retained sensitivity to MOPP in patients who stay in remission in excess of 1 year indicated that patients were almost cured by the induction program, and might benefit from future intensification of treatment. However, the failure of malignant cells in this population to develop resistance over several years following MOPP argues strongly against a spontaneous pressure toward mutations that would lead to resistance. This is suggested by the fact that 14 out of 15 patients who relapsed 1 year or more after the end of therapy achieved a durable second remission. The relative insensitivity of the tumor of patients who experience short remissions (<12 months) suggests that the primary cause of treatment failure in this group is the presence and overgrowth of cells resistant to the drugs in the MOPP program at the time of diagnosis. More importantly, the observation on retained sensitivity after long drug-induced remissions has carried over to virtually all types of advanced cancers where complete remissions in response to drug combinations are feasible and illustrate an important and general biologic principle that is under investigation (59,60).

By 1970, with the publication of the impressive survival curves in MOPP-treated patients, it was possible to state that advanced Hodgkin's disease was curable by combination chemotherapy. This made it ethically possible to proceed with the question of the use of chemotherapy alone to cure early Hodgkin's disease, when the tumor volume was low and presumably more vulnerable to chemotherapy, in a patient population where a significant fraction could be cured by radiotherapy alone.

Such a trial was initiated at the NCI in 1978, the first of its kind, and compared MOPP therapy alone, in laparotomy-staged patients, to subtotal nodal irradiation therapy (61). The results of that study showed that MOPP, in the original study group, was statistically superior to radiotherapy in both relapse-free and overall survival. This study confirmed that the inverse rule applied as well, in that the complete remission rate was 95% in MOPP-treated early-stage disease compared to 80% in the NCI studies of patients with advanced disease, and only 15% of MOPP-treated, complete-responding, early-stage patients relapsed compared to 35% of complete responders with advanced disease. When the early-stage study was reanalyzed with patients with large mediastinal masses removed from both groups, the results of MOPP and radiotherapy were equivalent in relapse-free and overall survival, as the results of radiotherapy without patients with large mediastinal masses improved. Only one other similar trial has been done in the world, and although the results are conflicting (62), they have led some investigators to explore chemotherapy as an alternative to radiotherapy in early-stage patients as long-term toxic effects of radiotherapy, with the appearance of in-field solid tumors, continue to emerge as a major problem (63).

Thus, virtually every observation thought to be important to the chemotherapy of Hodgkin's disease was made in some form in these initial MOPP studies (47). In addition to those prognostic and biologic factors mentioned above, they include the first evidence of the long-term carcinogenic effects of cancer chemotherapeutic agents in cured humans (64,65); the first evidence of male sterility from cytotoxic drugs (66), and the impact of chemotherapy on ovarian function (67); the first evidence of the recovery of the immune defect unique to Hodgkin's disease with therapy that was in itself immunosuppressive (68); and the identification of infectious complications unique to cancer patients at that time, including the first successful diagnosis and treatment of *Pneumocystis carinii* pneumonia in an adult (69).

This saga of clinical investigation, conducted by a single group at one institution, took 29 years, as measured by the time it took to completely publish the results of all the studies designed in the 1960s and 1970s, and is a testimony to the difficulties of clinical investigation. It also led to the first cure of diffuse large cell lymphomas with a variant of MOPP, which is another story in itself (70).

However, it remained to find ways to treat those who were not cured by MOPP. With the passage of the National Cancer Act in 1971, a long and enduring relationship developed with investigators in Milan, most especially between the two authors of this chapter, that was to lead to the next major advance in the chemotherapy of Hodgkin's disease, the development of a second drug combination not cross-resistant to MOPP—Adriamycin, bleomycin, vinblastine, and dacarbazine (ABVD). Other collaborations between the NCI and the Istituto Nazionale Tumori would also revolutionize the treatment of breast cancer, which is not unrelated to Hodgkin's disease, as it took evidence that drugs could cure some kinds of advanced cancers of major organ systems in adults, such as Hodgkin's disease, to overcome the extraordinary resistance to the concept of the use of toxic cancer drugs as an adjuvant to surgery in patients, some of whom were presumably cured by surgery alone, most especially in diseases like breast cancer. This proved impossible in the early years in the United States, and Italian investigators broke new ground.

THE RATIONALE FOR THE ABVD PROGRAM

Although the MOPP studies carried out at the NCI revolutionized the treatment of advanced Hodgkin's disease, 15% to 30% of patients did not achieve complete remission after MOPP and 20% to 30% of complete responders eventually relapsed. This indicated selective drug resistance in patients with primary treatment failure or early disease recurrence. Thus, at the beginning of the 1970s, these limits of MOPP or MOPP-derived combinations, as well as the availability of new compounds (71–74), induced many investigators to design and test new chemotherapeutic regimens to be delivered first in MOPP-resistant patients and then to potentially substitute for or complement the four drugs used in the MOPP combination (59). The ABVD program was the first and most effective. The four drugs included in the ABVD regimen (75) were selected based on pharmacologic and clinical rationales and built on the basic principles of chemotherapy reviewed above. Adriamycin, a new anticancer antibiotic, became available during the summer of 1968. It was first tested through phase I and II studies by the medical oncology group at the Milan Cancer Institute (72–75). During these studies, the most important properties of this new antibiotic were observed, namely its prompt therapeutic effects, the wide range of responsive tumors, the lack of cross-resistance to many standard drugs, as well as the problem of cardiac toxicity. In the experience of the Milan Cancer Institute, Adriamycin, delivered through five different schedules, was found particularly effective in malignant lymphomas previously treated with standard regimens (71).

In 1972, Frei et al. (78) reported that dacarbazine, administered intravenously in a 5-day course at the initial dose of 250 mg/m^2, was able to achieve objective remissions in 56% of previously treated patients with Hodgkin's disease. The selection of dacarbazine, like vincristine in MOPP, was in part because it is devoid of significant myelosuppression in the majority of adequately treated patients. When combined with Adriamycin, a synergism was found in experimental systems, with no additive toxicity.

Of the two remaining drugs, the antibiotic bleomycin was also devoid of myelosuppression and non–cross-resistant with the drugs included in the MOPP regimen, while vinblastine appeared to show little cross-resistance with vincristine in humans, despite evidence of cross-resistance in animal neoplasms.

Thus, the four drugs were combined. During the initial part of the first clinical trial (70), the dose schedule was as follows: Adriamycin (25 mg/m^2), bleomycin (10 mg/m^2), and vinblastine (6 mg/m^2) were administered on days 1 and 15 every 4 weeks, while dacarbazine was given during the first 5 days of each treatment cycle at the dose of 150 mg/m^2. All drugs were delivered by rapid intravenous injection. Subsequently, to reduce nausea and vomiting associated with prolonged exposure to dacarbazine, the treatment schedule was made simpler and dacarbazine was delivered on days 1 and 15 at the dose of 375 mg/m^2. The selected treatment schedule was similar to the MOPP program with rest intervals chosen to allow marrow recovery between the two drug courses of each cycle in the vast majority of patients. A sliding scale to adjust for dose-related marrow toxicity, however, was planned to permit the administration of each cycle on time and to preserve the dose rate. As in the MOPP program, subsequent cycles were delayed only if toxicity was severe enough to require omission of drugs from that cycle to preserve the integrity of the drug combination (36,75).

A pilot study was mounted in 1973 (75) to test in a randomized fashion whether ABVD chemotherapy could induce a complete remission rate comparable with that achieved with MOPP chemotherapy. The case series included 76 consecutive patients, 55 of whom were previously untreated and 21 in their first relapse in nodal or extranodal sites after primary radical radiotherapy. Six cycles of either regimen were delivered and complete plus partial responders were subsequently irradiated. In the presence of primary chemotherapy failure or treatment relapse, a crossover treatment was carried out between MOPP and ABVD. Table 1 summarizes the essential comparative results at 5 years. Overall, six cycles of either regimen yielded a comparable incidence of complete remissions, particularly in patients with extranodal disease, and this trend had an influence on the 5-year freedom from progression and relapse-free survival rates (79). The median time to achieve complete remission was similar to the original MOPP study, about 4 months for both treatments. The limited number of patients enrolled in this trial prevented any adequate assessment of treatment outcome in relation to main characteristics.

Treatment tolerance was, in general, fairly good for both regimens. No increased incidence of bacterial and viral infection was observed, and, during six cycles, more than 85% of the planned doses for each drug could be administered in both regimens. Myelosuppression represented the most common side effect, but during chemotherapy the incidence of severe myelosuppression, as determined at the time of intravenous drug injection, was negligible. Subsequent radiotherapy was found to be slightly more toxic to bone marrow in the MOPP group where, compared to ABVD, a higher number of patients had to delay or discontinue irradiation (79). There were major differences between MOPP and ABVD in reference to toxicity, however. During the first 5 years of follow-up, two patients in the MOPP group developed acute leukemias, while fatal radiation pneumonitis occurred in a patient given ABVD. One patient of the ABVD group developed cardiomegaly after 433 mg/m^2 of Adriamycin. Despite three episodes of congestive failure, the patient remained alive and disease-free 5 years from completion of the irradiation program, which included the mediastinal area (79).

This pilot study showed that ABVD chemotherapy was as effective as MOPP in inducing durable remissions in advanced Hodgkin's disease. Acute toxic effects were similar in both drug regimens, but the later sequelae were completely different. Radiation therapy contributed to the development of acute leukemias in patients given the alkylating-containing regimen, whereas the concomitant effect of Adriamycin, bleomycin, and irradiation to the heart and lungs proved to be of a concern with ABVD. Based on these results, in September 1974, investigators of the Milan Cancer Institute initiated a new multimodal study to compare treatment results and iatrogenic morbidity, especially sterility and carcinogenesis, in a large series of patients with pathologic stage IIB and III (A and B) (80). All patients were previously untreated and were randomly allocated to receive three cycles of MOPP or ABVD before and after irradiation. Both drug regimens were administered according to the classic dose schedule; subtotal nodal irradiation was delivered in patients with no retroperitoneal adenopathy, while all other patients received total nodal irradiation. Radiation therapy (35 Gy to involved lymphoid areas, 30 Gy to adjacent areas) was preceded and followed by a 4- to 6-week rest period. By July 1982, a total of 232 eligible patients were entered onto this study. Preliminary and intermediate results (80,81) showed that treatment started with ABVD induced a higher frequency of durable complete remissions (92%) compared with treatment including MOPP (81%, p <.02). Long-term results assessed after a median follow-up of 18 years are reported in Table 2. While the superiority of the Adriamycin-containing regimen in regard to remission duration and tumor mortality is apparent, there has been no significant effect on overall survival. Death due to progressive lymphoma occurred in one-third of the patients started on MOPP and in 14% of those started on ABVD, while treatment-related deaths accounted for 2% and 7% of cases, respectively.

In both treatment groups, other causes of death were mainly attributable to the development of second malignancies. The cumulative incidence of second malignancies 18 years from starting chemotherapy was 10% in the MOPP group and 14% in the ABVD group. Four cases of acute leukemia were documented in the alkylating-containing regimen, while in the ABVD group one patient developed overt leukemia and in another patient a myelodysplastic syndrome was documented. In a regression analysis aimed at assessing variables poten-

TABLE 1. *Essential comparative results of the first pilot study testing MOPP vs. ABVD*

	MOPP (41 patients)	ABVD (35 patients)
Complete response (%)		
After chemotherapy	63	71
After chemotherapy plus radiotherapy	71	80
Survival at 5 years in complete responders (%)		
Relapse-free	84	91
Total survival	88	90

ABVD, Adriamycin, bleomycin, vinblastine, and dacarbazine; MOPP, nitrogen mustard, Oncovin, procarbazine, and prednisone.

TABLE 2. *Essential comparative results after MOPP-RT-MOPP vs. ABVD-RT-ABVD in stage IIB and III*[a]

	MOPP group (114 patients)	ABVD group (118 patients)
Complete remission (%)	81*	92*
Freedom from progression (%)	60**	77**
Freedom from tumor mortality (%)	67**	86**
Total survival (%)	56	62

[a]Median follow-up, 18 years.
*p=.02; **p=.002.
RT, radiation therapy

tially able to increase the risk of second cancers, the only factor able to significantly influence the development of second tumors was age at start of the multimodal treatment, the relative risk being fivefold higher in patients older than 40 years of age compared with younger patients (p = .0001), an observation that has subsequently been confirmed by others. Cardiac and pulmonary functions were assessed in a selected subgroup of patients who were in continuous complete remission for more than 5 years and agreed to participate in the necessary tests (75). Parenchymal lung damage, as assessed through systematic reevaluation of chest roentgenograms, occurred in both treatment groups along with increased radiation doses delivered to the mediastinum. Although lesions were more frequently detected in the ABVD-treated group (59% vs. 30%, p = .001), no clear radiographic evidence of bleomycin-related toxicity was documented. During the subsequent follow-up, the radiologic patterns remained essentially unchanged. Nevertheless, 18 years from starting treatment, pulmonary toxicity was the cause of death in 2% of MOPP-treated patients and in 4% of ABVD-treated patients. Gonadal toxicity was assessed in a small subset of 38 male patients who were younger than 45 years of age at the time of gonadal evaluation and who had received only subtotal nodal irradiation. All 13 patients treated with MOPP were azoospermic, while in the 25 patients started on ABVD, azoospermia was documented in 9 (36%) and oligospermia in 5 (20%). Sperm counts could be repeated in only 23 patients. As reported by the NCI group (66), only 1 in 10 tested patients given MOPP had recovery of spermatogenesis 36 months after the first sperm analysis, whereas full recovery was documented within 18 months in all 13 patients on ABVD who were tested (79).

ABVD in MOPP-Resistant Patients

Since the initial study testing MOPP versus ABVD in advanced Hodgkin's disease (75), it was noticed that salvage treatment with ABVD in patients failing during or soon after MOPP yielded higher complete remission rates (46%), compared with the opposite sequence, i.e., salvage MOPP in ABVD-resistant patients (25%) (79). The study of ABVD as second-line therapy, therefore, was pursued also in other patients resistant to primary MOPP (79). Before and after treatment with ABVD, patients were thoroughly staged. The duration of chemotherapy was flexible and related to the achievement of complete remission, and a minimum of six treatment cycles were planned in responsive patients, while after the attainment of complete remission patients were to receive two additional cycles. Postchemotherapy irradiation was delivered as consolidation treatment in a limited number of patients, especially in those who could achieve only a good partial remission (tumor shrinkage >75%) after six or more cycles. Table 3 summarizes the main therapeutic results. Overall, ABVD alone was able to attain complete remission in 46% of the 56 treated patients (36). The likelihood of achieving complete remission was significantly influenced by type of resistance to MOPP (primary failures vs. short-lasting remission, p = .04), and by the absence of extranodal disease (p = .009). There was no statistical evidence that age, sex, systemic symptoms, and histologic characteristics affected the probability of attaining a complete response with ABVD. It is worth noting that consolidative irradiation was able to achieve complete remission in six patients who were classified as partial responders after ABVD. Nevertheless, median duration of complete remission was shorter in this subgroup of patients (14.5 months) compared with those who showed prompt response (24.5 months). From all the above-reported findings, ABVD chemotherapy was demonstrated to be an effective salvage regimen, potentially able to achieve cure in approximately one-third of MOPP-resistant patients.

TABLE 3. *Essential results with ABVD in MOPP-resistant patients*

	No.	Complete remission (%)	p
Total series	56	46	
Failing during MOPP	33	33	.04
Relapsing <12 months	23	65	
Systemic symptoms			
Absent	22	59	.19
Present	34	38	
Disease extent			
Nodal	23	70	.009
Extranodal ± nodal	33	30	
5-year results			
Relapse-free survival			37%
Total survival			44%
Survival in complete responders			53%

THE RATIONALE FOR THE ALTERNATING DELIVERY OF MOPP AND ABVD

Having established that both the MOPP regimen developed at the Medicine Branch of the NCI in Bethesda, Maryland, and the ABVD chemotherapy developed at the Milan Cancer Institute were highly effective combinations able to induce durable complete remission in approximately two-thirds of patients with advanced Hodgkin's disease, the next step toward the achievement of a potentially higher cure rate was to combine them in some way. Clinical observations from both case series confirmed that patients with resistance to either MOPP or ABVD showed lymphoma progression after the first few cycles of chemotherapy, or within a few months after an initial complete remission, and that a fraction of these patients could be salvaged by the alternative chemotherapy. Based on these observations, investigators at the Milan Cancer Institute empirically designed what was called the alternating MOPP and ABVD regimen (79).

The following major biologic and pharmacologic principles underlying the use of non–cross-resistant regimens in the primary treatment of advanced cancer, in particular of Hodgkin's disease, were also largely derived from studies by Skipper (81,82): (a) neoplastic cells were thought to mutate spontaneously to a state of specific resistance to a wide variety of anticancer drugs; (b) essentially all classes of anticancer drugs can select and allow overgrowth of specifically drug-resistant neoplastic cells; (c) the rate of selection of a drug-resistant subline of cancer cells is directly related to the rate of eradication of the drug-sensitive cells and is influenced by the tumor cell burden and the intensity and duration of treatment; (d) if the tumor population is large (e.g., stage III–IV malignant lymphomas), combination chemotherapy may select sublines that are resistant to two or more drugs; (e) the number of anticancer drugs that show little or no cross-resistance is larger than some realize.

The First MOPP/ABVD Program

The first study was started in September 1974, and by May 1982, 88 consecutive patients classified as stage IV according to the Ann Arbor criteria, and previously untreated with chemotherapy, were prospectively randomized to receive either 12 monthly cycles of MOPP, twice the number of cycles normally used, to match treatment duration in both arms of the study, or six cycles of MOPP monthly alternated with six cycles of ABVD (83). Patients with stage IV disease were selected because the high frequency of resistant cells in disseminated lymphoma provided the best test for assessing the effectiveness of a regimen that alternated singly effective combinations. In fact, in many untreated patients with nodal lymphoma, the rate of spontaneous mutation may be low, and this would explain the excellent results achieved in earlier stages with either MOPP or ABVD alone. In responsive patients, treatment duration in both arms was longer than usually planned with MOPP and was selected in the attempt to deliver an adequate treatment in all patient subsets and to decrease the frequency of late relapses, which can potentially be caused by undertreatment (57,84).

MOPP was delivered in the schedule designed at the NCI Medicine Branch (36) both when used alone or alternated with ABVD. Also ABVD was given at the classic dose schedule (75) and was started on day 29 from the initiation of the previous MOPP cycle; in the alternating regimen both regimens were recycled every other month. No consolidation radiotherapy was delivered to responsive patients.

The early findings demonstrated a superiority of the alternating regimen over MOPP alone in the achievement of complete remission (89% vs. 74%) (83), and this superiority was evident in those subsets known to be less affected by MOPP chemotherapy (Table 4). However, in this study, attempting to give MOPP for 12 months led to a marked reduction in dose intensity (59), which could have accounted for the differences. It has not proven possible to maintain the intensity of dosing particularly with vincristine for 12 months in a program as toxic as MOPP. A study of alternating chemotherapy at the NCI in Bethesda, compared MOPP alone in six cycles at full doses, with no vincristine capping, to three cycles of MOPP alternating with three cycles of a combination of cyclohexl-nitrosourea, Adriamycin, bleomycin, and streptozotocin (CABS). CABS had also been shown to be equally as effective as MOPP in untreated patients with advanced Hodgkin's disease and able to salvage MOPP failures as efficiently as ABVD (85). The results showed no advantage for alternating cyclical chemotherapy when MOPP was given at full doses. CABS, although effective, has proven too toxic for general use. A similar study in the United Kingdom using LOPP (leukeran, vincristine, procarbazine, prednisone), a much less dose-intensive version of MOPP, alone versus LOPP alternating with EVAP (etoposide, vinblastine, cytarabine, cifplatin)

TABLE 4. *Essential results of MOPP vs. alternating MOPP/ABVD in stage IV disease*[a]

	MOPP (43 patients)	MOPP/ABVD (45 patients)
Complete response (%)		
Total series	74	89
Age >40 years	67	100
Bulky lymphoma	57	89
Systemic symptoms	73	90
Freedom from tumor progression (%)	30*	61*
Freedom from tumor mortality (%)	53**	77**
Total survival (%)	43	53

[a]Median follow-up, 18 years.
*p=.002; **p=.04.

showed superiority of the alternating regime (86). Investigators from the Cancer and Acute Leukemia Group (CALGB) tested MOPP alone versus ABVD alone versus MOPP plus ABVD in stage III and IV patients (87). This study, as was the case in the NCI MOPP/CABS study (85), confirmed that a well-delivered four-drug combination program (ABVD in this case), given in adequate doses, can be as effective as alternating therapy. Again, as in the Milan trial, in this study MOPP doses were reduced far beyond the original NCI experience with MOPP, and vincristine doses were artificially capped (87). When dose intensity is taken into consideration, the balance of data favors a well-administered four-drug combination over two programs alternated.

The 18-year results from the Milan study, however, remain consistent. In that study, with its unique design, alternating two effective and non–cross-resistant drug combinations yielded a superior response rate, although there is no difference in overall survival. Over 18 years 47% of the patients in the MOPP alone group died because of disease progression as compared with 23% of the patients given the alternating regimen. The cumulative incidence of second malignancies was fairly similar in the two treatment groups (10% vs. 14%), and once more patients older than 40 years of age were at higher risk (relative risk 7.08, $p = .015$) to develop a second cancer as compared to their younger counterparts.

SUBSEQUENT STUDIES

As previously mentioned, the first alternating MOPP/ABVD program was empirically designed by investigators of the Milan Cancer Institute and was essentially based on clinical findings from their experience with MOPP and ABVD (79). The study design and its treatment results were subsequently interpreted in a mathematical model proposed by Goldie and Coldman (88) that related the drug sensitivity of tumors to their spontaneous mutation rate. As suggested by this model, based on somatic mutation theory, stable genetic alterations arise in tumor cells and result in phenotypic changes in drug sensitivity. In responsive tumors, such as malignant lymphomas, the proportion of drug-sensitive cells will almost always be much greater than the resistant fraction. For this reason, the tumor can be expected to exhibit temporary measurable remission to chemotherapy until the size of the fraction resistant to the drugs regrows. Two non–cross-resistant combinations offered the promise for a higher rate of continuous complete remission and possibly a higher rate of cure of advanced Hodgkin's disease compared to the continuous administration of a single multidrug regimen.

This fascinating hypothesis coupled with the early results of the first MOPP/ABVD program convinced investigators to test the alternating delivery of the two regimens in a variety of new ways.

Unlike the above-mentioned studies, later trials tested combining all the eight drugs into each cycle of chemotherapy rather than alternating each four-drug cycle monthly, and these regimens were called hybrid regimens. Canadian investigators first designed a regimen in which dacarbazine was deleted and Adriamycin, bleomycin, and vinblastine were delivered on day 8 of each monthly cycle (89). This regimen was able to achieve results similar to those achieved with the standard MOPP/ABVD regimen. A subsequent trial (90) was aimed at testing alternating MOPP/ABVD versus hybrid MOPP and ABV, and found no differences between the two regimens. In another trial, the Milan Cancer Institute randomly tested 415 patients with stage IIB, III, and IV disease with alternating MOPP/ABVD versus hybrid chemotherapy where a half-cycle of MOPP and a half-cycle of ABVD were delivered on days 1 and 15, respectively. At 10 years, the rates of complete remission (91% vs. 89%), freedom from progression (67% vs. 69%), and total survival (74% vs. 72%) were equivalent between the two treatment groups (79).

The 8-year results of U.S. Intergroup trial testing in 737 patients with stage III to IV disease the hybrid MOPP/ABV versus the sequential delivery of a version of MOPP, with the dose of vincristine capped and other significant dose reductions, followed by ABVD have recently been published (91). The hybrid regimen was significantly more effective than the sequential regimen. Rates of complete remission (83% vs. 75%, $p = .02$), failure-free survival (64% vs. 54%, $p = .01$) and total survival (79% vs. 71%, $p = .02$) were significantly improved in the hybrid arm, which was associated with a lower incidence of acute leukemia or myelodysplasia. Overall, results in the sequential administration were not dissimilar to those obtained with MOPP alone in the CALGB trial (87), and both studies had equivalent dose reductions. However, the Canadian study testing the hybrid combination versus standard MOPP/ABVD had to be stopped prematurely because of excessive mortality in the hybrid arm.

The Goldie-Coldman hypothesis has served as the basis for testing alternating combination chemotherapy in a number of other cancers as well, although, because of the lack of truly non–cross-resistant drug combinations in most cancers, adequate tests of the hypothesis have been difficult. With the availability of new data on what might be the basis of drug resistance as we know it (60), and the lack of efficacy of alternating drug combinations, the testing of this approach is no longer a high priority.

THE CONSEQUENCE OF CURE: THE DECLINE IN MORTALITY

MOPP chemotherapy of advanced Hodgkin's disease demonstrated that combination chemotherapy could cure a high proportion of patients with an advanced adult malignancy, using well-defined therapeutic principles. The most reliable indicator of the effectiveness of MOPP chemotherapy in the management of Hodgkin's disease is the decrease in the national mortality rate from Hodgkin's disease in the United States by over 60% once this regimen was extensively utilized in clinical practice, a process that in the United States took 11 years to complete (92).

The principles behind MOPP went beyond the treatment of Hodgkin's disease. The modern approach of intermittent (cyclical) combination chemotherapy with a full-dose regimen, as well as the concept of different dose attenuation schedules in the presence of various types and degrees of toxicity, and the importance of the delivered dose intensity were all derived from the initial trials with MOPP.

Most of the controversy about the treatment of Hodgkin's disease today centers on which approach to combination chemotherapy is the most effective and the impact of dose reductions (93); whether or not radiotherapy is beneficial in advanced disease as an adjunct to chemotherapy; and whether chemotherapy alone can be sufficient for the treatment of early-stage disease to avoid what has become a frightening incidence of solid tumors secondary to radiotherapy, especially breast cancers (63). New poly-drug regimens devised by American and European research institutions require additional follow-up time to document their real benefit as compared to conventional regimens. Actual choices in practice today, outside of a clinical trial, remain one of the standard four-drug programs and, in some cases, a program that combines two of the standard programs in an alternating or hybrid fashion.

Today, nearly one-third of patients with Hodgkin's disease die without evidence of lymphoma at autopsy. A significant number of patients, however, die of complications of therapy, both nonmalignant and malignant. This has led to the focus of new treatment programs on morbidity and the cost of delivery of treatment. Relatively few new programs are evaluating the use of either chemotherapy or radiotherapy alone as compared to combined approaches in all stages of disease.

The total conquest of Hodgkin's disease does not appear to be a too distant goal. To achieve this requires new treatment studies for high-risk groups as well as more consideration of overt and relatively occult treatment morbidity. Patients with Hodgkin's disease should continue to be referred to major research institutions where efforts in accurate diagnosis, proper staging, the discipline of controlled trials, and identification of complications will remain the essential ingredients of progress. It is of passing interest to note also that the cure of this disease has been achieved without the knowledge of the cell of origin of Hodgkin's disease.

REFERENCES

1. Osler W. *The principles and practice of medicine.* New York: D. Appleton, 1894.
2. Marshall EK. *Historical perspectives in chemotherapy.* New York: Academic Press 1964:1.
3. Hersh SM. *Chemical and biological warfare:* American's hidden arsenal. New York: Bobbs Merrill, 1968.
4. Alexander SF. *Final report of bari mustard casualties.* Allied Force Headquarters, Office of the Surgeon, APO 512, June 20, 1944.
5. Goodman LS, Wintrobe MM, Dameshek W, et al. Nitrogen mustard therapy. Use of methyl bis (B-chloroethyl) amine hydrochloride and tris (B-chloroethyl) amine hydrochloride for Hodgkin's disease lymphosarcoma, leukemia, certain allied and miscellaneous disorders. *JAMA* 1946;132:126–132.
6. Alpert LK, Petersen SK. The use of nitrogen mustard in the treatment of lymphomata. Bull US Army Med Dept 1947;7:187–194.
7. Dameshek W, Weisfuse L, Stein T. Nitrogen mustard therapy in Hodgkin's disease. Analysis of 50 consecutive cases. *Blood* 1949;4: 338–379.
8. Farber S, Diamond LK, Mercer RD, et al. Temporary remission in acute leukemia in children produced by folic acid antagonist, 4-aminopteroyl glutamic acid aminopterin. *N Engl J Med* 1948;738:787.
9. Goldin A, Schepartz SA, Venditti JM, DeVita VT. Historical development and current strategy of the National Cancer Institute's Drug Development Program. In: DeVita VT, Busch H, eds. *Methods of cancer research:* cancer drug development, vol 16A.New York: Academic Press 1979:165–247.
10. Scott JL. The effect of nitrogen mustard and maintenance chlorambucil in the treatment of advanced Hodgkin's disease. *Cancer Chemother Rep* 1963;27:27–32.
11. Jacobs EM, Peters FC, Luce JK, et al. Mechlorethamine HCL and cyclophosphamide in the treatment of Hodgkin's disease and the lymphomas. *JAMA* 1969;203:392–398.
12. Craft CB. Results with roentgen ray therapy in Hodgkin's disease. *Bull Staff Meet Univ Mim Hosp* 1940;11:391–409.
13. Johnson IS, Armstrong JG, Gorman M, et al. The vinca alkaloids: a new class of oncolytic agents. *Cancer Res* 1963;23:1390.
14. Carbone PP, Spurr C, Schneiderman M, et al. Management of patients with malignant lymphoma: a comparative study with cyclophosphamide and vinca alkaloids. *Cancer Res* 1963;28:811–822.
15. Bollag F, Grunberg E. Tumor inhibitory effects of a new class of cytotoxic agents: methyl hydrazine derivatives. *Experientia* 1963;19:75.
16. Mathe G, Schweisguth O, Schnieder M, et al. Methylhydrazine in treatment of Hodgkin's disease. *Lancet* 1963;2:1077.
17. Martz G, D'Alessandri A, Keel HJ, et al. Preliminary clinical results with a new antitumor agent RO 4-6467 (NSC 77213). *Cancer Chemother Rep* 1963;33:5–14.
18. DeVita VT, Hahn MA, Oliverio VT. Monoamine oxidase inhibition by a new carcinostatic agent, N-isopropyl-a-(2-methyl-hydrazine)-p-toluamide (MIH). *Proc Soc Exp Biol Med* 1965;120:561–565.
19. DeVita VT, Schein PS. The use of drugs in combination for the treatment of cancer: rationale and results. *N Engl J Med* 1973;288: 998–1006.
20. Li MC, Hertz R, Spencer DB. The effect of methotrexate upon choriocarcinoma and chorioadenoma. *Proc Soc Exp Biol Med* 1956;93: 361–366.
21. Nathanson L, Hall TC, Schilling AC, et al. Concurrent combination chemotherapy of human solid tumors: Experience with three-drug regimen and review of the literature. *Cancer Res* 1969;29:419–425.
22. Potter VR. Sequential blocking of metabolic pathways in vivo. *Proc Soc Exp Biol Med* 1951;76:41–46.
23. Satorelli AC. Approaches to the combination chemotherapy of transplantable neoplasms. *Prog Exp Tumor Res* 1965;6:228–288.
24. Skipper HE, Schabel FM Jr, Wilcox WS. Experimental evaluation of potential anticancer agents. VII. On the criteria and kinetics associated with "curability" of leukemia. *Cancer Chemother Rep* 1964;35:1–111.
25. Skipper HE, Schabel FM Jr, Mellet LB, et al. Implications of biochemical, cytokinetic, pharmacologic, and toxicologic relationships in the design of optimal therapeutic schedules. *Cancer Chemother Rep* 1950; 54:431–450.
26. Frei E II, Freireich EJ. Progress and perspectives in the chemotherapy of acute leukemia. *Adv Chemother* 1965;2:269–298.
27. DeVita VT. Cell kinetics and the chemotherapy of cancer. *Cancer Chemother Rep* 1971;2(part 3):230–233.
28. Young RC, DeVita VT. Cell cycle characteristics of human solid tumors in vivo. *Cell Tissue Kinet* 1970;3:285–295.
29. Yankee RA, DeVita VT, Perry S. The cell cycle of Leukemia L1210 cells in vivo. *Cancer Res* 1967;27:2381–2385.
30. Skipper HE. Reasons for success and failure in treatment of murine

leukemias with the drugs now employed in treating human leukemias. *Cancer Chemother* 1978;1:1–166. (Ann Arbor, MI, University Microfilms International.)
31. DeVita VT, Denham C, Perry S. Relationship of normal CDFI mouse leukocyte kinetics to growth characteristics of leukemia L1210. *Cancer Res* 1969;29:1067–1071.
32. DeVita VT, Moxley JH, Brace K, Frei E III. Intensive combination chemotherapy and x-irradiation in the treatment of Hodgkin's disease. *Proc Am Assoc Cancer Res* 1965;6:15.
33. Skipper HE, Schabel FM, Wilcox WS. Experimental evaluation of potential anticancer agents. XIII. On the criteria and kinetics associated with "curability" of experimental leukemia. *Cancer Chemother Rep* 1964;35:1–11.
34. Moxley JH III, DeVita VT, Brace K, et al. Intensive combination chemotherapy and x-irradiation in Hodgkin's disease. *Cancer Res* 1967;27:1258–1263.
35. Lacher MJ, Durant JR. Combined vinblastine and chlorambucil therapy of Hodgkin's disease. *Ann Intern Med* 1965;62:468–476.
36. DeVita VT, Serpick AA, Carbone PP. Combination chemotherapy in the treatment of advanced Hodgkin's disease. *Ann Intern Med* 1970;73:891–895.
37. DeVita VT, Serpick A. Combination chemotherapy in the treatment of advanced Hodgkin's disease. *Proc Am Assoc Cancer Res* 1967;8:13.
38. Canellos GP, Young RC, DeVita VT. Combination chemotherapy for advanced Hodgkin's disease in relapse following extensive radiotherapy. *Clin Pharmacol Ther* 1972;13:750–754.
39. Frei E III, Luce JK, Gamble JE, et al. Combination chemotherapy in advanced Hodgkin's disease in relapse following extensive radiotherapy. *Clin Pharmacol Ther* 1972;13:750–754.
40. Coltman CA, Frei E, Delaney FC. Effectiveness of actinomycin (A), methotrexate (MTX) and vinblastine (V) in prolonging the duration of combination chemotherapy (MOPP) induced remission in advanced Hodgkin's disease. *Proc ASCO* 1973;9:78.
41. Moore MR, Jones SE, Bull JM, et al. MOPP chemotherapy for advanced Hodgkin's disease. Prognostic factors in 81 patients. *Cancer* 1973;32:52–60.
42. Olweny CLM, Katon-Gole M, Biddie E, et al. Childhood Hodgkin's disease in Uganda: a ten year experience. *Cancer* 1978;42:787–792.
43. British National Lymphoma Investigation. Value of prednisone in combination chemotherapy of stage IV Hodgkin's disease. *Br J Med* 1975; 3:413–414.
44. Hugeley CM, Durant JR, Moores RR, Chank JK, Dorfman R, Johnson RA. A comparison of the effectiveness in advanced Hodgkin's disease of a combination of drugs and a single agent both given intensively over a six-month period. *Cancer* 1975;36:1227–1240.
45. Sutcliffe SB, Wrigley RF, Peto J, et al. MVPP chemotherapy regimen for advanced Hodgkin's disease. *Br Med J* 1978;6114:670–683.
46. Lowenbraun S, DeVita VT, Serpick AA. Combination chemotherapy with nitrogen mustard, vincristine, procarbazine, and prednisone in previously treated Hodgkin s disease. *Blood* 1970;36(6):704–717.
47. DeVita VT. Consequences of the chemotherapy of Hodgkin's disease. *Cancer* 1981;47:1–13.
48. DeVita VT, Simon RM, Hubbard SM, et al. Curability of advanced Hodgkin's disease with chemotherapy: long-term follow-up of MOPP treated patients at NCI. *Ann Intern Med* 1980;92(5):587–595.
49. Longo DL, Young RC, Wesley M, et al. Twenty years of MOPP therapy for Hodgkin's disease. *J Clin Oncol* 1986;4:1295–1305.
50. Young RC, Canellos GP, Chabner BA, et al. Maintenance chemotherapy for advanced Hodgkin's disease in remission. *Lancet* 1973;1: 1339–1343.
51. Durant JR, Gams RA, Velez-Garcia E, et al. BCNU, velban, cyclophosphamide, procarbazine, and prednisone (BVCPP) in advanced Hodgkin's disease. *Cancer* 1978;42(5):2101–2110.
52. Bennett JM, Bakemeier RF, Carbone PP, et al. Clinical trials with BCNU (NSC 409962) in malignant lymphomas by ECOG. *Cancer Treat Rev* 1976;60:737–745.
53. Coltman CA, Jones SE, Grozea RP, et al. Bleomycin in combination with MOPP for the management of Hodgkin's disease. SWOG experience. In: Carter SK, Crooke ST, Umezawa H, eds. *Bleomycins—current status and new developments.* New York: Academic Press;1978:227–242.
54. Morgenfeld M, Somoza N, Magnasco J, et al. Combined chemotherapy with cyclophosphamide, vinblastine, procarbazine, and prednisone (CVPP) vs CVPP plus CCNU (CCVPP) in Hodgkin's disease. *Cancer* 1979;43:1579–1586.
55. Coltman CA Jr, Frei E, Moon TE. MOPP maintenance (MM) vs (VMR) for MOPP induced complete remission (CR) of advanced Hodgkin's disease. *Proc ASCO* 1976;17:300.
56. Nissen NI, Stutzman L, Holland JF, et al. Chemotherapy of Hodgkin's disease in studies by Acute Leukemia Group B. *Arch Intern Med* 1973; 13:396–401.
57. Fisher RI, DeVita VT, Hubbard SM, et al. Prolonged disease-free survival in Hodgkin's disease with MOPP reinduction after first relapse. *Ann Intern Med* 1979;90(5):761–763.
58. Longo DL, Duffy PL, Young RC, Hubbard S, DeVita VT. Conventional dose salvage combination chemotherapy in patients relapsing with Hodgkin's disease after combination chemotherapy: The low probability for cure. *J Clin Oncol* 1992;10:210–218.
59. DeVita VT. The influence of information on drug resistance on protocol design. The Henry Kaplan Lecture 4th International Conference on Malignant Lymphomas, June 6–9, 1990, Lugano, Switzerland. *Ann Oncol* 1991;2:93.
60. Deisseroth AB. DeVita VT. The cell cycle: probing new molecular determinants of resistance and sensitivity to cytotoxic agents. *Cancer J (Sci Am)* 1995;1(1):15–23.
61. Longo DL, Glatstein E, Duffey PL, et al. Radiation therapy versus combination chemotherapy in the treatment of early-stage Hodgkin's disease: seven-year results of a prospective randomized trial. *J Clin Oncol* 1991;9:906.
62. Biti GP, Cimino G, Cartoni C, et al. Extended-field radiotherapy is superior to MOPP chemotherapy for the treatment of pathologic stage I-IIA Hodgkin's disease: eight-year update of an Italian prospective randomized study. *J Clin Oncol* 1992;10:378.
63. DeVita VT. Late sequelae of treatment of Hodgkin's disease. *Curr Opin Oncol* 1997;9:428–431.
64. Arseneau JC, Sponzo RW, Longo DL, Canellos GP, DeVita VT. Non lymphomatous malignant tumors complicating Hodgkin's disease: possible association with intensive therapy. *N Engl J Med* 1972;287: 1119–1122.
65. DeVita VT, Arseneau JC, Sherins RJ, Canellos GP, Young RC. Intensive chemotherapy for Hodgkin's disease: long-term complications. *NCI Monogr* 1973;36:447–454.
66. Sherins RJ, DeVita VT. Effects of drug treatment for treatment for lymphoma on male reproductive capacity: studies of men in remission after therapy. *Ann Intern Med* 1973;79:216–220.
67. Shilsky RL, Sherins RJ, Hubbard SM, DeVita VT. Long-term follow-up of ovarian function in women treated with MOPP chemotherapy for Hodgkin's disease. *Am J Med* 1982;93:109–114.
68. Fisher RI, DeVita VT, Bostick F, et al. Persistent immunologic abnormalities in long-term survivors of advanced Hodgkin's disease. *Ann Intern Med* 1980;92:595–599.
69. DeVita VT, Emmer M, Levine A, Jacobs B, Berard C. Pneumocystis carinii pneumonia: successful diagnosis and treatment of two patients with associated malignant processes. *N Engl J Med* 1969;280: 287–291.
70. DeVita VT, Canellos GB, Chabner BA, Schein PS, Young RC. Advanced diffuse histiocytic lymphomas, a potentially curable disease. *Lancet* 1975;1:248–254.
71. Bonadonna G, Beretta G, Tancini G, et al. Adriamycin (NSC-123127) studies at the Istituto Nazionale Tumori, Milan. *Cancer Chemother Rep* 1975;6(3):231–245.
72. Bonadonna G, Monfardini S, De Lena M, Fossati Bellani F, Beretta G. Phase I and preliminary phase II evaluation of adriamycin (NSC-123127). *Cancer Res* 1970;30:2572–2582.
73. Bonadonna G, Monfardini S, De Lena M, Fossati Bellani F. Clinical evaluation of adriamycin, a new antitumor antibiotic. *Br Med J* 1969; 3:503–506.
74. Skibba JL, Beal DD, Ramirez G, Bryan GT. N-demethylation of antineoplastic agent 4(5)-3,3-dimethyl-1-triazeno) imidazole-5(4) carboxamide by rats and man. *Cancer Res* 1970;30:147–150.
75. Bonadonna G, Zucali R, Monfardini S, De Lena M, Uslenghi C. Combination chemotherapy of Hodgkin's disease with Adriamycin, bleomycin, vinblastine and imidazole carboxamide versus MOPP. *Cancer* 1975;36:252–259.
76. Reference removed in page proofs.
77. Reference removen in page proofs.
78. Frei E III, Luce JK, Talley RW, Vaitkevicius VK, Wilson HE. 5-(3,3-dimethyl-triazeno) imidazole-4-carboxamide (NSC-45388) in the treatment of lymphoma. *Cancer Chemother Rep* 1972;56:667–670.

79. Bonadonna G. Chemotherapy strategies to improve the control of Hodgkin's disease. The Richard and Hinda Rosenthal Foundation Award Lecture. *Cancer Res* 1982;42:4309–4320.
80. Santoro A, Bonadonna G, Valagussa P, et al. Long-term results of combined chemotherapy-radiotherapy approach in Hodgkin's disease: superiority of ABVD plus radiotherapy versus MOPP plus radiotherapy. *J Clin Oncol* 1987;5:27–37.
81. Skipper HE. Concurrent comparisons of some 2-, 3-, and 4-drug combinations delivered simultaneously and sequentially (L1210 and P388 leukemia systems). *Cancer Chemotherapy* 1980:9. (Ann Arbor: University Microfilms International.)
82. Skipper HE. On reducing treatment failures due to overgrowth of specifically and permanently drug-resistant neoplastic cells. *Cancer Chemotherapy* 1979:2. (Ann Arbor: University Microfilms International.)
83. Bonadonna G, Valagussa P, Santoro A. Alternating non-cross-resistant combination chemotherapy or MOPP in stage IV Hodgkin's disease. A report of 8-year results. *Ann Intern Med* 1986;104:739–746.
84. Viviani S, Santoro A, Negretti E, Bonfante V, Valagussa P, Bonadonna G. Salvage chemotherapy in Hodgkin's disease. Results in patients relapsing more than twelve months after first complete remission. *Ann Oncol* 1990;1:123–127.
85. Longo DL, Duffey PL, DeVita VT, et al. Treatment of advanced stage Hodgkin's disease: alternating non-cross-resistant MOPP/CABS is not superior to MOPP. *J Clin Oncol* 1991;9:1409–1420.
86. Hancock BW, Vaughan Hudson G, Vaughan Hudson B, et al. LOPP alternating with EVAP is superior to LOPP alone in the initial treatment of advanced Hodgkin's disease: results of a British National Lymphoma Investigation trial. *J Clin Oncol* 1992;10:1252–1258.
87. Canellos GP, Anderson JR, Propert KJ, et al. Chemotherapy of advanced Hodgkin's disease with MOPP, ABVD or MOPP alternating with ABVD. *N Engl J Med* 1992;327:1478–1484.
88. Goldie JH, Coldman AJ. A mathematical model for relating the drug sensitivity of tumors to their spontaneous mutation rate. *Cancer Treat Rep* 1979;63:1727–1733.
89. Klimo P, Connors J. MOPP/ABV hybrid program: combination chemotherapy based on early introduction of seven effective drugs for advanced Hodgkin's disease. *J Clin Oncol* 1986;3:1174–1182.
90. Connors JM, Klimo P, Adams G, et al. MOPP/ABV hybrid versus alternating MOPP/ABVD for advanced Hodgkin's disease. *Am Soc Clin Oncol* 1992;11:317(abstr 1073).
91. Glick JH, Young ML, Harrington D, et al. MOPP/ABV hybrid chemotherapy for advanced Hodgkin's disease significantly improves failure-free and overall survival: the 8-year results of the Intergroup trial. *J Clin Oncol* 1998;16:19–26.
92. Feuer EJ, Kessler LG, Baker SG, et al. The impact of breakthrough clinical trials on survival in population based tumor registries. *J Clin Epidemiol* 1991;44(2):141–153.
93. Hryniuk WM. The importance of dose intensity in outcome of chemotherapy. In: DeVita VT, Hellman S, Rosenberg SA, eds. *Important advances in oncology.* Philadelphia: JB Lippincott, 1988:121–141.

Hodgkin's Disease, edited by P.M. Mauch,
J.O. Armitage, V. Diehl, R.T. Hoppe, and L.M. Weiss.
Lippincott Williams & Wilkins, Philadephia ©1999.

CHAPTER 3

Development of the Concept of Hodgkin's Disease as a Curable Illness: The European Experience

Maurice Tubiana

This chapter describes the evolution of ideas regarding the management of Hodgkin's disease from 1963 to the late 1980s in Europe. It may seem arbitrary to distinguish Western Europe from North America since there was close interaction between these two regions of the world during all this period. The concepts developed by the Stanford group [Henry Kaplan (1) and Saul Rosenberg (2)] and the Toronto group [Vera Peters (3–5)] had a profound influence on European thinking. In the 1960s and 1970s, several meetings were held in Western Europe and the United States [Paris (6), Rye (7), Ann Arbor (8), Stanford (9), London (10)], and large numbers of oncologists spent their sabbatical year on the other side of the Atlantic.

Nevertheless, there were differences in the philosophy of management. The large European groups were less innovative and more conservative, but also more concerned than their American counterparts with patients' body integrity and early and late side effects. For example, staging laparotomy, including splenectomy, or total nodal irradiation alone or associated with multiple chemotherapy, was always considered with suspicion in Europe (11), while as early as 1964 prognostic indicators were actively and prospectively studied by the European Organization for Research and Treatment of Cancer (EORTC) (12–14) with the clear purpose of tailoring the aggressiveness of the management to the characteristics of the disease.

The year 1963 was undoubtedly a turning point in the history of Hodgkin's disease with the dramatic claim by Easson and Russell (15) that this illness, previously considered inexorably fatal, could be cured. However, prior to 1963, a few authors had already shown that prolonged remission could be achieved following sufficiently high doses of radiotherapy, but the myth of incurability remained prevalent. During this period there were two conflicting approaches in the treatment of Hodgkin's disease. For most physicians, treatment was only palliative. Its aim was to relieve pain and to avoid cachexia, and the accepted philosophy was that no treatment was able to cure the disease but could, at best, only prolong life and reduce suffering. The concept of quality of life had not yet been introduced but was implied though unexpressed. In their book on Hodgkin's disease, Paul Chevalier and Jean Bernard (16) wrote in 1932: "The use of ionizing radiation raised great hopes for about a decade; the technique of irradiation became more sophisticated.... Currently radiotherapy is still used but it is no longer considered with curative intent; it can be only symptomatic because the nodes disappear but recur sooner or later. Our present thinking is directed toward biotherapy and chemotherapy." The strategy was to avoid any aggressive treatment that could interfere with the comfort of the patient and reduce his ability to cope with further treatment when relapse would occur.

In the late 1940s and early 1950s, this resigned attitude was still predominant. However some radiotherapists, in particular René Gilbert (17,18) from Geneva, advocated extended field radiation therapy with doses as high as possible. But with the 200 kV x-rays the tolerance was poor and doses were seldom higher than 20 or 27 Gy; even with these low doses the general status of the patients was altered, which may explain why many hematologists felt that radiation therapy could be harmful. Nevertheless, the data of Gilbert and also of Craft (19)

M. Tubiana: Centre Antoine Béclère, Faculté de Medecine, Paris, France.

indicating that prolonged remission could be achieved with sufficiently high doses had some impact. Hence, in the mid-1940s the treatment became more aggressive in some centers. Gilbert also advocated larger fields encompassing the palpable nodes and the surrounding areas in a segmental irradiation: "Many times I have seen...recurrence developing in the immediate vicinity of a field too narrowly irradiated" (18). Gilbert reported 5-year survival of 35% and Craft of 25%.

The advent in the late 1950s of high-energy radiation therapy markedly increased tolerance to high doses, and in the early 1960s a few radiotherapists started to deliver higher doses. However, it was still believed that Hodgkin's disease could not be cured and the intent remained palliative in most centers. The first attempts with chemotherapy were both spectacular in their immediate effects and disappointing because remissions were generally of short duration.

THE CURE OF HODGKIN'S DISEASE

In this context, the article by Easson and Russell (15) in the summer of 1963, claiming that patients with Hodgkin's disease had been cured, was met with great skepticism. Although it was recognized that long remission could be obtained following extensive radiotherapy (3,18), the dogma remained that recurrence was inevitable because it was believed that Hodgkin's disease was from the outset a multifocal disease. The conclusions of Easson and Russell concurred with those of a previous paper by Peters and Middlemiss (3) from Toronto that also indicated a long-term survival in a fair proportion of patients, but Easson and Russell's statistical methodology was more convincing. They analyzed the survival at 5, 10, and 15 years of 822 patients with Hodgkin's disease. They subdivided them into localized disease, which was called later (at the Rye meeting) (7) stages I_1 and I_2 and generalized disease (the other patients). The term *localized* implied that the lymphadenopathy was at the time of treatment confined to one lymph node region and was amenable to radical irradiation in one undivided volume of tissue (for example, one or both sides of the neck, one supraclavicular fossa and the mediastinum). Irradiation had been carried out with 250 kV up to a dose of 25 to 27.5 Gy. The overall age-corrected survival at 5, 10, and 15 years for patients with localized disease was 53%, 44%, and 41%, respectively, and for patients with generalized disease 17%, 11%, and 10% (15,20).

The rationale for using the word *cure* instead of *prolonged remission* was that the shape of the survival curve for Hodgkin's disease patients indicated that the rate of mortality progressively decreases after about the fifth year until between the 10th and the 15th year the death rate no longer exceeds that of the comparable normal population group. Another important point of this study was that there was no difference in survival between patients treated by radiation therapy alone or by radiation therapy and nitrogen mustard (at 10 years, 46.6% and 47.5%, respectively) (15,20).

In the late 1940s and 1950s, the Manchester Cancer Centre, under the strong leadership of Ralston Paterson (the predecessor of Eric Easson), was the world mecca of radiotherapy, and its medical statistics were of unchallenged value. Very few centers at that time were able to claim 15-year survival rates with only a few patients lost from view. Nevertheless, most internists and hematologists remained skeptical and believed that the so-called cures were due to either histologic mistakes or very benign histologic subtypes. On the other hand, many radiotherapists hailed Easson's data, which confirmed their own hopes. In the midst of this controversy I was able to convince the leading European hematologist, Jean Bernard, and the French societies of hematology and radiology to organize an international workshop in Paris (6) to check the validity of the Manchester data and those of Toronto and Stanford. Easson, Kaplan, and Peters reacted enthusiastically and within a few weeks it was decided that a panel of pathologists would conduct a blind review of the slides of the patients with long-term relapse-free survival mixed with an equal number of slides of patients of the same age and sex. A few hundred slides arrived from Manchester, Stanford, Toronto, and Paris. Three pathologists, R. Lukes (United States), Gompel (Belgium), and Nezelof (France), were designated to read them. When the meeting began in February 1965, no one, not even the pathologists, knew the results, which had been analyzed by a few statisticians. The results were unequivocal. The hypothesis of histologic mistakes could be rejected (21). The percentage of very favorable histologic types (paragranuloma) was only 7% among "cured" patients. Within a few months, oncologists' attitudes changed abruptly. Without any new techniques, but with the same old tools used more aggressively, the study had shown that it was possible to cure patients who were previously doomed to die. For the 60 participants, the Paris meeting was an enthusiastic brainstorming. All possible research avenues were envisaged and discussed. It was felt that, as Hodgkin's disease was curable, with better strategies the long-term survival could be improved and each participant hoped he could contribute to this progress.

A few prerequisites were clearly identified:

1. Strong interaction between research centers and periodic exchange of information were needed. In Paris it was decided that another meeting should be held the following year in the United States, which Kaplan offered to organize. This meeting was held in Rye, New York (7), and ample time was given to discussion and brainstorming.
2. To compare results of the coming studies, a common vocabulary was required. It was decided to set up

committees for international histologic classification and staging systems. These were briefly discussed in Paris (6), with a few amendments definitively accepted in Rye (7).
3. In 1964, there had been only a few controlled clinical trials in oncology. In Europe randomization had been accepted from an ethical point of view only in 1955. In 1964, EORTC was created with the purpose of setting up controlled clinical trials. In France, the first randomized trial had been launched at Villejuif in 1961.

In 1964 controversies remained regarding randomization, which was still considered as unethical by some physicians. The chief of the department of surgery of the Institut Gustave Roussy at Villejuif, who was a prominent surgeon, in a spectacular move resigned from his position and left the cancer center because he could not accept working in a hospital in which patients' treatments were determined by the throw of the dice. Nevertheless, most participants felt that to progress rapidly, controlled clinical trials were mandatory and urged hematologists and oncologists to organize them. One of the first trials launched by EORTC was the H_1 trial on Hodgkin's disease in 1964 (22,23).

However, in clear contrast with the optimistic and constructive attitude of the oncologists and hematologists, most general practitioners were skeptical and their views evolved very slowly. They did not realize the importance of an early diagnosis and the difficulties of treatment, which was required to be performed in highly specialized radiotherapy departments. Moreover, they had doubts about the validity of the aggressive treatment, since they had been taught when they were students or residents that aggressivity was detrimental because it reduced the capacity of the body to tolerate further treatment (16). A survey of French medical textbooks showed that although the possibility of a cure was evoked in the late 1960s, it was only at the beginning of the 1970s that the beneficial effect of high-dose therapy was clearly acknowledged (Guiomard, personal communication). In the United Kingdom the situation evolved similarly (Vaughan Hudson, personal communication).

Following the Rye meeting, several other meetings were organized in the United States [Ann Arbor 1971 (8), Stanford 1972 (9)] and in Europe [London (10), Lugano (24–26), Cotswold (27,28), Paris 1989 (29), and Köln 1987, 1991, 1995, 1998 (30,31)]. In all of them, as well as in the sessions devoted to the treatment of lymphoma in the oncology, hematology, and radiotherapy congresses, the results of recent investigations and clinical trials were critically reviewed. Thus, each year the groups that specialized in the treatment of Hodgkin's disease on both sides of the Atlantic had several opportunities to examine their data and to confront their points of view. Probably never before in the history of oncology was there such an open forum for the few dozen physicians committed to the treatment of a disease and such a good understanding of the avenues of research explored by each of the teams.

The History of the Hodgkin's Disease Staging System

One of the positive outcomes of these meetings was a continual refinement of the staging system and its wide acceptance. A clinical stage classification is mandatory for comparing results obtained with different types of treatment in various cancer centers, and it serves as a guide in determining prognosis and treatment. The Union International Contre le Cancer (UICC) TNM system is not applicable to lymphoma since it distinguished the primary tumor, the lymph nodes, and the metastases. The first recorded classification of Hodgkin's disease was proposed by Trousseau (32) in Paris and was based on three stages of the disease: latent, progressive, and cachectic. Reed (33) in 1902 termed lymph node enlargement as stage I and progressive cachexia as stage II. Easson and Russell in 1963 defined localized disease as confined to one or two contiguous lymph node regions and amenable to radical irradiation in one undivided volume of tissue (for example, two sides of the neck or one supraclavicular fossa and the related axilla); when the lymphadenopathy was not treatable in one volume (for example, the two axillae), it was a generalized disease. Whatever the anatomic extent, it was also classified as a generalized disease when systemic symptoms were present.

The M. V. Peters classification (3) distinguished three stages: I, involvement of one anatomic region; II, of two or three proximal regions; III, of distant lymphatic regions. Stage II was subdivided by the presence or absence of systemic symptoms. Kaplan, in 1962, proposed distinguishing a stage III for generalized lymphadenopathy from a stage IV when extranodal disease was present (1).

Oily contrast medium was directly injected in the dorsal lymphatic vessels for the exploration of retroperitoneal nodal involvement in 1961. This procedure showed the frequent involvement of these nodes and it rapidly became evident that staging and treatment had to take its results into account.

The Paris classification in February 1965 (6) comprised four stages [the only difference between the Paris and the Rye (September 1965) classifications concerns patients with two contiguous lymph node areas, which were classified stage II in Paris and stage I_2 in Rye]:

I. One anatomic region
II. Disease in two or more anatomic regions on the same side of the diaphragm
III. Disease on both sides of the diaphragm, but limited to involvement of lymphoid tissue (nodes or spleen)
IV. Any lymph node region with extranodal disease (lung, bone marrow, liver, etc.)

Any stage could be B (with systemic symptoms) or A (without symptoms). This classification subdivided Peters' stage III and introduced the A or B classification for each stage. Six months later it was decided at Rye (7) to amend the classification and to classify stage I_2 patients with two contiguous anatomic regions on the same side of the diaphragm. The Rye classification was widely accepted and used both in Europe and North America. It represented great progress. However, after a few years of use some problems became apparent (7), which were discussed at the Ann Arbor meeting (April 1971):

1. It was often difficult to differentiate two contiguous or noncontiguous anatomic regions. Therefore, it was decided to go back to the Paris system.
2. The classification did not distinguish localized extranodal disease by invasion of neighboring tissue, which can be treated by radiation therapy, from disseminated extralymphatic, which cannot be treated by radiation therapy and requires chemotherapy. At the Ann Arbor symposium (8), it was decided to classify as a local extranodal extension (E) patients with limited direct extension from an adjacent nodal site: patients are classified I E or II E (34). This classification was based on the work of Karl Musshof, who showed that the local extension has a prognosis equivalent to that of nodal disease of the same anatomic extent (35). Patients with several local nodal extensions remain as stage IV.
3. At the time of the Ann Arbor meeting, the staging laparotomy had become widely used in some hospitals. It had shown that splenic involvement could not be predicted with the imaging techniques available and that spleen size was a poor indicator of splenic involvement. Moreover, the equivocal lymphograms were more often indicative of negative rather than positive nodes histologically. Therefore, staging laparotomy provided useful information, although its results could not be taken into account in the definition of the stages because this procedure was not carried out in all centers.

I was one of the members of the group that had to propose the revision of the staging system (34). There was a long debate between the Americans, in particular Kaplan, who wanted to include staging laparotomy in the definition of stage, and the Europeans, who were reluctant. Finally, we proposed an association of two staging systems (34). The clinical stages (CS) are based on the results of physical examination and x-ray, including lymphography. They are identical to the previous Paris-Rye system with the small modifications discussed above. In view of the influence among CS II of the number of anatomic areas involved, it was advised to indicate this number by a subscript (CS II_2, CS II_3, CS II_4). The pathologic stages (PS) took into account the results of the staging laparotomy: splenectomy, liver biopsy, open marrow biopsy, and additional node biopsy. Thus, a CS II_3 patient with, for instance, a bilateral neck involvement plus one axilla can also be a PS III if the biopsy of paraaortic lymph nodes is positive despite an apparently normal lymphangiogram, or a PS IV if the liver biopsy is positive. To enable meaningful comparisons, each trial or publication must specify whether the stages are clinical or pathologic. This new classification was accompanied by detailed recommendations for evaluation procedures (36).

Another modification introduced by the Ann Arbor system regards the systemic symptoms. Generalized pruritus, which had been shown to be without prognostic significance in multivariate analysis (37), was dropped from the list of systemic symptoms. Conversely, unexplained loss of body weight (greater than 10%) is a significant variable (37) and was included in the systemic symptoms in addition to fever and night sweats. No biologic indicator was introduced in the classification because it was feared it would not be specific (1,36).

This dual approach of the Ann Arbor classification (34) explains why it remains valid despite the small number of patients currently submitted to laparotomy. However, in the light of experience gained in its use, a few recommendations were made at the Cotswold meeting (27,28). The usefulness of staging laparotomy had been questioned in Europe from the outset (11), in particular following the demonstration of an excellent prognosis for patients relapsing after initial radiation therapy when treated by multiple chemotherapy (23,38,39). Therefore, noninvasive methods, though less accurate, might be preferable for evaluating intraabdominal lymph nodes, in particular computed tomography (CT) and magnetic resonance imaging (MRI). Moreover, the bulk of disease was recognized to be of great importance (40). The bulk of palpable lymph nodes is defined by the largest dimension (in centimeters) of the single largest lymph node or conglomerate node mass in each region. A node or nodal mass of 10 cm or larger is recorded as bulky. For abdominal nodes the size of the node is measured using CT, MRI, or ultrasonography. Measurements of liver or spleen lesions by imaging techniques are too imprecise for staging purposes. A mediastinal mass is defined as bulky on posteroanterior chest radiographs when the maximum width is equal to or greater than one-third of the internal transverse diameter of the thorax at the level of T5/6. The chest radiograph should be taken with maximal inspiration in the upright position at a source-skin distance of 2 m (27,28).

The Search for Progress in Management

In 1964 in Europe, as in North America, radiotherapy was the main treatment, and an increase in the long-term survival was sought by two parallel avenues: the improvement in the techniques of irradiation and the combination of radiation therapy with chemotherapy.

In 1964, radiotherapy of Hodgkin's disease was still rather primitive in most radiation therapy departments. As the treatment was considered palliative, conventional 200 kV x-rays were still used. High-energy equipment (cobalt, betatron, and linear accelerators) was still rare, and it was reserved for patients treated with curative intent. The doses were low (25 to 30 Gy) and the irradiation field small, covering in most instances only the enlarged lymph nodes (15,37).

The Paris meeting had two consequences in Europe. First, conventional radiation therapy was abandoned and megavoltage therapy was introduced, which was better tolerated and allowed higher doses and larger irradiated fields. Second, the target volumes were enlarged. To avoid recurrences in the involved lymphatic area it was realized that at least the whole lymphatic area should be irradiated. The irradiation of the neighboring uninvolved lymphatic areas, as performed in Toronto by Peters (3,4), was controversial. Moreover, Kaplan in 1965 had developed an irradiation technique in which all the lymphatic areas located on the same side of the diaphragm were irradiated by single anterior and posterior fields (41,42). The rationale behind this technique was based on three assumptions: (a) the disease spreads via lymphatic channels to contiguous lymph node chains and other lymphatic structures; (b) the diaphragm represents a boundary between the upper and the lower torso; and (c) the progression from stage II (several lymph node areas involved on the same side of the diaphragm) to stage III (lymphatic areas involved on both sides of the diaphragm) corresponds to a marked increase in the seriousness of the disease, and in stage I and II without systemic symptoms it is sufficient to irradiate the areas located on the same side of the diaphragm. Kaplan showed that it is safe to irradiate all of these and simpler to irradiate them with a single field to avoid the errors in dosimetry that are likely to occur when multiple small fields are employed (42). This technique of mantle and inverted-Y fields was soon widely accepted in Europe despite the difficulties associated with execution (6). Irradiation of Hodgkin's disease was and remains technically difficult. It requires great skill and dosimetric rigor. The unfavorable results of radiation therapy and the high toxicity initially associated with radiation therapy in some centers were due in part to inadequate equipment but mainly to the insufficient experience of the team.

One of the advances associated with the first EORTC trial was to document the need for quality control of the radiotherapy techniques since all radiotherapy centers did not have sufficient expertise in the new method. Quality control was thus set up and became mandatory for all cooperating centers. Similarly, committees were set up for the rereading of lymphangiograms and pathologic slides as it became evident that the initial readings of some slides and lymphangiograms were controversial.

The First European Trial on Hodgkin's Disease: The H_1 EORTC Study for CS I and II

Several oncologists were not convinced of the advantages of large-field irradiation. However, since two trials were ongoing in the United States, at Stanford (42) and the Collaborative Study (43,44), comparing involved field (IF) and extended field in stage I and II, it was felt in most European centers that it was not useful to address this problem and that there were more urgent questions. In 1964–1965 chemotherapy of Hodgkin's disease was still in its infancy and limited to a few drugs given in monochemotherapy. Combination of chemotherapy and radiation therapy was considered by most radiotherapists, including Kaplan and Peters, as ineffective and possibly detrimental. Easson and Russell quoted previous Manchester data (20) in which full dosage of nitrogen mustard had not improved the survival: the age-corrected survival rates were at 5 and 10 years 55.2% and 47.5%, respectively, for the 35 patients treated from 1949 to 1952 by x-ray plus nitrogen mustard, and 60.9% and 46.6% for a similar series of 32 patients treated by radiotherapy alone. This lack of improvement provided by the combination with chemotherapy was interpreted as evidence against the supposed multifocal nature of the disease. The value of chemotherapy was therefore considered debatable.

It is in this context that in 1964 we discussed, within the EORTC, the protocol of the first controlled trial on Hodgkin's disease launched in Europe. The radiotherapists present (K. Breur, M. Tubiana, and B. van der Werf Messing) agreed that in view of the ongoing trials in the United States it was not useful to compare once again IF and extended field. On the other hand, the validity of the Manchester study on the combination of radiation therapy and chemotherapy was questioned because it was felt that the chemotherapy course had been much too short and the drugs not optimal. G. Mathé proposed instead a weekly injection of vinblastine for 2 years. Thus, regarding stages I and II, the question addressed in 1964 was: Could this monochemotherapy improve the results achieved with extended field therapy (mantle field or inverted-Y fields)? Most American colleagues were skeptical because they felt that chemotherapy would only delay the relapse and would be unable to control occult neoplastic tissue located outside the irradiated region. In fact, contrary to these expectations, the relapse-free survival was clearly higher in the arm treated with radiation therapy and vinblastine (at 15 years 60% versus 38% for radiation therapy alone, $p < .001$). Moreover, there was a small but not statistically significant advantage in overall survival (at 15 years 65% for radiation therapy and Velban vs. 58% for radiation therapy alone). However, the advantage in survival was significant in the unfavorable prognostic subgroup (22,23).

Despite relatively modest accrual (288 patients in 6 years), the analysis of the data led to several important conclusions:

1. Monochemotherapy with vinblastine is able to control in unirradiated lymphatic areas small neoplastic foci of up to 1 million malignant cells (45).
2. This 2-year course is well tolerated; surprisingly it did not increase the incidence of leukemia and solid tumors (23,46).
3. The incidence of relapse in the unirradiated paraaortic region was high, and influenced by the pattern of presentation—more frequent in patients without mediastinal involvement and in mixed-cellularity histologic type (22).
4. Salvage treatment after relapse was more successful in the group treated by radiation therapy alone than in patients who had received radiation therapy and vinblastine, thus progress in relapse-free survival did not necessarily yield a benefit in overall survival, an observation that was contrary to the common belief of that time.

These conclusions are consistent with the results of the trials and studies (29,47) that were later carried out with more aggressive multiple chemotherapy. A recent meta-analysis (48) that included 12 trials, but not the H_1, and 1,666 patients showed the risk of failure was also approximately halved in patients receiving adjuvant chemotherapy; however, due to the higher efficacy of salvage treatment in patients who initially had not received chemotherapy, the difference in survival was small and not significant (at 10 years 79.4% vs. 76.5%). Since radiation therapy carried out in the late 1960s was certainly much less satisfactory than that used in the later studies, H_1 data strongly suggest that in the adjuvant setting a simple and innocuous monochemotherapy could be about as beneficial as a much more noxious multiple chemotherapy, especially for low-risk patients.

The H_2 EORTC Trial for CS I and II

The results of the H_1 trial were taken into account in the subsequent H_2 study (49). The high incidence of relapse in the paraaortic region indicated that, despite a negative lymphangiogram, occult disease was often present in these lymph nodes. Contrary to what had been hypothesized, the diaphragm was not a barrier, and early disease was able to spread from the upper torso to the abdomen despite a flow of the lymph from the abdomen to the left supraclavicular lymph nodes. Moreover, in infradiaphragmatic disease, relapse occurred as often in the right as in the left supraclavicular and cervical areas. Thus it was decided to irradiate the paraaortic region in all CS I and II patients (49).

By that time the Stanford group had introduced staging laparotomy, and this method revealed a high incidence of occult splenic involvement (50). At Stanford, it had been assumed that spleen was a step toward liver involvement and that therefore colloidal gold (for liver irradiation) or chemotherapy should be administered to all patients with spleen involvement (1). This conclusion was challenged in Europe. Moreover, although staging laparotomy was acknowledged as a fascinating research tool, it was not widely accepted as a routine procedure in most European centers. The EORTC decided to address the question of its prognostic value. CS I and II patients were randomly assigned either to undergo a staging laparotomy and splenectomy or not. In the arm without laparotomy the spleen was irradiated. To assess the significance of splenic involvement, it was necessary to treat all patients similarly, whether or not the spleen was involved (49). At the first Lugano meeting in 1981 (no proceedings published) this protocol was criticized by Kaplan as unethical, but I pointed out that it was also unethical to give an aggressive treatment to all patients with spleen involvement without any certitude regarding its usefulness, and that, furthermore, when during the laparotomy a liver or a bone marrow involvement was discovered the patient was treated as a stage IV. In fact there was only one case of liver involvement among patients with splenic involvement. In patients treated by subtotal nodal irradiation and spleen irradiation or by staging laparotomy plus splenectomy and subtotal nodal irradiation, the relapse-free survival was 68% and 76%, respectively, and overall survival 77% and 79%, respectively; the differences were not significant. A positive laparotomy was very predictive of relapse (at 12-year follow-up, relapse-free survival was 85% for patients with a negative laparotomy vs. 53% for patients with a positive laparotomy) but the overall survival was essentially identical, 80% and 76%, respectively (22,23). However, the impact of positive laparotomy on relapse-free survival was observed only in patients with favorable prognostic indicators.

In 1970, multiple drug chemotherapy [mechlorethamine, Oncovin (vincristine), procarbazine, and prednisone (MOPP)] had been successfully introduced by DeVita et al. (51) in the treatment of Hodgkin's disease. This combination was still controversial in 1971 when the study was launched because of its toxicity (52), but it was recognized that multiple chemotherapy warranted investigation (53). Nevertheless, it was decided to compare vinblastine alone (as in H_1) to vinblastine plus procarbazine (49). This chemotherapy was restricted to patients with mixed-cellularity and lymphoid-depletion histologic subtypes since for the other histologic subgroups chemotherapy had not yielded any survival benefits in the H_1 study. The overall survival was identical in the two arms of the study (23).

This trial had considerable impact on the thinking regarding the treatment of Hodgkin's disease:

1. It was the first in which the aggressiveness of the treatment was modulated according to a prognostic factor (histologic subtype); before only the clinical or the pathologic stages influenced the treatment. Its overall results, which were excellent, confirmed the validity of modulation.
2. It definitively established the lack of consistency between relapse-free survival and overall survival (23,29).
3. It showed that staging laparotomy was a procedure that by itself did not improve overall survival and that, therefore, should be restricted to those patients in whom it could alter the strategy for treatment (22,23).

The Decrement in Treatment Aggressiveness

During the period from 1964 to 1975, there was a gradual increase in the aggressiveness of workup and treatment. One of the reasons for this tendency was the weight given to relapse-free survival as a criterion for assessing the value of a new therapeutic modality. Kaplan wrote in 1980 (1): "Data document the fact that patients who have had a relapse are much more likely to die.... Virtually all surviving patients at 10 or 20 years were those who encountered complete remission during the first course of treatment."

By the mid-1970s, it became clear that this increase in management aggressiveness was inducing side effects (54–57), which were not balanced by an improvement in survival (for discussion see refs. 22,23,29,58,59). The main point was that the efficacy of salvage therapy is high, in particular when chemotherapy is used for the second-line treatment in patients initially treated by radiation therapy alone. The efficacy of rescue was critically evaluated in several series (38,60), and it was shown that it varies with the characteristics of the initial treatment and of the disease (very high in favorable prognostic groups and less than 50% in unfavorable prognostic groups). Overall survival and disease-specific mortality at 8 or 10 years are therefore better end points than relapse-free survival (23). As discussed earlier in the H_1 and H_2 trials, despite a clear difference in relapse-free survival between the arms, the overall survival was the same, and the apparent superiority of the more aggressive arm vanished (23).

Besides the effectiveness of rescue, the change in strategy in the 1970s was made possible by the strong correlation between a few prognostic indicators and survival (1,37,61). The lymphoma group of the EORTC in 1972 advocated tailoring the treatment aggressiveness to patients' characteristics to reduce the side effects associated with staging laparotomy, extended radiation therapy, and multiple chemotherapy (13,22,49,62). It proposed a strategy based on the use of prognostic indicators to modulate the use of chemotherapy according to the histologic subtype. This approach initiated a debate that was raging in the mid-1970s but is still ongoing [see debate between Proctor and Specht (63)]. Briefly, the main argument of the opponents of the use of prognostic factors for the delineation of therapeutic subgroups was that when a treatment is more effective it should be used for all patients, because individual patients even with fairly good prognostic factors might relapse and die. Conversely, the proponents of the use of prognostic factors for tailoring treatment argued that overtreatment increases not only early but also late side effects. By and large the data that were accumulated during the past two decades support this second point of view, although further work is still required.

In the mid-1970s, in view of the high incidence of second cancers and the seriousness of treatment long-term side effects, a rollback strategy was advocated and became the basis of the H_5 trial that started in 1976 (22,39).

High death rates persist in patients cured of Hodgkin's disease, although the risk of death from Hodgkin's disease progression becomes virtually negligible after 15 years. In the EORTC cohort, which comprised 1,449 patients with CS I and II treated from 1963 to 1986, the standardized mortality ratio remained significantly increased 20 years after initial treatment (64). This was confirmed by the analysis of other series of patients (59,65–67). Besides second cancers (46,68–79, 74–77,79), the main causes of excess death are cardiac failure, infectious diseases, and late injuries in the irradiated tissues (80–87). In the 1970s it was shown that the incidence of radiation pneumonitis mainly depends on total dose delivered to the mediastinum and the size of the irradiated volume. Cosset et al. (88) reported an excess of death from ischemic heart disease relative to the general population in irradiated patients, while the risk was not increased in patients who were not irradiated. The higher the total dose to the anterior heart, and the larger the daily fractional dose over 2 Gy, the greater the risk of cardiac damage and other late effects (80,88,89).

By 20 years from initial treatment, the actuarial mortality from second cancer may exceed that from Hodgkin's disease (64–66). Data suggest that splenectomy and spleen irradiation increase the risk of second cancers (90). Several sets of data demonstrated a dose-effect relationship for second cancers (78,79). The risk of leukemia is correlated with the amount of alkylating agents given to patients, in particular in MOPP combinations (90), and the extent of radiation therapy when combined with MOPP. Limited-field radiation therapy or some drugs such as vinblastine do not seem to increase the leukemia risk (91).

For patients with follow-up longer than 15 years, some data suggest that the incidence of second cancers and the standardized mortality ratio (SMR) are higher in patients treated by multiple chemotherapy and radiation therapy than in patients treated by radiation therapy alone. However, other data do not show a clear correlation between the cumulative mortality due to deaths not caused by Hodgkin's disease and the type of treatment (29).

However, although overtreatment is hazardous, a too high relapse rate should also be avoided despite the remarkable efficacy of salvage treatment. It has been shown that in 1,057 patients aged 15 to 29 cured from Hodgkin's disease and entered into the British National Lymphoma Investigation (BLNI) from 1970 to 1992 and who had attained complete remission, the late mortality was higher in those who had remained disease free after the second-line treatment than in those who had remained disease free after the first-line treatment (overall survival at 15 and 20 years follow-up, 96% and 93% vs. 88% and 84%, respectively) (67). Although this late mortality is much lower than that due to Hodgkin's disease (25% in that series), these data evidence the toxicity of the more aggressive rescue treatments delivered after relapse. A balance should be sought between a relatively aggressive first-line treatment that achieves a high disease-free survival but at the expense of some late toxicity, and a milder first-line treatment that spares most of the patients from a toxic treatment but exposes those who relapse to a much more aggressive second-line treatment.

When in the late 1970s and the 1980s it became clear that there were several management strategies that could cure a very high proportion of patients, the attention was focused on the late toxicity. This attitude led to the reassessment of all the components of workup and treatment in CS I, II, and IIIA, and to the exploration by various European groups of three main research avenues:

1. In radiation therapy, reduction of the size of the target volumes and of the dose.
2. In chemotherapy, search for drugs as effective but less toxic and less carcinogenic.
3. Use of prognostic factors for tailoring the aggressiveness of the management according to the seriousness of the disease. Extensive prospective studies were carried out in Europe with the aim of identifying the simplest and the most reliable ones that could be used for this purpose.

Let us consider the European contribution to these various topics:

Reduction of the Radiation Dose and of the Target Volume

The results of the two U.S. trials comparing IF (involved field) and WF (wide field) including all lymphatic areas located on the same side of the diaphragm were not clear cut. The data of the Stanford trial revealed an advantage for extended field only in patients with systemic symptoms. The Stanford Group rapidly interrupted its trial because, as stated by Kaplan (1), the irradiation was limited to lymphatic areas located on the same side of the diaphragm, and the spleen was not irradiated. The other trial, the collaborative study, failed to reveal any significant difference in survival between the two arms; however, there was the suggestion of an advantage for WF primarily for the male patients (43,44).

In the 1970s, the BNLI launched two trials comparing limited to more extended radiation therapy. In CS IA and IIA, 40 Gy to IF in 4 weeks was compared to the same plus radiotherapy to contiguous regions (35 Gy in 4 weeks). No difference in 10-year survival was detected (92).

In CS IB and IIB WF mantle or inverted Y, up to 40 Gy was compared to the same plus radiation therapy on the other side of the diaphragm (mantle or inverted Y) up to 35 Gy. No advantage was derived from the more extensive radiation therapy since high relapse rates were observed in both arms. The conclusion was that patients with systemic symptoms require chemotherapy from the start of treatment (92).

However, in the meta-analysis that was carried out on eight trials (out of which six were European) that included 2,000 patients, reduction in the 10-year risk of failure was 12% and the proportional reduction was of broadly similar size for patients with or without systemic symptoms. However, more extensive radiation therapy did not improve overall survival, which was identical in the two arms (48).

In the EORTC H_5 trial (1977–1982) that we shall discuss later, PS I and II patients with favorable prognostic indicators (histologic subtypes of lymphocyte predominance and nodular sclerosis, age ≤40 years, erythrocyte sedimentation rate (ESR) ≤70, CS I whatever the nodal area involved or CS II with mediastinal involvement and negative laparotomy) were randomized between a mantle field irradiation or mantle field plus paraaortic lymph node irradiation.* There was no difference in relapse-free survival or total survival (39,23).

In the H_6 (93) and H_7 (94) EORTC trials, the dose to the uninvolved area was reduced to 36 Gy in patients treated by radiation therapy alone without any increase in the incidence of recurrence. In the HD4 German study, patients with PS IA and II_2 A or B without mediastinal mass were randomized between 40 Gy to a wide field or 40 Gy to the involved areas plus 30 Gy to uninvolved areas. The results do not show any difference in relapse-free survival or overall survival (S) (95).

*There was a misprint in the original article. It was stated that CS II patients without mediastinal involvement were included in the good prognostic group instead of patients with involvement. Subsequently, a letter was sent to the editor to correct this error (167). In the H_5 trial, the delineation of the good prognostic group had been made on the results of H_1 and H_2 trials that identified mediastinal involvement as a good prognostic factor. Subsequently, it was found that bulky mediastinal mass was of poor prognostic significance, and in the H_6 trial patients with bulky mediastinal involvement were excluded from the good prognostic group.

When radiation therapy is combined with chemotherapy, several groups have shown that the radiation therapy dose could be smaller. In the Pierre and Marie Curie CS I and II patients study, the reduction of the extent of radiation to involved fields combined with three cycles of MOPP did not diminish relapse-free survival (96). In children, more than two decades ago, the Stanford group (1) showed that a special approach was required to reduce the sequelae of irradiation, in particular the impact on bone growth; the dose was reduced from 40 to 20 Gy while chemotherapy by MOPP was administered to all patients. There was no increase in local recurrence. Subsequently, most pediatric oncology groups adopted similar strategies and moved away from the protocols used for adult patients (98–100). The aim was to find a balance between cure and a long-term toxicity that was felt to be difficult to accept in children (101,102). It should be acknowledged that interaction between pediatricians and oncologists was beneficial. Many concepts that were developed for children were subsequently found relevant for adults, and conversely efforts made in adults for reducing the burden of management, for example, the avoidance of staging laparotomy, inspired pediatricians. The German Group (GHSG) HD1 trial investigated the dose of radiation in nonbulky involved areas and noninvolved areas following only two double cycles of cyclophosphamide, Oncovin (vincristine), procarbazine, and prednisone (COPP) and Adriamycin, bleomycin, vinblastine, and dacarbazine (ABVD) in CS I, II, and IIIA patients. They found that 20, 30, or 40 Gy had similar effectiveness in nonbulky involved areas (95,97).

As the pediatricians did two decades ago, it is now time to reexamine radiation dose and target volumes, in particular because recent data show that the notable incidence of second solid tumors is correlated with such parameters (59). Thus, conversely to what was thought in the 1970s and early 1980s, the size of the irradiated volume and the dose should be restricted to what is really necessary. The above data show that a standard radiation therapy mantle field or subtotal nodal irradiation is no longer justified for all CS I and II patients, although it may be useful in some subsets. The radiation therapy technique should be modulated according to the prognostic factors and should differ depending whether or not radiation therapy is combined with chemotherapy. In particular, it should be recalled that the incidence of second cancers is higher in patients treated by a combination of radiation therapy and multiple chemotherapy.

The Search for Less Carcinogenic Multiple Chemotherapy

The introduction of the MOPP regimen by De Vita et al. (51) was a decisive advance. It soon became widely used throughout Europe despite the skepticism of some prominent European medical oncologists, such as Amiel et al. (52) and Hancock (103), who feared its toxicity: nausea, vomiting, and phlebitis leading to difficulty with venous access during later courses of treatment. This reluctance grew when the leukemogenicity of alkylating agents and of MOPP was shown (54). When a correlation between the leukemic risk and the amount of alkylating agents was demonstrated, efforts were made to reduce the dose and the number of cycles; for example, in the study of the Pierre and Marie Curie group there were three cycles instead of six (96).

However, most of the studies investigated MOPP-like regimens or other types of multiple chemotherapy. Nicholson et al. (104) proposed a slightly modified regimen, MVPP, in which vinblastine was substituted for vincristine and prednisone was used at lower dosage. The results were quite comparable to those of MOPP with less acute toxicity. In Germany, COPP was used because mechlorethamine was not available.

The BNLI investigated MOP, which is a MOPP without prednisone. MOPP was found to be clearly superior throughout follow-up and MOP was abandoned (92). In 1979, the BNLI initiated a randomized study comparing MOPP with LOPP in which mechlorethamine was replaced by Leukeran (chlorambucil). LOPP was found to be as effective and slightly less toxic, but only slightly less carcinogenic than MOPP (103,105).

The combination of epirubicin, bleomycin, vinblastine, and prednisone (EBVP) was introduced in 1987 by Zittoun's team (106,107). It is less carcinogenic than MOPP and was tested in the H_7 EORTC trial (94). It was found to be less effective than MOPP for unfavorable groups, but satisfactory as an adjuvant of radiation therapy in favorable subsets.

The most important advance in this field was made in 1975 by Bonadonna and the Milan group (108), who introduced Adriamycin, bleomycin, vinblastine, and dacarbazine (ABVD). In a small randomized trial, the Milan group showed that ABVD/radiation therapy is slightly more effective than MOPP/radiation therapy in patients with stages IIB, III, and IV. This was confirmed later in a subsequent larger randomized trial carried out in Milan (109) and in the EORTC H_6 trial (93). Thus, ABVD is more effective than MOPP and is definitely less carcinogenic (110). Its main drawbacks are its cardiac and lung toxicity, and one of the aims of the H_6 EORTC trial (see below) was to compare the relative merits of MOPP and ABVD (93).

The use of alternating potentially non–cross-resistant drug combinations MOPP and ABVD was investigated in 1978 in Milan and at the Memorial Hospital in New York. The Milan study demonstrated the superiority of MOPP/ABVD in stage IV disease (111,112). An EORTC trial comparing MOPP with MOPP/ABVD confirmed the superior results for the MOPP/ABVD arm (113). Similarly, a BNLI trial showed that the relapse-free survival and overall survival for alternating LOPP and etoposide, vinblastine, adriamycin (doxorubicin), and prednisone (EVAP) were superior to those of LOPP alone (114). However, the main criterion should be the long-term toxicity of these hybrid regimens and some data suggest that MOPP/ABVD might be more leukemogenic than ABVD alone.

One of the main conclusions of these studies is that long-term toxicity and side effects should be a main factor in the assessment of a chemotherapy regimen. This explains why a follow-up of at least 15 to 20 years is required.

Adjuvant Chemotherapy

As we have discussed above, the first trial on adjuvant chemotherapy, the EORTC H_1, started as early as 1964 (115). Several trials have since been carried out in Europe (22,39,92,116–123), and some of them were included in a meta-analysis including 12 trials comparing radiation therapy alone versus radiation therapy plus adjuvant multidrug chemotherapy (48,124). The combined results show that the recurrence rate was approximately halved in patients receiving combination therapy. The data do not provide evidence of the superiority of one chemotherapy regimen over the others, and the reduction of the risk of failure was similar in patients treated with involved field radiation therapy or more extensive radiation therapy. Due to the efficacy of salvage treatment, the effect on mortality rates was much smaller if any (23.2% vs. 25.5% with radiation therapy alone, P=NS). After a follow-up longer than 10 years, there were slightly more deaths in patients who had received chemotherapy. Thus, the small advantage in favor of adjuvant chemotherapy for mortality from Hodgkin's disease is partly counterbalanced by a small excess in death from other causes.

The lack of a clear advantage in favor of one of the treatment strategies is certainly disappointing, but confirms the data obtained for each of the trials. However, it should be pointed out that this meta-analysis did not attempt to subdivide patients according to prognostic factors. Therefore, its results do not exclude the possibility of a survival advantage for one of the strategies on subsets of patients delineated by means of prognostic indicators.

Finally, we must also mention the European trial by Biti et al. (125), who compared chemotherapy alone and radiation therapy alone in patients with early-stage disease. The results of radiation therapy alone are better than those of chemotherapy alone. However, this trial has been criticized because only 89 patients had been randomized; the low number of patients precludes the analysis of a possible impact of prognostic factors on the outcome.

Tailoring of the Treatment Aggressiveness According to Prognostic Indicators

This strategy is based on three assumptions:

1. With a proper modulation of the aggressiveness of initial treatment according to risk factors, the proportion of deaths due to Hodgkin's disease can be maintained as low as with the most intensive available treatment.
2. The number of deaths due to other causes, in particular second cancers and long-term toxicity, is lower in patients initially treated with a less extensive treatment despite a small increase in the incidence of relapse.
3. The quality of life is as good, or even better, in the group of patients in whom initial management is modulated, as when all patients receive the most effective treatment.

It should be recognized that of these three assumptions only the first has been consistently proved. Some data suggest that despite the higher incidence of relapse, the number of long-term deaths due to other causes can be lowered. However, further work is needed to get more data on the incidence of second cancers and late toxic and infectious deaths according to treatment age and pretreatment prognostic factors. In particular we need to know the cause of the persistent increase in the rate of mortality associated with infectious diseases: is it the impairment of immunity due to the disease or that due to the treatment? The high incidence of infectious disease in splenectomized patients, for whom the impact of treatment cannot be overlooked, should be quantified.

We have only indirect data on the third assumption (59). Obviously, relapse is associated with great anxiety and painful treatment, but on the other hand, aggressive initial management, including staging laparotomy and multiple chemotherapy, is also the source of suffering and severe sequelae such as sterility or impairment of gonadal function. This strategy requires a two-step procedure: (a) identification of relevant prognostic indicators, and (b) subdivision of patients according to the most relevant indicators and a search for the optimal treatment of each subset.

Studies Seeking Prognostic Factors

The analysis of the prognostic factors started early in Europe when it was realized that the malignancy of Hodgkin's disease was greater in some patients than in others, with a shorter time interval between diagnosis and death. Cachexia, fever, the extent of disease, and the histologic type were soon identified as variables having a major impact on the outcome and were introduced in the first staging systems during the 19th and the early 20th century. The search for prognostic factors was stimulated by the discovery of the disease's curability but hampered by statistical methodologic problems. In the first studies the variables were considered independently (126). Later, in the early 1970s, adjustment procedures were used to separate the individual contributions of the variables (37,38). Multivariate studies and the Cox model represented a major advance in the 1980s (14,92).

In the EORTC trials, from the outset in 1964, eight prognostic indicators, including ESR and the number of involved lymph node areas, were prospectively registered (115). The same methodology was adopted by the BNLI (92) and other groups. Thus, several multivariate analyses of prognostic factors were carried out in Europe (14,92, 127–129). Their results are not entirely concordant (58,130), probably due to different techniques of analysis, variable definitions of factors such as the number of regions involved or bulky disease, and variations in the intensity of staging or type of treatment. Nevertheless, the data concur on the following main points:

Age is associated with poor survival when deaths from all causes are included (14,38,131,132). It keeps its prognostic influence in studies when survival is corrected for age by matching with the general population, and in studies of cancer-specific mortality from Hodgkin's disease, excluding death from other causes. Age has a smaller impact on relapse-free survival, but is strongly related to survival after recurrence. Treatment results are slightly better in children than in adults. However, the age of the majority of patients with Hodgkin's disease ranges from 15 to 50 years, and in this age group the influence of age is reduced. The influence of age is partly due to lower tolerance to aggressive treatment, in particular during salvage therapy. Moreover, older patients commonly have underlying medical problems that may preclude adequate staging and treatment; illogical dose reductions are often made by clinicians solely in view of the patient's age, and this attitude could introduce a bias in the interpretation of the results. Nevertheless, the data suggest that age is by itself an adverse factor, as in many other cancer types. For example, there is a sharp difference in survival of patients with thyroid cancer after surgical treatment between those under or over 45 years of age (133). The source of age influence is not known and might be related to the lowering efficacy of the immune system.

Gender has a small but significant impact on both survival and relapse-free survival. The better prognosis of women with Hodgkin's disease had been reported by Epstein as early as 1939. However, gender and histology are not independent variables, and Kaplan (1) questioned the independent significance of gender in regionally localized cases. EORTC data show that this influence is modest but significant (14). Influence of gender is also observed in several other cancers, for example, thyroid cancer (133).

Stage has a strong prognostic value (1,4,5,8). The number of involved nodal regions has an influence on both survival and relapse-free survival (1,13,128). The *volume of disease* in individual regions was not considered in the Ann Arbor classification. In breast cancer it has been shown that disease remains localized when the tumor mass remains small until it reaches during its growth a critical mass at which the disease becomes generalized through hematologic dissemination (134). The tumor can also spread through the lymphatic channels and invade the contiguous lymphatic chains. Lymphatic involvement is not a cause of the hematologic dissemination; however, it is a reliable index of the propensity of the tumor cells to migrate, and although lymphatic dissemination occurs, on the average, earlier during the growth than hematologic dissemination, there is a good correlation between the two (135). In Hodgkin's disease, similarly, studies have shown the prognostic significance of tumor mass (40,128). This mass can be greater in some patients with stage II_2 or II_3 than in patients with stage III, which might explain the limited value of stage classification. The impact of tumor mass does not preclude a possible impact of the number of involved lymphatic areas, which might be an index of the propensities for lymphatic spread.

The natural history of Hodgkin's disease has raised much interest (1,14,38,58,136–138). For its understanding it would be important to distinguish lymphatic spread and hematologic spread (14,58). In the series of 1,139 patients with early stage that we reported in 1985 (14), among the 366 patients with CS II_2, two contiguous territories were involved in 345 patients, there was a mediastinal and an axillary territory involved in six, and the two areas were clearly separated in 14 patients. Thus, the proportion of CS II_2 patients with contiguous territories is approximately 96%, if one considers the mediastinum and axillary regions as contiguous, or more likely 94%, as there is no direct lymphatic pathway between the mediastinal and the axillary regions. The good results observed in these patients with limited radiation therapy support the concept that patients with two contiguous areas have a good prognosis, probably because in this case the extension occurred through lymphatic pathways. Conversely, among the 210 patients with three areas involved (CS II_3), there was a lymphatic contiguity in only two-thirds and this proportion was similar in the 67 patients with four territories involved (CS II_4). For CS II_3 and II_4 patients, limited radiation therapy gave much poorer results (13,14). Thus these results suggest that hematologic spread has occurred in only 6% of patients with stage II_2 but in 33% of stage II_3. Bulk of disease was not taken into consideration in this study and merits further investigation. The extent of disease at relapse has an impact on survival following rescue therapy (128).

A number of prospective or retrospective studies have identified large mediastinal adenopathy as a major factor for predicting an increased risk of relapse; however, it is not associated with a lower survival (28,85,139,140). It is noteworthy that in the first prognostic studies mediastinal involvement was associated with a good prognosis (38,141), and it may be hypothesized that it is because in most cases mediastinal involvement occurs in nodular sclerosis histologic types, which have a spread pattern different from that of mixed-cellularity histologic type (less frequent infradiaphragmatic involvement) (38,115).

From the outset, the presence of *systemic symptoms* (unexplained fever, night sweats, loss of body weight exceeding 10%) was considered as one of the main prognostic indicators (1). Tubiana et al. (37) showed that pruritus has no independent prognostic significance. However, more recent British data show that extremely severe pruritus, although rarely encountered, has adverse significance (27,28). There is a strong correlation between the percentage of patients with systemic symptoms and the stage and the number of involved lymph node areas. However, when these factors are taken into account in multivariate analysis, systemic symptoms retain significance (14). Recent studies have revealed correlations between total tumor burden and systemic symptoms; the more accurately the tumor mass is evaluated, the less prognostic importance systemic symptoms would appear to possess (128) (see Chapter 19).

Biologic Indicators

Erythrocyte sedimentation rate (ESR) is probably the best of the biologic indicators and it has the advantage of simplicity and low cost (12). Its value has been overlooked because it lacks specificity and sophistication. Moreover, its mechanism is still unknown (1). Nevertheless, of the large number of biologic indicators that have been proposed, it is one of the most sensitive and certainly the one with the best cost-effectiveness ratio. This is probably why it remains the most widely used in Europe since the 1950s. There is a strong correlation between ESR and the number of involved areas (58). ESR is also related to the bulk of the disease and loses most of its value when the bulk is taken into account (128); ESR might therefore provide an approximation of tumor burden. Systemic symptoms and ESR are correlated with each other but nevertheless have an independent significant prognostic impact. This prognostic significance is increased when they are combined (14). Vaughan Hudson et al. (142) have pointed out in their series of 840 patients that whereas 35% had systemic symptoms, an additional 53% of the patients had one or more abnormal blood values (ESR, haemoglobin, albumin, lymphocytes), though no systemic symptoms. Thus, only 12% of patients had no systemic disturbance as judged by these criteria. The data suggest that it is difficult to draw the boundary between what does or does not have significance. Currently, a combination of ESR and systemic symptoms is one of the simplest way to define the favorable and unfavorable groups (14,141). In the EORTC H_5 trial, which started in 1976, the ESR was used as a prognostic factor (39), whereas in the H_6 trial that started in 1982 (93) ESR and systemic symptoms were combined. During the follow-up, one of ESR's main interests is its correlation with the presence of residual disease after initial treatment and its ability to predict relapse in patients in complete remission (143—145).

Many other biologic indicators have been investigated in Europe (61,126), but only a few were tested in multivariate analyses. Only a few are still used. The blood lymphocyte count is related to the histologic type but not to the clinical stage or the presence of B symptoms, and lymphopenia has an independent significant prognostic value (37,126,142). However, it is of significance mainly in advanced disease (128). Low serum albumin also has an independent adverse prognostic significance (116). Anemia also possesses some independent significance, in particular in advanced stage. However, the prognostic impact of bone marrow involvement remains uncertain (146).

The prognostic significance of the *histologic subtype* was already underlined in 1932 by Chevalier and Bernard (16), who stressed the deleterious significance of mixed cellularity or of the sarcomatous type, and the favorable impact of fibrosis. The Lukes and Butler classification, which became at Paris-Rye the international one (147), was recognized from the outset for its predictive value; however, two limitations arose: (a) the prognostic significance of histologic subtype has been blurred by progress in management, and (b) a larger and increasing proportion of patients have nodular sclerosis histology (in industrialized countries about 70% of patients, whereas only 10% to 20% in developing countries). Proposals have been made to subdivide nodular sclerosis into two subtypes (148). The prognostic significance of this subdivision was confirmed in some studies but not in others (128).

Nodular sclerosis histology is strongly correlated with young age, female gender, and clinical presentation with mediastinal involvement; in multivariate analysis it has an independent significant favorable prognostic value, in particular in early stages. Some data suggest that it is associated with a slow course and an orderly spread to contiguous areas (38). Extralymphatic spread occurs preferentially in the mixed-cellularity type. Mixed cellularity and lymphoid depletion are associated with poor prognosis. Histologic subtype also has an influence on survival after relapse (38). However, histopathologic features are not currently considered a major prognostic indicator (14,128).

The correlation between the natural history and the histologic types underlines the heterogeneity of Hodgkin's disease, although the delineation of the various entities remains difficult despite progress in cell biology and membrane markers (149,150).

In Europe, as in North America, great expectations were placed on the prognostic information provided by immunologic tests. By and large they were disappointing (1). Patients with negative tuberculin tests have a lower survival (37). Complete anergy is present in 12% to 25% of untreated patients where six intradermal antigens are tested. However, it is generally considered that skin test reactivity cannot serve as a prognostic indicator. The same is true for cellular immune defects.

In Europe, the search for prognostic factors became more and more popular and sophisticated in the late 1980s. Multivariate analyses were performed on gradually larger numbers of patients, because, due to the efficacy of the treatments, the differences in survival during trials became smaller, and it was found that the prognostic factors pertaining to various types of treatment may be somewhat different. After the analysis of the 1,600 patients included in the EORTC trials from 1964 to 1987, the international database was set up in which 14,000 patients were registered (29). The results of the database studies are discussed in another chapter of this book.

In conclusion, besides age, the main indicators that influence the probability of survival are total tumor burden, and indicators associated with it such as number of involved extranodal organs, ESR above 80 mm/hour, a serum alkalin phosphatase above 230 IU/mL, and lymphopenia (151,128).

In the 1980s, the approaches in Europe and the United States diverged. For example, the Stanford group philosophy was that the advances in therapy would progressively render meaningless prognostic factors (2), whereas, as discussed above, in Europe most groups aimed at modulating the management according to the prognostic indicators. This topic is also discussed in Chapter 19. However, the selection of the prognostic variables on which the delineation of the various therapeutic subsets rests raises serious problems. Let us take age as an example. Age has a major impact on survival (14,38,131,132). If the aim of the patient stratification is to identify patients with poor prognosis for whom the treatment should be more aggressive, it is justified to take age into account if the disease is more malignant in patients over 50 years of age. However, this would be illogical if the poor prognosis of older patients is related to a reduced tolerance of older patients to treatment. As stated by Proctor and Specht, "Particular circumspection is needed when the results of prognostic factor studies are used as the rational basis for the selection of treatment for individual patients" (63). However, this legitimate circumspection should not lead to inaction but rather to clinical investigation. With regard to age, ongoing studies suggest that patients older than 50 can tolerate normal amounts of radiation and drugs during the frontline treatment but that their tolerance is reduced during rescue treatment after relapse; therefore, for them the aim should be to reduce the chance of relapse.

This pragmatic approach was the philosophy of the EORTC trials. The aim of these trials was to improve gradually the delineation of the various favorable and unfavorable subsets of patients and to find for each of these the optimal management. We shall first consider the early stage (CS I and II) (Table 1) and then advanced stages.

The H_5 EORTC Trial for CS I and II Patients (1976–1982) (39)

The trial was inspired by the results of the two previous trials, H_1 and H_2. Its aim was to further adapt the management strategy, taking into account its initial characteristics. As discussed above, the results available in 1976 had shown that in some subsets of patients wide field radiation therapy alone (mantle field or inverted Y) gave satisfactory results, while this same treatment gave poor results in other subsets among CS I and II patients. Thus two groups of patients (favorable and unfavorable) were delineated. Patients of the favorable group had all the following characteristics: age <40 years, ESR <70, lymphocyte-predominance or nodular sclerosis histology, and CS I or CS II with mediastinal involvement.

Patients belonging to this group underwent a staging laparotomy with splenectomy, since many studies, including the H_2 trial, had established the prognostic significance of splenic involvement. Patients with intraabdominal disease were included in the unfavorable group (H_5-u). Patients without intraabdominal disease were randomized between mantle field irradiation alone or mantle field plus paraaortic lymph node irradiation (subtotal nodal irradiation); 494 patients were included in this trial. After a 10-year follow-up there was no difference in disease-free survival or overall survival between the two arms (69%); the overall survival was slightly, but not significantly, higher in the mantle field arm (94% vs. 91%). Thus, a simple mantle field irradiation appeared to be sufficient for this subset of patients. The addition of infradiaphragmatic irradiation in this setting could be detrimental due to a possible increase in late gastrointestinal toxicity after the combination of laparotomy and abdominal irradiation.

In the unfavorable group, laparotomy was not performed since extensive treatment was thought to be necessary. This group also included favorable patients with positive laparotomy. Patients were randomized to receive either combined modality treatment (3 MOPP–radiation therapy–3 MOPP) or total nodal irradiation. The 9-year disease-free survival was markedly lower in the total nodal irradiation arm than in the MOPP plus Rt arm (66% vs. 83%, $p < .001$). The 9-year overall survival was also lower but the difference was small and only marginally significant (79% vs. 88%, $p = .06$). However, the main point of this trial was that the difference in overall survival was observed only in the subset of patients with the poorest prognostic indicators. For patients below 40 years of age there was no difference in overall survival between the two arms. Moreover, contrary to what was observed in patients over 40 years of age, in younger patients treated by radiation therapy alone no difference in overall survival was observed between patients without pelvic irradiation and patients with total nodal irradiation. Thus, subtotal total nodal irradiation could constitute for young

TABLE 1. *Subdivision of clinical stage (CS) I + II into various prognostic groups*[a]

Trial	Favorable	Intermediate	Unfavorable
H_2 (1972–76)	NS + LP histology		MC + LD histology
H_5	**All** of the following: Age <40 ESR <70 1st hour Histology: lymphocyte predominance or nodular sclerosis PS I or PS II but **with** mediastinal involvement		**Any** of the following: age ≥40 ESR ≥70 Histology mixed cellularity or lymphocyte depletion CS II **without** mediastinal involvement Patients with favorable prognostic indicators but with positive laparotomy
H_6 (1977–82)	**All** of the following: No B symptoms and ESR <50 or B symptoms and ESR <30 no bulky mediastinum PS I or PS II2 (randomization between staging lap or no lap)		All other CS I + CS II patients including patients with good prognostic factors but with positive staging laparotomy
H_7 (1988–93)	Female patients CS IA Age <40 LP or NS histology	Other patients	Age ≥50 CS II_4 or CS II_5 ESR ≥50 without B symptoms or ESR ≥30 with B symptoms
H_8 (1994–98)	Female patients CS IA Age <40 LP or NS histology	Other patients	Age ≥50 CS II_4 or CS II_5 ESR ≥50 without B symptoms or ESR ≥30 with B symptoms
GHSG	CS IA or IIA without unfavorable prognostic factors	At least one of the following risk factors: Massive mediastinal tumor Extranodal manifestation ESR >50 without B symptoms or ESR >30 with B symptoms 3 or more involved nodal areas	CS IIB with risk factors

[a]Criteria that have been used in the various European Organization for Research and Treatment of Cancer (EORTC) clinical trials on Hodgkin's disease for subdividing patients into favorable, intermediate, or unfavorable groups. The management protocol of patients is described in the text; the overall results of the trials are given in Figs. 1 and 2 and discussed in the text.

ESR, erythrocyte sedimentation rate; LD, lymphocyte depletion; LP, lymphocyte predominance; MC, mixed cellularity; PS, pathologic stage; GHSG, German Hodgkins Study Group.

patients a good therapeutic option when the preservation of reproductive potential is of importance (39,23).

H_6 EORTC Trial (93)

This trial included 578 CS I and II supradiaphragmatic patients from 1982 to 1988. The patients were divided into two subgroups on the basis of the main prognostic factors, which had been identified in the previous EORTC trials. The favorable group comprised patients with one or two lymph node areas involved on the upper side of the diaphragm, no bulky mediastinum, and either no B symptoms and ESR <50 or B symptoms and ESR <30. This favorable group (262 patients) was studied to address the question of the usefulness of staging laparotomy. In the first arm, the patients underwent a staging laparotomy, and the treatment was adapted to the pathology findings. If the laparotomy was negative, in patients with lymphocyte-predominance or nodular sclerosis histologic types, the treatment was mantle field irradiation alone. In patients with mixed-cellularity or lymphoid-depletion types, the treatment combined mantle field irradiation and paraaortic lymph node irradiation. When the laparotomy was positive, patients received a combination of chemotherapy and radiation therapy identical to the unfavorable group. In the other arm, no staging laparotomy was performed and, without any surgical exploration, patients received mantle field and paraaortic and spleen radiation therapy.

In this pragmatic trial, the end point was overall survival and not disease-free survival. As expected, the disease-free survival at 6 years was lower in the patients treated without staging laparotomy (80% vs. 84%). However, the overall survival was slightly but not significantly higher in the nonlaparotomized arm (93% vs. 89%) due to laparotomy related deaths.

In the unfavorable group, the aim was to compare two types of combinations of multiple chemotherapy and radiation therapy: 3 MOPP–radiation therapy–3 MOPP versus 3 ABVD–radiation therapy–3 ABVD. The overall results of ABVD were slightly better (6-year relapse-free survival 88% vs. 76%, $p = .01$, overall survival 91% vs. 85%, $p = .02$). The comparison of the long-term toxicity of MOPP and ABVD is still ongoing. However, the preliminary data showed that ABVD was superior to MOPP in terms of hematologic toxicity (7.3% vs. 14.5% for MOPP) and for gonadal toxicity. All ABVD patients recovered spermatogenesis, whereas practically all MOPP patients did not. However, early alteration of pulmonary vital capacity was observed more frequently after ABVD (12% vs. 2%, $p = .08$) with two cases of fatal respiratory failure in the ABVD arm. Also significant modifications of the isotopic left ventricular ejection fraction were detected.

Besides the advantage of ABVD over MOPP, the main conclusion of this trial was that, with a proper use of prognostic factors, a favorable group that comprised 45% of the entire cohort was defined. For this favorable group, when treated by radiation therapy alone, staging laparotomy gives only a small increase in relapse-free survival, which is not translated into a survival benefit (93).

Several conclusions emerged from these four EORTC trials concerning early stages (H_1, H_2, H_5, H_6):

1. The European studies had confirmed several of the findings of the Stanford group (50): the clinical size of the spleen and radiologic examinations are not predictive of spleen involvement, and laparotomy can detect unsuspected infradiaphragmatic involvement in about one-fourth of CS I and II patients (1). However, a positive laparotomy is predictive of liver involvement or of extranodal dissemination in only a very small proportion of patients (49).
2. The therapeutic efficacy of spleen irradiation is as good as that of splenectomy, and its immunologic sequelae are not greater and sometimes smaller. The effects of irradiation of the upper part of the left kidney were studied and found to be compensated by a hypertrophy of the left and right kidneys (86).
3. Since rescue treatments are extremely successful in patients under the age of 50 with good pretreatment prognostic factors and in whom initial treatment did not include multiple drug chemotherapy, splenic involvement does not mean that multiple chemotherapy should be delivered during initial treatment (H_2 and H_5 trials). Survival as high or higher can be achieved without laparotomy or initial chemotherapy (23).
4. Several prognostic indicators are good predictors of infradiaphragmatic involvement or abdominal relapse (14,137,138). In the H_2 cohort 26% of 144 patients were found to be PS III to IV (49). The selection of the H_5-f aimed to decrease this incidence, which fell to 16% (39). However, a main purpose of preselecting a subgroup is to reduce the risk of relapse following treatment by radiotherapy (subtotal nodal irradiation) alone. Indeed, the remodeling of the stratification prognostic indicators in the H_6-f trial halved the proportions of relapses in the laparotomized patients as compared to that of H_5-f (11% vs. 22%), although the proportion of positive laparotomy was twice as great (33% vs. 16%) (93). This promising achievement is consistent with previous data showing that predictors of paraaortic involvement are different from those of pelvic or extranodal involvement.
5. Staging laparotomy is not mandatory for identifying a good prognostic subset of patients who can be successfully treated by radiotherapy alone (11,23,39).

By this time, a retrospective analysis reported on behalf of BNLI by Worthy (152) and other BLNI studies (92) suggested also that laparotomy was no longer justified in female patients of all ages and in male patients under 45 years of age. Moreover, an attempt was made to find for each laparotomized patient a nonlaparotomized patient of the same age and gender, with the same mediastinal involvement, ESR, and pathologic grade; 75 such matched pairs were obtained. The survival curves were almost superimposed, which confirmed the conclusion from a Cox analysis that although laparotomy resulted in the initial treatment being changed because of more advanced staging, it did not contribute anything to improving survival (92). Hence, these retrospective BNLI studies are consistent with the EORTC prospective data. A few other European groups (62,137, 138) investigated the ability of selected prognostic factors to predict occult abdominal involvement in CS I and II patients. Hence, progressively during the 1980s a consensus was reached among European oncologists: the usefulness of systemic staging laparotomy is debatable and the procedure is justified only in a few clinical presentations (11,27,28).

On the other hand, by the end of the 1970s, most pediatric Hodgkin's study groups had abandoned laparotomy because of the high incidence of severe infection in splenectomized patients. Moreover, to protect skeletal growth, the dose of radiation therapy had been lowered and multiple chemotherapy was used (98,99). In the 1980s, a few groups adopted the same strategy for adult patients in Europe and in Canada (153). For example, in Paris, Andrieu et al. (118) compared in CS IA and IIA patients radiation therapy and three cycles of MOPP versus radiation therapy and three cycles of ABVD.

However, in all these studies the absence of staging laparotomy was compensated for by the administration of chemotherapy. In 1988, in the United States most groups still believed that a staging laparotomy was necessary when treatment by radiation therapy alone was envisaged, and that this treatment could be performed only when it was negative (66). The results of the H_6 trial gave a firm basis to the opposite point of view (93). It was thus decided in 1988 in the EORTC to give up staging laparotomy in the H_7 trial (94), a decision that markedly reduced the burden of the initial workup.

6. During the first 10 years of follow-up, there is no marked difference in survival between the H_2, H_5, and H_6 trials (Figs. 1 and 2) despite a continual decrease in the proportion of patients having received chemotherapy during initial treatment or at relapse (64). During this period, from 1972 to 1988, the main aim of the EORTC group was to reduce the proportion of patients receiving multiple chemotherapy or total nodal irradiation in order to reduce the late effects (23). It is difficult to know at present whether there will be a difference in late toxicity between these trials since the follow-up is still too short for the H_5 and H_6 trials. However, we can hope that it will be reduced because the chemotherapy was either less aggressive or given to a smaller proportion of patients, while the size of the fields and the dose to uninvolved lymphatic areas was slightly reduced. In the meantime, information about late effects should be gathered. This was the purpose of the International Database on Hodgkin's Disease, which was set up in Paris in 1989 (29) and is discussed in chapter 42 of this book.

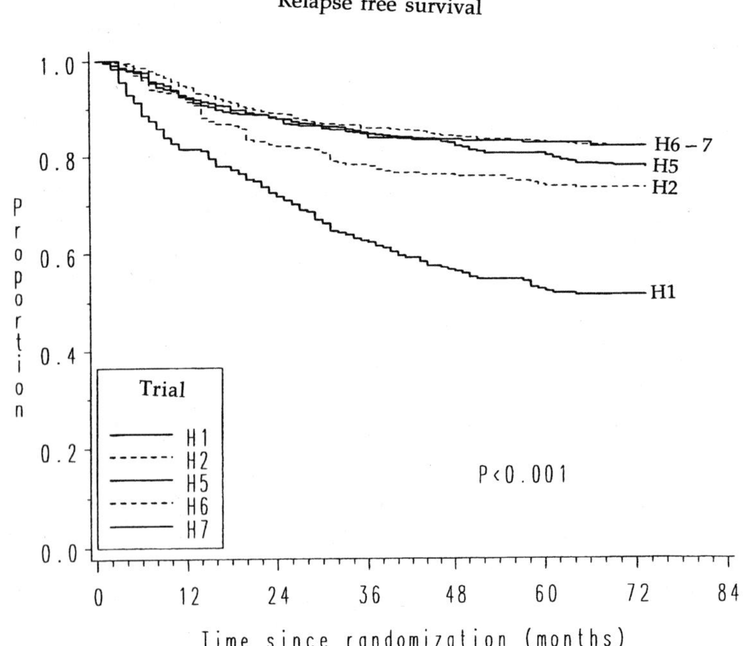

FIG. 1. Relapse-free survival of all patients included in the various EORTC trials, whatever the treatment and the prognostic subgroup. Great progress was made between the H_1 and H_2 trials. Progress has continued since but is less marked. (Data updated in 1998. Courtesy of P. Carde and S. Koscielny.)

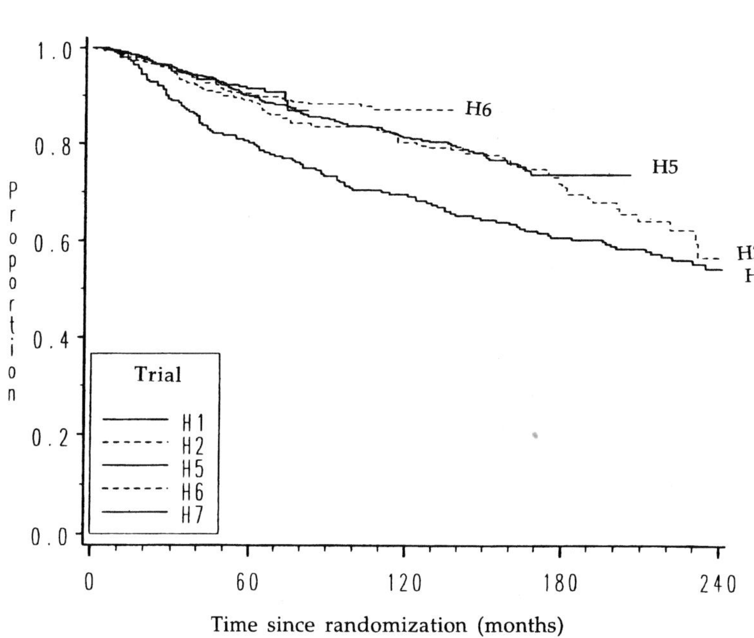

FIG. 2. Overall survival of all patients included in the various EORTC clinical trials (whatever the prognostic subgroup and the treatment). Great progress was made between the H_1 and H_2 trials. In the subsequent trials, the long-term survival rates are similar. It is only in the last trial (H_8) that overall survival seems to have slightly improved. (Data updated in 1998. Courtesy of P. Carde and S. Koscielny.)

7. The data of H_5 and H_6 trials show that CS I and II patients can be subdivided into three groups (23,39, 93,94):

   a. A *very favorable* subset, which can be defined without the help of a staging laparotomy and can be treated by limited-field radiation therapy. In the H_7 EORTC trial, which was launched in 1988 and closed in 1993, 770 patients, ages 15 to 70 years, were included (94). The very favorable subset was defined as follows: CS IA female patients younger than 40 years with ESR <50, and with lymphocyte-predominance or nodular sclerosis histology. It comprised 5% of the total cohort and was treated by a mantle field radiation therapy at a dose of 40 Gy in the involved lymph node area and 36 Gy in the other. The 6-year event-free survival was 66% (with 9 relapses out of 40 patients); the 6-year survival was 96% due to the efficacy of salvage treatment. For this subgroup the same definition and treatment were maintained in the following H_8 trial.
   b. An *unfavorable* subgroup, which comprised patients who must be treated aggressively by multiple chemotherapy combined with IF radiation therapy. Several options can be envisaged for the definition of this group (23). For the H_7 trial it was patients aged 50 years or over, or with four or five involved nodal sites, or no B symptoms and ESR ≥50 or B and ESR ≥30. It comprised about 50% of the patients. In the H_7 trial the patients of this subgroup were randomized between 6 MOPP–ABV and IF radiation therapy or 6 EBVP and IF radiation therapy. Preliminary data indicated that EBVP was better tolerated but that relapse-free survival was clearly superior in the MOPP–ABV arm. The EBVP arm was therefore closed. At 6 years the relapse-free survival was 79% in the EBVP-radiation therapy arm versus 94% in the MOPP/ABV-radiation therapy arm ($p = .001$). Due to the efficacy of salvage the difference in survival was much smaller (82% vs. 89%, $p = .09$) (94).
   c. A favorable subgroup, which is an intermediary subset that comprises all the patients who are not in either the very favorable or the unfavorable groups. In the H_7 trials they were randomized between subtotal nodal irradiation and splenic radiation therapy (involved area 40 Gy, uninvolved—including spleen—35 Gy) or to six cycles of EBVP followed by IF radiation therapy 36 to 40 Gy. In this favorable subgroup the relapse-free survival of the EBVP-radiation therapy arm was good and superior to that achieved by subtotal nodal irradiation (relapse-free survival 92% vs. 81% for subtotal nodal irradiation, $p = .004$). However, the 6-year overall survival rates were satisfactory in both arms (96% for subtotal nodal irradiation vs. 98% for EBVP-radiation therapy, P=NS). Subtotal nodal irradiation can therefore remain a reference arm. The main point will be, of course, late toxicity (94).

The division between these three subgroups was kept unchanged in the subsequent H_8 trial (1993–1998), which will not be discussed here. The German Group (GHSG) also subdivided patients into three groups that form the basis of the subsequent treatment modalities (97). As is, group I consisted of CS or PS IA or IIA without unfavorable prognostic factors. Group II was CS I or CS II with at least one of the following risk factors: massive mediastinal tumor, extranodal manifestation, massive spleen infiltration, no B symptoms and ESR ≥50 or B and ESR ≥30, and three or more involved lymph node areas. CS IIB with some of the risk factors and III A without risk factors belong to this group. These patients are treated by combined chemotherapy and radiation therapy. Group III consisted of CS IIB and CS IIIA with the above risk factors. CS IIIB and IV belong to this group, which is treated by extensive chemotherapy with radiation therapy for initially bulky disease.

In the future the boundary between the subgroups will certainly be changed to better take into account the results of the investigation on prognostic indicators. Hence, four or five subgroups instead of three might be envisaged to further tailor the treatment to the individual characteristics of the patients. The various types of treatment might also be altered to alleviate the late effects, but the use of prognostic factors for delineating subgroups will probably be kept. A reduction of the dose or of the size of the field might be envisaged for protecting the heart.

ADVANCED STAGES

Patients with stage IIIA comprise a heterogeneous clinical group varying from those with minimal disease below the diaphragm and only two or three involved areas above the diaphragm to those with extensive nodal disease or gross splenic involvement. Some groups have concluded that patients with extensive abdominal disease require chemotherapy in the initial management.

The BNLI (154) compared in a randomized study total nodal irradiation versus chemotherapy for PS IIIA (confirmed by laparotomy) patients and concluded that there was no significant difference in the overall survival rate for patients without splenic involvement. The comparison in PS IIIA of total nodal irradiation versus six cycles of MVPP (mustine, vinblastine, procarbazine, and prednisone) did not evidence any significant difference in survival (154).

A few groups aimed at delineating the subsets of IIIA patients that do or do not require combinations of multiple chemotherapy and radiation therapy. The precise definition of these subsets varies between trial groups (155), while the drug combination, the number of chemotherapy cycles, the field size, and the dose of radiation remain subject to debate (156). The data of the HD_1 trial of the GHSG suggests that a large proportion of IIIA patients can be treated by total nodal irradiation and 2 LOPP/ABVD cycles (97).

During the period 1964 to 1980, in contrast to the large number of clinical trials devoted to early stages, there were only a small number of studies in Europe for advanced stages (IIIB and IV), probably because it was felt that for these there were much fewer possible strategies. In the 1960s, some centers used radiation therapy alone. It was soon discovered that in most patients relapses occurred rapidly after the completion of radiation therapy, suggesting that the disease had already disseminated to areas other than those with overt clinical disease (157). Therefore, two other treatments were used (52). The first was chemotherapy alone, delivered during several months or even years (53,157,158). It was recognized that monochemotherapy, either by vinblastine (VBL) or methylhydrazine, was ineffective with less than 25% of complete remission. The combination of VBL and methylhydrazine did not yield better results. In contrast, multiple chemotherapy (MOPP or ABVD) achieved much higher rates of complete remission and survival; the regimen was used in a large number of centers after the publication of the remarkable results reported by DeVita et al. (51). Moreover, it was shown that the control of advanced disease requires high doses of MOPP delivered during a short time interval (159). In the late 1980s, it was shown in several trials (111,112,160,161), in particular one carried out by EORTC (113), that hybrid regimen MOPP/ABVD is superior to MOPP in advanced stages, while the BNLI trial reported better results with LOPP and EVAP than with LOPP alone (103).

Another strategy was also explored: the combination of chemotherapy and radiation therapy (53). In 1970, Amiel et al. (162) reported the good results obtained by sequential combination chemotherapy–radiation therapy–chemotherapy. Chemotherapy was a combination of vinblastine and procarbazine, and radiation therapy was delivered up to a dose of 40 Gy to all initially involved areas and eventually to bone lesions. In 1986 the EORTC launched the H3B4 trial in which 192 patients with CS IIIB or IV Hodgkin's disease were randomized between two arms—eight courses of MOPP or eight hybrid courses of MOPP/ABVD—and in which all patients received involved field radiation after chemotherapy therapy (113). As reported above, the DFS was significantly higher in the arm treated by the hybrid regimen. It demonstrated also that a rapid regression of the tumor mass under chemotherapy was a main prognostic factor. In multivariate analysis (Cox model) it was shown that the relative risk (RR) for death was doubled (RR = 2.08, $p = .01$) when a complete remission had not been achieved after four cycles of chemotherapy (whether it was MOPP or MOPP/ABVD). However, the patients for whom a complete remission was observed after eight cycles had also a much better 4-year and 8-year survival than those who were in partial remission or without remission. This study also showed that survival was inversely correlated with age (>50 years, RR for death of 1.66, $p = .1$, [NS]) and with the number of lymph node areas involved, and was poor when more than six areas were involved (RR = 1.9, $p = .01$). In some of the patients enrolled in the trial, radiation therapy was not carried out for various reasons; for these the death rate was substantially higher (in multivariate analysis RR = 2.17, $p < .005$). This result strongly suggested the beneficial effect of radiation therapy.

Prior to this H3B4 trial, several attempts had been unsuccessfully made within the EORTC to assess the contribution of radiation therapy in the treatment of IIIB in a randomized trial. However, it was difficult to persuade a sufficient number of collaborating centers to join this study, and it was only in 1986 that the H3B4 trial was launched in which after MOPP/ABVD courses patients in complete remission are randomized between no radiation therapy and a radiation therapy dose of 24 Gy on initially involved areas. Patients in whom only partial remission was achieved were irradiated and the preliminary data show that a complete remission was often achieved with subsequently a satisfactory survival. The arguments in favor of the systematic irradiation of the initially involved areas are presently supported only by nonrandomized studies (119). In the United States, Fabian et al. (163) observed a longer remission in patients receiving low-dose radiation therapy (10 to 20 Gy) to involved sites with bulky disease but no difference in survival. In the German study group patients with CS IIIB and IV are treated with extensive chemotherapy using an Adriamycin-containing regimen. Radiation therapy is delivered to initially bulky disease or residual disease after chemotherapy (97). A similar sequence of extensive chemotherapy and radiation therapy to involved areas has been recommended in poor prognosis early stages (164) or when a complete remission is not observed following treatment with chemotherapy alone or radiation therapy alone. However, optimal delivery of chemotherapy and radiation therapy is still debated.

A main problem in these CS IIIB and IV patients is identifying those who require an even more aggressive therapy. The high-dose therapy regimens are more effective when they are given early during the course of the disease. However, they cause bone marrow failure and require transplantation of hemopoietic stem cells. Identifying new modalities and the best way to utilize them has become one of the main questions of the late 1980s and 1990s (165–167). Two approaches have been envisaged: first, selecting based on pretreatment prognostic indicators, or second, taking into account the response to treatment assessed either clinically as in the H3B4 trial (113) or by monitoring biologic indicators such as ESR at the end of treatment. An elevated ESR after completion of treatment has proved to provide reliable information on the subsequent course of the disease in early stages (144,145). It should be tested in the advanced stage. Several prospective studies were launched in the late 1980s but their analysis is out of the scope of this chapter. In the 1990s, dose intensification and the use of hemopoietic growth factors have been investigated. They will probably play a main role in further progress.

CONCLUSION

From the early 1960s to the late 1980s, the history of Hodgkin's disease was one of the most fascinating in medicine during the 20th century, and progress in treatment led to spectacular successes. The improvement in the initial workup technique and treatment methods has resulted in long-term cause-specific survival rates as high as 90% in early stages and over 75% in advanced stages. But this success revealed another problem: the mortality of cured patients remains two- to threefold higher than that of the normal population. The demonstration by Easson of the curability of Hodgkin's disease was based on the parallelism of the survival curve of patients who have been treated and of the normal population for follow-up longer than 10 years. Unfortunately, we no longer observe such a parallelism, and this late toxicity has become one of the main topics for Hodgkin's disease clinical investigation and for many other cancers as well. Hence, during both phases Hodgkin's disease was a model for oncologic research.

North American and European therapeutic research were intermingled and their goals were similar; nevertheless, their philosophies were distinct. In the 1960s and the early 1970s the emphasis was put on greater therapeutic effectiveness. The radiation therapy technique that had been developed in North America (linear accelerator, wide field shaped by lead blocks) inspired European radiotherapy departments. However, very early European oncologists explored combinations of radiotherapy and chemotherapy, despite the relatively low efficacy of chemotherapy at the time, and started to register prospectively prognostic factors. They also recognized that relapse-free survival is not a reliable indicator for assessing management efficacy, and that survival after recurrence is influenced by several prognostic factors and by the aggressiveness of the initial treatment. In multicenter trials, the comparison between the results of the cooperating centers evidenced the necessity of quality assurance.

In the late 1970s, it became apparent that, despite more radical management, survival was at a standstill. Moreover, the high efficacy of rescue treatment when patients had not received initially multiple chemotherapy and the severity of side effects were demonstrated. Thus several European groups started to explore strategies in which the initial management was less radical, accepting a higher incidence of relapse in order to lower the number of patients receiving a potentially harmful treatment. This decrement in management aggressiveness was based on the use of prognostic factors for subdividing patients into subsets with the hope of tailoring the aggressiveness of management to the severity of the disease and therefore to lower late mortality in the favorable subgroups and to improve the quality of life by reducing the sequelae of treatment. Efforts should be pursued to demonstrate the benefits associated with this approach and to assess on more objective criteria the quality of life.

During the first period, Hodgkin's disease became a model for oncology because it proved the efficacy of a multidisciplinary approach and of multicenter clinical trials. It showed also the increase of survival that can be achieved by a better use of existing tools, by associating several chemical agents in multiple chemotherapy, and by combining radiotherapy and chemotherapy. In the second period it demonstrated the importance that should be given to long-term side effects and second cancers in a therapeutic strategy. It also strongly suggested the advantages when a disease is heterogeneous of adapting treatment protocol to the disease heterogeneity either by a proper use of validated prognostic indicators or by monitoring the course of the disease under treatment. It should be emphasized that one of the prerequisites to these advances is the long-term follow-up of patients. In the early 1970s many oncologists believed that a therapeutic strategy could be assessed by the analysis of the 5-year survival. We know today, and Hodgkin's disease has been instrumental in this progress, that 15- to 25-year follow-up is mandatory because it enables the assessment of the long-term effect of the treatment not only on the tumor but also on the normal tissues.

The history of the management of Hodgkin's disease during this early period has also taught us that an optimistic attitude of a few leaders may change the pace of progress. During this first decade, pioneers such as Kaplan, Easson, Peters, David Smithers, and Karl Musshof, and their close cooperation, had a key role in the victory over Hodgkin's disease. The early part of this saga also showed the need for large controlled trials and a global strategy with frequent joint meetings of the leaders of the trials. It demonstrated the impact of quality control, in particular regarding the radiotherapeutic techniques, the interpretation of the histologic slides, and the amount of drugs given to the patients. These comparisons, which were carried out, could not be published. They illustrated the risks associated with treatment carried out in small centers treating an insufficient number of patients annually. The comparison between the remarkable results achieved in some of the highly specialized centers and the end results calculated at regional levels by means of cancer registries documented this disparity in cure rates. Hodgkin's disease, with its complex management strategy, was instrumental in showing the need for continuing medical education, the role of specialized centers, the necessity of quality assurance, and long-term follow-up associated with a proper statistical survey.

REFERENCES

1. Kaplan HS. *Hodgkin's disease,* 2nd ed. Cambridge, MA: Harvard University Press, 1980.
2. Rosenberg SA. The management of Hodgkin's disease: half a century of change. *Ann Oncol* 1996;7:555.
3. Peters MV, Middlemiss KCH. A study of Hodgkin's disease treated by irradiation. *Am J Roentgenol* 1958;79:114.
4. Peters MV, Alison RE, Bush RS. Natural history of Hodgkin's disease as related to staging. *Cancer* 1966;19:308.
5. Peters MV. The need for a new clinical classification in Hodgkin's disease. *Cancer Res* 1971;31:1713.
6. La radiothérapie de la maladie d'Hodgkin. (Presidents Bernard J, Tubiana M, Symposium du 15-2-1965) *Nouv Rev Fr Hematol* 1966;6:7.
7. Symposium: obstacles to the control of Hodgkin's disease (Rye-NY). *Cancer Res* 1966;26:1044.
8. Symposium on staging in Hodgkin's disease. (Ann Arbor, April 26–28, 1971). *Cancer Res* 1971;31:1707.
9. Kaplan HS. Clinical trials in Hodgkin's disease (Proceedings of a Symposium held in Stanford 1974). *NCI Monogr* 1973;36:587.
10. Symposium on non-Hodgkin lymphoma. *Br J Cancer* 1975;31(suppl 2).
11. Carde P. Diagnostic procedures. In: Diehl V, ed. *Hodgkin's disease—Baillière's clinical haematology.* London: Baillière Tindall, 1996;9: 479.
12. Tubiana M, Henry-Amar M, Burgers M V, van der Werf Messing B, Hayat M. Prognostic significance of erythrocyte sedimentation rate in clinical stages I-II of Hodgkin's disease. *J Clin Oncol* 1984;2:194.
13. Tubiana M, Henry-Amar M, Hayat M, et al. Prognostic significance of the number of involved areas in the early stages of Hodgkin's disease. *Cancer* 1984;54:885.
14. Tubiana M, Henry-Amar M, van der Werf-Messing B, et al. A multivariate analysis of prognostic factors in early stage Hodgkin's disease. *Int J Radiat Oncol Biol Phys* 1985;11:23.
15. Easson EC, Russell MH. The cure of Hodgkin's disease. *Br Med J* 1963;1:1704.
16. Chevalier P, Bernard J. *La maladie de Hodgkin-lymphogranulomatose maligne.* Paris: Masson et Cie, 1932.
17. Gilbert R. La roentgenthérapie de la granulomatose maligne. *J Radiol Electrol* 1925;9:509.
18. Gilbert R. Radiotherapy in Hodgkin's disease (malignant granulomatosis); anatomic and clinical foundations; governing principles; results. *Am J Roentgenol* 1939;41:198.
19. Craft CB. Results with roentgen ray therapy in Hodgkin's disease. *Bulletin of Staff Meeting at the University of Minnesota Hospital* 1940;11:391.
20. Paterson E. Evaluation of chemotherapeutic compounds in the reticuloses. *Br J Cancer* 1958;12:332.
21. Lukes R, Gompel C, Nezelof C. Le diagnostic histopathologique de la maladie d'Hodgkin (analyse préliminaire d'une étude conduite à l' aveugle sur 395 observations par trois pathologistes de nationalité différente). *Nouv Rev Fr Hematol* 1966;6:11.
22. Tubiana M, Henry-Amar M, Hayat M, et al. The EORTC treatment of early stages of Hodgkin's disease. The role of radiotherapy. *Int J Radiat Oncol Biol Phys* 1984;10:197.
23. Tubiana M, Henry-Amar M, Carde P, et al. Toward comprehensive management tailored to prognostic factors of patients with clinical stages I and II in Hodgkin's disease. The EORTC Lymphoma Group controlled clinical trials: 1964–1987. *Blood* 1989;73:47.
24. International Conference on Malignant Lymphoma (Second) June 13–16, 1984, Lugano, Switzerland.In: Cavalli F, Bonadonna G, Rozencweig M, eds. *Proceedings:* malignant lymphoma and Hodgkin's disease: experimental and therapeutic advances. Boston, MA: Martinus Nijhoff, 1985.
25. International Conference on Malignant Lymphoma (Fourth) June 6-9, 1990, Lugano, Switzerland: proceedings. *Kluwer Publ Ann Oncol Suppl* 1991;2(part 1–2).
26. International Conference on Malignant Lymphoma (Fifth) June 9–12, 1993, Lugano, Switzerland: proceedings. *Kluwer Publ Ann Oncol Suppl* 1994;5(part 1–2).
27. Lister TA, Crowther D, Sutcliffe SB, et al. Report of a committee convened to discuss the evaluation and staging of patients with Hodgkin's disease: Cotswold meeting. *J Clin Oncol* 1989;7:1630.
28. Lister TA, Crowther D. Staging for Hodgkin's disease. *Semin Oncol* 1990;17:696.
29. Somers R, Henry-Amar M, Meerwaldt JH & Carde P, eds. *Treatment strategy in Hodgkin's disease. Colloque INSERM.* London, Paris: Les Editions INSERM/John Libbey Eurotext, 1990:196.

30. Diehl V, Pfreundschuh M, Loeffler M. New aspects in the diagnosis and treatment of Hodgkin's disease. Köln, Germany Oct 1–3, 1987. *Rec Results Cancer Res* 1989.
31. The Second International Symposium on Hodgkin's Disease (Oct. 3-5, 1991, Guest Editor Diehl V, Engert A). Ann Oncol 1992;3:suppl 4.
32. Trousseau A. De l'adenie. Clin Med Hôtel-Dieu (Paris) 1863;3:355.
33. Reed DM. On the pathological changes in Hodgkin's disease with especial reference to its relation to tuberculosis. *John Hopkins Hosp Rep* 1902;10:133.
34. Carbone PP, Kaplan HS, Musshoff K, Smithers D, Tubiana M. Report of the Committee on Hodgkin's Disease Staging Classification. *Cancer Res* 1971;31:1860.
35. Musshoff K. Therapy and prognosis of two different forms of organ involvement in cases of malignant lymphoma (Hodgkin's disease, reticulum cell sarcoma, lymphosarcoma) as well as a report about stage division in these diseases. *Klin Wochenschr* 1970;48:673.
36. Rosenberg SA, Boiron M, DeVita VT, et al. Report of the committee on Hodgkin's disease staging procedures. *Cancer Res* 1971;31:1864.
37. Tubiana M, Attié E, Flamant R, et al. Prognostic factors in 454 cases of Hodgkin's disease. *Cancer Res* 1971;31:1801.
38. Tubiana M, Van der Werf-Messing B, Laugier A, et al. Survival after recurrence: prognostic factors and spread patterns in clinical stages I and II of Hodgkin's disease. *NCI Monogr* 1973;36:513.
39. Carde P, Burgers JMV, Henry-Amar M, et al. Clinical stages I and II Hodgkin's disease: a specifically tailored therapy according to prognostic factors. *J Clin Oncol* 1988;6:239.
40. Specht L. Tumour burden as the main indicator of prognosis in Hodgkin's disease. *Eur J Cancer* 1992;28A:1982.
41. Kaplan HS. The radical radiotherapy of regionally localized Hodgkin's disease. *Radiology* 1962;78:553.
42. Kaplan HS, Rosenberg SA. Extended-field radical radiotherapy in advanced Hodgkin's disease: short-term results of 2 randomized clinical trials. *Cancer Res* 1966;26:1268.
43. A Collaborative Study. Survival and complications of radiotherapy following involved and extended field therapy of Hodgkin's disease, stages I and II. *Cancer* 1976;38:288.
44. A Collaborative Study. Radiotherapy of stage I and II Hodgkin's disease. *Cancer* 1984;541928.
45. Guiguet M, Valleron AJ, Tubiana M. Distribution des tailles de la metastase à la detection et traitement adjuvant: approche biomathematique. *Comptes Rendus Acad Sc (Paris)* 1982;294:15.
46. Henry-Amar M, Pellae-Cosset B, Bayle-Weisgerber C, et al. Risk of secondary acute leukemia and pre-leukemia after Hodgkin's disease: the Institut Gustave Roussy experience. *Recent Results Cancer Res* 1989;117:270.
47. Horwich A, Specht L, Ashley S. Survival analysis of patients with clinical stages I or II Hodgkin's disease who have relapsed after initial treatment with radiotherapy alone. *Eur J Cancer* 1997;33:848.
48. Specht L, Gray RG, Clarke MJ, Peto R. The influence of more extensive radiotherapy and adjuvant chemotherapy on long-term outcome of early stage Hodgkin's disease. A meta-analysis of 23 randomized trials involving 3,888 patients. *J Clin Oncol* 1998;16:830.
49. Tubiana M, Hayat M, Henry-Amar M, Breur K, van der Werf-Messing B, Burgers M. Five-year results of EORTC randomized study of splenectomy and spleen irradiation in clinical stages I - II Hodgkin's disease. *Eur J Cancer* 1981;17:355.
50. Glatstein E, Guernsey JM, Rosenberg SA, Kaplan HS. The value of laparotomy and splenectomy in the staging of Hodgkin's disease. *Cancer* 1969;24:709.
51. DeVita VT, Serpick A, Carbone PP. Combination chemotherapy in the treatment of advanced Hodgkin's disease. *Ann Intern Med* 1970;73:881.
52. Amiel JL, Mathé G, Tubiana M, Schlumberger JR, Rouëssé J, Pouillart P. Traitement des maladies de Hodgkin'stades III B et IV, par la séquence chimiothérapie, radiothérapie, chimiothérapie. *Bull Cancer (Paris)* 1971;58:191.
53. Bernard J, Boiron M, Goguel A, Jacquillat C, Tanzer J, Weil M. Traitement de la maladie de Hodgkin par une polychimiothérapie associant moutarde à l azote, vincristine, méthylhydrazine et prednisone. *Presse Med* 1967;75:2647.
54. Belpomme D, Carde P, Oldham RK, et al. Malignancies possibly secondary to anticancer therapy. *Recent Results Cancer Res* 1974;49:115.
55. Slanina J, Musshoff K, Rahner T, Stiasny R. Long-term side effects in irradiated patients with Hodgkin's disease. *Int J Radiat Oncol Biol Phys* 1977;2:1.
56. Romanelli R, Ciampelli L, Mungai V. Severe heart disease induced by radiation and chemotherapy for Hodgkin's disease. *Tumori* 1981;67:361.
57. Zucali R, Pagnoni AM, Zanini M, et al. Radiological and spirometric evaluation of mediastinal and pulmonary late effects after radiotherapy and chemotherapy for Hodgkin's disease. *Eur J Cancer (Paris)* 1981;2:169.
58. Tubiana M. Hodgkin's disease: historical perspective and clinical presentation. In: Diehl V, ed. *Hodgkin's disease—Baillière's clinical haematology.* London: Baillière Tindall, 1996;9:503.
59. Henry-Amar M. Treatment sequelae and quality of life. In: Diehl V, ed. *Hodgkin's disease—Baillière's clinical haematology.* London: Baillière Tindall, 1996;9:595.
60. Musshoff K, Harmann C, Niklaus B, Rossner R. The prognostic significance of first and second remission after first and second relapse radiotherapy in Hodgkin's disease. *Z Krebsforsch* 1976;85:243.
61. Teillet F, Boiron M, Bernard J. Reappraisal of clinical and biological signs in staging of Hodgkin's disease. *Cancer Res* 1971;31:1723.
62. Rutherford C, Desforges J, Davies D, Barnett A. The decision to perform staging laparotomy in symptomatic Hodgkin's disease. *Br J Haematol* 1980;44:347.
63. Proctor SJ, Specht L. Hodgkin's disease: a challenge to the classical staging system. A debate. *Leukemia* 1993;11:1910.
64. Henry-Amar M, Somers R. Long-term survival in early in early stage Hodgkin's disease: the EORTC experience. In: Somers R, Henry-Amar M, Meerweldt JH, Carde P, eds. *Treatment strategy in Hodgkin's disease. Colloque INSERM.* London, Paris: Les Editions INSERM/John Libbey Eurotext, 1990;196:151.
65. Henry-Amar M, Somers R. Survival outcome after Hodgkin's disease: a report from the international data base on Hodgkin's disease. *Semin Oncol* 1991;17:758.
66. Mauch PM, Kalish LA, Marcus KC, et al. Long-term survival in Hodgkin's Disease. Relative impact of mortality, second tumors, infection and cardiovascular disease. *Cancer J Sci Am* 1995;1:33.
67. Vaughan Hudson B, Vaughan Hudson G, Linch DC, Anderson L. Late mortality in young patients cured of Hodgkin's disease. *Ann Oncol* 1994;5(suppl 2):S65.
68. Andrieu JM, Ifrah N, Payen C, et al. Increased risk of secondary acute nonlymphocytic leukemia after extended-field radiation therapy combined with MOPP chemotherapy for Hodgkin's disease. *J Clin Oncol* 1990;8:1148.
69. Bennett MH, MacLennan KA, Vaughan Hudson G, et al. Non-Hodgkin's lymphoma arising in patients treated for Hodgkin's disease in the BNLI: a 20-year experience. *Ann Oncol* 1991;2(suppl 2):83.
70. Biti G, Cellai E, Magrini S, et al. Second solid tumors and leukemia after treatment for Hodgkin's disease: an analysis of 1121 patients from a single institution. *Int J Radiat Oncol Biol Phys* 1994;29:25.
71. Boffetta P, Kaldor JM. Secondary malignancies following cancer chemotherapy. *Acta Oncol* 1994;33:591.
72. Devereux S, Selassie TG, Vaughan Hudson G, Vaughan Hudson B, Linch DC. Leukaemia complicating treatment for Hodgkin's disease; the experience of the British National Lymphoma Investigation. *Br Med J* 1990;301:1077.
73. Henry-Amar M. Second cancer after treatment for Hodgkin's disease: a report from the International Data Base on Hodgkin's Disease. *Ann Oncol* 1992;3:117.
74. Henry-Amar M, Dietrich PY. Acute leukemia after the treatment of Hodgkin's disease. *Hematol Oncol Clin North Am* 1993;7:369.
75. Jacquillat C, Khayat D, Desprez-Curely J, et al. Non-Hodgkin's lymphoma occurring after Hodgkin's disease. *Cancer* 1984;53:459.
76. Kaldor JM, Day NE, Band P, et al. Second malignancies following testicular cancer, ovarian cancer, and Hodgkin's disease: an international collaborative study among cancer registries. *Int J Cancer* 1987; 39:571.
77. Swerdlow AJ, Douglas AJ, Vaughan Hudson G, Vaughan Hudson B, MacLennan KA. Risk of second primary cancer after Hodgkin's disease in patients in the British National Lymphoma Investigation: relationships to host factors, histology and stage of Hodgkin's disease, and splenectomy. *Br J Cancer* 1993;68:1006.
78. van Leeuwen FE, Chorus AMJ, van den Belt-Dusebout AW, et al. Leukemia risk following Hodgkin's disease: relation to cumulative dose of alkylating agents, treatment with tenisposide combinations, number of episodes of chemotherapy, and bone marrow damage. *J Clin Oncol* 1994;12:1063.

79. van Leeuwen FE, Klokman WJ, Hagenbeek A, et al. Second cancer risk following Hodgkin's disease: a 20-year follow-up study. *J Clin Oncol* 1994;12:312.
80. Cosset JM, Henry-Amar M, Burgers JMV, et al. Late injuries of the gastrointestinal tract in the H2 and H5 EORTC Hodgkin's disease trials: emphasis on the role of exploratory laparotomy and fractionation. *Radiother Oncol* 1988;13:61.
81. Cosset JM, Henry-Amar M, Girinski T. Late toxicity of radiotherapy in Hodgkin's disease: the role of fraction size. *Acta Oncol* 1988;27: 123.
82. Cosset JM, Henry-Amar M, Meerwaldt JH. Long-term toxicity of early stages of Hodgkin's disease therapy: the EORTC experience. *Ann Oncol* 1991;2:77.
83. Gustavsson A, Eskilsson J, Landberg T, et al. Late cardiac effects after mantle radiotherapy in patients with Hodgkin's disease. *Ann Oncol* 1990;1:355.
84. Gustavsson A, Eskilsson J, Landberg T, et al. Long-term effects on pulmonary function of mantle radiotherapy in patients with Hodgkin's disease. *Ann Oncol* 1992;3:455.
85. Lagrange JL, Thyss A, Caldani C, et al. Toxicity of a combination of ABVD chemotherapy and mediastinal irradiation for Hodgkin's disease patients with massive initial mediastinal involvement. *Bull Cancer (Paris)* 1988;75:801.
86. Le Bourgeois JP, Meignan M, Parmentier C, Tubiana M. Renal consequences of irradiation of the spleen in lymphoma patients. *Br J Radiol* 1979;52:56.
87. Peerboom PF, Hassink EAM, Melkert R, et al. Thyroid function 10–18 years after mantle field irradiation for Hodgkin's disease. *Eur J Cancer* 1992;28A:1716.
88. Cosset JM, Henry-Amar M, Pellae-Cosset B, et al. Pericarditis and myocardial infarctions after Hodgkin's disease therapy at the Institut Gustave-Roussy. *Int J Radiat Oncol Biol Phys* 1991;21:447.
89. Dubray B, Henry-Amar M, Meerwaldt JH, et al. radiation-induced lung damage after thoracic irradiation for Hodgkin's disease: the role of fractionation. *Radiother Oncol* 1995;36:211.
90. Dietrich PY, Henry-Amar M, Cosset JM, et al. Second primary cancers in patients continuously disease-free from Hodgkin's disease: a protective role for the spleen? *Blood* 1994,84.1209.
91. Henry-Amar M, Hayat M, Meerwaldt JH. Causes of death for early stages Hodgkin's disease entered in EORTC protocols. *Int J Radiat Oncol Biol Phys* 1990;19:1155.
92. Haybittle JL, Hayhoe FGJ, Easterling MJ, et al. Review of British National Lymphoma Investigation studies of Hodgkin's disease and development of prognostic index. *Lancet* 1985;1:967.
93. Carde P, Hagenbeek A, Hayat M, et al. Clinical staging versus laparotomy and combined modality with MOPP versus ABVD in early stage Hodgkin's disease. The H6 twin trials from the European Organization for Research and Treatment of Cancer Lymphoma Cooperating Group. *J Clin Oncol* 1993;11:2258.
94. Noordijk EM, Carde P, Mandard AM, et al. Preliminary results of the EORTC-GPMC controlled clinical trial H7 in early-stage Hodgkin's disease. *Ann Oncol* 1994;5:S107.
95. Löffler M, Diehl V, Pfreundschuh M, et al. Low dose radiotherapy following four cycles of alternating poly chemotherapy in intermediate stage Hodgkin's disease. *J Clin Oncol* 1997;15:2275.
96. Zittoun R, Audebert A, Hoerni V, et al. Extended versus involved field irradiation combined with MOPP chemotherapy in early clinical stages of Hodgkin's disease. *J Clin Oncol* 1985;3:207.
97. Tesch H, Sieber M, Diehl V. Treatment of intermediate stages. In: Diehl V, ed. *Hodgkin's disease—Baillière's clinical haematology*. London: Baillière Tindall, 1996;9:543.
98. Lemerle J, Oberlin O, Schaison G, et al. Hodgkin's disease in children: adaptation of treatment to risk factors. *Recent Results Cancer Res* 1989;117:214.
99. Oberlin O, Leverger G, Pacquement H, et al. Low-dose radiation therapy and reduced chemotherapy in childhood Hodgkin's disease: the experience of the French Society of Pediatric Oncology. *J Clin Oncol* 1992;10:1602.
100. Schellong G, Brämswig JH, Hörnig-Franz I. Treatment of children with Hodgkin's disease- results of the German Pediatric Oncology Group. *Ann Oncol* 1992;3:73.
101. Brämswig JH, Hörnig-Franz I, Riepenhausen M, et al. The challenge of pediatric Hodgkin's disease—where is the balance between cure and long-term toxicity? A report of the West German multicenter studies DAL-Hodgkin's Disease-78, DAL-Hodgkin's Disease-82, and DAL-Hodgkin's Disease-85. *Leukemia Lymphoma* 1990;2:183.
102. Schellong G. Treatment of children and adolescents with Hodgkin's disease: the experience of the German-Austrian Pediatric Study Group. In: Diehl V, ed. *Hodgkin's disease—Baillière's clinical haematology*. London: Baillière Tindall 1996;9:619.
103. Hancock BW. Randomized study of MOPP against LOPP in advanced Hodgkin's disease. *Radiother Oncol* 1986;7:215.
104. Nicholson WM, Beard MEJ, Crowther D, et al. Combination chemotherapy in generalized Hodgkin's disease. *Br Med J* 1970;3:7.
105. Hancock BW, Vaughan Hudson G, Vaughan Hudson B, et al. British National Lymphoma Investigation randomized study of MOPP (mustine, Oncovin, procarbazine, prednisone) against LOPP (Leukeran substituted for mustine) in advanced Hodgkin's disease. Long-term results. *Br J Cancer* 1991;63:579.
106. Zittoun R, Eghbali H, Audebert A, et al. Groupe Pierre et Marie Curie: association d'épirubicine, bléomycine, vinblastine et prednisone (EBVP). *Bull Cancer (Paris)* 1987;74:151.
107. Hoerni B, Orgerie MB, Eghbali H, et al. Nouvelle association d'épirubicine, bléomycine, vinblastine et prednisone (EBVP II) avant radiothérapie dans les stades localisés de Maladie de Hodgkin: essai de phase II chez 50 malades. *Bull Cancer (Paris)* 1988;8:789.
108. Bonadonna G, Zucali R, Monfardini S, et al. Combination therapy of Hodgkin's disease with adriamycin, bleomycin, vinblastine and imidazole carboxamide versus MOPP. *Cancer* 1975;36:252.
109. Santoro A, Bonadonna G, Valagussa P. Long-term results of combined chemotherapy approach in Hodgkin's disease: superiority of ABVD - radiotherapy versus MOPP plus radiotherapy. *J Clin Oncol* 1987;5:27.
110. Bonfante V, Santoro A, Viviani S, et al. ABVD in the treatment of Hodgkin's disease. *Semin Oncol* 1992;19(suppl 5):38.
111. Santoro A, Bonadonna G, Bonfante V, Valagusso P. Alternating drug combinations in the treatment of advanced Hodgkin's disease. *N Engl J Med* 1982;306:770.
112. Bonadonna G, Valagussa P, Santoro A. Alternating non-cross-resistant combination chemotherapy or MOPP in stage IV Hodgkin's disease: a report of 8-year results. *Ann Intern Med* 1986;104:739.
113. Somers R, Carde P, Henry-Amar M, et al. A randomized study in stage IIIB and IV Hodgkin's disease comparing eight courses of MOPP versus an alternation of MOPP with ABVD: a European Organization for Research and Treatment of Cancer Lymphoma Cooperative Group and Groupe Pierre-et-Marie-Curie controlled clinical trial. *J Clin Oncol* 1994;12:279.
114. Hancock BW, Vaughan Hudson G & Vaughan Hudson B. LOPP alternating with EVAP is superior to LOPP alone in the initial treatment of advanced Hodgkin's disease: the results of a British National Lymphoma Investigation Trial. *J Clin Oncol* 1992;10:1252.
115. Tubiana M, Henry-Amar M, Hayat M, Breur K, van der Werf-Messing B, Burgers M. Long-term results of the EORTC randomized study of irradiation and vinblastine in clinical stages I and II Hodgkin's disease. *Eur J Cancer* 1975;15:645.
116. Anderson H, Crowther D, Deakin D, et al. A randomized study of adjuvant MVPP chemotherapy after mantle radiotherapy in pathologically staged IA-IIB Hodgkin's disease: 10-year follow-up. *Ann Oncol* 1991;2:49.
117. Andrieu JM, Coscas Y, Cramer P, et al. Chemotherapy plus radiotherapy in clinical stages I A to III B. Results of the H77 trial (1977-1980). In: Cavalli F, Bonadonna G, Rozencweig M, eds. *Malignant lymphoma and Hodgkin's disease.* Boston, MA: Martinus Nijhoff 1985.
118. Andrieu JM, Montagnon B, Asselain B, et al. Chemotherapy-radiotherapy associations in Hodgkin's disease, clinical stages IA, II2A. Results of a prospective clinical trial with 166 patients. *Cancer* 1980; 46:2126.
119. Brizel DM, Winer EP, Prosnitz LR, et al. Improved survival with the use of combined modality therapy. *Int J Radiat Oncol Biol Phys* 1990; 19:535.
120. Brusamolino E, Lazzarino M, Orlandi E. Early stage Hodgkin's disease: long-term results with radiotherapy alone or combined radiotherapy and chemotherapy. *Ann Oncol* 1994;5(suppl 2):S101.
121. Diehl V, Pfreundschuh M, Löffler M, et al. Therapiestudien der deutschen Hodgkin-Stediengruppe. Zwischenergebnisse der Studienprotokolle Hodgkin's Disease-1, Hodgkin's Disease-2 and Hodgkin's Disease-3. *Onkologie* 1987;10:62.

122. Fermé C, Teillet F, d'Agay MF. Combined modality in Hodgkin's disease: comparison of six versus three courses of MOPP with clinical and surgical restaging. *Cancer* 1984;54:2324.
123. Nissen NI, Nordentoft AM. Radiotherapy versus combined modality treatment of stage I + II Hodgkin's disease. *Cancer Treat Rep* 1992; 66:799.
124. Specht L, Carde P, Mauch P, Magrini SM, Santarelli MT. Radiotherapy versus combined modality in early stages. *Ann Oncol* 1992;3:577.
125. Biti G, Cimino G, Cartoni C, et al. Extended-field radiotherapy is superior to MOPP chemotherapy for the treatment of pathologic stage I-IIA Hodgkin's disease: eight-year update of an Italian prospective randomized study. *J Clin Oncol* 1992;10:378.
126. Westling P. Studies of the prognosis in Hodgkin's disease. *Acta Radiol* 1965;245(suppl):5.
127. Horwich A, Easton D, Nogueira-Costa R, et al. An analysis of prognostic factors in early stage Hodgkin's disease. *Radiother Oncol* 1986; 7:95.
128. Specht L. Prognostic factors in Hodgkin's disease. *Semin Radiat Oncol* 1996;6:146.
129. Meerwaldt J H, Van Glabbeke M & Vaughan Hudson B. Prognostic factors for stage I and II Hodgkin's disease. In: Somers R, Henry-Amar M, Meerwaldt J K, Carde P, eds. *Treatment strategy in Hodgkin's disease.* Proceedings of the Paris International Workshop and Symposium held on June 28–30, 1989. Colloque INSERM No. 196. London, Paris: INSERM/John Libbey Eurotext, 1990:37.
130. Specht L. Prognostic factor studies in Hodgkin's disease, problems and pitfalls. *Leukemia* 1993;7:1915.
131. Vaughan Hudson B, MacLennan K A, Easterling M J, et al. The prognostic significance of age in Hodgkin's disease: examination of 1500 patients (BNLI report No. 23). *Clin Radiol* 1983;34:503.
132. Specht L, Nissen NI. Hodgkin's disease and age. *Eur J Haematol* 1989;43:127.
133. Tubiana M, Schlumberger M, Rougier P, et al. Long-term results and prognostic factors in patients with thyroid carcinoma. *Cancer* 1985; 55:794.
134. Koscielny S, Tubiana M, Le MG, et al. Relationship between the size of primary tumour and the probability of metastatic dissemination. *Br J Cancer* 1984;49:709.
135. Tubiana M, Koscielny S. Natural history of human breast cancer: recent data and clinical implications. *Breast Cancer Res Treat* 1991; 18:125.
136. Banfi A, Bonadonna G, Carnevali G, et al. Preferential sites of involvement and spread in malignant lymphomas. *Eur J Cancer* 1968; 4:319.
137. Brada M, Easton D, Horwich A, et al. Clinical presentation as a predictor of laparotomy findings in supradiaphragmatic stage I and II Hodgkin's disease. *Radiother Oncol* 1986;5:15.
138. Aragon de la Cruz G, Cardenes H, Otero J, et al. Individual risk of abdominal disease in patients with stages I and II supradiaphragmatic Hodgkin's disease. *Cancer* 1989;63:1799.
139. Yarnold JR, Jelliffe AM, Vaughan Hudson G. Patterns of relapse following radiotherapy for Hodgkin's disease. *Clin Radiol* 1982;33:137.
140. Cosset JM, Henry-Amar M, Carde P, Clarke D, Le Bourgeois JP, Tubiana M. The prognostic significance of large mediastinal masses in the treatment of Hodgkin's Disease. The experience of the Institut Gustave-Roussy. *Hematol Oncol* 1984;2:33.
141. Papillon J, Croizat P, Revol L, et al. Les survies de plus de 10 ans dans la maladie de Hodgkin. *Nouv Rev Fr Hematol* 1966;6:79.
142. Vaughan Hudson B, MacLennan KA, Bennett MH, Easterling MJ, Vaughan Hudson G, Jelliffe AM. Systemic disturbance in Hodgkin's disease and its relation to histopathology and prognosis (BNLI report No. 30). *Clin Radiol* 1987;38:257.
143. Le Bourgeois JP, Tubiana M. The erythrocyte sedimentation rate as a monitor for relapse in patients with previously treated Hodgkin's disease. *Int J Radiat Oncol Biol Phys* 1977;2:241.
144. Friedman S, Henry-Amar M, Cosset JM, et al. Evolution of erythrocyte sedimentation rate as predictor of early relapse in post-therapy early-stage Hodgkin's disease. *J Clin Oncol* 1988;6:596.
145. Henry-Amar M, Friedman S, Hayat M, et al. Erythrocyte sedimentation rate predicts early relapse and survival in early-stage Hodgkin's disease. *Ann Intern Med* 1991;114:361.
146. Munker R, Hasenclever D, Brosteanu O, Hiller E, Diehl V. Bone marrow involvement in Hodgkin's disease: an analysis of 135 consecutive cases. *J Clin Oncol* 1995;13:403.
147. Lukes RJ, Craver LF, Hall TC, et al. Report of the Nomenclature Committee. *Cancer Res* 1966;26:1311.
148. MacLennan KA, Bennett MH, Tu A, et al. Relationship of histopathologic features to survival and relapse in nodular sclerosing Hodgkin's disease. A study of 1659 patients. *Cancer* 1989;64:1686.
149. MacLennan KA, Bennett MH, Bosq J, et al. The histology and immunohistology of Hodgkin's disease: its relationship to prognosis and clinical behaviour. In: Somers R, Henry-Amar M, Meerwaldt JK, Carde P, eds. *Treatment strategy in Hodgkin's disease.* Proceedings of the Paris International Workshop and Symposium held on June 28-30, 1989. Colloque INSERM No. 196. London, Paris: INSERM/John Libbey Eurotext, 1990:35.
150. Diehl V, Tesch H. Hodgkin's disease: environmental or genetic. *N Engl J Med* 1995;332:461.
151. Löffler M, Dixon DO, Swindell R. Prognostic factors of stage III and IV Hodgkin's disease. In: Somers R, Henry-Amar M, Meerwaldt JK, Carde P, eds. *Treatment strategy in Hodgkin's disease.* Proceedings of the Paris International Workshop and Symposium held on June 28–30, 1989. Colloque INSERM No. 196. London, Paris: INSERM/John Libbey Eurotext, 1990:89.
152. Worthy TS. Evaluation of diagnostic laparotomy and splenectomy in Hodgkin's disease. *Clin Radiol* 1981;32:523.
153. Bergsagel DE, Alison RE, Bean HA, et al. Results of treating Hodgkin's disease without a policy of laparotomy staging. *Cancer Treat Rep* 1982;66:717.
154. Timothy AR, Sutcliffe SB, Lister A, et al. The management of stage III A Hodgkin's disease. *Int J Radiat Oncol Biol Phys* 1980;6:135.
155. Loeffler M, Mauch P, MacLennan K, et al. Review on prognostic factors. *Ann Oncol* 1992;3(suppl 4):63.
156. Pfreundschuh P, Lathan B, Loeffler M, et al. Recommendations for future clinical trials on Hodgkin's disease. *Ann Oncol* 1992;3(suppl 4):101.
157. Amiel JL, Berumen L, Schwarzenberg L, et al. Essai de traitement de la maladie d'Hodgkin généralisée par une chimiothérapie multiple. *Semaine Hôpitaux (Paris)* 1966;24:2970.
158. Jacquillat C, Weill M, Gogual A, et al. Chimiothérapie de la Maladie d'Hodgkin par des associations médicamenteuses. *Presse Med* 1971; 79:513.
159. Carde P, Mackintosh FR, Rosenberg SA. A dose and time response analysis of the treatment of Hodgkin's Disease with MOPP chemotherapy. *J Clin Oncol* 1983;1:146.
160. Viviani S, Bonadonna G, Santoro A, et al. Alternating versus hybrid MOPP-ABVD in Hodgkin's disease: the Milan experience. *Ann Oncol* 1991;2:55.
161. Gobbi PG, Pieresca C, Federico M, et al. MOPP/EBV/CAD hybrid chemotherapy with or without limited radiotherapy in advanced or unfavorably presenting Hodgkin's disease: a report from the Italian Lymphoma Study Group. *J Clin Oncol* 1993;11:712.
162. Amiel JL, Schlienger M, Laugier A, et al. Essai de traitement de la maladie d'Hodgkin généralisée ou disséminée (Stade III et IV) par la séquence chimiothérapie-radiothérapie. Association éventuelle à splenectomie et chimiothérapie supplémentaire. *Nouv Rev Fr Hematol* 1970;10:597.
163. Fabian CJ, Mansfield CM, Dahlberg S, et al. Low dose involved field radiation in advanced Hodgkin's disease. A SWOG randomized study. *Ann Intern Med* 1994;120:903.
164. Cosset JM, Fermé C, Noordijk EM, Dubray BM, Thirion P, Henry-Amar M. Combined modality treatment for poor prognosis stages I and II Hodgkin's disease. *Semin Oncol* 1996;6:185.
165. Gribben J, Linch DC, Vaughan Hudson B. The potential value of intensive therapy with autologous bone marrow rescue in the treatment of malignant lymphoma. *Hematol Oncol* 1987;5:281.
166. Linch DC, Winfield D, Goldston AH, et al. Dose intensification with autologous bone marrow transplantation in relapsed and resistant Hodgkin's disease: results of a BNLI randomized trial. *Lancet* 1993; 341:1051.
167. Carde P. Clarification of entry criteria for the EORTC H_5 favorable trial of early stage Hodgkin's disease. *J Clin Oncol* 1994;12:1739.

Hodgkin's Disease, edited by P. M. Mauch,
J. O. Armitage, V. Diehl, R. T. Hoppe, and L. M. Weiss.
Lippincott Williams & Wilkins, Philadephia ©1999.

CHAPTER 4

Development of the Concept of Hodgkin's Disease as a Curable Illness: The American Experience

Saul A. Rosenberg

THE RESULTS OF PETERS AND KAPLAN

The successful management of Hodgkin's disease has been one of the most significant achievements in oncology of the past century. This once uniformly fatal disease is now one of the most curable of human neoplasms. Though the clinical investigators and developments that have led to this success have come from international efforts, North Americans have contributed very significantly.

Important advances in radiotherapy equipment, techniques, and concepts resulted from the pioneering work of the late M. Vera Peters and the late Henry S. Kaplan. Both of these radiotherapists advocated the use of radiation fields in adequate dose to irradiate the Hodgkin's disease where it was evident, and to administer irradiation to adjacent regions where Hodgkin's disease might be occult.

Peters' results at the Princess Margaret Hospital in Toronto were reported in a classic paper in 1950 (1). She subsequently compared 5- and 10-year survival results in four groups of patients, as shown in Figure 1 (2). Patients with Hodgkin's disease, who were treated with high doses to both the involved sites and adjacent sites, had improved survival when compared to those who received lower doses to involved sites and/or did not receive irradiation to adjacent sites. Her patients, however, were not concurrent and, of course, were not randomly assigned to the various treatment plans.

S. A. Rosenberg: Department of Medicine and Radiation Oncology, Stanford University School of Medicine, Stanford, California.

Kaplan's results were equally provocative. He had the great advantage and major contribution of the Stanford Medical Linear Accelerator. Kaplan recognized the potential value of the klystron tube and other physics developments of Stanford colleagues working in the high-energy physics department. Along with Edward Ginzton, a physicist, the Stanford group invented and built the first medical linear accelerator in the United States. It revolutionized radiation therapy because it could deliver x-irradiation in the supervoltage range (1 MeV or greater) with a field size and dose intensity practical for treating patients with cancer.

The availability of the Stanford Medical Linear Accelerator allowed Kaplan to treat patients with relatively localized Hodgkin's disease with so-called radical techniques. He reported his results in 1962 (3) and at the Rye, New York, conference (4), comparing the survival of patients treated with previously standard or palliative techniques and those treated with orthovoltage equipment (Fig. 2). Kaplan's results were excellent and unprecedented. However, as with Peters' results, patients in the comparison groups were nonconcurrent and not randomly selected. On the other hand, the results could not be ignored and a completely new era of the irradiation of Hodgkin's disease resulted from the experience of Peters and Kaplan, and the availability of supervoltage irradiation.

THE RYE CONFERENCE

One of the most significant events in the history of the understanding and management of Hodgkin's was the conference, "Obstacles to the Control of Hodgkin's Disease,"

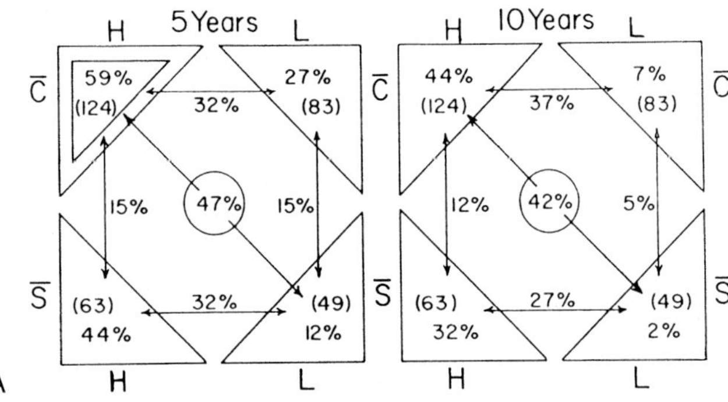

A

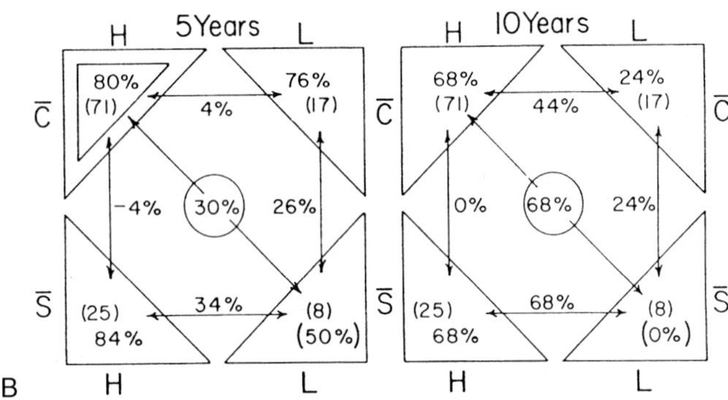

B

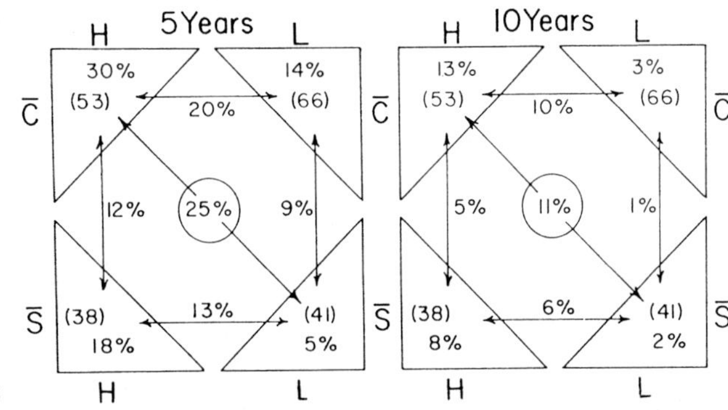

C

FIG. 1. The effect of various radiation treatment methods on 5- and 10-year survivals of patients with early **(B)** or late **(C)** stages of Hodgkin's disease as shown in the 1966 report by Peters. **A:** All stages of Hodgkin's disease: radiotherapy response according to method of treatment, 1928–1954, at 5 years *(left)* and 10 years *(right)*. **B:** Early stages (I and IIA) of Hodgkin's disease: radiotherapy response according to method of treatment, 1928–1954, at 5 years *(left)* and 10 years *(right)*. **C:** Late stages (IIB and III) of Hodgkin's disease: radiotherapy response according to method of treatment, 1928–1954, at 5 years *(left)* and 10 years *(right)*. H, high tumor dose to involvement; L, low tumor dose to involvement; C, with radiation of adjacent areas; S, without radiation of adjacent areas. (From ref. 2, with permission.)

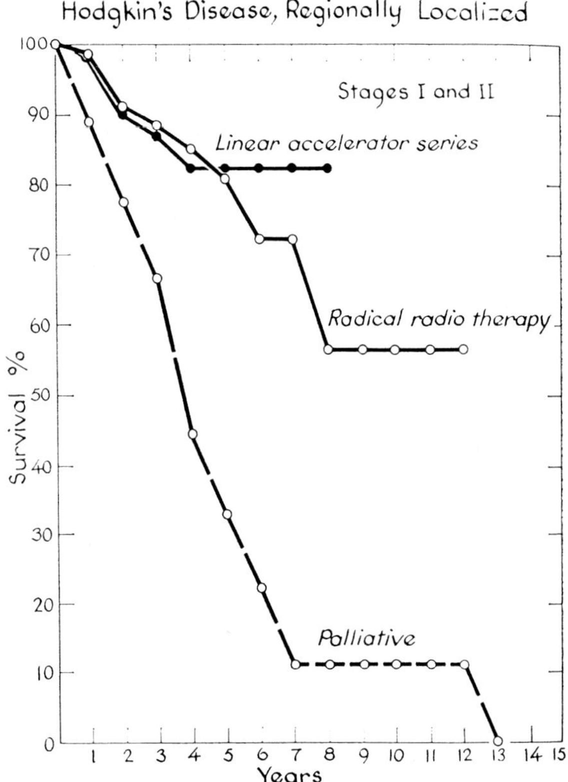

FIG. 2. The results of treating localized stages I and II Hodgkin's disease with different radiation treatment methods as shown in the 1966 report by Kaplan. Actuarial analysis of survival in 88 regionally localized (stage I and II) cases of Hodgkin's disease treated radically (3,500–4,000 rad in 4 weeks) with megavoltage radiotherapy, compared with survival in a small series of similarly staged cases treated palliatively (400–1,000 rad in 1 to 2 weeks) with kilovoltage radiotherapy. (From ref. 4, with permission.)

held at the Westchester Country Club in Rye, New York, September 13 to 15, 1965. This followed a similar conference held in Paris, France, on February 15, 1965. The conference was sponsored jointly by the American Cancer Society and the U.S. National Cancer Institute. The program committee and staff representatives are shown, from the original program publication, in Figures 3 and 4.

This conference, subsequently referred to as the Rye conference, brought together 45 leaders in the field, 40 from the United States, one from Canada (Peters), and four from Europe (including Eric Easson and Maurice Tubiana). The meeting occurred at an exciting time for the participants. Radiotherapists had new equipment and techniques available, which they argued could cure Hodgkin's disease. Chemotherapists were beginning to observe clinical responsiveness, which was unprecedented. New diagnostic methods, particularly lower extremity lymphangiography, enlightened clinicians to the extent and patterns of Hodgkin's disease at its onset. Pathologists proposed significant changes in the classification of Hodgkin's disease

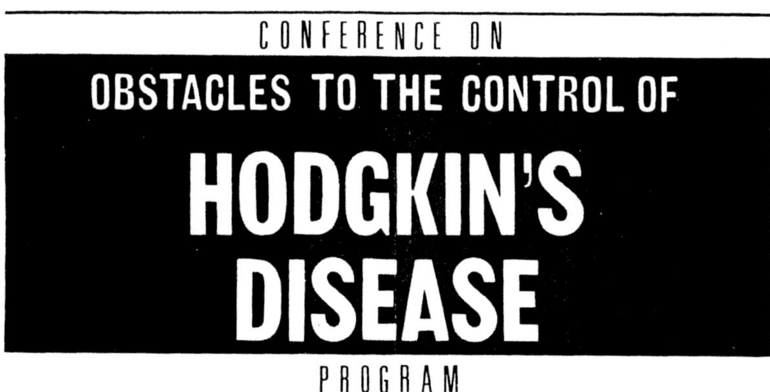

CONFERENCE ON
OBSTACLES TO THE CONTROL OF
HODGKIN'S
DISEASE
PROGRAM

Westchester Room
WESTCHESTER COUNTRY CLUB
Rye, New York

September 13, 14, 15, 1965

FIG. 3. The cover page from the 1965 Rye conference on obstacles to the control of Hodgkin's Disease.

THIS CONFERENCE IS BEING SPONSORED BY THE AMERICAN CANCER SOCIETY THROUGH FUNDS MADE AVAILABLE BY APPROPRIATION #R-16 AND THE NATIONAL CANCER INSTITUTE THROUGH FUNDS MADE AVAILABLE BY CONTRACT #PH43-66-1

* * * *

PROGRAM COMMITTEE

DR. SIDNEY FARBER, *Chairman*
Director, Children's Cancer Research Foundation

DR. JOSEPH H. BURCHENAL
Sloan-Kettering Institute for Cancer Research

DR. JAMES T. GRACE
Roswell Park Memorial Institute

DR. HENRY S. KAPLAN
Stanford University

DR. HOWARD E. SKIPPER
Southern Research Institute

DR. C. GORDON ZUBROD
National Cancer Institute

STAFF REPRESENTATIVES

DR. JACK W. MILDER
American Cancer Society

DR. ARTHUR SERPICK
National Cancer Institute

FIG. 4. The program committee and credits appearing in the original program from the 1965 Rye conference.

with important clinical relevance. Immunologists, virologists, and epidemiologists were applying new techniques and methodologies to understanding the etiology and pathogenesis of the disease.

Of most importance, the Rye conference was a unique experience and opportunity, for rapid communication of results and ideas from a relatively small group of leaders from diverse fields to interact, discuss, and debate the scientific issues. The sponsors and organizers of the Paris and Rye conferences could not have known the great impact they had on the subsequent advances that have led to the virtual control and cure of the great majority of patients with Hodgkin's disease.

The proceedings and discussion, and eventual committee reports of the Rye conference, were published in a special June 1966 issue of *Cancer Research,* volume 26, number 6. Every student of Hodgkin's disease should read these proceedings. The most significant contributions presented at the Rye conference are as follows:

- The epidemiology of Hodgkin's disease (MacMahon) (5): MacMahon was able to distinguish three age periods (0–14, 15–34, and 50+) with distinctive clinical features. The bimodal age-specific incidence and mortality rates were identified, with postulates for their cause.
- Pathologic classification (Lukes, Rappaport) (6,7): The six subtypes of the Lukes-Collins classification were described, and, by committee consensus, were eventually described as a four-subtype Rye classification, replacing the less useful Jackson-Parker scheme.

- Diagnostic methods of lymphangiography and bone marrow biopsy (Lee, Rosenberg) (8,9): Lower extremity lymphangiography was shown to be much more sensitive in demonstrating retroperitoneal lymph node involvement than any previously used method. Bone marrow biopsy could demonstrate Hodgkin's disease involvement not detectable by any other method.
- Staging classification (Rosenberg) (9): A four-stage clinical classification, made necessary by the diagnostic value of lymphangiography, was a committee recommendation and widely utilized thereafter.
- Orderly progression (Rosenberg, Kaplan) (10): Patterns of disease at presentation, and at first relapse, which are more accurate because of better diagnostic methods and attention to involved sites, clearly demonstrated the probability of unicentric origin and orderly progression of Hodgkin's disease.
- Radiation therapy results (Easson, Peters, Kaplan) (2,4,11): The radiotherapists presented convincing evidence that a significant proportion of patients with relatively localized disease could be rendered free of disease recurrence for prolonged periods and considered cured of Hodgkin's disease.
- Chemotherapy results (Frei, DeVita, Carbone) (12): For the first time clinical investigators utilizing multiple drugs in combination were able to achieve high response rates of surprising durability.
- Immunologic abnormalities (Chase, Aisenberg) (13,14): The basic immunologic defects of anergy, parallel with sarcoidosis, was more fully described utilizing the best immunologic methods of the time. The real etiologic role of the immunologic defect, however, remained obscure.

In addition to these presentations, a very important aspect of the Rye conference (and also of the earlier Paris conference) was the presentation and discussion of new clinical trials being considered and initiated in the United States, Canada, and Europe. For the first time, cure was considered an appropriate goal. Equally important was the appreciation that controlled clinical trials were necessary to establish the superiority of promising new treatment strategies.

Though the Paris conference preceded the Rye conference by 7 months, and was stimulated in part by it, the Rye conference can be considered the opening salvo of the scientific revolution that has transformed Hodgkin's disease from a fatal to a curable disease.

THE ANN ARBOR CONFERENCE

The success of the 1965 Rye conference and developments in the clinical management of Hodgkin's disease led to a major conference on the staging of Hodgkin's disease, held at the University of Michigan in Ann Arbor, April 26 to 28, 1971. The conference was sponsored by the American Cancer Society (ACS) and the U.S. National Cancer Institute (NCI) with financial assistance of the Whiting Foundation of Flint, Michigan. The meeting was held in Michigan and called the Ann Arbor conference, to honor the 1971 president of the ACS, H.M. Pollard, a Michigan physician. There were 29 invited speakers at the meeting, 23 from the United States, five from Europe, and one (Peters) from Canada. The proceedings of the symposium were published, as a November 1971 supplement to *Cancer Research,* volume 31.

The program committee for the Ann Arbor Symposium included Paul Carbone (chair), Henry Rappaport, Saul A. Rosenberg, and Jack W. Milder (staff). The chairs and subject areas of the symposium were:

- Staging procedures in Hodgkin's disease: Maurice Trubiana (Paris, France).
- Histologic criteria for diagnosis of the extent of Hodgkin's disease: Louis B. Thomas (NCI, Bethesda, Maryland).
- Prognostic and therapeutic implications of staging in Hodgkin's disease: M. Vera Peters (Toronto, Canada).
- Other considerations: David W. Smithers (London, England).

The most important accomplishments of the Ann Arbor conference could be summarized as follows:

Exploratory laparotomy and splenectomy provided considerable information of the extent and patterns of Hodgkin's disease in untreated patients (15). Occult disease was found in abdominal sites, not detectable by the diagnostic methods available at that time. This was especially the case for involvement of the spleen with Hodgkin's disease. Normal-sized spleens were involved in almost one-third of the cases, and some spleens thought to be, or proved to be, enlarged did not contain the disease. Liver involvement was poorly correlated with clinical parameters, and almost always associated with splenic disease. Equivocal abnormalities in the paraaortic lymph nodes were clarified by appropriate biopsies.

This greater accuracy in defining the extent of Hodgkin's disease, in untreated patients, provided further support for the orderly progression of Hodgkin's disease in its initial presentation.

The prognostic significance of the stage designations had to consider the use of staging laparotomy (16). Because exploratory laparotomy was not performed in all patients, nor in many medical centers, the staging classification had to be modified. Therefore, the Ann Arbor staging classification was developed, which distinguished patients evaluated without laparotomy as clinical stage (CS) or with laparotomy as pathologic stage (PS).

The staging classification and clinical significance of limited extension of Hodgkin's disease to extranodal sites had to be considered. This led to the concept of the

E-lesion, as proposed by Karl Musshoff (17). Disease that extended directly to extranodal sites and closely related to lymph node involvement did not carry the same prognosis as widespread extranodal distributions. Though difficult to define, the concept was clear, distinguishing the E substages from stage IV.

Dramatic improvements in the control of Hodgkin's disease were being achieved by radiotherapists utilizing supervoltage and very wide treatment fields (18). Radiotherapists were able to deliver so-called total nodal irradiation in adequate dosage to patients with localized and intermediate stages of the disease. Short-term follow-up indicated control and possible cure rates of 80% or greater.

The combination chemotherapy [mechlorethamine, Oncovin (vincristine), procarbazine, and prednisone (MOPP)] resulted in a significant probability of sustained complete remission in a phase II trial of 43 patients treated at the NCI by DeVita and Carbone (19). The longer follow-up of this important initial series of patients treated in the mid-1960s established the important role of combination chemotherapy in the management of Hodgkin's disease.

AMERICAN CLINICAL TRIALS

The conferences described above, held in Paris and Rye in 1965 and in Ann Arbor in 1971, had a major impact on clinical investigators of Hodgkin's disease, worldwide. From an historical perspective, the American trials of great significance and impact can be divided into early (1960s and 1970s) and later (1980s and 1990s), periods.

Among the clinical investigations during the early period, several were noteworthy. The results of Peters at the Princess Margaret Hospital in Toronto have already been referred to. She adapted some of the principles of the Swiss radiotherapist, Renee Gilbert (20) and the concept of unicentric origin and orderly progression and treated patients with extended fields of irradiation. Her results were very good, but were not subjected to the rigorous requirements of the controlled clinical trial. Peters, in her early efforts, did not have supervoltage radiation equipment, which became available in the 1960s. However, she was a student of the disease, and her insights and results had a significant impact on the acceptance of proper radiation therapy for the treatment of relatively localized Hodgkin's disease.

Clinical trials of the treatment of Hodgkin's disease were initiated by Kaplan and Rosenberg at Stanford in 1962. These were among the first randomized studies of the management of Hodgkin's disease. Though the Manchester group carried out several randomized clinical trials in the treatment of Hodgkin's disease, the Stanford studies were unique in the United States. Kaplan and I realized that patient selection and other biases could greatly influence the outcome of disease-free and eventual survival statistics. The two senior investigators (Kaplan and Rosenberg) philosophically disagreed on the necessary aggressiveness of the proper treatment, but to their credit respected each other sufficiently to test hypotheses in controlled trials. Throughout the Stanford trials, no control group or relatively conservative treatment arm of a study was less than a very good standard of care. Secondary or salvage therapy was always given promptly for recurrences, so that survival disadvantages were rarely if ever seen over the 35 years of the Stanford trials.

Colleagues found the randomized trial design acceptable, but more formal approvals by granting agencies or institutional officers were not required in the 1960s. Patients were informed as fully as possible, and usually accepted randomization, often because of the awe and respect they and their personal physicians felt for Kaplan. Kaplan would often say that he could not accept a randomized control treatment arm because he would not be able to sleep at night. This proved to be an effective ethical and scientific review procedure.

The Stanford clinical trials of Hodgkin's disease have continued uninterrupted for over 35 years, and have been summarized from time to time (21). The earliest Stanford studies, randomly compared limited versus extended fields of irradiation for Hodgkin's disease stages I and II. Stage III patients were treated with low-dose (palliative) irradiation versus previously untested total nodal irradiation to full dose (3,600–4,400 rad). In 1962, when these studies were initiated, modern successful chemotherapy was not available for Hodgkin's disease. These Stanford trials (1962–1967) demonstrated the tolerance of patients to relatively high-dose, extended fields of supervoltage radiotherapy, and very good treatment results. However, the relative superiority of various treatment plans was not proved in these small initial studies.

After 1968 and throughout the 1970s, Stanford's randomized clinical trials utilized exploratory laparotomy and splenectomy, routinely, in staging patients. Studies used total nodal irradiation (the mantle and inverted-Y fields) as the standard of radiotherapy for stages I, II, and III patients, comparing lesser fields of irradiation for favorable patients, and combined modality therapy, with MOPP chemotherapy, for intermediate and advanced stages of the disease. The results were interesting and often provocative. Considerable differences in progression-free survival could be demonstrated, but overall survival results were not different, but excellent for the times.

During the 1960s and 1970s, very important advances in the use of combination chemotherapy of Hodgkin's disease were reported by Vincent DeVita and colleagues from the NCI in Bethesda. The MOPP regimen resulted not only in clinical complete remissions of advanced and recurrent Hodgkin's disease but also in significant numbers of patients achieving prolonged progression-free survival (Fig. 5). This was a breakthrough in the manage-

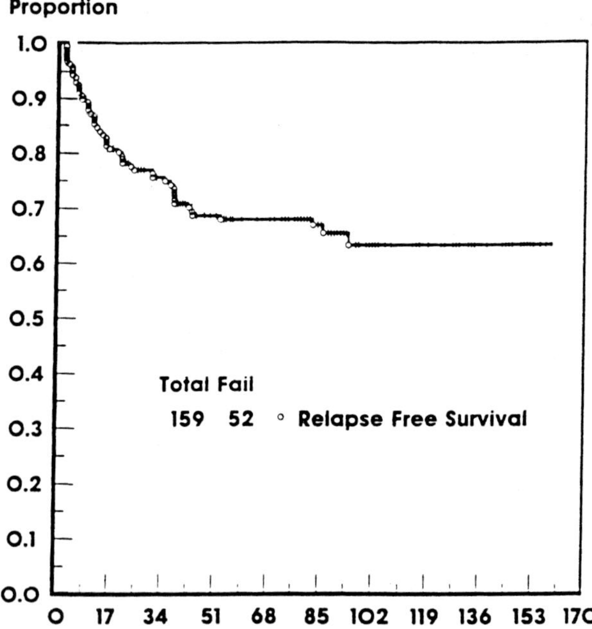

FIG. 5. The relapse-free survival curve of 159 complete responders of 188 patients treated for Hodgkin's disease by DeVita and colleagues (38), published in 1980; the patients attained complete remission with mechlorethamine, Oncovin (vincristine), procarbazine, and prednisone (MOPP) treatment. One hundred seven patients have been continuously disease free from the time of discontinuation of treatment. (From ref. 38, with permission.)

ment of Hodgkin's disease, influencing subsequent studies and the treatment of patients worldwide (22).

The NCI investigators also studied relatively radical irradiation management of Hodgkin's disease, and their colleagues at the Baltimore branch of the NCI were among the first to study combined irradiation and chemotherapy in randomized trials (Fig. 6) (23).

In 1967, a collaborative clinical trial was initiated in North America, testing in a randomized study the relative value of extended-field versus involved-field radiotherapy. This study accrued 460 patients and closed for entry in 1973. The results have been reported at various times, most recently in 1984 (24). This study enrolled patients with localized (stage I and II) disease from 22 collaborating centers. The steering committee for the study included George Hutchinson, chairman, Ruth E. Alison, Lillian Fuller, Peters, Kaplan, Burton Lee, James J. Nickson, Rappaport, Rosenberg, Robert J. Shalek, and Manuel Viamonte. The results and final conclusions of this study are complex, since staging methods (laparotomy and splenectomy) and radical treatment methods changed during the course of the trial, and were carried out differently at different centers. Nonetheless, progression-free survival was improved by extending the fields of irradiation, but eventual survival differences were minimal, because of the success of subsequent salvage therapies (Tables 1 and 2).

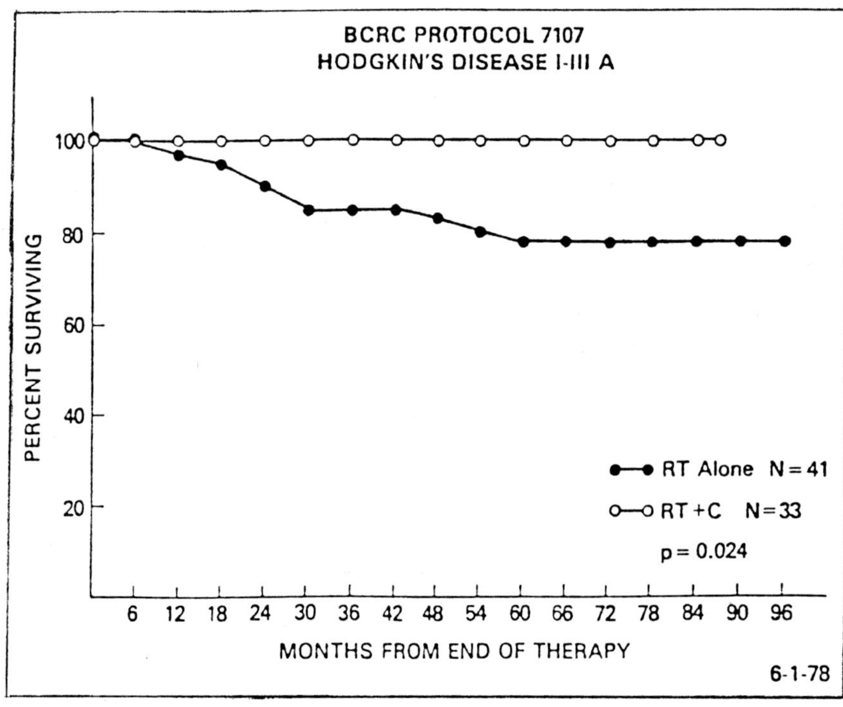

FIG. 6. The results of a randomized trial comparing radiotherapy alone (RT) and combined modality therapy (RT+C) in 74 patients, stages I to IIIA by Wiernick et al., reported in 1979. Survival curves compare all patients receiving combined modality therapy with those receiving radiotherapy alone. If the censored data described in Fig. 10 are not censored, the *p* value for this figure becomes .086. (From ref. 23, with permission.)

TABLE 1. *Survival by treatment*[a]

	No. at risk		Percent survival[b]		No. of deaths in interval	
Months	IF	EF	IF	EF	IF	EF
0	220	240	100	100	4	7
12	216	233	98	97	17	16
36	199	216	90	90	12	9
60	186	205	85	87	5	7
72	173	194	83 (3)	84 (2)	10	3
84	150	175	78 (3)	82 (2)	2	3
96	121	134	77 (3)	81 (3)	3	1
108	83	93	74 (3)	80 (3)	2	2
120	52	51	72 (4)	78 (3)	1	2
132	30	25	70 (4)	74 (4)	1	2
144	7	3	64 (7)	65 (7)	0	0
156	0	1	64 (7)	65 (7)	—	0
Total deaths					57	52

[a]Results from the North American Cooperative Clinical Trial initiated in 1967 reported in 1984 comparing involved field (IF) and extended field (EF) radiation therapy of localized (stages I and II) Hodgkin's disease. From ref. 24, with permission.

[b]Numbers in parentheses are standard errors.

SRR (standardized risk ratio): risk in IF/risk in EF = 1.3 95%; confidence limits of SRR (0.9, 1.9).

TABLE 2. *Extension-free survival by treatment*

	No. at risk		Percentage extension-free survival[b]		No. of extensions or deaths free of extension in interval[c]	
Months	IF	EF	IF	EF	IF	EF
0	220	240	100	100	54	36 (2)
12	166	204	75	85	58 (3)	40 (5)
36	108	163	49	68	15 (3)	10 (1)
60	92	151	42	64	1	7 (1)
72	87	142	42 (3)	61 (3)	4 (2)	2 (1)
84	77	128	40 (3)	60 (3)	0	4 (2)
96	61	96	40 (3)	58 (3)	0	1 (1)
108	38	70	40 (3)	57 (3)	0	2 (2)
120	26	39	40 (3)	55 (4)	0	2 (1)
132	14	17	40 (3)	52 (4)	0	1 (1)
144	4	1	40 (3)	48 (5)	0	0
156	0	1	40 (3)	48 (5)	—	0
Total					132	105

[a]Results from the North American Cooperative Clinical Trial initiated in 1967 reported in 1984 comparing involved field (IF) and extended field (EF) radiation therapy of localized (stages I and II) Hodgkin's disease. From ref. 24, with permission.

[b]Numbers in parenthesis are standard errors.

[c]Numbers in parentheses are deaths without known extension.

Standardized risk ratio: risk in IF/risk in EF = 1.7 95% confidence limits, (1.3, 2.1).

LATER TRIALS (1980–1990)

The Stanford randomized clinical trials continued into the 1980s and 1990s. Sequentially various chemotherapy programs [Adriamycin, bleomycin, vinblastine, and dacarbazine (ABVD); procarbazine, Alkeran (melphalan), and Velban (vinblastine sulfate) (PAVe); vinblastine, bleomycin, and methotrexate (VBM)] were compared to the MOPP regimen in randomized trials. Often the irradiation fields were reduced in volume and dose. Children were managed in nonrandomized trials with combined modality programs and reduced dose of irradiation, after unacceptable bone and muscle growth abnormalities were observed in children passing through puberty; results were excellent.

In the late 1980s and 1990s Stanford studies eliminated staging laparotomy with splenectomy, utilizing combined modality treatment plans routinely and modified chemotherapy regimens. The Stanford V chemotherapy program, an intensive 12-week schedule, emerged as remarkably successful, with minimal long-term morbidity, for patients with unfavorable and advanced disease (25). An even shorter course of intensive chemotherapy is being studied, with further reduction in irradiation dose and fields, for even the most favorable disease setting. This approach is being adapted and studied worldwide in the 1990s. The Stanford studies began to recognize the serious treatment complications in patients treated and apparently cured of Hodgkin's disease in the earlier periods. Secondary malignancies were among the most serious treatment complications, but cardiac, vascular, and pulmonary complications were increasingly recognized (26).

It is interesting to look at the sequential results of the Stanford studies over a 35-year period. They are representative of results obtained by other investigators. The actuarial freedom from recurrence (Fig. 7), disease-specific survival (Fig. 8), and overall survival (Fig. 9) are shown for over 1,100 patients enrolled in randomized clinical trials.

The L studies randomized patients, stages I, II, and III only, to various irradiation plans, usually involved fields versus extended fields. The H, K, R studies generally compared radiation alone to radiation followed by MOPP chemotherapy. The S studies reduced the radiation fields to involved fields followed by MOPP for favorable stages I and II patients, or compared MOPP to a better tolerated modification, PAVe, in combined modality plans for advanced stages III and IV. The C studies employed a completely new chemotherapy, VBM, to preserve fertility and avoid leukemia, as an adjuvant in favorable patients, and compared ABVD to PAVe in more advanced patients. PAVe and irradiation in combined modality plans was compared to alternating chemotherapy only for stages IIIB and IV patients. The G studies have utilized the dose-intensive Stanford V chemotherapy regimen, usually with adjuvant radiotherapy, for patients with advanced disease, initiated in 1988, and in favorable patients, initiated in 1995.

The Stanford results (Figs. 7 to 9) show progressive improvement in all measures of outcome, despite the practice of almost always employing a control group receiving the standard best therapy of the time in randomized studies.

During the later period (1980–1990) investigators at the M. D. Anderson Hospital studied combined modality treatment regimens, usually employing the MOPP program. They were among the first to show the value of even several cycles of chemotherapy, combined with irradiation for patients with intermediate stages of the disease (Fig. 10) (27).

Clinicians at Yale University, under the leadership of Leonard Prosnitz, reported excellent results of combined modality therapy employing a modification of the MOPP program and reduced irradiation dose to most sites of disease (28). This phase II study was among the first to demonstrate the probable value of this approach (Fig. 11).

Connors and colleagues in Vancouver at the British Columbia Cancer Institute made important modifications of the chemotherapy regimen for Hodgkin's disease in the 1980s. Modifying the approach of alternating therapy of the Milan Group, they developed the MOPP/ABV hybrid chemotherapy, which remains one of the current standards of treatment for Hodgkin's disease (29). The Vancouver group has also reported on early results of treating patients

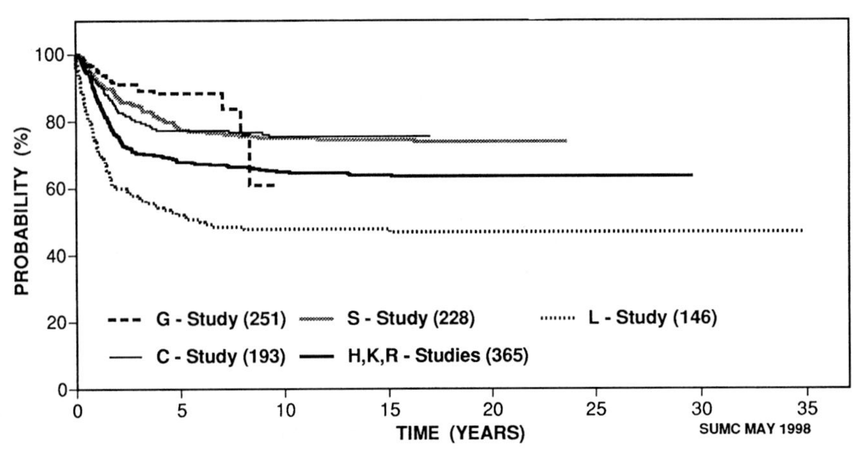

FIG. 7. The actuarial freedom from progression of 1,183 patients with Hodgkin's disease treated on sequential clinical trials at Stanford, initiated in 1962.

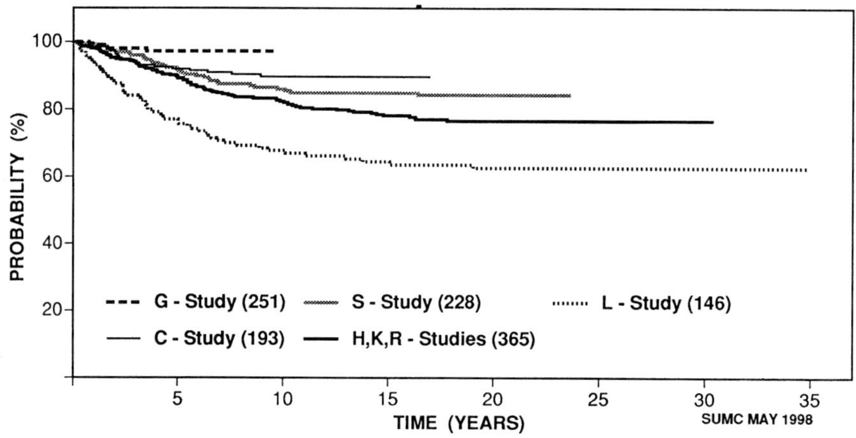

FIG. 8. The actuarial disease-specific survival of 1,183 patients with Hodgkin's disease treated on sequential clinical trials at Stanford, initiated in 1962.

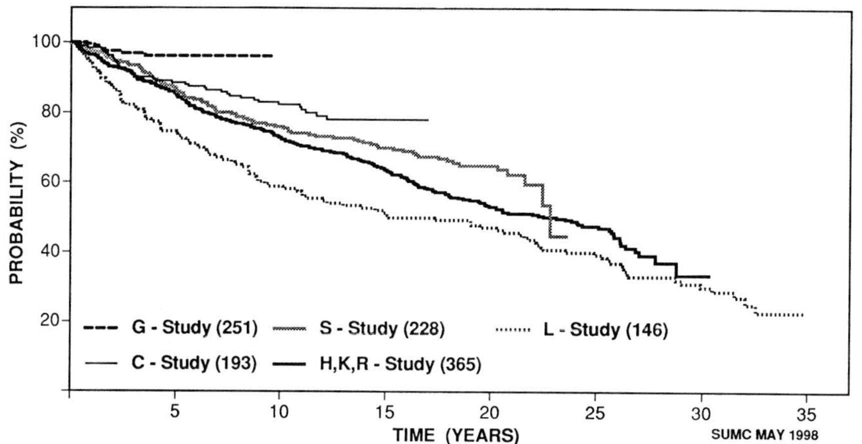

FIG. 9. The actuarial overall survival of 1,183 patients with Hodgkin's disease treated on sequential clinical trials at Stanford, initiated in 1962.

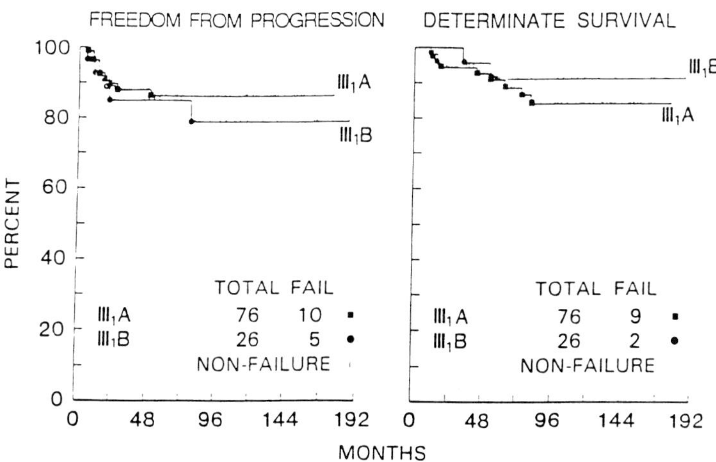

FIG. 10. The results of a nonrandomized study at the M. D. Anderson Hospital treating stage III patients with Hodgkin's disease with two cycles of MOPP and radiation therapy, reported in 1988. Comparison of freedom from progression (FFP) and determinate survival rates for patients with stage IIIA Hodgkin's disease with those for patients with stage IIIB Hodgkin's disease. (From ref. 27, with permission.)

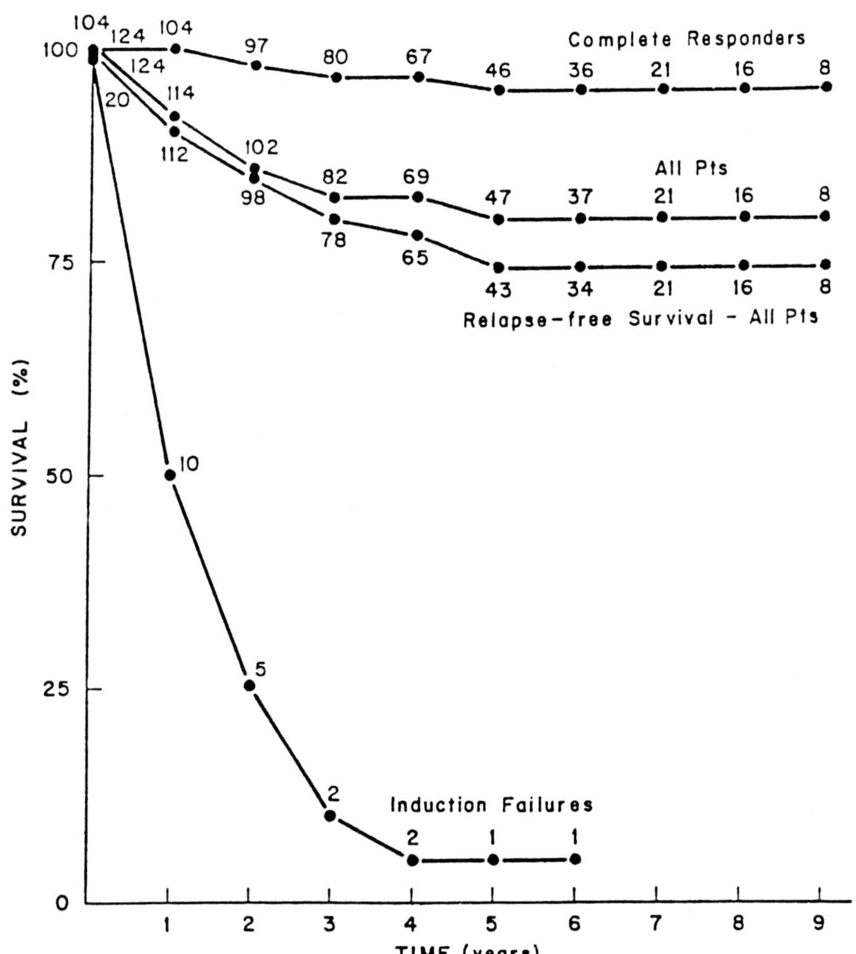

FIG. 11. The results of a nonrandomized study by the Yale group treating various stages of Hodgkin's disease with reduced doses of irradiation in a combined modality program, reported by Prosnitz et al. (28) in 1980. Cumulative survival curves for 118 Hodgkin's disease patients undergoing combined-modality therapy. (From ref. 28, with permission.)

with relatively short courses of intensive chemotherapy and limited radiation fields for relatively favorable patients. The results have been excellent.

During the 1980s and 1990s the U.S. and Canadian National Cooperative Groups have gradually completed studies of significant magnitude to help establish the relative value of the major chemotherapy regimens for Hodgkin's disease. As a result of this summary of many studies, it is now accepted, because of these controlled trials, that an anthracycline-based regimen is preferred to the MOPP-type regimen because of its greater effectiveness and lesser toxicity (30).

The Southwest Oncology Group (SWOG) has completed and reported the results of two of the major clinical trials, testing the value of adjuvant radiotherapy after MOPP (31) or MOP–bleomycin, Adriamycin, and prednisone (BAP) (32) chemotherapy. Though the results are difficult to interpret, in general relapse-free survival was improved for patients with combined modality therapy, especially for those with nodular sclerosis and large mediastinal masses. But survival differences were minimal. The Eastern Cooperative Group (ECOG) failed to show the value of adjuvant radiotherapy after various chemotherapy regimens, including the BCNU, cyclophosphamide, vinblastine, procarbazine, prednisone (BCVPP) program (33). A multicenter Canadian study, of complicated design, has also reported borderline improvement in relapse-free survival utilizing combined-modality therapy compared to a prolonged chemotherapy regimen. No survival benefit was demonstrated in the Canadian study (34).

NATIONAL UNITED STATES SURVIVAL DATA

The improved cure and survival rates for patients with Hodgkin's disease have been documented in the United States by the end results data of the Surveillance Epidemiology and End Results (SEER) program of the NCI. Between 1960 and 1992, the 5-year survival of patients with Hodgkin's disease in the United States rose from 40% to 82% (35). This represents one of the most successful translations of new therapeutic approaches from centers of clinical investigations to standard practice in the field of oncology.

The American College of Radiology through its Patterns of Care Study (PCS) has had an excellent program of documenting management standards of Hodgkin's disease in the United States since 1973 (36). These have been summarized from time to time, most recently in 1997 (37).

Changes have occurred in the United States patterns of care since 1973, including the following:

- Decreased use of staging laparotomy and splenectomy.
- Decreased use of lower extremity lymphangiography.
- Increased use of computed tomography (CT).
- Increased use of the gallium scan.
- Increased use of combined modality therapy.
- Decreased use of MOPP, in favor of ABVD or alternating regimens.
- Increased use of chemotherapy, prior to irradiation.

Relapse-free survival and overall survival have increased for all stages of disease. The failure-free survival was superior at academic versus community or free-standing facilities in 1973, though this could not be demonstrated in the 1983 survey (37).

SUMMARY

It is gratifying to appreciate that both U.S. and Canadian clinical investigators have contributed so significantly to the important advances achieved in the management of Hodgkin's disease. Interactions with their European colleagues, especially from the Milan Group, the European Organization for Research and Treatment of Cancer (EORTC), and, in the 1990s, the German Group, have been very beneficial. The cure of Hodgkin's disease, now quite probable in over 80% of all patients, can be predicted to improve even more, and most significantly with reduced acute and late toxicity. These achievements have resulted from international studies, but none more important than those carried out in the United States and Canada.

REFERENCES

1. Peters MV. A study of survivals In Hodgkin's disease treated radiologically. *Am J Roentgenol Radium Ther Nucl Med* 1950;63:299–311.
2. Peters MV. Prophylactic treatment of adjacent areas in Hodgkin's disease. *Cancer Res* 1966;26:1232–1243.
3. Kaplan HS. The radical radiotherapy of regionally localized Hodgkin's disease. *Radiology* 1962;78:553–561.
4. Kaplan HS. Long-term results of palliative and radical radiotherapy of Hodgkin's disease. *Cancer Res* 1966;26:1250–1252.
5. MacMahon B. Epidemiology of Hodgkin's disease. *Cancer Res* 1966; 26:1189–1200.
6. Lukes RJ, Butler JJ. The pathology and nomenclature of Hodgkin's disease. *Cancer Res* 1966;26:1063–1081.
7. Rappaport H. Discussion on: the pathology and nomenclature of Hodgkin's disease. *Cancer Res* 1966;26:1082–1083.
8. Lee BJ. Lymphangiography in Hodgkin's disease: indications and contraindications. *Cancer Res* 1966;26:1084–1089.
9. Rosenberg SA. Report of the Committee on the Staging of Hodgkin's Disease. *Cancer Res* 1966;26:1310.
10. Rosenberg SA, Kaplan HS. Evidence for an orderly progression in the spread of Hodgkin's disease. *Cancer Res* 1966;26:1225–1231.
11. Easson EC. Long-term results of radical radiotherapy in Hodgkin's disease. *Cancer Res* 1966;26:1244–1247.
12. Frei E III, DeVita VT, Moxley JH III, Carbone PP. Approaches to improving the chemotherapy of Hodgkin's disease. *Cancer Res* 1966; 26:1284–1289.
13. Chase MW. Delayed-type hypersensitivity and the immunology of Hodgkin's disease, with a parallel examination of sarcoidosis. *Cancer Res* 1966;26:1097–1120.
14. Aisenberg AC. Manifestations of immunologic unresponsiveness in Hodgkin's disease. *Cancer Res* 1966;26:1152–1160.
15. Rosenberg SA. A critique of the value of laparotomy and splenectomy in the evaluation of patients with Hodgkin's disease. *Cancer Res* 1971; 31:1737–1740.
16. Carbone PP, Kaplan HS, Musshoff K, Smithers DW, Tubiana M. Report of the Committee on Hodgkin's Disease Staging Classification. *Cancer Res* 1971;31:1860–1861.
17. Musshoff K. Prognostic and therapeutic implications of staging in extranodal Hodgkin's disease. *Cancer Res* 1971;31:1814–1827.
18. Smithers DW. Summary of papers delivered at the Conference on Staging in Hodgkin's Disease (Ann Arbor). *Cancer Res* 1971;31:1869–1870.
19. DeVita VT Jr, Carbone PP. Chemotherapeutic implications of staging in Hodgkin's disease. *Cancer Res* 1971;31:1838–1844.
20. Gilbert R. Radiotherapy in Hodgkin's disease (malignant granulomatosis): anatomic and clinical foundations; governing principles: results. *Am J Roentgenol Radium Ther Nucl Med* 1939;41:198–241.
21. Rosenberg SA, Kaplan HS. The evolution and summary results of the Stanford randomized clinical trials of the management of Hodgkin's disease: 1962–1984. *Int J Radiat Oncol Biol Phys* 1985;11:5–22.
22. DeVita VT Jr, Serpick AA, Carbone PP. Combination chemotherapy in the treatment of advanced Hodgkin's disease. *Ann Intern Med* 1970;73: 881–895.
23. Wiernik PH, Gustafson J, Schimpff SC, Diggs C. Combined modality treatment of Hodgkin's disease confined to lymph nodes. *Am J Med* 1979;67:183–193.
24. Hutchison GB, Alison RE, Fuller LM, et al. Radiotherapy of stage I and II Hodgkin's disease. *Cancer* 1984;54:1928–1942.
25. Bartlett NL, Rosenberg SA, Hoppe RT, Hancock SL, Horning SJ. Brief chemotherapy (Stanford V) and adjuvant radiotherapy for bulky and advanced Hodgkin's disease: a preliminary report. *J Clin Oncol* 1995; 13:1080–1088.
26. Tucker MA, Coleman CN, Cox RS, Varghese A, Rosenberg SA. Risk of second cancers after treatment for Hodgkin's disease. *N Engl J Med* 1988;318:76–81.
27. Henkelmann GC, Hagemeister FB, Fuller LM. Two cycles of MOPP and radiotherapy for stage III_1A and stage III_1B Hodgkin's disease. *J Clin Oncol* 1988;6:1293–1302.
28. Prosnitz LR, Wu JJ, Yahalom J. The case for adjuvant radiation therapy in advanced Hodgkin's disease. *Cancer Invest* 1996;14:361–370.
29. Klimo P, Connors JM. MOPP/ABV hybrid program: combination chemotherapy based on early introduction of seven effective drugs for advanced Hodgkin's disease. *J Clin Oncol* 1985;3:1174–1182.
30. Canellos G, Anderson JR, Propert KJ, et al. Chemotherapy of advanced Hodgkin's disease with MOPP/ABVD, or MOPP alternating with ABVD. *N Engl J Med* 1992;327:1478–1484.
31. Grozea PN, Depersio EJ, Coltman CA Jr, et al. Chemotherapy alone versus combined modality therapy for stage III Hodgkin's disease: a five-year follow-up of a Southwest Oncology Group Study. In: Cavalli F, Bonadonna G, Rozencweig M, eds. *Malignant lymphomas and Hodgkin's disease:* experimental and therapeutic advances. Boston, Martinus Nijhoff, 1985:345–351.
32. Fabian CJ, Mansfield CM, Dahlberg S, et al. Low-dose involved field radiation after chemotherapy in advanced Hodgkin's disease. *Ann Intern Med* 1994;120:901–912.
33. Glick J, Tsiatis A, Chen M, et al. Improved survival with MOPP-ABVD compared to BCVPP ± radiotherapy (RT) for advanced Hodgkin's disease: 6-year ECOG results. *Blood* 1990;76(suppl 1):350a(abst 1392).
34. Yelle L, Bergsagel D, Basco V, et al. Combined modality therapy of Hodgkin's disease: 10-year results of National Cancer Institute of Canada Clinical Trials Group Multicenter Clinical Trial. *J Clin Oncol* 1991;9:1983–1993.
35. Parker SL, Tong T, Bolden S, Wingo PA. Cancer statistics, 1997. *CA* 1997;47:5–27.
36. Hanks GE, Kinzie JJ, White RL, et al. Patterns of care outcome studies. Results of the National Practice in Hodgkin's Disease. *Cancer* 1983;51:569–573.
37. Smitt MC, Buzydlowski J, Hoppe RT. Over 20 years of progress in radiation oncology: Hodgkin's disease. *Semin Radiat Oncol* 1977;7:127–134.
38. DeVita VT Jr, Simon RM, Hubbard SM, et al. Curability of Advanced Hodgkin's disease with chemotherapy. *Ann Intern Med* 1980;92: 587–595.

SECTION II

Etiology and Epidemiology

Hodgkin's Disease, edited by P. M. Mauch, J. O. Armitage, V. Diehl, R. T. Hoppe, and L. M. Weiss. Lippincott Williams & Wilkins, Philadephia ©1999.

CHAPTER 5

The Epidemiology of Hodgkin's Disease

Nancy E. Mueller and Seymour Grufferman

HISTORICAL PERSPECTIVE

The early history of Hodgkin's disease is immensely rich as documented in an extensive and comprehensive literature. In 1948, Hoster and Dratman (1,2) wrote one of the most extensive and thorough early reviews of Hodgkin's disease, which covered a bibliography of 572 late 19th to mid–20th century publications, clearly indicating that numerous physicians and scientists shared a great interest in the disease. Why has this disease, which is relatively uncommon, been of such great interest to generations of pathologists, oncologists, epidemiologists, and other researchers?

There are many answers to this question. First, the disease was initially described in 1832 by the British physician Thomas Hodgkin, who was as eccentric as he was brilliant (3). In addition to Hodgkin's many contributions to 19th century medicine, he was a Quaker (when it was highly unfashionable to be one) who was devout to a fault, a social activist on behalf of the underprivileged, particularly the Aborigines and the Jews, and a good friend of Sir Moses Montefiore. His productive, creative, and colorful life has been chronicled in several biographies (4–8).

Second, the disease has many clinical features that suggest it might be caused by infectious agents. The frequent fever, often in recurrent cycles (Pel-Ebstein fever); night sweats; and lymphadenopathy, which sometimes has a dramatic sudden onset and often appears in previously healthy young adults, has led many clinicians to suspect an infectious cause. Hodgkin himself thought the disease to be a sort of hypertrophy of the lymphatic system rather than a cancer (8). Other great figures in the debate over the etiology of Hodgkin's disease include Sternberg, who believed it was a form of tuberculosis, and Reed, who thought it was an inflammatory process rather than a malignancy (1,2,8). As a result, the literature is replete with scientific publications on suspected infectious causes of Hodgkin's disease. In the first part of the 20th century there were reports of bacterial agents such as *Bacillus hodgkini* and *Corynebacterium granulomatis maligni* (9,10). At present the Epstein-Barr virus, first isolated from a Burkitt's lymphoma specimen, is actively being investigated as a cause of the disease. Generations of leading investigators of their times have believed that Hodgkin's disease is caused by an infectious agent and this belief has persisted.

A third compelling feature of Hodgkin's disease is the amazing therapeutic success story of the disease. Hodgkin's disease was a largely incurable disease until the midpoint of the 20th century when extended-field, high-dose radiation therapy was found to result in permanent disease remission (8). The addition of multiagent chemotherapy to the therapeutic armamentarium against Hodgkin's disease led to further dramatic survival improvements. Today, Hodgkin's disease is a largely curable disease with upward of 90% 5-year survival from localized disease. Hodgkin's disease is often held up as the prototype of progress toward the cure of cancer in general.

The epidemiology of Hodgkin's disease is another source of fascination to students of the disease and also points to an infectious etiology. The landmark observations of MacMahon (11) regarding the bimodality of Hodgkin's disease incidence launched a whole new era of epidemiologic investigation of cancer causation. He was the first to recognize the bimodality in age-incidence patterns of the disease and suggested that the young adult form of the disease may be the result of an infectious process. Other investigators went on to liken the epidemiologic features of the disease to paralytic poliomyelitis and hypothesized that Hodgkin's disease was due to late age of first infection with a common infectious agent (12–15). Several studies have provided confirmation of this hypothesis (16,17). The notion of an infectious etiology for the disease was accelerated by two

N. E. Mueller: Department of Epidemiology, Harvard University School of Public Health, Boston, Massachusetts.

S. Grufferman: Department of Family Medicine and Clinical Epidemiology, University of Pittsburgh School of Medicine, Pittsburgh, Pennsylvania.

startling reports that suggested that the disease might be transmitted from person to person in schools (18,19). While these findings could not be confirmed by others, they led to another outpouring of publications on the possibly infectious nature of the disease (20–22).

More recently, renewed interest in the disease has been generated by the use of molecular methods to identify the frequent presence of the Epstein-Barr virus in tumor specimens from patients with Hodgkin's disease (23). Prior to this, it was shown that persons with documented infectious mononucleosis (caused by the Epstein-Barr virus) had about a threefold increased risk of Hodgkin's disease (24). Later studies showed that patients with Hodgkin's disease more frequently had elevated anti–Epstein-Barr virus antibody titers years in advance of the onset of the disease (25,26). Thus, it now seems likely that an infectious agent, the Epstein-Barr virus, does play a role in the etiology of Hodgkin's disease. The intuition of generations of astute researchers may well be proven valid.

DESCRIPTIVE EPIDEMIOLOGY

Incidence, Mortality, and Variation with Age

The distinguishing epidemiologic feature of Hodgkin's disease is its bimodal age-incidence curve that is characteristically seen in economically advantaged populations such as in the United States (Fig. 1) (27), where the majority of patients are young adults. With relatively few cases occurring among children, there is a rapid increase of incidence rates among teenagers that peaks at about age 25. Thereafter, incidence rates decline to a plateau through middle-age, after which they increase again with advancing age. There is a male excess of cases, especially in children and in the middle and late decades of life.

In interpreting this unusual variation with age, MacMahon (28) proposed in 1957 that the bimodality results from the overlap of distributions of two diseases with differing age peaks. He further suggested that among young adults, Hodgkin's disease is caused by a biologic agent of low infectivity, while among the elderly the cause is similar to those of the other lymphomas (11). As discussed below, the evolving epidemiology and viral evidence has generally supported his hypothesis for the origin of young adult Hodgkin's disease, while the pronounced bimodality is still unexplained.

Currently, about 7,500 new cases and about 1,500 deaths occur in the United States annually (27). The age-adjusted incidence rate in 1993 was 2.7 per 100,000 person-years and that for mortality, 0.5 per 100,000 person-years. In 1989, the 5-year relative survival of Hodgkin's disease cases was 81.0%. The incidence rates for American men and women in 1994 were 2.9 and 2.5 per 100,000 person-years, respectively. The 5-year relative survival was higher for women (85.3%) than for men (77.5%), mirroring the fact that women more com-

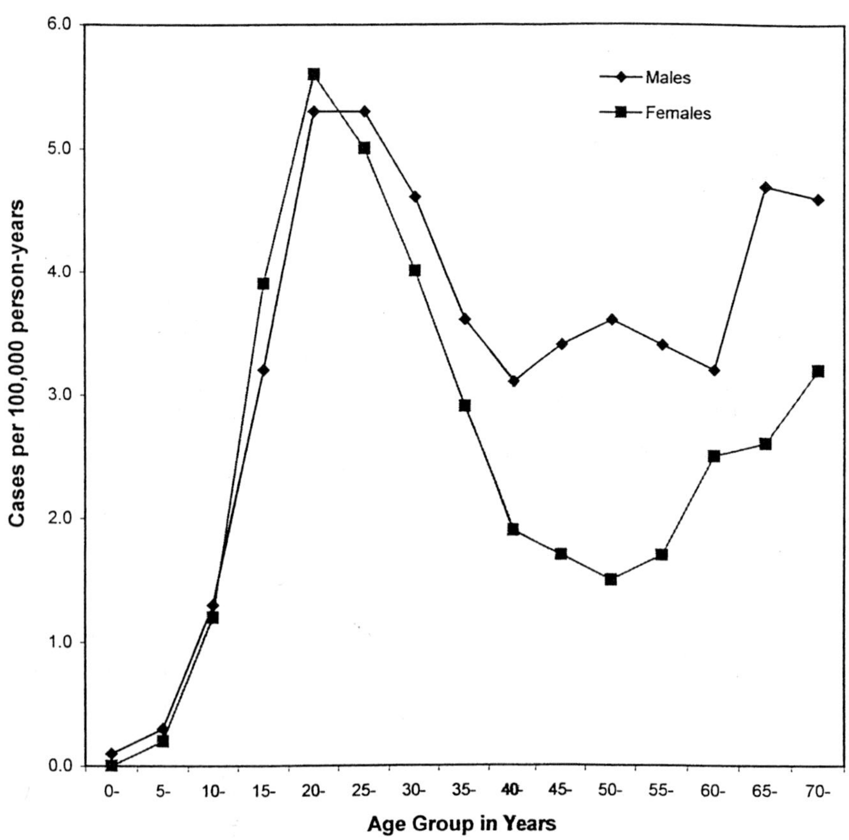

FIG. 1. Age-specific average annual incidence rates of Hodgkin's disease for all races by sex per 100,000 population, 1990–1994, in the SEER program. (Adapted from ref. 27.)

monly present with the nodular sclerosis subtype of Hodgkin's disease and more favorable stage. Five-year relative survival (1986–1993) diminishes with increasing age: 87.7% for patients younger than 45 years at diagnosis, 76.7% for those 45 to 54, 67.1% for those 55 to 64, 50.1% for those 65 to 74, and only 37.5% for those 75 and older (27).

American whites have higher incidence rates of Hodgkin's disease than do other racial and ethnic subgroups as shown in Table 1 (29). This observation reflects the role of socioeconomic status in modifying the risk of the disease in young adulthood, as well as the generally low rates in Asian populations. The current lifetime risk of developing Hodgkin's disease for American whites is 0.26% (1 in 385) and 0.23% (1 in 435) for males and females, respectively. That for American blacks is 0.19% (1 in 526) and 0.16% (1 in 625) for males and females, respectively. The relative differences between blacks and whites in their cumulative risk of developing Hodgkin's disease are greater than for the age-adjusted rates because of the current longer life expectancy for whites.

Secular Trends

Between 1973 and 1994, the incidence of Hodgkin's disease has decreased for both American blacks (–2.9%) and whites (–13.1%). Most of this decrease occurred among the population ages 65 years and older—a total of 37.2% (27). Glaser and Swartz (30) analyzed national data collected by the National Cancer Institute for the period 1969 to 1980 with correction for diagnostic error, based on time, age, and histology-specific confirmation rates from the Repository Center for Lymphoma Clinical Studies. Upon adjustment, they found that the incidence rates for older adults were lower than previously observed and showed no secular trend. Further, they found a slight increase for nodular sclerosis Hodgkin's disease among young adults. An analysis of time trends and age-period-cohort patterns for the incidence in Hodgkin's disease in Connecticut between 1935 and 1992 concluded that the incidence has increased among young adults aged 20 to 44 years. This increase was greater for women and primarily seen in the nodular sclerosis subtype of Hodgkin's disease (31).

TABLE 1. *Incidence rates of Hodgkin's disease, 1977–1983, in major ethnic subgroups in the United States*

Group	Incidence per 100,000 person-years	
	Males	Females
White	1.1	0.7
Black	0.9	0.5
Chinese	0.5	0.1
Japanese	0.1	0.0
Filipino	0.3	0.2
American Indian	0.5	0.1

International Variation

The bimodality in the age-specific incidence rates of Hodgkin's disease, first noted in the late 1950s, continues to characterize populations living in economically advantaged, Westernized populations. Since that time, the peak incidence in the first (young adult) mode has increased from about 3 to 6 cases per 100,000 person-years. In 1971, Correa and O'Conor (32) reported that a different age pattern is evident among economically disadvantaged populations. In these populations, there is an initial peak in childhood but only for boys, relatively low rates among young adults, followed by the late peak among those of advanced age. They further described an intermediate pattern, contrasting data from rural and urban Norwegians in the 1960s. The shift from the developing to an intermediate pattern in parallel with economic development has been noted by others (33,34).

Currently, essentially all majority populations in Europe and North America have a well-defined developed pattern of Hodgkin's disease incidence. The height of peak occurrence in young adulthood varies within this set of countries, being high in Canada, the United States, Switzerland, and France, and lower in southern Europe. The pattern within Eastern Europe is variable. In contrast, the pattern in Asia and Africa is generally intermediate or developing. Figure 2 shows characteristic age-incidence curves for males from various populations (35).

Variation with Socioeconomic Status

The association of the incidence of Hodgkin's disease in young adults and socioeconomic status has been found within populations based on the analysis of small-area socioeconomic status indices (15,36). This association appears to be specific for the nodular sclerosis subtype of Hodgkin's disease. Henderson et al. (37) computed histologic-specific incidence rates for Hodgkin's disease in Los Angeles County from 1972 to 1975 by socioeconomic status. They found that the incidence of the nodular sclerosis type was directly related to socioeconomic status, but there was no consistent association for the other histologic types. These data were confirmed and extended through 1985 by Cozen et al. (38), who also found that the increase in incidence between 1972 and 1985 occurred only among cases of the nodular sclerosis subtype. They further reported that the risk pattern for mixed-cellularity Hodgkin's disease was quite distinct and negatively associated with socioeconomic status.

These findings are consistent with national data. Using the United States Surveillance, Epidemiology, and End Results Registry (SEER) incidence data from 1969 to 1980, Glaser (39) reported that incidence rates for young adults were positively correlated with community-level socioeconomic status indicators and that the incidence of the nodular sclerosis subtype increased in parallel with regional socioeconomic status indices. In general, the

A

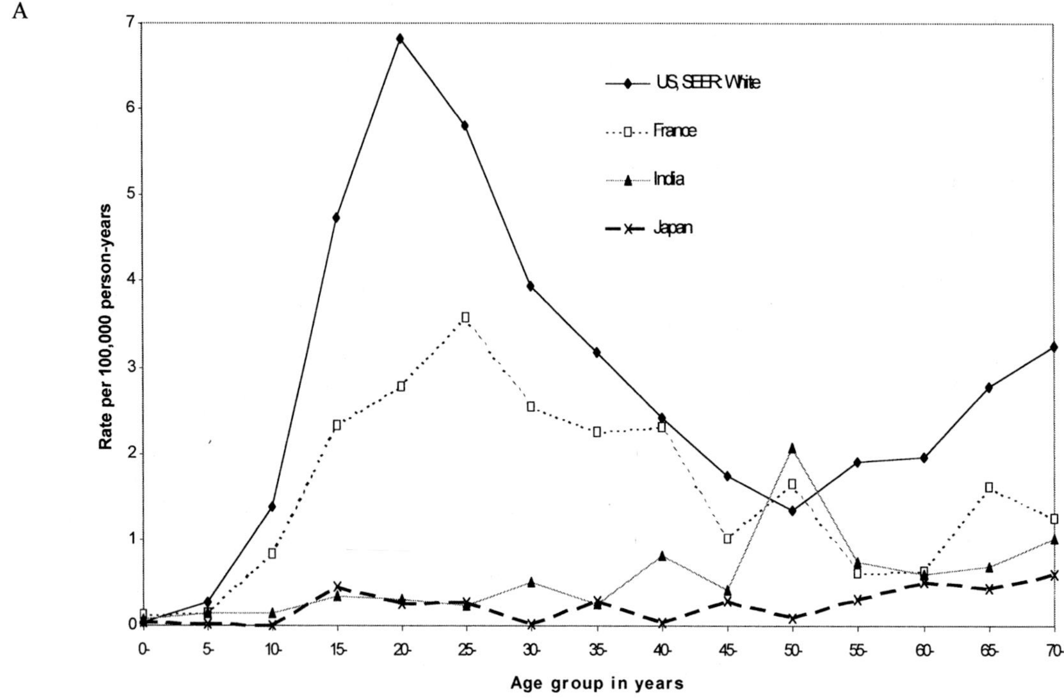

B

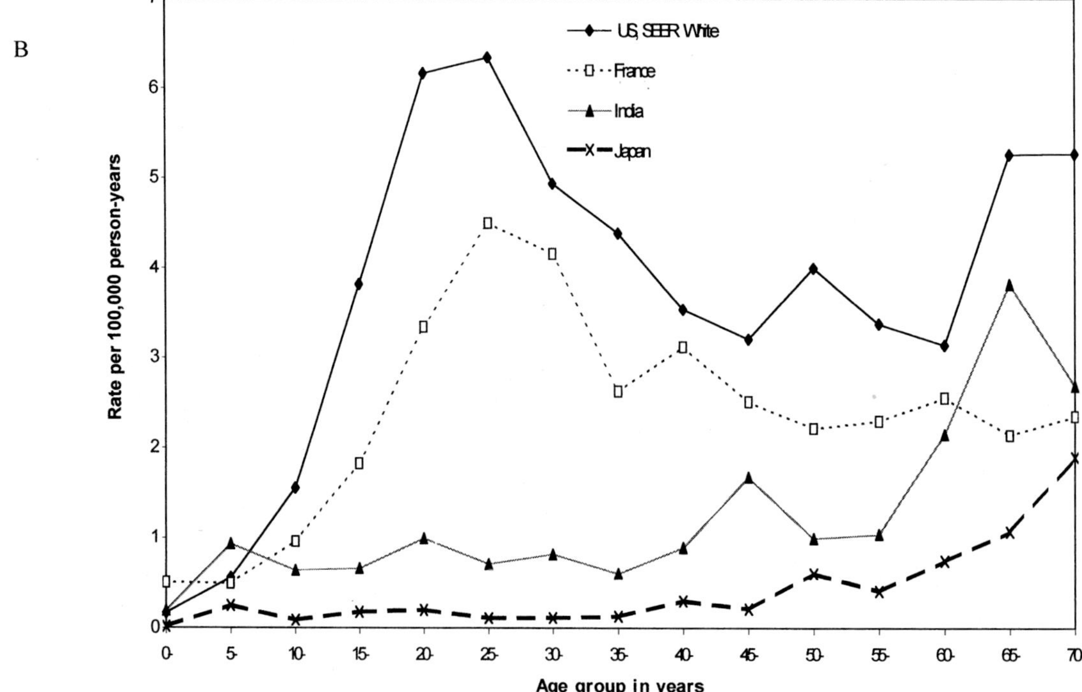

FIG. 2. Female **(A)** and male **(B)** age-specific incidence rates of Hodgkin's disease in various countries per 100,000 population. (Adapted from ref. 35.)

Hodgkin's disease cases occurring in economically developing populations and among lower socioeconomic status groups in developed populations are predominantly of the mixed-cellularity and lymphocyte-depletion subtypes (40), and are more frequently Epstein-Barr virus–positive as discussed below.

CLUSTERING

Given the long-standing notion of an infectious etiology for Hodgkin's disease, reports of clustering of cases have generated great interest. Clustering, which can be defined as the occurrence of cases close together in time and place at the time of their diagnosis, is a characteristic of infectious diseases. This is particularly the case for infectious diseases transmitted by direct person-to-person contact. It must be recognized that clusters of cases could also be due to common source exposure to noninfectious environmental agents.

It should also be noted that many apparent clusters of cases are chance occurrences that often become highlighted because of concerns about possibly causal environmental hazards. Frequently, a cluster that may just simply be the random closeness in time and space of several cases due to chance, ends up being inappropriately analyzed in a manner leading to false results. Many cluster investigations use what has been termed the "Texas sharpshooter approach" (20). This name is based on an old joke about a traveler in Texas driving through a farming area, where she notices that on each of the barns in the region there is a large target with a single bullet hole passing through the exact center of the bull's-eye. When she stopped at a local gas station, she asked the owner about the remarkable sharpshooter. She then learned that it was the handiwork of a man named Old Joe who would shoot at the side of a barn and then paint a target over the hole so that the bullet hole invariably passed through the center of the bull's-eye. In many investigations of apparent clusters, the time frame and geographic area for study are usually selected in a post hoc manner analogous to the Texas sharpshooter. Often, the time frame for study is selected on the basis of when the first and last cases occurred and the geographic area is selected on the basis of the cases that lived farthest apart. When statistical analyses are done comparing the observed frequency of cases in the cluster with that expected in the region during the time studied, almost always there is a remarkably high incidence of the clustered disease.

In 1971, Vianna and colleagues (18,41) reported an extraordinary cluster of Hodgkin's disease cases centered around a single graduating class (1954) of a high school in Albany, New York. This reported cluster was noteworthy in several ways. First, the cluster was much larger than most previously reported cancer clusters, involving 31 cases of Hodgkin's disease. Second, the analysis of the cluster utilized epidemiologic methods more typical of infectious disease investigations. Third, cases were linked to one another both directly and indirectly through intermediate personal healthy contacts. This report generated a great deal of interest in the scientific community and in the lay media as evidence that an etiologic agent for Hodgkin's disease might be transmitted from person to person. Unfortunately, the Albany report did not employ appropriate control groups and thus the significance of the findings remain undefined.

Perhaps the most important contribution of the Albany study is that it looked at disease clustering in a novel way. Traditional studies of time-space clustering have focused on interaction of these variables at the time of the cases diagnosis. The approach used in the Albany study was to look at the closeness of contacts between cases at the time of a possibly shared causal exposure with the disease occurring at different later times following direct or indirect contact with a case. The term *aggregation of exposures* has been used to describe this latter approach to the study of time-place interactions in Hodgkin's disease occurrence (20). The term *clustering* should be used to cover closeness in time and space of cases at the time of diagnosis. The difficulty with assessing aggregation of exposures arises when diseases have long and/or variable latency periods between etiologic exposure and disease diagnosis. Thus, patients may have had shared exposures while they were students in high school, but their disease may be diagnosed at various later times when they are in college or have migrated out of the area of first exposure.

The Albany report was criticized for lack of a valid comparison group. As a result, Vianna and Polan (19) conducted another study on Long Island, near New York City. Here they used several infectious disease methods to assess whether students attending high schools in which diagnosed patients had been in attendance had an increased risk of developing Hodgkin's disease themselves. The first approach they used was a two–time period method. In this approach, schools were classified as positive or negative based on whether or not a student with Hodgkin's disease had been in attendance during an initial 5-year period. Students at high schools with cases (positive schools) and without cases (negative schools) during the first 5-year period were observed for a subsequent 5-year period. Comparisons were then made between the occurrence of Hodgkin's disease in positive schools and negative schools during the second period. Five of eight positive schools and none of 16 matched negative schools had cases diagnosed during the second period, a truly remarkable finding. The second approach they used was an index–secondary case method. The risk of Hodgkin's disease was assessed in those students and teachers who had overlapped in attendance with a diagnosed case for a period of a year. Comparison was then made between the expected occurrence of Hodgkin's disease in those subjects exposed to cases and that observed. There were 21 Hodgkin's disease cases observed in students versus 9.3 cases expected. For teachers, 7 Hodgkin's disease cases were observed versus 0.9 expected secondary cases. Both approaches yielded strong evidence of an increased risk of Hodgkin's disease in children, and to a lesser extent teachers, exposed to cases in the high school setting.

Several studies attempted to replicate the Long Island findings. Smith et al. (21) conducted a case-control study of Hodgkin's disease in Oxford, England, in which links between subjects were assessed. They found no evidence of person-to-person transmission. We performed a close replication of the Long Island study in the greater Boston area. Using two–time period approaches with varying time intervals and index–secondary case approaches, no increased risk of Hodgkin's disease was observed in students who had contact with Hodgkin's disease cases or attended positive schools in the Boston area (22). Thus, the Long Island study findings could not be confirmed in other settings.

It is possible that the Long Island study findings are an artifact of cancer treatment referral patterns, since cases were identified via hospital and other treatment facility records (22). Long Island is in close proximity to New York City, where there are several major cancer treatment centers. In contrast, Long Island at the time did not have any major cancer treatment centers. Attempts were made by the researchers to identify Long Island Hodgkin's disease cases in a search of selected hospitals in New York City. However the hospitals surveyed were not the major cancer treatment centers. If patients living in close proximity to New York City were frequently referred to hospitals in the city and not entered into the study, whereas those patients residing further from New York City received their treatment locally, this could produce an artifact of clustering. Support for this interpretation is provided by the observation that the annual incidence rate of Hodgkin's disease on Long Island reported by Vianna and Polan was lower than the mortality rate for Hodgkin's disease reported by the National Cancer Institute for the same area at the same time (22).

Newer statistical methods have been developed for assessing time-space clustering. Earlier methods were available for statistically assessing whether cases were closer together in time and space than would be expected by chance (42–44). These very clever methods, such as the method of all possible pairs, are of value primarily for assessing clustering at the time of diagnosis. More recently, simpler methods have been developed that rely on closeness at time of diagnosis without need to consider the geographic frame. While the earlier statistical methods of assessing time-space clustering essentially proved negative, some of the newer approaches suggest that there might be weak clustering of cases (45).

In summary, at present there is little strong or persuasive evidence of clustering of Hodgkin's disease or of aggregations of exposures of the disease. This is important for clinical management in that patients can be reassured that there is no risk of their transmitting the disease to others. Relatives and friends may recall media reports of transmissibility of the disease and unnecessarily alarm patients about their possible contagiousness. Patients should be informed that this is definitely not the case.

GENETIC FACTORS

Familial Aggregation

Familial aggregation and genetic susceptibility appear to play important roles in the causation of Hodgkin's disease. There are numerous anecdotal reports in the early literature of the occurrence of multiple cases of Hodgkin's disease in families. Razis et al. (46) were the first to quantify the magnitude of increased risk to close relatives of Hodgkin's disease cases. Using medical records from Memorial Hospital in New York City, they found a significantly increased risk of Hodgkin's disease in first-degree relatives of Hodgkin's disease cases. When their data were reanalyzed, there were 13 proved and 5 unproved cases of Hodgkin's disease in first-degree relatives of 1,102 Hodgkin's disease cases. There was a total of two confirmed Hodgkin's disease cases and eight unconfirmed cases in similar relatives of 2,925 hospital controls, most of whom had other malignancies. This yields a relative risk* of 4.8 [95% confidence interval (CI), 2.1–11.3] when both confirmed and unconfirmed cases in relatives are included. In a population-based study in the greater Boston area, we found an increased Hodgkin's disease risk in siblings of young adult patients but no increased risk in siblings of old adults with the disease (47). Siblings of young adult patients appeared to have a sevenfold increased risk of the disease. Curiously, siblings of the same sex as the patient were at higher risk of the disease (ninefold) than were opposite-sex siblings (fivefold). We hypothesized that this might be due to sex-concordant sibling pairs having more shared environmental exposures (for example, shared bedrooms or friends) than did sex-discordant sibling pairs. We reviewed the world literature on reported sibling pairs with Hodgkin's disease and found confirmation of our findings. A second, later review of the literature also found an excess of reported same-sex sibling pairs (48). Similar significant excesses of same-sex sibling pairs were found in the literature for sarcoidosis, Behçet's disease and multiple sclerosis, a group of diseases that are also suspected of having infectious etiologies (48).

More recently, Mack et al. (49) reported a remarkably increased risk in monozygotic twins of Hodgkin's disease cases. They reported 10 of 179 identical twins of a twin with Hodgkin's disease also had the disease, compared to none of 187 dizygotic twins, relative risk = 99 (95% CI,

*Relative risk refers to measures of association including the odds ratio, rate ratio, relative incidence and risk ratio.

48–182). The authors indicated that the absence of an increased risk of Hodgkin's disease in the dizygous twins of cases was probably due to a much lesser genetic predisposition and to a very low risk of the disease in their small population of twins. Nevertheless, it is curious that a remarkably increased risk was observed for monozygous twins, with no increased risk for the heterozygous twins. This is an unusual study in that the subjects were identified via advertisements in newspapers and other media soliciting participation in the study of twins with cancer. The question arises as to whether the use of advertising to identify twin pairs might not have led to selective reporting of doubly affected pairs or of monozygous twin pairs. Nevertheless, it is hard to imagine that such bias would lead to the extremely high relative risk observed. The earlier Boston study of sibling pairs with the disease suggested an interaction between genetic susceptibility and shared childhood exposures. The Mack et al. observation of a remarkably increased risk of Hodgkin's disease in monozygous twins, but not in heterozygous twins, would argue in favor of a purely genetic basis for this susceptibility to this disease.

Other researchers have also concerned themselves with genetic issues relating to Hodgkin's disease. Chakravarti et al. (50) identified 41 pedigrees from a variety of sources and performed linkage analyses on these pedigrees. They found strong evidence of a recessive susceptibility gene tightly linked to the human leukocyte antigen (HLA) complex and responsible for 60% of cases in multiplex families. The residual 40% was suggested to be due to other familial and/or environmental factors. They found no increase in sex concordance, but an increased concordance for histologic type. He concluded that there is etiologic heterogeneity in Hodgkin's disease with at least three independent determinants: an HLA-linked gene, an HLA-unlinked factor, and an environmental/genetic factor determining concordance in histologic type.

Preliminary results from a large case-control study of childhood Hodgkin's disease currently in progress suggests that first-degree relatives of patients younger than 15 years of age at diagnosis had a 2.7-fold increased risk of *all* cancers. In a series of 464 Hodgkin's disease cases and 699 individual matched controls, 29 cases and 17 controls had a first-degree relative with a diagnosis of cancer. Four cases had parents with Hodgkin's disease but none of the controls did, and there appeared to be an increased occurrence of all lymphoreticular malignancies, melanoma, and testicular cancer in case families (51). A previous study by Olsen et al. (52) examined the risks of cancer in parents of childhood cancer cases from Denmark. Overall, they found no increased occurrence of cancer in case parents and they specifically observed no increased risk of cancer in parents of childhood Hodgkin's disease patients. This discrepancy may be accounted for by the fact that the case-control study from the United States and Canada obtained data by direct interview of parents of patients, whereas the Scandinavian study relied upon linkage of registry records.

Human Leukocyte Antigen

There have been many investigations of associations between HLA types and risk of Hodgkin's disease. Early case-control studies from Scandinavia identified a slightly increased risk of Hodgkin's disease associated with the HLA antigens A1, B5, B8, and B18. It was found that persons with these HLA types had relative risks of Hodgkin's disease ranging from 1.3 to 1.5 (53,54). Subsequent studies of HLA and Hodgkin's disease risk have led to a good deal of confusion, some of which relates to the fact that some studies found HLA associations with only certain histologic subtypes of the disease and others did not. Nevertheless, there appears to be consistency in the findings of an association between Hodgkin's disease and HLA-A1 and to a lesser degree HLA-B5, -B8, and -B18 (54). More recently, Oza et al. (54) pooled data from 17 centers to obtain HLA data for 741 Hodgkin's disease patients and 686 controls. Using more modern approaches defining specific alleles, they found a relative risk of 1.95 (p <.01) for HLA-DPB1*0301 in white patients. There were significant reductions in the frequency of HLA-DBP1*0401 in patients from Japan and Taiwan (relative risk = 0.15, p <.01). They also found decreased duration of remission in patients with HLA-DPB1*0901 overall (p <.05) and particularly in Japan and Taiwan (p = .02) where this type is most prevalent. There have also been attempts to relate Epstein-Barr virus positivity of tumors from Hodgkin's disease patients with HLA types. This was done because HLA-A*0201 in healthy seropositive individuals is known to be associated with cytotoxic T-cell response to the LMP-2 protein of the virus (55). However, no associations could be found between Epstein-Barr virus status and HLA-A2 in two studies (55,56). Thus, there appears to be definite, but weak, associations between HLA type and risk of Hodgkin's disease, which appears to be independent of Epstein-Barr virus status. However, Chakravarti et al. (50) did find evidence of a recessive susceptibility gene tightly linked to the HLA complex.

Increased Risk Among Jews

It has been noted (but often overlooked) that Jews are at somewhat higher risk of Hodgkin's disease. MacMahon (28), in an early population-based case-control study conducted in Brooklyn, New York in the 1940s and 1950s, found that older—but not younger—Jews were at increased risk. However, in our population-based case-control study conducted in eastern Massachusetts in the 1970s, both young adult and older Jews had notably higher rates of the disease (17). The level of affluence increased substantially between these two generations; it is likely that in the earlier study, most subjects were infected with Epstein-Barr virus in childhood due to more crowded living conditions and larger families, which reduced their risk for young adult Hodgkin's disease. In our later study, the risk related to being Jewish, with control for all the socioeconomic status indices, was still two to three times higher for all age groups (57). This finding was confirmed by later population-based studies in Great Britain (58,59) and in Los Angeles (38).

In summary, Hodgkin's disease in some patients appears to have a genetic basis but there is likely etiologic heterogeneity. The increased risk of Hodgkin's disease in close relatives of patients appears to be about three- to fivefold, and the risk to identical twins appears to be about 100-fold. The increased Hodgkin's disease risk in relatives is most marked for young adult patients' relatives. Additionally, first-degree relatives of childhood patients appear to be at increased risk of a variety of malignancies. These findings suggest that Hodgkin's disease patients' families represent a high-risk group for Hodgkin's disease and perhaps other cancers. However, it must be remembered that Hodgkin's disease is a relatively uncommon disease and three to five times an uncommon risk is still within the realm of uncommon; thus, patients' families need not be unduly alarmed. It is important to counsel patients that although their family members might be at slight increased risk, the likelihood of their family members ever developing the disease is still remote and they need not take any special precautions.

Additional research is needed to further clarify the genetics of Hodgkin's disease and whether or not there are genetic-environmental interactions that lead to familial aggregation. There is need to confirm or refute the findings of Mack et al. as well as our earlier findings of higher risk in same-sex siblings. Further evaluation of HLA types with linkage to Hodgkin's disease may prove valuable. The explanation for the increased risk among Jews begs discovery. It would also be of great interest to identify heritable factors related to the immune response to the Epstein-Barr virus, which might underlie the genetic susceptibility to the disease of Hodgkin's disease patients' relatives.

ENVIRONMENTAL/LIFESTYLE RISK FACTORS

Risk Factors Related to Age at Infection

There is a consistent body of evidence that risk of Hodgkin's disease is associated with factors in the childhood social environment that influence age at infection with the Epstein-Barr virus or very similar viruses. These associations pertain to risk of the disease occurring from early childhood through middle age, that is, within the first incidence peak. Among patients who are diagnosed in their 50s or later, there is no apparent or consistent association with indicators of childhood socioeconomic status (Fig. 3).

Children

While a great deal is known about environmental risk factors for adult-onset Hodgkin's disease, relatively little is known about such factors for childhood Hodgkin's disease. This is not surprising, given the extreme rarity of this lymphoma diagnosed in children younger than 15 years of age. We conducted a population-based case-control study of Hodgkin's disease in the greater Boston area in which limited demographic data were collected from the annual town registers (60). We found that the 14 very young children (less than age 10) with Hodgkin's disease came from lower socioeconomic status backgrounds than did the population controls. However, no socioeconomic status differences were observed for the 52 children who were 10 to 14 years of age at diagnosis. This finding suggests a transition in socioeconomic status of Hodgkin's disease patients from early to later childhood, in parallel with their probable age at infection with the Epstein-Barr virus.

We are currently conducting a large multiinstitutional case-control study of childhood Hodgkin's disease in the United States and Canada at the University of Pittsburgh. Over 500 cases of this very rare disease and individually matched controls are being studied for environmental and lifestyle factors. Thus far, preliminary results have been published on two findings from this study, one of which relates to an environmental factor (51,61). A statistically significant 40% protective effect of breast-feeding was found in this study. This finding confirms an earlier finding by Davis et al. (62) and by Schwartzbaum et al. (63). Whether it is exposure of the child to viruses or other infectious agents transmitted in mother's milk, or due to a protective effect of antibodies, cytokines, or other substances in the milk that protects the child against Hodgkin's disease risk, is unknown. This association between breast-feeding status and Hodgkin's disease is not modified by Epstein-Barr virus status of the tumor specimens. Of interest here is the report of Kusuhara et al. (64) that no differences were observed in the acquisition of Epstein-Barr virus infection between breast-fed and non–breast-fed Japanese infants.

In summary, little is known about environmental or lifestyle factors associated with the risk of Hodgkin's disease in children. This is an intriguing area for investigation since the poliomyelitis hypothesis of Hodgkin's disease etiology would suggest that these cases, should they be due to infection by a common virus, would be analogous to the widespread inapparent infections or perhaps to the sporadic paralytic cases of the disease observed in countries with poor hygiene. The limited data that are available are consistent in suggesting that the youngest children who develop Hodgkin's disease are those at increased risk of early infections.

A very interesting feature of Hodgkin's disease in childhood is the marked male preponderance in very young cases. This observation was first made by MacMahon (11)

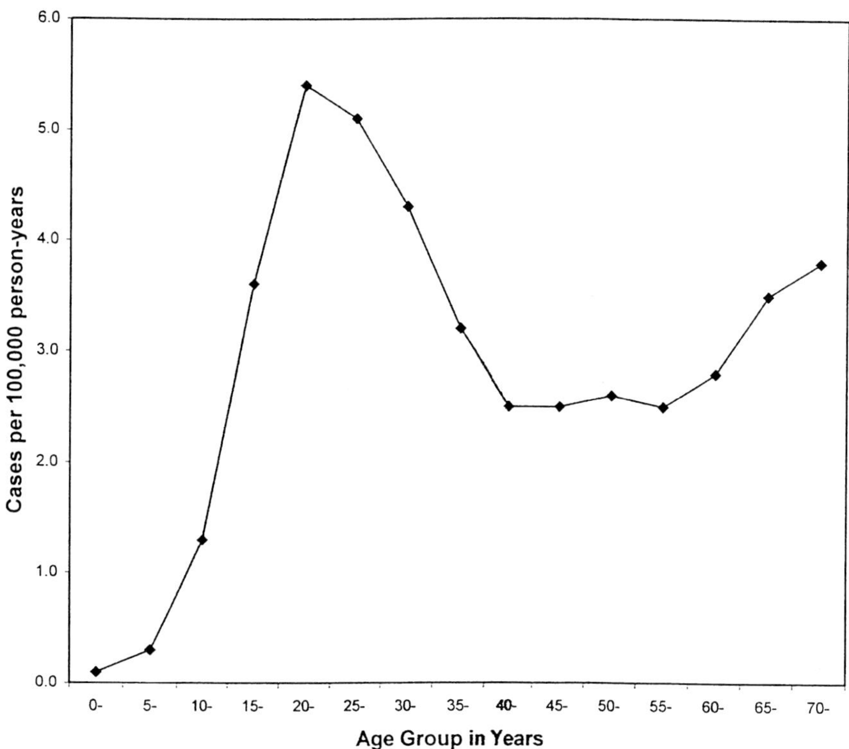

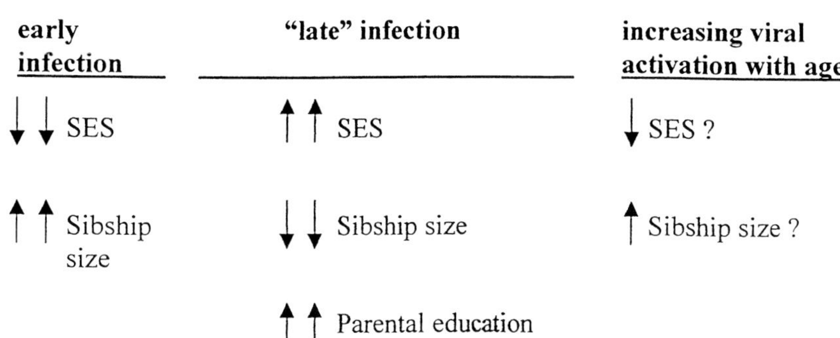

FIG. 3. Childhood social environment risk factors by age at diagnosis. Age-specific average annual incidence rate of Hodgkin's disease for all races and sexes combined per 100,000 population, 1990–1994, in the SEER program. (From refs. 27 and 57.)

and later confirmed by other investigators. Fraumeni and Li (65) found a 3:1 male excess in children with Hodgkin's disease. In children diagnosed before the age of 4 there is a 19-fold excess of affected males over females (66). In another series examining children diagnosed before the age of 7, a high sex ratio of 4.6:1 was also observed (67). This finding is consistent with the notion of an infectious etiology of the disease. It is well known that males are far more susceptible to infections during childhood than are females (68–71). This is true for bacterial, viral, and even parasitic diseases. This extreme male excess appears to diminish in Hodgkin's disease patients after age 10 (65), and suggests that the early childhood form of the disease might be quite different epidemiologically from other forms of the disease.

This notion of the childhood disease being different from young adult disease received impetus from an early paper by Correa and O'Conor (32), who, while using international registry data, observed that there was an inverse relationship in the relative frequencies of childhood- and young adult–onset Hodgkin's disease. In less developed countries such as Colombia, there was a relatively high incidence of Hodgkin's disease in children, and reciprocally there was a relatively low incidence rate for young adult Hodgkin's disease. Conversely, in developed countries like Denmark, the authors observed high incidence rates for young adult disease and reciprocally low rates for childhood-onset Hodgkin's disease. This intriguing finding was reassessed recently by Macfarlane and colleagues (72). Using later data from the same source, they found that this inverse relationship no longer was present. Incidence rates for young adult Hodgkin's disease had risen in developing countries while remaining fairly constant in more developed countries. These new findings suggest that environmental factors might be changing in Third World countries to more closely approximate those in the rest of the world.

Adults

Among young adults (mid-teens through the 30s), the occurrence of Hodgkin's disease is consistently associated with factors fostering escape from Epstein-Barr virus infection in childhood (13). In this age group, there is generally a twofold or greater increased risk in persons with a higher socioeconomic status and educational level (13,17,59,73–75). More interestingly, there is an inverse association of risk with sibship size, with the risk among persons from larger families only half that of persons from the smallest (13,17,59,76). In addition, those persons in the later birth-order positions of large families are at lower risk than those born earlier (13,17).

Most recently, the sibship size and birth-order findings have been replicated in a population-based cohort study involving over 2 million Danes whose mothers were born in Denmark since 1935 (77). In this cohort, 72 children and 306 young adults were diagnosed with Hodgkin's disease, and their characteristics (sibship size, birth order, parental age at birth, and year of diagnosis) were contrasted to that of the remaining cohort. For those cases diagnosed as young adults, there was a decrease in risk with increasing sibship *size (Table 2)*. This decrease was not statistically significant, primarily because of the lower risk observed among only children versus those with one sibling. A possible explanation for this heterogeneity could be that only children in Denmark are more likely to attend day care than those with siblings. However, for those in the largest families (5+ children), the relative risk of Hodgkin's disease was 0.57 (95% CI, 0.30–1.1) compared to those with only one sibling. There is a parallel graded relationship with birth order—*p* value for trend is .07. In contrast, these associations were reversed for the children who developed Hodgkin's disease, where being from a large family carried relative risk of 3.3 (1.4–8.0).

In a population-based case-control study conducted in eastern Massachusetts, we evaluated whether the inverse sibship size association was explainable by its mixture with other risk factors including higher maternal education and parental socioeconomic status, lower housing density, Jewish religion, smaller number of playmates, and self-reported history of infectious mononucleosis. However, adjustment for these correlated factors had little effect on the significant association with sibship size (relative risk for >5 versus 1–2 = 0.56), indicating that reduced exposure to infectious agents within the family was associated with increased risk of Hodgkin's disease as an young adult. Similarly, living in a single-family house during childhood, as opposed to multiple-family housing, was a primary risk factor for the malignancy (relative risk for three units versus single family = 0.56).

A large number of studies have evaluated the risk of Hodgkin's disease among young adults with a history of infectious mononucleosis. These include six cohort studies that evaluated the risk of Hodgkin's disease following the diagnosis of infectious mononucleosis (78–83). These involved nearly 42,000 young adults with serologically confirmed infectious mononucleosis, with the expected number of cases based on population data. Overall, there was about a threefold increased risk of Hodgkin's disease following a diagnosis of infectious mononucleosis. This finding has been replicated in multiple case-control studies (84). A question that can be raised is whether this finding simply reflects confounding by other risk factors

TABLE 2. *Relative risk (RR) and 95% confidence interval (CI) of developing Hodgkin's disease in a Danish cohort of children by sibship size and birth order for diagnosis in childhood and young adulthood*

	Age			
	<15 years		≥15 years	
	RR (95% CI)	Trend[a] (95% CI)	RR (95% CI)	Trend (95% CI)
Sibship size[b]				
1	0.71 (0.31–1.61)		0.80 (0.50–1.28)	
2	1 ref.	1.28 (1.00–1.63)	1 ref.	0.91 (0.81–1.03)
3	0.94 (0.53–1.68)	$p = .06$	0.94 (0.73–1.22)	$p = .12$
4	1.11 (0.46–2.66)		0.74 (0.50–1.09)	
5+	3.31 (1.36–8.02)		0.57 (0.30–1.08)	
Birth order[c]				
1	1 ref.		1 ref.	
2	0.93 (0.50–1.70)	1.26 (0.92–1.73)	0.98 (0.74–1.28)	0.85 (0.71–1.01)
3	2.04 (0.97–4.26)	$p = .17$	0.78 (0.50–1.22)	$p = .07$
4+	1.50 (0.42–5.33)		0.30 (0.10–0.97)	

[a] Trend is the relative increase in risk of Hodgkin's disease per increase in sibship size or birth order.
[b] Adjusted for age, gender, year of diagnosis, and maternal age at birth of children.
[c] Adjusted for age, gender, year of diagnosis, maternal age at birth of child, and number of younger siblings.
Adapted from ref. 77.

related to susceptibility to late infection. However, in our study conducted in eastern Massachusetts, where the effect of other related risk factors (sibship size, birth order, density of childhood housing) was adjusted for, history of infectious mononucleosis was still significantly associated with Hodgkin's disease, relative risk = 1.8 (17).

Among middle-aged persons (40 to 54 years) in the Massachusetts study, increased risk of Hodgkin's disease was found also to be associated with factors that reflect susceptibility to late infections (Fig. 3) (57). However, the mix of these factors differed somewhat from that seen among the young adults. In the middle-aged group there was a threefold inverse gradient of risk associated with family size, a somewhat greater range than that among young adults. However, the gradient of risk was lost when the confounding effects of other factors were controlled. In contrast to the young adults, neither birth order nor number of playmates in childhood was a risk factor for the middle-aged subjects. Although patients were more likely to have lived in a single-family or two-family home than were controls, the association was much weaker among the middle-aged than among young adults. However, whether the patient had shared his or her bedroom with other children was of some importance; 57% of the Hodgkin's disease patients had their own bedrooms when they were 11 years old, as compared to 33% of controls. When controlled for sibship size, the association of risk with having one's own bedroom was evident only among subjects in families with three to five children with relative risk of 5.2 (95% CI, 1.9–14.3). Few patients in this age group reported a history of infectious mononucleosis: the unadjusted relative risk being 2.1; the adjusted risk being 1.3.

The most important risk factor in this middle-age group was maternal education. Risk among people whose mothers had more than a high school education was five times that of people whose mothers had not attended high school. Although maternal education was clearly associated with the other socioeconomic status factors, its association with disease risk was quite primary. Higher paternal socioeconomic status was also associated with Hodgkin's disease risk; however, it had no independent effect once maternal education was taken into account. The findings from a similar study in Israel (74) that provided data for this age group were consistent with the observation that middle-aged patients appear to be individuals whose childhood provided some protection from early infection. These observations suggest that these patients in this age group may be susceptible individuals who were infected as adults, perhaps by their children.

Among the oldest persons (55+ years) in the Massachusetts study, risk was not directly associated with socioeconomic status. If anything, patients came from a somewhat lower socioeconomic status than did controls. However, within the Israeli population (74), older patients appeared to come from somewhat higher socioeconomic status. Whether this latter observation is confounded by the apparent general increased risk of Hodgkin's disease among adult Jews (see above) is unknown.

In summary, children living under relatively poor conditions are at risk of Hodgkin's disease. For both young adult and middle-aged persons, there is evidence that Hodgkin's disease may be a rare consequence of Epstein-Barr virus infection, which is strongly influenced by age at infection. The role of age at infection is not apparent for risk in the oldest ages, but the data are too sparse to reach a firm conclusion. The variation in known risk factors for the three epidemiologic types of Hodgkin's disease—childhood, young adult, and older adult—is perhaps unique in cancer epidemiology and underscores an important role for environmental/social factors in the etiology of the disease.

Epstein-Barr Virus

Multiple case-control studies conducted in the 1970s and 1980s evaluated whether Hodgkin's disease patients had a different profile of antibodies to the major Epstein-Barr virus antigens compared to healthy controls, as had been documented in both Burkitt's lymphoma and nasopharyngeal carcinoma, which are other Epstein-Barr virus–associated malignancies. In interpreting antibody profiles, it is important to note that host control of latent Epstein-Barr virus infection is primarily accomplished by virus-specific cytotoxic T cells, not antibodies. Rather, the relative level of specific antibodies appears to reflect the level of viral antigen. Seroepidemiologic studies have documented that Hodgkin's disease patients as a group differ from controls in having elevated titers against the viral capsid antigen (VCA) and the early antigen (EA)—indicative of viral activation (85). Those studies that had also tested for antibodies against the Epstein-Barr nuclear antigen (EBNA) complex had mixed findings (86). However two cohort studies have been reported on Epstein-Barr virus serology preceding Hodgkin's disease diagnosis. In both, the elevated antibodies to the VCA and EA were confirmed. In addition, both found that elevated titers to the EBNA complex predicted subsequent Hodgkin's disease (26,87). In the earlier study, multivariate analysis controlling for all antibodies measured, histology, age, and sex found the strongest predictors were the prevalence of high titers against EBNA, relative risk = 6.7 (90% CI, 1.8–24.5) and an inverse association for immunoglobulin M (IgM) antibodies against the VCA, relative risk = 0.07 (90% CI, 0.01–0.53). This antibody profile is in itself paradoxical as it suggests an enhanced level of Epstein-Barr virus replication *and* of immune response to the latent cycle antigens. These findings point to a protracted interaction between the host and the latent Epstein-Barr virus infection.

As detailed in Chapter 6, there is now overwhelming evidence that the Epstein-Barr virus plays a central role in the etiology of some Hodgkin's disease patients (86). This conclusion is based on the molecular analysis of multiple case series by numerous laboratories on patients from a range of populations throughout the world (84). These studies document that about in a third to a half of Hodgkin's disease patients, monoclonal Epstein-Barr virus genome is detectable in the Reed-Sternberg cells in affected lymph nodes. Further, the virus consistently expresses a restricted latent phenotype signature. Of note, Epstein-Barr virus positivity of tumor specimens is more common for children and among the oldest cases.

Glaser et al. (88) recently reported a combined analysis of data from 14 such studies involving a total of 1,546 Hodgkin's disease patients. Using multivariate analysis, they found that patients with Epstein-Barr virus–positive Hodgkin's disease were significantly more likely to have mixed cellularity versus nodular sclerosis histology; the relative risk varied by age group: 7.3 (95% CI, 3.8–14.2) for children; 13.4 (9.0–19.9) for ages 15 to 49; 4.9 (2.8–8.7) for those older. Cases with Epstein-Barr virus–positive disease were more likely to be male among young adults, relative risk = 2.5 (1.7–3.3), and, among children, from less economically developed areas, relative risk = 6.0 (2.0–18.0). In addition, patients of Hispanic background were more likely to have Epstein-Barr virus–positive disease, relative risk = 4.1 (1.8–9.6), an association first reported by Gulley et al. (89). Since essentially all adult Hodgkin's disease patients have antibodies against the Epstein-Barr virus, these risk factors relate not to whether a patient has been infected with the virus but how. The finding that children with Hodgkin's disease who come from economically underdeveloped areas were six times more likely to have Epstein-Barr virus–positive disease would suggest that their earlier age at infection was related. However, among young adults—where susceptibility to late Epstein-Barr virus infection is a consistent risk factor of Hodgkin's disease itself--those with a history of infectious mononucleosis are not more likely to have Epstein-Barr virus–positive Hodgkin's disease (90). Thus given that a patient has Hodgkin's disease, the likelihood that the tumor itself tests positive for Epstein-Barr virus genes or gene products appears to be related to factors indicative of somewhat poorer host response; namely, male sex, living under somewhat poorer conditions, and having mixed cellularity histology.

Jarrett et al. (91) have proposed that infection with another oncogenic virus is responsible for Epstein-Barr virus–negative Hodgkin's disease. An alternative hypothesis to reconcile these paradoxical findings is that the Epstein-Barr virus is involved in the etiology of essentially all of Hodgkin's disease cases, but the viral genome itself is somehow lost from the Reed-Sternberg cells in patients with a stronger host response (92). In support of this latter proposal, several factors related to immune function have been reported to be associated with Epstein-Barr virus–positive Hodgkin's disease. The most striking observation is by Frisan et al. (93). In this study, cultures of Epstein-Barr virus–specific cytotoxic T lymphocytes from nine patients were derived from tumor-infiltrating lymphocytes and expanded in interleukin-2 (IL-2) conditioned medium. These cytotoxic T lymphocytes were then tested for killing of autologous Epstein-Barr virus–transformed lymphoblastic cell lines. None of six cultures from Epstein-Barr virus–positive subjects exhibited HLA class 1–restricted Epstein-Barr virus–specific cytotoxicity, while all of three cultures from Epstein-Barr virus–negative patients did. It has been reported that levels of expression of both IL-6 and IL-10—cytokines that downregulate cellular immunity—are significantly higher in Epstein-Barr virus–positive Reed-Sternberg cells than in negative Reed-Sternberg cells (94,95).

Few data are available on the relationship of Epstein-Barr virus status and Epstein-Barr virus antibody profiles. Ohshima et al. (96) reported a single case of a 8-year-old boy with Epstein-Barr virus–positive Hodgkin's disease. His detailed serologic pattern (VCA-IgG 1:1280, -IgA 1:10, -IgM 1:10; anti-EA 1:160; anti-EBNA 1:40) was consistent with an active Epstein-Barr virus infection. In an overlapping series of 107 cases, Brousset et al. (97) and Delsol et al. (98) concluded there was no association with Epstein-Barr virus positivity and a serologic pattern of reactivation, which they defined as anti-VCA >1:640, anti-EA >1:40, anti-EBNA >1:160. However, only 1 of 35 Epstein-Barr virus–negative and none of 16 –positive cases had this rather extreme pattern. Levine et al. (99) assessed the relation of Epstein-Barr virus status for 39 cases with previously published serology. In this series, there were no differences between the Epstein-Barr virus–positive and –negative cases for either anti-VCA or anti-EA. Enblad et al. (100) compared detailed Epstein-Barr virus serology between 27 Epstein-Barr virus–positive Hodgkin's disease cases and 80 –negative cases. They reported only one significant difference: Epstein-Barr virus–positive cases were more likely to have IgG antibodies against the respected component of the E.A.

There is some evidence that risk of Hodgkin's disease is increased among patients with certain primary immunodeficiencies. Although there is a substantial risk of non-Hodgkin's lymphoma associated with loss of immunologic control of Epstein-Barr virus among such patients (101), the number diagnosed with Hodgkin's disease is relatively small, about 9% of all malignancies (and 15% of all lymphomas) reported in a special registry (102). These include children with ataxia telangiectasia (16 of 150 malignancies) (103). In Wiskott-Aldrich syndrome, of 78 cancers diagnosed, three were Hodgkin's disease. Eight Hodgkin's disease cases among 120 malignancies diagnosed in patients with common variable immunodeficiency have been reported.

Hodgkin's disease is even less common among the malignancies occurring in renal transplant patients, in whom it makes up about 2% of all lymphomas (103,104). Whether this is greater than expected is not clear, as generally the number of patients and length of follow-up is not stated. In one report that did calculate the expected value, no Hodgkin's disease case occurred, with 0.2 case expected (105).

As reviewed in Chapter 39, Hodgkin's disease has become recognized as part of the spectrum of opportunistic malignancies occurring in the natural history of human immunodeficiency virus-1 (HIV-1) infection (106). In general, these HIV-1–infected patients present with advanced Hodgkin's disease with poor prognosis; the great majority have Epstein-Barr virus–positive tumors. In many, Hodgkin's disease appears to spread noncontiguously without mediastinal or splenic involvement (107). This alteration in the natural history of Hodgkin's disease has been attributed to the loss of T-helper cells in HIV-1 infection.

Thus, there is a substantial amount of evidence that age at infection, immune function, and the Epstein-Barr virus are central to the etiology of Hodgkin's disease. However, the enigma of Epstein-Barr virus–negative Hodgkin's disease remains, and the relation of individual risk factors and serologic status to the Epstein-Barr virus–positive status has yet to be knitted together.

Nonviral Factors

Occupation

There have been numerous cohort studies and fewer case-control studies that have examined possible associations between occupational exposures and Hodgkin's disease risk. These results have been summarized in two earlier reviews (24,84). The study of the possible etiologic role of occupational and environmental exposures in a relatively uncommon disease like Hodgkin's disease poses several basic methodologic problems. In case-control approaches to the study of occupation, it is usually difficult to identify large-enough numbers of subjects with a particular job title or occupational exposure to perform proper analyses. Typical case-control studies have fewer than 500 cases and thus on a simple probabilistic basis are unlikely to observe many cases with the same occupational exposures, particularly if the exposure of interest is uncommon. On the other hand, cohort studies are efficient for the study of rare occupational exposures but inefficient for assessing Hodgkin's disease as an end point, since it is a relatively uncommon disease and very large cohorts would be necessary to generate sufficient numbers of Hodgkin's disease cases for conducting proper analyses. This is the basic dilemma faced in studying occupational risk factors for Hodgkin's disease.

Several occupational exposures have been associated with Hodgkin's disease. Many reports center on occupational exposure to wood, herbicides, and other chemicals (24,84). Unfortunately, the results of most studies have been inconsistent and few findings reach statistical significance, let alone support a causal association. For example, in a recent report from the Institute of Medicine on the health effects of Agent Orange exposure during the Vietnam War, associations were observed between the chemical constituents of Agent Orange (particularly contaminants of the compound) and Hodgkin's disease (108). While this report suggests an association between Agent Orange exposure and Hodgkin's disease, the committee that produced the report did not attempt to interpret the results to assess causality; rather, they simply reported that statistical associations exist for these exposures in the literature. The findings regarding woodworking and risk of Hodgkin's disease are subject to yet another potential limitation. Over the past decades, particleboard increasingly has been used in furniture making and construction. As a result, wood-processing companies find it profitable to place vacuum hoods over woodworking sites to collect particulates resulting from the manufacturing process. As a result, the workplace has become cleaner and workers exposures have probably diminished.

A problem with cohort studies is that most such studies can assess associations between occupational exposures and many different outcomes, including Hodgkin's disease and other malignancies. Given the large array of outcomes assessed, many of the associations observed for Hodgkin's disease might be due to chance. The general lack of consistency of findings in occupational cohort studies of Hodgkin's disease risk would suggest that chance may account for most of these positive findings. Furthermore, null findings tend to be underreported in the literature.

As a result, there are no well-established occupational risk factors for Hodgkin's disease. High on the suspected, but not proven, list would be woodworking, herbicides, and other chemical exposures. Additional studies are needed to address this important research question. It is probably more advantageous to approach this topic by cohort studies than by case-control studies, unless extremely large case-control studies are conducted. Cohort studies to address this question would need to have extremely large numbers of subjects followed; would need to use incidence rather than mortality data, since survival in the disease is relatively excellent; and would need to have precise measurements of worker's exposures to the suspected causal agents. Thus, any attempt to study occupational risk factors for Hodgkin's disease would necessarily involve very expensive and very large studies. It is perhaps for that reason, as well as the weak associations previously observed, that we are left in a quandary of not knowing what role occupational exposures might play if any in the causation of Hodgkin's disease.

Parity

As Glaser (109) has pointed out, there appears to be a deficit of cases among women in their late 1930s and 1940s in recent data from the United States and elsewhere. She proposes that this may represent a protective effect from childbearing, perhaps mediated by estrogen exposure. Kravdal and Hansen (110) evaluated the association of parity and Hodgkin's disease in the Norwegian population for the cohorts born between 1935 and 1974 using linkage to population registries. Most of these cases were diagnosed among young adults. In their analysis, there was no association of risk for parity for men, but an increasing protective effect for women; for women with at least three births, the relative risk was 0.46. Adjustment for socioeconomic status as indexed by either the patients' or their fathers' educational level did not modify this finding, although each of these socioeconomic status measures were positively associated with risk, as would be predicted. The relationship between Hodgkin's disease risk in women and parity was also examined by Franceschi et al. (111) using data from an earlier hospital-based case-control study in northern Italy (112). They found a small nonsignificant protective association with at least three pregnancies, relative risk = 0.77, and a nearly significant effect for ever having an abortion, relative risk = 0.4 (95% CI, 0.20–1.1). In a population-based case-control study conducted in Slovenia, no association between parity and Hodgkin's disease was apparent (113).

Tonsillectomy

A considerable number of epidemiologic studies have addressed the question of whether tonsillectomy is a risk factor for Hodgkin's disease. This relates to the broader question of the role of a virus in the etiology of the disease. Tonsillectomy is a risk factor for two diseases that share epidemiologic characteristics with Hodgkin's disease, paralytic poliomyelitis (114) and multiple sclerosis (115). The relative risk of Hodgkin's disease among persons with prior tonsillectomy relative to those without has ranged from 0.46 to 3.6 in published studies (84,113,116). There is also great variation in the prevalence of tonsillectomy among the populations studied, from 9% in Denmark to 74% among Boston area cases (117), which does not correlate with Hodgkin's disease incidence rates.

In all four of the published studies using sibling controls, a positive association was found. However, in two of the three of these that involved adult cases, the association was not uniformly present within all family-size groups (118). This lack of uniform association suggests either that tonsillectomy is not a causal factor or, if it is, its effect is complex and modified by factors related to family size. The former explanation is favored by our findings from two companion population-based case-control studies on this question (119). These studies involved 556 cases and 1,499 siblings from the metropolitan areas of Boston and Worcester, Massachusetts, and Detroit, Michigan. There was no evidence among young adults that prior tonsillectomy was a risk factor, relative risk = 1.0. Among middle-aged persons, the relative risk was 1.5 and not significant. Among older persons, the relative risk, 3.0, was significantly elevated, but the data are sparse. Taken together, the variability of findings, the variability of the practice of tonsillectomy, and the potential confounding with known risk factors for Hodgkin's disease argue against a causal association.

Other Factors

There are few other oncogenic exposures that appear to be related to risk of Hodgkin's disease. It is one of a handful of cancers that is clearly *not* associated with radiation exposure (120,121). The role of diet, physical activity, smoking, and alcohol use have had little attention.

SUMMARY

Hodgkin's disease continues to be an exceptional malignancy in its epidemiology and its biology. Few risk factors—other than those related to viral exposure and immune function—have been identified (Table 3). The

TABLE 3. *Summary: risk factors for Hodgkin's disease*

Factor	Strength of association	Consistency of association	Variation by subgroup
Epstein-Barr virus in Reed-Sternberg cells	Strong	Consistent	Mixed cellularity; males; children/older adults; Hispanics
Family history of Hodgkin's disease	Moderate to strong	Consistent	Younger cases
Demographic characteristics	Moderate to strong	Consistent	Males; adults in Westernized populations; children in economically disadvantaged populations
Childhood social environment	Moderate	Consistent	Favors early infection in children; favors late infection in young adults (and middle-aged adults?)
History of infectious mononucleosis	Moderate	Consistent	Young adults
Jewish religion	Moderate	Consistent	(May be conditional on age of infection)
Immunodeficiency syndromes	Weak to moderate	Fairly consistent	
HLA genotypes	Weak	Fairly consistent	
Occupation	Weak	Inconsistent	
Low parity	Weak	Inconsistent	Women only
Tonsillectomy	Weak	Inconsistent	

HLA, human leukocyte antigen.

major unexplored area concerns genetic risk. The molecular breakthrough of the detection of the Epstein-Barr virus genes and gene products within the Reed-Sternberg cells has opened new avenues for inquiry. The question of how the virus plays a role in pathogenesis and why it is less frequently found in those cases most suggestive of an infectious etiology—young women with nodular sclerosis disease—is a challenge for epidemiologists, virologists, clinicians, and pathologists alike. Where these new clues lead us remains to be seen. Thomas Hodgkin indeed started us all on a merry chase.

REFERENCES

1. Hoster HA, Dratman MB. Hodgkin's disease (part I) 1832–1947. *Cancer Res* 1948;8:1.
2. Hoster HA, Dratman MB. Hodgkin's disease (part II) 1832–1947. *Cancer Res* 1948;8:49.
3. Hodgkin T. On some morbid appearances of the absorbent glands and spleen. *Med Chir Trans* 1832;17:68.
4. Kass AM. Doctors afield: Dr. Thomas Hodgkin's friendship with Sir Moses Montefiore. *N Engl J Med* 1984;310:401.
5. Kass AM, Kass EH. *Perfecting the world: the life and times of Dr. Thomas Hodgkin 1798–1866.* New York: Harcourt Brace Javanovich, 1988.
6. Rosenfeld L. *Thomas Hodgkin: morbid anatomist and social activist.* Lanham, MD: Madison, 1993.
7. Aterman K. Thomas Hodgkin (1798–1866). *Am J Dermatopathol* 1986; 8:157.
8. Kaplan HS. *Hodgkin's disease,* 2nd ed. Cambridge, MA: Harvard University Press, 1980.
9. Cunningham WF. The status of diphtheroids with special reference to Hodgkin's disease. *Am J Med Sci* 1917;153:406.
10. Yates JL, Bunting CH. The rational treatment of Hodgkin's disease. *JAMA* 1915;64:1953.
11. MacMahon B. Epidemiology of Hodgkin's disease. *Cancer Res* 1966; 26:1189.
12. Newell GR. Etiology of multiple sclerosis and Hodgkin's disease. *Am J Epidemiol* 1970;91:119.
13. Gutensohn (Mueller) N, Cole P. Epidemiology of Hodgkin's disease in the young. *Int J Cancer* 1977;19:595.
14. Gutensohn (Mueller) NM, Cole P. Epidemiology of Hodgkin's disease. *Semin Oncol* 1980;7:92.
15. Alexander FE, McKinney PA, Williams J, Ricketts TJ, Cartwright RA. Epidemiological evidence for the two-disease hypothesis in Hodgkin's disease. *Int J Epidemiol* 1991;20:354.
16. Paffenbarger RS Jr, Wing AL, Hyde RT. Characteristics in youth indicative of adult onset Hodgkin's disease. *J Natl Cancer Inst* 1977;58:1489.
17. Gutensohn (Mueller) NM, Cole P. Childhood social environment and Hodgkin's disease. *N Engl J Med* 1981;304:135.
18. Vianna NJ, Greenwald P, Davies JNP. Extended epidemic of Hodgkin's disease in high school students. *Lancet* 1971;1:1209.
19. Vianna NJ, Polan AK. Epidemiologic evidence for transmission of Hodgkin's disease. *N Engl J Med* 1973;289:499.
20. Grufferman S. Clustering and aggregation of exposures in Hodgkin's disease. *Cancer* 1977;39:1829.
21. Smith PG, Pike MC, Kinlen LJ, Jones A, Harris R. Contacts between young patients with Hodgkin's disease. A case-control study. *Lancet* 1977;2:59.
22. Grufferman S, Cole P, Levitan TR. Evidence against transmission of Hodgkin's disease in high schools. *N Engl J Med* 1979;300:1006.
23. Weiss LM, Strickler JG, Warnke RA, Purtilo DT, Sklar J. Epstein-Barr viral DNA in tissues of Hodgkin's disease. *Am J Pathol* 1987;129:86.
24. Grufferman S, Delzell E. Epidemiology of Hodgkin's disease. *Epidemiol Rev* 1984;6:76.
25. Evans AS, Comstock GW. Presence of elevated antibody titers to Epstein-Barr virus before Hodgkin's disease. *Lancet* 1981;1:1183.
26. Mueller N, Evans A, Harris NL, et al. Hodgkin's disease and Epstein-Barr virus. Altered antibody pattern before diagnosis. *N Engl J Med* 1989;320:689.
27. Ries LAG, Kosary CL, Hankey BF, Miller BA, Harras A, Edwards BK, eds. *SEER cancer statistics review: 1973–1994.* NIH publ. no. 97-2789. Bethesda: National Cancer Institute, 1997.
28. MacMahon B. Epidemiological evidence on the nature of Hodgkin's disease. *Cancer* 1957;10:1045.
29. Horn JW, Devesa SS, Burhansstipanov L. Cancer incidence, mortality and survival among racial and ethnic minority groups in the United States. In: Schottenfeld D, Fraumeni JF Jr, eds. *Cancer epidemiology and prevention,* 2nd ed. New York: Oxford University Press, 1996:192.
30. Glaser SL, Swartz WG. Time trends in Hodgkin's disease incidence: the role of diagnostic accuracy. *Cancer* 1990;66:2196.
31. Chen YT, Zheng T, Chou MC, Boyle P, Holford TR. The increase of Hodgkin's disease incidence among young adults. Experience in Connecticut, 1935–1992. *Cancer* 1997;79:2209.
32. Correa P, O'Conor GT. Epidemiologic patterns of Hodgkin's disease. *Int J Cancer* 1971;8:192.
33. Hartge P, Devesa SS, Fraumeni JF Jr. Hodgkin's disease and non-Hodgkin's lymphomas. *Cancer Surv* 1994;19/20:423.
34. Glaser SL. Hodgkin's disease in black populations: a review of the epidemiologic literature. *Semin Oncol* 1990;17:643.
35. Parkin DM, Whelan SL, Ferlay J, Raymond L, Young J, eds. *Cancer incidence in five continents,* vol 7. IARC Scientific publ. no. 143. Lyon, France: International Agency for Research on Cancer, 1997.
36. Alexander FE, Ricketts TJ, McKinney PA, Cartwright RA. Community lifestyle characteristics and incidence of Hodgkin's disease in young people. *Int J Cancer* 1991;48:10.
37. Henderson BE, Dworsky R, Pike MC, et al. Risk factors for nodular sclerosis and other types of Hodgkin's disease. *Cancer Res* 1979;39: 4507.
38. Cozen W, Katz J, Mack T. Risk patterns of Hodgkin's disease in Los Angeles vary by cell type. *Cancer Epidemiol Biomarkers Prev* 1992; 1:261.
39. Glaser SL. Regional variation in Hodgkin's disease incidence by histologic subtype in the US. *Cancer* 1987;60:2841.
40. Hu E, Hufford S, Lukes R, et al. Third-world Hodgkin's disease at Los Angeles County-University of Southern California Medical Center. *J Clin Oncol* 1988;6:1285.
41. Vianna NJ, Greenwald P, Brady, et al. Hodgkin's disease: cases with features of a community outbreak. *Ann Intern Med* 1972;77:169.
42. Greenberg RS, Grufferman S, Cole P. An evaluation of space-time clustering in Hodgkin's disease. *J Chronic Dis* 1983;36:257.
43. Knox G. Detection of low intensity epidemicity: application to cleft lip and palate. *Br J Prev Soc Med* 1963;17:121.
44. Ederer F, Myers MH, Mantel N. A statistical problem in space and time: do leukemia cases come in clusters? *Biometrics* 1964;20:626.
45. Alexander FE, Daniel CP, Armstrong AA, et al. Case clustering, Epstein-Barr virus Reed-Sternberg cell status and herpes virus serology in Hodgkin's disease: results of a case-control study. *Eur J Cancer* 1995;31A:1479.
46. Razis DV, Diamond HD, Craver LF. Familial Hodgkin's disease: its significance and implications. *Ann Intern Med* 1959;51:933.
47. Grufferman S, Cole P, Smith PG, Lukes RJ. Hodgkin's disease in siblings. *N Engl J Med* 1977;296:248.
48. Grufferman S, Barton JW, Eby NL. Increased sex concordance of sibling pairs with Behçet's disease, Hodgkin's disease, multiple sclerosis and sarcoidosis. *Am J Epidemiol* 1987;126:365.
49. Mack TM, Cozen W, Shibata DK, et al. Concordance for Hodgkin's disease in identical twins suggesting genetic susceptibility to the young-adult form of the disease. *N Engl J Med* 1995;332:413.
50. Chakravarti A, Halloran SL, Bale SJ, Tucker MA. Etiological heterogeneity in Hodgkin's disease: HLA linked and unlinked determinants of susceptibility independent of histological concordance. *Genet Epidemiol* 1986;3:407.
51. Grufferman S, Ambinder RF, Shugart YY, Brecher ML, Gilchrist GS. Increased cancer risk in families of children with Hodgkin's disease. *Am J Epidemiol* 1998;147(11):S8(abst).
52. Olsen JH, Boice JD, Seersholm N, Bautz A, Fraumeni JF Jr. Cancer in the parents of children with cancer. *N Engl J Med* 1995;333:1594.
53. Hors J, Dausset J. HLA and susceptibility to Hodgkin's disease. *Immunol Rev* 1983;70:167.
54. Oza AM, Tonks S, Lim J, Fleetwood MA, Lister TA, Bodmer JG, and Collaborating Centers. A clinical epidemiological study of human leukocyte antigen-DPB alleles in Hodgkin's disease. *Cancer Res* 1994;54:5101.
55. Bryden H, MacKenzi J, Andrew L, et al. Determination of HLA-A*02

antigen status in Hodgkin's disease and analysis of an HLA-A*02-restricted epitope of the Epstein-Barr virus LMP-2 protein. *Int J Cancer* 1997;72:614.
56. Poppema S, Visser L. Epstein-Barr virus positivity in Hodgkin's disease does not correlate with an HLA A2-negative phenotype. *Cancer* 1994;73:3059.
57. Gutensohn (Mueller) N. Social class and age at diagnosis of Hodgkin's disease: new epidemiologic evidence on the two-disease hypothesis. *Cancer Treat Rep* 1982;66:689.
58. Bernard SM, Cartwright RA, Bird CC, et al. Aetiologic factors in lymphoid malignancies: a case-control epidemiological study. *Leuk Res* 1984;8:681.
59. Bernard SM, Cartwright RA, Darwin CM, et al. Hodgkin's Disease: case control epidemiological study in Yorkshire. *Br J Cancer* 1987; 55:85.
60. Gutensohn (Mueller) N, Shapiro D. Social class risk factors among children with Hodgkin's disease. *Int J Cancer* 1982;30:433.
61. Grufferman S, Davis MK, Ambinder RF, Shugart YY, Gilchrist GS, Brecher ML. A protective effect of breast-feeding on risk of Hodgkin's disease in children. *Paediatr Perinat Epidemiol* 1998;12: A13.
62. Davis MK, Savitz DA, Graubard BI. Infant feeding and childhood cancer. *Lancet* 1988;2:365.
63. Schwartzbaum JA, George SL, Pratt CB, David B. An exploratory study of environmental medical factors potentially related to childhood cancer. *Med Pediatr Oncol* 1991;19:115.
64. Kusuhara K, Takabayashi A, Ueda K, et al. Breast milk is not a significant source for early Epstein-Barr virus or human herpesvirus 6 infection in infants: a seroepidemiologic study in 2 endemic areas of human T-cell lymphotropic virus type I in Japan. *Microbiol Immunol* 1997;41:309.
65. Fraumeni JF Jr, Li FP. Hodgkin's disease in childhood: an epidemiologic study. *J Natl Cancer Inst* 1969;42:681.
66. Kung FH. Hodgkin's disease in children 4 years of age or younger. *Cancer* 1991;67:1428.
67. White L, McCourt BA, Isaacs H, Siegel SE, Stowe SM, Higgins GR. Patterns of Hodgkin's disease at diagnosis in young children. *Am J Pediatr Hematol Oncol* 1983;5:251.
68. Green MS. The male predominance in the incidence of infectious diseases in children: a postulated explanation for disparities in the literature. *Int J Epidemiol* 1992;21:381.
69. Melnick JL. Enteroviruses. In: Evans AS, ed. *Viral infections of humans:* epidemiology and control, 3rd ed. New York: Plenum, 1989: 214.
70. Washburn TC, Medearis DN, Childs B. Sex differences in susceptibility to infections. *Pediatrics* 1965;35:57.
71. Schlegel RJ, Bellanti JA. Increased susceptibility of males to infection. *Lancet* 1969;2:826.
72. Macfarlane GJ, Evstifeeva TV, Boyle P, Grufferman S. International patterns in the occurrence of Hodgkin's disease in children and young adult males. *Int J Cancer* 1995;61:165.
73. Cohen BM, Smetana HE, Miller RW. Hodgkin's disease: long survival in a study of 388 World War II army cases. *Cancer* 1964;17:856.
74. Abramson JH, Pridan H, Sacks MI, Avitzour M, Peritz E. A case-control study of Hodgkin's disease in Israel. *J Natl Cancer Inst* 1978; 61:307.
75. Serraino D, Franceschi S, Talamini R, et al. Socioeconomic indicators, infectious diseases and Hodgkin's disease. *Int J Cancer* 1991;47:352.
76. Bonelli L, Vitale V, Bistolfi F, Landucci M, Bruzzi P. Hodgkin's disease in adults: association with social factors and age at tonsillectomy. A case-control study. *Int J Cancer* 1990;45:423.
77. Westergaard T, Melbye M, Pedersen JB, Frisch M, Olsen JH, Andersen PK. Birth order, sibship size and risk of Hodgkin's disease in children and young adults: a population-based study of 31 million person-years. *Int J Cancer* 1997;72:977.
78. Miller RW, Beebe GW. Infectious mononucleosis and the empirical risk of cancer. *J Natl Cancer Inst* 1973;50:315.
79. Rosdahl N, Larsen SO, Clemmesen J. Hodgkin's disease in patients with previous infectious mononucleosis: 30 years experience. *Br Med J* 1974;2:253.
80. Connelly RR, Christine BW. A cohort study of cancer following infectious mononucleosis. *Cancer Res* 1974;34:1172.
81. Carter CD, Brown TM Jr, Herbert JT, et al. Cancer incidence following infectious mononucleosis. *Am J Epidemiol* 1977;105:30.
82. Muñoz N, Davidson RJL, Witthoff B, et al. Infectious mononucleosis and Hodgkin's disease. *Int J Cancer* 1978;22:10.
83. Kvåle G, Hoiby EA, Pedersen E. Hodgkin's disease in patients with previous infectious mononucleosis. *Int J Cancer* 1979;23:593.
84. Mueller NE. Hodgkin's disease. In: Schottenfeld D, Fraumeni JF Jr, eds. *Cancer epidemiology and prevention,* 2nd ed. New York: Oxford University Press, 1996:893.
85. Evans AS, Gutensohn (Mueller) N. A population-based case-control study of EBV and other viral antibodies among persons with Hodgkin's disease and their siblings. *Int J Cancer* 1984;34:149.
86. IARC. IARC monographs on the evaluation of carcinogenic risks to humans. Epstein-Barr virus and Kaposi's sarcoma herpesvirus/human herpesvirus 8. *IARC Monogr Carcinog Risks Hum* 1997;70:157.
87. Lehtinen T, Lumio J, Dillner J, et al. Increased risk of malignant lymphoma indicated by elevated Epstein-Barr virus antibodies a prospective study. *Cancer Causes Control* 1993;4:187.
88. Glaser SL, Lin RJ, Stewart SL, et al. Epstein-Barr virus-associated Hodgkin's disease: epidemiologic characteristics in international data. *Int J Cancer* 1997;70:375.
89. Gulley ML, Eagan PA, Quintanilla-Martinez L, et al. Epstein-Barr virus DNA is abundant and monoclonal in the Reed-Sternberg cells of Hodgkin's disease: association mixed cellularity subtype and Hispanic American ethnicity. *Blood* 1994;83;1595.
90. Sleckman B, Mauch PM, Ambinder RF, et al. Epstein-Barr virus in Hodgkin's disease: Correlation of risk factors and disease characteristics with molecular evidence of viral infection. *Cancer Epidemiol Biomarkers Prev* 1998;7:1117.
91. Jarrett AF, Armstrong AA, Alexander E. Epidemiology of EBV and Hodgkin's lymphoma. *Ann Oncol* 1996;7:S5.
92. Mueller NE. Epstein-Barr virus and Hodgkin's disease: an epidemiological paradox. *Epstein-Barr Virus Report* 1997;4:1.
93. Frisan T, Sjoberg J, Dolcetti R, et al. Local suppression of Epstein-Barr virus (EBV)-specifically cytotoxicity in biopsies of EBV-positive Hodgkin's disease. *Blood* 1995;86:1493.
94. Herbst H, Samol J, Foss HD, Raff T, Niedobitek G. Modulation of interleukin-6 expression in Hodgkin and Reed-Sternberg cells by Epstein-Barr virus. *J Pathol* 1997;182:299.
95. Dukers DF, Jaspars LH, Vos W, Hayes D, Cillessen S, Meijer CJLM. *Quantitative immunohistochemical analysis of cytokine profiles and T-cell infiltrate in Epstein-Barr virus positive and negative cases of Hodgkin's disease.* Stockholm: Eight International Meeting of the EBV Association, June 1998:abst 4.
96. Ohshima K, Kikuchi M, Eguchi F, et al. Analysis of Epstein-Barr viral genomes in lymphoid malignancy using southern blotting, polymerase chain reaction and in situ hybridization. *Virchows Arch [B]* 1990;59:383.
97. Brousset P, Chittal S, Schlaifer D, et al. Detection of Epstein-Barr virus messenger RNA in Reed-Sternberg cells of Hodgkin's disease by in situ hybridization with biotinylated probes on specially modified acetone methyl benzoate xylene (ModAmex) sections. *Blood* 1991; 77:1781.
98. Delsol G, Brousset P, Chittal S, Rigal-Huguet F. Correlation of the expression of Epstein-Barr virus latent membrane protein and in Situ hybridization with biotinylated Bam HI-W probes in Hodgkin's disease. *Am J Pathol* 1992;140:247.
99. Levine P, Pallesen G, Ebbesen P, Harris N, Evans AS, Mueller N. Evaluation of Epstein-Barr virus antibody patterns and detection of viral markers in the biopsies of patients with Hodgkin's disease. *Int J Cancer* 1994;59:48.
100. Enblad G, Sandvej K, Lennette E, et al. Lack of correlation between EBV serology and presence of EBV in the Hodgkin and Reed-Sternberg cells of patients with Hodgkin's disease. *Int J Cancer* 1997;72:394.
101. List AF, Greco FA, Vogler LB. Lymphoproliferative diseases in immunocompromised hosts: the role of Epstein-Barr virus. *J Clin Oncol* 1987;5:1673.
102. Filipovich AH, Mathur A, Kamat D, Shapiro RS. Primary immunodeficiencies: genetic risk factors for lymphoma. *Cancer Res* 1992;52:5465s.
103. Sheil AGR. Cancer in organ transplant recipients: part of an induced immune deficiency syndrome. *Br Med J* 1984;288:659.
104. Doyle TJ, Kumarapuram KV, Maeda K, et al. Hodgkin's disease in renal transplant recipients. *Cancer* 1983;51:245.
105. Kinlen LJ, Sheil AGR, Peto J, et al. Collaborative United Kingdom-Australasian study of cancer in patients treated with immunosuppressive drugs. *Br Med J* 1979;ii:1461.

106. Schulz TF, Boshoff CH, Weiss RA. HIV infection and neoplasia. *Lancet* 1996;348:587.
107. Knowles DM, Chamulak GA, Subar M, et al. Lymphoid neoplasia associated with the Acquired Immunodeficiency Syndrome (AIDS). The New York University Medical Center experience with 105 patients (1981–1986). *Ann Intern Med* 1988;108:744.
108. Institute of Medicine (U.S.). *Committee to Review the Health Effects in Vietnam Veterans of Exposure to Herbicides.* Veterans and Agent Orange, Update 1996. Washington DC: National Academy Press, 1996.
109. Glaser SL. Reproductive factors in Hodgkin's disease in women: a review. *Am J Epidemiol* 1994;139:237.
110. Kravdal , Hansen S. Hodgkin's disease: the protective effect of childbearing. *Int J Cancer* 1993;55:909.
111. Franceschi S, Bidoli E, La Vecchia C. Pregnancy and Hodgkin's disease. *Int J Cancer* 1994;58:465.
112. Franceschi S, Serraino D, LaVecchia C, et al. Occupation and risk of Hodgkin's disease in north-east Italy. *Int J Cancer* 1991;48:831.
113. Zwitter M, Primic Zakelj M, Kosmelj K. A case-control study of Hodgkin's disease and pregnancy. *Br J Cancer* 1996;73:246.
114. Paffenbarger RS Jr, Wilson VO. Previous tonsillectomy and current pregnancy as they affect risk of poliomyelitis attack. *Ann NY Acad Sci* 1955;61:856.
115. Poskanzer DC. Tonsillectomy and multiple sclerosis. *Lancet* 1965; 2:1264.
116. Liaw KL, Adami J, Gridley G, Nyren O, Linet MS. Risk of Hodgkin's disease subsequent to tonsillectomy: a population-based cohort study in Sweden. *Int J Cancer* 1997;72:711.
117. Mueller NE. The epidemiology of Hodgkin's disease. In: Selby D, McElwain TJ, eds. *Hodgkin's disease.* Oxford: Blackwell Scientific, 1987:68.
118. Gutensohn (Mueller) N, Li FP, Johnson RE, et al. Hodgkin's disease, tonsillectomy and family size. *N Engl J Med* 1975;292:22.
119. Mueller N, Swanson GM, Hsieh C-C, Cole P. Tonsillectomy and Hodgkin's disease: results from companion population-based studies. *J Natl Cancer Inst* 1987;78:1.
120. Boice JD Jr, Land CE, Preston DL. Ionizing radiation. In: Schottenfeld D, Fraumeni JF Jr, eds. *Cancer epidemiology and prevention,* 2nd ed. New York: Oxford University Press, 1996:319.
121. Halnan, KE. Failure to substantiate two cases of alleged occupational radiation carcinogenesis. *Lancet* 1988;1:639.

Hodgkin's Disease, edited by P. M. Mauch,
J. O. Armitage, V. Diehl, R. T. Hoppe, and L. M. Weiss.
Lippincott Williams & Wilkins, Philadephia ©1999.

CHAPTER 6

Association of Epstein-Barr Virus with Hodgkin's Disease

Richard F. Ambinder and Lawrence M. Weiss

Variation in the incidence of Hodgkin's disease with age suggests that Hodgkin's disease in young adults might be a rare consequence of a common infection (1) (see Chapter 5). Case reports document Hodgkin's disease developing in close association with primary Epstein-Barr viral (EBV) infection (2). Furthermore, cohort studies of patients with serologically confirmed infectious mononucleosis have consistently documented a threefold excess of Hodgkin's disease (3,4). Serologic studies show higher mean antibody titers to the viral capsid antigen (VCA) in patients with Hodgkin's disease than in controls and more patients with detectable antibody to early antigen than in controls. Furthermore, elevations in titer precede the diagnosis of Hodgkin's disease by several years (5). Thus, with the discovery of EBV infection in Reed-Sternberg cells, it might seem that the relationship between virus and tumor would be straightforward. It is not. Although EBV infection is ubiquitous, viral infection of Reed-Sternberg cells is present in only about half of cases of Hodgkin's disease, and the frequency with which it is present varies dramatically between populations. To those who would dismiss the association as an epiphenomenon, it must be pointed out that clonality studies indicate that infection precedes expansion of the tumor cell population and that infected Reed-Sternberg cells express high levels of a transforming viral protein. In this chapter, the biology of EBV and its association with other malignancies is reviewed, along with the evidence directly linking the virus to Hodgkin's disease.

R. F. Ambinder: Department of Oncology, Pharmacology, and Pathology, Johns Hopkins University School of Medicine, Baltimore, Maryland.

L. M. Weiss: Department of Pathology, City of Hope National Medical Center, Duarte, California.

BIOLOGY OF EPSTEIN-BARR VIRUS

Certain structural and biologic features are characteristic of EBV. The icosahedral capsid contains a large genome (171 kb) of linear, double-stranded DNA (6). Although infection with EBV, like infection with other herpesviruses, is generally controlled in the immunocompetent host, infected cells persist, and infections are lifelong. There are two alternative states of infection: lytic and latent (7). Lytic infection, which is synonymous with productive infection, is characterized by expression of the viral enzymes involved in replicating viral DNA and proteins that are incorporated into new virions. Latent infection denotes persistence of the viral genome but not the production of new virions.

Epstein-Barr Viral Infection

Although most human herpesviruses are widespread, EBV is perhaps the most ubiquitous. Serologic studies suggest that more than 90% of the adult population worldwide is infected by the virus (8). Serologic evidence of infection is found in all racial, ethnic, and geographic groups. Primary infection is usually asymptomatic in childhood, but when it is delayed to adolescence or young adulthood, as is common in affluent western societies, it is associated with the syndrome of infectious mononucleosis in approximately a third of cases (9,10).

The virus is transmitted in the saliva (8,11). Initial replication of virus in the oropharyngeal epithelium may account for the pharyngitis that accompanies infectious mononucleosis (Fig. 1) (12,13). Infected B cells are driven to proliferate and thus expand the pool of latently infected cells throughout the B-cell compartment (14). Early in infection, as many as several percent of lymphocytes may be infected by virus as visualized in lymph node biopsy specimens (typically obtained to exclude a

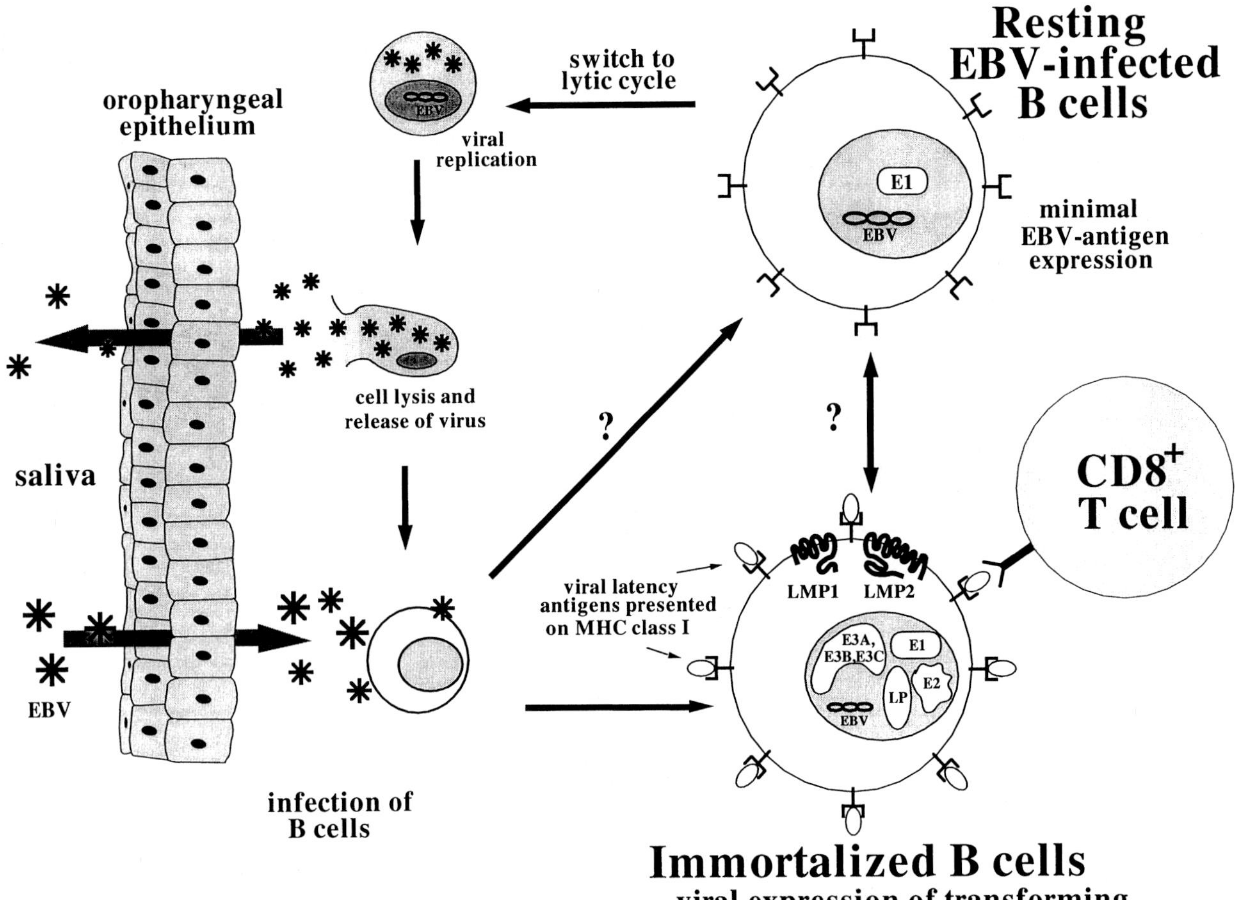

FIG. 1. The viral life cycle. Epstein-Barr virus (EBV) (*) is transmitted in saliva. Mucosal B cells become infected, giving rise to immortalized B cells. The immortalized B cells harbor virion DNA in episomal form (∞) and express Epstein-Barr viral nuclear antigen 1 (EBNA1), EBNA2, EBNA3A, EBNA3B, EBNA3C, EBNA-LP, and latent membrane protein 1 (LMP1) and LMP2. These proteins drive proliferation. The proliferating cells present viral antigens and are susceptible to killing by CD8+ cytotoxic T cells. Some EBV-infected cells elude this immune surveillance. Viral antigen expression is limited to EBNA1, which is not processed for presentation in MHC class I molecules. The antigens that drive proliferation are not expressed. These infected cells are resting and are believed to constitute the major latent reservoir of infection. Intermittently, such resting EBV-infected B cells may switch to lytic cycle and produce new virions. These virions may be released into saliva through the oropharyngeal epithelium or may infect more B cells. Artwork courtesy of M. Victor Lemas.

malignant disorder) or peripheral blood smears when *in situ* hybridization or antigen detection procedures are carried out (15–17). By polymerase chain reaction (PCR), as many as 2×10^4 copies of the genome per 10^4 peripheral blood mononuclear cells may be present (18).

The localization of latent infection in B cells and the capacity to proliferate and expand the infected cell pool by several orders of magnitude without further cycles of infection are features that distinguish EBV from other common human herpesviruses, such as herpes simplex virus, varicella-zoster virus, and cytomegalovirus (8). Latency established by herpes simplex virus in sensory ganglia is not associated with any disease manifestation except on reactivation. Proliferative or neoplastic diseases are not associated with these viruses. In contrast, EBV may induce proliferation of latently infected cells, and all the neoplastic and proliferative diseases associated with EBV are associated with latent infection. An important consequence of this association of neoplasia with latent infection is that although lytic herpesvirus infections and their associated diseases may be controlled by antiviral agents that inhibit viral DNA polymerase, EBV-associated neoplasms are impervious to these agents.

Following primary infection, latency proteins drive proliferation of the infected lymphocytes. However, with time, as the cellular immune response is established, expression of immunodominant viral antigens serves to target these proliferating B cells for destruction by virus-specific cytotoxic T lymphocytes (19,20). A subset of the infected cells persists for life. Their presence can be demonstrated by cultivation of peripheral blood mononuclear cells to give rise to spontaneous EBV-immortalized B-cell lines (21,22). Spontaneous transformation assays typically involve culture of peripheral blood mononuclear cells in the presence of a pharmacologic agent such as cyclosporine, which prevents T-cell activation. A lower limit on the frequency of infected B cells can be inferred from the minimum number of B cells that must be cultured to yield an immortalized B-cell line. In healthy EBV-seropositive donors, this is usually in the range of 10^4 to 10^6 B cells (23). PCR yields similar estimates of the frequency of infected cells (19,24).

Epstein-Barr Virus and Lymphocyte Immortalization

To understand better the relationship between EBV and malignancy, it is useful to consider the effects of EBV infection of B lymphocytes *in vitro*. B cells are infected through an interaction between the viral envelope glycoprotein gp350/220 and CD21, a component of the complement receptor on the surface of B cells (25). Major histocompatibility complex (MHC) class II may serve as a cofactor (26,27). Endocytosis, fusion with the host cell membrane, and transport to the nucleus follow. In the nucleus, linear viral genomes circularize to form episomes. Six nuclear proteins, three membrane proteins, and two small polymerase III transcripts (the EBERs) are expressed (7). The infected lymphocytes become immortalized, meaning that they will proliferate indefinitely in culture. They will also form human B-cell tumors in mice with severe combined immunodeficiency (SCID) (28). No other agent, viral or chemical, so readily transforms primary human cells. One of the consequences of the ease with which such lymphocytes can be cultured is that they are the most thoroughly studied form of EBV latency.

The coordinated expression of five viral genes is required for immortalization (Fig. 2) (7). The best-studied latency proteins are Epstein-Barr virus nuclear antigen 1 (EBNA1), EBNA2, and latent membrane protein 1 (LMP1). EBNA1, a sequence-specific DNA-binding protein, is required for maintenance of the viral episome (29,30). EBNA2, which interacts with a cellular DNA-binding protein, acts as a transcriptional transactivator, turning on expression of a variety of viral and cellular genes important in regulating cell growth (31–33). Two strains or biotypes of EBV have been recognized that differ mainly in EBNA2 coding sequence. These differences are associated with biologic differences in terms of the efficiency of immortalization (34). LMP1, an intrinsic membrane protein that resembles a constitutively activated member of the tumor necrosis factor receptor (TNFR) superfamily, interacts with TNFR-associated factors (TRAFs) that lead to activation of NFκB and modulation of a variety of apoptotic and growth pathways (35). In some but not all cell lines, LMP1 expression is associated with upregulation of cellular bcl2, interleukin-10 (IL-10), and MHC class I proteins (36–38). LMP1 expression in murine cell lines leads to loss of contact inhibition, anchorage independence, and tumorigenicity in nude mice (39). Deletions in the carboxyl terminus of LMP1 that interfere with TRAF signaling and a variety of other point mutations have been recognized, but their biologic importance is uncertain (40,41).

Two families of transcripts expressed in immortalized lymphocytes but not required for immortalization deserve further comment. LMP2A is an intrinsic membrane protein that inhibits lytic cycle activation by blocking normal B-cell transduction mechanisms (42–44). LMP2B is encoded by an overlapping transcript and differs only in that it lacks the amino terminal sequence of LMP2A. Transcripts for the LMP2 proteins are spliced across the terminal repeats of the circularized viral genome.

EBER1 and EBER2 are also not required for immortalization (45). These short RNA polymerase III transcripts, which do not code for proteins, have emerged as important markers of EBV latent infection by virtue of their abundance. Whereas most of the viral genome is silent in latency and even those viral genes required for immortalization are expressed at relatively low copy numbers, the EBERs are expressed at copy numbers estimated at 10^7 copies per cell (46–48).

Not every cell in an EBV-immortalized cell line is latently infected. A small minority of cells, fewer than 1%, are productively infected. Phorbol esters, butyrate, and other agents will increase the fraction of lytically infected cells, but even with such treatment the percentage remains very low (49). ZTA is the first viral protein to be expressed in lytic cycle (50,51). A sequence-specific DNA-binding protein and transcriptional transactivator, its expression initiates a cascade of events that leads to expression of delayed early genes, late genes, and ultimately packaging and release of infectious virus. Among the delayed early genes are two with sequence and functional homology to cellular genes implicated in tumorigenesis. These are BHRF1, a viral bcl2 homolog, and BCRF1, a viral IL-10 homolog. Both viral proteins share functional properties with their cellular homologs (52–54). The final steps of the lytic cascade of events, the synthesis of viral DNA and of the late proteins, can be blocked with antiviral agents such as acyclovir and ganciclovir. However, the growth of the latently infected cells and maintenance of the viral genome are not inhibited by these agents.

Alternative Patterns of Viral Gene Expression in Tumors and Normal B Cells

Although viral gene expression and many other aspects of EBV biology have been most thoroughly studied in

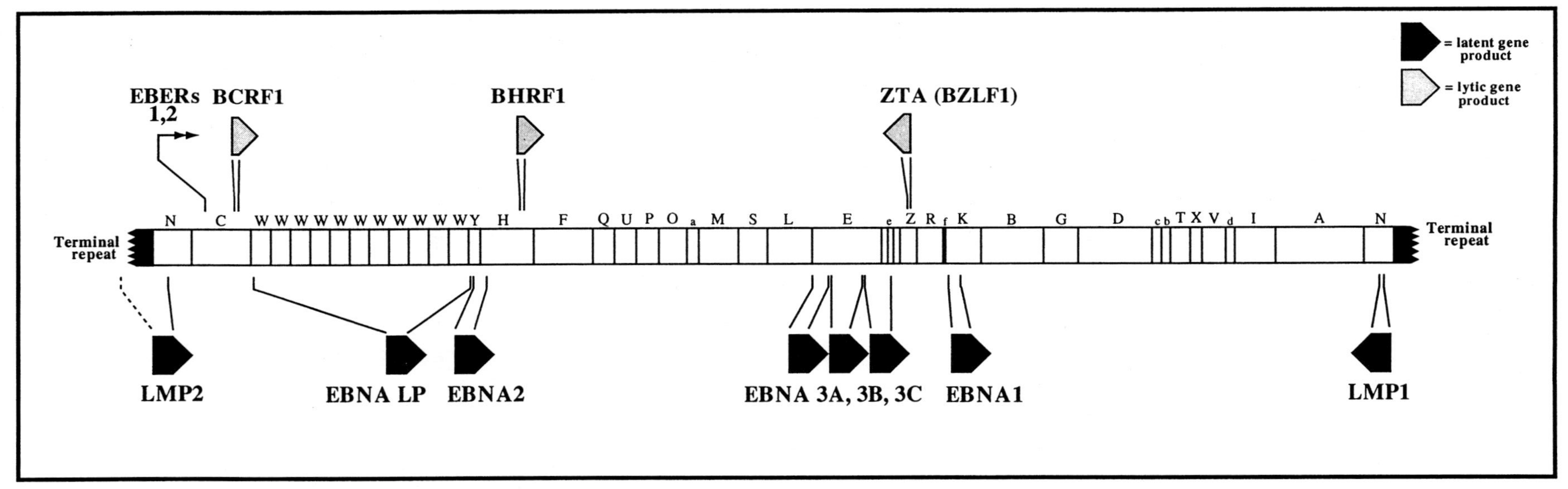

FIG. 2. Schematic map of the linear viral genome. Proteins discussed in the text are indicated. *Vertical lines* indicate Bam HI restriction sites. Restriction fragments are designated by *letters*. A variable number of terminal repeats are present at either end of the genome. Artwork courtesy of M. Victor Lemas.

immortalized lymphoblastoid cell lines, these cell lines represent only one end of a spectrum of patterns of viral gene expression detected in latency. This pattern of viral gene expression, often referred to as latency III, is similar to the pattern of viral gene expression detected in some B-cell tumors arising in immunocompromised patients, particularly organ and bone marrow transplant recipients with EBV-associated lymphoproliferative disease (Fig. 3) (55). In a variety of other tumors, including those of Hodgkin's disease, a more restricted pattern of viral gene expression, referred to as latency II, has been recognized. EBNA1, LMP1, LMP2A, LMP2B, and the EBERs are expressed (56–58). The most restricted pattern of viral gene expression, termed latency I, is found in African Burkitt's lymphoma. In this tumor and some of its derivative cell lines, most cells express only EBNA1 and the EBERs, although heterogeneity within tumors has been recognized (59). In Hodgkin's disease and in Burkitt's lymphoma, the failure to express EBNAs other than EBNA1 has been correlated with methylation of the C promoter, the promoter that drives all the EBNAs in latency III cells (60).

The latently infected B cells in the reservoir of EBV-seropositive persons resemble Burkitt's lymphoma cells more than EBV-immortalized lymphoblastoid cell lines with regard to patterns of viral gene expression (Figs. 1 and 3). Differences between latently infected lymphocytes *in vivo* and EBV-immortalized lymphoblastoid cell lines established *in vitro* were first suggested when it was shown that inhibitors of lytic viral infection added to peripheral blood mononuclear cells blocked spontaneous outgrowth of EBV-immortalized B cell lines but had no effect on immortalized cell lines established *in vitro* (21). This study suggested that infected lymphocytes *in vivo* are not already immortalized and that establishment of immortalized cell lines in the spontaneous outgrowth assay requires a cycle of lytic viral replication and infection of lymphocytes *in vitro*. Differences between EBV-immortalized lymphocytes *in vitro* and latently infected lymphocytes *in vivo* were also detected by reverse transcriptase PCR. Viral RNAs expressed in EBV-immortalized lymphocytes such as EBNA2 and LMP1 are not expressed *in vivo* (19,61,62). Transcripts that are detected *in vivo* include EBNA1 and the EBERs. LMP2A transcripts have not been consistently detected. Furthermore, the pattern of expression of cellular surface antigens by the cells that harbor virus also differs from the expression pattern in EBV-immortalized cell lines. These cells express the B-cell marker CD20, but not the activation markers such as CD23 that are expressed by EBV-immortalized cell lines (24,63). As in tumors, this restricted pattern of viral gene expression in latently infected lymphocytes *in vivo* has been correlated with methylation of the C promoter (64).

Immune Response to Epstein-Barr Viral Infection

Primary infection is associated with the appearance of immunoglobulin M (IgM) titers to VCA and rising IgG titers to VCA and early antigen (EA). During several months, IgM titers to VCA disappear, whereas IgG titers rise and then persist indefinitely. Titers to EBNA appear late but also persist. Antigen complexes rather than individual antigens are being measured in these assays. For instance, anti-EBNA detected in the traditional immunofluorescence assay measures six EBNAs. Specific assays for particular antigens or peptides have been developed (65,66), but most of the literature relating to Hodgkin's disease has utilized the traditional assays. Although neu-

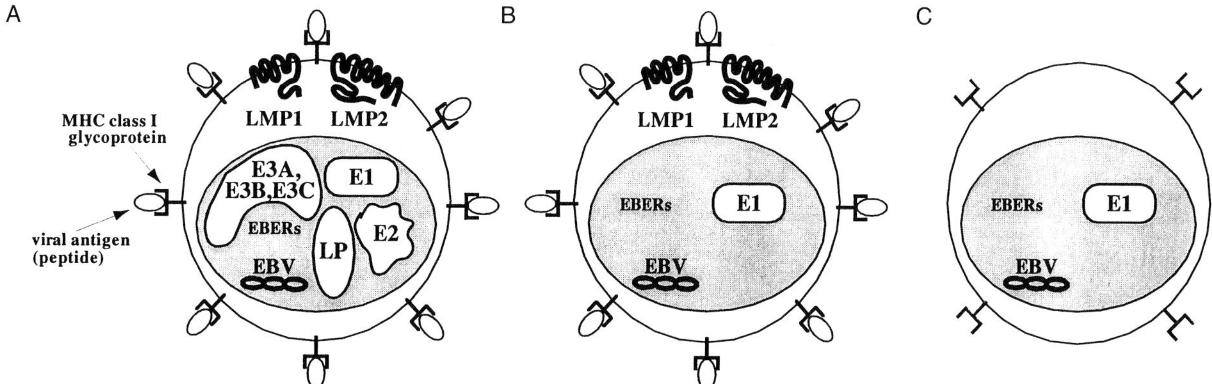

FIG. 3. Epstein-Barr virus (EBV) in three types of lymphoma. Posttransplant lymphoproliferative disease is associated with expression of the full range of viral latency antigens in immortalized B cells (latency I). Hodgkin's disease is associated with a more restricted pattern (latency II). Burkitt's lymphoma is associated with the most restricted pattern (latency III). In Burkitt's lymphoma, MHC class I molecules are often downregulated, and antigens are not processed for presentation. Artwork courtesy of M. Victor Lemas.

tralizing antibodies directed against gp350/220 are recognized, the humoral response is thought to have little impact on latent infection, as the target antigens are either nuclear and therefore not accessible or are not expressed in latently infected cells. For the diagnosis of primary EBV infection in the clinical setting, the most commonly used diagnostic assays detect heterophil antibodies that agglutinate sheep and horse erythrocytes. Their appearance coincides with the early phase of infectious mononucleosis, when polyclonal activation of B cells leads to a general elevation of total IgM, IgG, and IgA. Within weeks or months after the resolution of acute symptoms, these heterophil antibodies cease to be detectable. The explanation for their appearance and peculiar specificity remains elusive, and diagnostic use is entirely empiric.

Several of the manifestations of infectious mononucleosis, including lymphocytosis, lymphadenopathy, and splenomegaly, reflect an active cellular immune response (17). There is a peripheral lymphocytosis that typically consists of more than 60% CD8+ cells. Most of these cells are activated, and a proportion of CD4+ cells are activated as well. These cells directly lyse EBV+ B-cell lines and natural killer (NK) targets as well (67). Infection of peripheral blood mononuclear cells from EBV-naïve or immune donors *in vitro* shows that CD16+ NK cells, interferon-α (INF-α), and INF-γ can slow the outgrowth of EBV-immortalized lymphocytes. T cells from healthy EBV-seropositive donors completely block outgrowth. The cells that mediate this effect are mainly CD8+ human leukocyte antigen (HLA) class I restricted, although CD4+ HLA class II restricted cells have also been recognized (68). EBV-specific cytotoxic precursors are detected in a limiting dilution assay at frequencies of $1/10^3$ to $1/10^4$ circulating T cells (69).

The targets of these cytotoxic T-cell responses have been studied in healthy volunteers (70,71). Individuals show clear differences in target antigen choice, but the the most frequently targeted antigens are EBNA3A, EBNA3B, and EBNA3C. Other latency antigens, including EBNA2, EBNA-LP, LMP1, and LMP2, are sometimes targeted. Cells expressing EBNA1, even when targeted, are not killed because a *cis*-acting glycine-alanine repetitive sequence within EBNA1 inhibits its antigen processing and MHC class I presentation (72,73). Considered in the context of the cellular immune response, the highly restricted pattern of viral gene expression in latently infected lymphocytes (EBNA1 and LMP2A) makes sense. Cells with broad expression of EBV latency antigens would be expected to be killed rapidly by cytotoxic T lymphocytes. Limited antigen expression and the resting state of the infected B cells in the latency reservoir may combine to make these cells relatively invisible to cytotoxic T cells.

Animal Models of Epstein-Barr Viral Lymphomagenesis

There are a variety of animal models with relevance to EBV and tumorigenesis. Most Old World nonhuman primates harbor their own EBV-like herpesviruses. Like humans, most are infected early in life. Infection of seropositive animals with EBV is generally unsuccessful, probably because of cross-reactive immunity. However, New World primates, such as cottontop marmosets, are not naturally infected by similar viruses, and parenteral inoculation leads to polyclonal B-cell lymphoproliferative disease (74). In mice with severe combined immunodeficiency (SCID), EBV-associated B-cell tumors develop following any of a variety of manipulations. These include transfer of peripheral blood mononuclear cells from EBV-seropositive donors, or transfer of peripheral blood mononuclear cells from EBV-seronegative donors followed by inoculation with EBV, or simply transfer of EBV-immortalized B-cell lines (28,75). A transgenic murine model in which EBNA1 expression is associated with lymphomagenesis has also been reported, although EBNA1 expression is not detected in resultant tumors (76).

EPSTEIN-BARR VIRUS IN HUMAN NEOPLASMS

Aspects of Characterization of Epstein-Barr Virus in Tumor Specimens

Before discussing the association of EBV with tumors, it is useful to consider the distinctive aspects of the application of Southern blot hybridization and *in situ* hybridization to the detection and characterization of EBV in tumor specimens. Southern blot hybridization in a variety of tumor virus systems has provided important insights into tumorigenesis. Thus, integration of retroviral genomic DNA into the host genome is a critical step in the viral life cycle and plays an important part in tumorigenesis in various model systems. Similarly, the transition from episome to integrated genome is important in cervical cancer pathogenesis. In both retroviral and papillomavirus-associated tumorigenesis, viral integration serves to mark clonal expansions of tumor cells. As noted above, integration of the EBV genome does not occur in lymphocyte immortalization, and integrated viral genomes are not commonly detected in tumors, although they have often been recognized in some tumor-derived cell lines (77). Nonetheless, the state of the viral genome has allowed insights into clonality. Indeed, some of the evidence that Reed-Sternberg cells are clonal is inferred from analysis of the state of the EBV genome in tumor tissue, discussed below. To understand the analysis of clonality as it relates to EBV, it is necessary to understand how episomes (closed, circular DNA molecules) are formed from the linear viral genomes present in virions (Fig. 4). Genomes in virions are bounded at either

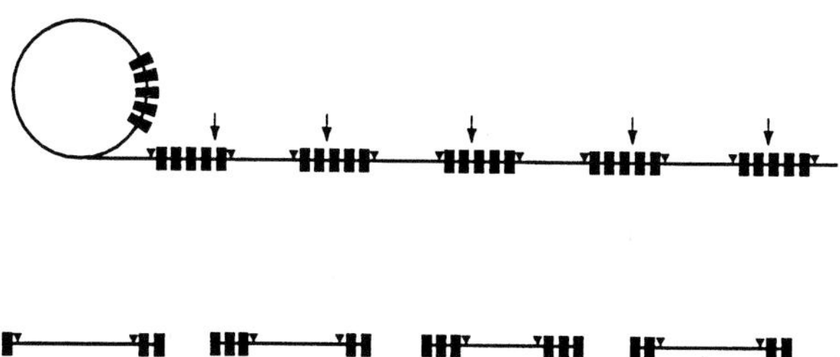

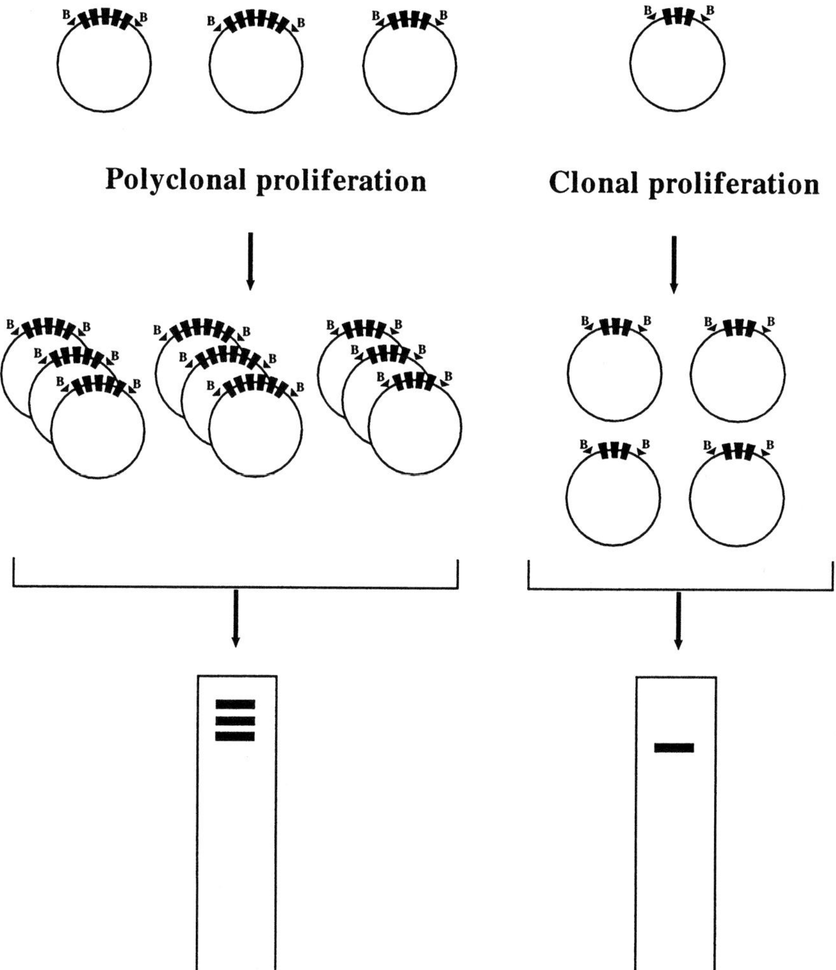

FIG. 4. Analysis of clonality by Southern blot hybridization. Characterization of the state of the terminal repeats of the viral genome distinguishes polyclonal from monoclonal infected cell expansions. Rolling circle replication, illustrated at the top, leads to the generation of multiple-genome-length concatameric intermediates. These are cleaved semirandomly to yield single-genome-length linear DNA molecules with variable numbers of terminal repeats at the left and right ends of the viral genome. On infection, these linear genomes fuse to form episomes. The fusion joints carry variable numbers of terminal repeats. The size of the fusion joint reflecting the number of terminal repeats can be assessed by digestion with a restriction enzyme such as Bam HI followed by Southern blot hybridization with a terminal repeat probe. Bam HI restriction sites (*B*) are shown. Because each infectious event leads to the circularization of a linear viral genome with a particular number of terminal repeats, and because the number of repeats is preserved in latently infected daughter cells, the occurrence of one or many infectious events may be distinguished by the presence of one or more bands corresponding to the fused terminal repeats. Thus, in a polyclonal proliferation of cells, several bands will be detected (*bottom left*), whereas in a monoclonal proliferation of cells, only a single band will be detected. Artwork courtesy of M. Victor Lemas.

end by tandem direct repeats of approximately 0.5 kb. On infection, these linear genomes circularize to form episomes, during which process the terminal repeats at either end are fused. These episomes in turn serve as templates for the generation of multigenome length concatamers that are cleaved to form linear viral genomes (78). Cleavage occurs semirandomly within the terminal repeat sequences, such that linear genomes generated from the same parental template differ in their numbers of terminal repeats. When these linear genomes circularize, the resultant episomes also differ from one another in terms of the number of terminal repeats. In latent infection, the episomes are replicated as such rather than through concatameric intermediates. Thus, numbers of terminal repeats in the episome are perpetuated from generation to generation. These different forms of the viral genome may be recognized by analysis of the terminal repeat fragments by Southern blot hybridization. The fused terminal repeats of episomes are readily distinguished from the shorter left and right terminal repeat fragments associated with linear genomes. Separate infectious events (i.e., different virions infecting different cells) give rise to latent episomes with varying numbers of terminal repeats. On the other hand, when only a single infectious event gives rise to the latent episomes in a tissue (through proliferation of the infected cell), then all the episomes in the tissue will carry a fixed number of terminal repeats. With appropriate restriction enzymes and probe, separate infectious events can be distinguished from a single infectious event by the appearance of multiple versus single bands corresponding to the fused terminal repeats of viral genomes in an infected tissue.

In situ hybridization has played an important role in the characterization of viral infection in many systems. However, the application of *in situ* hybridization to the detection of latent virus in tumor tissue is generally limited by the sensitivity of the technique. The EBERs, in contrast to other latency targets, are very readily detected by virtue of their abundance (79,80). The first application of EBER *in situ* hybridization to clinical specimens was to localize the site of EBV infection in Hodgkin's tumor tissue (81). An example of EBER *in situ* hybridization is shown in Figure 5.

Epstein-Barr Virus in Non-Hodgkin's Tumors

EBV is associated with a number of human neoplasms, including malignant lymphoma, carcinoma, and even mesenchymal neoplasms. Specifically, EBV is associated with almost 100% of cases of nasopharyngeal carcinoma, regardless of the geographic location (82,83). In addition, EBV can be identified in a subset of cases of gastric carcinoma, probably representing 5% to 10% of cases overall, with a particular predilection for cases of gastric carcinoma with a high content of lymphoid cells (so-called lymphoepithelioma) (84,85). EBV is associated with lymphoepitheliomas occurring at other sites, particularly foregut sites such as the salivary gland (especially in Eskimos), thymus, and nasal region (82). Mesenchymal neoplasms that have been associated with EBV include smooth-muscle neoplasms occurring in immunocompromised patients, particularly children with AIDS (86), and inflammatory pseudotumors of the liver and spleen, tumors that may represent a peculiar subset of follicular dendritic neoplasm (87).

Both B-cell and T-cell lymphomas are associated with EBV (88). B-cell lymphomas that are associated with EBV include Burkitt's lymphoma, lymphoproliferations arising in cases of acquired or congenital immunodeficiencies, pulmonary lymphomatoid granulomatosis, and pyothorax-associated pleural lymphoma. Burkitt's lymphoma was the first neoplasm found to have an association with EBV, as EBV viral particles were first identified in cell lines derived from African Burkitt's lymphoma (89). As is well-known, Burkitt's lymphoma is endemic in equatorial Africa, a high incidence zone for malaria; it occurs only rarely the United States and Europe and has an intermediate rate of occurrence in northern Africa and South America (90). The association of Burkitt's lymphoma with EBV varies similarly, with a nearly 100% association in endemic areas, about a 15% association in low-incidence areas, and an intermediate association in northern Africa and South America (91–95). In the large majority of EBV-associated cases, a restricted type I latency pattern is seen (59,96). However, cultured Burkitt's lymphoma cells may convert to a less restricted pattern of latency (97). Variation in the sequence of the EBNA1 gene is found in EBV-associated Burkitt's lymphoma, raising the possibility that some EBNA1 subtypes are more likely to lead to oncogenesis (98). In endemic cases, either type A or type B EBV is found, whereas primarily type A EBV is found in sporadic cases.

It is still not clear what role EBV plays in the etiology or pathogenesis of Burkitt's lymphoma. It is clear that an important factor in the pathogenesis of Burkitt's lymphoma is deregulation of the c-myc proto-oncogene, which is important in the control of cellular growth. Although the specific site of the chromosomal break point differs in sporadic versus endemic cases, virtually all cases of Burkitt's lymphoma are associated with a chromosomal translocation involving the immunoblo-globulin heavy or κ or λ light chain gene and the c-myc locus on chromosome 8 (91). The possibility that EBV may play a role in sporadic tumors apparently lacking the virus has been entertained. Several hypotheses are proposed involving loss of viral episomes, integration of viral fragments into the host cell genome, or integration of the viral genome followed by deletion of the viral genome. Ongoing loss of viral episomes from a Burkitt's lymphoma cell line in culture has been demonstrated (99). Loss is evident only when the cell line is cloned because cells retaining episomes have a growth advantage over those that do not. Although in this system EBV clearly contributes to tumor cell growth, it is certainly possible in other circumstances that accumulated mutations in Burkitt's tumors may render the growth advantage associated with EBV episomes irrelevant and that episomes may be lost. One group analyzed a series of sporadic cases of Burkitt's lymphoma by using multiple probes from different regions of the EBV genome and was able to demonstrate evidence of integrated, defective viral genome in three of nine cases shown to be negative for EBV by EBNA1 immunostaining (100). Another group has reported a lymphoma cell line in which integration of EBV into the host genome leads to an achromatic gap, leading in turn to a region of enhanced chromosomal instability (101). In hybrid cells, loss of integrated EBV, together with an adjacent chromosomal fragment, occurs during long-term cultivation; the inte-

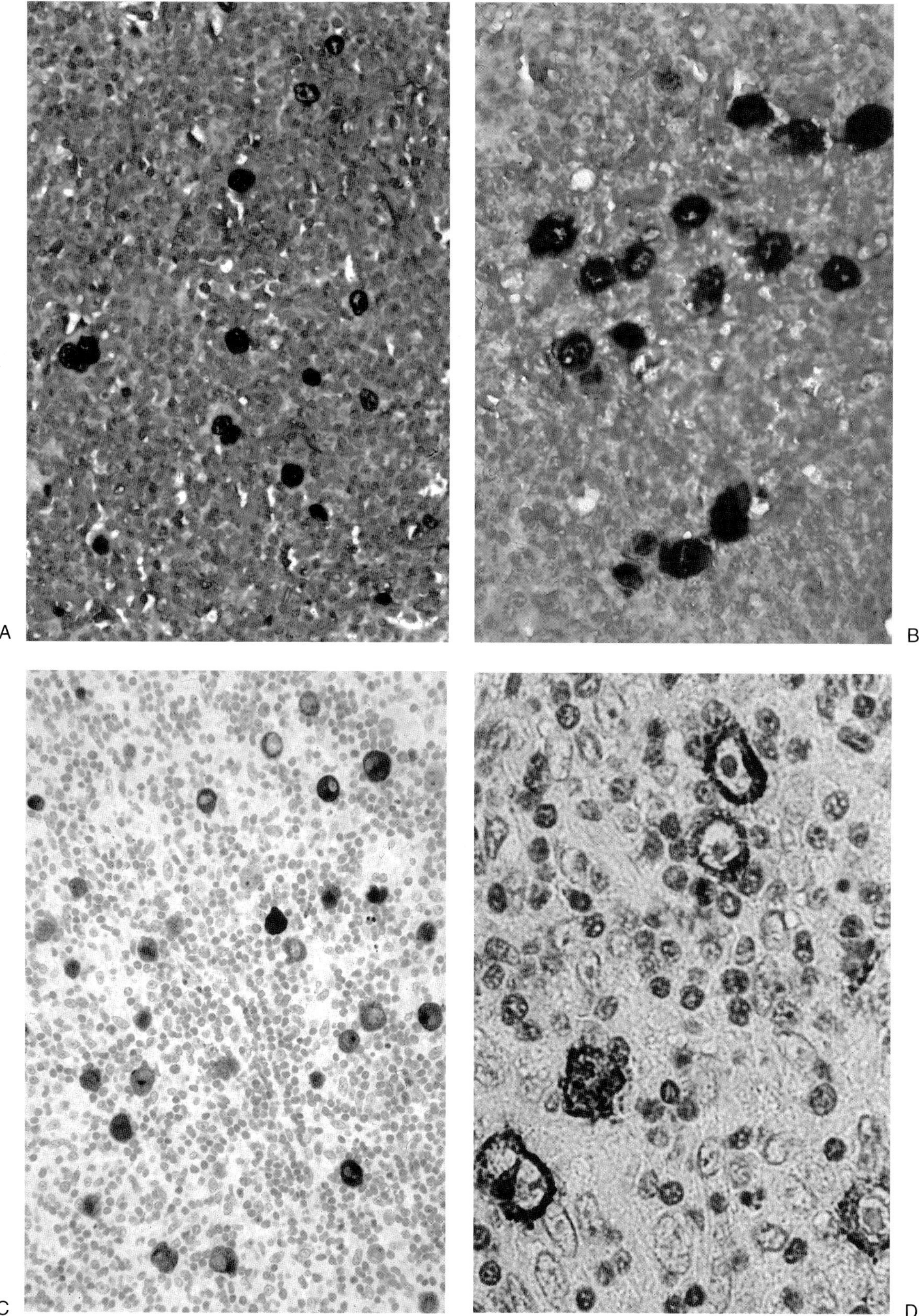

FIG. 5. Epstein-Barr viral (EBV) gene expression in Reed-Sternberg cells. **A:** Polymerase III transcript (EBER) *in situ* hybridization. **B:** EBER *in situ* hybridization with CD15 labeling of Hodgkin's cells. **C:** Latent membrane protein 1 (LMP1) immunohistochemistry. **D:** LMP2 immunohistochemistry. (These figures are printed in color as Plates 1 through 4.)

grated EBV genome becomes partially deleted. Interestingly, the LMP and EBER genes are among the genes that are deleted.

Lymphoproliferative disorders in patients with iatrogenically induced immunodeficiencies (such as lymphoproliferative disorders following transplantation), AIDS-associated malignant lymphomas, and lymphomas arising in patients with congenital immunodeficiencies have all been associated with EBV (88,102). EBV-associated posttransplantation lymphoproliferative disorders have been studied the longest and represent a relatively well-understood model of EBV tumor pathogenesis. Depending on the organ transplanted, the immunosuppressive regimen, and patient characteristics (age, whether the recipient is EBV-seronegative, and HLA differences between donor and recipient), lymphoproliferative disorders develop in approximately 1% to 10% of organ transplant recipients after transplantation. These cases show a range of histologic features, from clearly benign hyperplasia, to polymorphic proliferations, through monomorphic histologies that are indistinguishable from de novo malignant lymphoma. The hyperplasia is usually polyclonal or oligoclonal. The polymorphic proliferations are usually monoclonal but usually do not have additional genetic alterations. The monomorphic proliferations are usually monoclonal and are associated with additional alterations in either cellular proto-oncogenes or tumor suppressor genes. Approximately 95% of cases of posttransplantation lymphoproliferative disorders are associated with EBV (103–105). There is usually a high copy number of EBV genomes, usually of type A, which in *in situ* hybridization studies is demonstrable in all or virtually all the proliferating B cells. The EBV-infected cells usually show a type III latency pattern, probably because of the relatively immunocompromised status of the patient, although individual cells may show type I or type II latency patterns within the same case. LMP1 gene deletions, when they occur, are an early occurrence and do not correlate with aggressiveness of the proliferation (106).

It is been hypothesized that a posttransplantation lymphoproliferation arises from a polyclonal proliferation of EBV-infected cells that progresses to a clinical mass in patients with a relatively compromised immune system. Individual clones become dominant, leading to oligoclonal and then monoclonal proliferations. These proliferations may regress if immunosuppressive therapy is withdrawn or reduced. In other instances, monoclonal proliferations do not regress. This resistance to changes in immunosuppression may reflect the accumulation of additional genetic alterations, such as p53 mutations, rearrangements of c-myc, mutations of N-ras, or alterations in bcl6, that confer autonomy on the monoclonal proliferation, so that it is no longer affected by a mere reduction in immunosuppression (105). Alternatively, resistance to cytotoxic T cells may result from downregulation of immunodominant EBV genes commonly targeted by cytotoxic T cells (107,108). Accumulation of genetic mutations may occur simultaneously with downregulation of immunodominant EBV genes, so that accumulated mutations may render the viral genes that drive proliferation superfluous, while their immunodominance renders them a liability in a patient with a functioning immune system such that they are at a selective disadvantage.

It is thought that T-cell immunodeficiency, particularly in regard to the number of EBV-specific cytotoxic cells, is the most critical factor in the development of posttransplantation lymphoproliferations (109). For example, in bone marrow transplantation, the period when the patient is at greatest risk for lymphoproliferations coincides with the nadir for EBV-specific cytotoxic T cells (110). However, helper T cells may also play a role, as lymphoproliferations occur more often in patients with lower counts of CD4+ cells. Given this hypothesis of pathogenesis, several groups have attempted to treat posttransplantation lymphoproliferative disorders in human marrow allograft recipients with small populations of donor-derived lymphocytes, with impressive success (111). The limitation of this therapy is the possibility that, in addition to providing EBV-specific cytotoxic T cells, the infusions may also contain alloresponsive T cells capable of causing severe graft-versus-host disease. For this reason, several groups are exploring the use of virus-specific T-cell lines or antigen-specific T-cell lines (112, 113). Although the studies are preliminary, the results obtained to date are encouraging and provide additional evidence that virus-specific T cells are of critical importance in the pathogenesis of these lymphoproliferations.

In AIDS, T-cell surveillance is also defective, leading to abnormally high numbers of EBV-infected B cells in the peripheral blood and nonneoplastic lymphoid tissue (114). Approximately 40% to 67% of AIDS-associated lymphomas are EBV-associated (88). The association is higher in systemic and central nervous system immunoblastic lymphomas, neoplasms that tend to occur in persons with longstanding AIDS who have extremely low T-cell counts; the association is lower in small noncleaved or large-cell lymphomas, which tend to occur in nodal sites in persons with earlier-stage AIDS (115,116). One unusual AIDS-associated lymphoma is primary effusion lymphoma, in which tumor cells are found in serosal cavities without the formation of tumor masses (117,118). This neoplasm has been closely linked to Kaposi's sarcoma-related herpesvirus (KSHV, alternatively known as HHV-8), but EBV can also be identified in a majority of cases. EBV gene expression is very limited in these tumors (119).

In addition to B-cell lymphomas, a variety of peripheral T-cell or T/NK-cell lymphomas have been associated with EBV (88). The lymphoma with the highest association with EBV is the nasal-type T/NK-cell lymphoma. This is a relatively rare lymphoma in Western populations, but it has a high frequency of occurrence in Asian populations. This neoplasm has been associated with EBV in virtually all cases and in all populations studied (120). EBV can be identified by *in situ* hybridization in all or virtually all neoplastic cells. In contrast, in most other EBV-associated peripheral T-cell lymphomas, including angioimmunoblastic-like peripheral T-cell lymphoma, EBV is usually identified in only a subset of the neoplastic population (as well as in nonneoplastic B cells) (121,122). Detection of EBV in only a subset of tumor cells is consistent with EBV infection of cells in the early stages of tumor development, with loss of the viral genome from some cells during tumor progression, or with EBV infection and disease of established cells in association with tumor progression.

Epstein-Barr Virus in Hodgkin's Disease

Viral Nucleic Acid in Hodgkin's Disease

The presence of EBV genomic DNA in Hodgkin's disease was first reported by dot blot and Southern blot hybridization studies in 1987 (123) and was soon confirmed in several other reports (124–126). By means of these techniques, about 20% to 30% of cases of Hodgkin's disease were shown to be associated with EBV. With a probe directed against DNA sequences adjacent to the EBV terminus, the EBV genome has been shown to be present in a monoclonal population of cells in most cases, implying that the EBV is present before clonal expansion (123–127). The EBV genome has been estimated to be amplified at least 50-fold in the EBV+ Reed-Sternberg cells (128).

In situ hybridization studies localize the virus to Reed-Sternberg cells and variants (Hodgkin cells) (125,126, 129–132). *In situ* hybridization studies, most often utilizing probes to EBER RNA, have demonstrated that approximately 40% to 50% of cases of classic Hodgkin's disease occurring in immunocompetent persons in Western countries are EBV-associated (129,133–136). In almost all EBER+ cases, all or nearly all Reed-Sternberg cells are EBV+. EBV is detected in rare small lymphocytes by means of this methodology, both in cases of Hodgkin's disease in which the Reed-Sternberg cells are EBV+ and in cases in which the Reed-Sternberg cells are EBV- (133,136–140). As shown in double-labeling *in situ* hybridization/immunohistochemistry studies, these small lymphocytes are predominantly B-lineage (CD20+) lymphocytes, and a minority are T lymphocytes (CD3+ and CD43+). A small percentage of lymphocytes are unlabeled in these studies (133). These cells presumably reflect the presence of EBV-infected B and T lymphocytes in EBV-negative seropositive persons, as similar EBV+ cells can be identified in lymph nodes from normal controls. In two cases of EBV-associated Hodgkin's disease, the EBV infecting the Reed-Sternberg cells had a different BNLF1 gene than did the EBV infecting the reservoir lymphocytes, suggesting that the two populations were infected by different EBV strains (141). However, one group has speculated that these EBV+ small cells may be related to Reed-Sternberg cells; possibly they are precursors (137).

In approximately 50% to 80% of cases of Hodgkin's disease, whole-section extracts studied by PCR show evidence of EBV genomes (131,133,134,138,142–146). This incidence is a much higher than in results of *in situ* hybridization studies. However, the PCR-amplifiable EBV DNA undoubtedly includes EBV within the Reed-Sternberg cells and variants and also within latently infected lymphocytes of EBV-seropositive persons. Because of the overly high sensitivity of PCR studies, it has been recommended that *in situ* hybridization be utilized as the "gold standard" in determining whether a case of Hodgkin's disease is truly EBV-associated (147). EBV DNA also has been detected in individual Reed-Sternberg cells by using the technique of single-cell PCR (148,149).

Immunohistochemistry

Immunohistochemical studies have yielded additional data regarding the nature of EBV infection in Hodgkin's disease. Poppema and associates (150) were the first investigators to report immunohistochemical detection of a latent EBV gene product in Reed-Sternberg–like cells from a patient with chronic lymphadenopathy resembling Hodgkin's disease. EBNA1 protein has been demonstrated in paraffin sections in a majority of EBV+ cases (57). In 1991, Pallesen et al. (151) and Herbst et al. (152) used monoclonal antibody frozen section immunohistochemistry to identify abundant expression of LMP1 in Reed-Sternberg cells in approximately 50% of cases of Hodgkin's disease. Subsequent studies, particularly those using modern immunohistochemical techniques, have confirmed their findings. In addition, recent studies show that LMP1 paraffin-based immunohistochemistry studies and EBER *in situ* hybridization studies yield nearly identical results in Reed-Sternberg cells (116,134–136). In a given EBV+ case, approximately 50% to 90% of the Reed-Sternberg cells are usually LMP1+, although one study found a range from 7% to 100% (average, 69%) (153). However, in contrast to EBER antibodies, LMP1 antibodies do not stain small lymphocytes. In some cases, LMP1 protein may be detected in EBER– follicular dendritic cells, suggesting that it may have been taken up as an immune complex (154). LMP1 transcription in Hodgkin's disease resembles that seen in nasopharyngeal carcinoma. Immunoblotting reveals full-length LMP1 protein in Hodgkin's disease tissue extracts and a variable size of the LMP1 band, which are thought to be consistent with the presence of a different viral isolate in each of the cases.

EBV+ Reed-Sternberg cells also express the LMP2A antigen, and both LMP2A and LMP2B mRNAs have been identified by reverse transcription PCR studies

(56,58). The EBNA1 transcripts are driven from Qp. The Cp, which drives expression of EBNA2, EBNA3A, EBNA3B, and EBNA3C (the immunodominant EBNAs), is silent. As is true in other EBV-associated tumors in which the Cp is silent, the Cp region is heavily methylated. Reed-Sternberg cells lack the lytic proteins gp350/220, VCA, and early membrane antigen, and only a small minority of cells in a minority of cases express ZTA (also referred to as BZLF1) (138,155–157). Rare cases may express EA-R and BLLF1 transcripts (which encode for the membrane antigen gp350/220), consistent with active viral replication (158). These observations are consistent with a latent infection, with a coexisting abortive lytic infection present in a small number of cases and actual viral replication in rare cases. Even in Hodgkin's specimens from patients with HIV infection, latent rather than lytic infection predominates (157).

Correlates of the Viral Association with Hodgkin's Disease

Histologic type, age, sex, ethnicity, and the physiologic effects of poverty all affect the association of EBV with Hodgkin's disease. In one compilation of data from 1,546 patients with Hodgkin's disease in 14 studies, the risk for EBV+ disease was examined with logistic regression (159). The odds ratios for EBV-associated Hodgkin's disease were significantly elevated for mixed-cellularity versus nodular sclerosis histologic subtypes, male versus female young adults, Hispanics versus whites, and children from economically underdeveloped versus better-developed regions. EBV is most commonly associated with the mixed-cellularity and lymphocyte depletion subtypes of Hodgkin's disease (128,130,133,136,151, 160) and less frequently with the nodular sclerosis subtype of Hodgkin's disease. Nodular lymphocyte predominant cases virtually never contain EBV in the lymphocytic and histiocytic (L&H) cells (57,130,133,156), although rare cases of EBV+ cases have been reported (161). Age is also associated with EBV positivity in Hodgkin's disease. Several studies have found an increased incidence in children (defined as 0 to 15 years of age for Hodgkin's disease) in both developed and developing countries (162–164). Some studies suggest an increased incidence of EBV positivity in cases in adults more than 50 years of age as opposed to cases in patients between the ages of 15 and 50 years (162). In one study, it was demonstrated that age and histologic type are more predictive than geographic region in determining the association of EBV with Hodgkin's disease (165).

EBV positivity appears to correlate with geographic, cultural, genetic, and/or socioeconomic influences, all of which are difficult to separate. Among persons from the United States, most parts of Europe, and Israel, approximately 40% to 50% of cases of Hodgkin's disease have been shown to contain EBV+ Reed-Sternberg cells (133, 134,137,159,166). In contrast, among populations from less developed regions, particularly those with large numbers of pediatric cases of Hodgkin's disease (e.g., populations from Central and South America), a very high prevalence of EBV has been found. One study found an EBV prevalence rate of 94% in the Reed-Sternberg cells of cases of Hodgkin's disease among an indigenous Indian population from an underdeveloped area of Peru (167). In this study, the demographic features of the patient population were typical of those described for "third world" patients with Hodgkin's disease: a young median age (9 years), male predominance (male-female ratio of 3.5:1), and a predominance of the mixed cellularity subtype. EBV RNA was identified in all or nearly all the Reed-Sternberg cells and variants in 30 of the 32 cases. This high rate of EBV positivity was statistically significantly higher than that found in typical Western cases, even after control for age and histologic subtype. Another study found a 100% incidence of EBV positivity in a series of pediatric cases of Hodgkin's disease from Honduras (160). High rates of EBV positivity have also been reported in Brazilian (163), Mexican (168), and Argentine (169,170) series. The stronger association of EBV with Hodgkin's disease in Hispanics versus whites holds true even in U.S. series (128,160).

Cases of Hodgkin's disease in Africa also have a very high incidence of EBV positivity. In one study, 100% of 53 pediatric cases of Hodgkin's disease and 66% of 48 adult cases of Hodgkin's disease occurring in Kenya were associated with EBV (164); in another study, EBV positivity was found in 92% of Kenyan cases, in comparison with 48% of Italian cases (171). These results suggest that at least in Kenya, EBV may play a role similar to its role in endemic Burkitt's lymphoma. Other countries with a very high prevalence of EBV positivity in Hodgkin's disease include Iran and Greece (90% of pediatric cases) (164).

The incidence of EBV positivity in Asian populations may also be higher than that of Western populations. Zhou and colleagues (138) found an incidence of EBV EBER/LMP1 positivity in 61% of 28 cases from the People's Republic of China, and Chan and colleagues (172) found an incidence of EBV EBER positivity in 65% of 23 cases from Hong Kong. In a Maylasian series, the association of EBV with Hodgkin's disease was 61%, with a 93% association in childhood cases (173). In addition, seven of eight cases of pediatric Hodgkin's disease from Saudi Arabia and more than 70% of pediatric cases of Hodgkin's disease from Australia were EBV-associated (163,164). However, one study of Hodgkin's disease in the Philippines reported an EBV prevalence of 43%, a percentage similar to that of Western industrialized countries (174).

The incidence of EBV positivity in Hodgkin's disease occurring in HIV-infected patients is nearly 100%, which is higher than the rate of EBV positivity in HIV-associated non-Hodgkin's lymphomas (156,157,175). In contrast to Hodgkin's disease in immunocompetent persons, HIV-associated Hodgkin's disease is associated with both type 1 and type 2 EBV (176,177). In one study, the only EBV− case showed the histology of nodular lymphocyte predominance (175). In addition, cases of HIV-associated Hodgkin's disease have a very high prevalence of gene deletions at the 3' end of the LMP1 gene (10 of 10 cases and 10 of 12 cases in two reported series) (178,179).

Cases of familial Hodgkin's disease are less likely to be EBV-associated than are sporadic cases (180–182). In one large series of 60 patients from 27 families with familial Hodgkin's disease, the EBV association was 28%, with no excess of positive concordance (180). There was no correlation between EBV serology and EBV positivity in the series.

To date, univariate analyses have shown no correlation between the presence or absence of EBV and patient serology (183–185) or stage of disease (146). One study showed no correlation between the presence of EBV genomes and patient survival, but another recent study found that EBV positivity, as assessed by LMP1 immunostaining, was a favorable prognostic marker in a multivariate analysis (186). In patients with stage I Hodgkin's disease, EBV positivity has been associated with presentation in cervical lymph nodes (187). The relationship of EBV with bcl2 expression in Hodgkin's disease is somewhat controversial; Khan and colleagues found a 30% incidence of both bcl2 protein positivity and EBV positivity, but coexpression was found in only 4% of cases (188). The authors speculated that EBV infection and bcl2 expression may both have a pathogenetic role in Hodgkin's disease, with each representing different and exclusive events in a multistep pathway of oncogenesis. However, work by other groups does not support these conclusions (189–191). The different findings of Khan's group may be explained by the fact that most of their EBV+ cases were found in the category of MC, whereas most of the bcl2+ cases were found in the category of nodular sclerosis. Regardless of whether an inverse correlation between bcl2 and EBV exists, it is clear that EBV LMP1 expression in Reed-Sternberg cells does not lead to induction of the bcl2 protein in Hodgkin's cells, as may occur in B lymphocytes.

Cellular Gene Expression and Epstein-Barr Virus

Although there is no relationship between EBV and p53 expression (192,193), there may be an inverse correlation between EBV positivity and the identification of p53 mutations (193). It has been suggested that one EBV protein, EBNA-LP (also referred to as EBNA5), can form a complex with p53, providing one possible alternative means for p53 protein inactivation in the absence of mutation (194). However, others have presented evidence that latent viral gene expression does not inactivate p53, and the biologic significance of the *in vitro* interaction remains unresolved (195).

EBV positivity in Hodgkin's disease does not correlate with B-cell phenotype, the presence of clonal immunoglobulin heavy chain and T-cell receptor γ chain rearrangements (123,196), β_2-microglobulin, HLA-A2 or HLA-DR positivity (197,198), CD23 expression (189), or cytokine profile (199). However, there may be a decreased expression of lineage markers in EBV+ Reed-Sternberg cells (200).

Epstein-Barr Viral Strain

PCR studies have been useful in determining that type 1 EBV is detected in most cases occurring in immunocompetent persons (127,201). Partial deletions of the LMP1 gene were found in approximately 10% of cases, particularly those associated with numerous Reed-Sternberg cells, necrosis, and/or anaplasia, in at least one series (40,202). These deletions are consistently found in a region near the 3' end of the LMP1 gene, identical to deletions seen in cases of nasopharyngeal carcinoma that behave aggressively when transplanted into nude mice (203). These gene deletions lead to a loss of 10 amino acids near the carboxyl terminus of the protein, extending the half-life of the protein. Our studies show a high prevalence of LMP1 gene deletions in cases from the United States and Brazil (33% and 46%, respectively) (204). However, we found no correlation between LMP1 gene deletions and numbers or anaplasia of Reed-Sternberg cells, and we found an even higher frequency of LMP1 gene deletions in reactive lymphoid tissues, which suggests that LMP1 gene deletions may not be relevant to the pathogenesis of Hodgkin's disease outside the setting of HIV infection.

When multiple sites of disease have been studied, EBV-associated cases contain EBV+ Reed-Sternberg cells at all sites; similarly, recurrences of EBV-associated cases are usually EBV+ (132,205,206). However, there is one case report of a patient with EBV+ nodular sclerosing Hodgkin's disease who was found to be EBV− in the relapse of the tumor (207). Southern blotting studies in which a probe is directed against DNA near the EBV terminus have demonstrated EBV in the same clonal population at all involved sites (206,208). Furthermore, analysis of the EBV LMP1 gene has revealed identical deletions in both the diagnostic and relapse specimens of Hodgkin's disease (208). However, we have found that the presence or absence of EBV LMP1 deletions is not always consistent between all sites of disease, suggesting that some LMP1 gene deletions may be acquired after neoplastic transformation (205).

Association of Epstein-Barr Virus with Tumors Preceding, Coexisting with, or Following Hodgkin's Disease

EBV is infrequently identified in non-Hodgkin's lymphomas that precede, develop simultaneously with, or follow the development of Hodgkin's disease. However, several cases of composite Hodgkin's/non-Hodgkin's lymphoma have been reported in which both the Reed-Sternberg cells and B-cell lymphoma cells contained EBV (209). EBV has not been identified in cases of large-cell lymphoma associated with nodular lymphocyte predominance (210).

In situ hybridization studies were used to localize EBV to Hodgkin's-like cells in the extremely rare entity of chronic lymphocytic leukemia/small lymphocytic lymphoma with Reed-Sternberg–like cells (211). In addition to a low-grade B-cell lymphoproliferative disorder, all cases demonstrated occasional cells with cytologic features indistinguishable from those of Reed-Sternberg cells and variants, but without the typical background cells of Hodgkin's disease. The Reed-Sternberg–like cells of some cases had immunologic features of B cells, whereas in other cases, the Hodgkin's-like cells had immunologic features typical of Hodgkin's cells. In yet other cases, the Reed-Sternberg–like cells had a transitional phenotype. EBV was not found in the neoplastic small lymphocytes in any of the cases. Regardless of their phenotype, the Reed-Sternberg–like cells were shown to contain EBV in 12 of 13 cases. In some of the patients with this disease, disseminated Hodgkin's disease subsequently developed; the Reed-Sternberg cells in the subsequent Hodgkin's disease were also EBV+. Similar cases have been reported by other investigators (212).

Immunologic Aspects

Cytotoxic T-lymphocyte responses to LMP1 and LMP2 have been demonstrated in the blood of EBV-seropositive persons, yet the apparent failure of the cytotoxic T-cell response to eliminate tumor cells expressing LMP1 and LMP2 in Hodgkin's disease *in vivo* has given rise to the suggestion that Hodgkin's disease may be characterized by the presence of defects in antigen processing and presentation or in cytotoxic T-lymphocyte function. Several possible explanations for tumor resistance have been investigated: CD8+ cytotoxic T cells targeting EBV antigens might be ineffective because viral antigens are not presented by target cells, perhaps because of MHC class I downregulation or defects in antigen processing; viral antigens might not be recognized by CD8+ cytotoxic T cells because of strain variation or mutation; or effector cells might be rendered ineffective by the local cytokine milieu.

The discovery that Reed-Sternberg cells in many cases of Hodgkin's disease do not express MHC class I antigens suggested the possibility that virus-infected tumor cells might escape CD8+ immune surveillance (213). However, subsequent investigations yielded the curious finding that MHC class I downregulation is characteristic of EBV– Hodgkin's disease but rare in EBV+ Hodgkin's disease (214,215). Indeed, a high level of MHC class I expression may even be a consequence of EBV, insofar as LMP1 upregulates class I expression when transfected into EBV– B-cell lines (38).

Cells that express MHC class I might nonetheless fail to process antigen for presentation. Failure to process antigen for presentation is well established in endemic Burkitt's lymphoma cell lines that retain the type 1 phenotype. These lack the peptide transporter proteins TAP1 and TAP2. In contrast, investigation of a Hodgkin's disease cell line, HDLM2, shows antigen-processing pathways to be intact, such that following infection of these with recombinant vaccinia leading to the expression of EBV proteins, cells are efficiently lysed by antigen-specific CD8+ T cells (216). Immunohistochemistry demonstrates expression of TAP1 and TAP2 in tested Hodgkin's disease cell lines (HDLM2, L428, HS445 and Km-H2) and in Reed-Sternberg cells in paraffin-embedded or snap-frozen tumor tissue in almost every case (215).

Mutation or variation in expressed viral protein epitopes might also explain resistance to tumor killing. In healthy volunteers of HLA-A2.1 subtype, CD8+ cytotoxic T-cell precursors specific for an LMP2 epitope are readily demonstrated (71). One might anticipate that this epitope sequence in LMP2 would be a locus for such escape mutation. However, investigation of the LMP2 epitope sequence in tumor tissue from patients of HLA-A2.1 subtype with Hodgkin's disease shows little variation (215,217,218).

Evidence has been presented for local suppression of EBV-specific immunity in the vicinity of tumor. A study of EBV-specific responses in patients with EBV+ and EBV– Hodgkin's disease demonstrated virus-specific cytotoxicity in the tumor-infiltrating lymphocytes from EBV– but not EBV+ cases (219). The finding that precursors of cytotoxic T lymphocytes were detected in the blood of one of the EBV+ patients may be indicative of local immune suppression. One explanation of this finding might relate to the observation that a significantly higher proportion of EBV+ cases of Hodgkin's disease contained tumor cells expressing IL-10 in comparison with EBV- cases, suggesting that IL-10 production by tumor cells may be responsible for local downregulation of the cytotoxic T-lymphocyte response in EBV+ cases (220).

Therapeutic Aspects

Evidence that Reed-Sternberg cells express viral antigens and process these antigens for presentation has implications not only for the pathogenesis of Hodgkin's disease but also possibly for its treatment. Adoptive cellular immunotherapy has proved effective in the prevention and treatment of lymphoproliferative disease in the setting of bone marrow transplantation (111–113). Similar strategies for the treatment of Hodgkin's disease that specifically target tumor cells by virtue of their expression of viral antigens are presently being explored (112). Selective destruction of cells carrying viral genomes with viral antigen-specific T cells promises to make treatment of Hodgkin's disease more effective and less toxic.

Other Viruses

In contrast to EBV, other viruses have not been consistently implicated in Hodgkin's disease. Serologic studies of herpes simplex virus, varicella-zoster virus, cytomegalovirus, HHV-7, rubella virus, measles virus, and parainfluenza virus have all been negative (221). Elevated HHV-6 titers have been reported, but direct-detection studies using Southern blot hybridization have generally failed to detect viral DNA (222). In rare cases in which virus has been detected, there has been no evidence to support its localization to Reed-Sternberg cells (223,224). A recent study failed to detect adenovirus type 5 or 12, simian virus 40 (SV40), HHV-6, or HHV-8 (225).

CONCLUSION

Epidemiologic, serologic, and direct-detection studies all independently point to EBV as a potential etiologic cofactor. Clonality studies show that viral infection precedes clonal expansion of tumor cells. The ability of the virus to immortalize lymphocytes in tissue culture and other properties of the viral genome lend biologic plausibility to the theory of virus as cofactor, as does the viral association with many other tumor types. However, as with other human tumor viruses, the relationship between infection and tumorigenesis remains complex and poorly understood. Even before these questions are completely resolved, it is possible that the presence of viral antigens may provide tumor-specific targets for new therapeutic strategies.

REFERENCES

1. MacMahon B. Epidemiological evidence on the nature of Hodgkin's disease. *Cancer* 1957;10:1045–1054.
2. Veltri RW, Shah SH, McClung JE, Klingberg WG, Sprinkle PM. Epstein-Barr virus, fatal infectious mononucleosis, and Hodgkin's disease in siblings. *Cancer* 1983;51:509–520.
3. Miller RW, Beebe GW. Infectious mononucleosis and the empirical risk of cancer. *J Natl Cancer Inst* 1973;50:315–321.
4. Kvale G, Hoiby EA, Pedersen E. Hodgkin's disease in patients with previous infectious mononucleosis. *Int J Cancer* 1979;23:593–597.
5. Mueller N, Evans A, Harris NL, et al. Hodgkin's disease and Epstein-Barr virus. Altered antibody pattern before diagnosis. *N Engl J Med* 1989;320:689–695.
6. Baer B, Bankier A, Biggin MD, et al. DNA sequence and expression of the B95-8 Epstein-Barr virus genome. *Nature* 1984;310:207–211.
7. Kieff E. Epstein-Barr virus and its replication. In: Fields BN, Knipe DM, Howley PM, et al., eds. *Fields virology*. Philadelphia: Lippincott–Raven Publishers, 1996:2343–2396.
8. Rickinson AB, Kieff E. Epstein-Barr Virus. In: Fields BN, Knipe DM, Howley PM, et al., eds. *Fields virology*. Philadelphia: Lippincott–Raven Publishers, 1996:2397–2446.
9. Evans AS, Niederman JC, McCollum RW. Seroepidemiologic studies of infectious mononucleosis with EB virus. *N Engl J Med* 1968;279: 1121–1127.
10. Henle G, Henle W, Diehl V. Relation of Burkitt's tumor-associated herpes-type virus to infectious mononucleosis. *Proc Natl Acad Sci U S A* 1968;59:94–101.
11. Yao Q, Rickinson A, Epstein M. Oropharyngeal shedding of infectious Epstein-Barr virus in healthy virus immune donors: a prospective study. *Chin Med J* 1988;98:191–196.
12. Lemon SM, Hutt LM, Shaw JE, Li J-LH, Pagano JS. Replication of EBV in epithelial cells during infectious mononucleosis. *Nature* 1977; 268:268–270.
13. Sixbey JW, Nedrud JG, Raab-Traub N, Hanes RA, Pagano JS. Epstein-Barr virus replication in oropharyngeal epithelial cells. *N Engl J Med* 1984;310:1225–1230.
14. Diehl V, Henle G, Henle W, Kohn G. Demonstration of a herpes group virus in cultures of peripheral leukocytes from patients with infectious mononucleosis. *J Virol* 1968;2:663–669.
15. Klein G, Svedmyr E, Jondal M, Persson PO. EBV-determined nuclear antigen (EBNA)-positive cells in the peripheral blood of infectious mononucleosis patients. *Int J Cancer* 1976;17:21–26.
16. Ryon JJ, Hayward SD, MacMahon EME, et al. *In situ* detection of lytic Epstein-Barr virus infection: expression of the Not1 early gene and vIL-10 late gene in clinical specimens. *J Infect Dis* 1993;168: 345–351.
17. Reynolds DJ, Banks PM, Gulley ML. New characterization of infectious mononucleosis and a phenotypic comparison with Hodgkin's disease. *Am J Pathol* 1995;146:379–388.
18. Laroche C, Drouet EB, Brousset P, et al. Measurement by the polymerase chain reaction of the Epstein-Barr virus load in infectious mononucleosis and AIDS-related non-Hodgkin's lymphomas. *J Med Virol* 1995;46:66–74.
19. Tierney RJ, Steven N, Young LS, Rickinson AB. Epstein-Barr virus latency in blood mononuclear cells—analysis of viral gene transcription during primary infection and in the carrier state. *J Virol* 1994; 68:7374–7385.
20. Callan MF, Steven N, Krausa P, et al. Large clonal expansions of CD8+ T cells in acute infectious mononucleosis. *Nat Med* 1996;2:906–911.
21. Rickinson AB, Finerty S, Epstein MA. Mechanism of the establishment of Epstein-Barr virus genome containing lymphoid cell lines from infectious mononucleosis patients: studies with phosphonoacetate. *Int J Cancer* 1977;20:861–868.
22. Rickinson AB, Rowe M, Hart IJ, et al. T-cell-mediated regression of "spontaneous" and of Epstein-Barr virus-induced B-cell transformation *in vitro*: studies with cyclosporin A. *Cell Immunol* 1984;87:646–658.
23. Yao QY, Rickinson AB, Epstein MA. A re-examination of the Epstein-Barr virus carrier state in healthy seropositive individuals. *Int J Cancer* 1985;35:35–43.
24. Miyashita EM, Yang B, Lam KM, Crawford DH, Thorley-Lawson DA. A novel form of Epstein-Barr virus latency in normal B cells *in vivo*. *Cell* 1995;80:593–601.
25. Martin DR, Marlowe RL, Ahearn JM. Determination of the role for CD21 during Epstein-Barr virus infection of B-lymphoblastoid cells. *J Virol* 1994;68:4716–4726.
26. Li Q, Spriggs MK, Kovats S, et al. Epstein-Barr virus uses HLA class II as a cofactor for infection of B lymphocytes. *J Virol* 1997;71: 4657–4662.
27. Kurilla MG, Heineman T, Davenport LC, Kieff E, Hutt-Fletcher LM. A novel Epstein-Barr virus glycoprotein gp150 expressed from the BDLF3 open reading frame. *Virology* 1995;209:108–121.
28. Rowe M, Young LS, Crocker J, Stokes H, Henderson S, Rickinson AB. Epstein-Barr virus (EBV)-associated lymphoproliferative disease in the SCID mouse model: implications for the pathogenesis of EBV-positive lymphomas in man. *J Exp Med* 1991;173:147–158.
29. Yates JL, Warren N, Sugden B. Stable replication of plasmids derived from Epstein-Barr virus in various mammalian cells. *Nature* 1985; 313:812–815.
30. Rawlins DR, Milman G, Hayward SD, Hayward GS. Sequence-specific DNA binding of the Epstein-Barr virus nuclear antigen (EBNA-1) to clustered sites in the plasmid maintenance region. *Cell* 1985; 42:859–868.
31. Grossman SR, Johannsen E, Tong X, Yalamanchili R, Kieff E. The Epstein-Barr virus nuclear antigen 2 transactivator is directed to response elements by the J kappa recombination signal binding protein. *Proc Natl Acad Sci U S A* 1994;91:7568–7572.
32. Henkel T, Ling PD, Hayward SD, Peterson MG. Mediation of Epstein-Barr virus EBNA2 transactivation by recombination signal-binding protein J kappa. *Science* 1994;265:92–95.
33. Hsieh JJ, Hayward SD. Masking of the CBF1/RBPJ kappa transcriptional repression domain by Epstein-Barr virus EBNA2. *Science* 1995;268:560–563.

34. Cohen JI, Wang F, Mannick J, Kieff E. Epstein-Barr virus nuclear protein 2 is a key determinant of lymphocyte transformation. *Proc Natl Acad Sci U S A* 1989;86:9558–9562.
35. Izumi KM, Kaye KM, Kieff ED. The Epstein-Barr virus LMP1 amino acid sequence that engages tumor necrosis factor receptor associated factors is critical for primary B lymphocyte growth transformation. *Proc Natl Acad Sci U S A* 1997;94:1447–1452.
36. Henderson S, Rowe M, Gregory C, et al. Induction of *bcl*-2 expression by Epstein-Barr virus latent membrane protein 1 protects infected B cells from programmed cell death. *Cell* 1991;65:1107–1115.
37. Nakagomi H, Dolcetti R, Bejarano MT, Pisa P, Kiessling R, Masucci MG. The Epstein-Barr virus latent membrane protein-1 (LMP1) induces interleukin-10 production in Burkitt lymphoma lines. *Int J Cancer* 1994;57:240–244.
38. Cuomo L, Trivedi P, Wang F, Wimberg G, Klein G, Masucci M. Expression of the Epstein-Barr virus (EBV)-encoded membrane antigen LMP increases the stimulatory capacity of EBV negative B lymphoma lines in allogeneic mixed lymphocyte cultures. *Eur J Immunol* 1990;20:2293–2299.
39. Wang D, Liebowitz D, Kieff E. An EBV membrane protein expressed in immortalized lymphocytes transforms established rodent cells. *Cell* 1985;43:831–840.
40. Knecht H, Bachmann E, Brousset P, et al. Deletions within the LMP1 oncogene of Epstein-Barr virus are clustered in Hodgkin's disease and identical to those observed in nasopharyngeal carcinoma. *Blood* 1993;82:2937–2942.
41. Miller WE, Edwards RH, Walling DM, Raab-Traub N. Sequence variation in the Epstein-Barr virus latent membrane protein 1. *J Gen Virol* 1994;75:2729–2740.
42. Longnecker R, Kieff E. A second Epstein-Barr virus membrane protein (LMP2) is expressed in latent infection and colocalizes with LMP1. *J Virol* 1990;64:2319–2326.
43. Miller CL, Longnecker R, Kieff E. Epstein-Barr virus latent membrane protein 2A blocks calcium mobilization in B lymphocytes. *J Virol* 1993;67:3087–3094.
44. Miller CL, Burkhardt AL, Lee JH, et al. Integral membrane protein 2 of Epstein-Barr virus regulates reactivation from latency through dominant negative effects on protein-tyrosine kinases. *Immunity* 1995;2:155–166.
45. Swaminathan S, Tomkinson B, Kieff E. Recombinant Epstein-Barr virus with small RNA (EBER) genes deleted transforms lymphocytes and replicates *in vitro*. *Proc Natl Acad Sci U S A* 1991;88:1546–1550.
46. Arrand JR, Rymo L. Characterization of the major Epstein-Barr virus-specific RNA in Burkitt lymphoma-derived cells. *J Virol* 1982;41:376–389.
47. Howe JG, Steitz JA. Localization of Epstein-Barr virus-encoded small RNAs by *in situ* hybridization. *Proc Natl Acad Sci U S A* 1986;83:9006–9010.
48. Howe JG, Shu MD. Epstein-Barr virus small RNA (EBER) genes: unique transcription units that combine RNA polymerase II and III promoter elements. *Cell* 1989;57:825–834.
49. Davies AH, Grand RJA, Evans FJ, Rickinson AB. Induction of Epstein-Barr virus lytic cycle by tumor-promoting and non–tumor-promoting phorbol esters requires active protein kinase C. *J Virol* 1991;65:6838–6844.
50. Countryman J, Miller G. Activation of expression of latent Epstein-Barr herpesvirus after gene transfer with a small cloned subfragment of heterogeneous viral DNA. *Proc Natl Acad Sci U S A* 1985;82:4085–4089.
51. Sarisky RT, Gao Z, Lieberman PM, Fixman ED, Hayward GS, Hayward SD. A replication function associated with the activation domain of the Epstein-Barr virus Zta transactivator. *J Virol* 1996;70:8340–8347.
52. Henderson S, Huen D, Rowe M, Dawson C, Johnson G, Rickinson A. Epstein-Barr virus-coded BHRF1 protein, a viral homologue of Bcl-2, protects human B cells from programmed cell death. *Proc Natl Acad Sci U S A* 1993;90:8479–8483.
53. Vieira P, de Waal-Malefyt R, Dang MN, et al. Isolation and expression of human cytokine synthesis inhibitory factor cDNA clones: homology to Epstein-Barr virus open reading frame BCRFI. *Proc Natl Acad Sci U S A* 1991;88:1172–1176.
54. Gesser B, Leffers H, Jinquan T, et al. Identification of functional domains on human interleukin 10. *Proc Natl Acad Sci U S A* 1997;94:14620–14625.
55. Young L, Alfieri C, Hennessy K, et al. Expression of Epstein-Barr virus transformation-associated genes in tissues of patients with EBV lymphoproliferative disease. *N Engl J Med* 1989;321:1080–1085.
56. Deacon EM, Pallesen G, Niedobitek G, et al. Epstein-Barr virus and Hodgkin's disease: transcriptional analysis of virus latency in the malignant cells. *J Exp Med* 1993;177:339–349.
57. Grasser FA, Murray PG, Kremmer E, et al. Monoclonal antibodies directed against the Epstein-Barr virus-encoded nuclear antigen 1 (EBNA1): immunohistologic detection of EBNA1 in the malignant cells of Hodgkin's disease. *Blood* 1994;84:3792–3798.
58. Niedobitek G, Kremmer E, Herbst H, et al. Immunohistochemical detection of the Epstein-Barr virus-encoded latent membrane protein 2A in Hodgkin's disease and infectious mononucleosis. *Blood* 1997;90:1664–1672.
59. Niedobitek G, Agathanggelou A, Rowe M, et al. Heterogeneous expression of Epstein-Barr virus latent proteins in endemic Burkitt's lymphoma. *Blood* 1995;86:659–665.
60. Robertson KD, Manns A, Swinnen LJ, Zong JC, Gulley ML, Ambinder RF. CpG methylation of the major Epstein-Barr virus latency promoter in Burkitt's lymphoma and Hodgkin's disease. *Blood* 1996;88:3129–3136.
61. Qu L, Rowe DT. Epstein-Barr virus latent gene expression in uncultured peripheral blood lymphocytes. *J Virol* 1992;66:3715–3724.
62. Chen F, Zou JZ, di Renzo L, et al. A subpopulation of normal B cells latently infected with Epstein-Barr virus resembles Burkitt lymphoma cells in expressing EBNA-1 but not EBNA-2 or LMP1. *J Virol* 1995;69:3752–3758.
63. Miyashita EM, Yang B, Babcock GJ, Thorley-Lawson DA. Identification of the site of Epstein-Barr virus persistence *in vivo* as a resting B cell. *J Virol* 1997;71:4882–4891.
64. Robertson KD, Ambinder RF. Methylation of the Epstein-Barr virus genome in normal lymphocytes. *Blood* 1997;90:4480–4484.
65. Milman G, Scott AL, Cho MS, et al. Carboxyl-terminal domain of the Epstein-Barr virus nuclear antigen is highly immunogenic in man. *Proc Natl Acad Sci U S A* 1985;82:6300–6304.
66. van Grunsven WM, Spaan WJ, Middeldorp JM. Localization and diagnostic application of immunodominant domains of the BFRF3-encoded Epstein-Barr virus capsid protein. *J Infect Dis* 1994;170:13–19.
67. Tomkinson BE, Maziarz R, Sullivan JL. Characterization of the T cell-mediated cellular cytotoxicity during acute infectious mononucleosis. *J Immunol* 1989;143:660–670.
68. Misko IS, Pope JH, Hutter R, Soszynski TD, Kane RG. HLA-DR-antigen-associated restriction of EBV-specific cytotoxic T-cell colonies. *Int J Cancer* 1984;33:239–243.
69. Bourgault I, Gomez A, Gomard E, Levy JP. Limiting-dilution analysis of the HLA restriction of anti-Epstein-Barr virus-specific cytolytic T lymphocytes. *Clin Exp Immunol* 1991;84:501–507.
70. Khanna R, Burrows SR, Kurilla MG, et al. Localization of Epstein-Barr virus cytotoxic T cell epitopes using recombinant vaccinia: implications for vaccine development. *J Exp Med* 1992;176:169–176.
71. Murray RJ, Kurilla MG, Brooks JM, et al. Identification of target antigens for the human cytotoxic T cell response to Epstein-Barr virus (EBV): implications for the immune control of EBV-positive malignancies. *J Exp Med* 1992;176:157–168.
72. Blake N, Lee S, Redchenko I, et al. Human CD8+ T cell responses to EBV EBNA1: HLA class I presentation of the (Gly-Ala)-containing protein requires exogenous processing. *Immunity* 1997;7:791–802.
73. Levitskaya J, Coram M, Levitsky V, et al. Inhibition of antigen processing by the internal repeat region of the Epstein-Barr virus nuclear antigen-1. *Nature* 1995;375:685–688.
74. Shope T, Dechairo D, Miller G. Malignant lymphoma in cottontop marmosets after inoculation with Epstein-Barr virus. *Proc Natl Acad Sci U S A* 1973;70:2487–2491.
75. Mosier DE, Baird SM, Kirven MB, et al. EBV-associated B-cell lymphomas following transfer of human peripheral blood lymphocytes to mice with severe combined immune deficiency. *Curr Top Microbiol Immunol* 1990;166:317–323.
76. Wilson JB, Bell JL, Levine AJ. Expression of Epstein-Barr virus nuclear antigen-1 induces B cell neoplasia in transgenic mice. *EMBO J* 1996;15:3117–3126.
77. Gulley ML, Raphael M, Lutz CT, Ross DW, Raab-Traub N. Epstein-Barr virus integration in human lymphomas and lymphoid cell lines. *Cancer* 1992;70:185–191.
78. Sato H, Takimoto T, Tanaka S, Tanaka J, Raab-Traub N. Concatameric

replication of Epstein-Barr virus: structure of the termini in virus-producer and newly transformed cell lines. *J Virol* 1990;64:5295–5300.
79. Ambinder R, Mann R. Epstein-Barr-encoded RNA *in situ* hybridization. *Hum Pathol* 1994;25:602–605.
80. Ambinder R, Mann R. Detection and characterization of Epstein-Barr virus in clinical specimens. *Am J Pathol* 1994;149:235–252.
81. Wu TC, Mann RB, Epstein J, et al. Abundant expression of EBER1 small nuclear RNA in nasopharyngeal carcinoma: a morphologically distinctive target for detection of Epstein-Barr virus in formalin-fixed paraffin-embedded carcinoma specimens. *Am J Pathol* 1991;138:1461–1469.
82. Iezzoni JC, Gaffey MJ, Weiss LM. The role of Epstein-Barr virus in lymphoepithelioma-like carcinomas. *Am J Clin Pathol* 1995;103:308–315.
83. Niedobitek G, Herbst H. Epstein-Barr virus-associated carcinomas. *EBV Rep* 1994;1994:81–85.
84. Shibata D, Weiss LM. Epstein-Barr virus-associated gastric adenocarcinoma. *Am J Pathol* 1992;140:769–774.
85. Shibata D, Tokunaga M, Uemura Y, Sato E, Tanaka S, Weiss LM. Association of Epstein-Barr virus with undifferentiated gastric carcinoma with intense lymphoid infiltration. *Am J Pathol* 1991;139:469–474.
86. Lee ES, Locker JL, Nalesnik M, et al. The association of Epstein-Barr virus with smooth-muscle tumors occurring after organ transplantation. *N Engl J Med* 1995;332:19–25.
87. Arber DA, Kamel OW, van de Rijn M, et al. Frequent presence of the Epstein-Barr virus in inflammatory pseudotumor. *Hum Pathol* 1995;26:1093–1098.
88. Weiss LM, Chang KL. Association of the Epstein-Barr virus with hematolymphoid neoplasia. *Adv Anat Pathol* 1996;3:1–15.
89. Epstein MA, Achong BG, Barr YM. Virus particles in cultured lymphoblasts from Burkitt's lymphoma. *Lancet* 1964;1:702–703.
90. Lenoir GM, Philip T, Sohler R. EBV association and cytogenetic markers in cases from various geographic locations. In: Magrath I, O'Conor G, eds. *Pathogenesis of leukemias and lymphomas: environmental influences*. New York: Raven Press, 1984:283.
91. Shiramizu B, Barriga F, Neequaye J, et al. Patterns of chromosomal breakpoint locations in Burkitt's lymphoma: relevance to geography and Epstein-Barr virus association. *Blood* 1991;77:1516–1526.
92. Bacchi MM, Bacchi CE, Alvarenga M, Miranda R, Chen YY, Weiss LM. Burkitt's lymphoma in Brazil: strong association with Epstein-Barr virus. *Mod Pathol* 1996;9:63–67.
93. Gutierrez MI, Bhatia K, Barriga F, et al. Molecular epidemiology of Burkitt's lymphoma from South America: differences in breakpoint location and Epstein-Barr virus association from tumors in other world regions. *Blood* 1992;79:3261–3266.
94. Hummel M, Anagnostopoulos I, Korbjuhn P, Stein H. Epstein-Barr virus in B-cell non-Hodgkin's lymphomas: unexpected infection patterns and different infection incidence in low- and high-grade types. *J Pathol* 1995;175:263–271.
95. Chan JK, Tsang WY, Ng CS, Wong CS, Lo ES. A study of the association of Epstein-Barr virus with Burkitt's lymphoma occurring in a Chinese population. *Histopathology* 1995;26:239–245.
96. Tao Q, Robertson KD, Manns A, Hildesheim A, Ambinder RF. Epstein-Barr virus (EBV) in endemic Burkitt's lymphoma: molecular analysis of primary tumor tissue. *Blood* 1998;91:1373–1381.
97. Rowe M, Rowe DT, Gregory CD, et al. Differences in B cell growth phenotype reflect novel patterns of Epstein-Barr virus latent gene expression in Burkitt's lymphoma cells. *EMBO J* 1987;6:2743–2751.
98. Bhatia K, Raj A, Gutierrez MI, et al. Variation in the sequence of Epstein-Barr virus nuclear antigen 1 in normal peripheral blood lymphocytes and in Burkitt's lymphomas. *Oncogene* 1996;13:177–181.
99. Shimizu N, Tanabetochikura A, Kuroiwa Y, Takada K. Isolation of Epstein-Barr virus (EBV)-negative cell clones from the EBV-positive Burkitt's lymphoma (BL) line. Akata-malignant phenotypes of BL cells are dependent on EBV. *J Virol* 1994;68:6069–6073.
100. Razzouk BI, Srinivas S, Sample CE, Singh V, Sixbey JW. Epstein-Barr virus DNA recombination and loss in sporadic Burkitt's lymphoma. J Infect Dis 1996;173:529–535.
101. Jox A, Rohen C, Belge G, et al. Integration of Epstein-Barr virus in Burkitt's lymphoma cells leads to a region of enhanced chromosome instability. *Ann Oncol* 1997;8(Suppl 2):131–135.
102. Filipovich AH, Mertens A, Robison L, Ambinder RF, Shapiro RS, Frizzera G. Lymphoproliferative disorders associated with primary immunodeficiencies. In: Magrath I, ed. *The non-Hodgkin's lymphomas*, 2nd ed. New York: Oxford University Press, 1995:459–471.
103. Randhawa PS, Jaffe R, Demetris AJ, et al. The systemic distribution of Epstein-Barr virus genomes in fatal post-transplantation lymphoproliferative disorders. *Am* J Pathol 1991;138:1027–1033.
104. Cleary ML, Nalesnik MA, Shearer WT, Sklar J. Clonal analysis of transplant-associated lymphoproliferations based on the structure of the genomic termini of the Epstein-Barr virus. *Blood* 1988;72:349–352.
105. Knowles DM, Cesarman E, Chadburn A, et al. Correlative morphologic and molecular genetic analysis demonstrates three distinct categories of posttransplantation lymphoproliferative disorders. *Blood* 1995;85:552–565.
106. Scheinfeld AG, Nador RG, Cesarman E, Chadburn A, Knowles DM. Epstein-Barr virus latent membrane protein-1 oncogene deletion in post-transplantation lymphoproliferative disorders. *Am* J Pathol 1997;151:805–812.
107. Cen H, Williams PA, McWilliams HP, Breinig MC, Ho M, McKnight JL. Evidence for restricted Epstein-Barr virus latent gene expression and anti-EBNA antibody response in solid organ transplant recipients with posttransplant lymphoproliferative disorders. *Blood* 1993;81:1393–1403.
108. Oudejans JJ, Jiwa M, Vandenbrule AJC, et al. Detection of heterogeneous Epstein-Barr virus gene expression patterns within individual post-transplantation lymphoproliferative disorders. *Am* J Pathol 1995;147:923–933.
109. O'Reilly RJ, Small TN, Papadopoulos E, Lucas K, Lacerda J, Koulova L. Biology and adoptive cell therapy of Epstein-Barr virus-associated lymphoproliferative disorders in recipients of marrow allografts. *Immunol Rev* 1997;157:195–216.
110. Lucas KG, Small TN, Heller G, Dupont B, O'Reilly RJ. The development of cellular immunity to Epstein-Barr virus after allogeneic bone marrow transplantation. *Blood* 1996;87:2594–2603.
111. Papadopoulos EB, Ladanyi M, Emanuel D, et al. Infusions of donor leukocytes to treat Epstein-Barr virus-associated lymphoproliferative disorders after allogeneic bone marrow transplantation. *N Engl J Med* 1994;33:1185–1191.
112. Rooney CM, Smith CA, Ng CY, et al. Use of gene-modified virus-specific T lymphocytes to control Epstein-Barr-virus-related lymphoproliferation. Lancet 1995;345:9–13.
113. Heslop HE, Ng CY, Li C, et al. Long-term restoration of immunity against Epstein-Barr virus infection by adoptive transfer of gene-modified virus-specific T lymphocytes. *Nat Med* 1996;2:551–555.
114. Arber DA, Shibata D, Chen YY, Weiss LM. Characterization of the topography of Epstein-Barr virus infection in human immunodeficiency virus-associated lymphoid tissues. *Mod Pathol* 1992;5:559–566.
115. Raphael MM, Audouin J, Lamine M, et al. Immunophenotypic and genotypic analysis of acquired immunodeficiency syndrome-related non-Hodgkin's lymphomas. Correlation with histologic features in 36 cases. French Study Group of Pathology for HIV-associated Tumors. *Am J Clin Pathol* 1994;101:773–782.
116. Hamilton-Dutoit SJ, Pallesen G, Franzmann MB, et al. AIDS-related lymphoma: histopathology, immunophenotype, and association with Epstein-Barr virus as demonstrated by *in situ* nucleic acid hybridization. *Am* J Pathol 1991;138:149–163.
117. Nador RG, Cesarman E, Chadburn A, et al. Primary effusion lymphoma: a distinct clinicopathologic entity associated with the Kaposi's sarcoma-associated herpes virus. *Blood* 1996;88:645–656.
118. Cesarman E, Chang Y, Moore PS, Said JW, Knowles DM. Kaposi's sarcoma-associated herpesvirus-like DNA sequences in AIDS-related body-cavity-based lymphomas. *N Engl J Med* 1995;332:1186–1191.
119. Horenstein MG, Nador RG, Chadburn A, et al. Epstein-Barr virus latent gene expression in primary effusion lymphomas containing Kaposi's sarcoma-associated herpesvirus/human herpesvirus- 8. *Blood* 1997;90:1186–1191.
120. Weiss LM, Gaffey MJ, Chen Y-Y, Frierson HF Jr. Frequency of EBV DNA in "Western" sinonasal and Waldeyer's ring non-Hodgkin's (T and B cell) lymphomas. *Am J Surg Pathol* 1992;16:156–162.
121. Weiss LM, Jaffe ES, Liu XF, Chen YY, Shibata D, Medeiros LJ. Detection and localization of Epstein-Barr viral genomes in angioimmunoblastic lymphadenopathy and angioimmunoblastic lymphadenopathy-like lymphoma. *Blood* 1992;79:1789–1795.
122. Anagnostopoulos I, Hummel M, Finn T, et al. Heterogeneous Epstein-Barr virus infection patterns in peripheral T-cell lymphoma of angioimmunoblastic lymphadenopathy type. *Blood* 1992;80:1804–1812.
123. Weiss LM, Strickler JG, Warnke RA, Purtilo DT, Sklar J. Epstein-Barr

viral DNA in tissues of Hodgkin's disease. *Am* J Pathol 1987;129: 86–91.
124. Staal SP, Ambinder R, Beschorner WE, Hayward GS, Mann R. A survey of Epstein-Barr virus DNA in lymphoid tissue: frequent detection in Hodgkin's disease. *Am J Clin Pathol* 1989;91:1–5.
125. Weiss LM, Movahed LA, Warnke RA, Sklar J. Detection of Epstein-Barr viral genomes in Reed-Sternberg cells of Hodgkin's disease. *N Engl J Med* 1989;320:502–506.
126. Anagnostopoulos I, Herbst H, Niedobitek G, Stein H. Demonstration of monoclonal EBV genomes in Hodgkin's disease and Ki-1 positive anaplastic large cell lymphoma by combined Southern blot and *in situ* hybridization. *Blood* 1989;74:810–816.
127. Gledhill S, Gallagher A, Jones DB, et al. Viral involvement in Hodgkin's disease: detection of clonal type A Epstein-Barr virus genomes in tumour samples. *Br J Cancer* 1991;64:227–232.
128. Gulley ML, Eagan PA, Quintanilla-Martinez L, et al. Epstein-Barr virus DNA is abundant and monoclonal in the Reed-Sternberg cells of Hodgkin's disease: association with mixed cellularity subtype and Hispanic American ethnicity. *Blood* 1994;83:1595–1602.
129. Wu TC, Mann RB, Charache P, et al. Detection of EBV gene expression in Reed-Sternberg cells of Hodgkin's disease. *Int J Cancer* 1990; 46:801–804.
130. Brousset PB, Chittal S, Schlaifer D, et al. Detection of Epstein-Barr virus messenger RNA in Reed-Sternberg cells of Hodgkin's disease by *in situ* hybridization with biotinylated probes on specially processed modified acetone methyl benzoate xylene (ModAMeX) sections. *Blood* 1991;77:1781–1786.
131. Uhara H, Sato Y, Mukai K, et al. Detection of Epstein-Barr virus DNA in Reed-Sternberg cells of Hodgkin's disease using the polymerase chain reaction and *in situ* hybridization. *Jpn J Cancer Res* 1990;81: 272–278.
132. Coates PJ, Slavin G, d'Ardenne AJ. Persistence of Epstein-Barr virus in Reed-Sternberg cells throughout the course of Hodgkin's disease. *J Pathol* 1991;164:291–297.
133. Weiss LM, Chen YY, Liu XF, Shibata D. Epstein-Barr virus and Hodgkin's disease: a correlative *in situ* hybridization and polymerase chain reaction study. *Am* J Pathol 1991;139:1259–1265.
134. Lauritzen AF, Hording U, Nielsen HW. Epstein-Barr virus and Hodgkin's disease: a comparative immunological, *in situ* hybridization, and polymerase chain reaction study. *APMIS* 1994;102:495–500.
135. Khan G, Coates PJ, Gupta RK, Kangro HO, Slavin G. Presence of Epstein-Barr virus in Hodgkin's disease is not exclusive to Reed-Sternberg cells. *Am* J Pathol 1992;140:757–762.
136. Herbst H, Steinbrecher E, Niedobitek G, et al. Distribution and phenotype of Epstein-Barr virus-harboring cells in Hodgkin's disease. *Blood* 1992;80:484–491.
137. Jiwa NM, Kanavaros P, De Bruin PC, et al. Presence of Epstein-Barr virus harbouring small and intermediate-sized cells in Hodgkin's disease. Is there a relationship with Reed-Sternberg cells? *J Pathol* 1993; 170:129–136.
138. Zhou XG, Hamilton-Dutoit SJ, Yan QH, Pallesen G. The association between Epstein-Barr virus and Chinese Hodgkin's disease. *Int J Cancer* 1993;55:359–363.
139. Hummel M, Anagnostopoulos I, Dallenbach F, Korbjuhn P, Dimmler C, Stein H. EBV infection patterns in Hodgkin's disease and normal lymphoid tissue: expression and cellular localization of EBV gene products. *Br J Haematol* 1992;82:689–694.
140. Bellas C, Mampaso F, Fraile G, Molina A, Bricio T, Cuesta C. Detection of Epstein-Barr genome in the lymph nodes of Hodgkin's disease. *Postgrad Med J* 1993;69:916–919.
141. Meggetto F, Brousset P, Selves J, Delsol G, Mariame B. Reed-Sternberg cells and "bystander" lymphocytes in lymph nodes affected by Hodgkin's disease are infected with different strains of Epstein-Barr virus. *J Virol* 1997;71:2547–2549.
142. Herbst H, Niedobitek G, Kneba M, et al. High incidence of Epstein-Barr virus genomes in Hodgkin's disease. *Am* J Pathol 1990;137:13–18.
143. Bignon Y-V, Bernard D, Cure H, et al. Detection of Epstein-Barr viral genomes in lymph nodes of Hodgkin's disease patients. *Mol Carcinog* 1990;3:9–11.
144. Knecht H, Odermatt BF, Bachmann E, et al. Frequent detection of Epstein-Barr virus DNA by the polymerase chain reaction in lymph node biopsies from patients with Hodgkin's disease without genomic evidence of B- or T-cell clonality. *Blood* 1991;78:760–767.
145. Wright CF, Reid AH, Tsai MM, et al. Detection of Epstein-Barr virus sequences in Hodgkin's disease by the polymerase chain reaction. *Am* J Pathol 1991;139:393–398.
146. Fellbaum C, Hansmann ML, Niedermeyer H, et al. Influence of Epstein-Barr virus genomes on patient survival in Hodgkin's disease. *Am J Clin Pathol* 1992;98:319–323.
147. Armstrong AA, Weiss LM, Gallagher A. Criteria for the definition of Epstein-Barr virus association in Hodgkin's disease. *Leukemia* 1992;6:869–874.
148. Roth J, Daus H, Gause A, Trumper L, Pfreundschuh M. Detection of Epstein-Barr virus DNA in Hodgkin and Reed-Sternberg cells by single cell PCR. *Leuk Lymphoma* 1994;13:137–142.
149. Teramoto N, Akagi T, Yoshino T, Takahashi K, Jeon HJ. Direct detection of Epstein-Barr virus DNA from a single Reed-Sternberg cell of Hodgkin's disease by polymerase chain reaction. *Jpn J Cancer Res* 1992;83:329–333.
150. Poppema S, van Imhoff G, Torensma R, Smit J. Lymphadenopathy morphologically consistent with Hodgkin's disease associated with Epstein-Barr virus infection. *Am J Clin Pathol* 1985;84:385–390.
151. Pallesen G, Hamilton-Dutoit SJ, Rowe M, Young LS. Expression of Epstein-Barr virus (EBV) latent gene products in tumour cells of Hodgkin's disease. Lancet 1991;337:320–322.
152. Herbst H, Dallenbach F, Hummel M, et al. Epstein-Barr virus latent membrane protein expression in Hodgkin and Reed-Sternberg cells. *Proc Natl Acad Sci U S A* 1991;88:4766–4770.
153. Teramoto N, Cao L, Kawasaki N, et al. Variable expression of Epstein-Barr virus latent membrane protein I in Reed-Sternberg cells of Hodgkin's disease. *Acta Med Okayama* 1996;50:267–270.
154. van Gorp J, Jacobse KC, Broekhuizen R, Alers J, van den Tweel JG, de Weger RA. Encoded latent membrane protein 1 of Epstein-Barr virus on follicular dendritic cells in residual germinal centres in Hodgkin's disease. *J Clin Pathol* 1994;47:29–32.
155. Pallesen G, Sandvej K, Hamilton-Dutoit SJ, Rowe M, Young LS. Activation of Epstein-Barr virus replication in Hodgkin and Reed-Sternberg cells. *Blood* 1991;78:1162–1165.
156. Uccini S, Monardo F, Stoppacciaro A, et al. High frequency of Epstein-Barr virus genome detection in Hodgkin's disease of HIV-positive patients. *Int J Cancer* 1990;46:581–585.
157. Siebert JD, Ambinder RF, Napoli VM, Quintanilla-Martinez L, Banks PM, Gulley ML. Human immunodeficiency virus-associated Hodgkin's disease contains latent, not replicative, Epstein-Barr virus. *Hum Pathol* 1995;26:1191–1195.
158. Bibeau F, Brousset P, Knecht H, et al. Epstein-Barr virus replication in Hodgkin disease. *Bull Cancer (Paris)* 1994;81:114–118.
159. Glaser SL, Lin RJ, Stewart SL, et al. Epstein-Barr virus-associated Hodgkin's disease: epidemiologic characteristics in international data. *Int J Cancer* 1997;70:375–382.
160. Ambinder RF, Browning PJ, Lorenzana I, et al. Epstein-Barr virus and childhood Hodgkin's disease in Honduras and the United States. *Blood* 1993;81:462–467.
161. Khalidi HS, Lones MA, Zhou Y, Weiss LM, Medeiros LJ. Detection of Epstein-Barr virus in the L & H cells of nodular lymphocyte predominance Hodgkin's disease: report of a case documented by immunohistochemical, *in situ* hybridization, and polymerase chain reaction methods. *Am J Clin Pathol* 1997;108:687–692.
162. Jarrett RF, Gallagher A, Jones DB, et al. Detection of Epstein-Barr virus genomes in Hodgkin's disease: relation to age. *J Clin Pathol* 1991;44:844–848.
163. Armstrong AA, Alexander FE, Paes RP, et al. Association of Epstein-Barr virus with pediatric Hodgkin's disease. *Am* J Pathol 1993;142: 1683–1688.
164. Weinreb M, Day PJ, Niggli F, et al. The consistent association between Epstein-Barr virus and Hodgkin's disease in children in Kenya. *Blood* 1996;87:3828–3836.
165. Razzouk BI, Gan YJ, Mendonca C, et al. Epstein-Barr virus in pediatric Hodgkin disease: age and histiotype are more predictive than geographic region. *Med Pediatr Oncol* 1997;28:248–254.
166. Benharroch D, Brousset P, Goldstein J, et al. Association of the Epstein-Barr virus with Hodgkin's disease in Southern Israel. *Int J Cancer* 1997;71:138–141.
167. Chang KL, Albújar PF, Chen YY, Johnson RM, Weiss LM. High prevalence of Epstein-Barr virus in the Reed-Sternberg cells of Hodgkin's disease occurring in Peru. *Blood* 1993;81:496–501.
168. Quintanilla-Martinez L, Gamboa-Domnquez A, Gamez-Ledesma I, Dominque F, Angeles-Angeles A, Mohar A. Association of Epstein-

SECTION III

Pathology

Hodgkin's Disease, edited by P. M. Mauch,
J. O. Armitage, V. Diehl, R.T. Hoppe, and L. M. Weiss.
Lippincott Williams & Wilkins, Philadephia ©1999.

CHAPTER 7

Pathology of Classical Hodgkin's Disease

Lawrence M. Weiss, John K. C. Chan, Kenneth MacLennan, and Roger A. Warnke

HISTORICAL ASPECTS OF PATHOLOGY AND CLASSIFICATION

The earliest descriptions of the disease process we now know as Hodgkin's disease are provided by Malpighi (1). In his book *De Viscerum Structura*, he describes the appearances of enlarged lymph nodes and splenic lesions found at postmortem examination [quoted by Hodgkin (2) and by Hoster and Dratman (2)]. Similar findings were also described by Craigie (4).

In 1832, Thomas Hodgkin described his findings in six cases of pathologic enlargement of lymph nodes and spleen that first came to his attention in 1826 (2). A seventh case, recognized from a watercolor painted by his friend Robert Carswell of a postmortem examination that Carswell performed while working in Paris, was added to the series with his permission. Hodgkin noted the similar macroscopic appearances of these seven cases and regarded the process as a "primitive (primary) affection of these bodies," and he thought the condition to be an "idiopathic interstitial enlargement of the absorbent glandular structure throughout the body." He also noted the distribution of enlarged lymph nodes adjacent to major arteries.

In 1856, Wilks (5) described a series of cases that he termed "lardaceous" disease. These were further classified into five subtypes, many representing examples of amyloidosis. One subtype, of which there were 10 cases that he termed "cases of a peculiar enlargement of the lymphatic glands frequently associated with enlargement of the spleen," appeared to be heterogeneous. Four cases were associated with tuberculosis, but he stated that the remaining six "appear to constitute a special form of malady." Unwittingly, Wilks included the first four cases from Hodgkin's original series, which he obtained from the museum at Guy's Hospital, in this latter group (6). In 1865, Wilks published a definitive study, "Cases of enlargement of the lymphatic glands and spleen (or, Hodgkin's disease), with remarks" (6). In this article, Wilks stated, "Although my own observations were at the time original, I had been forestalled by Dr. Hodgkin, who was the first, as far as I am aware, to call attention to this peculiar form of disease." The generous attachment of the eponymous term Hodgkin's disease to this process has spared future generations "non-Wilk's lymphoma."

The delineation of Hodgkin's disease by Thomas Hodgkin and Samuel Wilks was based solely on the macroscopic appearances of the disease, although Wilks provided some brief microscopic descriptions. An American pathologist, Herbert Fox, while visiting Guy's Hospital identified the cases of Thomas Hodgkin through the papers of Bright and Wilks. He prepared material for histologic examination from cases 2, 4, and 6 (7). Cases 2 and 4 displayed histologic features we recognize today as Hodgkin's disease; case 6 was felt to be an example of non-Hodgkin's lymphoma or leukemia—interestingly, case 6 was also regarded as being slightly different from the others by Hodgkin (2). These findings were reproduced by other expert hematopathologists (8).

Shortly after the publication of Wilks' second article, the first detailed microscopic descriptions of Hodgkin's disease were reported by Ollivier and Ranvier in 1867 (9). These were followed by other descriptions, by Tuckwell in 1870 (10), Bristowe and Pick, also in 1870 (11), Langhans in 1872 (12), Greenfield in 1873 (13), and Gowers in 1879 (14). In each report, cells with large nuclei approximately 10 times the size of a small lymphocyte and prominent nucleoli were noted, as well as giant multinucleated cells. The first illustrations of Reed-Sternberg cells were provided by Greenfield in 1878 (13). Drs. Carl Sternberg in 1898 (15) and Dorothy Reed in 1902 (16) provided the

L. M. Weiss: Department of Pathology, City of Hope National Medical Center, Duarte, California.

J. K. C. Chan: Department of Pathology, Queen Elizabeth Hospital, Kowloon, Hong Kong.

K. MacLennan: I.C.R.F. Cancer Medicine Research Unit, St. James University Hospital, Leeds, United Kingdom.

R. A. Warnke: Department of Pathology, Stanford University Medical Center, Stanford, California.

most through descriptions of the large multilobated cells, with excellent illustrations provided by Reed, which is perhaps why their names, and not those of their predecessors, have become associated with these cells.

Ewing (17), in his classic monograph on cancer published in 1919, was perhaps the first to attempt to subdivide cases of Hodgkin's disease, recognizing a variant he described as Hodgkin's sarcoma. Hodgkin's sarcoma was clinically extremely aggressive, and histologically it contained numerous pleomorphic mononuclear and multinucleated Reed-Sternberg cells. In retrospect, some of these cases probably represented high-grade non-Hodgkin's lymphoma. Although Ewing had recognized a morphologically distinctive and biologically aggressive form of Hodgkin's disease, a morphologic separation of prognostically distinct groups was not attempted before Rosenthal's article of 1936 (18). This study was initially undertaken to evaluate the histologic changes in irradiated lymph nodes, particularly those affected by lymphogranuloma. As the work progressed, Rosenthal found a relationship between the duration of disease and the number of lymphocytes and lymph nodules in lymph nodes. Based on the histologic appearances of 39 lymph node biopsy specimens obtained before treatment, Rosenthal recognized three subtypes of lymphogranuloma with an inverse relationship between the number of lymphocytes and abnormal reticular cells. It was in the lymphocyte-rich forms of lymphogranuloma that orthovoltage radiotherapy proved to be of clinical value and improved survival.

Using many of the ideas proposed by Rosenthal, Jackson in 1937 (19) described an indolent form of Hodgkin's disease, referring to it initially as early Hodgkin's disease; when it was later realized that the disease might persist for many years, the name was changed to Hodgkin's paragranuloma (20). The Jackson and Parker classification was to dominate thinking for nearly two decades (20,21). Three types were recognized: paragranuloma, granuloma, and sarcoma (Table 1). Paragranuloma was considered to be a disease of lymph nodes with a high incidence of primary cervical involvement. Histologically, this subtype was defined as partial or complete effacement of the normal lymph node architecture by a proliferative process composed predominantly of small round lymphocytes. Reed-Sternberg cells, although regarded as essential for the diagnosis, were generally scanty. Capsular invasion, necrosis, and numerous eosinophils and granulocytes were never seen in this subtype; when present, these features were regarded as indicating progression to the granuloma subtype. Histologically, Hodgkin's granuloma was characterized by the presence of Reed-Sternberg cells and by a high degree of pleomorphism. The lymph node architecture was generally completely obliterated, and lymphocytes, eosinophils, and plasma cells were frequently found in large numbers. The Reed-Sternberg cells varied widely in numbers and density, from a few scattered cells to aggregates containing large numbers. Although Hodgkin's granuloma was considered to be a disease primarily of lymph nodes, Jackson and Parker were impressed by the diversity of symptomatology and the degree and extent of extranodal disease (22). Hodgkin's sarcoma frequently presented with retroperitoneal lymph node disease; bulky lymphadenopathy with capsular invasion led to the formation of "large, irregularly shaped, conglomerate masses" (22). The normal lymph node architecture was diffusely replaced by a destructive proliferation of cells that were two to three times the size of a normal lymphocyte and possessed round or ovoid nuclei with prominent nucleoli: these were regarded as anaplastic variants of Reed-Sternberg cells. Extranodal disease was common, with a high frequency of gastrointestinal involvement. It seems that many of the cases classified as Hodgkin's sarcoma were probably examples of high-grade non-Hodgkin's lymphoma.

TABLE 1. *Classification of Jackson and Parker*

Subtype	Number	Percentage	5-Year survival (%)
Paragranuloma	28	10.2	55.0
Granuloma	213	78.1	15.6
Sarcoma	32	11.7	0
Total	**273**	**100**	**23.8**

From refs. 20–22.

In the three subtypes within the Jackson and Parker classification, histologic evidence of malignancy increased from paragranuloma to sarcoma, with corresponding changes in clinical behavior. The major problem was that the vast majority of cases fell into the clinically heterogeneous granuloma subtype, which displayed a wide range of presentations and prognoses. This fact severely affected the clinical value of the Jackson and Parker classification and prompted many clinicians to believe that histologic classification offered little prognostic guidance and that the extent of disease spread was far more important (23–25). Histologic review of other large series of cases of Hodgkin's disease showed a similar numeric predominance of the granuloma subtype (26–29). In the study of Smetana and Cohen (28), a sclerosing variant of Hodgkin's granuloma was described that was associated with a more favorable prognosis. From their description and illustration (Fig. 5 in their article), most modern pathologists would recognize their case as one of nodular sclerosis. Harrison, in his description of "benign Hodgkin's disease," also appears to have recognized nodular sclerosis, as did others from this period (29–33). The accurate definition of this subtype awaited the detailed histologic studies of Lukes and coworkers (34–36).

CURRENT CLASSIFICATION SYSTEMS

The major criticism of the classification of Jackson and Parker was that although the categories of paragranuloma and sarcoma appeared to be of prognostic value, nearly 80% of cases fell into the "wastebasket" category of granuloma. In addition, the classification did not seem to have a biologic basis—that is, it did not provide insight into the nature of the process (37). In 1963, Lukes published his classification (35), which was further refined several years later with Butler and colleagues (34,36,37). Lukes and Butler recognized six major types of Hodgkin's disease: lymphocytic and/or histiocytic (L&H) nodular, L&H diffuse, nodular sclerosis, mixed, diffuse fibrosis, and reticular (Table 2). This classification attempted to provide a categorization that was both biologically and prognostically significant. It was based on two main principles: that an inverse relationship exists between the number of mature lymphocytes and Reed-Sternberg cells and that this relationship is reflected in clinical stage and survival (as proposed by Rosenthal) (18); and that a distinctive type of sclerosis, termed nodular sclerosis, defines an important prognostic group and shows a regional preference for the anterior superior mediastinum.

The two L&H types of Hodgkin's disease were distinguished from other types of Hodgkin's disease by the predominance of variable proportions of small mature lymphocytes and histiocytes. The lymphocytic component usually, but not always, predominated, and the histiocytes appeared either singly or in small aggregates. Two types of Hodgkin's cells were present. The predominant cells were large with folded, twisted, lobated pale nuclei that had fine, lacy, delicate chromatin and small nucleoli; these are now known as L&H variants. The second type, the true Reed-Sternberg cell, was said to be extremely infrequent, often requiring a vigorous search. In L&H types of Hodgkin's disease, eosinophils and plasma cells were few, fibrosis was typically absent, and necrosis was always absent. The diffuse variant showed a uniform diffuse proliferation throughout the lymph node, whereas in the nodular variant, the cellular proliferation was aggregated into vague nodules. Lukes and Butler believed the diffuse form evolved from the nodular type and could evolve to the mixed type. The lymphocyte-rich forms of the L&H Hodgkin's disease were thought to correspond best to paragranuloma, whereas the histiocyte-rich forms were thought to correspond to Jackson and Parker's granuloma.

Nodular sclerosis was characterized by orderly bands of interconnecting collagenous connective tissue that subdivided the lymphoid tissue partially or entirely into isolated cellular nodules and lacunar cells, although classic Reed-Sternberg cells were still required for the diagnosis. Lukes and Butler believed that the process essentially started as a proliferation of lacunar cells before the formation of collagen bands. Lukes and Butler were unable to find cases in which nodular sclerosis evolved from or to other subtypes of Hodgkin's disease, and regarded this variant as biologically separate.

The mixed type was felt to represent an intermediate state between the L&H forms of Hodgkin's disease on the one hand and diffuse fibrosis and reticular forms on the other. Reed-Sternberg cells and variants were usually numerous and prominent, and the background was composed of a heterogeneous mixture of histiocytes, neutrophils, eosinophils, plasma cells, and lymphocytes, in variable proportions. Fibrosis could be present, but organized collagenous bands were not found. In diffuse fibrosis, a cellular depletion involved all cell types, particularly lymphocytes. Fibrosis was variable in appearance but generally comprised compact, amorphous, hypocellular material, without organization into discrete fibrous bands. This type was commonly observed at autopsy. In the reticular type, a predominant component of Reed-Sternberg cells was associated with a mixture of cell types. This type corresponded best with the sarcoma subtype of Jackson and Parker.

The Lukes and Butler classification of Hodgkin's disease appeared to be highly relevant for pathologists and clinicians, and also to be relevant from a biologic standpoint. In addition, initial studies suggested that this classification system resulted in a better distribution of cases among the various types, and that these types also correlated well with prognosis (Table 2) (37). However, it was thought that the classification was a little too cumbersome for most clinicians and pathologists. Thus, the four categories with the fewest cases were combined into two new categories—L&H nodular and L&H diffuse were combined into lymphocyte predominance, and diffuse fibrosis and reticular were combined into lymphocyte depletion (Table 3) (38). This Rye classification, as it came to be known because it was adopted at a confer-

TABLE 2. *Classification of Lukes*

Subtype	Number	Percentage	15-Year survival (%)
L&H nodular	23	6.1	43.5
L&H diffuse	40	10.6	27.5
Nodular sclerosis	149	39.5	15.4
Mixed	97	25.7	10.3
Diffuse fibrosis	47	12.5	2.1
Reticular	21	5.6	4.8
Total	**377**	**100**	**14.9**

L&H, lymphocytic and histiocytic.
From refs. 34–37.

TABLE 3. *Rye classification*

	Number	Percentage	5-Year survival (%)
Lymphocyte predominance	77	6.7	84
Nodular sclerosis	820	71.8	70
Mixed cellularity	223	19.6	96
Lymphocyte depletion	22	1.9	26
Total	**1,142**	**100**	**75**

From refs. 38, 212.

ence in Rye, New York, was a very practical way to subdivide cases of Hodgkin's disease, with numerous studies attesting to its reproducibility and ability to separate patients according to clinical presentation and prognosis (the latter now obscured by successful modern treatment protocols).

The Rye classification has been essentially the only classification used for Hodgkin's disease during the last 25 years, being accepted throughout the world. Nonetheless, ongoing biologic, pathologic, and clinical studies have suggested a need for further modifications. The International Lymphoma Study Group has introduced a revised European-American classification of malignant lymphomas, including some modifications in the classification of Hodgkin's disease (39). Even more recently, the Society for Hematopathology and the European Society of Hematopathology convened a committee under the auspices of the World Health Organization (WHO) as part of their sponsorship of a series of books on the histologic typing of tumors. The WHO classification, which encompasses both leukemias and lymphomas, has suggested similar changes in the subtyping of Hodgkin's disease (Table 4). Specifically, it recognizes Hodgkin's disease as a lymphoma (i.e., a neoplasm of lymphoid lineage), with the designation Hodgkin lymphoma to be used synonymously with Hodgkin's disease. In addition, nodular lymphocyte predominant Hodgkin's disease (with or without diffuse areas) is clearly separated from other types of Hodgkin's disease, in view of its distinct biologic, histologic, and clinical features. Other forms of Hodgkin's disease formerly recognized as lymphocyte predominant are now given the designation lymphocyte-rich (nodular or diffuse) within the category of classical Hodgkin's disease. The categories of nodular sclerosis, mixed cellularity, and lymphocyte depletion remain unchanged.

The remainder of this chapter is devoted to a discussion of the pathology of classical Hodgkin's disease. Chapter 11 covers in depth the pathology of nodular lymphocyte predominance Hodgkin's disease and the lymphocyte-rich forms of classical Hodgkin's disease, and Chapter 12, on the interrelationships of Hodgkin's disease and non-Hodgkin's lymphomas, covers anaplastic large-cell lymphoma-like Hodgkin's disease.

TABLE 4. *New proposed World Health Organization classification (1999)*

Nodular lymphocyte predominance Hodgkin lymphoma
Classical Hodgkin lymphoma
Nodular sclerosis (grades 1 and 2)
Lymphocyte-rich
Mixed cellularity
Lymphocyte depletion

CONSIDERATIONS IN TISSUE HANDLING

Optimally, the largest abnormal lymph node should be excised intact. It should be submitted fresh, preferably sterile, to allow the pathologist as many options as possible in pursuing special studies. It is best to place the node inside a capped empty container, and not on a dry towel or sponge, for these may introduce artifacts at the edge of the tissue. If there is a chance that the tissue will dry before the pathologist receives it, then the tissue may be placed in some sterile saline solution, although even this may make the subsequent preparation of frozen sections suboptimal. The pathologist may prepare touch preparations or, as we prefer, scrape preparations, which permit subsequent cytochemical studies and provide excellent preservation of cytologic characteristics. The differential diagnosis generally guides the allocation of tissue by the pathologist. The pathologist will always fix a generous aliquot in one or more fixatives, generally formalin and in North America a metal-based fixative such as B5. This provides for excellent morphology and allows virtually all immunohistochemical studies useful in the diagnosis of Hodgkin's disease to be performed. If non-Hodgkin's lymphoma is in the differential diagnosis, then some tissue should be frozen and/or submitted for flow cytometric studies. The frozen tissue may be used for either immunohistochemical or molecular studies. Fresh tissue is required for conventional cytogenetic studies, which may be useful if these are readily available, and tissue may also be sent for microbiologic studies if an infectious process is a possibility.

Sometimes, a formal lymph node excisional biopsy specimen cannot be obtained, particularly from sites not easily accessible to the surgeon, such as the mediastinum. Hodgkin's disease may be diagnosed in small biopsy specimens, although immunohistochemical studies are often required to confirm the diagnosis. Fine needle aspiration biopsy is being increasingly used for the diagnosis of lymphoid lesions (40). Although a primary diagnosis of Hodgkin's disease can be rendered on fine needle aspiration specimens by experts (41), usually with the aid of immunohistochemistry, it is generally prudent for most pathologists without extensive experience to defer the diagnosis. However, fine needle aspiration may still play a role in the diagnosis of a non-Hodgkin's lymphoma or a specific type of reactive lymphadenopathy, particularly an infectious lymphadenopathy. Fine needle aspiration biopsy is more reliable in the diagnosis of recurrent Hodgkin's disease and in staging cases of known Hodgkin's disease, although even in these circumstances, it must be used with great caution and by those experienced in using the technique (42).

Frozen sections are usually not very reliable in the primary diagnosis of Hodgkin's disease, except when used by those with extensive experience. The diagnosis of Hodgkin's disease by frozen section is most accurate when frozen section is combined with a cytologic preparation, such as a touch or scrape preparation. Frozen sections are excellent for assessing lymph node architecture but are poor in revealing cytologic characteristics, whereas the opposite is true of touch or scrape preparations. Frozen section may still have an important role in the workup apart from determination of a specific diagnosis—it is most useful in determining the adequacy of a biopsy specimen and may prompt the pathologist to request additional tissue specimens from the surgeon.

GROSS APPEARANCE

Excised lymph nodes involved by classical Hodgkin's disease generally range in diameter from 2 to 5 cm. In cases of MC or LD, the lymph nodes generally do not adhere to adjacent tissues and are soft to moderately firm. The cut section usually reveals a vague nodularity with a tan color. In cases of nodular sclerosis, the lymph node often adheres to adjacent tissues and is generally firm. The cut section usually reveals a distinct nodularity, gray-white to tan in color; foci of necrosis may be apparent.

HISTOPATHOLOGY

The diagnosis of classical Hodgkin's disease is established with the identification of Hodgkin's cells in the appropriate cellular milieu. Hodgkin's cells encompass either diagnostic Reed-Sternberg cells or their variants (Figs. 1–3). For many years, the identification of so-called diagnostic Reed-Sternberg cells was required for the definitive diagnosis of classical Hodgkin's disease, and this was probably a prudent policy. However, it might have led to underdiagnosis of Hodgkin's disease—for example, when the tissue sampling was suboptimal. This policy might have also led to overdiagnosis of Hodgkin's disease, if the pathologist concentrated only on the identification of diagnostic Reed-Sternberg cells to the exclusion of the cellular milieu, as cells closely resembling diagnostic Reed-Sternberg cells can be found in a wide variety of reactive and neoplastic diseases. At the current time, the definitive diagnosis of Hodgkin's disease can be made either by morphologic assessment alone, or by morphologic assessment combined with immunohistochemical studies, thus diminishing the importance of the definitive identification of diagnostic Reed-Sternberg cells.

Diagnostic Reed-Sternberg cells are large cells, either with a large polyploid nucleus or multinucleated (Figs. 1 and 2). Each lobe or nucleus contains one large inclusion-like eosinophilic nucleolus, ranging in size up to about 10 μm, the diameter of a small lymphocyte nucleus. The chromatin immediately surrounding the nucleolus often shows a clear zone. The remaining chromatin is generally vesicular but usually shows some degree of coarse clumping. The nuclear membrane is usually thick, and

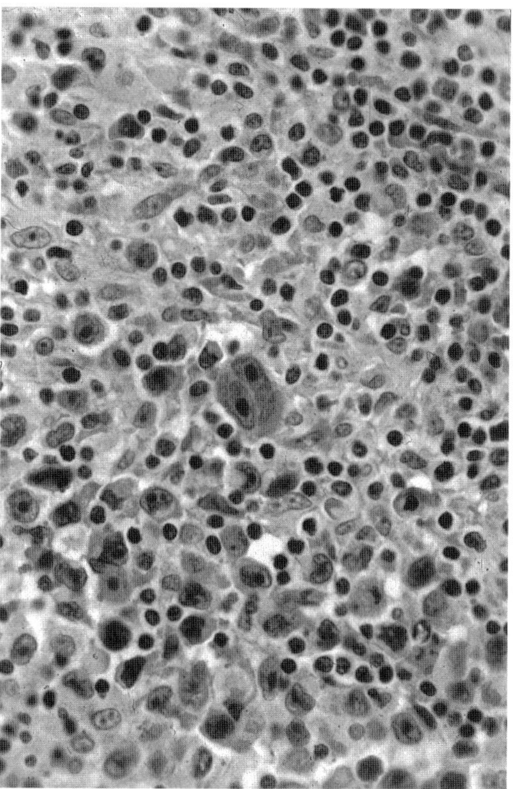

FIG 1. A diagnostic Reed-Sternberg cell with two nuclei is seen in the center, with a prominent eosinophilic nucleolus present in each nucleus. There is some chromatin clearing around each nucleolus. Several mononuclear Reed-Sternberg variants are also present in the bottom half of the field. (This figure is printed in color as Plate 5.)

often chromatin is clumped against it. The nuclear outlines are usually rounded, but highly irregular nuclear outlines can be seen in some cases. Mitotic figures can be identified but are usually not as frequently encountered as in large-cell non-Hodgkin's lymphoma. The cytoplasm is usually relatively abundant, so that an overall diameter of about 20 to 50 μm yields an area ranging from four to 25 times that of adjacent small lymphocytes. In sections stained with hematoxylin and eosin, the cytoplasm may be acidophilic, amphophilic, or basophilic, but it lacks the deep basophilia or paranuclear hof characteristic of immunoblasts. Most mononuclear Reed-Sternberg cell variants are similar to diagnostic Reed-Sternberg cells, but they are not multilobated or multinucleated. Lacunar cells are mononuclear Reed-Sternberg cell variants with abundant amphophilic cytoplasm (at least in metal-based fixatives) that is usually retracted to the nuclei in formalin-fixed sections (Fig. 3). Often, their nuclei have smaller lobes with more irregularities and the eosinophilic nucleoli may be less prominent. Occasionally, apoptotic Hodgkin's cells, sometimes termed mummified or zombie cells, are present. These cells contain pyknotic chromatin, often with barely recognizable nucleoli having fuzzy outlines, and deeply eosinophilic retracted cytoplasm.

The background infiltrate in Hodgkin's disease consists of a mixture of cell types (Fig. 4). Small lymphocytes usually predominate numerically, but scattered eosinophils, neutrophils, histiocytes, plasma cells, and fibroblasts are usually also present in variable numbers. Eosinophils vary from rare to extremely numerous, even to the extent of forming eosinophilic abscesses, although they are most often moderate in number. In most cases, there are far fewer neutrophils than eosinophils, but neutrophils may predominate in rare cases, often associated with severe B symptoms. Histiocytes may have the appearance of tissue histiocytes or epithelioid histiocytes, or they may rarely be foamy. They most often occur singly but occasionally form well-defined granulomas, and multinucleated giant cells may also be seen. In rare cases, histiocytes may be so numerous as to give an appearance reminiscent of Lennert's lymphoma (non-Hodgkin's lymphoma with a high content of epithelioid cells), xanthogranulomatous inflammation, or lipid storage disease (43). Plasma cells are usually present in scattered numbers, and if they are present in very large numbers or sheets, the diagnosis of Hodgkin's disease should be doubted. One rare manifestation is the appearance of Hodgkin's cells in the midst of a reactive monocytoid B-cell proliferation (44,45).

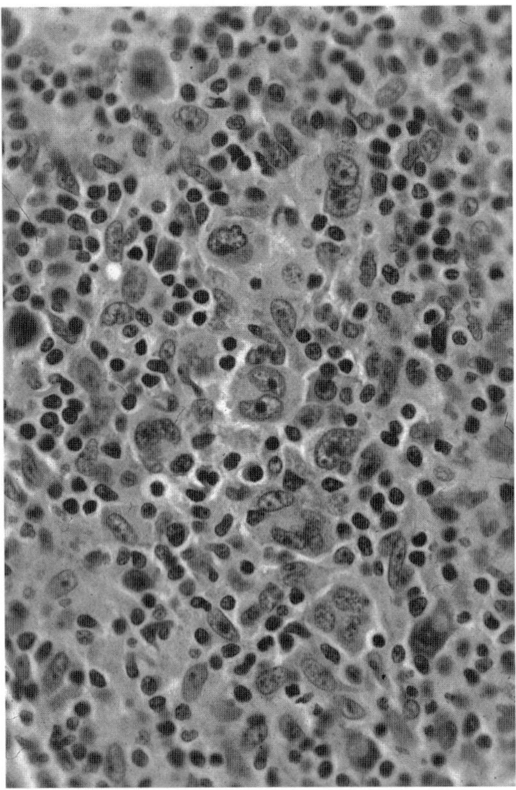

FIG 2. A diagnostic Reed-Sternberg cell is seen in the center, and many mononucleated and multinucleated Reed-Sternberg variants are seen throughout the field. (This figure is printed in color as Plate 6.)

FIG 3. Several lacunar cells are present. A "mummified" Reed-Sternberg cell is in the upper left corner. (This figure is printed in color as Plate 7.)

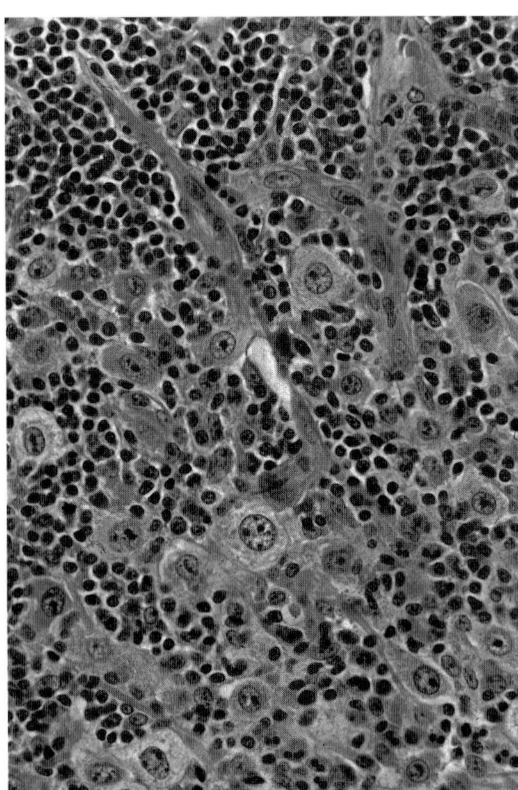

FIG 4. The background cells consist predominantly of small lymphocytes, along with scattered eosinophils, histiocytes, and plasma cells. (This figure is printed in color as Plate 8.)

Fibroblasts vary from isolated spindle cells, seen in typical cases, to widespread proliferation with areas resembling fibrous histiocytoma (46,47). Rarely, small foci of Langerhans cell histiocytosis may be found in tissues involved by Hodgkin's disease (48).

Histologic Subtyping

Nodular Sclerosis

As discussed above, the nodular sclerosis subtype is characterized by collagenous bands and lacunar cells (Fig. 5). However, in practice, the presence of one or more sclerotic bands is the defining feature. These bands usually radiate from a thickened lymph node capsule, often following the course of a penetrating artery. The bands are composed of mature, laminated, relatively acellular collagen. They are described in textbooks as showing birefringence in polarized light, but in practice polarization is rarely carried out. In most cases, several broad collagenous bands can be identified, but a single band may be present, or fibrosis can be so extensive that only isolated nodules of lymphoid tissue remain. Can one recognize cases of nodular sclerosis in which bands are not yet present? This situation has been described by some as the cellular phase of nodular sclerosis, although in Lukes' original description of the cellular phase of nodular sclerosis, at least one intranodal collagen band was required for the diagnosis (36). Some of these cases probably fit the recent description of "follicular" Hodgkin's disease (49), and others may represent the follicular variant of lymphocyte-rich classical Hodgkin's disease (see Chapter 11). Clinical studies of small numbers of cases of the cellular phase of nodular sclerosis have demonstrated some clinical features and an overall survival rate similar to those of MC, but a relapse-free survival rate similar to that of nodular sclerosis (50).

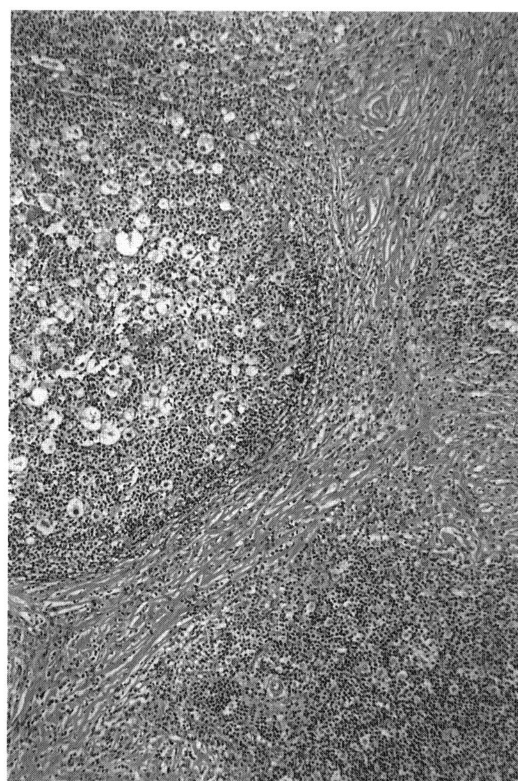

FIG 5. Nodular sclerosis Hodgkin's disease. Broad bands of fibrosis separate several nodules. (This figure is printed in color as Plate 9.)

The collagenous bands of nodular sclerosis enclose nodules of lymphoid tissue containing variable numbers of Hodgkin's cells and reactive infiltrate. Lacunar cells are the most common type of Hodgkin's cell present and may be found in large numbers or in sheets. They tend to aggregate at the center of nodules, sometimes forming a rim around central areas of necrosis. Diagnostic Reed-Sternberg cells are usually not easily identified and may not be found in small biopsy specimens. Eosinophils and neutrophils are often numerous, but histiocytes and plasma cells usually less conspicuous in nodular sclerosis. Fibrohistiocytic foci are sometimes found in the centers of nodules or extensively replacing the tissue.

In the practice of most Western centers, nodular sclerosis is by far the most common type of Hodgkin's disease, accounting for greater than two-thirds of all cases (50). Therefore, various investigators have attempted to subclassify nodular sclerosis into prognostic groups (51). The most successful effort has come from the British National Lymphoma Investigation (52–55). These investigators have proposed the subclassification of nodular sclerosis into two grades. Cases are classified as grade 2 if (a) more than 25% percent of the cellular nodules show reticular or pleomorphic lymphocyte depletion, (b) more than 80% of the cellular nodules show the fibrohistiocytic variant of lymphocyte depletion, or (c) more than 25% of the nodules contain numerous bizarre and highly anaplastic-appearing Hodgkin's cells without depletion of lymphocytes. All cases of nodular sclerosis not meeting these criteria are considered to be grade 1. Although this system appears to be somewhat hard to learn, some additional studies have demonstrated that cases classified as grade 2 have a significantly worse prognosis than those classified as grade 1 (56,57); other studies have failed to demonstrate a difference between these grades of nodular sclerosis (58,59).

Mixed Cellularity

The subtype of MC comprises approximately 30% of cases of Hodgkin's disease in Western populations, but it may comprise 50% or more of cases in developing countries (60). This intermediate subtype falls between lymphocyte-rich classical Hodgkin's disease and lymphocyte depletion. The capsule is usually intact and of normal thickness. A vague nodularity may be present at low magnification, but the presence of any definite fibrous bands would warrant classification as nodular sclerosis rather than mixed cellularity. At high magnification, a heterogeneous mixture of Hodgkin's cells, small lymphocytes, eosinophils, neutrophils, epithelioid and nonepithelioid histiocytes, plasma cells, and fibroblasts is present (Fig. 6). Diagnostic Reed-Sternberg cells and mononuclear variants are usually easy to find. Small foci of necrosis may be present, but the extent is much less than that seen in nodular sclerosis.

Lymphocyte Depletion

As explained above, lymphocyte depletion encompasses two types of Hodgkin's disease in the Lukes and Butler classification: diffuse fibrosis and reticular. In diffuse fibrosis, the most characteristic features are a marked degree of reticulin fibrosis surrounding single cells along with lymphocyte depletion (Fig. 7). In contrast to nodular sclerosis, this subtype is not characterized by the presence of thick fibrous bands, and the fibrosis envelops individual cells, not nodules of cells. Hodgkin's cells are usually easily identified, but increased numbers of Hodgkin's cells are not essential to the diagnosis. In the reticular variant, sheets of Hodgkin's cells, often showing pleomorphic features, are found. Obviously, distinction from a large-cell non-Hodgkin's lymphoma, particularly immunoblastic lymphoma, can be difficult, and immunohistochemical studies are essential to confirm the diagnosis of the reticular subtype. In some cases of lymphocyte depletion, features of both diffuse fibrosis and the reticular subtype may be present in different areas of the biopsy specimen.

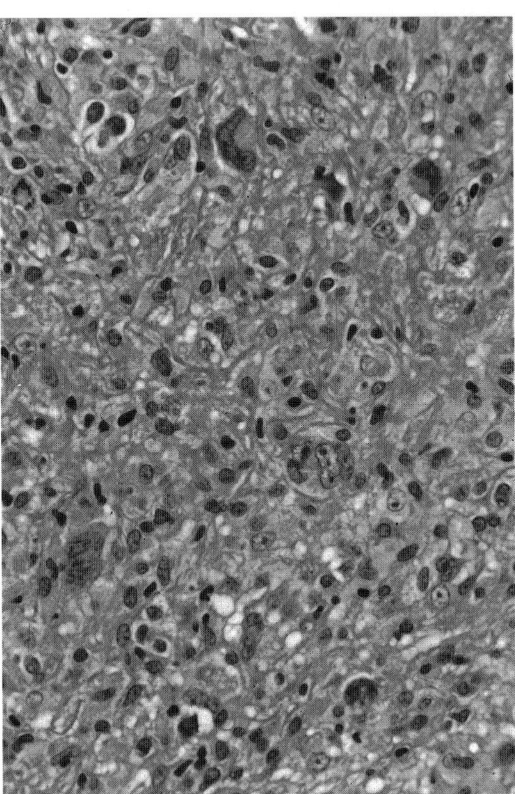

FIG 7. Lymphocyte depletion, diffuse fibrosis type. There is a reticulin collagen fibrosis around single cells. Although the Hodgkin's cells appear atypical, results of immunophenotyping studies were characteristic of Hodgkin's disease in this case. (This figure is printed in color as Plate 11.)

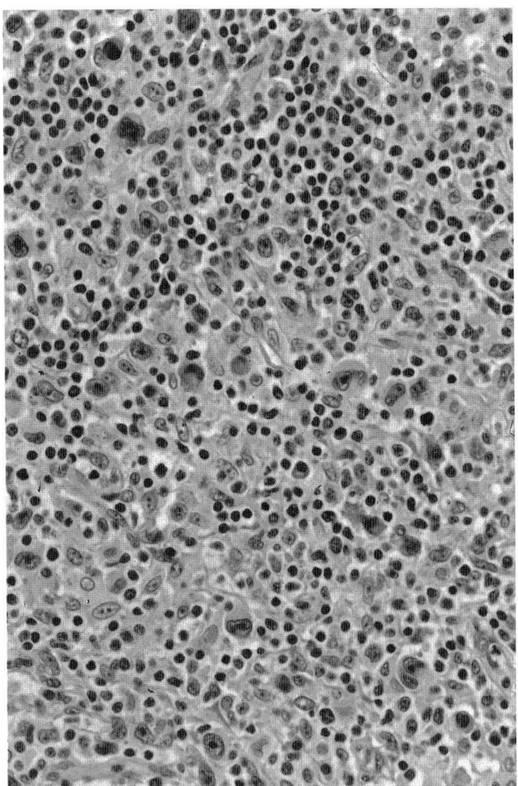

FIG 6. Mixed-cellularity Hodgkin's disease. There is an absence of fibrous bands. (This figure is printed in color as Plate 10.)

Other Histologic Types

Strickler and colleagues (61) described the syncytial variant of nodular sclerosis, in which cohesive aggregates of lacunar cells and other variants are seen, closely resembling non-Hodgkin's lymphoma, carcinoma, or malignant melanoma (Fig. 8). Often, the centers of the aggregates are necrotic, rimmed by sheets of lacunar cells. Immunohistochemical studies are often necessary for accurate diagnosis. These cases probably represent a subset of the grade 2 nodular sclerosis cases according to the British National Lymphoma Investigation; therefore, this histologic appearance may be associated with an adverse prognosis.

Doggett and colleagues (62) described interfollicular Hodgkin's disease, in which Hodgkin's cells are present in interfollicular regions between reactive follicles (Fig. 9). This variant of Hodgkin's disease can be easily dismissed as reactive hyperplasia, such as can be seen in a viral infection. This variant probably represents focal nodal involvement by Hodgkin's disease rather than a

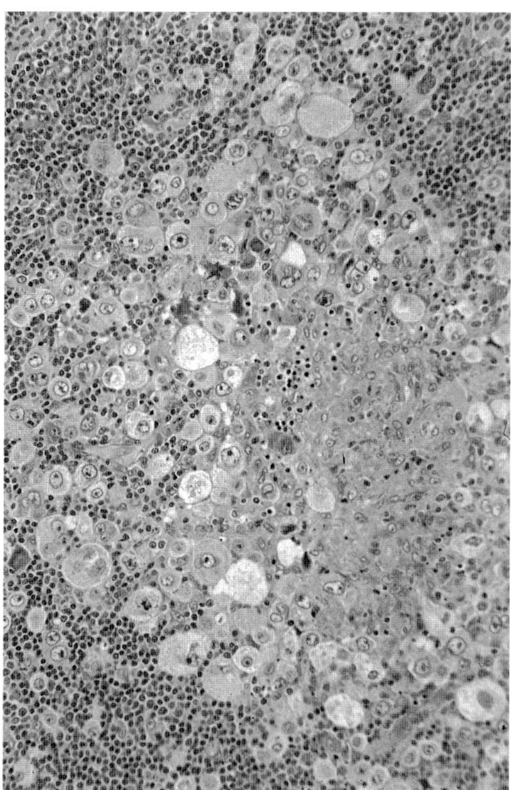

FIG 8. Syncytial form of nodular sclerosis Hodgkin's disease; sheets of lacunar cells are clustered around a central area of necrosis. (This figure is printed in color as Plate 12.)

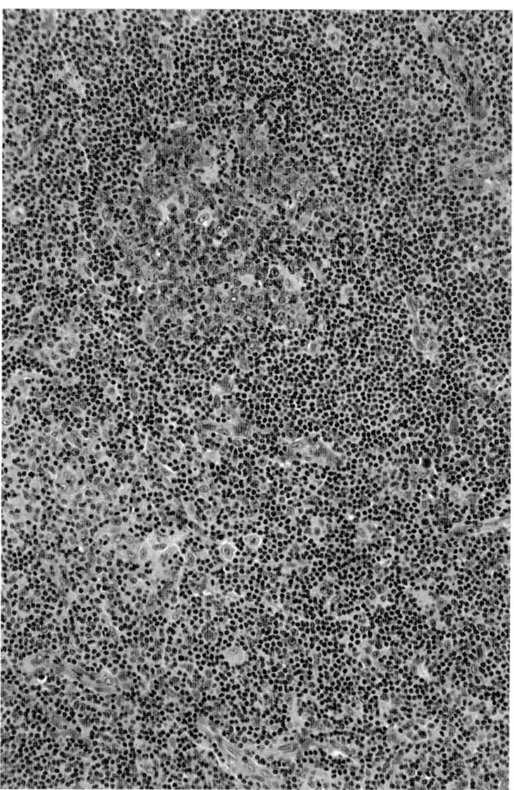

FIG 9. Interfollicular Hodgkin's disease. At the top is a reactive follicle. Several Hodgkin's cells are seen in the interfollicular region in the bottom half of the field. (This figure is printed in color as Plate 13.)

specific subtype, as other lymph nodes from the same patient, or even other foci in the same biopsy specimen, often show classic features of either nodular sclerosis or mixed cellularity Hodgkin's disease.

In a large study of cases of Hodgkin's disease, a fibroblastic variant was recognized (50). In this variant, increased numbers of fibroblasts are present, without significant collagen deposition. Many of these cases probably correspond to the fibrohistiocytic areas described by the British National Lymphoma Investigation in some cases of grade 2 nodular sclerosis. In the original description, the fibroblastic variant was associated with a shorter relapse-free survival period than were other types of Hodgkin's disease.

Finally, a small number of cases of Hodgkin's disease with a purely follicular pattern have been described; these have been termed follicular Hodgkin's disease (49). In these cases, the Hodgkin's cells had the phenotype of classical Hodgkin's disease but also expressed B-lineage antigens. In each case, the Hodgkin's cells were confined to the follicles, which consisted mainly of mantle zone B cells. The follicle centers were atrophic and usually eccentrically placed, and did not contain Hodgkin's cells. Some or all of these cases may correspond to the follicular variant of lymphocyte-rich classical Hodgkin's disease (see Chapter 11).

Fine Needle Aspiration Biopsy Studies

Fine needle aspiration smears of Hodgkin's disease show a dispersed population of lymphoid and other cells in which scattered large cells are evident (40,41). As expected, the lymphocytes are small with a mature chromatin pattern. The Hodgkin's cells are recognizable as large cells with bilobed or multilobated nuclei and prominent nucleoli. Often, these cells appear to have more abundant cytoplasm than is generally appreciated in tissue sections. Immunohistochemical studies, particularly those employing an alkaline phosphatase detection (to circumvent interpretive problems associated with the pseudoperoxidase in red cells), may be very useful in confirming a presumptive fine needle aspiration diagnosis of Hodgkin's disease.

Extranodal Disease and Staging Specimens

The same modern principles used to diagnose Hodgkin's disease in the lymph nodes should be applied to diagnosing it in extranodal sites. The diagnosis rests on the definitive identification of Hodgkin's cells, either by histopathology or histopathology combined with immunohistochemical studies, in the appropriate cellular milieu (63). Primary extranodal Hodgkin's disease is very uncommon outside the setting of HIV infection, but it is relatively common as a secondary phenomenon. Once a diagnosis of Hodgkin's disease has been established in a primary site, it is probably best not to provide a typing on staging biopsies of extranodal sites, where sclerosis may not be type-specific feature.

Hodgkin's disease usually manifests in bone marrow as scattered foci of fibrosis in which Hodgkin's cells can be identified (64,65). Therefore, the aspirated specimen is rarely helpful in establishing a diagnosis, even in cases with extensive involvement. In the biopsy specimen, the patchy areas of fibrosis can usually be appreciated at low magnification. It is in these areas that a search for the Hodgkin's cells should be made at high magnification; a search made in areas of normal marrow can lead to misidentification of hematopoietic precursors or megakaryocytes as Hodgkin's cells. If Hodgkin's cells are not seen in the areas of patchy fibrosis, serial levels should be obtained. If Hodgkin's cells cannot be demonstrated after serial levels have been obtained in a focal area of fibrosis in a random bone marrow biopsy specimen from patient with known Hodgkin's disease, these areas should still be suspected of harboring Hodgkin's disease, provided that another cause for the fibrosis cannot be discovered. The uninvolved marrow may show myeloid hyperplasia, eosinophilia, or increased numbers of plasma cells (66). It is best to confirm a primary diagnosis of Hodgkin's disease in a bone marrow biopsy specimen with immunohistochemical studies.

Splenic involvement by Hodgkin's disease begins in the periarterial lymphoid sheath and the marginal B-cell zone and progresses to involve all the malpighian bodies of the white pulp (67). In time, adjacent involved malpighian bodies may coalesce. Grossly, splenic involvement takes the form of discrete nodules ranging in size from 1 to 2 mm up to several centimeters; thus, splenic involvement may easily be missed by conventional radiologic studies. The pathologist who examines a spleen needs to section the organ very thinly and make a special effort to identify splenic hilar lymph nodes. Splenic hilar fat may yield small, grossly inapparent lymph nodes. The number of gross nodules should be recorded, and at least five, if present, should be documented histologically. Random sections of grossly normal spleen essentially never reveal evidence of Hodgkin's disease. Histologically, the splenic nodules of Hodgkin's disease usually resemble the nodules at other sites, although it is best not to try to type the disease, as nonspecific areas of fibrosis may be seen even in cases of mixed cellularity.

Liver involvement by Hodgkin's disease is rarely seen in the absence of splenic involvement outside the setting of HIV infection. The portal areas are affected at first, showing microscopic involvement, but in advanced cases, gross nodules can be seen in a portal distribution (68,69). It is usually prudent to obtain immunohistochemical confirmation to distinguish Hodgkin's disease from nonspecific periportal lymphocytic infiltration in cases of early involvement.

The thymus is a common site of primary Hodgkin's disease and probably is the site of origin in a significant percentage of cases of Hodgkin's disease presenting in the mediastinum, particularly the nodular sclerosis type. At one time, involvement of the thymus by Hodgkin's disease was mistakenly labeled as granulomatous thymoma (70). Thymic involvement by Hodgkin's disease often leads to cystic formations; these may persist as a residual mass following therapy, as may areas of sclerosis.

The lung is a relatively common site of secondary involvement and only rarely is the site of primary disease (71). Secondary involvement manifests in two ways. Most commonly, it results from contiguous involvement by mediastinal disease, but it also may manifest as miliary involvement, reflective of vascular dissemination. Both primary and secondary involvement of the gastrointestinal tract and tonsillar tissue are very rare but have been reported (72–74). Similarly, both primary and secondary involvement of the skin are unusual, except by contiguous spread from an underlying lesion. A diagnosis of primary Hodgkin's disease in the skin should be made with great caution and with confirmation by immunohistochemical studies, as CD30+ lymphoproliferative disease (including lymphomatoid papulosis), a much more common skin lymphoma, can closely mimic Hodgkin's disease (75–77). Virtually every extranodal site, including the central nervous system, has been described as a primary or secondary site of Hodgkin's disease, but such cases are fortunately extremely rare (78–80).

In addition, or more commonly, instead of disclosing evidence of Hodgkin's disease, staging biopsies may show sarcoidlike noncaseating epithelioid granulomas (81). On rare occasions, these granulomas may coalesce to form gross nodules. Unless definite evidence of concurrent Hodgkin's disease is demonstrated, the finding of noncaseating granulomas should not be considered evidence of involvement by Hodgkin's disease. In the past, the presence of epithelioid granulomas in the liver or spleen of patients with Hodgkin's disease had been reported to be associated with a better 5-year overall and relapse-free survival (82,83); however, this survival advantage may not be seen with long-term follow-up or with modern therapies (84).

Posttreatment, Relapse, and Autopsy Findings

Sites of successful treatment for Hodgkin's disease usually show dense collagenous scars, with only a few lymphocytes and fibroblasts and no identifiable Hodgkin's cells; foamy macrophages may also be present (85). Occasionally, the centers contain an amorphous eosinophilic necrotic debris surrounded by a poorly cellular fibrous rim, resembling an old infectious granuloma. These scars are most often found in lymph nodes, but they may also be encountered in liver, lung, bone marrow, and spleen. Large scars up to 4 cm in size may be evident on gross examination, and occasionally they may cause a clinically apparent mass—for example, in the mediastinum following successful treatment.

The histology of recurrent Hodgkin's disease is different, depending on whether the site of recurrence falls within or outside the treatment area. When the site of relapse is outside the treatment area, there is an impressive maintenance of the histologic appearance in the relapse biopsy specimens, with a change in histology seen in only a small percentage of cases (86,87). When an unusual histologic pattern of Hodgkin's disease, such as extensive necrosis or large numbers of epithelioid histiocytes, has been present in the initial biopsy, it is often also present in the relapse specimen. The same histologic type is usually present in the initial and relapse specimens, although progression from one type to another, most commonly lymphocyte-rich classical Hodgkin's disease to mixed cellularity, or mixed cellularity to lymphocyte depletion, occasionally occurs. Cases of nodular sclerosis tend to remain nodular sclerosis, although even this type can manifest as another type, usually mixed cellularity. However, there is a tendency for the number of eosinophils, histiocytes, and Hodgkin's cells to increase in the relapse specimens. The increase in eosinophils is more marked in those patients who relapse 2 years or more after the initial diagnosis, whereas an increase in the number of Hodgkin's cells is more often seen in patients who relapse early. Lymphocytes and reactive follicles appear to decrease in number between initial and relapse biopsy specimens. Those patients with a relapse-free interval longer than 1 year more often have a granulomatous reaction, in contrast to those who relapse in a shorter period of time.

When Hodgkin's disease recurs in irradiated sites, the tendency toward retention of the same histologic appearance is much smaller (88). Recurrences may have an unusual appearance, often with a marked decrease in the number of lymphocytes, a decrease in the number of eosinophils, and increased numbers of Hodgkin's cells with a greater range of cytologic atypia. Recurrent cases of nodular sclerosis frequently exhibit fewer nodules and less sclerosis than formerly, and they are often difficult to subclassify. Nonetheless, histologic features of recurrence specimens cannot be used to identify those patients who will later die of Hodgkin's disease versus those who can be successfully retreated. The histologic appearance of Hodgkin's disease at autopsy is somewhat similar to that in treated sites but is often even more exaggerated (89,90). Although in some patients the pretherapy histologic appearance is maintained, in many cases a marked increase in the number and atypia of Hodgkin's cells is noted. Occasionally, sheets of Hodgkin's cells may be present at autopsy. Most cases of nodular sclerosis lose their nodularity and sclerosis by the time of autopsy. Evidence of vascular dissemination of disease, to noncontiguous sites and to multiple extranodal sites, is common.

Patients successfully and unsuccessfully treated for Hodgkin's disease may show a wide range of other changes at autopsy, undoubtedly reflective of treatment effects (89,90). Fibrosis and atrophy are common findings in multiple organs, including the lungs, gastrointestinal tract, liver, kidneys, endocrine organs (particularly the thyroid gland and gonads), and bone marrow. In addition, patients treated for Hodgkin's disease may show evidence of second neoplasms, most commonly acute nonlymphocytic leukemia and non-Hodgkin's lymphoma, but also other neoplasms, such as breast carcinoma and malignant melanoma (see Chapter 33) (91,92).

ULTRASTRUCTURAL FINDINGS

Electron microscopic study is generally not useful in the diagnosis of Hodgkin's disease. The ultrastructural appearance of Hodgkin's cells is similar to that of transformed lymphocytes (93). As expected from the light microscopic findings, the nuclei of Hodgkin's cells are large and multilobated, with uniformly dispersed chromatin. Nucleoli are very prominent and have well-developed nucleolonemata. The cytoplasm is abundant and shows evidence of synthetic activity, usually with numerous polyribosomes and prominent Golgi regions composed of numerous vesicles. Variable numbers of mitochondria are present, and lysosomes (a prominent constituent of macrophages) are usually few in number.

IMMUNOPHENOTYPING STUDIES

Immunophenotyping studies with frozen sections are of limited utility in the immunodiagnosis of Hodgkin's disease. With the suboptimal cytologic features of frozen sections and the relative rarity of Hodgkin's cells, it is often difficult to ascertain staining results on Hodgkin's cells with certainty. Similarly, flow cytometric studies, although useful in ruling out the presence of a non-Hodgkin's lymphoma, particularly a B-cell lymphoma, are also of limited usefulness in making a positive diagnosis of Hodgkin's disease. Conventional flow cytometric studies are unable to gate easily on such an infrequent cell type as the Hodgkin's cell in Hodgkin's disease, so that the results generally reflect the background cell population and not the Hodgkin's cells. In fact, flow cytometric studies may even be misleading, as the profile usually seen—polyclonal B cells with numerous immunophenotypically normal T cells—is identical to that seen in a reactive lymph node.

Fortunately, immunohistochemical studies with paraffin sections are of great use in the diagnosis of Hodgkin's disease (94–102). Rather than any one marker being both highly sensitive and specific for Hodgkin's cells, a relatively limited panel of monoclonal antibodies, when analyzed in the aggregate, can provide very useful informa-

TABLE 5. *Immunophenotype of Reed-Sternberg cells in paraffin sections*

	CD45 (%)	CD15 (%)	CD30 (%)	CD20 (%)
Classical Hodgkin's disease	7	87	89	24
Nodular lymphocyte predominance	65[a]	37[b]	38[c]	92
B-cell lymphoma	97	4	18	94
T-cell lymphoma	89	21	42	0

CD, cluster of differentiation.
[a]Results are skewed by the inclusion of one large study in which all the cases were said to be CD45-negative.
[b]Results given may include cases of lymphocyte-rich classical Hodgkin's disease.
[c]Positive cells may be immunoblasts rather than lymphocytes and histiocytes (L&H cells).
From refs. 103, 105, 106, 113.

tion. The phenotype of Hodgkin's cells is summarized in Table 5. The percentages given are derived from compiled reviews of the literature (103–106) and therefore may differ from laboratory to laboratory. The data suggest, however, that CD45 may be the most useful marker in the immunodiagnosis of Hodgkin's disease. CD45 (or CD45RB, which is commonly assessed in paraffin sections) represents a group of antibodies directed against a family of related molecules present on virtually all hematolymphoid cells, with the exception of maturing erythroid cells and megakaryocytes; therefore, the antigen has been called leukocyte common antigen (106). Its utility as a negative marker for Hodgkin's cells (expressed in only 7% of cases) is enhanced by the finding that about 97% of B-cell lymphomas and 89% of T-cell lymphomas express CD45 (98,101,102,106–112). The category of non-Hodgkin's lymphoma that is most likely to be confused histologically with Hodgkin's disease and that may lack CD45 expression is anaplastic large-cell lymphoma (negative for CD45 in about 33% of cases). Diffuse large B-cell lymphomas with immunoblastic features may also be nonreactive for CD45 on occasion. The interpretation of CD45 staining may be difficult because it is important not to mistake membranous reactivity on adjacent cells as positivity of Hodgkin's cells—not a trivial task, as Hodgkin's cells are typically surrounded by T cells. Staining results should be regarded as positive only if a clear, strong rim is observed entirely circling the cell (best assessed when two Hodgkin's cells are adjacent to each other).

The CD30 cluster of antibodies is directed against the Ki-1 antigen (113). In reactive tissues, these antibodies stain scattered large activated B and T lymphoid cells. Staining of the Reed-Sternberg cells and variants is seen in about 89% of cases of classical Hodgkin's disease (98, 113–119). The staining pattern for CD30 in Hodgkin's disease is usually strong and membranous and/or paranuclear in distribution, often associated with a weaker diffuse cytoplasmic positivity (Fig. 10). In addition to labeling Hodgkin's cells, CD30 antibodies will also stain virtually all cases of anaplastic large-cell lymphoma and CD30+ cutaneous lymphoproliferative disease (including lymphomatoid papulosis), about 15% of B-lineage large-cell lymphomas, and about 40% of peripheral T-cell lymphomas. In most non-anaplastic non-Hodgkin's lymphomas that show reactivity for CD30, the CD30 staining is usually seen on a subset of the neoplastic cells. In addition to their reactivity on lymphoid cells, CD30 antibodies also label embryonal carcinoma, and they may label some other carcinomas as well as sarcomas (113,120).

The CD15 cluster of antibodies is directed against the carbohydrate X hapten (103). CD15 antibodies generally stain mature neutrophils, many macrophages, and a subset of T cells, particularly after activation. Staining of the Reed-Sternberg cells and variants is seen in about 87% of cases of classical Hodgkin's disease (Fig. 11) (101–103,

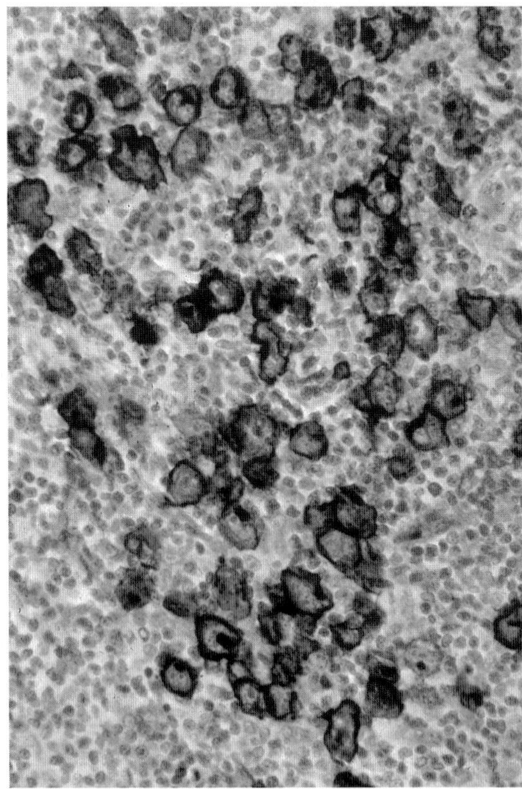

FIG 10. Immunostaining for CD30. There is strong membrane and paranuclear staining, and weaker cytoplasmic staining, of the Hodgkin's cells. (This figure is printed in color as Plate 14.)

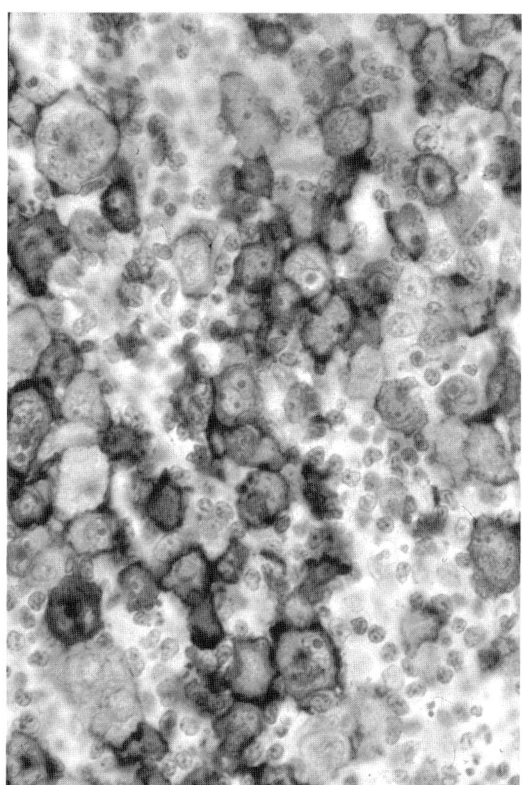

FIG 11. Immunostaining for CD15. There is strong membrane and paranuclear staining of the Hodgkin's cells. (This figure is printed in color as Plate 15.)

109,115,119,121–127). The staining pattern on Hodgkin's cells is similar to that seen for CD30. Patients whose Hodgkin's cells are CD15– are older and predominantly male, and their clinical stage at diagnosis is more advanced than that of patients whose Hodgkin's cells are CD15+; mixed cellularity is more common than nodular sclerosis among CD15– cases (119). Cases that are CD30+, CD20–, and CD15– have significantly less freedom from treatment failure and poorer overall survival in comparison with cases that are CD30+, CD20–, and CD15+. Multivariate analysis has shown that lack of CD15 staining is an independent adverse prognostic indicator (119). In addition to staining most cases of classical Hodgkin's disease, CD15 antibodies also stain about two-thirds of cases of acute myeloid leukemia, 5% of B-cell lymphomas, and 20% of T-cell lymphomas. Often, the staining pattern in non-Hodgkin's lymphoma is different from that seen in Hodgkin's disease, being cytoplasmic and granular, although staining patterns indistinguishable from those of Hodgkin's cells may also be seen. In addition, CD15 antibodies label many carcinomas, particularly adenocarcinomas of the lung (103,128).

The CD20 cluster of antibodies detects a mature B-cell antigen (105). CD20 antibodies stain the vast majority of B-cell neoplasms, except the most immature cases of B-lineage acute lymphoblastic leukemia and plasma cell neoplasms. CD20 may rarely show reactivity with nonhematolymphoid cells, such as the epithelial cells in a subset of thymomas. There is a wide range of reported reactivity for CD20 in Hodgkin's disease, ranging from fewer than 5% to a majority of cases; the overall average is about 25% (99,105,119,122,129–131). Typically, when a case of Hodgkin's disease is CD20+, only a subset of the Hodgkin's cells stain, and these in a heterogeneous pattern (some cells strongly positive, some weakly positive, and some negative). This pattern contrasts with the consistently strong staining typically seen in B-cell non-Hodgkin's lymphomas. Despite the positivity for CD20 in some cases, Hodgkin's cells lack functional transcripts of immunoglobulin light and heavy chains (132–134). Therefore, Hodgkin's cells either lack detectable immunoglobulin light and heavy chain or, more commonly, stain for both κ and λ light chains as a consequence of passive absorption of immunoglobulin from tissue fluid (135). The immunoglobulin-associated molecule CD79a may be expressed by Hodgkin's cells in a manner similar to CD20. Thus, one study found a small proportion of the neoplastic cells staining for CD79a in 20% of non-LP cases, in contrast to a small proportion of cells staining for CD20 in 30% of these cases (136). Labeling of more than 50% of cells for CD79a was seen less frequently than for CD20 (1% vs. 7% of cases). Similarly, CD45RA represents another B-lineage marker for which Hodgkin's cells are usually negative (106).

CD3, CD45RO, and CD43 are T cell-related markers of varying specificity, with CD3 the most specific and CD43 the least specific. Hodgkin's cells are rarely reported to stain for these markers in paraffin sections (106,137). However, some expression of T-cell antigens, including the T-cell receptor chain antigen, has been reported in frozen sections as well as in plastic-embedded sections, in up to 40% of cases in one series (96,97, 138–141).

Some laboratories perform additional paraffin section immunohistochemical studies to aid in the diagnosis of Hodgkin's disease, particularly in difficult cases in which the results derived from more commonly used markers are ambiguous. Antibodies against Epstein-Barr virus latent membrane protein (EBV LMP) consistently stain Hodgkin's cells in the subset of cases of Hodgkin's disease that are EBV-related (Fig. 12) (142–144). Because cases of mixed cellularity and lymphocyte depletion as well as cases seen in the setting of HIV infection are most likely to be EBV-associated, this stain is most useful when the differential diagnosis includes these types. Antibodies against CD40 recognize an antigen that, like CD30, is a member of the tumor necrosis/nerve growth receptor family. CD40 is expressed in 70% to 100% of cases of Hodgkin's disease, but in only 20% of cases of anaplastic large-cell lymphoma (145). In addition, the pattern of staining in Hodgkin's cells is somewhat different than in anaplastic large-cell lymphoma, resembling

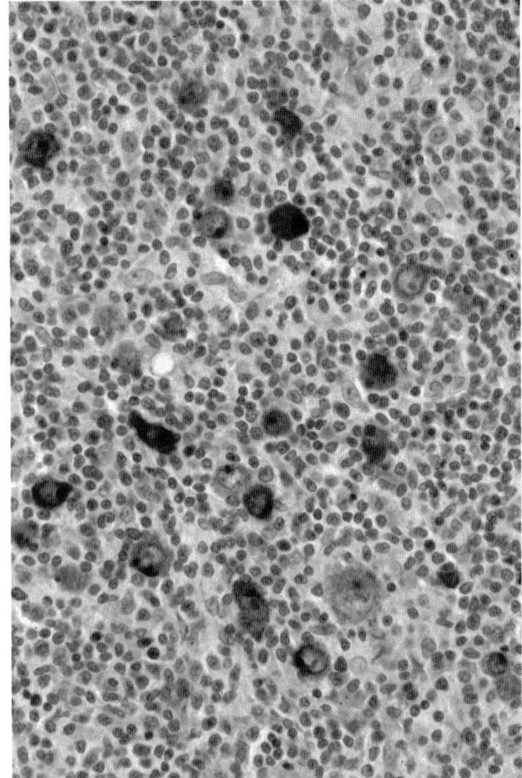

FIG 12. Immunostaining for Epstein-Barr virus (EBV) latent membrane protein (LMP) in a case of EBV-associated Hodgkin's disease. There is strong cytoplasmic staining, with paranuclear accentuation in the Hodgkin's cells. EBV+ small lymphocytes do not stain for LMP in Hodgkin's disease. (This figure is printed in color as Plate 16.)

that of CD30 in Hodgkin's disease. Epithelial membrane antigen may be useful in the differential diagnosis of Hodgkin's disease versus anaplastic large-cell lymphoma, as it is expressed in a majority of cases of anaplastic large-cell lymphoma, but in fewer than 5% of cases of classical Hodgkin's disease (98). Hodgkin's cells also stain with the lectins peanut agglutinin and Bauhinia purpurea in a majority of cases (124,146).

We recommend the use of a panel of CD45RB, CD30, CD15, CD20, and CD3 in the routine immunodiagnosis of Hodgkin's disease. Additional, second-line markers that may be utilized in particularly difficult or immunohistochemically confusing cases may EBV LMP, CD40, epithelial membrane antigen, and other B- and T-cell markers.

One study has reported expression of the follicular dendritic cell marker CD21 in a significant percentage of cases (147), but others have not confirmed this observation; differences in fixation and processing may explain the discrepancy. Other markers of dendritic cells, including fascin and CD83, have been identified in Hodgkin's cells in a high percentage of cases (148,149). Fascin is a 55-kd actin-bundling protein that is highly selective for dendritic cells in nonneoplastic tissues, although viral induction of fascin expression has been reported in EBV-infected B cells (150). Among neoplasms, fascin is a consistent marker for the Hodgkin's cells of classical Hodgkin's disease, showing a strong diffuse cytoplasmic staining that frequently highlights dendritic shapes (148). In contrast, no staining for fascin is seen in the L&H cells of nodular lymphocyte predominance Hodgkin's disease, and only about 15% of non-Hodgkin's lymphomas are positive for fascin. When more experience is accumulated with fascin, it may become a routine marker for the immunodiagnosis of Hodgkin's disease.

Other markers reactive in Hodgkin's cells include CD74 (most cases); the intermediate filament-associated protein restin (most cases), HLA-DR (Ia), class I antigens (variable expression, associated with EBV expression), CD25 (the interleukin-2 receptor), and CD71 (the transferrin receptor) (96,118,138,151–154). Most Hodgkin's cells are positive for Ki-67, a nuclear proliferation marker expressed in cycling cells, as well as proliferating cell nuclear antigen (PCNA) and p34, the protein product of the cell cycle control cdc2 gene (155–161). Hodgkin's cells are positive for p53 by immunohistochemistry, indicating the presence of higher-than-normal levels of the protein (162–165). There is also variable expression of bcl2 and the p53-complexing protein mdm2, although there are no strong correlations between levels of the three proteins (157,162,164).

Immunohistochemical studies have shown that most of the background lymphoid cells in Hodgkin's disease represent T cells, with CD4+ helper cells predominating over CD8+ cytotoxic/suppressor cells (147,152,166–169). In addition, numerous macrophages can be identified. In many cases of Hodgkin's disease, expanded and disrupted networks of follicular dendritic cells can be identified, with Hodgkin's cells often found embedded within them. This pattern is particularly well developed in cases of follicular Hodgkin's disease. One study has found that cases of Hodgkin's disease with prominent numbers of follicular dendritic cells have a better prognosis than other cases (170).

DIAGNOSTIC MOLECULAR AND CYTOGENETIC FINDINGS

The molecular biology of Hodgkin's cells is covered in Chapter 8, and the cytogenetics of Hodgkin's disease is covered in Chapter 13. From a diagnostic standpoint, the most important use of molecular studies is to rule out a non-Hodgkin's lymphoma. Results of Southern blot studies for the detection of antigen receptor gene rearrangements are generally negative unless extremely large numbers of Hodgkin's cells are present (171–181). In the latter situation, light-rearranged bands of immunoglobulin light and/or heavy chains may be present; however, they can usually be distinguished from the more sizable bands observed in typical cases of non-Hodgkin's lymphoma. Similarly, results of Southern blot studies to detect chromosomal translocations usually associated with subsets of non-Hodgkin's lymphomas, such as t(14;18) and t(2;5), are also usually negative (182–191). Caution needs to be exercised in the interpretation of the results of polymerase chain reaction (PCR) studies in Hodgkin's disease, as some of these translocations can rarely be detected by this methodology, and clonal immunoglobulin gene rearrangements may also be found in some cases, particularly those with large numbers of Hodgkin's cells (192–199).

DIFFERENTIAL DIAGNOSIS

The differential diagnosis of classical Hodgkin's disease is extremely broad, including carcinoma, malignant melanoma, sarcoma, reactive lymphoid lesions, non-Hodgkin's lymphoma, and nodular lymphocyte predominance Hodgkin's disease (200); the differential diagnosis of classical Hodgkin's disease and the latter is covered in Chapter 11. Cases of the syncytial variant of nodular sclerosis Hodgkin's disease in particular may simulate carcinoma, melanoma, or a germ cell tumor, whereas cases of undifferentiated nasopharyngeal carcinoma presenting in a cervical lymph node may closely simulate mixed cellularity or nodular sclerosis Hodgkin's disease. When carcinoma is in the differential diagnosis, a keratin stain should either confirm or rule out that possibility (Table 6). Although embryonal carcinomas may be CD30+, they are also strongly positive for keratin. Germinomas (seminoma or dysgerminoma) are commonly negative for keratin, but they lack CD30 and CD15 and are positive for placental alkaline phosphatase. Similarly, if malignant melanoma is in the differential diagnosis, an S100 protein stain and possibly also an HMB-45 stain should be performed. Virtually all cases of malignant melanoma (as well as a wide variety of other neoplasms) are S100+, but Hodgkin's cells are consistently negative, although large numbers of S100+ dendritic cells may be seen in some cases. HMB-45 is a much more specific marker for malignant melanoma, but about 10% of cases may be negative. Rarely, fibroblastic areas in Hodgkin's disease can be confused with a spindle cell sarcoma. Attention to the cytologic features of the most spindled cells is important; they are bland in Hodgkin's disease, but atypical in sarcoma.

Two main patterns of reactive lymphoid proliferation can be easily confused with Hodgkin's disease. Cases of nodular sclerosis Hodgkin's disease in which necrosis is present in the center of one or more nodules may be misdiagnosed as a necrotizing granulomatous lymphadenitis or suppurative granulomatous lymphadenitis (the prototype being cat scratch disease). Attention should be given to the cells immediately rimming the areas of coagulative or suppurative necrosis. In necrotizing granulomatous lymphadenitis, the cells lining the areas of necrosis are epithelioid histiocytes. In suppurative granulomatous lymphadenitis, the rimming cells are monocytoid cells and histiocytes with or without epithelioid features. In contrast, in Hodgkin's disease, at least some Hodgkin's cells, usually lacunar cells, will be present. Hodgkin's cells can be distinguished from histiocytes and monocytoid cells by the presence of at least some prominent nucleoli, and by the frequently multilobated nuclei. In cases of difficulty, immunohistochemical studies are of great help. Although histiocytes may occasionally show a granular cytoplasmic staining with CD15, they do not show membrane staining with CD15, they are always CD30-, and they are CD45+.

The second pattern of reactive lymphoid proliferation that can be easily confused with Hodgkin's disease is a reactive immunoblastic proliferation, including so-called interfollicular Hodgkinoid lymphadenitis (201). In this setting, scattered immunoblasts or sheets of immunoblasts are present in the paracortical regions, either with or without hyperplastic follicles. When follicles are absent, the appearance can be easily confused with mixed cellularity Hodgkin's disease; when follicles are present, the appearance can be easily confused with interfollicular Hodgkin's disease. Immunoblasts can closely resemble Hodgkin's cells, as they have large nuclei, a vesicular chromatin pattern, and prominent nucleoli. Occasionally, they may be multilobated or multinucleated; cells resembling diagnostic Reed-Sternberg cells are well-known to occur in virally induced reactive immunoblastic proliferations such as EBV-associated acute infectious mononucleosis. However, in contrast to Hodgkin's cells, reactive immunoblasts usually have a basophilic cytoplasm, often with a distinct paranuclear hof. They are usually associated with marked plasmacytosis, and transitional forms between frank plasma cells and immunoblasts are usually present. In addition, the immunoblasts are usually more evenly dispersed throughout the lymphoid proliferation;

TABLE 6. *Immunohistologic differential of Hodgkin's disease versus nonhematolymphoid neoplasms*

	Keratin	S100	Alkaline phosphatase	CD30
Hodgkin's disease	–	–	–	+
Carcinoma	+	–/+	–	–
Embryonal carcinoma	+	–	+	+
Germinoma	–/+	–	+	–
Malignant melanoma	–	+	–	–

CD, cluster of differentiation.

in contrast, Hodgkin's cells in Hodgkin's disease are more irregularly clustered. Immunohistochemical studies are again of great help. Like Hodgkin's cells, immunoblasts are often CD30+, but the intensity of staining is often variable from cell to cell. In contrast to Hodgkin's cells, they are usually CD45+ and stain with either B- or T-cell markers. In addition, immunoblasts are usually CD15-, although the immunoblasts found in cytomegalovirus-associated lymphadenitis have been reported to be CD15+.

Many types of non-Hodgkin's lymphoma can be easily confused with Hodgkin's disease. Lymphocyte-rich classical Hodgkin's disease must be distinguished from lymph node involvement by B-cell chronic lymphocytic leukemia/small-lymphocyte lymphoma. The latter often contains scattered cells with large nuclei, termed prolymphocytes and paraimmunoblasts, but does not usually contain eosinophils. Rarely, the phenomenon of chronic lymphocytic leukemia with Reed-Sternberg–like cells has been described (see Chapter 12) (202,203). Histologically, lymph nodes involved by chronic lymphocytic leukemia/small-lymphocyte lymphoma usually show pale staining areas at low magnification (termed pseudofollicular growth centers), which is a highly characteristic feature of this neoplasm. The prolymphocytes and paraimmunoblasts do not possess nucleoli as large as those of Hodgkin's cells. The differential diagnosis may be easily resolved by immunohistochemical studies, as the dominant small-lymphocytic cell type in chronic lymphocytic leukemia/small-lymphocyte lymphoma is a B lymphocyte that shows aberrant coexpression of CD43 and CD5 and is usually also CD23+, whereas the dominant small-lymphocytic cell type is usually a T lymphocyte in classical Hodgkin's disease.

T cell-rich or histiocyte-rich B-cell lymphoma may be quite difficult to distinguish from MC Hodgkin's disease (204,205). In the first case, the predominant cell type is a small lymphocyte that is a reactive T-cell component, whereas in the second case, large numbers of both reactive histiocytes and T cells are present. In both lymphomas, which may represent variants of the same entity, a minority population of large cells represents the neoplastic B-cell component. The large-cell population can have nuclear features virtually indistinguishable from those of Hodgkin's cells. Many cases of T cell-rich B-cell lymphoma have other areas more consistent with a diffuse large B-cell lymphoma, but this is by no means always the case. In interpreting the results of immunohistochemical studies, one must remember that Hodgkin's cells may express the B-lineage marker CD20 (albeit often in a heterogeneous pattern), but they usually lack expression of CD45RA, another B-lineage marker. The large cells in T cell-rich B-cell lymphoma are CD45+, CD20+ (with all large cells showing the same intensity of staining), usually CD45RA+, and usually CD15- and CD30-. In addition, they are often positive for epithelial membrane antigen (a marker rarely present in Hodgkin's disease), and restriction of light chains can sometimes be demonstrated. Distinction between diffuse large-cell lymphoma of the mediastinum and the syncytial variant of nodular sclerosis Hodgkin's disease can also be extremely difficult. The sclerosis in mediastinal large B-cell lymphoma usually consists of thin rather than the thick fibrous bands of nodular sclerosis Hodgkin's disease, and it usually compartmentalizes small groups of cells; however, this distinction may be very difficult to appreciate in the small biopsy specimens often obtained at this site. Immunohistochemical studies are often necessary for the distinction to be made (Table 5).

Peripheral T-cell lymphomas, particularly polymorphic examples, may also be difficult to distinguish from mixed cellularity Hodgkin's disease (206). Both neoplasms can demonstrate a mixed reactive infiltrate sometimes containing many eosinophils, and Hodgkin's-like cells are not uncommonly seen in peripheral T-cell lymphoma. Cytologically, one tries to identify a range of cellular atypia in peripheral T-cell lymphoma, from atypical small to atypical medium to atypical large-sized lymphoid cells. The mitotic rate in peripheral T-cell lymphoma is also generally higher than that seen in Hodgkin's disease (207). Immunohistochemical studies are of great use, as the large cells in peripheral T-cell lymphoma should stain with CD45 as well as one or more T-lineage markers, a rare phenomenon in Hodgkin's cells. If necessary, immunophenotyping studies of frozen sections often can demonstrate an aberrant T-cell phenotype in peripheral T-cell lymphoma (208–210). Molecular studies, with the demonstration of a sizable rearrangement of the β or γ T-cell receptor genes, would obviously favor a diagnosis of peripheral T-cell lymphoma. Anaplastic large-cell lymphoma may be extremely difficult to distinguish from Hodgkin's disease—so much so that terms such as anaplastic large-cell–like Hodgkin's disease and Hodgkin's disease-like anaplastic large-cell lymphoma have been introduced into the literature. This topic is discussed in more detail in Chapter 12.

Cases of lymphocyte depletion Hodgkin's disease are virtually always difficult to distinguish from non-Hodgkin's lymphoma. Immunohistochemical studies should be performed to confirm the diagnosis of this rare type of Hodgkin's disease. In addition to the other immunohistochemical studies already mentioned to be helpful in the differential diagnosis of Hodgkin's disease versus non-Hodgkin's lymphoma, EBV LMP may be of use, as cases of lymphocyte depletion Hodgkin's disease are often associated with EBV (see Chapter 6), whereas fewer than 5% of cases of non-Hodgkin's lymphoma occurring outside the setting of HIV infection are EBV+ (211).

REFERENCES

1. Malpighi. *De viscerum structura exercitatio anatomica.* Bologna: Omnia Opera, 1666 (English translation in *Ann Med History* 1925; 7:245).

2. Hodgkin T. On some morbid appearances of the absorbent glands and spleen. *Med Chir Soc Trans* 1832;17:68.
3. Hoster HA, Dratman MB. Hodgkin's disease 1832–1947, parts I and II. *Cancer Res* 1948;8:1.
4. Craigie D. *Elements of general and pathological anatomy*. Edinburgh: Adam Black, 1828.
5. Wilks SS. Cases of lardaceous disease and some allied affections, with remarks. *Guy's Hosp Rep* 1856;17(Ser II, Vol 2):103.
6. Wilks S. Cases of enlargement of the lymphatic glands and spleen (or, Hodgkin's disease), with remarks. *Guy's Hosp Rep* 1865;11:56.
7. Fox H. Remarks on microscopical preparations made from some of the original tissue described by Thomas Hodgkin, 1832. *Ann Med History* 1926;8:370.
8. Symmers WS. Museum piece. *Pathol Annu* 1984;19(Pt 1):375.
9. Ollivier A, Ranvier L. Observation pour servir à l'histoire de l'adénite. In: Mémoires lus à la société de biologie, 1867:99.
10. Tuckwell HM. Enlargement of lymph glands in the abdomen, with formation of peculiar morbid growths in the spleen and peritoneum. *Trans Pathol Soc London* 1870;21:362.
11. Bristowe JS, Pick TP. Report of the committee on morbid growth on Dr. Tuckwell's case. *Trans Pathol Soc London* 1870;21:365.
12. Langhans T. Das maligne Lymphosarkom (Pseudoleukämie). *Virchows Arch Pathol Anat* 1872;54:509.
13. Greenfield WS. Specimens illustrative of the pathology of lymphadenoma and leucocythemia. *Trans Pathol Soc London* 1878;29:272.
14. Gowers WR. Hodgkin's disease. In: Reynolds JR, ed. *A system of medicine*. London: Macmillan, 1879:306.
15. Sternberg C. Uber eine eigenartige unter dem Bilde der Pseudoleukamie verlaufende Tuberculose des lymphatischen Apparates. *Z Heilk* 1898;19:21.
16. Reed DM. On the pathological changes in Hodgkin's disease, with especial reference to its relation to tuberculosis. *Johns Hopkins Hosp Rep* 1902;10:133.
17. Ewing J. *Neoplastic diseases*. Philadelphia: WB Saunders, 1928.
18. Rosenthal SR. Significance of tissue lymphocytes in the prognosis of lymphogranulomatosis. *Arch Pathol* 1936;21:628.
19. Jackson H Jr. Classification and prognosis of Hodgkin's disease and allied disorders. *Surg Gynecol Obstet* 1937;64:465.
20. Jackson H Jr, Parker F Jr. Hodgkin's disease II. Pathology. *N Engl J Med* 1944;231:35.
21. Jackson H Jr, Parker F Jr. Hodgkin's disease I. General Considerations. *New Engl J Med* 1944;230:1.
22. Jackson JH, Parker JF. *Hodgkin's disease and allied disorders*. New York: Oxford University Press, 1947.
23. Peters MV, Middlemiss KCH. A study of Hodgkin's disease treated by irradiation. *Am J Roentgenol* 1958;79:114.
24. Peters MV. A study of survivals in Hodgkin's disease treated radiologically. *Roentgenol Radiat Ther* 1950;63:299.
25. Jelliffe AM, Thompson AD. The prognosis in Hodgkin's disease. *Br J Cancer* 1955;9:21.
26. Lumb G. Reticular lymphoma. In: *Tumours of lymphoid tissue*. Edinburgh: E & S Livingstone, 1954:71.
27. Lumb G, Newton KA. Prognosis in tumours of lymphoid tissue: an analysis of 602 cases. *Cancer* 1957;10:976.
28. Smetana HF, Cohen BM. Mortality in relation to histologic type in Hodgkin's disease. *Blood* 1956;11:211.
29. Wright CJE. The benign form of Hodgkin's disease (Hodgkin's paragranuloma). *J Pathol Bacteriol* 1960;80:157.
30. Rappaport H. Tumors of the hematopoietic system, Section III, Fascicle 8, *Atlas of tumor pathology*. Washington, DC: Armed Forces Institute of Pathology, 1966.
31. Wright CJE. Hodgkin's paragranuloma. *Cancer* 1956;9:773.
32. Harrison CV. Benign Hodgkin's disease (Hodgkin's paragranuloma). *J Pathol Bacteriol* 1952;64:513.
33. Hanson TAS. Histological classification and survival in Hodgkin's disease. A study of 251 cases with special reference to nodular sclerosing Hodgkin's disease. *Cancer* 1964;17:1595.
34. Lukes RJ, Butler JJ. The pathology and nomenclature of Hodgkin's disease. *Cancer Res* 1966;26:1063.
35. Lukes RJ. Relationship of histologic features to clinical stages in Hodgkin's disease. *Am J Roentgenol* 1963;90:944.
36. Lukes RJ. Criteria for involvement of lymph node, bone marrow, spleen, and liver in Hodgkin's disease. *Cancer Res* 1971;31:1755.
37. Lukes RJ, Butler JJ, Hicks EB. Natural history of Hodgkin's disease as related to its pathologic picture. *Cancer* 1966;19:317.
38. Lukes RJ, Craver LF, Hall TC, Rappaport H, Ruben P. Report of the nomenclature committee. *Cancer Res* 1966;26:1311.
39. Harris NL, Jaffe ES, Stein H, et al. A revised European-American classification of lymphoid neoplasms. A proposal from the International Lymphoma Study Group. *Blood* 1994;84:1361.
40. Pitts WC, Weiss LM. The role of fine needle aspiration biopsy in diagnosis and management of hematopoietic neoplasms. In: Knowles DM, ed. *Neoplastic hematopathology*. Baltimore: Williams & Wilkins, 1992:385.
41. Das DK, Gupta SK, Datta BM, Sharma SC. Fine needle aspiration cytodiagnosis of Hodgkin's disease and its subtypes. I. Scope and limitations. *Acta Cytol* 1989;34:329.
42. Friedman M, Kim U, Shimaoka K, Panahon A, Han T, Stutzman L. Appraisal of aspiration cytology in management of Hodgkin's disease. *Cancer* 1980;45:1653–1663.
43. Variakojis D, Strum SB, Rappaport H. The foamy macrophages in Hodgkin's disease. *Arch Pathol* 1972;93:453.
44. Mohrmann RL, Nathwani BN, Brynes RK, Sheibani K. Hodgkin's disease occurring in monocytoid B-cell clusters. *Am J Clin Pathol* 1991;95:802.
45. Plank L, Hansmann ML, Fisher R. Monocytoid B-cells occurring in Hodgkin's disease. *Virchows Arch* 1994;424:321.
46. Khalidi HS, Singleton TP, Weiss SW. Inflammatory malignant fibrous histiocytoma: distinction from Hodgkin's disease and non-Hodgkin's lymphoma by a panel of leukocyte markers. *Mod Pathol* 1997;10:438.
47. Suster S. Transformation of Hodgkin's disease into malignant fibrous histiocytoma. *Cancer* 1986;57:264.
48. Burns BF, Colby TV, Dorfman RF. Langerhans' cell granulomatosis (histiocytosis X) associated with malignant lymphomas. *Am J Surg Pathol* 1983;7:529.
49. Ashton-Key M, Thorpe PA, Allen JP, Isaacson PG. Follicular Hodgkin's disease. *Am J Surg Pathol* 1995;19:1294.
50. Colby TV, Hoppe RT, Warnke RA. Hodgkin's disease: a clinicopathologic study of 659 cases. *Cancer* 1981;49:1848.
51. Mann RB, Jaffe ES, Berard CW. Malignant lymphomas—a conceptual understanding of morphologic diversity. A review. *Am J Pathol* 1979;94:105.
52. Bennett MH, MacLennan KA, Easterling MJ, Vaughan HB, Jelliffe AM, Vaughan HG. The prognostic significance of cellular subtypes in nodular sclerosing Hodgkin's disease: an analysis of 271 non-laparotomised cases (BNLI report no. 22). *Clin Radiol* 1983;34:497.
53. MacLennan KA, Bennett MH, Vaughan HB, Vaughan HG. Diagnosis and grading of nodular sclerosing Hodgkin's disease: a study of 2190 patients. *Int Rev Exp Pathol* 1992;33:27.
54. MacLennan KA, Bennett MH, Tu A, et al. Relationship of histopathologic features to survival and relapse in nodular sclerosing Hodgkin's disease: a study of 1,659 patients. *Cancer* 1989;64:1686.
55. Haybittle JL, Hayhoe FGJ, Easterling MJ, et al. Review of British National Lymphoma Investigation studies of Hodgkin's disease and development of prognostic index. *Lancet* 1985;1:967.
56. Ferry JA, Linggood RM, Convery KM, Efird JT, Eliseo R, Harris NL. Hodgkin's disease, nodular sclerosis type: implications of histologic subclassification. *Cancer* 1993;71:457.
57. Wijlhuizen TJ, Vrints LW, Jairam R, et al. Grades of nodular sclerosis (NSI–NSII) in Hodgkin's disease: are they of independent prognostic value? *Cancer* 1989;63:1150.
58. Masih AS, Weisenburger DD, Vose JM, Bast MA, Armitage JO. Histologic grade does not predict prognosis in optimally treated, advanced-stage nodular sclerosing Hodgkin's disease. *Cancer* 1992;69:228.
59. Hess JL, Bodis S, Pinkus G, Silver B, Mauch P. Histopathologic grading of nodular sclerosis Hodgkin's disease. Lack of prognostic significance in 254 surgically staged patients. *Cancer* 1994;74:708.
60. Correa P, O'Conor GT. Epidemiologic patterns of Hodgkin's disease. *Int J Cancer* 1971;8:192.
61. Strickler JG, Michie SA, Warnke RA, Dorfman RF. The "syncytial variant" of nodular sclerosing Hodgkin's disease. *Am J Surg Pathol* 1986;10:470.
62. Doggett RS, Colby TV, Dorfman RF. Interfollicular Hodgkin's disease. *Am J Med* 1983;78:22.
63. Rappaport H, Berard CW, Butler JJ, Dorfman TF, Lukes RJ, Thomas LB. Report of the committee on histopathological criteria contributing to staging of Hodgkin's disease. *Cancer Res* 1971;31:1864.
64. O'Carroll DI, McKenna RW, Brunning RD. Bone marrow manifestations of Hodgkin's disease. *Cancer* 1976;38:1717.
65. Bartl R, Frisch B, Burkhardt R, Huhn D, Pappenberger R. Assessment

of bone marrow histology in Hodgkin's disease: correlation with clinical factors. *Br J Haematol* 1982;51:345.
66. Te Velde J, Den Ottolander GJ, Spaander PJ, Van Den Berg C, Hartgrink-Groenveld CA. The bone marrow in Hodgkin's disease: the non-involved marrow. *Histopathology* 1978;2:31.
67. Dorfman RF, Colby TV. The pathologist's role in management of patients with Hodgkin's disease. *Cancer Treat Rep* 1982;66:675.
68. Dich NH, Goodman ZD, Klein MA. Hepatic involvement in Hodgkin's disease: clues to histologic diagnosis. *Cancer* 1989;64:2121.
69. Bagley CM Jr, Roth JA, Thomas LB, Devita VT Jr. Liver biopsy in Hodgkin's disease: clinicopathologic correlations in 127 patients. *Ann Intern Med* 1972;76:219.
70. Katz A, Lattes R. Granulomatous thymoma or Hodgkin's disease of the thymus? A clinical and histological study and a re-evaluation. *Cancer* 1969;23:1.
71. Kern WH, Crepeau A, Jones JC. Primary Hodgkin's disease of the lung: report of four cases and review of the literature. *Cancer* 1961; 14:1151.
72. Söderström K-O, Joensuu H. Primary Hodgkin's disease of the stomach. *Am J Clin Pathol* 1988;89:806.
73. Todd GB, Michaels L. Hodgkin's disease involving Waldeyer's lymphoid ring. *Cancer* 1974;34:1769.
74. Devaney K, Jaffe ES. The surgical pathology of gastrointestinal Hodgkin's disease. *Am J Clin Pathol* 1991;95:794.
75. Kaudewitz P, Stein H, Dallenbach F. Primary and secondary Ki-1+ (CD30+) anaplastic large cell lmphomas. *Am J Pathol* 1989;135:359.
76. Sioutos N, Kerl H, Murphy SB, Kadin ME. Primary cutaneous Hodgkin's disease. Unique clinical, morphologic, and immunophenotypic findings. *Am J Dermatopathol* 1994;16:2.
77. Smith JLJ, Butler JJ. Skin involvement in Hodgkin's disease. *Cancer* 1980;45:345.
78. Ashby MA, Barber PC, Holmes AE, Freer CEL, Collins RD. Primary intracranial Hodgkin's disease: a case report and discussion. *Am J Surg Pathol* 1988;12:294.
79. Meis JM, Butler JJ, Osborne BM. Hodgkin's disease involving the breast and chest wall. *Cancer* 1986;57:1859.
80. Saponzink MD, Kaplan HS. Intracranial Hodgkin's disease: a report of 12 cases and review of the literature. *Cancer* 1983;14:1151.
81. Kadin ME, Donaldson S, Dorfman RF. Isolated granulomas in Hodgkin's disease. *N Engl J Med* 1970;283:859.
82. O'Connell MJ, Schimpff SC, Kirschner RH, Abt AB, Wiernik PH. Epithelioid granulomas in Hodgkin's disease. A favorable prognostic sign? *JAMA* 1975;233:886.
83. Sacks EL, Donaldson SS, Gordon J, Dorfman RF. Epithelioid granulomas associated with Hodgkin's disease: clinical correlations in 55 previously untreated patients. *Cancer* 1978;41:562.
84. Abrams J, Pearl P, Moody M, Schimpff SC. Epithelioid grnaulomas revisited: long-term follow-up in Hodgkin's disease. *Am J Clin Oncol* 1988;11:456.
85. Chen JL, Osborne BM, Butler JJ. Residual fibrous masses in treated Hodgkin's disease. *Cancer* 1987;60:407.
86. Colby TV, Warnke RA. The histology of the initial relapse of Hodgkin's disease. *Cancer* 1980;45:289.
87. Strum SB, Rappaport H. Consistency of histologic subtypes in Hodgkin's disease in simultaneous and sequential biopsy specimens. *Natl Cancer Inst Monogr* 1973;36:253.
88. Dolginow D, Colby TV. Recurrent Hodgkin's disease in treated sites. *Cancer* 1981;48:1124.
89. Colby TV, Hoppe RT, Warnke RA. Hodgkin's disease at autopsy: 1972–1977. *Cancer* 1981;47:1852.
90. Grogan TM, Berard CW, Steinhorn SC, et al. Changing patterns of Hodgkin's disease at autopsy: a 25-year experience at the National Cancer Institute, 1953–1978. *Cancer Treat Rep* 1982;66:653.
91. Krikorian JG, Burke JS, Rosenberg SA, Kaplan HS. Occurrence of non-Hodgkin's lymphoma after therapy for Hodgkin's disease. *N Engl J Med* 1979;300:452.
92. Bookman MA, Longo DL. Concomitant illness in patients treated for Hodgkin's disease. *Cancer Treat Rev* 1986;13:77.
93. Glick AD, Leech JH, Flexner JM, Collins RD. Ultrastructural study of Reed-Sternberg cells. Comparison with transformed lymphocytes and histiocytes. *Am J Pathol* 1976;85:195.
94. Giffler RF, Gillespie JJ, Ayala AG, Newlang JR. Lymphoepithelioma in cervical lymph nodes of children and young adults. *Am J Surg Pathol* 1977;1:293.
95. Angel C, Warford A, Campbell A, Pringle J, Lauder I. The immunohistology of Hodgkin's disease—Reed-Sternberg cells and their variants. *J Pathol* 1987;153:21.
96. Agnarsson BA, Kadin ME. The immunophenotype of Reed-Sternberg cells. A study of 50 cases of Hodgkin's disease using fixed frozen tissues. *Cancer* 1989;63:2083.
97. Casey TT, Olson SJ, Cousar JB, Collins RD. Immunophenotypes of Reed-Sternberg cells: a study of 19 cases of Hodgkin's disease in plastic-embedded sections. *Blood* 1989;74:2624.
98. Chittal SM, Caveriviere P, Schwarting R, et al. Monoclonal antibodies in the diagnosis of Hodgkin's disease: the search for a rational panel. *Am J Surg Pathol* 1988;12:9.
99. Chu W-S, Abbondanzo SL, Frizzera G. Inconsistency of the immunophenotype of Reed-Sternberg cells in simultaneous and consecutive specimens from the same patients. A paraffin section evaluation in 56 patients. *Am J Pathol* 1992;141:11.
100. Strauchen JA, Dimitriu-Bona A. Immunopathology of Hodgkin's disease. Characterization of Reed-Sternberg cells with monoclonal antibodies. *Am J Pathol* 1989;123:293.
101. Vasef MA, Alsabeh R, Medeiros LJ, Weiss LM. Immunophenotype of Reed-Sternberg and Hodgkin's cells in sequential biopsy specimens of Hodgkin's disease. A HIER-based study. *Am J Clin Pathol* 1997; 108:54.
102. Hall PA, D'Ardenne AJ, Stansfeld AG. Paraffin section immunohistochemistry. II. Hodgkin's disease and large cell anaplastic (Ki1) lymphoma. *Histopathology* 1988;13:161.
103. Arber DA, Weiss LM. CD15: a review. *Appl Immunohistochem* 1993; 1:17.
104. Chang KL, Chen Y-Y, Shibata D, Weiss LM. *In situ* hybridization methodology for the detection of EBV EBER-1 RNA in paraffin-embedded tissues, as applied to normal and neoplastic tissues. *Diagn Mol Pathol* 1992;1:246.
105. Chang KL, Arber DA, Weiss LM. CD20: a review. *Appl Immunohistochem* 1996;4:1.
106. Weiss LM, Arber DA, Chang KL. CD45: a review. *Appl Immunohistochem* 1993;1:166.
107. Pinkus GS, Said JW. Hodgkin's disease, lymphocyte predominance type, nodular—a distinct entity? Unique staining profile of L&H variants of Reed-Sternberg cells defined by monoclonal antibodies to leukocyte common antigen, granulocyte specific antigen, and B-cell specific antigen. *Am J Pathol* 1985;116:1.
108. Warnke RA, Gatter KC, Falini B, et al. Diagnosis of human lymphoma with monoclonal antileukocyte antibodies. *N Engl J Med* 1983;309: 1275.
109. Dorfman RF, Gatter KC, Pulford KAF, Mason DY. An evaluation of the utility of anti-granulocyte and anti-leukocyte monoclonal antibodies in the diagnosis of Hodgkin's disease. *Am J Pathol* 1986;123: 508.
110. Medeiros LJ, Weiss LM, Warnke RA, Dorfman RF. Utility of combining antigranulocyte with antileukocyte antibodies in differentiating Hodgkin's disease from non-Hodgkin's lymphoma. *Cancer* 1988; 62:2475.
111. Strickler J, Weiss L, Copenhaver C, et al. Monoclonal antibodes reactive in routinely processed tissue sections of malignant lymphoma, with emphasis on T-cell lymphomas. *Hum Pathol* 1987;18:808.
112. Wieczorek R, Burke JS, Knowles DM. Leu-M1 antigen expression in T-cell neoplasia. *Am J Pathol* 1985;121:374.
113. Chang KL, Arber DA, Weiss LM. CD30: a review. *Appl Immunohistochem* 1993;1:244.
114. Miettinen M. Immunohistochemical study on formaldehyde-fixed, paraffin-embedded Hodgkin's and non-Hodgkin's lymphomas. *Arch Pathol Lab Med* 1992;116:1197.
115. De Mascarel I, Trojani M, Eghbali H, Coindre JM, Bonichon F. Prognostic value of phenotyping by Ber-H2, Leu-M1, EMA in Hodgkin's disease. *Arch Pathol Lab Med* 1990;114:953.
116. Ree HJ, Neiman RS, Martin AW, Dallenbach F, Stein H. Paraffin section markers for Reed-Sternberg cells. A comparative study of peanut agglutinin, Leu-M1, LN-2, and Ber H2. *Cancer* 1989;63:2030.
117. Schwarting R, Gerdes J, Durkop H, Falini B, Pileri S, Stein H. BER-H2: a new anti-Ki-1 (CD30) monoclonal antibody directed at a formol-resistant epitope. *Blood* 1989;74:1678.
118. Stein H, Mason DY, Gerdes J, et al. The expression of the Hodgkin's disease associated antigen Ki-1 in reactive and neoplastic lymphoid tissue: evidence that Reed-Sternberg cells and histiocytic malignancies are derived from activated lymphoid cells. *Blood* 1985;66:848.
119. von Wasielewski R, Mengel M, Fischer R, et al. Classical Hodgkin's

disease: clinical impact of the immunophenotype. *Am J Pathol* 1997; 151:1123.

120. Pallesen G, Hamilton DS. Ki-1 (CD30) antigen is regularly expressed by tumor cells of embryonal carcinoma. *Am J Pathol* 1988;133:446.
121. Stein H, Hansmann ML, Lennert K, Brandtzaeg P, Gatter KC, Mason DY. Reed-Sternberg and Hodgkin cells in lymphocyte-predominant Hodgkin's disease of nodular subtype contain J chain. *Am J Clin Pathol* 1986;86:292.
122. Pinkus GS, Said JW. Hodgkin's disease, lymphocyte predominance type, nodular—further evidence for a B cell derivation: L&H variants of Reed-Sternberg cells express L26, a pan B cell marker. *Am J Pathol* 1988;133:211.
123. Frierson HF, Innes DJ. Sensitivity of anti-Leu-M1 as a marker in Hodgkin's disease. *Arch Pathol Lab Med* 1985;109:1024.
124. Hsu SM, Jaffe ES. Leu-M1 and peanut agglutinin stain the neoplastic cells of Hodgkin's disease. *Am J Clin Pathol* 1984;82:29.
125. Fellbaum C, Hansmann ML, Parwaresch MR, Lennert K. Monoclonal antibodies Ki-B3 and Leu M1 discriminate giant cells of infectious mononucleosis and of Hodgkin's disease. *Hum Pathol* 1988;19:1168.
126. Hyder DM, Schnitzer B. Utility of Leu M1 monoclonal antibody in the differential diagnosis of Hodgkin's disease. *Arch Pathol Lab Med* 1986;110:416.
127. Hall PA, D'Ardenne AJ. Value of CD15 immunostaining in diagnosing Hodgkin's disease: a review of published literature. *J Clin Pathol* 1987;40:1298.
128. Sheibani K, Battifora H, Burke JS, Rappaport H. Leu-M1 antigen in human neoplasms: an immunohistologic study of 400 cases. *Am J Surg Pathol* 1986;10:227.
129. Zukerberg L, Collins A, Ferry J, Harris N. Coexpression of CD15 and CD20 by Reed-Sternberg cells in Hodgkin's disease. *Am J Pathol* 1991;139:475.
130. Enblad G, Sundstrom C, Glimerlius B. Immunohistochemical characteristics of Hodgkin and Reed-Sternberg cells in relation to age and clinical outcome. *Histopathology* 1993;22:535.
131. Bai MC, Jiwa NM, Horstman A, et al. Decreased expression of cellular markers in Epstein-Barr virus-positive Hodgkin's disease. *J Pathol* 1994;174:49.
132. Hummel M, Ziemann K, Lammert H, Pileri S, Sabattini E, Stein H. Hodgkin's disease with monoclonal and polyclonal populations of Reed-Sternberg cells. *N Engl J Med* 1995;333:901.
133. Küppers R, Rajewsky K, Zhao M, et al. Hodgkin disease: Hodgkin and Reed-Sternberg cells picked from histological sections show clonal immunoglobulin gene rearrangements and appear to be derived from B cells at various stages of development. *Proc Natl Acad Sci U S A* 1994;91:10962.
134. Ruprai AK, Pringle JH, Angel CA, Kind CN, Lauder I. Localization of immunoglobulin light chain mRNA expression in Hodgkin's disease by *in situ* hybridization. *J Pathol* 1991;164:37.
135. Kadin ME, Stites DP, Levy R, Warnke R. Exogenous immunoglobulin and the macrophage origin of Reed-Sternberg cells in Hodgkin's disease. *N Engl J Med* 1978;299:1208.
136. Korkolopoulou P, Cordell J, Jones M, et al. The expression of the B-cell marker mb-1 (CD79a) in Hodgkin's disease. *Histopathology* 1994; 24:511.
137. Arber DA, Weiss LM. CD43: a review. *Appl Immunohistochem* 1993; 1:88.
138. Kadin M, Muramoto L, Said J. Expression of T cell antigens on Reed-Sternberg cells in a subset of patients with nodular sclerosis and mixed cellularity Hodgkin's disease. *Am* J Pathol 1988;130:345.
139. Falini B, Stein H, Pileri S, et al. Expression of T-cell antigens on Hodgkin's and Sternberg-Reed cells of Hodgkin's disease. A combined immunocytochemical and immunohistological study using monoclonal antibodies. *Histopathology* 1987;12:129.
140. Falini B, Stein H, Pileri S, et al. Expression of lymphoid-associated antigens on Hodgkin's and Reed-Sternberg cells of Hogdkin's disease. An immunocytochemical study on lymph node cytospins using monoclonal antibodies. *Histopathology* 1987;11:1229.
141. Dallenbach FE, Stein H. Expression of T-cell-receptor chain in Reed-Sternberg cells. *Lancet* 1989;2:828.
142. Chang KL, Albujar PF, Chen Y-Y, Johnson RM, Weiss LM. High prevalence of Epstein-Barr virus in the Reed-Sternberg cells of Hodgkin's disease occurring in Peru. *Blood* 1993;81:496.
143. Pallesen G, Hamilton-Dutoit SJ, Rowe M, Young S. Expression of Epstein-Barr virus latent gene products in tumour cells of Hodgkin's disease. *Lancet* 1991;337:320.
144. Herbst H, Dallenbach F, Hummel M, et al. Epstein-Barr virus latent membrane protein expression in Hodgkin and Reed-Sternberg cells. *Proc Natl Acad Sci U S A* 1991;88:4766.
145. O'Grady JT, Stewart S, Lowrey J, Howie SEM, Krajewski AS. CD40 expression in Hodgkin's disease. *Am* J Pathol 1994;144:21.
146. Chang KL, Curtis CM, Momose H, Lopategui J, Weiss LM. Sensitivity and specificity of Bauhinia purpurea as a paraffin section marker for the Reed-Sternberg cells of Hodgkin's disease. *Appl Immunohistochem* 1993;1:208.
147. Delsol G, Meggetto F, Brousset P, et al. Relation of follicular dendritic reticulum cells to Reed-Sternberg cells of Hodgkin's disease with emphasis on the expression of CD21 antigen. *Am* J Pathol 1993; 142:1729.
148. Pinkus GS, Pinkus JL, Langhoff E, et al. Fascin, a sensitive new marker for Reed-Sternberg cells of Hodgkin's disease. Evidence for a dendritic or B cell derivation? *Am* J Pathol 1997;150:543.
149. Sorg UR, Morse TM, Patton WN, et al. Hodgkin's cells express CD83, a dendritic cell lineage associated antigen. *Pathology* 1997;29:294.
150. Mosialos G, Yamashiro S, Baughman RW, et al. Epstein-Barr virus infection induces expression in B lymphocytes of a novel gene encoding an evolutionarily conserved 55-kilodalton actin-bundling protein. *J Virol* 1994;68:7320.
151. Sherrod AE, Felder B, Levy JN, et al. Immunohistologic identification of phenotypic antigens associated with Hodgkin and Reed-Sternberg cells. A paraffin section study. *Cancer* 1986;57:2135.
152. Poppema S, Visser L. Absence of HLC class I expression by Reed-Sternberg cells. *Am* J Pathol 1994;145:37.
153. Delabie J, Shipman R, Bruggen J, et al. Expression of the novel intermediate filament-associated protein restin in Hodgkin's disease and anaplastic large-cell lymphoma. *Blood* 1992;80:2891.
154. Hsu S, Yang K, Jaffe E. Phenotypic expression of Hodgkin's and Reed-Sternberg cells in Hodgkin's disease. *Am* J Pathol 1985;118:209.
155. Gerdes J, van Baarlen J, Pileri S, Schwarting R, van Unnik JAM, Stein H. Tumor cell growth fraction in Hodgkin's disease. *Am* J Pathol 1987;128:390.
156. Sabattini E, Gerdes J, Gherlinzoni F, et al. Comparison between the monoclonal antibodies Ki-67 and PC10 in 125 malignant lymphomas. *J Pathol* 1993;169:397.
157. LeBrun DP, Ngan BY, Weiss LM, Warnke RA, Cleary ML. Involvement of the bcl-2 oncogene in the origin of Hodgkin's disease from follicular non-Hodgkin's lymphoma. *Blood* 1994;83:223.
158. Freeman J, Kellock DB, Yu CCW, Crocker J, Levison DA, Hall PA. Proliferating cell nuclear nuclear antigen (PCNA) and nucleolar organiser regions in Hodgkin's disease: correlation with morphology. *J Clin Pathol* 1993;46:446.
159. Hell K, Lorenzen J, Hansmann ML, Fellbaum C, Busch R, Fischer R. Expression of the proliferating cell nuclear antigen in the different types of Hodgkin's disease. *Am J Clin Pathol* 1993;99:598.
160. Schmid C, Sweeney E, Isaacson PG. Proliferating cell nuclear antigen (PCNA) expression in Hodgkin's disease. *J Pathol* 1992;168:1.
161. Gupta RK, Lister TA, Bodmer JG. Proliferation of Reed-Sternberg cells and variants in Hodgkin's disease. *Ann Oncol* 1994;5(Suppl 1): S117.
162. Chen W-G, Chen Y-Y, Kamel OW, Koo CH, Weiss LM. p53 mutations in Hodgkin's disease. *Lab Invest* 1996;75:519.
163. Gupta RK, Norton AJ, Thompson IW, Lister TA, Bodmer JG. p53 expression in Reed-Sternberg cells of Hodgkin's disease. Br J *Cancer* 1992;66:649.
164. Doussis IA, Pezzella F, Lane DP, Gatter KC, Mason DY. An immunocytochemical study of p53 and bcl-2 protein expression in Hodgkin's disease. *Am J Clin Pathol* 1993;99:663.
165. Doglioni C, Pelosio P, Mombello A, Scarpa A, Chilosi M. Immunohistochemical evidence of abnormal expression of the antioncogene-encoded p53 phosphoprotein in Hodgkin's disease and CD30+ anaplastic lymphomas. *Hematol Pathol* 1991;5:67.
166. Pinkus GS, Barbuto D, Said J, Churchill WH. Lymphocyte subpopulations of lymph nodes and spleens in Hodgkin's disease. *Cancer* 1978;42:1270.
167. Abdulaziz Z, Mason D, Stein H, Gatter K, Nash J. An immunohistological study of the cellular constituents of Hodgkin's disease using a monoclonal antibody panel. *Histopathology* 1984;8:1.
168. Valente G, Ferrara P, Stramignoni A. Lymphocyte populations of non-scleronodular Hodgkin's disease subtypes in different stages of lymphocyte depletion. An immunophenotypic and quantitative study. *Virchows Arch B* 1990;58:289.

169. Alavaikko JF, Hansmann ML, Nebendahl C, Parwaresch MR, Lennert K. Follicular dendritic cells in Hodgkin's disease. *Am J Clin Pathol* 1991;95:194.
170. Alavaikko MJ, Blanco G, Aine R. Follicular dendritic cells have prognostic relevance in Hodgkin's disease. *Am J Clin Pathol* 1994;101:761.
171. Jacobson JO, Wilkes BM, Harris NL. Polyclonal rearrangement of the T-cell antigen receptor genes in Hodgkin's disease: implications for diagnosis. *Mod Pathol* 1991;4:172.
172. Roth MS, Schnitzer B, Bingham EL, Harnden CE, Hyder DM, Ginsburg D. Rearrangement of immunoglobulin and T-cell receptor genes in Hodgkin's disease. *Am J Clin Pathol* 1988;131:331.
173. Brinker MGL, Poppema S, Buys CHCM, Timens W, Osinga J, Visser L. Clonal immunoglobulin gene rearrangements in tissues involved by Hodgkin's disease. *Blood* 1987;70:186.
174. Griesser H, Feller AC, Mak TW, Lennert K. Clonal rearrangements of T-cell receptor and immunoglobulin genes and immunophenotypic antigen expression in different subclasses of Hodgkin's disease. *Int J Cancer* 1987;40:157.
175. Herbst H, Tippelmann G, Anagnostopoulos I, et al. Immunoglobulin and T cell receptor gene rearrangements in Hodgkin's disease and Ki-1-positive anaplastic large cell lymphoma: dissociation between phenotype and genotype. *Leuk Res* 1989;13:103.
176. Hu EHL, Ellison D, Zovich D, Nichols P, Pattengale P. Molecular analysis of Hodgkin's disease with abundant Reed-Sternberg cells. *Hematol Pathol* 1990;4:27.
177. O'Connor N, Crick J, Gatter K, Mason D, Falini B, Stein H. Cell lineage in Hodgkin's disease. *Lancet* 1987;1:158.
178. Weiss LM, Strickler JG, Hu E, Warnke RA, Sklar J. Immunoglobulin gene rearrangements in tissues involved by Hodgkin's disease. *Hum Pathol* 1986;17:1006.
179. Weiss LM, Warnke RA, Sklar J. Clonal antigen receptor gene rearrangements and Epstein-Barr viral DNA in tissues in Hodgkin's disease. *Hematol Oncol* 1988;6:233.
180. Knowles D, Neri A, Pelicci P, et al. Immunoglobulin and T-cell receptor beta-chain gene rearrangement analysis of Hodgkin's disease: implications for lineage determination and differential diagnosis. *Proc Natl Acad Sci U S A* 1986;83:7942.
181. Sundeen J, Lipford E, Uppenkamp J, et al. Rearranged antigen receptor genes in Hodgkin's disease. *Blood* 1987;70:96.
182. Chan WC, Elmberger G, Lozano MD, Sanger W, Weisenburger DD. Large-cell anaplastic lymphoma-specific translocation in Hodgkin's disease. *Lancet* 1994;345:920.
183. Weiss LM, Lopategui JR, Sun L-H, Kamel OW, Koo CH, Glackin C. Absence of the t(2;5) in Hodgkin's disease. *Blood* 1995;85:2845.
184. Weiss LM, Warnke RA, Sklar J, Cleary ML. Molecular analysis of the t(14;18) chromosomal translocation in malignant lymphomas. *N Engl J Med* 1987;317:1185.
185. Wellmann A, Otsuki T, Vogelbruch M, Clark HM, Jaffe ES, Raffeld M. Analysis of the t(2;5)(p23;q35) by RT-PCR in CD30+ anaplastic large cell lymphomas, in other non-Hodgkin's lymphomas of T-cell phenotype, and in Hodgkin's disease. *Blood* 1995;86:2321.
186. Ladanyi M, Cavalchire G, Morris SW, Downing J, Filippa DA. Reverse transcriptase polymerase chain reaction for the Ki-1 anaplastic large cell lymphoma-associated t(2;5) translocation in Hodgkin's disease. *Am* J Pathol 1994;145:1296.
187. Lamant L, Meggetto F, Al Saati T, et al. High incidence of the t(2;5)(p23;q35) translocation in anaplastic large cell lymphoma and its lack of detection in Hodgkin's disease. Comparison of cytogenetic analysis, RT-PCR and P-80 immunostaining. *Blood* 1996;87:284.
188. Koduru PRK, Susin M, Schulman P, et al. Phenotypic and genotypic characterization of Hodgkin's disease. *Am J Hematol* 1993;44:117.
189. Shibata D, Hu E, Weiss LM, Brynes RK, Nathwani BN. Detection of specific t(14;18) chromosomal translocations in fixed tissues. *Hum Pathol* 1990;21:199.
190. Athan E, Chadburn A, Knowles DM. The bcl-2 gene translocation is undetectable in Hodgkin's disease by Southern blot hybridization and polymerase chain reaction. *Am* J Pathol 1992;141:193.
191. Louie DC, Kant JA, Brooks JJ, Reed JC. Absence of t(14;18) major and minor breakpoints and of bcl-2 protein overproduction in Reed-Sternberg cells of Hodgkin's disease. *Am* J Pathol 1991;139:1231.
192. Orscheschek K, Mere H, Hell J, Binder T, Bartels H, Feller AC. Large-cell anaplastic lymphoma-specific translocation (t[2;5][p23;q35]) in Hodgkin's disease—indication of a common pathogenesis? *Lancet* 1995;345:87.
193. Stetler-Stevenson M, Crush-Stanton S, Cossman J. Involvement of the bcl-2 gene in Hodgkin's disease. *J Natl Cancer Inst* 1990;82:855.
194. Gupta RK, Whelan JS, Lister TA, Young BD, Bodmer JG. Direct sequence analysis of the t(14;18) chromosomal translocation in Hodgkin's disease. *Blood* 1992;79:2084.
195. Reid AH, Cunningham RE, Frizzera G, O'Leary TJ. bcl-2 rearrangement in Hodgkin's disease. Results of polymerase chain reaction, flow cytometry, and sequencing on formalin-fixed, paraffin-embedded tissue. *Am* J Pathol 1993;142:395.
196. LeBrun DP, Ngan BY, Weiss LM, Huie P, Warnke RA, Cleary ML. The bcl-2 oncogene in Hodgkin's disease arising in the setting of follicular non-Hodgkin's lymphoma. *Blood* 1994;83:223.
197. Tamaru J, Hummel M, Zemlin M, Kalvelage B, Stein H. Hodgkin's disease with a B-cell phenotype often shows a VDJ rearrangement and somatic mutations in the V_H genes. *Blood* 1994;84:708.
198. Orazi A, Jiang B, Lee CH, et al. Correlation between presence of clonal rearrangements of immunogloublin heavy chain genes and B-cell antigen expression in Hodgkin's disease. *Am J Clin Pathol* 1995; 104:413.
199. Kamel OW, Chang PP, Hsu FS, Dolezal MV, Warnke RA, van de Rijn M. Clonal VDJ recombination of the immunoglobulin heavy chain gene by PCR in classical Hodgkin's disease. *Am J Clin Pathol* 1995;104:419.
200. Warnke RA, Weiss LM, Chan JKC, Cleary ML, Dorfman RF. Tumors of the lymph nodes and spleen. In: Rosai J, ed. *Atlas of tumor pathology*, vol 14. Washington DC: Armed Forces Institute of Pathology, 1995.
201. Fellbaum CH, Hansmann M-L, Lennert K. Lymphadenitis mimicking Hodgkin's disease. *Histopathology* 1988;12:253.
202. Williams J, Schned A, Cotelingam JD, Jaffe ES. Chronic lymphocytic leukemia with coexistent Hodgkin's disease. Implications for the origin of the Reed-Sternberg cell. *Am J Surg Pathol* 1991;15:33.
203. Momose H, Jaffe ES, Shin SS, Chen Y-Y, Weiss LM. Chronic lymphocytic leukemia/small lymphocytic lymphoma with Reed-Sternberg–like cells and possible transformation to Hodgkin's disease. Mediation by Epstein-Barr virus. *Am J Surg Pathol* 1992;16:859.
204. Macon WR, Williams ME, Greer JP, Stein RS, Collins RD, Cousar JB. T-cell-rich B-cell lymphomas. A clinicopathologic study of 19 cases. *Am J Surg Pathol* 1992;16:351.
205. Delabie J, Vandenberghe E, Kennes C, et al. Histiocyte-rich B-cell lymphoma. A distinct clinicopathologic entity possibly related to lymphocyte predominant Hodgkin's disease, paragranuloma subtype. *Am J Surg Pathol* 1992;16:37.
206. Banks PM. The distinction of Hodgkin's disease from T-cell lymphoma. *Semin Diag Pathol* 1992;9:279.
207. Osborne BM, Uthman MO, Butler JJ, McLaughlin P. Differentiation of T-cell lymphoma from Hodgkin's disease: mitotic rate and S-phase analysis. *Am J Clin Pathol* 1990;93:227.
208. Picker LJ, Weiss LM, Medeiros LJ, Wood GS, Warnke RA. Immunophenotypic criteria for the diagnosis of non-Hodgkin's lymphma. *Am* J Pathol 1987;128:181.
209. Weiss LM, Crabtree GS, Rouse RV, Warnke RA. Morphologic and immunologic characterization of 50 peripheral T-cell lymphomas. *Am* J Pathol 1985;118:316.
210. Borowitz M, Reichert TA, Brynes RK, et al. The phenotypic diversity of peripheral T-cell lymphomas. The Southeastern Cancer Study Group experience. *Hum Pathol* 1986;17:567.
211. Weiss LM, Chang KL. Association of the Epstein-Barr virus with hematolymphoid neoplasia. *Adv Anat Pathol* 1996;3:1.
212. Kaplan HS. *Hodgkin's disease*, 2nd ed. Cambridge, MA: Harvard University Press, 1980.

Hodgkin's Disease, edited by P. M. Mauch,
J. O. Armitage, V. Diehl, R.T. Hoppe, and L.M. Weiss.
Lippincott Williams & Wilkins, Philadephia ©1999.

CHAPTER 8

The Nature of Reed-Sternberg Cells, Lymphocytic and Histiocytic Cells and Their Molecular Biology in Hodgkin's Disease

Harald Stein, Volker Diehl, Theresa Marafioti, Andrea Jox, Jürgen Wolf, and Michael Hummel

DISCOVERY OF REED-STERNBERG CELLS AND LYMPHOCYTIC AND/OR HISTIOCYTIC (L&H) CELLS

In 1832, Thomas Hodgkin (1) described the anatomic findings of seven patients with enormous lymph node swellings. Independently, Samuel Wilks (2) published an article in 1856 summarizing 10 cases (including four of the seven cases already investigated by Hodgkin) having the same anatomic features. As soon as he became aware of his mistake, he appended an appropriate comment to his article. In the following years, Wilks collected an additional 15 cases and interpreted them as pathognomonic for a new disease entity (3). Although it was Wilks who separated Hodgkin's disease from other diseases associated with lymph node swellings, he was sufficiently magnanimous to name the disease after Hodgkin in acknowledgment of Hodgkin's first report of some cases. The histopathologic features of this disease were initially described by Langhans in 1872 (4) and Greenfield in 1878 (5). However, Carl Sternberg in 1898 (6) and Dorothy Reed in 1902 (7) published, independently of each other, a more detailed description of the cytologic features of the multinucleated giant cells, which have since been known as Reed-Sternberg cells. The mononucleated blasts were later designated Hodgkin cells. In 1966, Lukes and Butler (8) described a multilobated variant of the Hodgkin and Reed-Sternberg cells that occurs mainly in the nodular lymphocyte-predominant type of Hodgkin's disease. These multilobated blasts were called L&H cells because in lymphocyte predominance Hodgkin's disease the cellular background consists of lymphocytes and histiocytes. Because of the multilobated nuclear morphology of these cells, Neiman (9) suggested that they be called popcorn cells.

Immunohistological studies of the last 20 years [reviewed in (10) and (11) and recently extended in (12)] have shown that two distinct immunophenotypes of the atypical blasts exist in Hodgkin's disease (Table 1). Immunophenotype I is characterized by the consistent expression of CD20 and J chain, and the constant absence

TABLE 1. *The two immunophenotypes of neoplastic cells encountered in Hodgkin's disease and their correlation with the morphologically distinct L&H cell and classical Hodgkin and Reed-Sternberg cell types*

	Immunophenotype I: lymphocyte-predominance Hodgkin's disease	Immunophenotype II: classical Hodgkin's disease
Antigen		
J chain	+(−)	−
CD20	+	−/+
CD79a	+	−/+
CD30	−	+
CD15	−	+/−
Cell type		
L&H	+	−
HRS	−	+

CD, cluster of differentiation; L&H, lymphocytic and histiocytic; HRS, Hodgkin and Reed-Sternberg.

H. Stein, T. Marafioti, and M. Hummel: Institute of Pathology, Universitätsklinikum Freien Universität Berlin, Berlin, Germany.

V. Diehl, A. Jox, and J. Wolf: Department of Internal Medicine, Klinik I für Innere Medizin der Universität zu Köln, Köln, Germany.

TABLE 2. *World Health Organization classification of Hodgkin's disease*

Nodular lymphocyte predominant Hodgkin lymphoma
+/– Diffuse areas
Classic Hodgkin's lymphoma
Lymphocyte-rich
Nodular sclerosis (grades I and II)
Mixed cellularity
Lymphocyte depletion

of CD30 and CD15; immunophenotype II is characterized by the constant expression of CD30, frequent expression of CD15, and constant absence of J chain. Combined histologic and immunohistologic investigations revealed that the L&H cells defined by Lukes and Butler have immunophenotype I, and the other HRS cells have immunophenotype II. These findings clearly demonstrate that (a) L&H cells and Hodgkin and Reed-Sternberg cells represent different cell populations and that (b) Hodgkin's disease therefore comprises two distinct diseases: lymphocyte predominance Hodgkin's disease and non-lymphocyte predominance Hodgkin's disease. This distinction correlates well with the clinical findings that the early stages of lymphocyte predominance Hodgkin's disease may be quite indolent, and that all other forms of Hodgkin's disease progress steadily without treatment and therefore require immediate treatment (13). In view of these findings, the International Lymphoma Study Group (11) proposed to subsume all Hodgkin's disease histotypes with immunophenotype II, which include nodular sclerosis, mixed cellularity, and lymphocyte depletion, under the generic term classical Hodgkin's disease, to emphasis their relationship to one other and their distinctness from lymphocyte predominance Hodgkin's disease.

In the past, the clear difference between lymphocyte predominance Hodgkin's disease and classical Hodgkin's disease was often not recognized. A recent multinational study of lymphocyte predominance Hodgkin's disease clarified the reason for this confusion by finding a Hodgkin's disease form that closely resembles, in growth pattern and cellular composition, nodular lymphocyte predominance Hodgkin's disease but that resembles, in the immunophenotype of its atypical blasts, classical Hodgkin's disease. In the new World Health Organization (WHO) classification of malignant lymphoma (14), this form of Hodgkin's disease is designated as nodular lymphocyte-rich classical Hodgkin's disease, a new histologic subtype of classical Hodgkin's disease (Table 2).

ELUCIDATION OF ORIGIN AND CLONALITY OF HODGKIN AND REED-STERNBERG CELLS AND L&H CELLS

Because Hodgkin and Reed-Sternberg cells and L&H cells are rare in the tissues affected by Hodgkin's disease, research has been hampered for decades. Recently, however, it has been possible to clarify the nature and origin of both Hodgkin and Reed-Sternberg cells and L&H cells by the combined application of different methods and reagents (Table 3) developed within the last 30 years. Outlined below are the most important steps that have led to new findings.

Immunohistology

As Hodgkin and Reed-Sternberg cells and L&H cells make up only a small minority of the cells present in the Hodgkin's disease tissue samples, a method was sought that allowed for the specific detection of certain molecules in tissue sections at the single-cell level. Between 1945 and 1955, a method was developed by Coons and colleagues (15) that combined morphologic analysis with specific antibody-binding reactions. For this purpose, tissue sections were stained with antibodies conjugated to a fluorescent dye. However, a disadvantage of this immunohistologic technique is that morphology is difficult to assess because the sections can be evaluated only by means of a fluorescent microscope, which results in a visible labeling of the cells that bind the antibody but leaves other cells and structures more or less invisible. To make the labeled and unlabeled cells simultaneously visible, the fluorescent label was replaced by enzymes such as horseradish peroxidase or alkaline phosphatase, which produce color precipitates detectable by common light microscopy, and counterstaining was carried out with haemalaun. One of the first applications of this enzyme-labeled immunohistology was the analysis of Hodgkin and Reed-Sternberg cells in formalin-fixed and paraffin-embedded tissue sections for the expression of immunoglobulin G (IgG) (16,17). The Hodgkin and Reed-Sternberg cells in all cases studied showed a strong cytoplasmic positivity, pointing to a relationship between Hodgkin and Reed-Sternberg cells and IgG-producing B cells. Further studies revealed, however,

TABLE 3. *Methods and reagents required for elucidation of origin and clonality of Hodgkin and Reed-Sternberg cells and L&H cells*

Immunohistology
Permanent cell lines established from Hodgkin's disease
Monoclonal antibody technology
CD30 cytokine receptor as a marker for Hodgkin and Reed-Sternberg cells
CD20 and J chains as characteristic as markers for L&H cells
Immunoglobulin gene rearrangements as a marker for B cells and clonality
Polymerase chain reaction
Isolation of single Hodgkin and Reed-Sternberg cells and L&H cells from tissue sections
Cytotoxic molecules as a marker for T cells

CD, cluster of differentiation; L&H, lymphocytic ad histiocytic.

that the individual Hodgkin and Reed-Sternberg cells not only bound antibodies to IgG but also antibodies to immunoglobulin κ and λ light chains (18–20). Because normal B cells produce either immunoglobulin κ or immunoglobulin λ light chains, but never both, the immunostaining of Hodgkin and Reed-Sternberg cells for immunoglobulin κ and immunoglobulin λ and IgG was thought to represent a technical artifact caused by uptake of immunoglobulins from the serum during the fixation process. This observation made it evident that immunohistologic detection of a molecule in a given cell does not necessarily indicate that it is synthesized by the labeled cell, especially if the molecule under investigation is present in the serum at a significant concentration. Therefore, attempts were made to produce antibodies against cell type-specific molecules that are absent from serum. These attempts to characterize Hodgkin and Reed-Sternberg cells succeeded when (a) permanent cell lines derived from Hodgkin and Reed-Sternberg cells as a source of Hodgkin's disease-associated antigens became available and (b) monoclonal antibody technology was established.

Permanent Hodgkin's Disease Cell Lines

To make pure populations of Hodgkin and Reed-Sternberg cells available for molecular studies, many attempts were made to establish permanently growing cell lines from these cells. Despite the development of efficient tissue culture methods in the 1960s, most attempts failed up until the late 1970s for various reasons: outgrowths of Epstein-Barr virus-positive (EBV+) lymphoblastoid cell lines derived from normal EBV-infected B cells, short-term cultures (21), or contamination with nonhuman monkey kidney cells (22). The first two permanent cell lines (designated L428 and L540) that were highly likely to be derived from Hodgkin and Reed-Sternberg cells were established in Diehl's laboratory in 1979 (23). Both cell lines were established from patients with advanced-stage Hodgkin's disease (CS IV B). The L428 line grew out from a pleural effusion and the L540 cell line from bone marrow. With few exceptions, all additional cell lines were also established from body fluids (bone marrow, pleural effusion, peripheral blood) of patients with advanced-stage disease. Possibly, this observation reflects an *in vivo* adaptation of the cells to the conditions of suspension culture as a prerequisite for *in vitro* outgrowth. These cell lines resembled *in situ* Hodgkin and Reed-Sternberg cells in morphology, ability to bind T cells to form rosettes, expression of major histocompatibility complex (MHC) class II molecules, and absence of immunoglobulin and macrophage characteristic enzymes (24). More than 10 *bona fide* Hodgkin's disease cell lines have now been established (Table 4) *(25–27)*. Despite the close resemblance in immunophenotype, these Hodgkin's disease cell lines are not generally accepted as being truly derived from Hodgkin and Reed-Sternberg cells. The reasons for the skepticism are (a) the Hodgkin's disease cell lines are not homogeneous in that two-thirds of them exhibit the immunophenotypic and genotypic features of

TABLE 4. *Immunophenotype and genotype of cell lines established from cases of classical Hodgkin's disease*

Cell lines	CD30	CD70	CD15	CD68	B-AG	T-AG	Rearranged AGR gene	AGR chain expression	EBV	Ref.
L428[a]	+	+	+	–*	–	–	IgH, L	–	–	23
L591[a]	+	+	+/–	–	CD19, 20	CD2	IgH, L	IgAλ	+	162
KM-H2[a]	+	+	+	–	–	–	IgH, L	–	–	163
L540[a]	+	+	(+)	–	–	–	TCRα,β,δ	–	–	162, 164
CO[a]	+	–	+	–	–	cyCD3, 7	TCRβ,δ	–	–	165, 23
HO[a]	+	+	–	–	–	CD3, 5, 7	TCRβ,δ	TCRβ?	–	166
HDLM2[a]	+	nd	+	–	–	CD2	TCRα,β,δ	–	–	167, 168
DEV[b]	+	nd	+	nd	CD20, 22	–	IgH, L	cyIgA	–	169, 170
HD-70[b]	+	nd	+	nd	–	–	IgH, L	cyIgAκ	–	171
ZO[b]	+	nd	+	nd	–	–	IgH, L	nd	–	170
SUP-HD1[b]	–	nd	+	–	–	–	IgH, L, TCRβ	κ	–	172
HD-MyZ[c]	–	–	–	+	–	–	–	–	–	30
L1236[a]	+	+	+	–	–	–	IgH, L	–	–	32

CD, cluster of differentiation; AG, antigen; AGR, antigen receptor; EBV, Epstein Barr virus; Ig, immunoglobulin; cy, cytoplasmic; TCR, T-cell receptor; +, constantly positive; (+), faintly positive; +/–, variably positive; –, constantly negative; nd, not done.

*In some sublines reported to be weakly positive.

[a]Permanently growing and available.

[b]It is not known whether these lines are still alive or whether the diagnosis of the primary material was correct; most of these cell lines have not been made available.

[c]This line has been established from a patient with nodular sclerosis Hodgkin's disease. However, it is highly unlikely that the cell line is derived from the Hodgkin and Reed-Sternberg cells because the Hodgkin and Reed-Sternberg cells in the tissue biopsy specimen proved to be CD30+, CD15+, CD68–, whereas the cell line cells are CD30–, CD15–, and CD68+ (24).

B cells, and the other third the characteristics of T cells; (b) the karyotype of the cell lines is grossly disordered without having consistent cytogenetic aberrations; and (c) among the 13 Hodgkin's disease lines, only one (L591) is EBV+, whereas *in vivo* the Hodgkin and Reed-Sternberg cells of 50% of classical Hodgkin's disease cases are infected with EBV (28,29). One of these so-called Hodgkin's disease cell lines, the HD-MyZ cell line, differs totally in immunophenotype and genotype from *in situ* Hodgkin and Reed-Sternberg cells (30). It expresses the macrophage-characteristic CD68 antigen and lacks CD30, CD15, CD70 and rearranged Ig genes (31). In summary, the findings obtained by analysis of these cell lines suggested the following: classical Hodgkin's disease may be derived from either B cells or T cells; a specific genetic defect common to all cases and types of classical Hodgkin's disease might be missing; and among the 13 Hodgkin's disease cell lines, those derived from EBV+ Hodgkin and Reed-Sternberg cells are greatly underrepresented.

It must be stressed that for only one of the above-mentioned 13 Hodgkin's disease cell lines was a direct derivation from Hodgkin and Reed-Sternberg cells proved. It was again work from the laboratory of Diehl that closed this gap. For the newly established (1996) cell line L1236, it could be shown that the cells harbor the same CDR3 sequence in the rearranged immunoglobulin gene as the *in situ* Hodgkin and Reed-Sternberg cells of the patient from whom the cell line was established (32).

The establishment of Hodgkin's disease cell lines represents a very important step in the progress of research on Hodgkin's disease; for example, the cell lines were used successfully for the discovery of Hodgkin and Reed-Sternberg cell-associated antigens that include CD30 (Ki-1) (33,34), CD70 (Ki-24) (35), and Ki-27 (35) for cloning the CD30 gene and for studying the CD30 signal transduction pathway. Moreover, they enabled the *in vitro* testing of new immunotherapeutic modalities like ricin A-linked anti-CD30 immunotoxins, saporin-linked anti-CD30 immunotoxins, anti-CD16/CD30 bi-specific antibodies, and CD30 anti-idiotype vaccine (36–39).

Animal Models for Hodgkin's Disease

The establishment of an animal model for Hodgkin's disease was desirable to circumvent some of the problems associated with analysis of primary tumor material (e.g., scarcity of tumor cells and their rare outgrowth *in vitro*). However, after subcutaneous transplantation in athymic T cell-deficient nude mice, neither primary Hodgkin's disease cells nor the Hodgkin's disease-derived cell lines were tumorigenic (40). Only after intracranial transplantation into nude mice was growth of two Hodgkin's disease-derived cell lines observed (41). Severe combined immunodeficient (SCID) mice lacking functional B and T lymphocytes were described in 1983 (42) and seemed to be a better alternative to nude mice, allowing the successful propagation of human lymphoma cells and even human untransformed B cells. To test whether SCID mice would also enable the establishment of an animal model for Hodgkin's disease, in a first attempt, Hodgkin's disease-derived cell lines were xenotransplanted subcutaneously. In contrast to what occurred in nude mice, all cell lines tested (L428, L540, L591, HD-LM2, KM-H2) did grow progressively and reproducibly after subcutaneous inoculation into SCID mice without prior treatment of the animals (40). Based on these observations, Hodgkin's disease cell lines were also inoculated intravenously into the tail veins of SCID mice to achieve disseminated growth resembling the growth pattern of Hodgkin's disease cells in humans. When this approach was used, of three cell lines tested (L540, L428, and KM-H2), only the L540 cell line gave rise to tumors (43). After intravenous inoculation, L540 cells showed progressive disseminated growth and preferentially localized to the lymph nodes, particularly the cervical, iliac, and inguinal nodes. Surprisingly, the spleen was found to be involved only rarely. This disseminated SCID mouse model for the growth of Hodgkin's disease cells was successfully used for preclinical *in vivo* testing of new immunotherapeutic modalities, such as ricin A-linked anti-CD25 immunotoxins and CD16/CD30 bi-specific antibodies (37,44). In the meantime, further Hodgkin's disease-derived cell lines showed disseminated growth in SCID mice. These observations encouraged us to transplant primary Hodgkin cells into this mouse strain (45). Thus, lymph node or spleen tissue affected by Hodgkin's disease was transplanted into the subrenal capsule of SCID mice. From the material of three patients (from a total of 13), tumors of human origin developed and spread predominantly into the lymph nodes. These tumors, however, did not consist of Hodgkin and Reed-Sternberg cells. Rather, an outgrowth of EBV+ B lymphocytes was observed. Surprisingly, these B cells growing out from xenografted Hodgkin's disease tissue displayed a high number of numeric as well as structural chromosomal aberrations compared with EBV+ B cells growing out in SCID mice after the transplantation of B cells from healthy donors. Possibly, this observation points to an inherent cytogenetic instability of the B lymphocytes in the surrounding Hodgkin and Reed-Sternberg cells. These cytogenetic aberrations might result in an *in vivo* growth advantage. Whether these cells also resemble tumor precursor cells of the Hodgkin and Reed-Sternberg cells remains speculative. The *in vivo* growth of established Hodgkin's disease cell lines in SCID mice provides a model for preclinical testing of new treatment modalities. Because of the lack of a Hodgkin's disease-specific growth pattern (i.e., the predominance of nonmalignant bystander cells in the tumors), this model is of limited usefulness for studying the biology of Hodgkin's disease. The problem also could not be circumvented by the transplantation of primary tumor material into SCID mice, as only very rarely was the outgrowth of HRS cells observed.

ANTIGENS ASSOCIATED WITH HODGKIN AND REED-STERNBERG CELLS AND L&H CELLS

CD15

The first antigen found to be commonly associated with Hodgkin and Reed-Sternberg cells was CD15. This association was first recognized by use of the antibodies Tü9 (46) and 3C4 (47), and later of Leu-M1 (48) and C3D1 (49). The CD15 antibodies are directed at the trisaccharide antigen lacto-*N*-fucipentaose III, also termed X-hapten (50). The detection of the CD15 moiety has achieved diagnostic significance because it is present in Hodgkin and Reed-Sternberg cells in most cases of classical Hodgkin's disease but is constantly absent from L&H cells of LP Hodgkin's disease. However, CD15 has no value as a marker of cell lineage because in normal subjects it is expressed on a variety of cells, including late cells of granulopoiesis, epithelioid-type macrophages, various epithelial cells, and a subset of B and T cells following activation and/or transformation by EBV. It may also be found on some Hodgkin and Reed-Sternberg-like cells in infectious mononucleosis, and on the neoplastic cells of some non-Hodgkin lymphomas (48,50,51,52).

CD30 and CD70

In search of viral antigens in Hodgkin and Reed-Sternberg cells, the research team of Stein in 1981 generated polyclonal antibodies (53), and 1 year later monoclonal antibodies (33,34), against the Hodgkin's disease cell line L428. These studies led to the discovery of the Ki-1 and Ki-24 molecules (33,35), which were clustered as CD30 in 1987 (54) and as CD70 in 1989 (55).

In 1993, the CD70 antigen was identified as the ligand of the CD27 receptor (56) and was thus found to be involved in the modulation of the T-cell immune response. Because there are no detailed studies on CD70 in relation to Hodgkin's disease, what follows is a description of the characteristics of the CD30 molecule.

By molecular cloning, the CD30 antigen was identified as a cytokine receptor of the tumor necrosis factor receptor family (57). Gene disruption and functional studies (58–60) revealed that CD30 is involved in the negative selection of thymocytes and in the regulation of apoptosis and proliferation of activated lymphoid cells. The CD30 antigen proved to be an ideal marker for Hodgkin and Reed-Sternberg cells because it selectively labels Hodgkin and Reed-Sternberg cells in tissues affected by classical Hodgkin's disease (33,34,61). The detection of the CD30 molecule on some large perifollicular and intrafollicular blasts in normal lymphoid tissue, and the finding that expression of this molecule can be induced on normal peripheral blood B and T cells by mitogens and viruses such as EBV and human T-cell leukemia virus (HTLV) I and II (61), indicate that the CD30 antigen does not represent a viral antigen but rather a differentiation antigen whose expression is associated with activation of lymphoid cells. The restriction of the occurrence of the CD30 antigen in normal subjects to occasional activated lymphoid cells strongly favors a lymphocytic origin of Hodgkin and Reed-Sternberg cells (61).

B-cell and T-cell Marker Molecules

Supporting the above conclusion was the detection of B-cell antigens (e.g., CD19, CD20, CD22, CD79a) or T-cell antigens (e.g., CD3, CD4, CD8, T-cell receptor β chain) on variable proportions of Hodgkin and Reed-Sternberg cells in approximately 40% of cases of classical Hodgkin's disease (61–72). Although these findings were in harmony in principle with the cell lineage characteristics of the Hodgkin's disease cell lines, they evoked much skepticism. Because the mentioned markers were not demonstrable in approximately 60% of cases of classical Hodgkin's disease cases and when so only on varying proportion of Hodgkin and Reed-Sternberg cells, it was widely believed that the detectability of B- and T-cell antigens on Hodgkin and Reed-Sternberg cells represents an aberrant antigen expression phenomenon that does not permit any conclusions to be drawn concerning the cellular origin of HRS cells. Fortunately, the situation proved to be clearer for L&H cells. These cells were shown to express constantly the B cell-associated molecules J chain (73,74), CD20 (64,75), and CD79a (67), and to lack CD30, CD15, and T-cell antigens (12), indicating their distinctness from Hodgkin and Reed-Sternberg cells and their derivation from B cells.

Molecules Associated with Dendritic Cells

An interesting but not yet fully understood finding is the expression of restin (77,78), fascin (79), and thymus and activation regulated chemokine (TARC) (80). All three molecules have in common that they are expressed in normal tissues on dendritic cells (79–81). This finding fits in well with the observation that the cells of the Hodgkin's disease cell lines are able to present antigen more efficiently to T cells than normal B cells. These properties prompted some authors to believe that Hodgkin and Reed-Sternberg cells are related to dendritic cells rather than to lymphoid cells. Beyond that, the expression of TARC could possibly explain the mechanism by which CD4+ T cells form rosettes around the Hodgkin and Reed-Sternberg cells. TARC is a chemokine that attracts CD4+

T cells by binding to chemokine receptor 4 (CCR4) and is expressed by the Hodgkin and Reed-Sternberg cells (80).

CD40

The CD40 molecule is a member of the tumor necrosis factor receptor family (82) that is constantly expressed on B cells, dendritic cells of interdigitating type, macrophages, thymic epithelium, and many carcinomas (83). CD40 is also regularly expressed on Hodgkin and Reed-Sternberg cells (84,85). Considering the broad cellular expression of CD40, its detection on Hodgkin and Reed-Sternberg cells is of no help regarding the lineage assignment of these cells. However, CD40 appears to be of interest functionally because its involvement in the deregulation of the cytokine network in Hodgkin's disease has been reported. Experiments with cultured Hodgkin's disease cells (84) showed that activation of CD40 by its ligand or anti-CD40 antibodies enhances the expression of co-stimulatory molecules such as the intracellular adhesion molecule 1 (ICAM-1) and B7-1.

Conclusions of the Immunophenotypic Studies

In summary, these studies agree that the L&H cells of lymphocyte predominance Hodgkin's disease constantly carry B-cell antigens, so that their derivation from B cells is generally accepted. For the Hodgkin and Reed-Sternberg cells of classical Hodgkin's disease, the situation is less clear because these cells in most instances lack lineage-specific antigens and express some unusual molecules, including those characteristic of dendritic antigen-presenting cells. However, on the whole, the antigen profile of the Hodgkin and Reed-Sternberg cells points toward a derivation from activated lymphoid cells of B-cell type (most commonly) and T-cell type (less commonly).

IMMUNOGLOBULIN GENES AS MARKERS FOR B CELLS AND CLONALITY

The clarification of the structure of the immunoglobulin gene locus led to the discovery that in B cells—in contrast to all other somatic cells—the immunoglobulin genes are rearranged [reviewed in (86)]. It could be further shown that this rearrangement takes place during the development of B cells, and that the recombination of the immunoglobulin gene segments is random and associated with a random incorporation of nucleotides (known as N segments) between the rearranged immunoglobulin gene segments in the IgH gene and the IgL gene (86). The result is that each single mature nonmalignant B cell contains distinct IgH and IgL gene rearrangements that are—like a fingerprint for a given human being—specific for an individual B cell (86). This specificity is predominantly located within the complementarity determining region 3 (CDR3). In contrast to reactive B cells, neoplastic cells from B-cell lymphomas have identically rearranged immunoglobulin genes and thus identical CDR3 sequences. This finding confirms that each B-cell lymphoma is derived from one single transformed B cell and so represents—in contrast to the polyclonal proliferation of reactive B cells—a monoclonal B-cell population. It was evident from these findings that analysis of the immunoglobulin gene locus in Hodgkin and Reed-Sternberg cells and L&H cells would unequivocally clarify whether they are B cell-derived and whether they are polyclonal, arisen from many (e.g., virally) transformed B cells, or monoclonal, derived from a single transformed B cell. Therefore, many research groups (87–95) analyzed DNA extracted from Hodgkin's disease biopsy specimens for the presence of monoclonal immunoglobulin rearrangements. The results of these investigations were heterogeneous, with the majority being negative (87–95). This was not surprising, considering the low sensitivity of the Southern blot technique initially used, which requires that more than 5% identical B cells be present in any given cell mixture for the demonstration of monoclonally rearranged immunoglobulin genes. As mentioned previously, Hodgkin and Reed-Sternberg cells or L&H cells rarely exceed 1% of the cell populations present in tissue samples affected by Hodgkin's disease.

Polymerase Chain Reaction Studies of Whole-tissue DNA

The development of polymerase chain reaction (PCR) in 1985 (96) and its subsequent simplification (through the use of a thermally stable polymerase) in 1988 (97) opened up a new dimension in the analysis of genes. By means of this method, it became possible to amplify nucleic acid sequences a million times. However, the application of PCR to the detection of monoclonally rearranged immunoglobulin genes in Hodgkin's disease biopsy specimens did not clarify the cellular origin and the clonality of Hodgkin and Reed-Sternberg cells and L&H cells because monoclonal immunoglobulin gene rearrangements were found in a varying proportion of cases (98–102). For example, in the hands of Stein's research group, an optimized PCR procedure led to the detection of monoclonally rearranged immunoglobulin genes in 28% of cases of classical Hodgkin's disease and in 67% of cases of nodular lymphocyte predominance Hodgkin's disease (98). These data were difficult to interpret. Because the results were obtained with whole-tissue DNA, it could not be determined whether the monoclonal rearrangements were really derived from Hodgkin and Reed-Sternberg cells or L&H cells and not from other cells [e.g., B-cell clones present in a germinal center]. In addition, the data obtained did not explain why the PCR assay demonstrated monoclonal immunoglobulin rearrangements in only a fraction of cases. The question to be answered was the following: Is the nondetectability of clonally rearranged immunoglobulin genes in the majority of cases a consequence of their really being absent from Hodgkin and Reed-Sternberg cells and L&H cells, or is it a consequence of a too-low specificity of the PCR method or of technical artifacts not yet considered? Because it was clear that the questions raised could not be answered by further studies of whole-tissue DNA, several research teams focused on developing methods to isolate Hodgkin and Reed-Sternberg cells and L&H cells.

Polymerase Chain Reaction Studies of Single Cells

Methods for Isolating Single Hodgkin and Reed-Sternberg Cells and L&H Cells

The incredibly high sensitivity of PCR made it possible to detect single-gene copies for the first time. Therefore, no further attempts were made to isolate populations of Hodgkin and Reed-Sternberg cells and L&H cells for molecular biologic investigations; instead, single exemplars of these cells were used. In the first attempt of this kind, fresh biopsy tissue was suspended and the putative Hodgkin and Reed-Sternberg cell selected by their large size and their negativity for CD3, CD14, and CD20 and their morphology were isolated by means of a pipette (103). However, no consistent pattern of gene expression was observed in this study, which might indicate that the reliable identification of Hodgkin and Reed-Sternberg cells in this way is difficult. The research team led by Pfreundschuh (104) tried to improve cell identification with the method described by precipitating the suspended cells onto slides with a cytocentrifuge and subsequently immunostaining them for CD30 or CD20. A second method of cell isolation—developed in the laboratory of Chan (105)—used thick paraffin sections, from which cells were suspended by means of enzymatic digestion and mechanical force. The suspended cells were immunostained in solution and then isolated by means of a pipette. A third method that was developed is the most straightforward procedure. From immunostained frozen sections, CD30+ Hodgkin and Reed-Sternberg cells or CD20+ L&H cells are extracted by means of two hydraulically driven pipettes. This method was established in the laboratories of Rajewsky and Hansmann (106). The great advantage of this method is that the cells to be isolated can be identified reliably based on their morphology, antigen expression, and tissue localization, as the architecture of the tissue is not destroyed. This technique also avoids the loss of certain cell types that regularly occurs when tissue is suspended. A further important advantage of this method is that the isolation procedure can be optically monitored in each of its phases.

Preliminary Results and Initial Problems

The first single-cell studies of Hodgkin and Reed-Sternberg cells and L&H cells provided heterogeneous results (Table 5). Pfreundschuh's group (104) failed to

TABLE 5. *Rearrangements of immunoglobulin-genes in Hodgkin and Reed-Sternberg cells and L&H cells: preliminary results and initial problems of single-cell analysis*

Research team (year) (ref.)	No. cases studied	Type of Hodgkin's disease	Cases without Ig-R	Cases with identical Ig-R only	Cases with identical and nonidentical Ig-R	Cases with nonidentical Ig-R only	Interpretation
Pfreundschuh et al. (1994) (104)	12	Classical	12	0	0	0	HRS cells are unrelated to B cells.
Pfreundschuh et al. (1994) (104)	1	LP	1	0	0	0	L&H cells are unrelated to B cells.
Rajewsky/Hansmann et al. (1994) (107)	2	Classical	0	0	2	0	HRS cells are clonal B cells.*
Rajewsky/Hansmann et al. (1994) (107)	1	LP	0	0	1	0	L&H cells are clonal B cells.*
Chan et al. (1994) (105)	4	LP	0	0	0	4	L&H cells are polyclonal B cells.
Chan et al. (1996) (108)	6	Classical	3	0	0	3	HRS cells are polyclonal B cells.
Stein et al. (1995) (109)	12	Classical	0	3	3	6	HRS cells are 3× clonal B cells. HRS cell are 6× polyclonal B cells. HRS cells are 3× a mixture of clonal and polyclonal B cells.

L&H, lymphocytic and histiocytic; Ig-R, immunoglobulin gene rearrangement; LP, lymphocyte predominance; HRS, Hodgkin and Reed-Sternberg.

*Nonidentical rearrangements were interpreted by the authors as cellular contamination since such rearrangements were amplified with the same frequency from T-cells.

demonstrate immunoglobulin gene rearrangements in single Hodgkin and Reed-Sternberg cells and L&H cells. In contrast, the research teams of Rajewsky/Hansmann, Chan (105,107), Chan (108), and Stein (109) found rearranged immunoglobulin genes in both Hodgkin and Reed-Sternberg cells and L&H cells. However, despite this agreement, the results of these groups differed in the rearrangement patterns. The L&H cell-derived and Hodgkin and Reed-Sternberg cell-derived immunoglobulin rearrangements reported by Chan's group were unrelated (i.e., polyclonal), whereas those found by Rajewsky's group were identical (i.e., monoclonal). Stein's group observed both rearrangement patterns in Hodgkin and Reed-Sternberg cells (i.e., cases with unrelated and cases with identical immunoglobulin gene rearrangements) (Table 6). The following possibilities for these discordant findings were considered: (a) isolation of cells other than Hodgkin and Reed-Sternberg cells; (b) nonbinding of the primers to the target gene sequences of the monoclonal immunoglobulin rearrangements because of hypermutations, but binding to contaminating DNA derived from B cells with few or no mutations, in cases in which only or additional polyclonal immunoglobulin rearrangements were demonstrated; (c) presence of reactive (i.e., polyclonal) CD30+ blasts among true monoclonal CD30+ Hodgkin and Reed-Sternberg cells, in cases in which both monoclonal and polyclonal immunoglobulin rearrangements were demonstrated. To clarify which of the possibilities was valid, Stein's team (110) undertook the following investigations. First, the monoclonal and polyclonal Hodgkin's disease cases were reanalyzed by using additional primer sets. This study confirmed the presence of monoclonal immunoglobulin rearrangements in the Hodgkin and Reed-Sternberg cells of all the cases of classical Hodgkin's disease already determined to be monoclonal. However, in two of the four cases with polyclonal rearrangements, the reinvestigation led to the detection of identical (monoclonal) rearrangements, showing that the monoclonal rearrangements had escaped detection with the consensus primers used in the first analysis. To clarify why in some cases only monoclonal immunoglobulin rearrangements and in others both monoclonal *and* polyclonal rearrangements were detectable in the Hodgkin and Reed-Sternberg cells, these rearrangement patterns were correlated with the cellular composition of the sections used for the isolation procedure. This analysis revealed that all sections that gave rise to polyclonal rearrangements in the single-cell assay contained a significant number of reactive B cells, whereas reactive B cells were rare or missing in the cases without polyclonal rearrangements. This strongly suggested that the polyclonal rearrangements stemmed from the contaminating DNA of reactive small B cells rather than from Hodgkin and Reed-Sternberg cells. The subsequent examination of the cell isolation procedure revealed that this was indeed the case. It was shown that the DNA of reactive B cells tend to float off into the buffer with which the frozen sections are covered during cell isolation, and that there is a great risk for including contaminating B cell-derived DNA in the PCR assay when the selected Hodgkin and Reed-Sternberg cell or L&H cell is transferred to the PCR tube with a large volume of covering buffer. By a 100-fold reduction of the volume of buffer

TABLE 6. *Rearrangements of immunoglobulin genes in Hodgkin and Reed-Sternberg cells and L&H cells: final results of single-cell analysis*

Research team (year) (ref.)	No. cases studied	Type of Hodgkin's disease	Cases without Ig-R	Cases with identical Ig-R only	Cases with identical and nonidentical Ig-R	Cases with nonidentical Ig-R only	Interpretation
Rajewsky/Hansmann et al. (1996) (110)	15	Classical	1	7	7	0	HRS cells are clonal B cells in 90% of the cases.
Stein et al. (1998) (113)	25	Classical	1	24	0	0	HRS cells are clonal B cells in >90% of cases.
Stein et al. (1997) (112)	11	LP	0	11	0	0	L&H cells are clonal B cells in all cases.
Rajewsky/Hansmann et al. (1996) (114)	5	LP	0	5	0	0	L&H cells are clonal B cells in all cases.
Chan et al. (1997) (115)	5	LP	0	0	5	0	L&H cells are clonal B cells in all cases.

L&H, lymphocytic and histiocytic; Ig-R, immunoglobulin rearrangement; LP, lymphocyte predominance; HRS, Hodgkin and Reed-Sternberg.

Nonindentical rearrangements were interpreted by the authors as cellular contamination since such arrangements were amplified with the same frequency from T-cells.

with which the isolated cells are transferred into the PCR test tube, the contamination rate was brought down to under 1% (111).

Final Results

With optimization of the cell isolation procedure, and the use of new sets of IgH gene and IgL gene primers, Stein's group investigated 1078 single Hodgkin and Reed-Sternberg cells and 615 single L&H cells from 25 classical Hodgkin's disease cases (112), and 11 LPHD cases (111). All analyzable cells of all lymphocyte predominance Hodgkin's disease cases and 24 of the 25 classical Hodgkin's disease cases showed identical Ig gene rearrangements in a given case. In the remaining classical Hodgkin's disease case no Ig rearrangement was detectable. An unrelated rearrangement was found in only one out of these 1693 cells. Since this cell did not harbor in contrast to all Hodgkin and Reed-Sternberg or L&H cell derived monoclonal rearrangements any somatic mutation in their rearranged Ig genes, it probably represented a contamination. These findings confirm that the Hodgkin and Reed-Sternberg cells and L&H cells of most classical Hodgkin's disease cases and all lymphocyte predominance Hodgkin's disease cases contain monoclonal Ig gene rearrangements, and also indicates that the detection of additional polyclonal rearrangements represents a technical artifact.

In Cologne and Frankfurt 15 additional cases of classical Hodgkin's disease and 5 additional cases of lymphocyte predominance Hodgkin's disease were analyzed (32a,113,114,114a,114b) (Table 6). In all but one of the cases clonal Ig gene rearrangements were detected (one case was negative in the analysis). In two of the cased CD30 positive cells were enriched by magnetic cell sorting from the lymph node biopsy (114a). It was demonstrated by molecular Ig gene analysis that the enriched cells indeed represent the primary Hodgkin and Reed-Sternberg cells of the patient. This shows that viable Hodgkin and Reed-Sternberg cells represent clonal populations throughout the involved lymph nodes (114a). Moreover, for three of the cases analyzed in Cologne the question of dissemination and persistence of the Hodgkin and Reed-Sternberg cells in the patient during the course of the disease was addressed (114b,116). Indeed for each of these cases, it was shown that the same Hodgkin and Reed-Sternberg tumor clone can be found in different lymphoid organs and that relapses of the disease were caused by the original lymphoma clone. Dissemination of lymphoma cells was also observed for two cases of lymphocyte predominance Hodgkin's disease (111,116). Chan s group analyzed five additional cases of lymphocyte predominance Hodgkin's disease and detected clonal and polyclonal Ig gene rearrangements in each of them (116).

Taken together, the results of the single-cell studies in Hodgkin's disease described above lead to the following conclusions:

- The failure to detect rearranged immunoglobulin genes in Hodgkin and Reed-Sternberg cells and L&H cells represents a false-negative finding.
- The reported detection of polyclonal rearrangements described so far in Hodgkin and Reed-Sternberg cells and L&H cells is caused by a technical artifact, making the existence of polyclonal Hodgkin and Reed-Sternberg cells and L&H cells highly unlikely.
- The demonstration of immunoglobulin gene rearrangements in Hodgkin and Reed-Sternberg cells in approximately 90% of cases of classical Hodgkin's disease and in L&H cells in all cases of LP Hodgkin's disease proves the B-cell nature of these cells in most or all instances, respectively.
- The presence of identical immunoglobulin gene rearrangements in Hodgkin and Reed-Sternberg cells and L&H cells indicates their origin from a single transformed B cell and a subsequent monoclonal expansion.

MAPPING OF HODGKIN AND REED-STERNBERG CELLS AND L&H CELLS ONTO NORMAL B-CELL DEVELOPMENT

According to current knowledge (86), somatic hypermutations are introduced into the rearranged immunoglobulin genes during the germinal center reaction. Therefore, germinal center B cells as well as post-germinal center B cells are characterized by base substitutions within the immunoglobulin genes when compared with germline V_H segments. Comparison of the sequences of rearranged immunoglobulin genes of Hodgkin and Reed-Sternberg cells and L&H cells with the corresponding germline segments revealed high loads of somatic mutations, indicating their derivation from germinal center B cells or post-germinal center B cells. In L&H cells of the majority of cases of LP Hodgkin's disease, the rearranged immunoglobulin genes in addition harbor diverse V_H mutations within the clonally rearranged tumor cell population. This clearly indicates that the somatic hypermutation process is still active, making a derivation of the L&H cells from germinal center B cells likely. This is supported by other germinal center cell features present on L&H cells which are their predominant localization within lymphoid follicles, their cytological similarity to centroblasts, and their expression of BCL-6 (117–119). In contrast, Hodgkin and Reed-Sternberg cells display features which resemble those of germinal center cells only in part. They harbor in their V-genes like some reactive germinal center cells stop codons and deletions, but in difference to germinal center cells, are devoid of ongoing mutations and express CD30 and CD15 and lack B cell antigens and BCL-6 and home to regions outside germinal centers. Thus the precise relationship of Hodgkin and Reed-Sternberg cells to germinal center cells remains to be elucidated.

MOLECULAR DIFFERENCES BETWEEN HODGKIN AND REED-STERNBERG CELLS, L&H CELLS, AND B-TYPE NON-HODGKIN'S LYMPHOMAS

Comparison of the sequence characteristics of rearranged immunoglobulin genes in Hodgkin and Reed-Sternberg cells, L&H cells, and tumor cells of B-type non-Hodgkin's lymphomas (Table 7) reveals that L&H cells closely resemble follicular lymphoma cells, which is in agreement with the germinal center origin of both neoplasms. In both, L&H cells and follicular lymphoma cells retain the capacity to express immunoglobulin chains, and in both lesions signs of ongoing mutations are present. This raises the question of why lymphocyte predominance Hodgkin's disease is still grouped with Hodgkin's disease and not with non-Hodgkin's lymphomas. The answer is that lymphocyte predominance Hodgkin's disease—despite the close resemblance of its L&H cells to centroblasts—possesses the specific features of Hodgkin's disease, which include (a) the abundant admixture of various nonmalignant cells to the few large neoplastic blasts, exceeding the latter 100-fold, (b) the binding of T cells to the neoplastic blasts, and (c) the separation of neoplastic blasts from each other by the admixed reactive cells.

The comparison of Hodgkin and Reed-Sternberg cells with tumor cells of other types of malignant B-cell lymphomas reveals that Hodgkin and Reed-Sternberg cells are different in several respects. They are consistently unable to express immunoglobulin chains; their rearranged immunoglobulin genes frequently contain stop codons, deletions, and/or frame shifts, disrupting the coding capacity of the immunoglobulin genes; and they lack ongoing mutations. In this respect, Hodgkin and Reed-Sternberg cells differ from the neoplastic cells of follicle center lymphoma, lymphocyte predominance Hodgkin's disease, and most, if not all, other lymphoid malignancies.

IMPLICATIONS OF IMMUNOGLOBULIN GENE ANALYSIS IN THE PATHOGENESIS OF HODGKIN'S DISEASE

Evidence for Blockage of the Apoptotic Pathway

For their long-term survival, normal B cells require contact with antigen, which is mediated by their membrane immunoglobulin receptors (86,120). If the immunoglobulin genes lose their ability to code for the immunoglobulin receptors that bind antigen, or the cells become unable to synthesize immunoglobulin, the B cell carrying such deficient genes dies of apoptosis. B cells without immunoglobulin expression or with low-affinity immunoglobulin receptors arise in germinal centers as a negative by-product of the affinity maturation process. The goal of this process is the generation of B cells that express high-affinity immunoglobulin receptors. This is achieved by the introduction of point mutations into the rearranged immunoglobulin gene segments and subsequent antigen selection. The antigen selection is necessary because the mutation process is, to a certain degree,

TABLE 7. *Pattern of somatic mutations in the rearranged immunoglobulin genes of normal B-cell populations, Hodgkin's disease, and B-cell non-Hodgkin lymphomas*

Cell type/lymphoma (refs.)	No. cells/ cases studied	No. cells/cases with mutations	Average mutation incidence (%)	Ongoing mutations	Loss of coding capacity (No. cells/cases)
Normal cells (106, 173, 174, 175)	Cells				
Mantle cells	58	0	0	No	0
Germinal center cells	97	56	7.9	Yes	15[a]
Memory B cells (IgM)	15	4	1.5	No	0
Memory B cells (IgG)	6	4	4	No	0
Lymphoma	Cases				
LPHD (107, 114)	17	17	13.1	10	1[b]
Classical HD (107, 109, 113)	17	17	10.7	1	6
DLBC (176, 176a))	19	19	11.2	1	16
Burkitt's (176)	10	8	5.4	No	0
B-CLL (177)	6	0	0	No	0
Mantle cell (177)	6	0	0	No	0
Follicle center (177)	6	6	11.8	6	0
Marginal zone (178)	4	4	5.2	2	0

LPHD, lymphocyte predominance Hodgkin's disease; DLBC, diffuse large B-cell lymphoma; B-CLL, B cell-type chronic lymphocytic leukemia.

*Included only stop codons in originally functional rearrangements.

[a]These cells will be eliminated by apoptosis in the course of antigen selection.

[b]Only in a proportion of cells.

random, resulting in favorable mutations that increase the affinity of the immunoglobulin receptors and unfavorable mutations that lead to the decrease of affinity, or to a complete loss of the coding capacity. The B cells with favorable mutations are selected for differentiation into memory B cells or plasma cells, whereas the B cells with unfavorable mutations are eliminated by apoptosis (86) (Fig. 1).

The sequence analysis of the rearranged Ig genes of the L&H and Hodgkin and Reed-Sternberg cells revealed somatic mutations in a number normally not found in germinal center or post-germinal center B cells indication that the L&H and Hodgkin and Reed-Sternberg cells have undergone several rounds of mutation and thus have probably stayed in the germinal center for a prolonged period of time. When compared to other types of lymphomas it became evident that only the tumor cells of follicular lymphomas and diffuse large B-cell lymphomas carry similarly high number of mutations (Table 7) for which an unusual long residence of the tumor cells of their precursors is well accepted.

In Hodgkin and Reed-Sternberg cells the acquisition of mutations is consistently associated with a loss of Ig production. This might be due to the presence of crippling mutations outside the coding region affecting the regulation of the Ig gene expression (as observed in one case) (123a) are responsible for the absence of Ig in the remaining cases of cellular HD remains to be clarified. Irrespective of what is the reason for the inability to express Ig, Hodgkin and Reed-Sternberg cells would normally die. The fact that this does not happen indicates that the Hodgkin and Reed-Sternberg cells are rescued from apoptosis by a (yet unknown) transforming event. In contrast to Hodgkin and Reed-Sternberg cells, L&H cells retain their Ig coding capacity in most instances. However, it seems likely the expressed Ig molecules are of low antigen affinity. The evidence is twofold: (a) Highly mutated V-regions have a high chance of harboring mutations, resulting in incorrectly folded heavy or light Ig chains, reducing or abolishing their antigen binding ability; (b) The L&H cell derived rearrangements frequently lack signs of antigen selection. We therefore speculate that due to the low or lost antigen binding capacity of the expressed Ig receptors, L&H cells would also die under normal conditions, and that they are rescued from death by a blockage of the apoptotic pathway. This is supported by the observation of L&H cells with disrupted V-genes in two cases, preventing Ig expression.

Possible Mechanism Preventing Apoptosis

It is tempting to assume that viruses such as EBV, genes monitoring the human genome for damaged DNA such as p53, and/or defects in the genes regulating apoptosis might be involved in the postulated hindrance of the apoptotic pathway. In this context, recent studies of the nuclear transcription factor NFκB in classical Hodgkin's disease may be of interest. This molecule proved to be constitutively expressed in Hodgkin and Reed-Sternberg cells (124). Cell physiologic studies with transfected

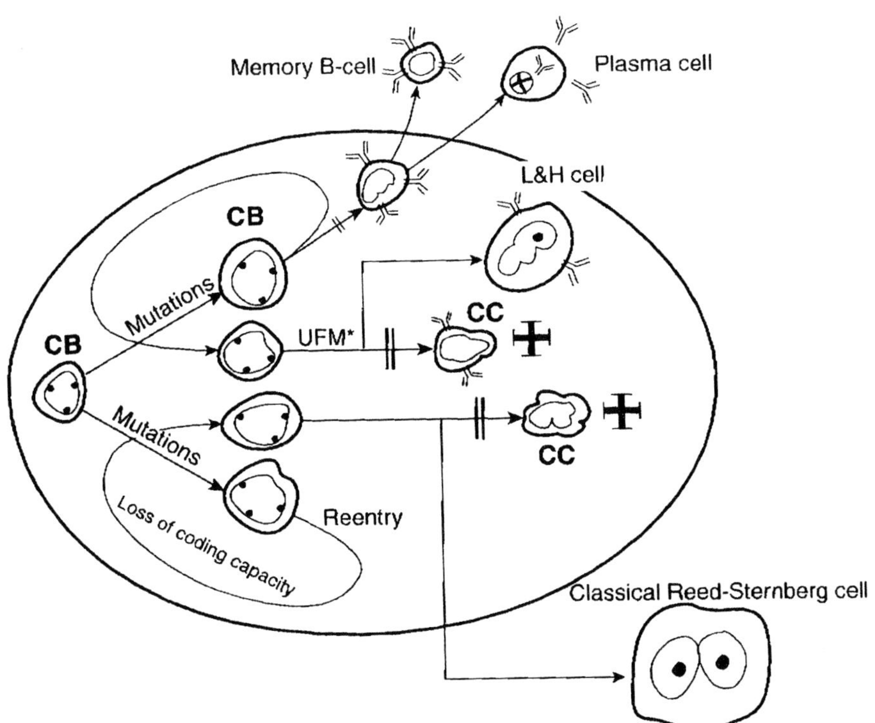

FIG. 1. Model of the putative events in a germinal center (GC) that may lead to the development of (L&H) cells and classical Hodgkin and Reed-Sternberg (HRS) cells (see text for details). *CB*, centroblast; *CC*, centrocyte; *FM*, favorable mutations; *UFM*, unfavorable mutations; ✝, apoptosis; Y, immunoglobulin receptor.

Hodgkin's disease cell lines suggest that inactivation of NFκB restores the sensitivity of Hodgkin and Reed-Sternberg cells to apoptosis, pointing to the possibility that NFκB plays an important role in obstruction of the apoptotic pathway. The deregulation of NFκB might be caused by defects in the IκBα molecule that is the natural inhibitor of NFκB (124,125). However, other molecules have also been shown to mediate the NFκB activation. A very prominent candidate in this respect is the TNFR-associated factor (TRAF) 1 molecule, which displayed a strong overexpression in the Hodgkin and Reed-Sternberg cells and L&H cells of all Hodgkin's disease cases studied (126). In view of the findings that TRAF1 overexpression in transgenic mice inhibits antigen-induced apoptosis in CD8+ T lymphocytes, it is tempting to speculate that a deregulation of the TRAF1 gene contributes to the blockage of apoptosis in Hodgkin and Reed-Sternberg cells and L&H cells (127).

Recently, the expression of the BCLX protein, a BCl2-related protein, was demonstrated in Hodgkin's disease (128,129). Whether this or other yet-unknown apoptosis-related proteins are also involved in the prevention of apoptosis in Hodgkin's disease remains to be established.

ROLE OF EPSTEIN-BARR VIRUS

The role of EBV in the pathogenesis of Hodgkin's disease is still an unsolved issue. Initial Southern blot experiments (130–132) as well as later investigations with PCR (133,134) provided evidence that EBV genomes are present in a significant proportion of cases. Because of the extractive nature of these techniques, however, it could not be determined which cells in the tissues under investigation were responsible for these positive results. Not until *in situ* hydridization for the detection of EBV-encoded small nuclear transcripts became available could it be demonstrated that Hodgkin and Reed-Sternberg cells are indeed infected by EBV (135,136). Results of the many investigations performed during recent years agree that about 50% of cases of Hodgkin's disease are EBV-associated. When these results were analyzed according to Hodgkin's disease subtypes, EBV was most frequently associated with mixed cellularity classical Hodgkin's disease (28); on the other hand, EBV has not been convincingly demonstrated in the L&H cells of lymphocyte predominance Hodgkin's disease thus far. The comparison of the EBV infection pattern of Hodgkin's disease with that of non-Hodgkin's lymphomas of B-cell or T-cell type led to the detection of at least two interesting differences. First, in contrast to what is observed in most other types of lymphoma, except for Burkitt's lymphoma, nearly all Hodgkin and Reed-Sternberg cells are EBV-infected. This finding is in harmony with former Southern blot results demonstrating monoclonal EBV episomes, which suggests that EBV infection takes places early in the development of Hodgkin's disease. The reason for only partial EBV infection in most other types of lymphoma remains to be elucidated. Second, EBV infection of Hodgkin and Reed-Sternberg cells is associated with the expression of EBV-encoded latent membrane protein 1 (LMP1) in the vast majority of cases (137–139). Because LMP1 is known to harbor transforming and anti-apoptotic potential (140), it was speculated that EBV is directly involved in the pathogenesis of Hodgkin's disease. However, EBV cannot be the transforming factor in all cases of Hodgkin's disease because it is detectable in only half of cases.

The frequent presence of EBV in Hodgkin and Reed-Sternberg cells is interesting not only in regard to the pathogenesis of Hodgkin's disease but also in regard to the determination of the nature of Hodgkin and Reed-Sternberg cells. As convincingly shown by several studies, EBV infection is restricted to certain cell types: neoplastic epithelial cells, neoplastic muscle cells, and normal as well as neoplastic B cells and T cells (141). A reliable and reproducible EBV infection of other cell types, such as myeloid cells, macrophages, interdigitating cells, and follicular dendritic cells, has not been found thus far. These observations, in conjunction with the constant absence of epithelial and myogenic markers such as cytokeratin, desmosomes, desmin, and others, are highly supportive of a derivation of Hodgkin and Reed-Sternberg cells from lymphoid cells of either B or T type.

DOES A T-CELL TYPE OF CLASSICAL HODGKIN'S DISEASE EXIST?

Repeated reports of the detection of T-cell antigens on Hodgkin and Reed-Sternberg cells (61,66,70,71,142), in conjunction with the establishment of Hodgkin's disease cell lines having immunophenotypic and genotypic features of T cells, point toward the existence of T cell-derived Hodgkin and Reed-Sternberg cells. To substantiate this possibility further, immunophenotypical studies were recently extended to the cytotoxic molecules perforin and granzyme B because they were found to be specific markers for cytotoxic T cells and natural killer cells (143–146). These studies showed that Hodgkin and Reed-Sternberg cells of 10% to 20% of cases of classical Hodgkin's disease express one or both cytotoxic molecules, and that the presence of the mentioned molecules is often associated with expression of the T-cell markers CD3, CD4, and CD8 and/or the T-cell receptor β chain. Although these findings underscore the existence of T cell-derived Hodgkin and Reed-Sternberg cells, they must not be regarded as conclusive. Conclusive proof can be provided only by the demonstration of clonally rearranged T-cell receptor genes in single Hodgkin and Reed-Sternberg cells. So far, results of such studies have not been positive (146a).

ONCOGENES AND TUMOR SUPPRESSOR GENES IN HODGKIN'S DISEASE

The scarcity of Hodgkin and Reed-Sternberg cells in tissue affected by Hodgkin's disease has hampered not only the elucidation of their lineage origin but also the detection of expression of a specific oncogene or inactivation of a tumor suppressor gene. This problem could not be solved even by analyzing the Hodgkin's disease-derived cell lines because no consistent pattern of oncogene expression could be detected in these cell lines (147). However, nearly all these cell lines were established from end-stage Hodgkin's disease. Thus, genetic alterations observed in cell culture, to some extent, might be related to the application of mutagenic agents in the course of therapy. When tissue sections of classical Hodgkin's disease were analyzed for genomic alterations or deregulated expression of oncogenes such as *myc, jun, raf,* and *ras,* no characteristic pattern could be detected (148,149). The same holds true for the investigation of tumor suppressor genes. The retinoblastoma (Rb) tumor suppressor gene, which is involved in cell cycle regulation, is mutated and/or deleted on both alleles in many malignancies, resulting in the absence of RNA and protein. However, in most of the Hodgkin's disease cases analyzed, expression of the Rb protein was found (150). Another tumor suppressor gene, p53, is also found to be expressed in most cases of classical Hodgkin's disease (151–153). The unmutated p53 gene codes for a protein involved in control of the cell cycle and induction of apoptosis after DNA damage. Mutations might result in nonexpression of the protein as well as in expression of an altered protein that is accumulated in nuclei. A nuclear accumulation of p53 is frequently observed in Hodgkin and Reed-Sternberg cells. However, mutations in the p53 gene were detected only in a subset of cases of Hodgkin's disease including one cell line (154,155). Thus, the significance of detection of p53 protein in Hodgkin and Reed-Sternberg cells remains unclear at present. Overexpression of p53 might be caused not only by mutations in the gene itself but also by inactivating interactions with p53-binding proteins. The protein encoded by the mouse double minute (*mdm*) 2 oncogene, for instance, can antagonize p53. Overexpression of the MDM2 gene product simultaneously with overexpression of p53 has been described in Hodgkin and Reed-Sternberg cells (156). Similarly other gene products interacting with p53 (e.g. p21 WAF1/CIP), involved in the regulation of the cell cycle, are also expressed in a proportion of Hodgkin and Reed-Sternberg cells and L&H cells of most Hodgkin's disease cases suggesting a preservation of the p53 functionality (149a).

In the search for a recurrent chromosomal alteration in Hodgkin and Reed-Sternberg cells, many attempts were made with PCR to detect break points in the major break point region (mbr) affected by the majority of t(14;18) chromosomal translocations. This translocation results in an overexpression of BCl2, which can prevent the apoptotic death of tumor cells. In several studies, the t(14;18) translocation was found in from 0 to 39% of Hodgkin's disease cases (150). However, in these positive cases, it remained unproven whether the translocation was localized in the Hodgkin and Reed-Sternberg cells, particularly because detection of the BCL2 protein by immunohistochemistry *in situ* was not congruent with detection of the translocation itself in all cases. In a recent study investigating isolated single Hodgkin and Reed-Sternberg cells for the presence of t(14;18), it was shown that this translocation was localized in nonmalignant bystander B cells and not in Hodgkin and Reed-Sternberg cells (157). Similarly, no pathogenetic role in Hodgkin's disease could be established for the chromosomal translocation t(2;5), which results in the oncogenic NPM/ALK fusion transcript. This translocation is consistently found in anaplastic large-cell lymphoma of T-cell origin and leads to the constant expression of the tyrosine kinase ALK. Although the presence of NPM/ALK fusion transcripts was described in Hodgkin's disease in one study (158), other studies could not reproduce these results (159,160). Recently, when single-cell PCR analysis of micromanipulated Hodgkin and Reed-Sternberg cells was performed, the NPM/ALK fusion RNA could be detected only in rare cases of Hodgkin's disease and only in occasional Hodgkin and Reed-Sternberg cells (161).

REFERENCES

1. Hodgkin T. On some morbid appearances of the absorbent glands and spleen. *Med Chir Soc Trans* 1832;17:68.
2. Wilks S. Cases of lardaceous disease and some allied affections, with remarks. *Guy's Hosp Rep* 1856;17:103.
3. Wilks S. Enlargement of the lymphatic glands and spleen (or, Hodgkin's disease), with remarks. *Guy's Hosp Rep* 1865;11:56.
4. Langhans T. Das maligne Lymphosarkom (Pseudoleukämie). *Virchows Arch Pathol Anat* 1872;54:509.
5. Greenfield WS. Specimens illustrative of the pathology of lymphadenoma and leucocythemia. *Trans Pathol Soc* 1878;20:272.
6. Sternberg C. Über eine eigenartige unter dem Bilde der Pseudoleukämie verlaufende Tuberculose des lymphatischen Apparates. *Z Heilk* 1898;19:21.
7. Reed D. On the pathological changes in Hodgkin's disease, with especial reference to its relation to tuberculosis. *Johns Hopkins Hosp Rep* 1902;10:133.
8. Lukes RJ, Butler JJ. The pathology and nomenclature of Hodgkin's disease. *Cancer Res* 1966;26:1063.
9. Neiman RS. Current problems in the histopathologic diagnosis and classification of Hodgkin's disease. *Pathol Annu* 1978;13:289.
10. Mason DY, Banks PM, Chan J, et al. Nodular lymphocyte predominance Hodgkin's disease: a distinct clinico-pathological entity. *Am J Surg Pathol* 1994;18:526.
11. Harris NL, Jaffe ES, Stein H, et al. A revised European-American classification of lymphoid neoplasms: a proposal from the International Lymphoma Study Group. *Blood* 1994;84:1361.
12. Anagnostopoulos I, Hansmann ML, Franssila K, et al. European Task Force on Lymphoma project on lymphocyte predominance Hodgkin's disease: histological and immonohistological analysis of submitted cases reveal two types of Hodgkin's disease with abundant lymphocytes. Submitted to *Blood,* 1999.
13. Hansmann ML, Zwingers T, Boske A, Loffler H, Lennert K. Clinical features of nodular paragranuloma (Hodgkin's disease, lymphocyte predominance type, nodular). *J Cancer Res Clin Oncol* 1984;108:21.

14. Stein H. Hodgkin's Disease: classification and biology. In: Perry MC, ed. *Educational book, American Association of Clinical Oncology*, 34th meeting, 1998:191.
15. Coons AH, Leduc EH, Connolly JM. Studies on antibody production. I. A method for the histochemical demonstration of specific antibody and its application to a study of the hyperimmune rabbit. *J Exp Med* 1955;102:49.
16. Garvin AJ, Spicer SS, Parmley RT, Munster AM. Immunohistochemical demonstration of IgG in Reed-Sternberg cells and other cells in Hodgkin's disease. *J Exp Med* 1974;139:1077.
17. Taylor CR. The nature of Reed-Sternberg cells and other malignant reticulum cells. *Lancet* 1974;2:802.
18. Taylor CR. An immunohistological study of follicular lymphoma, reticulum cell sarcoma and Hodgkin's disease. *Eur J Cancer* 1976; 12:61.
19. Mason DY, Stein H, Naiem M, Abdulaziz Z. Immunohistological analysis of human lymphoid tissue by double immunoenzymatic labelling. *J Cancer Res Clin Oncol* 1981;101:13.
20. Kadin M, Stites D, Levy R, Warnke R. Exogenous immunoglobulin and the macrophage origin of Reed-Sternberg cells in Hodgkin's disease. *N Engl J Med* 1978;299:1208.
21. Kaplan HS, Gartner S. Sternberg-Reed giant cells of Hodgkin's disease: cultivation *in vitro*, heterotransplantations, and characterization as neoplastic macrophages. *Int J Cancer* 1977;19:511.
22. Harris NL, Gang DL, Quay SC, et al. Contamination of Hodgkin's disease cell cultures. *Nature* 1981;289:228.
23. Schaadt M, Fonatsch C, Kirchner H, Diehl V. Establishment of a malignant Epstein-Barr-virus (EBV) negative cell-line from the pleura effusion of a patient with Hodgkin's disease. *Blut* 1979;38:185.
24. Schaadt M, Diehl V, Stein H, Fonatsch C, Kirchner H. Two neoplastic cell lines with unique features derived from Hodgkin's disease. *Int J Cancer* 1980;26:723.
25. Drexler HG. Recent results on the biology of Hodgkin and Reed-Sternberg cells. II—Continuous cell lines. *Leuk Lymphoma* 1993;9:1.
26. Schaadt M, Burrichter H, Pfreundschuh M, et al. Biology of Hodgkin cell lines. *Recent Results Cancer Res* 1989;117:53.
27. Stein H, Hummel M, Durkop H, Foss HD, Herbst H. Biology of Hodgkin's disease. In: Canellos GP, Lister AT, Sklar JL, eds. *The lymphomas*. Philadelphia: WB Saunders, 1998:287.
28. Hummel M, Anagnostopoulos I, Dallenbach F, Korbjuhn P, Dimmler C, Stein H. EBV infection patterns in Hodgkin's disease and normal lymphoid tissue: expression and cellular localization of EBV gene products. *Br J Haematol* 1992;82:689.
29. Herbst H, Steinbrecher E, Niedobitek G, et al. Distribution and phenotype of Epstein-Barr virus-harboring cells in Hodgkin's disease. *Blood* 1992;80:484.
30. Bargou RC, Mapara MY, Zugck C, et al. Characterization of a novel Hodgkin cell line, HD-MyZ, with myelomonocytic features mimicking Hodgkin's disease in severe combined immunodeficient mice. *J Exp Med* 1993;177:1257.
31. Stein H. Unpublished observation.
32. Wolf J, Kapp U, Bohlen H, et al. Peripheral blood mononuclear cells of a patient with advanced Hodgkin's lymphoma give rise to permanently growing Hodgkin-Reed Sternberg cells. *Blood* 1996;87:3418.
32a. Kanzler H, Hansmann ML, Kapp U, et al. Molecular single cell analysis demonstrates the derivation of a peripheral blood deprived cell line (L-1236) from the Hodgkin/Reed-Sternberg cells of a Hodgkin's lymphoma patient. *Blood* 1996;87:3429.
33. Schwab U, Stein H, Gerdes J, et al. Production of a monoclonal antibody specific for Hodgkin and Reed-Sternberg cells of Hodgkin's disease and a subset of normal lymphoid cells. *Nature* 1982;299:65.
34. Stein H, Gerdes J, Schwab U, et al. Identification of Hodgkin and Sternberg-Reed cells as a unique cell type derived from a newly detected small cell population. *Int J Cancer* 1982;30:445.
35. Stein H, Gerdes J, Schwab U, et al. Evidence for the detection of the normal counterpart of Hodgkin and Sternberg-Reed cells. *Haematol Oncol* 1983;1:21.
36. Engert A, Martin G, Pfreundschuh M, et al. Antitumor effects of ricin A chain immunotoxins prepared from intact antibodies and Fab fragments on solid human Hodgkin's disease tumors in mice. *Cancer Res* 1990;50:2929.
37. Hombach A, Jung W, Pohl C, et al. A CD16/CD30 bispecific monclonal antibody induces analysis of Hodgkin's cells by unstimulated natural killer cells *in vitro* and *in vivo*. *Int J Cancer* 1993;55:830.
38. Pohl C, Renner C, Schwonzen M, et al. CD30-specific AB1-AB2-AB3 internal image antibody network: potential use as an anti-idiotype vaccine against Hodgkin's lymphoma. *Int J Cancer* 1993;54:418.
39. Falini B, Bolognesi A, Flenghi L, et al. Response of Hodgkin's disease to monoclonal anti-CD30 immunotoxin. *Lancet* 1992;339:1195.
40. Kalle C, Wolf J, Becker A, et al. Growth of Hodgkin cell lines in severely combined immunodeficient mice. *Int J Cancer* 1992;52: 887.
41. Diehl V, Kirchner HH, Schaadt M, Fonatsch C, Stein H. Lymphoproliferation and heterotransplantation in nude mice: tumor cells in Hodgkin's disease. *Hamatol Bluttransfus* 1981;26:229.
42. Bosma G, Custer R, Bosma M. A severe combined immunodeficiency mutation in the mouse. *Nature* 1983;301:527.
43. Kapp U, Düx A, Schell-Frederick E, et al. Disseminated growth of Hodgkin's derived cell lines L540 and L540cy in immune-deficient SCID mice. *Ann Oncol* 1994;5(Suppl 1):121.
44. Winkler U, Gottstein C, Schön G, et al. Successful treatment of disseminated human Hodgkin's disease in SCID mice with deglycosylated ricin-A chain immunotoxins. *Blood* 1994;83:466.
45. Kapp U, Wolf J, Hummel M, et al. Hodgkin's lymphoma-derived tissue serially transplanted into severe combined immunodeficient mice. *Blood* 1993;82:1247.
46. Stein H, Uchanska-Ziegler B, Gerdes J, Ziegler A, Wernet P. Hodgkin and Sternberg-Reed cells contain antigens specific to late cells of granulopoiesis. *Int J Cancer* 1982;29:283.
47. Schienle HW, Stein H, Müller-Ruchholtz W. Neutrophil granulocytic cell antigen defined by a monoclonal antibody: its distribution within normal hematological and non-hematological tissue. *J Clin Pathol* 1982;35:959.
48. Pinkus GS, Thomas P, Said JW. Leu-M1—a marker for Reed-Sternberg cells in Hodgkin's disease. An immunoperoxidase study of paraffin-embedded tissues. *Am J Pathol* 1985;119:244.
49. Stein H, Hansmann ML, Lennert K, Brandtzaeg P, Gatter KC, Mason DY. Reed-Sternberg and Hodgkin cells in lymphocyte-predominant Hodgkin's disease of nodular subtype contain J chain. *Am J Clin Pathol* 1986;86:292.
50. Knapp W, Dörken B, Gilks WR, et al. (Organizing Committee of the Fourth International Workshop on Human Leucocyte Differentiation Antigens). Appendix A: CD guide. In: Knapp W, Dörken B, Gilks WR, et al., eds. *Leucocyte typing IV—activation antigens*. New York: Oxford University Press, 1989:1074.
51. Wieczorek R, Burke JS, Knowles DM. I. Leu-M1 antigen expression in T cell neoplasia. *Am J Pathol* 1985;121:374.
52. Sheibani K, Battifora H, Burke JS, Rappaport H. Leu-M1 antigen in human neoplasms. An immunohistological study of 400 cases. *Am J Surg Pathol* 1986;27:36.
53. Stein H, Gerdes J, Kirchner H, Schaadt M, Diehl V. Hodgkin and Sternberg-Reed cell antigen(s) detected by an antiserum to a cell line (L428) derived from Hodgkin's disease. *Int J Cancer* 1981;28:425.
54. Schwarting R, Gerdes J, Stein H. Ber-H2: a new monoclonal antibody of the Ki-1 family for the detection of Hodgkin's disease in formaldehyde-fixed tissue sections (A2.13). In: McMichael AJ, ed. *Leucocyte typing III—white cell differentiation antigens*. New York: Oxford University Press, 1987:74.
55. Stein H, Ferszt A, Dallenbach F, et al. CDw70mAb A 109 (Ki-24): expression by reactive and neoplastic lymphoid cells. In: Knapp W, Dörken B, Gilks WR, et al., eds. *Leucocyte typing IV—activation antigens*, New York: Oxford University Press, Oxford 1989:449.
56. Bowman MR, Crimmins MA, Yetz-Aldape J, Kriz R, Kelleher K, Hermann S. The cloning of CD70 and its identification as the ligand for CD27. *J Immunol* 1994;152:1756.
57. Durkop H, Latza U, Hummel M, Eitelbach F, Seed B, Stein H. Molecular cloning and expression of a new member of the nerve growth factor receptor family that is characteristic for Hodgkin's disease. *Cell* 1992;68:421.
58. Amakawa R, Hakem A, Kundig TM, et al. Impaired negative selection of T cells in Hodgkin's disease antigen CD30-deficient mice. *Cell* 1996;84:551.
59. Smith CA, Gruss HJ, Davis T, et al. CD30 antigen, a marker for Hodgkin's lymphoma, is a receptor whose ligand defines an emerging family of cytokines with homology to TNF. *Cell* 1993;73:1349.
60. Shanebeck KD, Maliszewski CR, Kennedy MK, et al. Regulation of murine B cell growth and differentiation by CD30 ligand. *Eur J Immunol* 1995;25:2147.

61. Stein H, Mason DY, Gerdes J, et al. The expression of the Hodgkin's disease-associated antigen Ki-1 in reactive and neoplastic lymphoid tissue. Evidence that Reed-Sternberg cells and histiocytic malignancies are derived from activated lymphoid cells. *Blood* 1985;66:848.
62. Stein H, Gerdes J, Lemke H, Gatter KC, Mason DY. Immunohistological classification of Hodgkin's disease and malignant histiocytosis. In: Ford RJ, Fuller LM, Hagermeister FB, Ut MD, eds. *New perspectives in human leukaemia*, vol 27. Anderson Clinical Conference on Cancer. New York: Raven Press, 1984:35.
63. Stein H, Herbst H, Anagnostopoulos I, Niedobitek G, Dallenbach F, Kratzsch H-C. The nature of Hodgkin and Reed-Sternberg cells, their association with EBV, and their relationship to anaplastic large-cell lymphoma. *Ann Oncol* 1991;12:33.
64. Chittal SM, Cavariviere P, Schwarting R, et al. Monoclonal antibodies in the diagnosis of Hodgkin's disease. *Am J Surg Pathol* 1988;12:9.
65. Casey TT, Olson SJ, Cousar JB, Collins RD. Immunophenotypes of Reed-Sternberg cells: a study of 19 cases of Hodgkin's disease in plastic embedded sections. *Blood* 1989;74:2624.
66. Agnarsson BA, Kadin ME. The immunophenotype of Reed-Sternberg cells. A study of 50 cases of Hodgkin's disease using fixed frozen tissues. *Cancer* 1989;63:2083.
67. Korkolopoulou P, Cordell JL, Jones M, et al. The expression of the B-cell marker mb-1 (CD79a) in Hodgkin's disease. *Histopathology* 1994;24:511.
68. Stein H, Gerdes J, Lemke H, Mason DY. Hodgkin's disease. A neoplasm of activated lymphoid cells of either T-cell or B-cell type. In: Grignani F, Martelli MF, Mason DY, eds. *Monoclonal antibodies in haematopathology*. Serono Symposia, vol 26. New York: Raven Press, 1985:265.
69. Angel CA, Warford A, Campbell AC, Pringle JH, Lauder I. The immunohistology of Hodgkin's disease—Reed-Sternberg cells and their variants. *J Pathol* 1987;153:21.
70. Dallenbach FE, Stein H. Expression of T-cell receptor β chain in Reed-Sternberg cells. *Lancet* 1989;2:828.
71. Falini B, Stein H, Pileri S, et al. Expression of lymphoid-associated antigens in Hodgkin's disease. An immunohistochemical study on lymph node cytopsins using monoclonal antibodies. *Histopathology* 1987;11:1229.
72. Cibull ML, Stein H, Gatter KC, Mason DY. The expression of the CD3 antigen in Hodgkin's disease. *Histopathology* 1989;15:599.
73. Poppema S. The diversity of the immunohistological staining pattern of Sternberg-Reed cells. *J Histochem Cytochem* 1980;28:788.
74. Stein H, Hansmann ML, Lennert K, Brandtzaeg P, Gatter KC, Mason DY. Reed-Sternberg and Hodgkin cells in lymphocyte-predominant Hodgkin's disease of nodular subtype contain J chain. *Am J Clin Pathol* 1986;86:292.
75. Said JS. The immunohistochemistry of Hodgkin's disease. *Semin Diagn Pathol* 1992;9:265.
76. Reference deleted in proofs.
77. Bilbe G, Delabie J, Bruggen J, et al. Restin: a novel intermediate filament-associated protein highly expressed in the Reed-Sternberg cells of Hodgkin's disease. *EMBO J* 1992;11:2103.
78. Delabie J, Shipman R, Bruggen J, et al. Expression of the novel intermediate filament-associated protein restin in Hodgkin's disease and anaplastic large-cell lymphoma. *Blood* 1992;80:2891.
79. Pinkus GS, Pinkus JL, Langhoff E, et al. Fascin, a sensitive new marker for Reed-Sternberg cells of Hodgkin's disease. Evidence for a dendritic or B cell derivation? *Am J Pathol* 1997;150:543.
80. Poppema S. Biology and nature of the admixed non-neoplastic cells in Hodgkin's disease. Fourth International Symposium on Hodgkin's Lymphomas, Cologne, Germany, 1998.
81. Said JW, Pinkus JL, Shintaku IP, et al. Alterations in fascin-expressing germinal center dendritic cells in neoplastic follicles of B-cell lymphomas. *Mod Pathol* 1998;11:1.
82. Stamenkovic I, Clark EA, Seed B. A B-lymphocyte activation molecule related to the nerve growth factor receptor and induced by cytokines in carcinomas. *EMBO J* 1989;8:1403.
83. Ledbetter JA, Clark EA, Norris NA, Shu G, Hellström I. Expression of a functional B-cell receptor CDw40(Bp50) on carcinomas (B3.7). In: McMichael AJ, ed. *Leucocyte typing III—white cell differentiation antigens*. New York: Oxford University Press, 1987:432.
84. Gruss HJ, Hirschstein D, Wright B, et al. Expression and function of CD40 on Hodgkin and Reed-Sternberg cells and the possible relevance for Hodgkin's disease. *Blood* 1994;84:2315.
85. O'Grady JT, Stewart S, Lowrey J, Howie SE, Krajewsky AS. CD40 expression in Hodgkin's disease. *Am J Pathol* 1994;144:21.
86. Rajewsky K. Clonal selection and learning in the antibody system. *Nature* 1996;381:751.
87. Knowles DM, Neri A, Pelicci PG, et al. Immunoglobulin and T-cell receptor beta-chain gene rearrangement analysis of Hodgkin's disease: implications for lineage determination and differential diagnosis. *Proc Natl Acad Sci U S A* 1986;83:7942.
88. Herbst H, Tippelmann G, Anagnostopoulos I, et al. Immunoglobulin and T-cell receptor gene rearrangements in Hodgkin's disease and Ki-1-positive anaplastic large cell lymphoma: dissociation between phenotype and genotype. *Leuk Res* 1989;13:103.
89. Weiss LM, Strickler JG, Hu E, et al. Immunoglobulin gene rearrangements in Hodgkin's disease. *Hum Pathol* 1986;17:1009.
90. Griesser H, Feller AC, Tak TW, Lennert K. Clonal rearrangements of T-cell receptor and immunoglobulin genes and immunophenotypic antigen expression in different subclasses of Hodgkin's disease. *Int J Cancer* 1987;40:157.
91. Sundeen J, Lipford E, Uppenkamp M, et al. Rearranged antigen receptor genes in Hodgkin's disease. *Blood* 1987;70:96.
92. Brinker M, Poppema S, Buys C, Timens W, Osinga J, Visser L. Clonal immunoglobulin rearrangement in tissues involved by Hodgkin's disease. *Blood* 1987;70:186.
93. O'Connor N, Crick J, Gatter K, Mason D, Falini B, Stein H. Cell lineage in Hodgkin's disease. *Lancet* 1987;1:158.
94. Roth M, Schnitzer B, Bingham E, Harnden C, Hyder D, Ginsburg D. Rearrangement of immunoglobulin and T-cell receptor genes in Hodgkin's disease. *Am J Pathol* 1988;131:331.
95. Cossman J, Sundeen J, Uppenkamp M, et al. Rearranging antigen-receptor genes in enriched Reed-Sternberg cell fractions of Hodgkin's disease. *Hematol Oncol* 1988;6:205.
96. Saiki RK, Scharf S, Faloona F, et al. Enzymatic amplification of beta-globin genomic sequences and restriction site analysis for diagnosis of sickle cell anemia. *Science* 1985;230:1350.
97. Saiki RK, Gelfland DH, Stoffel S, et al. Primer-directed enzymatic amplification of DNA with a thermostable DNA polymerase. *Science* 1988;239:487.
98. Tamaru J, Hummel M, Zemlin M, Kalvelage B, Stein H. Hodgkin's disease with B-cell phenotype often shows a VDJ rearrangement and somatic mutations in the V_H genes. *Blood* 1994;84:708.
99. Yatabe Y, Oka K, Asia J, Mori N. Poor correlation between clonal immunoglobulin gene rearrangement and immunoglobulin gene transcription in Hodgkin's disease. *Am J Pathol* 1996;149:1351.
100. Manzanal A, Sauton A, Oliva H, Bellas C. Evaluation of clonal immunoglobulin heavy chain rearrangements in Hodgkin's disease using the polymerase chain reaction (PCR). *Histopathology* 1995;27:21.
101. Orazi A, Jiang B, Lee C, et al. Correlation between presence of clonal rearrangements of immunoglobulin heavy chain genes and B-cell antigen expression in Hodgkin's disease. *Am J Clin Pathol* 1995;104:413.
102. Al Saati T, Galoin S, Gravel S, et al. IgH and TcR-gamma gene rearrangement identified in Hodgkin's disease by PCR demonstrate lack of correlation between genotype, phenotype and Epstein-Barr virus status. *J Pathol* 1997;181:387.
103. Trümper LH, Brady G, Bagg A, et al. Single-cell analysis of Hodgkin and Reed-Sternberg cells: molecular heterogeneity of gene expression and p53 mutations. *Blood* 1993;81:3097.
104. Roth J, Daus H, Trümper L, Gause A, Salamon-Looijen M, Pfreundschuh M. Detection of immunoglobulin heavy-chain gene rearrangement at the single-cell level in malignant lymphoma: no rearrangement is found in Hodgkin and Reed-Sternberg cells. *Int J Cancer* 1994;57:799.
105. Delabie J, Tierens A, Wu G, Weisenburger DD, Chan WC. Lymphocyte predominance in Hodgkin's disease: lineage and clonality determination using a single-cell assay. *Blood* 1994;84:3291.
106. Küppers R, Zhao M, Hansmann M-L, Rajewsky K. Tracing B cell development in human germinal centres by molecular analysis of single cells picked from histological section. *EMBO J* 1993;12:4955.
107. Küppers R, Rajewsky K, Zhao M, et al. Hodgkin and Reed-Sternberg cells picked from histological sections show clonal immunoglobulin rearrangements and appear to be derived from B cells at various stages of development. *Proc Natl Acad Sci U S A* 1994;91:10962.
108. Delabie J, Tierens A, Gavrill T, Wu G, Weisenburger DD, Chan WC.

Phenotype, genotype and clonality of Reed-Sternberg cells in nodular sclerosis Hodgkin's disease: results of a single-cell study. *Br J Haematol* 1996;94:198.
109. Hummel M, Ziemann K, Lammert H, Pileri S, Sabattini E, Stein H. Hodgkin's disease with monoclonal and polyclonal populations of Reed-Sternberg cells. *N Engl J Med* 1995;333:901.
110. Stein H, Hummel M, Marafioti T, Korbjuhn P, Anagnostopoulos I, Foss HD. Hodgkin's disease: its mystery is being revealed. *Verh Dtsch Ges Pathol* 1997;81:327.
111. Marafioti T, Hummel M, Anagnostopoulos I, et al. Origin of nodular lymphocyte-predominant Hodgkin's disease from a clonal expansion of highly mutated germinal-center B cells. *N Engl J Med* 1997;337:453.
112. Marafioti T, Hummel M, Foss HD, et al. Hodgkin and Reed-Sternberg cells represent an expansion of single clone originating from a germinal center B cell with functional immunoglobin gene rearrangements but defective immunoglobulin transcription. Submitted 1999.
113. Kanzler H, Küppers R, Hansmann ML, et al. Hodgkin and Reed-Sternberg cells in Hodgkin's disease represent the outgrowth of a dominant tumor clone derived from (crippled) germinal center B cells. *J Exp Med* 1996;184:1.
114. Braeuninger A, Küppers R, Strickler J, Wacker H-H, Rajewsky K, Hansmann M-L. Hodgkin and Reed-Sternberg cells in lymphocyte predominant Hodgkin disease represent clonal populations of germinal center-derived tumor cells. *Proc Natl Acad Sci U S A* 1997;94:9337.
114a. Irsch J, Nitsch S, Tesch H, et al. Hodgkin and Reed-Sternberg cells isolated from lymph nodes are clonal populations of highly differentiated B cells. *Proc Natl Acad Sci USA* 1998;95:10117.
114b. Vockerodt M, Soares M, Kanzler H, et al. Detection of clonal Hodgkin and Reed-Sternberg cells with identical somatically mutated and rearranged VH genes in different biopsies in relapsed Hodgkin's disease. *Blood* 1998;92:2899.
115. Ohno T, Stribley JA, Wu G, Hinrichs SH, Weisenburger DD, Chan WC. Clonality in nodular lymphocyte-predominant Hodgkin's disease. *N Engl J Med* 1997;337:459.
116. Jox A, Zander T, Kornacker M, et al. Detection of identical Hodgkin-Reed Sternberg cell specific immunoglobulin gene rearrangement in a patient with Hodgkin's disease of mixed cellularity subtype at primary diagnosis and in relapse two and a half years later. *Ann Oncol* 1998;9:283.
117. Hansmann ML, Fellbaum C, Hui PK, Moubayed P. Progressive transformation of germinal centers with and without association to Hodgkin's disease. *Am J Clin Pathol* 1990;93:219.
118. Ree HJ, Neiman RS, Martin AW, Dallenbach F, Stein H. Paraffin section markers for Reed-Sternberg cells. A comparative study of peanut agglutinin, Leu-M1, LN-2, and Ber-H2. *Cancer* 1989;63:2030.
119. Falini B, Bigerna B, Pasqualucci L, et al. Distinctive expression pattern of the BCL-6 protein in nodular lymphocyte predominance Hodgkin's disease. *Blood* 1996;87:465.
120. Lam K-P, Kühn R, Rajewsky K. *In vivo* ablation of surface immunoglobulin on mature B cells by inducible gene targeting results in rapid cell death. *Cell* 1997;90:1073.
121. Ruprai A, Pringle J, Angel C, Kind C, Lauder I. Localization of immunoglobulin light chain mRNA expression in Hodgkin's disease by *in situ* hybridization. *J Pathol* 1991;164:37.
122. Lauritzen A, Pluzek K, Kristensen L, Nielsen H. Detection of immunoglobulin light chain mRNA in nodular sclerosing Hodgkin's disease by *in situ* hybridization with biotinylated oligonucleotide probes compared with immunohistochemical staining with poly- and monoclonal antibodies. *Histopathology* 1992;21:353.
123. Hell K, Pringle J, Hansmann M, et al. Demonstration of light chain mRNA in Hodgkin's disease. *J Pathol* 1993;171:137.
123a. Jox A, Zander T, Kuppers R, et al. Somatic mutations within the untranslated regions of rearranged Ig genes in a case of classical Hodgkin's disease as a potential cause for the absence of immunoglobulin in the lymphoma cells. *Blood* 1999, in press.
124. Bargou R, Emmerich F, Krappmann D, et al. Constitutive nuclear factor-κ B-RelA activation is required for proliferation and survival of Hodgkin's disease tumor cells. *J Clin Invest* 1997;12:296.
125. Wood KM, Roff M, Hay RT. Defective IkappaBalpha in Hodgkin cell lines with constitutively active NF-kappaB. *Oncogene* 1998;16:2131.
126. Durkop H, Foss HD, Demel G, Klotzbach H, Hahn C, Stein H. Tumor necrosis factor receptor-associated factor 1 is overexpressed in Reed-Sternberg cells of Hodgkin's disease and Epstein-Barr virus-transformed lymphoid cells. *Blood* 1999;2:617–623.
127. Lee S, Park C, Choi Y. T-cell receptor-dependent cell death of T-cell hybridomas mediated by the CD30 cytoplasmic domain in association with tumor necrosis factor receptor-associated factors. *J Exp Med* 1996;183:669.
128. Schlaifer D, March M, Krajewski S, et al. High expression of the bcl-x gene in Reed-Sternberg cells of Hodgkin's disease. *Blood* 1995;85:2671.
129. Messineo C, Jamerson MH, Hunter E, et al. Gene expression by single Reed-Sternberg cells: pathways of apoptosis and activation. *Blood* 1998;91:2443.
130. Weiss LM, Movahed LA, Warnke RA, Sklar J. Detection of Epstein-Barr viral genomes in Reed-Sternberg cells of Hodgkin's disease. *N Engl J Med* 1989;320:502.
131. Weiss LM, Strickler JG, Warnke RA, Purtilo DT, Sklar J. Epstein-Barr viral DNA in tissues of Hodgkin's disease. *Am J Pathol* 1987;129:86.
132. Anagnostopoulos I, Herbst H, Niedobitek G, Stein H. Demonstration of monoclonal EBV genomes in Hodgkin's disease and Ki-1-positive anaplastic large cell lymphoma by combined Southern and *in situ* hybridization. *Blood* 1989;74:810.
133. Herbst H, Niedobitek G, Kneba M, et al. High incidence of Epstein-Barr virus genomes in Hodgkin's disease. *Am J Pathol* 1990;137:13.
134. Weiss LM, Chen YY, Lui XF, Shibata D. Epstein-Barr virus and Hodgkin's disease. A correlative *in situ* hybridization and polymerase chain reaction study. *Am J Pathol* 1991;139:1259.
135. Hummel M, Anagnostopoulos I, Dallenbach F, Korbjuhn P, Dimmler C, Stein H. EBV infection patterns in Hodgkin's disease and normal lymphoid tissue: expression and cellular localization of EBV gene products. *Br J Haematol* 1992;82:689.
136. Brousset P, Chittal S, Schlaifer D, et al. Detection of Epstein-Barr virus messenger RNA in Reed-Sternberg cells of Hodgkin's disease by *in situ* hybridization with biotinylated probes on specially processed modified acetone methyl benzoate xylene (ModAMeX) sections. *Blood* 1991;77:1871.
137. Herbst H, Dallenbach F, Hummel M, et al. Epstein-Barr virus latent membrane protein expression in Hodgkin- and Reed-Sternberg cells. *Proc Natl Acad Sci U S A* 1991;88:4766.
138. Pallesen G, Hamilton-Dutoit SJ, Rowe M, Young LS. Expression of Epstein-Barr virus latent gene products in tumor cells of Hodgkin's disease. *Lancet* 1991;337:320.
139. Delsol G, Brousset P, Chittal S, Rigal-Huguet F. Correlation of the expression of Epstein-Barr virus latent membrane protein and *in situ* hybridization with biotinylated Bam HI-W probes in Hodgkin's disease. *Am J Pathol* 1992;140:247.
140. Henderson S, Rowe M, Croom-Carter D, et al. Induction of bcl-2 expression by Epstein-Barr virus latent membrane protein 1 protects infected B cells from programmed cell death. *Cell* 1991;65:1107.
141. Anagnostopoulos I, Hummel M, Kreschel C, Stein H. Morphology, immunophenotype and distribution of latently and/or productively Epstein-Barr virus-infected cells in acute infectious mononucleosis: implications for the interindividual infection route of Epstein-Barr virus. *Blood* 1995;85:744.
142. Cibull ML, Stein H, Gatter KC, Mason DY. The expression of the CD3 antigen in Hodgkin's disease. *Histopathology* 1989;15:599.
143. Liu C-C, Walsh CM, Young JD-E. Perforin: structure and function. *Immunol Today* 1985;16:194.
144. Garcia-Sanz JA, MacDonald HR, Jenne DE, Tschopp J, Nabholz M. Cell specificity of granzyme gene expression. *J Immunol* 1990;145:3111.
145. Oudejans JJ, Kummer JA, Jiwa NM, et al. Granzyme B expression in Reed-Sternberg cells of Hodgkin's disease. *Am J Pathol* 1996;148:233.
146. Foss H-D, Anagnostopoulos I, Araujo A, et al. Anaplastic large-cell lymphomas of T-cell and null-cell phenotype express cytotoxic molecules. *Blood* 1996;88:4005.
146a. Daus H, Trumper L, Roth J, et al. Hodgkin and Reed-Sternberg cells do not carry T-cell receptor gamma gene arrangements: evidence from single-cell polymerase chain reaction examination. *Blood* 1995;85:1590.
147. Diehl V, von Kalle C, Fonatsch C, Tesch H, Jücker M, Schaadt M. The cell of origin of Hodgkin's disease. *Semin Oncol* 1990;17:660–672.
148. Steenvoorden AC, Janssen JW, Drexler HD, et al. Ras mutations in Hodgkin's disease. *Leukemia* 1988;2:325.

149. Mitani S, Sugawara I, Shiku H, Mori S. Expression of c-myc oncogene product and ras family oncogene product in various human malignant lymphomas defined by immunohistochemical techniques. *Cancer* 1988;62:2085.

149a. Sanchez-Beato M, Piris MA, Martinez-Montero JC, et al. MDM2 and p21WAF1/CIP1, wild-type p53-induced proteins, are regularly expressed by Sternberg-Reed cells in Hodgkin's disease. *J Pathol* 1996;180:58.

150. Weiss L. The pathogenesis of Hodgkin's disease: oncogene, tumor suppressor gene, and Epstein-Barr viral studies. In: Jarrett RF, ed. *Etiology of Hodgkin's disease*. New York: Plenum Publishing, 1995:197 (NATO ASI Series, vol 280).

151. Gupta RK, Norton AJ, Thompson IW, Lister TA, Bodmer JG. p53 expression in Reed-Sternberg cells of Hodgkin's disease. *Br J Cancer* 1992;66:649.

152. Dogliani C, Pelosie P, Mombello A, Scarpa A, Chilosi M. Immunohistochemical evidence of abnormal expression of the antioncogene-encoded p53 phosphoprotein in Hodgkin's disease and CD30+ anaplastic lymphomas. *Hematol Pathol* 1991;5:67.

153. Niedobitek G, Rowlands D, Young L, et al. Overexpression of p53 in Hodgkin's disease: lack of correlation with Epstein-Barr virus infection. *J Pathol* 1993;169:207.

154. Gupta RK, Patel K, Bodmer WF, Bodmer JH. Mutation of p53 in primary biopsy material and cell lines from Hodgkin disease. *Proc Natl Acad Sci U S A* 1993;90:2817.

155. Chen W-G, Chen Y-Y, Kamel OW, Koo CH, Weiss LM. p53 mutations in Hodgkin's disease. *Lab Invest* 1996;75:519.

156. Chilosi M, Doglioni C, Menestrina F et al. Abnormal expression of the p53-binding protein MDM2 in Hodgkin's disease. *Blood* 1994;84: 4295.

157. Gravel S, Delsol G, Al Saati T. Single-cell analysis of the t(14;18)(q32;q31) chromosomal translocation in Hodgkin's disease demonstrates the absence of this translocation in neoplastic Hodgkin and Reed-Sternberg cells. *Blood* 1998;91:2866.

158. Orscheschek K, Merz H, Hell J, Binder T, Bartels H, Feller AC. Large cell anaplastic lymphoma-specific translocation [t(2;5)(p23;q35)] in Hodgkin's disease: indication of a common pathogenesis? *Lancet* 1995;345:87.

159. Herbst H, Anagnostopoulos J, Heize B, Durkop H, Hummel M, Stein H. ALK gene products in anaplastic large cell lymphomas and Hodgkin's disease. *Blood* 1995;86:1694.

160. Elmberger PG, Lozano MD, Weisenburger DD, Sanger W, Chan WC. Transcripts of the npm-alk fusion gene in anaplastic large cell lymphoma, Hodgkin's disease, and reactive lymphoid lesions. *Blood* 1995;86:3517.

161. Trümper L, Daus H, Merz H, et al. NPM/ALK fusion mRNA expression in Hodgkin and Reed-Sternberg cells is rare but does occur: results from single-cell cDNA analysis. *Ann Oncol* 1997;8(Suppl 2): 83.

162. Diehl V, Kirchner HH, Burrichter H, et al. Characteristics of Hodgkin's disease-derived cell lines. *Cancer Treat Rep* 1982;66:615.

163. Kamesaki H, Fukuhara S, Tatsumi E, et al. Cytochemical, immunologic, chromosomal and molecular genetic analysis of a novel cell line derived from Hodgkin's disease. *Blood* 1986;68:285.

164. Diehl V, Kirchner HH, Schaadt M, et al. Hodgkin's disease: establishment and characterization of four *in vitro* cell lines. *J Cancer Res Clin Oncol* 1981;101:111.

165. Jones DB, Scott CS, Wright DH, et al. Phenotypic analysis of an established cell line derived from a patient with Hodgkin's disease (HD). *Hematol Oncol* 1985;3:133.

166. Jones DB, Furley AJW, Gerdes J, Greaves MF, Stein H, Wright DH. Phenotypic and genotypic analysis of two cell lines derived from Hodgkin's disease tissue biopsies. In: Diehl V, Pfreundschuh M, Loeffler M, eds. *New aspects in the diagnosis and treatment of Hodgkin's disease*. Berlin: Springer-Verlag, 1989:62.

167. Drexler HG, Gaedicke G, Lok MS, Diehl V, Minowada J. Hodgkin's disease derived cell lines HDLM-2 and L428: comparison of morphology, immunological and isoenzyme profiles. *Leuk Res* 1986;10: 487.

168. Drexler HG, Gignac SM, Hoffbrand AV, et al. Characterisation of Hodgkin's disease derived cell line HDLM-2. In Diehl V, Pfreundschuh M, Loeffler M, eds. *New aspects in the diagnosis and treatment of Hodgkin's disease*. Berlin: Springer-Verlag, 1989:75.

169. Poppema S, De Jong B, Atmosoerodjo J, Idenburg V, Visser L, De Ley L. Morphologic, immunologic, enzyme histochemical and chromosomal analysis of a cell line derived from Hodgkin's disease. Evidence for a B-cell origin of Reed-Sternberg cells. *Cancer* 1985;55:683.

170. Poppema S, Visser L, De Jong B, Brinker M, Atmosoerodjo J, Timens W. The typical Reed-Sternberg phenotype and Ig gene rearrangement of Hodgkin's disease derived cell line ZO indicating a B cell origin. In: Diehl V, Pfreundschuh M, Loeffler M, eds. *New aspects in the diagnosis and treatment of Hodgkin's disease*. Berlin: Springer-Verlag, 1989:67.

171. Kanzaki T, Kubonishi I, Eguchi T, et al. Establishment of a new Hodgkin's cell line (HD-70) of B-cell origin. *Cancer* 1992;69:1034.

172. Naumovski L, Lutz PJ, Bergstrom SK, et al. SUP-HD1: a new Hodgkin's disease-derived cell line with lymphoid features produces interferon-τ. *Blood* 1989;74:2733.

173. Klein U, Küppers R, Rajewsky K. Variable region gene analysis of B cell subsets derived from a 4-year-old child: somatically mutated memory B cells accumulate in the peripheral blood already at young age. *J Exp Med* 1994;180:1383.

174. Pascual V, Liu JY, Magalski A, de Bouteiller O, Banchereau J, Capra JD. Analysis of somatic mutation in five B cell subsets of human tonsil. *J Exp Med* 1994;180:329.

175. Dunn-Walters K, Isaacson PG, Spencer J. Analysis of mutations in immunoglobulin heavy chain variable region genes of microdissected marginal zone (MGZ) B cells suggests that the MGZ of human spleen is a reservoir of memory B cells. *J Exp Med* 1995;182:559.

176. Tamaru J, Hummel M, Marafioti T, et al. Burkitt's lymphomas express V_H genes with a moderate number of antigen-selected somatic mutations. *Am J Pathol* 1995;147:1398.

176a. Kuppers R, Rajewsky K, Hansmann ML. Diffuse large cell lymphomas are derived from mature B cells carrying V region genes with a high load of somatic mutation and evidence of selection for antibody expression. *Eur J Immunol* 1997;27:1398.

177. Hummel M, Tamaru J, Kalvelage B, Stein H. Mantle cell (previously centrocytic) lymphomas express V_H genes with no or very little somatic mutations like the physiologic cells of the follicle mantle. *Blood* 1994;84:403.

178. Hallas C, Greiner A, Peters K, Muller-Hermelink HK. Immunoglobulin V_H genes of high-grade mucosa-associated lymphoid tissue lymphomas show a high load of somatic mutations and evidence of antigen-dependent affinity maturation. *Lab Invest* 1998;78:277.

Hodgkin's Disease, edited by P. M. Mauch,
J. O. Armitage, V. Diehl, R.T. Hoppe, and L. M. Weiss.
Lippincott Williams & Wilkins, Philadephia ©1999.

CHAPTER 9

Cytokines and Cytokine Receptors in Hodgkin's Disease

Marshall E. Kadin and David N. Liebowitz

Hodgkin's disease is unique among lymphomas in that the malignant cell, known as the Hodgkin–Reed-Sternberg cell, comprises only a small minority of the tumor. The bulk of the tumor is composed of inflammatory cells (histiocytes, plasma cells, lymphocytes, eosinophils, neutrophils) and fibrosis. Evidence has accumulated to show that these reactive tissue elements are attracted or recruited by cytokines liberated first by Hodgkin–Reed-Sternberg cells and then by inflammatory cells, which, in turn, recruit additional inflammatory cells and stimulate collagen synthesis in a virtual cascade of reactivity. The importance of interactions between Hodgkin–Reed-Sternberg cells and host inflammatory cells is illustrated in murine xenografts of Hodgkin's disease, which resemble large-cell anaplastic lymphomas with few reactive murine cells in which the histologic types of Hodgkin's disease found in humans are not well represented (1). This disparity between Hodgkin's disease in the natural host and the murine model most likely reflects a lack of response of murine inflammatory cells to cytokines released by Hodgkin–Reed-Sternberg cells.

A variety of cytokines have been demonstrated in Hodgkin's disease tissues. These cytokines and their correlation with clinical features and histopathology of Hodgkin's disease are summarized in Table 1. Additional information concerning cytokine production and cytokine response of tumor cells in Hodgkin's disease has been obtained from neoplastic cell lines developed from tissues or effusions of patients with advanced clinical stages of Hodgkin's disease (2). Cytokines released by Hodgkin–Reed-Sternberg cells have numerous local and distal effects. A summary of the cytokines synthesized and released by Hodgkin–Reed-Sternberg cells in culture and in Hodgkin's disease tissues and patient sera is shown in Table 2.

M. E. Kadin: Department of Pathology, Beth Israel Deaconess Medical Center, Harvard Medical School, Boston, Massachusetts.

D. N. Liebowitz: Department of Medicine, University of Pennsylvania and Leonard and Madlyn Abramson Family Center Research Institute, University of Pennsylvania Cancer Center, Philadelphia, Pennsylvania.

TABLE 1. *Correlation of clinical and pathologic presentation Hodgkin's disease with detection of cytokines in Hodgkin's disease tumors: characteristics of a tumor of cytokine-producing cells*

Clinical and pathologic features of HD	Cytokines[a]
1. Constitutional "B" symptoms	TNF, LT-α, IL-1, IL-6
2. Polkyaron formation	IFN-γ, IL-4
3. Sclerosis	TGF-β, LIF, PDGF, IL-1, TNF
4. Acute phase reactions	IL-1, IL-6, IL-11, LIF
5. Eosinophilia	IL-5, GM-CSF, IL-2, IL-3
6. Plasmacytosis	IL-6, IL-11
7. Mild thrombocytosis	IL-6, IL-11, LIF
8. T/H-RS cell interaction	IL-1, IL-2, IL-6, IL-7, IL-9, TNF, LT-α, CD30L, CD40L, B7 Ligands (CD80 and CD86)
9. Immune deficiency	TGF-β, IL-10
10. Autocrine growth factors (?)	IL-6, IL-9, TNF, LT-α, CD30L, M-CSF
11. Increased alkaline phosphatase	M-CSF
12. Neutrophil accumulation/ activation	IL-8, TNF, TGF-β

[a]IL, interleukin; TNF, tumor necrosis factor; LT, lymphotoxin; IFN, interferon; PDGF, platelet-derived growth factor; TGF, transforming growth factor; LIF, leukemia inhibitory factor; GM-CSF, granulocyte–macrophage colony-stimulating factor; T, T cells; H-RS, Hodgkin and Reed-Sternberg cells; M-CSF, macrophage colony-stimulating factor.

From Gross HJ, Kadin ME. *Pharmacology of Hodgkin's disease.* Paris: Bailliere, 1996, with permission.

TABLE 2. *Summary of the expression and release of cytokines by cultured H-RS cells or HD-involved tissue and the detection of elevated serum concentrations for HD patients*[a]

Cytokine/ growth factor	Cultured H-RS cells[b]	HD-involved tissue: Overall % of + cases[c]	H-RS cells	Lymphoid cells	Histiocytes/ macro-phages	Others[d]	Serum levels[e]	Biological activities (correlation to features of HD)
IL-1α	4/5	70	+		+	+ (E)	↑ 3%	↑ B symptoms ↑ Cellular response
IL-1β	2/5	0[f]					↑ 2%	?
IL-1ra	2/2	N.D.					↑ 90%	↓ Immunosurveillance
IL-2	0/8	44	–	+	–	–	↑ 11%	↑ T cell activation Paracrine growth factor for H-RS cells
IL-3	0/3[g]	33	–	+	–	–	↑ 13%	Eosinophilia ↑ Cellular response
IL-4	1/8	15	–	+	–	–	0[f]	↑ T-cell activation and accumulation (? Th-2 immune response)
IL-5	4/7	84	+	+	–	–	N.D.	Eosinophilia ↑ Cellular response (? Th-2 immune response)
IL-6	7/8	82	+	+	+	+ (U)	↑ 51%	H-RS cell growth factor ↑ Acute phase response ↑ B symptoms ↑ Cellular response
IL-7	1/5	77	+	+	–	–	↑ 66%	↑ T-cell activation
IL-8	5/5	N.D.					↑ 46%	↑ Neutrophil activation and attraction
IL-9	1/4[g]	50	+	+	–	–	N.D.	Autocrine growth factor for H-RS cells ↑ T-cell activation
IL-10	2/4	46	+	+	–	–	↑ 32%	↓ Immune response Association with EBV
IL-12	N.D.	65	–	+			N.D.	↑ T-cell activation
TNF	7/8	64	+	+	+	+	↑ 50%	Autocrine and paracrine growth and activation factor for H-RS cells ↑ Cellular response ↑ B symptoms
LT-α	5/6	80	+	+	–	–	↑ 5%	Autocrine and paracrine growth and activation factor for H-RS cells ↑ Cellular response
CD27L	4/5	96	+	+	–	–	N.D.	↑ T-cell activation ↑ Cellular response
CD30L	0/4	100	+	+	+	+ (G)(E)	↑ 18%	Paracrine growth and avtivation factor for H-RS cells ↑ T-cell activation ↑ Cellular response
CD40L	0/4	100	–	+	–	–	↑ 42%	Paracrine activation factor for H-RS cells "Anti-apoptosis" factor
TGF-β	5/6	67	+	+	+	+	N.D.	↓ Immune response ↑ Sclerosis (NS HD) Involvement in cellular responses (↑ and ↓)
LIF	1/2[g]	87	–	–	+	–	↑ 3%	Paracrine activation factor for H-RS cells ↑ Cellular response
MCP-1	0/2	N.D.					N.D.	?
IFN-γ	2/6	50	+	+	–	–	0[5]	Paracrine activation factor for H-RS cells ↑ T-cell activation

TABLE 2. *Continued*

Cytokine/ growth factor	Cultured H-RS cells[b]	HD-involved tissue: Overall % of + cases[c]	H-RS cells	Lymphoid cells	Histiocytes/ macro-phages	Others[d]	Serum levels[e]	Biological activities (correlation to features of HD)
CD80 (B7-1)	4/4	98	+	–	–	+ (APC)	N.D.	↑ T-cell activation
CD86 (B7-2)	4/4	86	+	–	–	+ (APC)	N.D.	↑ T-cell activation
G-CSF	0/6	N.D.					↑ 59%	↑ Neutrophil counts
GM-CSF	2/7[g]	11	+				↑ 39%	↑ Neutrophil counts ↑ Cellular response
M-CSF	5/5	74	+	+	+	–	N.D.	Autocrine and paracrine growth factor for H-RS cells ↑ Bone metabolism ↑ Macrophage response
SCF (MGF)	0/5	N.D.					N.D.	Paracrine growth and activation factor for H-RS cells (?)

[a]H-RS, Hodgkin and Reed-Sternberg; HD, Hodgkin's disease; IL, interleukin; ↑ or ↓, increase or decrease; N.D., not determined; EBV, Epstein–Barr virus; TNF, tumor necrosis factor; LT, lymphotoxin; L, ligand; TGF, transforming growth factor; NS, nodular sclerosis; LIF, leukemia inhibitory factor; MCP, monocyte chemoattractant peptide; IFN, interferon; G, granulocyte; CSF, colony-stimulating factor; GM, granulocyte and macrophage; M, macrophage; SCF, stem-cell factor; MGF, mast cell growth factor.

[b]Cultured H-RS cells included the cell lines HDLM-2, HD-MyZ, KM-H2, L-428, L-540, L-591, L-1236, and SBH-1. Data are presented as number of positive cell lines for mRNA and/or protein expression of the indicated cytokine in relation to the total number of analyzed cell lines.

[c]Summarizes the percentage of HD cases with positive detection using immunohistochemistry (protein) and/or *in-situ* hybridization (mRNA) for the indicated cytokine in primary HD-involved tissue.

[d]Other cell types: E, endothelial cells; U, ubiquitous; G, granulocytes; E, eosinophils; and APC, antigen-presenting cells.

[e]Percentage of HD patients with elevated (↑) cytokine serum levels in comparison to normal control samples.

[f]0 indicates no detectable serum concentrations or tissue expression for HD patients.

[g]Most cell lines positive for indicated cytokine after activation.

From Gruss HJ, Kadin ME. *Pathophysiology of Hodgkin's disease.* Paris: Bailliere: functional and molecular aspects, 1996, with permission.

Cytokines can directly stimulate or suppress the growth of tumor cells. Because Hodgkin–Reed-Sternberg cells are derived from lymphocytes in most instances, cytokines that affect the growth of normal lymphocytes are candidates to modulate the growth of Hodgkin–Reed-Sternberg cells. Among the cytokines that appear to stimulate the growth of Hodgkin–Reed-Sternberg cells are CD40 ligand (CD40L) (3), IL-4 (4), IL-6 (5–7), and IL-9 (8). Several cytokines appear to act primarily on surrounding cells, which in turn release cytokines that affect the growth and survival of Hodgkin–Reed-Sternberg cells. For example, IL-8 released by Hodgkin–Reed-Sternberg cells (9,10) attracts neutrophils, which express CD30L (11); IL-5 synthesized by Hodgkin–Reed-Sternberg cells attracts eosinophils, which express both CD30L and TGF-β (12–14).

Cytokines can induce or upregulate the expression of cell surface adhesion molecules, which may determine the localization and metastatic potential of Hodgkin–Reed-Sternberg cells as well as their interaction with other cells, especially T lymphocytes, which are adherent to Hodgkin–Reed-Sternberg cells both *in vivo* and *in vitro* (15–19). Hodgkin–Reed-Sternberg–derived cell lines express adhesion molecules CD44, CD54, and CD58. Primary Hodgkin–Reed-Sternberg cells express adhesion molecules of the immunoglobulin superfamily, including ICAM-1, LDFA-3, the integrin family including CD15, and others (H-CAM, CD23, HD-lectin, and CD40). ICAM-1 (CD54), the ligand for LFA-1, mediates cell-to-cell and cellular matrix interactions (20). Elevated serum sICAM-1 has been detected in Hodgkin's disease patients with B symptoms, bulky and advanced stages of disease (21).

In order for cytokines to affect the behavior of Hodgkin–Reed-Sternberg cells, they must engage the cognate receptors on these cells. Hodgkin–Reed-Sternberg cells have been shown to display receptors for IL-2 (IL-2R) (22–25), CD30L (CD30) (26), and CD40L (CD40) (2,27,28). Receptors for some other cytokines such as IL-9 and TGF-β have not yet been demonstrated directly on Hodgkin–Reed-Sternberg cells; if present they appear to be few in number (29). This may be a result of the advanced-stage disease and consequently less differentiated state from which these cell lines are commonly derived.

Cytokines and/or cytokine receptors are often detected in the serum of Hodgkin's disease patients. Elevated sCD30, which is produced by Hodgkin–Reed-Sternberg cells, can also serve as an index of tumor burden in Hodgkin's disease (30).

Cytokine receptors expressed on the surface of Hodgkin–Reed-Sternberg cells can serve as targets for tailored immunotherapy directed against these cells. CD30 and IL-2R are the principal molecules that have been used as targets for antibodies conjugated to toxins or radionuclides (31–33).

METHODS FOR DETECTING AND MEASURING CYTOKINES AND CYTOKINE RECEPTORS

Several methods have been used to detect cytokines and their receptors in lymphomas. These include detection of mRNA in tissues or cell lines by Northern blots, RT-PCR, and *in situ* hybridization (ISH). Cytokine proteins can be detected in tissues by immunohistochemistry and in Hodgkin–Reed-Sternberg cell culture supernatants or patient sera by enzyme-linked immunosorbent assays (ELISA). Each method has its limitations, so a combination of methods is superior to any single method alone. For example, detection of mRNA in whole tissue extracts by Northern blots fails to localize synthesis of the message; this requires the use of ISH. Unfortunately, the small amount of cytokine mRNA is often difficult to detect, particularly by use of ISH in paraffin-embedded tissue sections. This may be overcome in some instances by the use of frozen paraformaldehyde-fixed tissues. Detection of cytokine mRNA does not ensure protein synthesis by the labeled cells, and immunohistochemistry or ELISA is necessary to confirm protein synthesis. However, immunohistochemistry is often inadequate to detect cytokines in tissues, presumably because of the low levels of tissue cytokine expression and rapid inactivation of cytokines. Moreover, some cytokines, such as TGF-β, require conformational change or activation from a latent precursor molecule for biologic activity and immunodetection (34). In Hodgkin's disease, there is evidence that a high-molecular-weight TGF-β active at physiologic pH is formed by L-428 cells (34). This might explain our lack of detection of TGF-β mRNA in Hodgkin–Reed-Sternberg cells with a probe for native TGF-β (35). Cytokine receptors are often expressed at levels below detection by routine immunohistochemistry. Their detection may require assessment of mRNA in tissues or binding of labeled ligand by cell lines using immunoprecipitation or Scatchard analysis (29,34). Measurement of cytokines and cytokine receptors in cell culture supernatants by ELISA is convenient and sensitive but may not reflect the true physiologic signficance of serum measurements *in vivo. In vivo* measurements integrate the effects of both cytokine and cytokine receptor synthesis and turnover, which ultimately produce the biological effects in the patient.

HETEROGENEITY OF CYTOKINE PRODUCTION

Clonal selection of tumor cells may eventuate in variable patterns of cytokine production at different anatomic sites of disease. We have demonstrated such differences in cell clones from related CD30$^+$ tumor cell lines (36; *unpublished data*). This may explain the different tissue reactions, such as presence or absence of collagen sclerosis, in different tissue specimens from the same patient.

THE TUMOR NECROSIS FACTOR RECEPTOR SUPERFAMILY

Members of the tumor necrosis factor receptor (TNFR) superfamily have a central role in Hodgkin–Reed-Sternberg cell signaling. This receptor family contains more than 10 cellular and viral open reading frames. Members of this receptor superfamily are characterized by multiple cysteine-rich domains in the extracellular (N-terminal) portion of the molecule that are involved in ligand binding (37). The cysteine-rich domains among the human TNFR superfamily members have between 25% and 30% homology on average (37,38). Some members of this family such as the nerve growth factor receptor (NGFR), TNF receptor-I (TNFR-I), TNFR-II, and FAS/APO-1 have an unrestricted tissue distribution, whereas other members of this family such as CD27, CD30, CD40, 4-1BB, and OX40 are restricted to cells of the lymphoid or hematopoietic systems (39,40). The ligands for the TNFR superfamily are a group of molecules that belong to the TNF ligand superfamily. Members of the TNF ligand superfamily share about 20% sequence homology in their extracellular domains and exist primarily as membrane-bound molecules (40). Molecular evidence suggests that most of these molecules form trimers or higher multimers in their biologically active state. Members of the TNF ligand superfamily include TNF, lymphotoxin-α (LT-α), LT-β, CD27 ligand (CD27L), CD30L, CD40L, 4-1BBL, OX40L, and FASL. Of these, only TNF, LT-α, and FASL have been found to have soluble forms. Members of the TNFR superfamily have significant variation in their cytoplasmic (C-terminal) domains. Over the past few years multiple signaling pathways that this receptor superfamily shares have been identified.

Tumor Necrosis Factor Receptor and Tumor Necrosis Factor Ligand Superfamily Expression in Hodgkin's disease

Immunophenotypic studies on Hodgkin's disease have identified many activation markers and Hodgkin's disease-associated antigens that are present on Hodgkin–Reed-Sternberg cells. The CD30 TNFR superfamily member, in fact, was initially identified as a Hodgkin's disease–associated antigen (41). CD30 expression has subsequently been shown not to be specific for Hodgkin–Reed-Sternberg cells; rather, it is a late activation marker for lymphoid cells, with normal CD30 expression being restricted to antigen-stimulated and memory T cells (42–45). Nearly all Hodgkin's disease-derived cell lines and approximately 85% to 90% of most types of Hodgkin's disease express CD30 in Hodgkin–Reed-Sternberg cells (24,26,41–43,46–52). An exception is the lymphocyte predominance subtype of Hodgkin's disease, in which only approximately one-third of the cases express CD30 (48,50). Soluble CD30 (sCD30) has been detected in the serum of patients with Hodgkin's disease under certain situations (53). High levels of sCD30 were found in the serum in a majority of Hodgkin's disease cases at diagnosis; they appear to correlate with advanced disease and thus are higher in patients with advanced-stage, bulky tumor and B symptoms (30,54–56). The level of sCD30 appears to be an independent prognostic factor, with high sCD30 levels being associated with a decreased disease free survival (30). Furthermore, sCD30 could not be detected in any Hodgkin's disease patient who was in complete remission.

In addition to being expressed on the majority of Hodgkin–Reed-Sternberg cells in most Hodgkin's disease subtypes, CD30 is also present on the tumor cells of the T-cell lineage CD30-positive anaplastic large-cell lymphoma (42). The Hodgkin–Reed-Sternberg cells also express several other members of the TNFR superfamily, including CD40, FAS, TNFR-I, TNFR-II, and 4-1BB (40,57). Additionally, primary Hodgkin–Reed-Sternberg cells express members of the TNFR ligand superfamily, including TNF, LT-α, CD27L, CD30L (40,57). The expression of multiple TNFR and TNF ligand superfamily members in Hodgkin–Reed-Sternberg cells with their potential shared signaling pathways is further complicated by the fact that in certain subtypes of Hodgkin's disease that are Epstein-Barr virus (EBV)–positive, the latent membrane protein 1 (LMP1) of EBV is also expressed in the Hodgkin–Reed-Sternberg cells (58,59). The EBV LMP1 is a signaling homolog of the TNFR superfamily (60–64). In the next few sections we attempt to describe the expression patterns of these different TNFR and TNF ligand superfamily members as well as their potential role in signal transduction in the pathogenesis of Hodgkin's disease. TNF ligand superfamily expression by Hodgkin–Reed-Sternberg cells may act to directly support the growth inactivation of these tumor cells by an autocrine mechanism and also has an effect on the surrounding reactive cells, particularly T lymphocytes, which are present in abundance in Hodgkin's tumor tissue. Although detailed functional information regarding the interactions of TNF ligand superfamily members and TNFR superfamily members in primary Hodgkin's disease lesions have yet to be confirmed, there are many predicted biologic activities of these molecules that can be inferred from their known function in other *in vivo* and *in vitro* systems.

Tumor Necrosis Factor Receptor Superfamily Signaling Pathways

Several signaling pathways that are involved in TNFR superfamily signaling have begun to be delineated and are depicted in Figure 1. There are multiple signal-transducing molecules that have been identified that interact with domains of TNFRs as well as with domains of other proteins that are directly involved in signal transduction. These so-called adapter molecules in most cases have more than one family member, each of which functions in a slightly different manner and ultimately leads to different signals being transduced. A complete description of all of the signaling molecules in each of these pathways is well beyond the scope of this chapter. Instead, we will focus on TNFR superfamily signaling pathways, which are shared with CD30, CD40, TNFR-I, TNFR-II as well as EBV LMP1. The family of adapter molecules called TNFR-associated factor (TRAF) has at least six members, TRAF1 through TRAF6 (60,65–76; for review see 77). Structural features of TRAF family members include a TRAF domain in the carboxyl terminal part of the protein, an N-terminal RING finger domain, a cluster of zinc fingers, and a coiled-coil domain (67,70,74). An exception to this is TRAF1, which lacks the RING finger domain. The TRAF domain is the defining structural feature of these molecules. The 230-bp TRAF domain mediates a number of specific protein–protein interactions (65,66,68,74,78–83). The genomic organization of TRAF1 indicated that the gene is approximately 12 kilobases (kb) and is separated into six exons, four of which encode parts of the TRAF domain (84). Preliminary information indicates that the TRAF domains of TRAF2 and TRAF3 are encoded by several exons.

TRAF2 mediates both NF-κB activation and activation of the *c-Jun* N-terminal kinase (JNK) pathway (67,78, 85–88). The activation of these two divergent pathways by TRAF molecules may begin to explain the pleiotropic effects of TNF receptor family signaling in cells. In addition, the specific mechanisms of activation of each of these pathways are beginning to be understood. TRAF2 mediates NF-κB activation by TNFR1, TNFR2, CD40, and CD30 (67,78,89–94). TRAF2 can mediate NF-κB activation by the EBV LMP1 protein as well (61,95,96). TRAF5 has been demonstrated to similarly activate NF-κB by members of the TNFR superfamily (72,73,97,98). The mechanism of activation of NF-κB signaling is through the recruitment and activation of a series of protein kinases, which leads to the translocation of activated NF-κB into the nucleus of the cell. Although TRAF molecules have no intrinsic catalytic capability, their interaction with certain

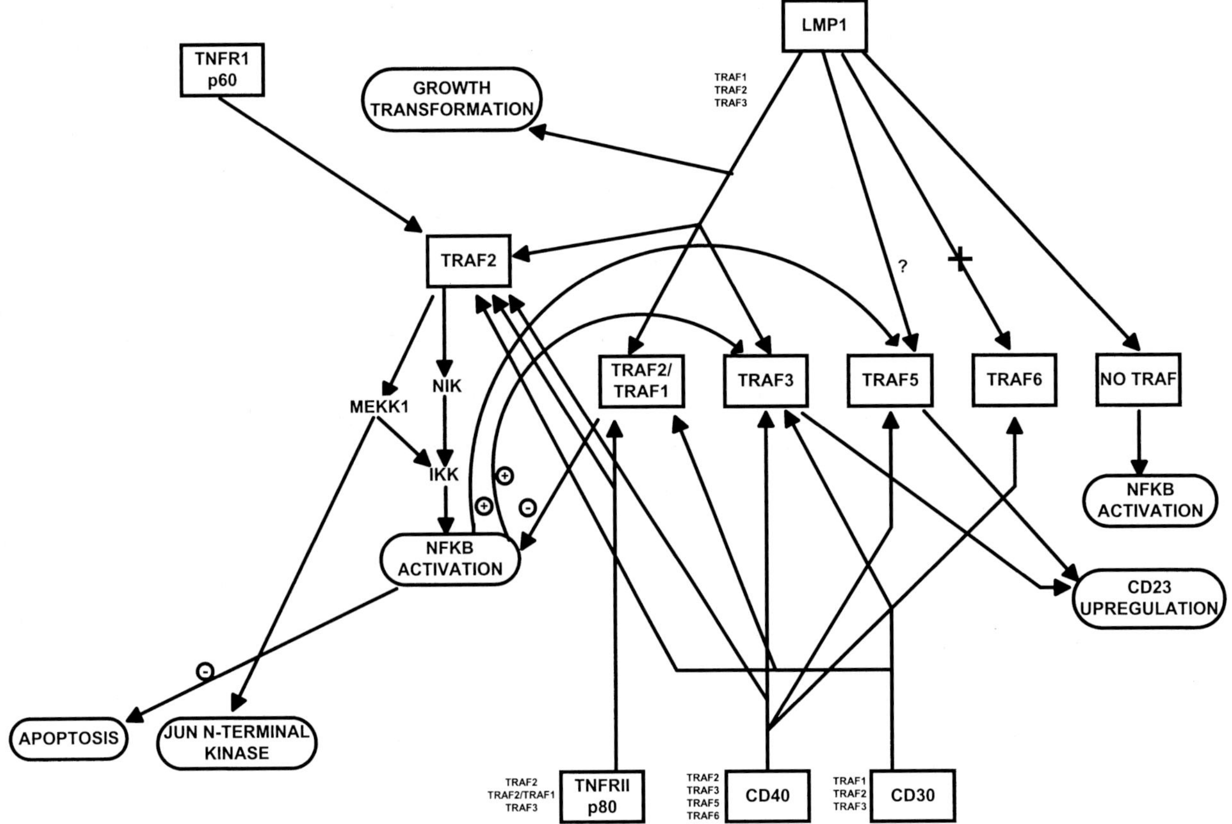

FIG. 1. Tumor necrosis factor receptor superfamily signaling pathways relevant to Hodgkin–Reed-Sternberg cells. The multiple signaling molecules that participate in the downstream signaling effects of TNF receptor signaling are depicted. Notice the participation of TRAF-2 in different signaling pathways. See text for details.

kinases appears to stimulate the activity of those molecules. The NF-κB–inducing kinase (NIK) is a mitogen-activated protein (MAP) kinase kinase kinase (MAP3K) (99). A substrate of NIK is the IκB complex (IKK), which consists of two subunits IKKα and IKKβ (100,101). The available data suggest that the IKK complex is essential for the phosphorylation and inactivation of the NF-κB inhibitor protein by IκB (100–104). IκB is found in the cytoplasm in association with NF-κB, keeping NF-κB in an inactivated state. On phosphorylation and degradation of IκB, NF-κB translocates into the nucleus in its activated state and can stimulate the transcription of a variety of cellular genes (for review, 105). Constitutive activation of NF-κB-RelA appears to be required for proliferation and survival of Hodgkin's disease tumor cells (106). Constitutive activation of NF-κB-RelA prevented Hodgkin's disease tumor cells from undergoing stress-induced apoptosis. Hodgkin's disease tumor cells depleted of constitutive NF-κB revealed strongly impaired tumor growth in severe combined immunodeficient mice.

In addition to binding NIK, TRAF2 has been shown to activate mitogen-activated protein kinase/ERK kinase kinase-1 (MEKK1) (85-87). MEKK1 is a central kinase in the c-Jun activation pathway. Additionally, there is a convergence of the two TRAF2-mediated pathways at MEKK1; MEKK1 has recently been shown to be able to phosphorylate IκBa, leading to the activation of NF-κB (107). Thus TRAF2 serves as an important branch point for the NF-κB and JNK pathways. Furthermore, the participation by MEKK1 in each of these signaling pathways provides the opportunity for these pathways to interact directly. The role of each of these pathways in mediating the downstream effects of TNF receptor family signaling is largely understood through experiments performed with dominant negative mutations of multiple members of the signaling molecules as well as in knock-out transgenic mice (108, 109). The results of these types of studies suggest that the activation of NF-κB can protect the cell against TNF induced apoptosis (106). Also JNK activation is not directly linked to the induction of TNFR1-mediated apoptosis (108,109). The expression of a TRAF2-dominant negative in transgenic mice *in vivo* suggests that TRAF2 is required for the activation of JNK, but not NF-κB, through TNFR or CD40 (109). These experiments also showed that TRAF2 has an antiapoptotic affect that is independent of its ability to activate NF-κB (108,109).

TRAF3 is unique among the TRAF family members thus far discovered in that this protein is capable is blocking TNF receptor family member–mediated activation of NF-κB (67). Furthermore, TRAF3 can block the ability of TRAF2 to activate this pathway. TRAF3 knockout mice do not show any significant defects in CD40 signaling (110). These mice, however, do show postnatal lethality and have defective T-cell–mediated immune responses (110). This suggests that TRAF3 is important in regulating certain cellular events during development. Although the effects of TRAF3 have not been directly studied regarding JNK activation, the ability of TRAF3 to block TRAF2-mediated NF-κB inactivation suggests that TRAF3 may play a role in determining the ability of TRAF2 to activate the NF-κB or JNK pathway.

The ability of multiple members of the TNF receptor superfamily such as CD30, CD40, or TNFR1 to interact with various members of the TRAF family of signal transduction molecules and their coexpression in Hodgkin–Reed-Sternberg cells may result in a complex cascade of signaling events in Hodgkin's disease. The ability of the EBV LMP1 protein to interact with TRAF family members and activate these pathways also adds a level of complexity to the potential signaling processes in EBV-positive cases of Hodgkin's disease. The notion that LMP1 may exert effects on H-RS cell growth *in vivo* through the TNF receptor signaling pathway is strengthened by the recent demonstration of TRAF-mediated LMP1 signaling *in vivo* in EBV-positive AIDS-related non-Hodgkin's lymphomas and posttransplant lymphoproliferative disease (64). The coexpression of multiple members of the TNF receptor superfamily, which all share components of the same signaling pathways, suggests that receptor cross-talk may be an important element to determining the phenotype of the Hodgkin–Reed-Sternberg cell and the microenvironment of Hodgkin's disease.

CD30 ligand

CD30L is expressed on activated T cells, macrophages, and granulocytes (111). All three cell types are found in Hodgkin's disease tissues and might therefore modulate the proliferation of primary Hodgkin–Reed-Sternberg cells by paracrine mechanisms. Pinto et al. showed that circulating and tissue eosinophils from patients with Hodgkin's disease and hypereosinophilic syndrome display CD30L mRNA and express CD30L protein at higher levels than healthy donors (13). Cytokines that regulate eosinophil proliferation and activation—IL-5, IL3, and GM-CSF—enhance cellular density of CD30L on purifed eosinophils from normal subjects. Native CD30L on human eosinophils is a functionally active surface molecule that can transduce proliferative signals on CD30$^+$ target cells; CD30 engagement by CD30L-expressing cells results in a dose-dependent proliferation of Hodgkin's disease derived cell line HDLM-2.

CD30L has pleiotropic effects on CD30-expressing cell lines (49). Recombinant CD30L and anti-CD30 antibodies (M44 and M67) enhanced proliferation of T-cell-like Hodgkin's disease–derived cell lines (HDLM-2 and L-540) and adult T-cell leukemia cell lines in a time- and dose-dependent manner but did not enhance proliferation of B-cell-like Hodgkin's disease–derived cell lines (KM-H2 and L-428). The enhanced proliferative effect of CD30L appeared specific because it could be blocked by addition of excess soluble CD30Fc protein. None of six Hodgkin's disease–derived cell lines examined showed CD30L mRNA or protein expression constitutively or after stimulation with TPA or cytokines (e.g., IL-1, IL-2, IL-4, IL-6, IL-9, TNF), indicating that these Hodgkin's disease–derived cell lines do not use CD30–CD30L interaction in an autocrine fashion.

CD40 ligand

CD40 is a 50-kd phosphoprotein expressed mainly on cells of B lineage, including most B-cell leukemias and lymphomas (112,113). CD40 acts as a receptor for a specific ligand (CD40L), which is a type II integral membrane glycoprotein that has homology to ligands for other receptors of the NGF/TNF receptor superfamily (37). CD40L is expressed primarily on activated CD4$^+$ helper T cells, including the cells that form rosettes around Hodgkin–Reed-Sternberg cells (2,114), and also is expressed on some mast cells and basophils (115). Engagement of CD40 antigen by CD40L or monoclonal antibodies results in the prevention of apoptosis of germinal center B cells (116,117). CD40L is directly mitogenic for human B cells (118). CD40L requires IL-3 as a costimulatory cytokine for human B-cell precursors, whereas IL-4 enhances proliferation of mature B cells in the CD40 system (119). CD40L-induced immunoglobulin secretion is also cytokine-dependent (120). CD40L is also stimulatory for human T cells; it induces CD25 and CD40L expression, and IFN-γ, TNF-α, and IL-2 secretion in the presence of submitogenic concentrations of phytohemagglutinin (121).

CD40 is expressed at high levels on primary and cultured Hodgkin–Reed-Sternberg cells (3,27,28) (Fig. 2). Therefore, engagement of CD40 might be expected to modulate the growth of Hodgkin–Reed-Sternberg cells. Whereas anti-CD40 antibodies and recombinant CD40L were found to inhibit the growth of cell lines derived from human Burkitt's and diffuse large B-cell lymphomas (122), engagement of CD40 by a soluble form of CD40L was found to enhance the clonogenic capacity and colony cell survival of Hodgkin's disease cell lines (3). Exposure of L-428 and KM-H2 cells to different concentrations of soluble human CD40L resulted in a dose-dependent enhancement of their clonogenic growth and a striking increase in their colony size. These effects were enhanced by addition of IL-9. CD40L also enhanced Hodgkin–Reed-Sternberg cell line expression

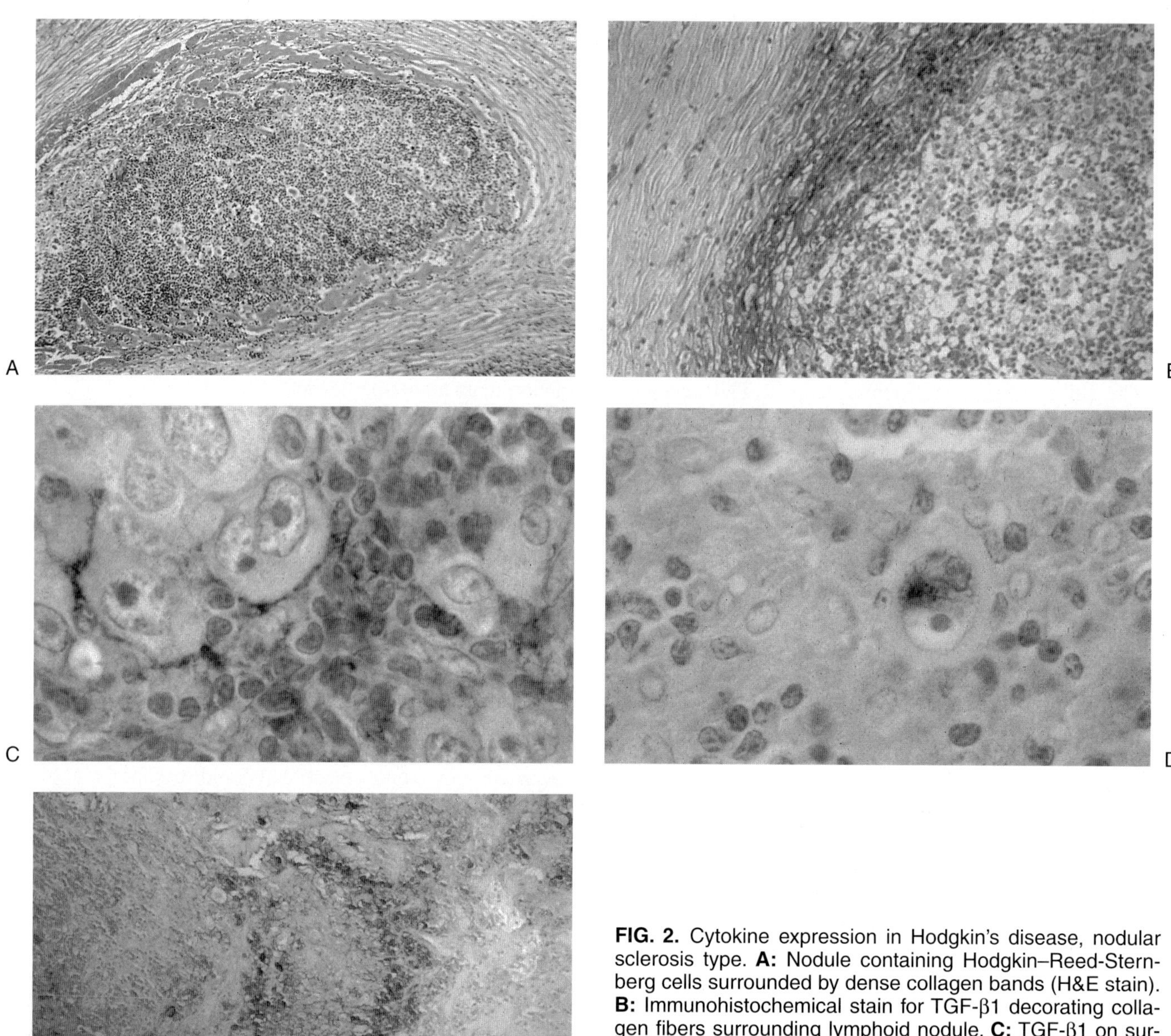

FIG. 2. Cytokine expression in Hodgkin's disease, nodular sclerosis type. **A:** Nodule containing Hodgkin–Reed-Sternberg cells surrounded by dense collagen bands (H&E stain). **B:** Immunohistochemical stain for TGF-β1 decorating collagen fibers surrounding lymphoid nodule. **C:** TGF-β1 on surface of Hodgkin–Reed-Sternberg cells and **D:** within cytoplasm of RS-cell, and **E:** CD40 expressed on surface of Hodgkin–Reed-Sternberg cells concentrated at the periphery of abnormal lymphoid nodule. (These figures are printed in color as Plates 17 through 21.)

of costimulatory and intercellular adhesion molecules ICAM-1/CD54 and B7-1/CD80 and induced their release of cytokines IL-8, IL-6, TNF, and lymphotoxin-α (28). Different effects of CD40L on B lymphoma cells have been observed when soluble CD40 antibodies were used, generally promoting B-cell growth and inhibition of apoptosis, in contrast to inhibition of cell growth when CD40 is cross-linked by immobilized antibody (122). Further studies of CD40L and agonistic anti-CD40 antibodies in animal models are needed to determine the *in vivo* consequences of engagement of CD40 on Hodgkin–Reed-Sternberg cells.

Other Cytokines as Growth Factors for Hodgkin–Reed-Sternberg Cells

Interleukin-6

Interleukin-6 (IL-6) is produced by activated B lymphocytes and neoplastic B cells in some non-Hodgkin's lymphomas and plasma cell myeloma (multiple myeloma) (123). Plasma cell tumors proliferate in response to IL-6, and this proliferation is specifically inhibited by IL-6 neutralizing antibodies, suggesting that IL-6 is an autocrine growth factor for terminally differentiated neoplastic plasma cells (124). Interleukin-6 is also a growth factor for

EBV-immortalized B lymphocytes (125). EBV is found in 40% to 50% of Hodgkin's disease cases, most commonly with mixed cellularity histology (60%), less frequently in nodular sclerosis (20%), and rarely, if ever, in lymphocyte predominance subtype (126,127).

Interleukin-6 and IL-6 receptor mRNA and protein have been found in Hodgkin's disease cell lines, and IL-6 mRNA can be localized to Hodgkin–Reed-Sternberg cells (5) and also to some reactive cells surrounding Hodgkin–Reed-Sternberg cells (7) in tissue sections of Hodgkin's disease. Merz et al. detected IL-6 mRNA expression in nine of 12 cases of Hodgkin's disease including nodular sclerosis, mixed cellularity, and lymphocyte predominance types (128). Interleukin-6 protein has been localized immunohistochemically to Hodgkin–Reed-Sternberg cells, reactive histiocytes, and endothelial cells in Hodgkin's disease (129). The IL-6 receptor (p80) has been detected on Hodgkin–Reed-Sternberg cells in some Hodgkin's disease cases and Hodgkin's disease cell lines (5), but not in others (129). Tesch et al. reported that IL-6R protein was expressed more commonly in mixed-cellularity than nodular sclerosis Hodgkin's disease (6). They proposed that coexpression of IL-6 and IL-6R could lead to an autocrine/paracrine loop for IL-6–dependent growth of Hodgkin–Reed-Sternberg cells. However, addition of IL-6 and antibodies against IL-6 or IL-6R could not be shown to affect the proliferation of Hodgkin's disease cell lines HDLM-2 or KM-H2. Thus, a definite role for IL-6 in the growth of Hodgkin–Reed-Sternberg cells has not yet been convincingly demonstrated.

Interleukin-4

Interleukin-4 is a pleiotropic factor that affects different steps of antigen-dependent maturation of human B cells. Following *in vitro* activation, IL-4 stimulates B-cell growth as well as the production of IgG and IgM (115). IL-4 can inhibit IL-2–dependent growth of freshly isolated non-Hodgkin's lymphoma malignant B cells (130).

Merz et al. observed IL-4 mRNA in only two of 12 cases of Hodgkin's disease, and the IL-4 message appeared to be confined to small lymphocytes (128). No studies of IL-4 receptor mRNA in Hodgkin's disease tissue sections have been reported. Hsu et al. were unable to detect IL-4 protein in cultures of HDLM or KM-H2 cells (129). They detected IL-4 immunohistochemically in 2% to 5% of small to medium-sized lymphoid cells and a small number of dendritic-like cells in all tissues involved by Hodgkin's disease; no staining for IL-4 was observed in Hodgkin–Reed-Sternberg cells.

A lymphokine with properties of IL-4 has been detected in culture supernatants of the cell line L-428 derived from a patient with clinically advanced nodular sclerosis Hodgkin's disease (4). The L-428–derived lymphokine has a molecular mass of 68 kd, identical to glycosylated recombinant IL-4, cross-reacts with the monoclonal antibody anti–IL-4 in Western immunoblotting, and competes for the IL-4 receptor. After acid elution, L-428 cells were found to have approximately 4,000 high-affinity receptors for IL-4. Recombinant IL-4 and the L-428–derived lymphokine equally induced DNA synthesis of L-428 cells. L-428 cells were also found to contain IL-4 mRNA, suggesting that IL-4 could be a secreted autocrine growth factor for L-428 cells. However, anti–IL-4 neutralizing antibody had no effect on sustained serum-free growth of L-428 cells. It remains possible that IL-4 interacts with its receptor intracellularly and is protected from exogenous specific antibody. However, there is presently insufficient experimental evidence to conclude that IL-4 is an autocrine growth factor for L-428 cells.

Interleukin-9

Interleukin-9 is the human homolog of the mouse T-cell growth factor P40, which causes antigen-independent proliferation and survival of some murine T-cell clones (131). Interleukin-9 is normally produced by activated $CD4^+$ T cells of the T_H2 subtype. Among human lymphomas, IL-9 appears to be expressed specifically by tumor cells in Hodgkin's disease and anaplastic large-cell lymphoma (8). Expression of IL-9 receptors by Hodgkin's disease cell lines and the role of IL-9 as a growth factor for these cells have not yet been confirmed.

Interleukin-2

Interleukin-2 is an important T-cell growth factor that is also implicated in the tumorigenicity of several T-cell malignancies and some nonhematopoietic tumors (132,133). The receptor for IL-2 is composed of α, β, and γ subunits; the high-affinity IL-2R is formed by the interaction of these three subunits (134). Hodgkin–Reed-Sternberg cells do not uniformly express IL-2R. Receptor analysis measured by immunofluoresence and binding of radiolabeled IL-2 indicated that L-428 cells lack measurable IL-2R (29). Consistent with this finding, L-428 cells showed no mitogenic response to IL-2 (29). Hsu and coworkers also failed to demonstrate a proliferative response of Hodgkin's disease cell lines to IL-2 (135).

A variable frequency of expression of IL-2R by Hodgkin–Reed-Sternberg cells has been detected in several studies, most likely as a result of differences in the type of tissues used (frozen versus paraffin-embedded tissues), the specific antibody and sensitivity of the detection system used, and the ability to distinguish staining of Hodgkin–Reed-Sternberg cells from that of surrounding inflammatory cells (22–25). Strauchen et al. reported expression of IL-2R in over 10% of RS cells in seven of 12 Hodgkin's disease cases (22). Sheibani et al. observed IL-2R expression in 37 of 41 cases but did not specify whether RS cells or surrounding lymphocytes expressed

IL-2R (23). Using paraformaldehyde-fixed frozen sections, which preserve antigen detection but in which it is sometimes difficult to distinguish staining of Hodgkin–Reed-Sternberg cells from surrounding cells, Agnarsson and Kadin found that of 50 cases of Hodgkin's disease, IL-2R appeared on cells in 72% of nodular sclerosis, 100% of mixed cellularity, and 80% of lymphocyte predominance cases (24). Recently, we used a sensitive biotinylated tyramine enhancement method in paraffin tissues to better localize the expression of IL-2R to tumor cells versus reactive lymphocytes in Hodgkin's disease (25) (Fig. 3). We found that expression of IL-2R by Hodgkin–Reed-Sternberg cells is not uniform within an individual case, and in Hodgkin's disease tissues from some cases, no IL-2R could be found on Hodgkin–Reed-Sternberg cells, whereas some surrounding small lymphocytes express IL-2R in all cases. By comparison, tumor cells in virtually all cases of $CD30^+$ anaplastic large-cell lymphomas were observed to express high levels of IL2R (25).

Effects of Cytokines on the Pathology of Hodgkin's disease

Interleukin-7

IL-7 is frequently expressed by Hodgkin–Reed-Sternberg cells in nodular sclerosis and mixed-cellularity Hodgkin's disease (137). Interleukin-7 could be responsible for some part of the inflammatory response and low-grade behavior of Hodgkin's disease because tumor cell lines of various cell lineages transfected with a functioning IL-7 gene and injected into mice were observed to evoke an antitumor response consisting of CD4+ and CD8+ T cells, macrophages, and eosinophils (138, 139).

Cytokine Induction of Adhesion Molecules

Cytokines have been shown to affect the expression and cell distribution of adhesion molecules in Hodgkin's disease tissues and reactive lymph nodes (140). Ruco and co-workers investigated expression of intercellular adhesion molecule (ICAM-1), vascular cell adhesion molecule (VCAM-1), endothelial leukocyte adhesion molecule (ELAM-1), and endothelial cell adhesion molecule (EndoCAM CD31) and HLA-DR antigens in tissue sections of reactive lymph nodes and Hodgkin's disease. EndoCAM (CD31) was constitutively expressed in all types of endothelial cells, sinus macrophages, and in epithelioid granulomas. ECAM-1 was selectively expressed by activated entothelial cells of high endothelial venules (HEVs). When expression of the cytokine-inducible adhesion molecules ICAM-1, VCAM-1, and ELAM-1 was comparatively evaluated in HEVs, it was

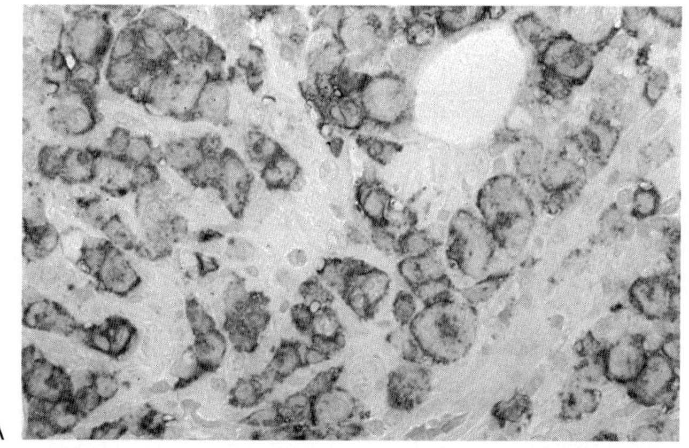
A

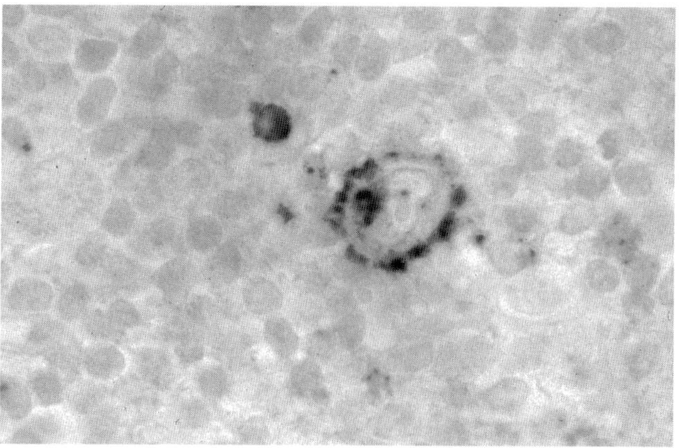
B

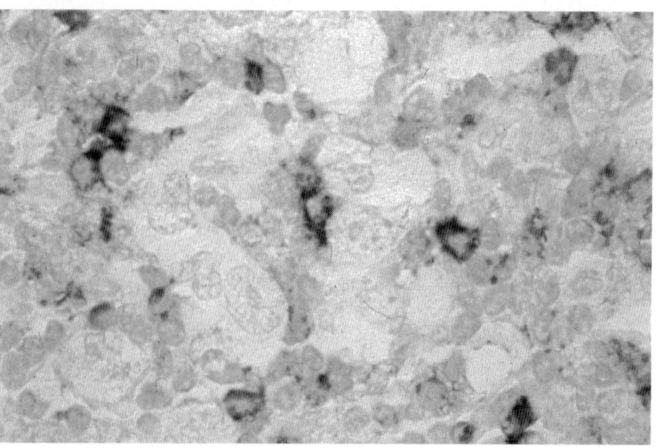
C

FIG. 3. Immunohistochemical demonstration of a subunit of IL-2 receptor (IL-2Rα) in **(A)** $CD30^+$ cutaneous anaplastic large-cell lymphoma (ALCL) and **(B** and **C)** Hodgkin's disease. Virtually all tumor cells stain for IL-2Rα in ALCL **(A);** large Reed-Sternberg cell shows cytoplasmic and surface staining **(B);** only small lymphocytes around Hodgkin–Reed-Sternberg cells are stained for IL-2Rα **(C).** Reproduced with permission from ref. 25. (These figures are printed in color as plates 22 through 24.)

found that ICAM-1+ HEVs were present in all reactive lymph nodes and Hodgkin's disease, whereas ELAM-1 and/or VCAM-1 were expressed only in those pathologic conditions characterized by high levels of interleukin-1 (IL-1) or tumor necrosis factor (TNF) production. Interleukin-1α and TNF-α are expressed by Hodgkin–Reed-Sternberg cells and macrophages (141). Interleukin-1α is also expressed by interdigitating reticulum cells and endothelial cells (141,142). In Hodgkin's disease, expression of ELAM-1/VCAM-1 was more pronounced in nodular sclerosis and was associated with accumulation of perivascular neutrophils. These findings support the hypothesis that cytokine-induced expression of adhesion molecules plays a role in the pathogenesis of Hodgkin's disease lesions and that different patterns of cytokine expression may contribute to the different histologic expressions of Hodgkin's disease.

Adhesion of T Lymphocytes to Hodgkin–Reed-Sternberg Cells

It has long been known that T lymphocytes adhere closely to RS cells both *in vivo* and *in vitro,* giving the appearance of a rosette of small lymphocytes around these giant cells (15,16). The T lymphocytes around Hodgkin–Reed-Sternberg cells are polyclonal (17). Hodgkin's cell lines express high levels of LFA-3 and ICAM-1, both of which are ligands for T-cell adhesion (18). The significance of these rosettes is poorly understood, but recent studies suggest a functional interaction of the Hodgkin–Reed-Sternberg cell as an antigen-presenting cell with T lymphocytes (143). Hodgkin–Reed-Sternberg cells express B7/BB1 (CD80), which is present on the membrane of professional antigen-presenting cells and is the natural ligand of CD28, a membrane receptor of T cells (144,145). CD28 ligation of T cells increases their secretion of IL-2, TNF-α, lymphotoxin, IFN-γ, and GM-CSF, thus potentially affecting the inflammatory infiltrate and histopathology of Hodgkin's disease (145).

The expression of accessory molecules involved in T-cell–Hodgkin–Reed-Sternberg-cell contact is regulated by interactions of CD30/CD30L and CD40/CD40L. CD40/CD40L interaction provides a critical signal for cell contact-dependent T-cell activation of B cells (38). CD40 ligation enhances other contact-dependent cell interactions following antigen-dependent stimulation such as CD11a/CD18/CD54 and B7 ligands (CD80 and CD86)/CD28 or CTLA4 for T- and B-cell interactions (120,144,145).

In addition to the role of adhesion molecules in the functional interaction between Hodgkin–Reed-Sternberg cells and T lymphocytes, certain adhesion molecules could be significant in the morphology and anatomic distribution of Hodgkin's disease. Ree and co-workers showed that cell adhesion molecules associated with germinal center formation are expressed in the large majority of cases of Hodgkin's disease (146). The expression of adhesion molecules CD54 on Hodgkin–Reed-Sternberg-cells and CD11a on T lymphocytes was associated with the occurrence of distinctive CD20+ B-cell aggregates. The extracellular matrices of these B-cell aggregates stained for adhesion molecules CD54 and VLA-4 and revealed follicular dendritic cell networks that formed germinal-center–related complexes and was correlated with formation of nodular sclerosis.

Hodgkin's disease initially is localized to lymph nodes and spreads in an orderly predictable manner (147, 148). Hodgkin–Reed-Sternberg cells appear fixed in tissues and rarely disseminate in the blood compared with frequent dissemination of tumor cells in non-Hodgkin's lymphomas. Kapp et al. devised a murine model for dissemination of Hodgkin's disease–derived cell lines (149). In this model, the adhesion molecule CD44 (Hermes) was found to be expressed on nondisseminating Hodgkin cell lines L-428 and KM-H2 but was not expressed on disseminating Hodgkin cell lines L540 and L540cy. CD44 is an adhesion molecule that undergoes alternative splicing, resulting in expression of different variant exons in diffuse large-cell lymphomas (150,151). Expression of CD44 variant exons is modulated by cytokines (152). We have detected expression of the hematopoietic form of CD44 (CD44H) on Hodgkin–Reed-Sternberg cells in nodular Hodgkin's disease *(unpublished data).* The expression of CD44 variant exons by Hodgkin–Reed-Sternberg cells in Hodgkin's disease has yet to be fully characterized.

Eosinophilia

Tissue and peripheral blood eosinophilia are common features of Hodgkin's disease and distinguish it from most non-Hodgkin's lymphoma. Samoszuk and Nansen have shown that eosinophilia in mixed-cellularity and nodular sclerosis Hodgkin's disease is associated with interleukin-5 mRNA detected in the cytoplasm of Hodgkin–Reed-Sternberg cells and their morphologic variants (12). Interleukin-5 normally is produced by activated T cells and, in murine systems, stimulates eosinopoiesis as well as B-cell growth and proliferation. Recently, Feldstein and co-workers reported a strong direct correlation of tissue eosinophilia with expression of eotaxin-1 mRNA expression in Hodgkin's disease tissues (153). Eotaxin-1 is an eosinophil-specific chemoattractant recently identified in rodent models of asthma and allergic inflammation. Its expression is induced by IL-3. A high expression of eotaxin-1 was found specifically in nodular sclerosis Hodgkin's disease compared to other subtypes. In contrast, significant expression was not found in B- or T-cell lymphomas with tissue eosinophilia, suggesting an independent pathway for eosinophilia in these disorders. Interleukin-3 mRNA expression was found in most but not all Hodgkin's disease cases with eosinophilia, and IL-5 expression was variable in Hodgkin's disease cases with eotaxin-1–associated eosinophilia.

Lymph nodes with nodular sclerosis show the heaviest infiltrate of eosinophils and the most pronounced extracellular depositis of eosinophil basic protein (154). Extracellular eosinophil peroxidase has been detected in a dendritic pattern in nodular sclerosis, suggesting that extensive eosinophil degranulation commonly occurs and may produce tissue damage that results in collagen bands and sclerosis (155). Sclerosis also may be associated with eosinophil secretion of TGF-β1, a product of activated eosinophils (14,35; see below).

Collagen Sclerosis

Bands of collagen surrounding and separating abnormal lymphoid nodules and surrounding blood vessels are characteristic of nodular sclerosis Hodgkin's disease, the most common histologic type of Hodgkin's disease (156). The mechanism for development of nodular sclerosis has become a subject of considerable interest. Newcom first showed that supernatants of cell cultures from nodular sclerosis potentiate the growth of fibroblasts *in vitro* (157). Ford and co-workers also found fibroblast-activating activity in Hodgkin's disease cell culture supernatants and attributed at least part of this activity to IL-1 (158). A subsequent study supported the production of IL-1-like activity constitutively in Hodgkin's disease–derived cell lines (159). Kretschmer suggested that TNF-α, detected in Hodgkin's disease cell lines and biopsy tissues, contributes to fibroblast growth in Hodgkin's disease (141, 160). However, the growth factor most consistently associated with nodular sclerosis has been transforming growth factor-β (TGF-β). TGF-β is known to stimulate fibroblast proliferation and collagen synthesis both *in vitro* and *in vivo* (161,162). Newcom characterized a high-molecular-weight transforming growth factor-β, active at physiologic pH, in supernants from the L-428 cell line derived from advanced nodular sclerosis (34). Kadin et al. confirmed the presence of activated TGF-β immunohistochemically in nodular sclerosis Hodgkin's disease (163). In Hodgkin's disease showing nodular sclerosis, TGF-β activity was associated with the extracellular matrix mainly around blood vessels, zones of necrosis, at the margins of bands of collagen sclerosis, and in areas containing syncytia of Hodgkin–Reed-Sternberg cells. The presence of activated TGF-β *in situ* on the cell membrane and within the cytoplasm of Hodgkin–Reed-Sternberg cells from patients with nodular sclerosis suggests that these Hodgkin–Reed-Sternberg-cells are secreting activated TGF-β continuously. *In situ* hybridization indicated that TGF-β mRNA can be localized to Hodgkin–Reed-Sternberg cells (164) and eosinophils (35), which are known to make TGF-β (14).

It is quite possible that TGF-β interacts with other cytokines, particularly basic fibroblast growth factor (bFGF) in causing the fibrosis in Hodgkin's disease. In a murine model of cutaneous fibrosis, simultaneous application of TGF-β and bFGF causes persistent fibrosis (165). Ohshima and co-workers recently demonstrated the presence of bFGF by immunohistochemistry and *in situ* hybridization in Hodgkin–Reed-Sternberg cells, histiocytes and stromal cells in nodular sclerosis Hodgkin's disease (166). Thus, both TGF-β and bFGF appear to contribute to the induction of collagen sclerosis in Hodgkin's disease.

In summary, various cytokines (IL-4, IL-5, eotaxin, IL-6, IL-7, TNF, lymphotoxin, TGF-β, and basic fibroblast growth factor) have been found in different histologic subtypes of Hodgkin's disease and appear to account for the distinctive histopathologic features of Hodgkin's disease, such as eosinophilia and collagen sclerosis.

Effects of Cytokines on the Clinical Manifestations of Hodgkin's Disease

B Symptoms

Hodgkin's disease patients often suffer from fever, weight loss, and night sweats, known as B symptoms. Ree found that fever was not associated specifically with inflammation or necrosis of tumors, and there was an absence of fever in most patients with nodular sclerosing Hodgkin's disease (167). The cause of B symptoms in Hodgkin's disease has been unknown, but there is good reason to suspect that certain cytokines are responsible.

Interleukin-1β, TNF-α, IFN-γ, and IL-6 are pyrogenic molecules that can also mediate inhibition of lipogenic enzymes and lead to development of anorexia and weight loss (168–174). Administration of these molecules to animals or humans can cause B symptoms. Thus, it was undertaken by several investigators to correlate B symptoms with detection of these molecules in patients with Hodgkin's disease.

Naumovski and co-workers derived a cell line, SUP-HD1, that produced IFN-γ mRNA and protein from the pleural effusion of a patient with nodular sclerosis Hodgkin's disease (175). They suggested that production of IFN-γ by the malignant cells might explain the clinical B symptoms of Hodgkin's disease. However, the patient from whom the cell line was developed lacked B symptoms despite advanced-stage disease.

Interleukin-1 was studied immunohistochemically in Hodgkin's disease biopsy specimens by Ree and co-workers, who found that Hodgkin–Reed-Sternberg cells, small to medium-sized cells of uncertain origin, and granulocytes often stained for IL-1. However, immunoreactivity for IL-1 could not be correlated with presence or absence of B symptoms in these Hodgkin's disease patients (176).

Ruco and co-workers detected IL-1α in macrophages, interdigitating reticulum cells, endothelial cells, and neoplastic cells in Hodgkin's disease (177). Cells positive for IL-1β were much fewer and consisted mainly of macrophages. Hodgkin–Reed-Sternberg cells were negative for

IL-1β, even after *in vitro* stimulation with bacterial endotoxin. TNF-α was present in macrophages and Hodgkin–Reed-Sternberg cells. Xerri and co-workers confirmed the presence of IL-1α and TNF-α mRNAs in Hodgkin–Reed-Sternberg cells but did not find a correlation with histologic type or clinical stage of Hodgkin's disease (142).

Hsu and co-workers extended the study of IL-1 to Hodgkin's disease cell lines in which they found heterogeneity of IL-1 production (178). Interleukin-1α was the major IL-1 secreted by HDLM-1 cells, and IL-1β the major cytokine secreted by KM-H2 cells. Sappino and co-workers found high levels of IL-1β mRNA in six of 23 Hodgkin's disease lymph nodes. They found very low amounts of TNF-α mRNA but elevated amounts of lymphotoxin mRNA in Northern blots from Hodgkin's tumors. The highest levels of lymphotoxin mRNA were found in lymphocyte predominance Hodgkin's disease and high grade non-Hodgkin's lymphomas (168). Although all nine samples from patients with systemic symptoms were associated with lymphotoxin mRNA expression, and three of nine were associated with IL-1β mRNA, no significant correlation was observed between lymphotoxin and or IL-1β gene expression and the presence of B symptoms.

Perfetti and co-workers found that IL-1β was increased about two to ten times in five of eight lymph nodes from Hodgkin's disease patients with B symptoms, whereas other cytokines (IL-1α, TNF-α, TNF-β, and IL-6) were expressed heterogeneously in both symptomatic and asymptomatic patients. Statistical analysis demonstrated that the difference in IL-1β expression between symptomatic and asymptomatic patients was significant ($p<.02$) (174).

Other workers have tried to correlate B symptoms with serum cytokine levels of patients with Hodgkin's disease. Gause and co-workers found elevated levels of GM-CSF (22/56, 39%), IL-3 (5/40, 13%), and IL-6 (32/56, 57%) in sera of Hodgkin's disease patients. TNF-α and IL-1β were detected in only 3/43 (7%), and G-CSF not at all. All patients with measurable IL-3 had both elevated IL-6 and GM-CSF levels, and most patients with elevated IL-6 also had elevated GM-CSF. Cytokine levels were independent of stage and B symptoms.

Kurzock et al. investigated serum levels of IL-1β, IFN-γ, TNF-α, and IL-6 in 28 Hodgkin's disease patients and 32 NHL patients with and without B symptoms as well as 20 normal volunteers (173). B symptoms were only infrequently associated with elevated levels of TNF-α and IL-1β, and IFN-γ was not elevated in sera of lymphoma patients (173). In contrast, measurable serum IL-6 (median level 28.9 pg/ml) was detected in 20 of 57 lymphoma patients (35%) and 17 of 29 patients (59%) with one or more B symptoms. There was no statistically significant difference between IL-6 levels in normal volunteers as compared with lymphoma patients without B symptoms. Nine of 15 (60%) Hodgkin's disease patients with B symptoms had detectable IL-6 levels versus only one of 11 without B symptoms ($p<.01$, X^2 test). The median survival of Hodgkin's disease patients with IL-6 levels over 22 pg/ml was 10 months, whereas the median survival of those with lower levels was not reached at median follow-up of 37.5 months (Wilcoxon p value .0012). Thus, it appears that elevated serum IL-6 was the cytokine best correlated with B symptoms in Hodgkin's disease. In this regard, it is puzzling that serum IL-6 levels are also elevated in plasma cell myeloma, where B symptoms such as fever are not a prominent feature (179). However, serum levels of IL-6 correlate with severity of disease in plasma cell dyscrasias (180).

At present, it is not clear which of several cytokine(s) (IL-1β, IFN-γ, TNF-α, lymphotoxin, and/or IL-6) are responsible for the B symptoms of patients with Hodgkin's disease, although the correlation of B symptoms is strongest with elevated serum levels of IL-6.

Immunosuppression

Most untreated patients with Hodgkin's disease, including those with limited-stage disease, have a defect in cell-mediated immunity (181–183). Defects in T-lymphocyte function include a depressed response to T-cell mitogens (183,184), decreased capacity of T lymphocytes to respond in an autologous or syngeneic mixed lymphocyte culture (185), and decreased *in vitro* synthesis of IL-2 and IFN-γ (186). Cytokines are thought to be responsible for impaired T-lymphocyte function in Hodgkin's disease. Among the cytokines described with potent immunomodulatory effects are TNF-α, lymphotoxin (TNF-β), IL-10, and TGF-β. TNF-α and lymphotoxin are active in the cyclooxygenase pathway and can potentiate prostaglandin synthesis (187). Enhanced prostaglandin-mediated suppressor activity by monocytes from Hodgkin's disease patients appears to contribute to depressed lymphocyte responses (188,189).

Interleukin-10 inhibits expression of interferon-γ and IL-2 by the T_H1 subset of T-helper cells and can directly inhibit T-cell growth (190). It also downregulates major histocompatibility complex class II molecules, causing reduced antigen-specific T-cell responses (191). Herbst and co-workers have shown frequent expression of IL-10 by EBV–harboring Hodgkin–Reed-Sternberg cells, which express LMP1 and suggested that upregulation of IL-10 by LMP1 may contribute to evasion of LMP1-positive Reed-Sternberg cells from cytotoxicity directed at EBV genes (192).

TGF-β suppresses the growth and differentiation of B and T lymphocytes (193,194), the cytolytic activity and interferon responsiveness of natural killer cells (195), and the proliferation and differentiation of precursors to natural killer cells (196). T lymphocytes of Hodgkin's disease patients have a defect in cytolytic function associated with downregulation of the T-cell receptor ζ-chain, possibly in response to TGF-β (197) (see below). Local TGF-β suppression of T-lymphocyte cytolytic activity in Hodgkin's disease lymph nodes may explain the findings of Frisan et al., who found an inverse correlation between the presence of EBV in Hodgkin–Reed-Sternberg cells and EBV-specific cytotoxic T lymphocytes in Hodgkin's disease lymph nodes while peripheral blood contained EBV specific cytotoxic T lymphocytes (198).

Potters et al. observed that the absence of effective T-lymphocyte activation in Hodgkin's disease may be the result of TGF-β production by Hodgkin–Reed-Sternberg cells (199). Supernatants from cultures of L-428 cells strongly inhibited CD3/CD28-induced activation of T lymphocytes, impairing their ability to undergo blastic transformation, to express CD25 activation antigen, or to produce IL-2 or IFN-γ. Depletion of TGF-β from L-428 culture supernatants abrogated T-lymphocyte inhibition, whereas removal of IL-10 had no effect. Thus, it appears more likely that L-428 cells inhibit T-lymphocyte activation through TGF-β production. The high-molecular-weight TGF-β isolated from L-428 cells is biologically active at physiogic pH and is almost completely destroyed by acidification, whereas native TGF-β occurs in a latent form that requires acidification to pH 2 or less for its activation (34). The high-molecular-weight TGF-β was detected in the urine of patients with active nodular sclerosis Hodgkin's disease but cleared from the urine of these patients following successful treatment (200). Both clinical and experimental evidence support a major role for TGF-β in the immune suppression of Hodgkin's disease, although IL-10 may also contribute to this important clinical feature.

Serum Levels of CD30 and IL-2R and Their Clinical Significance

The CD30 molecule is a 120-kd surface moiety consistently expressed by Hodgkin–Reed-Sternberg cells (41). A soluble 88-kd form of CD30 (sCD30) is released by CD30$^+$ cells *in vitro* and *in vivo,* probably as a result of proteolytic cleavage of the membrane-bound CD30 (53). Serum levels of soluble CD30 (sCD30) are elevated in most untreated patients with Hodgkin's disease and correlate with clinical features and prognosis. Elevated sCD30 is detected only in patients with active Hodgkin's disease and was never found in control sera or in sera of patients in remission from Hodgkin's disease (30). Serum levels of sCD30 are increased in most patients with Hodgkin's disease at presentation and correlate with advanced disease, being higher in patients with advanced stage, bulky tumors, and B symptoms. Patients with sCD30 levels greater than 100 U/mL at diagnosis have a significantly worse event-free survival in multivariate analysis. Besides reflecting tumor burden, sCD30 can decrease the availability of CD30L on peripheral blood lymphocytes of patients with CD30$^+$ tumors. Younes and co-workers have shown that elevated sCD30 can block membrane-bound CD30L-mediated apoptosis of CD30$^+$ tumor cells and suggested that this may be a mechanism by which CD30$^+$ tumors can escape immune surveillance (201).

Pizzolo and co-workers found that serum levels of sIL-2R (CD25) correlate significantly with severity of Hodgkin's disease and are significantly higher in patients with B symptoms (202). Patients with clinical stage IVB have the highest levels of sIL-2R (202–204). Low pretreatment sCD25 levels are associated with a favorable prognosis (203). However, sCD25 levels appear to have more value for prognosis than for measure of disease activity. Levels of sIL-2R may decrease in Hodgkin's disease patients even after progression of disease and are subject to modification by intercurrent infections and other tumor-unrelated causes, suggesting that sCD25 is released mostly from reactive cells instead of Hodgkin–Reed-Sternberg cells.

Cytokine Receptors and Their Potential Use as Targets for Immunotherapy

CD25 and CD30 can also serve as targets for immunotherapy of Hodgkin's disease. Falini and co-workers have shown a rapid and substantial reduction in Hodgkin's disease tumor mass (50–75%) in three of four patients with advanced refractory Hodgkin's disease when treated with an immunotoxin prepared by covalent linking of an anti-CD30 monoclonal antibody (Ber-H2) to saporin (S06), a type-1 ribosome-inactivating protein (31). Immunohistologic analysis showed that the Ber-H2 antibody specifically and strongly labeled Hodgkin–Reed-Sternberg cells, including those that were not imaged by immunoscintigraphy (32). Because there is no specific toxicity of the Ber-H2 immunotoxin to CD34$^+$ bone marrow precursors, this immunotoxin is also useful for *ex vivo* purging of bone marrow in Hodgkin's disease and CD30$^+$ lymphomas (205).

CD30 antigen also has been used as one of the targets for bispecific monoclonal antibodies in immunotherapy. Bispecific monoclonal antibodies directed against CD30 and the T-cell–triggering molecules CD3 and CD28, respectively, together with human T cells prestimulated *in vitro* with bispecific monoclonal antibodies in the presence of CD30$^+$ cells, could be used to cure mice of disseminated xenografted human Hodgkin's disease tumors (206). Applying this principle, Hartmann and co-workers treated 15 patients with refractory Hodgkin's disease in a phase I/II trial with a natural killer cell–activating bispecific monoclonal antibody directed against the Fcg-receptor II (CD16 antigen) and the CD30 antigen (207). The treatment was well tolerated, and side effects were rare, consisting of fever, pain in involved lymph nodes, and a maculopapular rash. A total of one complete and one partial remission, three minor responses, and one mixed response was achieved.

CD25 has also been used as a target for novel immunotherapies. Tepler and co-workers obtained a complete remission in a patient with refractory Hodgkin's disease treated with an IL-2 diphtheria fusion toxin in a phase I trial (208). Engert and co-workers conducted a phase I study of an anti-CD25 ricin A-chain immunotoxin in patients with refractory Hodgkin's disease (33). Two patients obtained partial remissions, one had a minor response, three had stable disease, and nine had progression of their Hodgkin's disease. Unlike CD30, which is expressed on virtually all Hodgkin–Reed-Sternberg cells, the variable expression of CD25 by Hodgkin–Reed-Sternberg cells may permit some tumor cells to escape the effects of immunotherapies directed against this molecule (25).

SUMMARY AND CONCLUSIONS

Hodgkin's disease is a tumor of cytokine-producing and cytokine-responding cells. Hodgkin's disease tumor cells express high levels of CD30 and CD40, members of the TNF receptor superfamily. Through adapter TRAF molecules, CD30, CD40, or EBV LMP1 can activate NF-κB and *c-Jun* N-terminal kinase (JNK) pathways, which may affect Hodgkin–Reed-Sternberg cell proliferation, apoptosis, expression of adhesion molecules and secretion of cytokines. The coexpression of multiple members of the TNF receptor superfamily, which all share components of the same signaling pathways, suggests that receptor cross-talk may be an important element in determining the phenotype of the Hodgkin–Reed-Sternberg cell and the microenvironment of Hodgkin's disease. Evidence for such receptor cross-talk exists for other EBV-positive malignancies, which express EBV LMP1, CD40, and CD30, such as AIDS-related lymphoma and post-transplant lymphoproliferative disease. It remains to be formally demonstrated whether these same pathways are utilized in Hodgkin's disease.

Different quantities of cytokines (IL-4, IL-5, eotaxin, IL-6, IL-7, TNF, lymphotoxin, TGF-β, and basic fibroblast growth factor) have been found in different histologic subtypes of Hodgkin's disease and appear to account for the distinctive histopathologic features of Hodgkin's disease, such as eosinophilia and collagen sclerosis. Adhesion molecules modulated by cytokines affect the interaction of Hodgkin–Reed-Sternberg cells with surrounding T lymphocytes and probably affect the spread of Hodgkin's disease. Systemic (B) symptoms of Hodgkin's disease are best correlated with elevated serum levels of IL-6. The immunosuppression characteristic of untreated patients with Hodgkin's disease has been associated with a unique high-molecular-weight form of TGF-β. High serum levels of CD30 and CD25 are correlated with advanced stage, B symptoms, and poor prognosis. The unusual expression of CD30 and CD25 on Hodgkin's disease tumor cells has been used to devise novel immunotherapies that bring tumor cells together with lethal toxins or effector immune cells.

REFERENCES

1. Winkler U, Gottstein C, Schon G, et al. Successful treatment of disseminated human Hodgkin's disease in SCID mice with deglycosylated ricin A-chain immunotoxins. *Blood* 1994;83:466–475.
2. Drexler HG. Recent results on the biology of Hodgkin and Reed-Sternberg cells. II. Continuous cell lines. *Leuk Lymphoma* 1993; 9:1–25.
3. Carbone A, Gloghini A, Gattei V, et al. Expression of functional CD40 antigen on Reed-Sternberg cells and Hodgkin's disease cell lines. *Blood* 1995;85:780–789.
4. Newcom SR, Ansari AA, Gu L. Interleukin-4 is an autocrine growth factor secreted by the L-428 Reed-Sternberg cell. *Blood* 1992;79: 191–197.
5. Jucker M, Abts H, Li W, et al. Expression of interleukin-6 and interleukin-6 receptor in Hodgkin's disease. *Blood* 1991;77:2413–2418.
6. Tesch H, Jucker M, Klein S, et al. Hodgkin and Reed-Sternberg cells express interleukin 6 and interleukin 6 receptors. *Leuk Lymphoma* 1992;7:297–303.
7. Foss HD, Herbst H, Oelmann E, et al. Lymphotoxin, tumour necrosis factor and interleukin-6 gene transcripts are present in Hodgkin and Reed-Sternberg cells of most Hodgkin's disease cases. *Br J Haematol* 1993;84:627–635.
8. Merz H, Houssiau FA, Orscheschek K, et al. Interleukin-9 expression in human malignant lymphomas: unique association with Hodgkin's disease and large cell anaplastic lymphoma. *Blood* 1991;78: 1311–1317.
9. Klein S, Jucker M, Diehl V, Tesch H. Production of multiple cytokines by Hodgkin's disease derived cell lines. *Hematol Oncol* 1992;10: 319–329.
10. Gruss HJ, Ulrich D, Braddy S, Armitage RJ, Dower SK. Recombinant CD30 ligand and CD40 ligand share common biological activities on Hodgkin and Reed-Sternberg cells. *Eur J Immunol* 1995;25: 2083–2089.
11. Gruss HJ, Pinto A, Gloghini A, et al. CD30 ligand expression in nonmalignant and Hodgkin's disease-involved lymphoid tissues. *Am J Pathol* 1996;149:469–481.
12. Samoszuk M, Nansen L. Detection of interleukin-5 messenger RNA in Reed-Sternberg cells of Hodgkin's disease with eosinophilia. *Blood* 1990;75:13–16.
13. Pinto A, Aldinucci D, Gloghini A, et al. Human eosinophils express functional CD30 ligand and stimulate proliferation of a Hodgkin's disease cell line. *Blood* 1996;88:3299–3305.
14. Wong DT, Elovic A, Matossian K, et al. Eosinophils from patients with blood eosinophilia express transforming growth factor beta 1. *Blood* 1991;78:2702–2707.
15. Kadin ME, Newcom SR, Gold SB, Stites DP. Origin of Hodgkin's cell. *Lancet* 1974;2:167.
16. Stuart AE, Williams AR, Habeshaw JA. Rosetting and other reactions of the Reed-Sternberg cell. *J Pathol* 1977;122:81.
17. Roers A, Montesinos-Rongen M, Hansmann ML, Rajewsky K, Kuppers R. T cells rosetting around Hodgkin and Reed-Sternberg cells in Hodgkin's disease are polyclonal. *Leuk Lymphoma* 1998;29(suppl 1): P-20.
18. Sanders ME, Makgoba MW, Sussman EH, Luce GE, Cossman J, Shaw S. Molecular pathways of adhesion in spontaneous rosetting of T-lymphocytes to the Hodgkin's cell line L428 [see comments]. *Cancer Res* 1988;48:37–40.
19. Paietta E, Stockert RJ, McManus M, Thompson D, Schmidt S, Wiernik PH. Hodgkin's cell lectin, a lymphocyte adhesion molecule and mitogen. *J Immunol* 1989;143:2850–2857.
20. Springer TA. Traffic signals for lymphocyte recirculation and leukocyte emigration: the multistep paradigm. *Cell* 1994;76:301–314.
21. Pizzolo G, Vinante F, Nadalli G, et al. ICAM-1 tissue overexpression associated with increased serum levels of its soluble form in Hodgkin's disease. *Br J Haematol* 1993;84:161–162.
22. Strauchen JA, Breakstone BA. IL-2 receptor expression in human lymphoid lesions. Immunohistochemical study of 166 cases. *Am J Pathol* 1987;126:506–512.

23. Sheibani K, Winberg CD, van de Velde S, Blayney DW, Rappaport H. Distribution of lymphocytes with interleukin-2 receptors (TAC antigens) in reactive lymphoproliferative processes, Hodgkin's disease, and non-Hodgkin's lymphomas. An immunohistologic study of 300 cases. *Am J Pathol* 1987;127:27–37.
24. Agnarsson BA, Kadin ME. The immunophenotype of Reed-Sternberg cells. A study of 50 cases of Hodgkin's disease using fixed frozen tissues. *Cancer* 1989;63:2083–2087.
25. Levi E, Butmarc J, Kourea HP, Kadin ME. Detection of interleukin-2 receptors on tumor cells in formalin-fixed, paraffin-embedded tissues. *Appl Immunohistochem* 1997;5:234–238.
26. Durkop H, Latza U, Hummel M, Eitelbach F, Seed B, Stein H. Molecular cloning and expression of a new member of the nerve growth factor receptor family that is characteristic for Hodgkin's disease. *Cell* 1992;68:421–427.
27. O'Grady JT, Stewart S, Lowrey J, Howie SE, Krajewski AS. CD40 expression in Hodgkin's disease [see comments]. *Am J Pathol* 1994; 144:21–26.
28. Gruss HJ, Hirschstein D, Wright B, et al. Expression and function of CD40 on Hodgkin and Reed-Sternberg cells and the possible relevance for Hodgkin's disease. *Blood* 1994;84:2305–2314.
29. Newcom SR, Kadin ME, Ansari AA. Production of transforming growth factor-beta activity by Ki-1 positive lymphoma cells and analysis of its role in the regulation of Ki-1 positive lymphoma growth. *Am J Pathol* 1988;131:569–577.
30. Nadali G, Vinante F, Ambrosetti A, et al. Serum levels of soluble CD30 are elevated in the majority of untreated patients with Hodgkin's disease and correlate with clinical features and prognosis. *J Clin Oncol* 1994;12:793–797.
31. Falini B, Bolognesi A, Flenghi L, et al. Response of refractory Hodgkin's disease to monoclonal anti-CD30 immunotoxin. *Lancet* 1992;339:1195–1196.
32. Falini B, Flenghi L, Fedeli L, et al. *In vivo* targeting of Hodgkin and Reed-Sternberg cells of Hodgkin's disease with monoclonal antibody Ber-H2 (CD30): immunohistological evidence. *Br J Haematol* 1992; 82:38–45.
33. Engert A, Diehl V, Schnell R, et al. A phase-I study of an anti-CD25 ricin A-chain immunotoxin (RFT5-SMPT-dgA) in patients with refractory Hodgkin's lymphoma. *Blood* 1997;89:403–410.
34. Newcom SR, Kadin ME, Ansari AA, Diehl V. L-428 nodular sclerosing Hodgkin's cell secretes a unique transforming growth factor-beta active at physiologic pH. *J Clin Invest* 1988;82:1915–1921.
35. Kadin M, Butmarc J, Elovic A, Wong D. Eosinophils are the major source of transforming growth factor-beta 1 in nodular sclerosing Hodgkin's disease. *Am J Pathol* 1993;142:11–16.
36. Chott A, Vonderheid EC, Olbricht S, Miao NN, Balk SP, Kadin ME. The dominant T cell clone is present in multiple regressing skin lesions and associated T cell lymphomas of patients with lymphomatoid papulosis. *J Invest Dermatol* 1996;106:696–700.
37. Smith CA, Farrah T, Goodwin RG. The TNF receptor superfamily of cellular and viral proteins: activation, costimulation, and death. *Cell* 1994;76:959–962.
38. Banchereau J, Bazan F, Blanchard D, et al. The CD40 antigen and its ligand. *Annu Rev Immunol* 1994;12:881–922.
39. Armitage RJ. Tumor necrosis factor receptor superfamily members and their ligands. *Curr Opin Immunol* 1994;6:407–413.
40. Gruss HJ, Dower SK. Tumor necrosis factor ligand superfamily: involvement in the pathology of malignant lymphomas. *Blood* 1995; 85:3378–3404.
41. Schwab U, Stein H, Gerdes J, et al. Production of a monoclonal antibody specific for Hodgkin and Sternberg-Reed cells of Hodgkin's disease and a subset of normal lymphoid cells. *Nature* 1982;299:65–67.
42. Stein H, Mason DY, Gerdes J, et al. The expression of the Hodgkin's disease associated antigen Ki-1 in reactive and neoplastic lymphoid tissue: evidence that Reed-Sternberg cells and histiocytic malignancies are derived from activated lymphoid cells. *Blood* 1985;66:848–858.
43. Schwarting R, Gerdes J, Durkop H, Falini B, Pileri S, Stein H. BER-H2: a new anti-Ki-1 (CD30) monoclonal antibody directed at a formol-resistant epitope. *Blood* 1989;74:1678–1689.
44. Ellis TM, Simms PE, Slivnick DJ, Jack HM, Fisher RI. CD30 is a signal-transducing molecule that defines a subset of human activated CD45RO[+] T cells. *J Immunol* 1993;151:2380–2389.
45. Andreesen R, Osterholz J, Lohr GW, Bross KJ. A Hodgkin cell-specific antigen is expressed on a subset of auto- and alloactivated T (helper) lymphoblasts. *Blood* 1984;63:1299–1302.
46. Drexler HG, Leber BF, Norton J, et al. Genotypes and immunophenotypes of Hodgkin's disease-derived cell lines. *Leukemia* 1988;2: 371–376.
47. Drexler HG, Minowada J. Hodgkin's disease derived cell lines: a review. *Hum Cell* 1992;5:42–53.
48. Herbst H, Stein H, Niedobitek G. Epstein-Barr virus and CD30[+] malignant lymphomas. *Crit Rev Oncog* 1993;4:191–239.
49. Gruss HJ, Boiani N, Williams DE, Armitage RJ, Smith CA, Goodwin RG. Pleiotropic effects of the CD30 ligand on CD30-expressing cells and lymphoma cell lines. *Blood* 1994;83:2045–2056.
50. Drexler HG. Recent results on the biology of Hodgkin and Reed-Sternberg cells. I. Biopsy material. *Leuk Lymphoma* 1992;8:283–313.
51. Miettinen M. CD30 distribution. Immunohistochemical study on formaldehyde-fixed, paraffin-embedded Hodgkin's and non-Hodgkin's lymphomas. *Arch Pathol Lab Med* 1992;116:1197–1201.
52. Pallesen G. The diagnostic significance of the CD30 (Ki-1) antigen [see comments]. *Histopathology* 1990;16:409–413.
53. Josimovic Alasevic O, Durkop H, Schwarting R, Backe E, Stein H, Diamantstein T. Ki-1 (CD30) antigen is released by Ki-1-positive tumor cells *in vitro* and *in vivo*. I. Partial characterization of soluble Ki-1 antigen and detection of the antigen in cell culture supernatants and in serum by an enzyme-linked immunosorbent assay. *Eur J Immunol* 1989;19:157–162.
54. Pfreundschuh M, Pohl C, Berenbeck C, et al. Detection of a soluble form of the CD30 antigen in sera of patients with lymphoma, adult T-cell leukemia and infectious mononucleosis. *Int J Cancer* 1990;45: 869–874.
55. Pizzolo G, Vinante F, Chilosi M, et al. Serum levels of soluble CD30 molecule (Ki-1 antigen) in Hodgkin's disease: relationship with disease activity and clinical stage. *Br J Haematol* 1990;75:282–284.
56. Gause A, Pohl C, Tschiersch A, et al. Clinical significance of soluble CD30 antigen in the sera of patients with untreated Hodgkin's disease. *Blood* 1991;77:1983–1988.
57. Gruss HJ, Duyster J, Herrmann F. Structural and biological features of the TNF receptor and TNF ligand superfamilies: interactive signals in the pathobiology of Hodgkin's disease. *Ann Oncol* 1996;4:19–26.
58. Herbst H, Dallenbach F, Hummel M, et al. Epstein-Barr virus latent membrane protein expression in Hodgkin and Reed-Sternberg cells. *Proc Natl Acad Sci USA* 1991;88:4766–4770.
59. Pallesen G, Hamilton Dutoit SJ, Rowe M, Young LS. Expression of Epstein-Barr virus latent gene products in tumour cells of Hodgkin's disease [see comments]. *Lancet* 1991;337:320–322.
60. Mosialos G, Birkenbach M, Yalamanchili R, VanArsdale T, Ware C, Kieff E. The Epstein-Barr virus transforming protein LMP1 engages signaling proteins for the tumor necrosis factor receptor family. *Cell* 1995;80:389–399.
61. Devergne O, Hatzivassiliou E, Izumi KM, et al. Association of TRAF1, TRAF2, and TRAF3 with an Epstein-Barr virus LMP1 domain important for B-lymphocyte transformation: role in NF-κB activation. *Mol Cell Biol* 1996;16:7098–7108.
62. Kaye KM, Devergne O, Harada JN, et al. Tumor necrosis factor receptor associated factor 2 is a mediator of NF-κB activation by latent infection membrane protein 1, the Epstein-Barr virus transforming protein. *Proc Natl Acad Sci USA* 1996;93:11085–11090.
63. Izumi KM, Kaye KM, Kieff ED. The Epstein-Barr virus LMP1 amino acid sequence that engages tumor necrosis factor receptor associated factors is critical for primary B lymphocyte growth transformation. *Proc Natl Acad Sci USA* 1997;94:1447–1452.
64. Liebowitz D. Epstein-Barr virus and a cellular signaling pathway in lymphomas from immunosuppressed patients. *N Engl J Med* 1998; 338:1413–1421.
65. Hu HM, O'Rourke K, Boguski MS, Dixit VM. A novel RING finger protein interacts with the cytoplasmic domain of CD40. *J Biol Chem* 1994;269:30069–30072.
66. Rothe M, Wong SC, Henzel WJ, Goeddel DV. A novel family of putative signal transducers associated with the cytoplasmic domain of the 75 kDa tumor necrosis factor receptor. *Cell* 1994;78:681–692.
67. Rothe M, Sarma V, Dixit VM, Goeddel DV. TRAF2-mediated activation of NF-κB by TNF receptor 2 and CD40. *Science* 1995;269:1424–1427.
68. Cheng G, Cleary AM, Ye ZS, Hong DI, Lederman S, Baltimore D. Involvement of CRAF1, a relative of TRAF, in CD40 signaling. *Science* 1995;267:1494–1498.
69. Regnier CH, Tomasetto C, Moog Lutz C, et al. Presence of a new conserved domain in CART1, a novel member of the tumor necrosis fac-

tor receptor-associated protein family, which is expressed in breast carcinoma. *J Biol Chem* 1995;270:25715–25721.
70. Cao Z, Xiong J, Takeuchi M, Kurama T, Goeddel DV. TRAF6 is a signal transducer for interleukin-1. *Nature* 1996;383:443–446.
71. Ishida T, Mizushima S, Azuma S, et al. Identification of TRAF6, a novel tumor necrosis factor receptor-associated factor protein that mediates signaling from an amino-terminal domain of the CD40 cytoplasmic region. *J Biol Chem* 1996;271:28745–28748.
72. Ishida TK, Tojo T, Aoki T, et al. TRAF5, a novel tumor necrosis factor receptor-associated factor family protein, mediates CD40 signaling. *Proc Natl Acad Sci USA* 1996;93:9437–9442.
73. Nakano H, Oshima H, Chung W, et al. TRAF5, an activator of NF-κB and putative signal transducer for the lymphotoxin-beta receptor. *J Biol Chem* 1996;271:14661–14664.
74. Takeuchi M, Rothe M, Goeddel DV. Anatomy of TRAF2. Distinct domains for nuclear factor-κB activation and association with tumor necrosis factor signaling proteins. *J Biol Chem* 1996;271: 19935–19942.
75. Sato T, Irie S, Reed JC. A novel member of the TRAF family of putative signal transducing proteins binds to the cytosolic domain of CD40. *FEBS Lett* 1995;358:113–118.
76. Song HY, Donner DB. Association of a RING finger protein with the cytoplasmic domain of the human type-2 tumour necrosis factor receptor. *Biochem J* 1995;309:825–829.
77. Baker SJ, Reddy EP. Transducers of life and death: TNF receptor superfamily and associated proteins. *Oncogene* 1996;12:1–9.
78. Hsu H, Shu HB, Pan MG, Goeddel DV. TRADD–TRAF2 and TRADD–FADD interactions define two distinct TNF receptor 1 signal transduction pathways. *Cell* 1996;84:299–308.
79. Rothe M, Pan MG, Henzel WJ, Ayres TM, Goeddel DV. The TNFR2–TRAF signaling complex contains two novel proteins related to baculoviral inhibitor of apoptosis proteins. *Cell* 1995;83: 1243–1252.
80. Song HY, Rothe M, Goeddel DV. The tumor necrosis factor-inducible zinc finger protein A20 interacts with TRAF1/TRAF2 and inhibits NF-κB activation. *Proc Natl Acad Sci USA* 1996;93:6721–6725.
81. Cheng G, Baltimore D. TANK, a co-inducer with TRAF2 of TNF- and CD 40L-mediated NF-κB activation. *Genes Dev* 1996;10:963–973.
82. Rothe M, Xiong J, Shu HB, Williamson K, Goddard A, Goeddel DV. I-TRAF is a novel TRAF-interacting protein that regulates TRAF-mediated signal transduction. *Proc Natl Acad Sci USA* 1996;93: 8241–8246.
83. Lee SY, Lee SY, Choi Y. TRAF-interacting protein (TRIP): a novel component of the tumor necrosis factor receptor (TNFR)- and CD30–TRAF signaling complexes that inhibits TRAF2-mediated NF-κB activation. *J Exp Med* 1997;185:1275–1285.
84. Siemienski K, Peters N, Scheurich P, Wajant H. Organization of the human tumour necrosis factor receptor-associated factor 1 (TRAF1) gene and mapping to chromosome 9q33-34. *Gene* 1997;195:35–39.
85. Liu ZG, Hsu H, Goeddel DV, Karin M. Dissection of TNF receptor 1 effector functions: JNK activation is not linked to apoptosis while NF-κB activation prevents cell death. *Cell* 1996;87:565–576.
86. Natoli G, Costanzo A, Ianni A, et al. Activation of SAPK/JNK by TNF receptor 1 through a noncytotoxic TRAF2-dependent pathway. *Science* 1997;275:200–203.
87. Reinhard C, Shamoon B, Shyamala V, Williams LT. Tumor necrosis factor alpha–induced activation of *c-jun* N-terminal kinase is mediated by TRAF2. *EMBO J* 1997;16:1080–1092.
88. Song HY, Regnier CH, Kirschning CJ, Goeddel DV, Rothe M. Tumor necrosis factor (TNF)-mediated kinase cascades: bifurcation of nuclear factor-κB and *c-jun* N-terminal kinase (JNK/SAPK) pathways at TNF receptor-associated factor 2. *Proc Natl Acad Sci USA* 1997;94: 9792–9796.
89. Ansieau S, Scheffrahn I, Mosialos G, et al. Tumor necrosis factor receptor-associated factor (TRAF)-1, TRAF-2, and TRAF-3 interact *in vivo* with the CD30 cytoplasmic domain; TRAF-2 mediates CD30-induced nuclear factor κ B activation. *Proc Natl Acad Sci USA* 1996;93:14053–14058.
90. Gedrich RW, Gilfillan MC, Duckett CS, Van Dongen JL, Thompson CB. CD30 contains two binding sites with different specificities for members of the tumor necrosis factor receptor-associated factor family of signal transducing proteins. *J Biol Chem* 1996;271:12852–12858.
91. Lee SY, Lee SY, Kandala G, Liou ML, Liou HC, Choi Y. CD30/TNF receptor-associated factor interaction: NF-κB activation and binding specificity. *Proc Natl Acad Sci USA* 1996;93:9699–9703.
92. Aizawa S, Nakano H, Ishida T, et al. Tumor necrosis factor receptor-associated factor (TRAF) 5 and TRAF2 are involved in CD30-mediated NFκB activation. *J Biol Chem* 1997;272:2042–2045.
93. Duckett CS, Gedrich RW, Gilfillan MC, Thompson CB. Induction of nuclear factor κB by the CD30 receptor is mediated by TRAF1 and TRAF2. *Mol Cell Biol* 1997;17:1535–1542.
94. Tsitsikov EN, Wright DA, Geha RS. CD30 induction of human immunodeficiency virus gene transcription is mediated by TRAF2. *Proc Natl Acad Sci USA* 1997;94:1390–1395.
95. Brodeur SR, Cheng G, Baltimore D, Thorley Lawson DA. Localization of the major NF-κB-activating site and the sole TRAF3 binding site of LMP-1 defines two distinct signaling motifs. *J Biol Chem* 1997;272:19777–19784.
96. Sandberg M, Hammerschmidt W, Sugden B. Characterization of LMP-1's association with TRAF1, TRAF2, and TRAF3. *J Virol* 1997; 71:4649–4656.
97. Hsu H, Solovyev I, Colombero A, Elliott R, Kelley M, Boyle WJ. ATAR, a novel tumor necrosis factor receptor family member, signals through TRAF2 and TRAF5. *J Biol Chem* 1997;272:13471–13474.
98. Marsters SA, Ayres TM, Skubatch M, Gray CL, Rothe M, Ashkenazi A. Herpesvirus entry mediator, a member of the tumor necrosis factor receptor (TNFR) family, interacts with members of the TNFR-associated factor family and activates the transcription factors NF-κB and AP-1. *J Biol Chem* 1997;272:14029–14032.
99. Malinin NL, Boldin MP, Kovalenko AV, Wallach D. MAP3K-related kinase involved in NF-κB induction by TNF, CD95 and IL-1. *Nature* 1997;385:540–544.
100. Regnier CH, Song HY, Gao X, Goeddel DV, Cao Z, Rothe M. Identification and characterization of an IκB kinase. *Cell* 1997;90:373–383.
101. Woronicz JD, Gao X, Cao Z, Rothe M, Goeddel DV. IκB kinase-beta: NF-κB activation and complex formation with IκB kinase-alpha and NIK [see comments]. *Science* 1997;278:866–869.
102. DiDonato JA, Hayakawa M, Rothwarf DM, Zandi E, Karin M. A cytokine-responsive IκB kinase that activates the transcription factor NF-κB [see comments]. *Nature* 1997;388:548–554.
103. Zandi E, Rothwarf DM, Delhase M, Hayakawa M, Karin M. The IκB kinase complex (IKK) contains two kinase subunits, IKKαlpha and IKKβeta, necessary for IκB phosphorylation and NF-κB activation. *Cell* 1997;91:243–252.
104. Mercurio F, Zhu H, Murray BW, et al. IKK-1 and IKK-2: cytokine-activated IκB kinases essential for NF-κB activation [see comments]. *Science* 1997;278:860–866.
105. Baldwin AS Jr. The NF-κB and I κB proteins: new discoveries and insights. *Annu Rev Immunol* 1996;14:649–683.
106. Bargou RC, Emmerich F, Krappmann D, et al. Constitutive nuclear factor-κB-RelA activation is required for proliferation and survival of Hodgkin's disease tumor cells. *J Clin Invest* 1997;100:2961–2969.
107. Lee FS, Hagler J, Chen ZJ, Maniatis T. Activation of the IκB alpha kinase complex by MEKK1, a kinase of the JNK pathway. *Cell* 1997; 88:213–222.
108. Yeh W-C, Shahinian A, Speiser D, et al. Early lethality, Functional NF-κB activation, and increased sensitivity to TNF-induced cell death in TRAF2-deficient mice. *Immunity* 1997;7:715–725.
109. Lee SY, Reichlin A, Santana A, Sokol KA, Nussenzweig MC, Choi Y. TRAF2 is essential for JNK but not NF-κB activation and regulates lymphocyte proliferation and survival. *Immunity* 1991;7:703–713.
110. Xu Y, Cheng G, Baltimore D. Targeted disruption of TRAF3 leads to postnatal lethality and defective T-dependent immune responses. *Immunity* 1996;5:407–415.
111. Smith CA, Gruss HJ, Davis T, et al. CD30 antigen, a marker for Hodgkin's lymphoma, is a receptor whose ligand defines an emerging family of cytokines with homology to TNF. *Cell* 1993;73:1349–1360.
112. Stamenkovic I, Clark EA, Seed B. A B-lymphocyte activation molecule related to the nerve growth factor receptor and induced by cytokines in carcinomas. *EMBO J* 1989;8:1403–1410.
113. Law CL, Wormann B, LeBien TW. Analysis of expression and function of CD40 on normal and leukemic human B cell precursors. *Leukemia* 1990;4:732–738.
114. Lane P, Traunecker A, Hubele S, Inui S, Lanzavecchia A, Gray D. Activated human T cells express a ligand for the human B cell-associated antigen CD40 which participates in T cell-dependent activation of B lymphocytes. *Eur J Immunol* 1992;22:2573–2578.
115. Gauchat JF, Henchoz S, Mazzei G, et al. Induction of human IgE synthesis in B cells by mast cells and basophils. *Nature* 1993;365: 340–343.

116. Banchereau J, de Paoli P, Valle A, Garcia E, Rousset F. Long-term human B cell lines dependent on interleukin-4 and antibody to CD40. *Science* 1991;251:70–72.
117. Liu YJ, Mason DY, Johnson GD, et al. Germinal center cells express *bcl-2* protein after activation by signals which prevent their entry into apoptosis. *Eur J Immunol* 1991;21:1905–1910.
118. Spriggs MK, Armitage RJ, Strockbine L, et al. Recombinant human CD40 ligand stimulates B cell proliferation and immunoglobulin E secretion. *J Exp Med* 1992;176:1543–1550.
119. Saeland S, Duvert V, Moreau I, Banchereau J. Human B cell precursors proliferate and express CD23 after CD40 ligation. *J Exp Med* 1993;178:113–120.
120. Armitage RJ, Macduff BM, Spriggs MK, Fanslow WC. Human B cell proliferation and Ig secretion induced by recombinant CD40 ligand are modulated by soluble cytokines. *J Immunol* 1993;150:3671–3680.
121. Armitage RJ, Tough TW, Macduff BM, et al. CD40 ligand is a T cell growth factor. *Eur J Immunol* 1993;23:2326–2331.
122. Funakoshi S, Longo DL, Beckwith M, et al. Inhibition of human B-cell lymphoma growth by CD40 stimulation. *Blood* 1994;83: 2787–2794.
123. Freeman GJ, Freedman AS, Rabinowe SN, et al. Interleukin 6 gene expression in normal and neoplastic B cells. *J Clin Invest* 1989;83: 1512–1518.
124. Kawano M, Hirano T, Matsuda T, et al. Autocrine generation and requirement of BSF-2/IL-6 for human multiple myelomas. *Nature* 1988;332:83–85.
125. Tosato G, Tanner J, Jones KD, Revel M, Pike SE. Identification of interleukin-6 as an autocrine growth factor for Epstein-Barr virus-immortalized B cells. *J Virol* 1990;64:3033–3041.
126. Weiss LM, Chang KL. Association of the Epstein-Barr virus with hematolymphoid neoplasia. *Adv Anat Pathol* 1996;3:1–15.
127. Delsol G, Brousset P, Chittal S, Rigal-Huguet F. Correlation of the expression of Epstein-Barr virus latent membrane protein and in situ hybridization with biotinylated BamHI-W probes in Hodgkin's disease. *Am J Pathol* 1992;140:247–253.
128. Merz H, Fliedner A, Orscheschek K, et al. Cytokine expression in T-cell lymphomas and Hodgkin's disease. Its possible implication in autocrine or paracrine production as a potential basis for neoplastic growth. *Am J Pathol* 1991;139:1173–1180.
129. Hsu SM, Xie SS, Hsu PL, Waldron JA Jr. Interleukin-6, but not interleukin-4, is expressed by Reed-Sternberg cells in Hodgkin's disease with or without histologic features of Castleman's disease. *Am J Pathol* 1992;141:129–138.
130. Defrance T, Fluckiger AC, Rossi JF, Magaud JP, Sotto JJ, Banchereau J. Antiproliferative effects of interleukin-4 on freshly isolated non-Hodcells. *Blood* 1992;79:990–996.
131. Uyttenhove C, Simpson RJ, Van Snick J. Functional and structural characterization of P40, a mouse glycoprotein with T-cell growth factor activity. *Proc Natl Acad Sci USA* 1988;85:6934–6938.
132. Nagarkatti M, Hassuneh M, Seth A, Manickasundari K, Nagarkatti PS. Constitutive activation of the interleukin 2 gene in the induction of spontaneous *in vitro* transformation and tumorigenicity of T cells. *Proc Natl Acad Sci USA* 1994;91:7638–7642.
133. Hassuneh MR, Nagarkatti PS, Nagarkatti M. Evidence for the participation of interleukin-2 (IL-2) and IL-4 in the regulation of autonomous growth and tumorigenesis of transformed cells of lymphoid origin. *Blood* 1997;89:610–620.
134. Taniguchi T, Minami Y. The IL-2/IL-2 receptor system: a current overview. *Cell* 1993;73:5–8.
135. Hsu SM, Hsu PL. Lack of effect of colony-stimulating factors, interleukins, interferons, and tumor necrosis factor on the growth and differentiation of cultured Reed-Sternberg cells. Comparison with effects of phorbol ester and retinoic acid. *Am J Pathol* 1990;136:181–189.
136. Tesch H, Herrmann T, Abts H, Diamantstein T, Diehl V. High affinity IL-2 receptors on a Hodgkin's derived cell line. *Leuk Res* 1990;14: 953–960.
137. Foss HD, Hummel M, Gottstein S, et al. Frequent expression of IL-7 gene transcripts in tumor cells of classical Hodgkin's disease. *Am J Pathol* 1995;146:33–39.
138. McBride WH, Thacker JD, Comora S, et al. Genetic modification of a murine fibrosarcoma to produce interleukin 7 stimulates host cell infiltration and tumor immunity. *Cancer Res* 1992;52:3931–3937.
139. Hock H, Dorsch M, Diamantstein T, Blankenstein T. Interleukin 7 induces CD4+ T cell-dependent tumor rejection. *J Exp Med* 1991;174: 1291–1298.
140. Ruco LP, Pomponi D, Pigott R, Gearing AJ, Baiocchini A, Baroni CD. Expression and cell distribution of the intercellular adhesion molecule, vascular cell adhesion molecule, endothelial leukocyte adhesion molecule, and endothelial cell adhesion molecule (CD31) in reactive human lymph nodes and in Hodgkin's disease. *Am J Pathol* 1992;140: 1337–1344.
141. Kretschmer C, Jones DB, Morrison K, et al. Tumor necrosis factor alpha and lymphotoxin production in Hodgkin's disease. *Am J Pathol* 1990;137:341–351.
142. Xerri L, Birg F, Guigou V, Bouabdallah R, Poizot Martin I, Hassoun J. *In situ* expression of the IL-1α and TNF-α genes by Reed-Sternberg cells in Hodgkin's disease. *Int J Cancer* 1992;50:689–693.
143. Fisher RI, Bostick Bruton F, Sauder DN, Scala G, Diehl V. Neoplastic cells obtained from Hodgkin's disease are potent stimulators of human primary mixed lymphocyte cultures. *J Immunol* 1983;130: 2666–2670.
144. Delabie J, Ceuppens JL, Vandenberghe P, de Boer M, Coorevits L, De Wolf Peeters C. The B7/BB1 antigen is expressed by Reed-Sternberg cells of Hodgkin's disease and contributes to the stimulating capacity of Hodgkin's disease-derived cell lines. *Blood* 1993;82:2845–2852.
145. Thompson CB, Lindsten T, Ledbetter JA, et al. CD28 activation pathway regulates the production of multiple T-cell-derived lymphokines/ cytokines. *Proc Natl Acad Sci USA* 1989;86:1333–1337.
146. Ree HJ, Khan AA, Qureshi MN, Teplitz C. Expression of cell adhesion molecules with germinal center in Hodgkin's disease: an immunohistochemical study. The germinal center related complex and histologic types. *Cancer* 1994;73:1257–1266.
147. Rosenberg SA, Kaplan HS. Evidence for an orderly progression in the spread of Hodgkin's disease. *Cancer Res* 1966;26:1225–1230.
148. Mauch PM, Kalish LA, Kadin M, Coleman CN, Osteen R, Hellman S. Patterns of presentation of Hodgkin disease. Implications for etiology and pathogenesis [see comments]. *Cancer* 1993;71:2062–2071.
149. Kapp U, Dux A, Schell Frederick E, et al. Disseminated growth of Hodgkin's-derived cell lines L540 and L540cy in immune-deficient SCID mice. *Ann Oncol* 1994;1:121–126.
150. DeCoteau JF, Winpenny R, Butmarc J, Kadin ME. Alterations in CD44 expression correlate with malignant progression and tissue of origin of cell lines from Ki-1+ anaplastic large cell lymphoma. *Proc Annu Meet Am Assoc Cancer Res* 1995;36:abstr 487.
151. Salles G, Zain M, Jiang WM, Boussiotis VA, Shipp MA. Alternatively spliced CD44 transcripts in diffuse large-cell lymphomas: characterization and comparison with normal activated B cells and epithelial malignancies. *Blood* 1993;82:3539–3547.
152. Mackay CR, Terpe HJ, Stauder R, Marston WL, Stark H, Gunthert U. Expression and modulation of CD44 variant isoforms in humans. *J Cell Biol* 1994;124:71–82.
153. Feldstein JT, Jaffe ES, Berkowitz JR, Burd PR, Tosato G. Eotaxin-1, a specific chemoattractant for eosinophils in Hodgkin's tissues. *Blood* 1997;90:388a.
154. Butterfield JH, Kephart GM, Banks PM, Gleich GJ. Extracellular deposition of eosinophil granule major basic protein in lymph nodes of patients with Hodgkin's disease. *Blood* 1986;68:1250–1256.
155. Samoszuk M, Sholly S, Epstein AL. Eosinophil peroxidase is detectable with a monoclonal antibody in collagen bands of nodular sclerosis Hodgkin's disease. *Lab Invest* 1987;56:394–400.
156. Kadin ME, Glatstein E, Dorfman RF. Clinicopathologic studies of 117 untreated patients subjected to laporatomy for staging of Hodgkin's disease. *Cancer* 1971;27:1277–1287.
157. Newcom SR, O'Rourke L. Potentiation of fibroblast growth by nodular sclerosing Hodgkin's disease cell cultures. *Blood* 1982;60:228–237.
158. Ford RJ, Mehta S, Davis F, Maizel AL. Growth factors in Hodgkin's disease. *Cancer Treat Rep* 1982;66:633–638.
159. Kortmann C, Burrichter H, Monner D, Jahn G, Diehl V, Peter HH. Interleukin-1-like activity constitutively generated by Hodgkin derived cell lines. I. Measurement in a human lymphocyte co-stimulator assay. *Immunobiology* 1984;166:318–333.
160. Sugarman BJ, Aggarwal BB, Hass PE, Figari IS, Palladino MA Jr, Shepard HM. Recombinant human tumor necrosis factor-alpha: effects on proliferation of normal and transformed cells *in vitro*. *Science* 1985;230:943–945.
161. Roberts AB, Sporn MB, Assoian RK, et al. Transforming growth factor type beta: rapid induction of fibrosis and angiogenesis *in vivo* and stimulation of collagen formation *in vitro*. *Proc Natl Acad Sci USA* 1986;83:4167–4171.
162. Mustoe TA, Pierce GF, Thomason A, Gramates P, Sporn MB, Deuel

TF. Accelerated healing of incisional wounds in rats induced by transforming growth factor-beta. *Science* 1987;237:1333–1336.
163. Kadin ME, Agnarsson BA, Ellingsworth LR, Newcom SR. Immunohistochemical evidence of a role for transforming growth factor beta in the pathogenesis of nodular sclerosing Hodgkin's disease. *Am J Pathol* 1990;136:1209–1214.
164. Newcom SR, Gu L. Transforming growth factor beta 1 messenger RNA in Reed-Sternberg cells in nodular sclerosing Hodgkin's disease. *J Clin Pathol* 1995;48:160–163.
165. Shinozaki M, Kawara HN, Kakinuma T, Igarashia, Takehara K. Induction of subcutaneous tissue fibrosis in newborn mice by transforming growth factor-β—simultaneous application with basic fibroblast growth factor causes persistent fibrosis. *Biochem Biophys Res Commun* 1997;237:292–296.
166. Ohshima K, Sugihara M, Suzumiya J, et al. Basic fibroblast growth factor and fibrosis in Hodgkin's disease. *Am J Hematol* (in press).
167. Ree HJ, Pezzullo JC. Inflammation and/or necrosis of tumors cannot account for fever in most febrile patients with Hodgkin's disease. *Cancer* 1987;60:1787–1789.
168. Sappino AP, Seelentag W, Pelte MF, Alberto P, Vassalli P. Tumor necrosis factor/cachectin and lymphotoxin gene expression in lymph nodes from lymphoma patients. *Blood* 1990;75:958–962.
169. Quesada JR, Talpaz M, Rios A, Kurzrock R, Gutterman JU. Clinical toxicity of interferons in cancer patients: a review. *J Clin Oncol* 1986; 4:234–243.
170. Feinberg B, Kurzrock R, Talpaz M, Blick M, Saks S, Gutterman JU. A phase I trial of intravenously-administered recombinant tumor necrosis factor-alpha in cancer patients. *J Clin Oncol* 1988;6:1328–1334.
171. Lahdevirta J, Maury CP, Teppo AM, Repo H. Elevated levels of circulating cachectin/tumor necrosis factor in patients with acquired immunodeficiency syndrome. *Am J Med* 1988;85:289–291.
172. Opp M, Obal F Jr, Cady AB, Johannsen L, Krueger JM. Interleukin-6 is pyrogenic but not somnogenic. *Physiol Behav* 1989;45:1069–1072.
173. Kurzrock R, Redman J, Cabanillas F, Jones D, Rothberg J, Talpaz M. Serum interleukin 6 levels are elevated in lymphoma patients and correlate with survival in advanced Hodgkin's disease and with B symptoms. *Cancer Res* 1993;53:2118–2122.
174. Perfetti V, Dragani TA, Paulli M, et al. Gene expression of pyrogenic cytokines in Hodgkin's disease lymph nodes. *Haematologica* 1992;77: 221–225.
175. Naumovski L, Utz PJ, Bergstrom SK, et al. SUP-HD1: a new Hodgkin's disease-derived cell line with lymphoid features produces interferon-gamma [see comments]. *Blood* 1989;74:2733–2742.
176. Ree HJ, Crowley JP, Dinarello CA. Anti-interleukin-1 reactive cells in Hodgkin's disease. *Cancer* 1987;59:1717–1720.
177. Ruco LP, Pomponi D, Pigott R, et al. Cytokine production (IL-1α, IL-1β, TNFα) and endothelial cell activation (ELAM-1 and HLA-DR) in reactive lymphadenitis, Hodgkin's disease, and in non-Hodgkin's lymphomas. An immunocytochemical study. *Am J Pathol* 1990;137: 1163–1171.
178. Hsu S-M, Krupen K, Lachman LB. Heterogeneity of interleukin 1 production in cultured Reed-Sternberg cell lines HDLM-1, HDLM-1d and KM-H2. *Am J Pathol* 1989;135:33–38.
179. Kyle RA. Multiple myeloma and other plasma cell disorders. In: Hoffman R, Benz EJ Jr, Shattil EJ, Furie B, Cohen HJ, Silberstein LE, eds. *Hematology. Basic principles and practice.* New York: Churchill Livingstone, 1995:1354–1374.
180. Bataille R, Jourdan M, Zhang XG, Klein B. Serum levels of interleukin 6, a potent myeloma cell growth factor, as a reflect of disease severity in plasma cell dyscrasias. *J Clin Invest* 1989;84:2008–2011.
181. Levy RA, Kaplan HS. Impaired lymphocyte function in untreated Hodgkin's disease. *N Engl J Med* 1974;290:181–186.
182. Twomey JJ, Rice L. Impact of Hodgkin's disease upon the immune system. *Semin Oncol* 1980;7:114–125.
183. Romagnani S, Ferrini PL, Ricci M. The immune derangement in Hodgkin's disease. *Semin Hematol* 1985;22:41–55.
184. Romagnani S, Amadori A, Biti G, et al. *In vitro* lymphocyte response to phytomitogens in untreated and treated patients with Hodgkin's disease. *Int Arch Allergy Appl Immunol* 1976;51:378–389.
185. Engleman EG, Benike CH, Hoppe RT, Kaplan HS, Berberich FR. Autologous mixed lymphocyte reaction in patients with Hodgklin's disease. Evidence for a T cell defect. *J Clin Invest* 1980;66:149–158.
186 Ford RJ, Tsao J, Kouttab NM, Sahasrabuddhe CG, Mehta SR. Association of an interleukin abnormality with the T cell defect in Hodgkin's disease. *Blood* 1984;64:386–392.
187. Bendstzen K. Interleukin-1, interleukin-6 and tumor necrosis factor in infection, inflammation and immunity. *Immunol Lett* 1988;9:183–199.
188. Schecter GS, Soehnlen F. Monocyte-mediated inhibition of lymphocyte blastogenesis in Hodgkin's disease. *Blood* 1978;52:261–271.
189. Bockman RS. Stage-dependent recution in T-colony formation in Hodgkin's disease. Coincidence with monocyte synthesis of prostaglandins. *J Clin Invest* 1980;66:523–531.
190. Fiorentino DF, Zlotnik A, Vieira P, et al. IL-10 acts on the antigen presenting cell to inhibit cytokine production by Th1 cells. *J Immunol* 1991;146:3444.
191. Taga K, Mostowski H, Tosato G. Human interleukin-10 can directly nhibit T cell growth. *Blood* 1993;81:2964.
192. Herbst H, Foss H-D, Samol J, et al. Frequent expression of interleukin-10 by Epstein-Barr virus–harboring tumor cells of Hodgkin's disease. *Blood* 1996;87:2918–2929.
193. Kehrl JH, Roberts AB, Wakefield LM, Jakowlew S, Sporn MB, Fauci AS. Transforming growth factor beta is an important immunomodulatory protein for human B lymphocytes. *J Immunol* 1986;137: 3855–3860.
194. Kehrl JH, Wakefield LM, Roberts AB, et al. Production of transforming growth factor beta by human T lymphocytes and its potential role in the regulation of T cell growth. *J Exp Med* 1986;163:1037–1050.
195. Rook AH, Kehrl JH, Wakefield LM, et al. Effects of transforming growth factor beta on the functions of natural killer cells: depressed cytolytic activity and blunting of interferon responsiveness. *J Immunol* 1986;136:3916–3920.
196. Kasid A, Bell GI, Director EP. Effects of transforming growth factor-beta on human lymphokine-activated killer cell precursors. Autocrine inhibition of cellular proliferation and differentiation to immune killer cells. *J Immunol* 1988;141:690–698.
197. Renner C, Ohnesorge S, Held G, et al. T cells from patients with Hodgkin's disease have a defective T-cell receptor zeta chain expression that is reversible by T-cell stimulation with CD3 and CD28. *Blood* 1996;88:236–241.
198. Frisan T, Sjoberg J, Dolcetti R, et al. Local suppression of Epstein-Barr virus (EBV)-specific cytotoxicity in biopsies of EBV-positive Hodgkin's disease. *Blood* 1995;86:1493–1501.
199. Potters M, Diepstra A, Meulenaar R, Visser L, Poppema S. The absence of effective T cell activation in Hodgkin's disease may be the result of TGF-β production by Reed-Sternberg cells. *Blood* 1997;90;(Suppl 1.): 2656.
200. Newcom SR, Tagra KK. High molecular weight transforming growth factor beta is excreted in the urine in active nodular sclerosing Hodgkin's disease. *Cancer Res* 1992;52:6768–6773.
201. Younes A, Consoli U, Snell V, et al. CD30 ligand in patients with CD30[+] tumors. *J Clin Oncol* 1997;15:3355–3362.
202. Pizzolo G, Chilosi M, Vinante F, et al. Soluble interleukin-2 receptors in the serum of patients with Hodgkin's disease. *Br J Cancer* 1987;55: 427–428.
203. Pui CH, Hudson M, Luo X, Wilimas J, Evans W, Crist WM. Serum interleukin-2 receptor levels in Hodgkin disease and other solid tumors of childhood. *Leukemia* 1993;7:1242–1244.
204. Hamon MD, Unal E, Macdonald I, Shamim F, Boesen E, Prentice HG. Plasma soluble interleukin 2 receptor levels in patients with malignant lymphoma are correlated with disease activity but not cellular immunosuppression. *Leuk Lymphoma* 1993;10:111–115.
205. Tazzari PL, Bolognesi A, de Totero D, et al. Ber-H2 (anti-CD30)-saporin immunotoxin: a new tool for the treatment of Hodgkin's disease and CD30[+] lymphoma: *in vitro* evaluation. *Br J Haematol* 1992; 81:203–211.
206. Renner C, Bauer S, Sahin U, et al. Cure of disseminated xenografted human Hodgkin's tumors by bispecific monoclonal antibodies and human T cells: the role of human T-cell subsets in a preclinical model. *Blood* 1996;87:2930–2937.
207. Hartmann F, Renner C, Jung W, et al. Treatment of refractory Hodgkin's disease with an anti-CD16/CD30 bispecific antibody. *Blood* 1997;89:2042–2047.
208. Tepler I, Schwartz G, Parker K, et al. Phase I trial of an interleukin-2 fusion toxin (DAB486IL-2) in hematologic malignancies: complete response in a patient with Hodgkin's disease refractory to chemotherapy. *Cancer* 1994;73:1276–1285.

Hodgkin's Disease, edited by P. M. Mauch,
J. O. Armitage, V. Diehl, R. T. Hoppe, and L. M. Weiss.
Lippincott Williams & Wilkins, Philadephia ©1999.

CHAPTER 10

Dysregulated Immune Response in Hodgkin's Disease

Sibrand Poppema and Marc Potters

Hodgkin's disease is a malignant lymphoma characterized by the presence of multinucleated giant cells, the Reed-Sternberg cells, and their mononuclear variants, sometimes termed the Hodgkin cells. These are now generally believed to be a clonal neoplastic population that derives from transformed B lymphocytes. The malignant cells usually comprise less than 1% of the total cell population and are surrounded by a prominent infiltrate of reactive cells. These are mostly T lymphocytes with variable admixtures of eosinophils, histiocytes, plasma cells, and, in cases of nodular lymphocyte predominance, also considerable numbers of small B lymphocytes.

IMPAIRED IMMUNE RESPONSE IN HODGKIN'S DISEASE PATIENTS

In the late 19th century, Hodgkin's disease was believed to be a granulomatous inflammatory lesion because Hodgkin's disease and tuberculosis were found to coexist in many autopsies. Sternberg even stated that it was simply an atypical form of tuberculosis (1). Some years later, evidence emerged that the two diseases were different, and in this context the precise definition of the morphologic features of the Reed-Sternberg cells was an important step (2–6). The coexistence of the two diseases remained, however, and in 1947 Jackson and Parker reported a frequency of 20% tuberculoses in autopsies of patients with Hodgkin's disease (7). Better treatment of tuberculosis led to a reduced incidence, and in 1969 Harris and co-workers reported that only four of 768 patients with Hodgkin's disease seen in the period 1944 through 1966 at the M. D. Anderson Hospital had tuberculosis (8).

S. Poppema and M. Potters: Department of Pathology and Laboratory Medicine, University Hospital Groningen, Groningen, The Netherlands.

Dorothy Reed was the first to document that Hodgkin's patients have an impaired immune response (3). She demonstrated the absence of a reaction to tuberculin in Hodgkin's patients. In the early 1930s, Parker and Steiner provided further evidence that an immunologic defect might be the cause of the increased susceptibility to tuberculosis because the tuberculin reaction was negative in a majority of patients with Hodgkin's disease even while some of these patients had active tuberculosis (9,10). In 1947, Dubin found only one positive tuberculin reaction among 38 patients with Hodgkin's disease, while at that time the positivity rate in the general population was over 52% (11). He also noted that the positivity of serologic reactions for syphilis was less than expected and that some patients with coexisting brucellosis were unable to produce anti-*Brucella* antibody titers. Based on this, Dubin postulated that the immunologic deficiency of Hodgkin's disease was not restricted to tuberculosis but was generalized (11).

Schier and co-workers conducted systematic tests of the capacity of 43 patients with Hodgkin's disease to react to tuberculoprotein, *Trychophyton gypseum, Candida albicans,* and mumps skin test antigen and found the delayed-type responses to be severely depressed as compared to control individuals (12). From that moment on, numerous reports confirmed an impairment of the immune response in Hodgkin's disease (Table 1). This lack of response has also been described as "anergy." Lamb et al. reported that this anergy was also present in patients with Hodgkin's disease in good condition, in contrast to the anergy of other malignancies, which was virtually restricted to patients in poor condition (13). In other words, it was concluded that the anergy of Hodgkin's disease is a primary attribute of the disease. However, in a carefully performed study, Brown et al. showed that patients in clinical stage I were comparable to those of

TABLE 1. *Nature of the immune response in patients with Hodgkin's disease*[a]

	In vitro	*In vivo*
T cells	Increased spontaneous proliferation	Reduced response against tuberculin
	Decreased mitogen-induced proliferation	Reduced response against DNCB
	Reduced response to recall antigens	
	Reduced mixed leukocyte reaction	
	Normal allogenic leukocyte reaction	
	Increased spontaneous cytokine production	Increased shedding of CD25, CD8, CD95
	Reduced mitogen/antigen induced cytokine production	
	Decreased CD3 ζ-chain expression	
B-cells	Increased mitogen-induced Ig production	Increased total Ig titer
	Reduced antigen-induced Ig production	Increased antiviral Ig titer

[a]DNCB, dinitrochlorobenzene; Ig, Immunoglobulin.

normal controls and that the frequency of anergy increased with advancing stage (14). This suggested that the disease needs to have a certain extent before it is reflected in a general reduction of delayed-type responses. Sokal and Primikinirios observed that two patients who had a long remission from Hodgkin's disease recovered the ability to react to tuberculin (15). This was confirmed in a later study that also suggested that the tuberculin test might serve as a prognostic index (16).

The major clinical importance of these observations is that individuals with Hodgkin's disease have greater susceptibility to infections with bacteria, viruses, fungi, and parasites (17). Before chemotherapy and radiotherapy were available, infectious diseases were a major cause of death in patients with Hodgkin's disease. Even now, infections account for a major part of deaths in patients with treated Hodgkin's disease. The most commonly observed infections after treatment are pneumonia, bacteremia, skin infections, and meningitis (18). *Streptococcus pneumoniae, Staphylococcus aureus,* and *Staphylococcus epidermidis* are the microorganisms most often isolated from Hodgkin's patients. Herpes zoster infections, which are commonly observed in immune-comprised individuals, are also frequently seen in individuals with Hodgkin's disease. Infections with gram-negative bacteria are less frequently observed. The infections in treated patients are partly also the result of therapy-induced immune deficiency.

Skin testing with natural antigens such as tuberculin does not really distinguish between true anergy in a previously sensitized individual and the lack of response in individuals never previously exposed to the antigen. Certain chemicals, like the extremely potent contact allergen 2,4-dinitrochlorobenzene (DNCB), elicit a tuberculin-type reaction, the delayed-type hypersensitivity reaction. In the early 1960s it was shown that patients with Hodgkin's disease had a reduced response toward dinitrochlorobenzene and that on remission there was a transition toward a normal reaction (Table 1) (19,20). In a study by Aisenberg, one of the patients relapsed, and this was accompanied by a transition toward unresponsiveness. Aisenberg concluded that the immunologic defect manifested by anergy for 2,4-dinitrochlorobenzene and other delayed-type hypersensitivity antigens is an early manifestation of Hodgkin's disease and is closely correlated with disease activity (19).

Attempts to convert anergic patients with Hodgkin's disease by active immunization with the bacillus of Calmette-Guérin (BCG) were found to show a good correlation between the inability to respond and poor prognosis (15). This suggested that the test was a measure of the activity of the mechanism responsible for resistance to the disease. The question whether there is indeed an effective antitumor response in some cases is still unresolved.

IMPAIRED PERIPHERAL BLOOD CELL RESPONSES *IN VITRO*

Lymphocyte counts in patients with Hodgkin's disease were found to be only slightly lower than normal in early stages but significantly lower in the higher stages and severely depressed in late stages (14). *In vitro,* a reduced proliferative response of lymphocytes from patients with Hodgkin's disease to phytohemagglutinin (PHA) was first demonstrated by Hersh and Oppenheim in 1961, and in 1965 Aisenberg used ^{14}C-labeled thymidine to quantify the blastoid transformation (21,22). The response to other mitogens such as concanavalin A and pokeweed mitogen and to recall antigens such as dinitrochlorobenzene or tuberculin was also found to be reduced (Table 1) (23). The response in an autologous mixed leukocyte reaction (MLR) was depressed as well (24). In contrast, the response in an allogeneic mixed leukocyte reaction was observed as normal (25). There was a reduction in the production of cytokines and a decreased immunoglobulin production on stimulation with mitogens or antigens (26,27). In contrast, increased spontaneous production of immunoglobulins (28) and an increased proportion of peripheral T cells that spontaneously synthesize DNA have been observed (29). In particular, an increase of IgE has been noted in up to 50% of the patients (30). These results indicate that there is a population of activated lymphocytes present in the peripheral blood of patients with Hodgkin's disease that do not have normal antigen responsiveness.

Recently it was discovered that peripheral blood T cells from patients with untreated Hodgkin's disease have decreased T-cell receptor (TCR) ζ-chain expression (Table 1) (31). This defect resulted in an altered signal transduction, as was shown by an impaired Ca^{2+} mobilization. Adequate stimulation with anti-CD3 and anti-CD28 antibodies resulted in normal expression of the ζ-chain and in the restoration of IL-2 production and cytotoxicity to normal values. Surprisingly, in the lymphocytes in the involved tissues of Hodgkin's disease, this reduction in TCR ζ-chain expression is much less pronounced than in the peripheral blood cells (S. Poppema, *unpublished observations*).

CD30, a member of the tumor necrosis factor receptor (TNFR) superfamily, is consistently detected on Hodgkin and Reed-Sternberg cells, and a soluble form of CD30 (sCD30) is found in the serum of Hodgkin's patients (32,33). The level of sCD30 correlates with the tumor burden, suggesting that the Hodgkin–Reed-Sternberg-cells are the major source of sCD30. The sCD30 has been found to have prognostic value for the outcome of treatment in Hodgkin's disease (33). CD30 can interact with its natural ligand CD30L, expressed on most hematopoietic cell types, and this interaction is associated with enhanced shedding of sCD30. Also, increased levels of sCD95, sCD8, and sCD25 are observed in patients with Hodgkin's disease (33,34). It is very likely that these and perhaps other soluble factors, including the so-called E-rosette–inhibiting factor, influence the immune response in patients with Hodgkin's disease by inhibiting interactions between antigen-presenting cells and T cells or otherwise by interfering with T-cell activation (35).

ABSENCE OF IMMUNE RESPONSE AGAINST EPSTEIN-BARR VIRUS–POSITIVE HODGKIN–REED-STERNBERG CELLS

The presence of an extensive population of reactive lymphocytes and plasma cells in the lymph nodes from patients with Hodgkin's disease suggests that there is an immunologic reaction in progress. An impairment of the local immune response is suggested by the absence of an effective cytotoxic response against Epstein-Barr virus (EBV) antigens by lymphocytes derived from EBV-positive Hodgkin's lymph nodes (Table 1). Most Hodgkin's patients have overcome an EBV infection earlier in life, and specific cytotoxic T cells can be found in the peripheral blood of these same patients (36). The absence of a cytotoxic response in EBV-positive cases is probably relevant because there is a cytotoxic response against EBV antigens by lymphocytes derived from EBV-negative Hodgkin's lymph nodes (36,37). The EBV latent membrane proteins LMP-1 and LMP-2 in association with human leukocyte antigen (HLA) class I serve as potential targets for specific $CD8^+$ T cells (38). The presentation of LMP-2 is restricted through the HLA class I antigen A2, and therefore, it has been hypothesized that HLA-A2-positive individuals would be underrepresented among Caucasians with EBV-associated Hodgkin's disease. However, there was no significant difference between the frequency of HLA A2 positivity in Hodgkin's disease cases and controls and between EBV-associated and -nonassociated cases of Hodgkin's disease (39,40). However, HLA class I was frequently found to be absent altogether from Hodgkin and Reed-Sternberg cells in the classical forms of Hodgkin's disease, although some cases of mixed cellularity Hodgkin's disease and all cases of nodular lymphocyte predominance Hodgkin's disease were positive (41). Interestingly, others have reported HLA class I to be usually present in EBV-positive cases and absent in EBV-negative cases of Hodgkin's disease (42). HLA class II is consistently highly expressed on Hodgkin and Reed-Sternberg cells in all cases of Hodgkin's disease. Absence of HLA class I presents a mechanism to escape the specific cytotoxic immune response. In EBV-positive Hodgkin's disease, normal expression of HLA class I and transporters associated with antigen processing can be found (43). Therefore, there are probably several other factors involved in the impaired cytotoxic response in Hodgkin's disease (Table 2, Fig. 1).

Whether the observed impaired systemic cellular immunity is the result of, or constitutes a predisposition for, Hodgkin's disease remains unclear. Some studies from Scandinavia found immunologic defects in unaffected siblings of patients with Hodgkin's disease, but this could not be confirmed in other studies (44,45). The data mentioned earlier on the presence or absence of a normal response to delayed-type antigens in early versus later stages of the disease suggest that most of the immunologic abnormalities are secondary phenomena. Obviously, the currently available radiotherapy and chemotherapy also contribute to the short-term and long-term immunodeficiency in patients treated for Hodgkin's disease, but there are no exact data on the precise contributions of the disease and its therapy.

TABLE 2. *Possible interactions between H-RS cells and T lymphocytes*[a]

	H-RS cells	Interaction	T-cells
Antigen recognition	Antigen?	?	TCR/CD3
	HLA class I (some)	±	CD8
	HLA class II	+	CD4
Co-stimulation	CD80	+	CD28
	CD86	+	CD28
	CD30	?	CD30L ?
	CD40	+	CD40L
Cell-cell contact	CD58	+	CD2
	CD54	+	CD11a/CD18

[a]TCR, T-cell receptor; HLA, human leukocyte antigen.

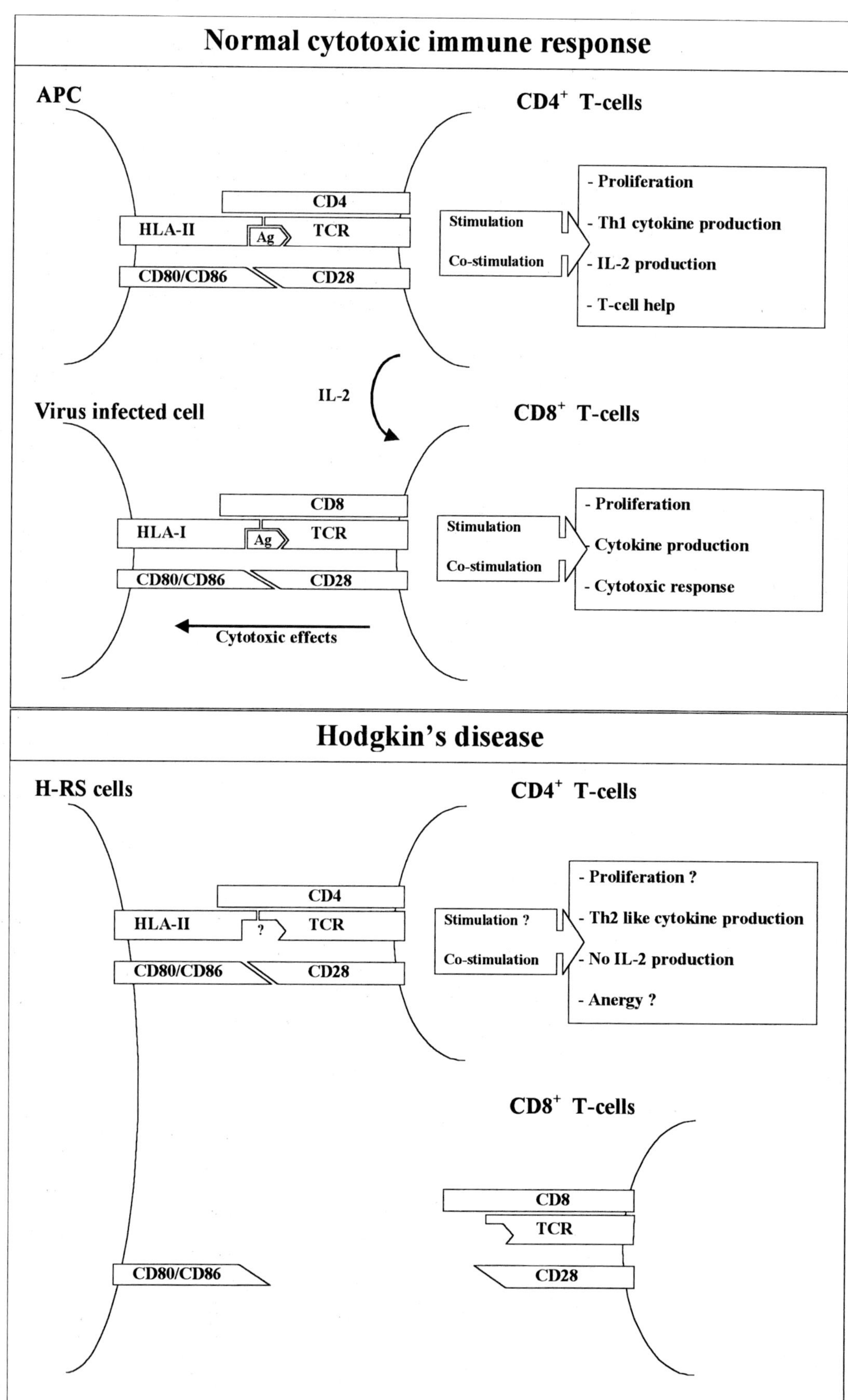

Normal cytotoxic immune response
APC
CD4+ T-cells
CD4
HLA-II
Ag
TCR
CD80/CD86
CD28
Stimulation
Co-stimulation
- Proliferation
- Th1 cytokine production
- IL-2 production
- T-cell help
IL-2
Virus infected cell
CD8+ T-cells
CD8
HLA-I
Ag
TCR
CD80/CD86
CD28
Stimulation
Co-stimulation
- Proliferation
- Cytokine production
- Cytotoxic response
Cytotoxic effects
Hodgkin's disease
H-RS cells
CD4+ T-cells
CD4
HLA-II
?
TCR
CD80/CD86
CD28
Stimulation ?
Co-stimulation
- Proliferation ?
- Th2 like cytokine production
- No IL-2 production
- Anergy ?
CD8+ T-cells
CD8
TCR
CD80/CD86
CD28

ACTIVATED CD4-POSITIVE T CELLS SURROUNDING THE HODGKIN AND REED-STERNBERG CELLS

The lymphocytes in close vicinity to Hodgkin and Reed-Sternberg cells are almost exclusively positive for CD4, whereas only very few $CD8^+$ or natural killer (NK) cells are usually present in this area (Tables 3 and 4) (46). In patients who are HIV positive, however, $CD8^+$ cells predominate, but it is not known whether these $CD8^+$ cells are cytotoxic. The generally observed increase of $CD4^+$ cells in Hodgkin's nodes is associated with a decrease in $CD4^+$ cells in the circulation and predominantly reflects increased influx of mature $CD4^+$ T lymphocytes into the involved tissues (47). Results of imaging with indium-111–labeled lymphocytes showing positivity in involved nodes support this concept (48). Activated $CD8^+$ T cells, as determined by granzyme positivity, have been described in some cases but not immediately surrounding the Hodgkin–Reed-Sternberg cells. Surprisingly, the presence of these granzyme-positive lymphocytes was associated with an unfavorable prognosis (49).

The $CD4^+$ T cells that surround the Hodgkin and Reed-Sternberg cells are in a state of activation, as indicated by the presence of several activation-associated surface markers, including CD38, CD69, CD71, and HLA class II (Tables 3 and 4) (50,51). A proportion of these $CD4^+$ cells also stain for the cytotoxic granule-associated molecule TIA-1, but the significance of this staining is not known. There are no indications that the lymphocytes are of clonal origin or have a restricted TCRβ-chain gene variable region repertoire (52,53). The lymphocytes lack expression of another activation marker, CD26 (dipeptidylpeptidase IV) (50), a surface molecule involved in co-stimulation of T lymphocytes (54,55).

Further characterization of $CD4^+$ T cells derived from lymph nodes of classical as well as the nodular lymphocyte predominance subtype of Hodgkin's disease, by flow cytometry, has revealed that they are predominantly $CD45RO^+/CD45RB^{dim}$, suggesting an activated/memory T_H2 phenotype (Tables 3 and 4) (50,56). The T_H1/T_H2 paradigm was originally described by Mossman et al. in mice (57) and allowed the distinction of T_H1 cells that supported inflammatory responses by producing interleukin-2 (IL-2) and interferon-γ (IFN-γ) from T_H2 cells that support humoral responses by producing cytokines such as interleukin-4 (IL-4), IL-5, IL-6, and IL-10. When a single-cell suspension is prepared from lymph nodes involved by Hodgkin's disease, and these cells are optimally stimulated *in vitro* with phorbol ester and ionomycin, they produce IL-2, IFN-γ, and IL-4. When the $CD4^+/CD26^-$ lymphocytes that immediately surround the Reed-Sternberg cells are sorted from Hodgkin's lymph nodes, these do not produce IL-2 but, when optimally stimulated *in vitro,* secrete increased amounts of IL-4. This cytokine profile also suggests a T_H2 phenotype of

TABLE 3. *Immunophenotype of lymphocytes surrounding the Hodgkin–Reed-Sternberg cells in Hodgkin's disease*[a]

	Nodular lymphocyte predominance Hodgkin's disease	Classical Hodgkin's disease
CD3	+	+
TCRαβ	+	+
CD4	+	+
CD8	–	–
CD57	+	–
CD26	–	–
CD28	+	+
CTLA-4	+	+
CD40L	–	+
CD69	+	+
CD45RA	–	–
CD45R0	+	+
CD45RB	dim	dim

[a]TCR, T-cell receptor; CTLA-4, cutaneous T-lymphocyte antigen.

TABLE 4. *The immune response in the Hodgkin's disease–involved lymph nodes*[a]

Lymphocyte subtypes	Predominance of activated $CD4^+$ cells
	Few $CD8^+$ cells
	Absence of NK cells
	Absence of $CD26^+$ cells
Immune response characteristics	CD45 isotype expression indicative of Th2 cells
	Absence of IL-2 production by $CD4^+/CD26^-$ cells
	Lymphocytes have characteristics of anergy
	No specific cytotoxic response against EBV in EBV^+ cases

[a]NK, natural killer; EBV, Epstein–Barr virus.

FIG. 1. Immune response toward virus-infected cells and Hodgkin's disease. Virus antigens are presented by HLA class I to $CD8^+$ T cells, which results in stimulation and co-stimulation, followed by proliferation and a cytotoxic response toward the virus-infected cells. The APC-activated $CD4^+$ T cells can give $CD8^+$ T cells help by producing IL-2 and several other T_H1-associated cytokines. In Hodgkin's disease there are only $CD4^+$ T cells present in the vicinity of the Hodgkin–Reed-Sternberg cells, and no $CD8^+$ T cells. This could be the result of the absence of HLA class I molecules on the Hodgkin–Reed-Sternberg cells. Moreover, the $CD4^+$ T cells that surround the Hodgkin–Reed-Sternberg cells seem to be activated but do not produce IL-2. They do, however, produce T_H2-associated cytokines. This cytokine profile could lead to an inappropriate response and may be the result of the absence of adequate stimulation. APC, antigen-presenting cells.

these T cells (50). The notion that the response in Hodgkin's disease is of T_H2 type is consistent with the finding that Hodgkin's patients have elevated serum levels of T_H2-type cytokine IL-6 and frequently have elevated levels of IgG and also IgE (30,58).

CD57$^+$ T CELLS SURROUNDING HODGKIN–REED-STERNBERG CELLS IN NLP HODGKIN'S DISEASE ARE A SPECIAL T_H2 SUBSET

The CD4$^+$ lymphocytes surrounding the lymphotic and/or histiocytic (L&H)-type Reed-Sternberg cells in the nodular lymphocyte predominance subtype express CD57 on their surface, in contrast to those surrounding Hodgkin and Reed-Sternberg cells in the classical subtypes of Hodgkin's disease, which do not express CD57 (Table 3) (51). The CD57-positive cells do not express CD40L. CD4 and CD57 coexpression is normally almost exclusively seen on T cells in the light zone of reactive germinal centers, and these cells also lack CD40L expression (59). In germinal centers there are at least two CD4 T-cell subsets: CD4$^+$/CD40L$^+$ cells are located at the rim of germinal center light zone and mantle zone; and CD4$^+$/CD57$^+$ cells are distributed within the light zone. The CD4$^+$/CD57$^+$ cells are similar to murine CD4$^+$/NK1.1$^+$ cells in their tissue distribution and cytokine production, indicating a possible similar function for both lymphocyte subpopulations. The murine CD4$^+$/NK1.1$^+$ cells are known to produce IL-4 early in the immune response and direct it toward a T_H2-type response (60). In human tonsillar germinal centers, the CD4$^+$/CD57$^+$ cells also express IL-4 mRNA (61).

In vitro, naive CD4$^+$ T cells can be primed for a T_H2 response by anti-CD28 without anti-CD3 in the presence of IL-2. Approximately 30% of T cells primed in this way express CD57 (62). CD57$^+$ T_H2-primed clones produced three times more IL-4 and IL-5 than the CD57$^-$ T_H2-primed clones and also produced IFN-γ. This cytokine pattern (IL-4 and IFN-γ but not IL-2) is also produced by sorted CD4$^+$/CD26$^-$ lymphocytes from Hodgkin's lymph nodes (50).

It has been suggested that CD57 expression is a marker of activation (63). Improper stimulation of the surrounding T cells or an arrest in the activation stage could lead to the unusual T_H2-like cytokine production. This may explain not only the observed T_H2 immunophenotype of the T cells in Hodgkin's disease (CD45RB^{dim}/CD26$^-$) but also the absence of a cytotoxic response against Reed-Sternberg cells (Fig. 1).

ANERGY OF SURROUNDING T CELLS AS A POSSIBLE CAUSE FOR IMPAIRED CYTOTOXICITY

As mentioned earlier, the T cells surrounding the Hodgkin–Reed-Sternberg cells in the classical types of Hodgkin's disease do not express CD26 (Tables 3 and 4), although more than 60% of normal peripheral blood and lymph node T cells are CD26$^+$ (64,65). CD26 physically interacts with adenosine deaminase (ADA) and with CD45R0, both of which are important in the immune response (66,67). CD26$^-$ T cells become CD26$^+$ by stimulation with antigens/mitogens under physiologic conditions (65), but the CD26$^-$ cells from Hodgkin's lesions remain negative after stimulation (50). This indicates that the absence of CD26 is potentially relevant with respect to the impaired immune response observed in Hodgkin's disease. Sorted CD26$^-$ lymphocytes from cases of classical Hodgkin's disease can be stimulated *in vitro* to produce IFN-γ and IL-4, but not IL-2 (50). Inability to produce IL-2 and reduced proliferation are the hallmarks of anergic T cells (Fig. 1).

Anergic T cells can be obtained by several mechanisms: lack of co-stimulation (68,69), activation by superantigens (70), or the effect of certain cytokines (IL-10, TGF-β) (71,72). Thus, a possible way for Reed-Sternberg cells to escape cytotoxic killing is by induction of anergy in T cells. The anergic state of the lymphocytes is probably not the result of lack of co-stimulation by CD80 (B7.1), CD86 (B7.2), and other adhesion/co-stimulatory molecules such as CD58 (LFA-3) and CD54 (ICAM-1), because these are highly expressed on Hodgkin and Reed-Sternberg cells (Fig. 1, Table 2) (32,73).

Reed-Sternberg cells are capable of producing a wide variety of cytokines, including IL-1, IL-5, IL-6, IL-9, IL-10, and TGF-β (74,75), and it is suspected that constitutive nuclear expression of NF-κB is responsible for this phenomenon (76). The cytokines produced by Reed-Sternberg cells also include IL-10 and TGF-β (77–79), which are indeed known to be capable of anergy induction (80). Supernatant from Hodgkin cell line L-428 was found to inhibit CD25 expression and IL-2 production when peripheral blood mononuclear cells were stimulated with anti-CD3, although the cells still became CD69 positive. This indicates that a soluble factor is responsible for the improper activation (81). L-428 is known to produce TGF-β and IL-10 (82), and depletion of TGF-β from L-428 supernatant was found to completely prevent the inhibitory effect. Adding the removed TGF to RPMI resulted in a similar reduced CD25 and IL-2 expression pattern as with L-428 supernatant (81). IL-10 depletion did not affect the inhibitory effect of L-428 supernatant. These findings strongly suggest that TGF-β is the T cell inhibitory factor in the L-428 cell line.

TGF-β is generally produced in a latent, inactive complex composed of the bioactive TGF-β homodimer (25 kd) and a noncovalently bonded precursor protein (83). Often a latent TGF-β binding protein is associated with this complex. Bioactive TGF-β homodimer can be released from the complex after very strong acidification. The TGF-β produced by the L-428 cell line was found to be active at physiologic pH and had a much higher molecular weight than the usual active form (82). By SDS-PAGE, the L-428 TGF-β was shown to contain a 25-kd molecule that cross-reacted with antibodies against TGF-β. High-molecular-weight TGF-β was also observed in the urine of patients with Hodgkin's disease, although it was absent from healthy controls, suggesting that it is also produced *in vivo* by the tumor (84). Production of TGF-β that is already active at physiologic pH by Reed-Sternberg cells might enable them to (de)regulate the immune response in their favor. TGF-β is also a potent growth factor for fibroblasts and is known to promote the formation of extracellular matrix and fibrosis (75,83). The L-428 cell line was derived from a patient with nodular sclerosis subtype of Hodgkin's disease and is EBV negative. By *in situ* hybridization we have demonstrated the presence of TGF-β mRNA in the Reed-Sternberg cells of nodular sclerosis cases. Therefore, TGF-β may shape the environment for Reed-Sternberg cells by suppressing the T-cell response and inducing the collagen formation in the nodular sclerosis subtype. There are indications that EBV–positive Hodgkin–Reed-Sternberg cells as frequently found in mixed cellularity relatively frequently produce IL-10, and this may result in the different environment in this subtype.

POSSIBLE ROLE FOR MEMBERS OF THE TNFR/NGFR AND TNFL SUPERFAMILIES IN HODGKIN'S DISEASE

CD30, now identified as a member of the tumor necrosis factor receptor (TNFR) family, was first discovered with a monoclonal antibody prepared against the cell line L-428 that showed a consistently high expression on Reed-Sternberg cells (85). Further investigations revealed that CD30 expression is not restricted to these cells alone but is also expressed on activated T and B lymphocytes. The abundant presence of CD30 on Reed-Sternberg cells and its absence in most non-Hodgkin's lymphomas suggest that it might play an important role in the development of Hodgkin's disease. However, it is not quite clear how CD30 might be involved because the CD30 ligand can not be demonstrated on the T cells surrounding the Reed-Sternberg cells, although it has been found on the eosinophils (86). The known TNF receptor superfamily has gradually grown in recent years (87). Their natural ligands form two superfamilies, the neutrophins [nerve growth factor (NGF) ligand superfamily] and the tumor necrosis factor (TNF) ligand superfamily. Several other members of both the TNF receptor and TNF ligand superfamily have also been observed in Hodgkin's disease: CD27L (CD70), CD40, and CD95 (Fas/Apo) are all highly expressed on Reed-Sternberg cells (88). Some of their ligands, notably CD40L, are expressed on the surrounding activated T cells (89). These T cells also express Fas (CD95) but only minimal amounts of Fas ligand (CD95L). Somewhat surprisingly, CD40L is absent from the $CD57^+$ lymphocytes in the nodular lymphocyte predominance subtype of Hodgkin's disease (89). Several members of these superfamilies have an important role in the regulation of proliferation and apoptosis, and CD40/CD40L interaction is extremely important in B-cell activation (90).

CD95/CD95L interaction is capable of apoptosis induction and is involved in the maintenance of immune privilege and peripheral tolerance (91). It is also one of the mechanisms used in the cytotoxic response by T cells. It is therefore interesting that there is no adequate cytotoxic response toward Hodgkin and Reed-Sternberg cells, although they express substantial amounts of CD95.

A possible mechanism for tumor cells to escape a cytotoxic response is deletion of the T_H1 cells, resulting in the absence of help to the effector cells. T_H1 cells, cytotoxic T cells, and NK cells are more sensitive than T_H2 cells to CD95-mediated activation–induced cell death (92). This difference in susceptibility is already present in T_H0 cells (93). In Hodgkin's disease, the lymphocytes surrounding the tumor cells predominantly express a T_H2 phenotype. A polyclonal antibody reactive with membrane-bound as well as secreted CD95L and a monoclonal antibody reactive with a cytoplasmic determinant of CD95L both give strong staining of Reed-Sternberg cells, whereas the surrounding lymphocytes have a very low expression of CD95L and relatively high expression of CD95 (S. Poppema, *unpublished results*). CD95L expression has also been detected on malignant cells in several other malignancies, giving these malignant cells yet another possible mechanism to escape the immune response (94). It is therefore possible that Reed-Sternberg cells escape a cytotoxic and T_H1 immune response through the induction of apoptosis in surrounding cytotoxic T and NK lymphocytes and T_H1 cells.

Traditionally, starting from the early observations that low numbers of lymphocytes were associated with a poor prognosis and normal numbers with a better prognosis, it has been accepted that the lymphocytes present a more or less effective immune response against the tumor cells or an associated etiologic agent. An alternative explanation for the specific phenotype of Hodgkin's disease is offered by our recent finding that the tumor cells of the classical subtypes of Hodgkin's disease produce high quantities of the CC chemokine TARC (95). As mentioned before, constitutive nuclear NF-κB expression may induce the production of several chemokines by Reed-Sternberg cells. NF-κB activation caused by the HTLV-1–encoded transactivator Tax can lead to the expression of several chemokines (96). It is therefore possible that the upregulation of TARC also results from NF-κB activation. This chemokine is normally produced in much smaller amounts by a subset of antigen-presenting cells and strongly attracts T lymphocytes expressing the CCR4 receptor (97–99). The activated T_H2 lymphocytes of Hodgkin's tissue indeed express the CCR4 receptor, whereas T_H1 lymphocytes do not but express the CCR5 receptor (100). The production of TARC by Reed-Sternberg cells may therefore result in specific attraction of T_H2-type T lymphocytes. The paradox of an extensive but apparently ineffective immune infiltrate may thus reflect chemotactic attraction of T_H2 cells by an aberrantly produced chemokine instead of an antitumor response. The upside of this may be that Hodgkin's disease leads to an exaggerated lymph node swelling and, as a result, may be diagnosed early. The downside may be that the very presence of a T_H2-type infiltrate may prevent the induction of an effective immune response.

SUMMARY

Hodgkin's disease is characterized by the presence of Reed-Sternberg cells surrounded by predominantly $CD4^+$ T lymphocytes. These lymphocytes express a variety of activation markers but are incapable of mounting an effective immune response against the tumor cells. The lymphocytes typically are $CD45RO^+/CD45RB^{dim}$, lack the expression of CD26, can be stimulated *in vitro* to produce IFN-γ and IL-4 but not IL-2, but do not spontaneously produce cytokines. The CD45 isotype expression, the absence of CD26, and the potential for IL-4 production suggest that these lymphocytes have a T_H2 phenotype. Activation of T cells via the CD28 coreceptor in a cytokine-rich environment without appropriate stimulation via the TCR may lead to the IL-4– and IFN-γ–producing cytokine profile found in the T cells in Hodgkin's tissues. Absence of IL-2 production is a characteristic not only of T_H2 cells but also of anergic cells, indicating that the lymphocytes also could be in a state of anergy. Lack of IL-2 production, the induction of a predominant T_H2 response, or the induction of anergy would each contribute to an ineffective immune response. Another factor involved in the lack of an effective immune response may be the cytokine TGF-β that is produced in an active form by Hodgkin and Reed-Sternberg cells and has potent immunosuppressive effects on T cells as well as a fibrosis-promoting effect. Interleukin-10, which is also produced by some Hodgkin and Reed-Sternberg cells, may also modulate the immune response toward a T_H2 type.

The production of the CC chemokine TARC by the Reed-Sternberg cells of the classical subtypes of Hodgkin's disease may also strongly contribute to the predominance of T_H2 cells in the lesions because TARC strongly binds to CCR4, a chemokine receptor that is expressed on activated T_H2 cells. In this manner, Reed-Sternberg cells are able to create a T_H2-type environment that benefits their own survival because it supports the proliferation of (abnormal) B cells and prevents the development of a cytotoxic immune response.

The TNF/TNFR superfamilies probably play an important role in Hodgkin's disease, as several members of these families, notably CD30, CD40, CD70, CD95, and also CD95L, are highly expressed on the Reed-Sternberg cells. Moreover, their natural ligands are expressed on the surrounding lymphocytes. A general feature of members of the TNF/TNFR family is their involvement in cell activation and/or apoptosis, and therefore, they may play a crucial role in improper activation of the lymphocytes. Unequal susceptibility of lymphocyte subpopulations to Fas-mediated cell death could result in absence of effector cells such as $CD8^+$ T cells and NK cells, or appropriate helper cells such as T_H1 $CD4^+$ cells.

In conclusion, there are a range of factors present in Hodgkin's disease that may contribute to the paradox of an extensive inflammatory infiltrate and concomitant ineffectiveness of the host antitumor response as well as the generalized cellular immune deficiency in patients with active Hodgkin's disease.

REFERENCES

1. Sternberg C. Über einem eigenartige unter dem bilde der pseudoleukämie verlaufende tuberculose des lymphatischen apparates. *Z Heilkd* 1898;19:21.
2. Clarke JM. Discussion on lymphadenoma. *Br Med J* 1901;2:701.
3. Reed DM. On the pathological changes in Hodgkin's disease; with especial reference to its relation to tuberculosis. *Johns Hopkins Hosp Rep* 1902;10:133.
4. Longcope WT. On the pathological histology of Hodgkin's disease, with a report of a series of cases. *Bull Ayer Clin Lab Penn Hosp* 1903;1:1.
5. Hoster HA, Dratman MV, Craver LF, Rolnick HA. Hodgkin's disease 1832–1947. *Cancer Res* 1948;8:1,49.
6. Waldhauser A. Hodgkin's disease. *Arch Pathol* 1933;16:522,672.
7. Jackson H Jr, Parker F Jr. *Hodgkin's disease and allied disorders.* New York: Oxford University Press, 1947.
8. Harris NL, Jaffe ES, Stein H, et al. A revised European-American classification of lymphoid neoplasms: a proposal from the International Lymphoma Study Group. *Blood* 1994;84:1361.
9. Parker F, Jackson H, Green H, Spies Y. Studies of diseases of the lymphoid and myeloid tissues. IV. Skin reaction to human and avian tuberculin. *J Immunol* 1932;22:277.
10. Steiner PE. Etiology of Hodgkin's disease. *Arch Intern Med* 1934; 54:11.
11. Dubin IN. The poverty of the immunological mechanism in patients with Hodgkin's disease. *Ann Intern Med* 1947;27:898.
12. Schier WW, Roth A, Ostroff G, Schrift MH. Hodgkin's disease and immunity. *Am J Med* 1956;20:94.
13. Lamb D, Pilney F, Kelly WD, Good RA. A comparative study of the incidence of anergy in patients with carcinoma, leukemia, Hodgkin's disease and other lymphomas. *J Immunol* 1962;89:555.
14. Brown RS, Haynes HA, Foley HT, Godwin HA, Berard CW, Carbone PP. Hodgkin's disease. Immunologic, clinical and histologic features of 50 untreated patients. *Ann Intern Med* 1967;67:291.
15. Sokal JE, Primikirios M. The delayed skin test response in Hodgkin's disease and lymphosarcoma. *Cancer* 1961;14:597.
16. Ciampelli E, Pelu G. Compartamento dello intradermoreazione alla tubercolina nei pazienti affetti da morbo di Hodgkin trattati radiologicamente. *Radiol Med* 1963;48:683.
17. Armstrong D, Minamoto GY. Infectious complications of infections of Hodgkin's disease. In: Lacher MJ, Redmann JR, eds. *Hodgkin's disease: The consequences of survival.* Philadelphia: Lea & Febiger, 1990:151.
18. Bookman MA, Longo DL. Concomitant illness in patients treated for Hodgkin's disease. *Cancer Treat Rev* 1986;13:77.
19. Aisenberg AC. Studies on the delayed hypersensitivity in Hodgkin's disease. *J Clin Invest* 1962;41:1964.
20. Sokal JE, Primikirios A. The delayed skin test response in Hodgkin's disease and lymphosarcoma. *Cancer* 1961;14:597.
21. Aisenberg AC. Quantitative estimation of the reactivity of normal and Hodgkin's disease lymphocytes with thymidine-2-C^{14}. *Nature* 1965; 205:1233.
22. Hersh EM, Oppenheim JJ. Impaired *in vitro* lymphocyte transformation in Hodgkin's disease. *N Engl J Med* 1965;273:1006.

23. Clerici M, Ferrario E, Trabattoni D, et al. Multiple defects of T helper cell function in newly diagnosed patients with Hodgkin's disease. *Eur J Cancer* 1994;30A:1464.
24. Gaines JD, Gilmer MA, Remington JS. Deficiency of lymphocyte antigen recognition in Hodgkin's disease. *Natl Cancer Inst Monogr* 1973;36:117
25. Engleman EG, Benike CJ, Hoppe RT, Kaplan HS, Berberich FR. Autologous mixed lymphocyte reaction in patients with Hodgkin's disease. *J Clin Invest* 1980;66:149.
26. Bjorkholm M, Holm G, Mellstedt H, et al. Immunological capacity of lymphocytes with Hodgkin's disease evaluated in mixed lymphocyte culture. *Clin Exp Immunol* 1977;22:373.
27. Ford RJ, Tsao J, Kouttab NM, Sahasrabuddhe CG, Mehta SR. Association of an interleukin abnormality with the T cell defect in Hodgkin's disease. *Blood* 1984;64:386.
28. Longmire RL, McMillan R, Yelenosky R, Armstrong S, Lang JE, Craddock CG. *In vitro* splenic IgG synthesis in Hodgkin's disease. *N Engl J Med* 1973;289:763.
29. Huber C, Michlmayr G, Falkensamer M, et al. Increased proliferation of T lymphocytes in the blood of patients with Hodgkin's disease. *Clin Exp Immunol* 1973;21:47.
30. Amlot PL, Slaney J. Hypergammaglobulinaemia E in Hodgkin's disease and its relationship to atopy or a familial predisposition to atopy. *Int Arch Allergy Appl Immunol* 1981;64:138
31. Renner C, Ohnesorge S, Held G, et al. T cells from patients with Hodgkin's disease have a defective T-cell receptor chain expression that is reversible by T-cell stimulation with CD3 and CD28. *Blood* 1996;88:236.
32. Gruss H-J, Pinto A, Duyster J, Poppema S. Hodgkin's disease: a tumor with disturbed immunological pathways. *Immunol Today* 1997;18:156.
33. Gause A, Jung W, Schmits R, et al. Soluble CD8, CD25 and CD30 antigens as prognostic markers in patients with untreated Hodgkin's lymphoma. *Ann Oncol* 1992;3:S49.
34. Nadali G, Vinante F, Chilosi M, Pizzolo G. Soluble molecules as biological markers in Hodgkin's disease. *Leuk Lymphoma* 1997;26 (suppl 1):99
35. Katay I, Wirnitzer U, Burrichter H, et al. L-428 cells derived from Hodgkin's disease produce E-rosette inhibiting factor. *Blood* 1990; 76:791.
36. Frisan T, Sjoberg J, Dolcetti R, et al. Local suppression of Epstein-Barr (EBV)-specific cytotoxicity in biopsies of EBV-positive Hodgkin's disease. *Blood* 1995;86:1493.
37. Dolcetti R, Frisan T, Sjoberg J, et al. Identification and characterization of an Epstein-Barr virus-specific T-cell response in the pathologic tissue of a patient with Hodgkin's disease. *Cancer Res* 1995;55:3675.
38. Khanna R, Burrows SR, Nichols J, Poulsen LM. Identification of cytotoxic T cell epitopes within Epstein-Barr virus (EBV) oncogene latent membrane protein 1 (LMP1): evidence for HLA A2 supertype-restricted immune recognition of EBV- infected cells by LMP-1 specific cytotoxic T lymphocytes. *Eur J Immunol* 1998;28:451.
39. Poppema S, Visser L. Epstein-Barr virus positivity in Hodgkin's disease does not correlate with HLA A2 negative phenotype. *Cancer* 1994;73:3059.
40. Bryden H, MacKenzie J, Andrew L, et al. Determination of HLA-A*02 antigen status in Hodgkin's disease and analysis of an HLA-A*02 restricted epitope of the Epstein-Barr virus LMP-2 protein. *Int J Cancer* 1997;72:614.
41. Poppema S, Visser L. Absence of HLA class I expression by Reed-Sternberg cells. *Am J Pathol* 1994;145:37.
42. Oudejans JJ, Jiwa NM, Kummer JA, et al. Analysis of major histocompatibility complex class I expression on Reed-Sternberg cells in relation to the cytotoxic T-cell response in Epstein-Barr virus-positive and -negative Hodgkin's disease. *Blood* 1996;87:3844.
43. Lee SP, Constandinou CM, Thomas WA, et al. Antigen presenting phenotype of Hodgkin Reed-Sternberg cells: analysis of the HLA class I processing pathway and the effects of interleukin-10 on Epstein-Barr virus-specific cytotoxic T-cell recognition. *Blood* 1998; 92:1020–1030.
44. Bjorkholm M, Holm G, De Faire U, Mellstedt H. Immunological defects in healthy twin siblings to patients with Hodgkin's disease. *Scand J Haematol* 1977;19:396.
45. Ricci M, Romagnani S. Immune status in Hodgkin's disease. In: Doria G, Eskol A, eds. *The immune system: function and therapy of dysfunction.* New York: Academic Press, 1980:105
46. Poppema S, Bhan AK, Reinherz EL, Posner MR, Schlossman SF. *In situ* immunologic characterization of cellular constituents in lymph nodes and spleens involved by Hodgkins's disease. *Blood* 1982;59:226.
47. Romagnani S, Del Prete GF, Maggi E, et al. Displacement of T lymphocytes with the helper/inducer phenotype from peripheral blood to lymphoid organs in untreated patients with Hodgkin's disease. *Scand J Haematol* 1983;31:305.
48. Lavender P, Goldman JM, Arnot RN, Thakur ML. Kinetics of indium-111 labeled lymphocytes in normal subjects and patients with Hodgkin's disease. *Br Med J* 1977;2:797
49. Oudejans JJ, Jiwa NM, Kummer JA, et al. Activated cytotoxic T cells as prognostic marker in Hodgkin's disease. *Blood* 1997;89:1376.
50. Poppema S. Immunology of Hodgkin's disease. *Baillieres Clin Haematol* 1996;9:447.
51. Poppema S. The nature of the lymphocytes surrounding Reed-Sternberg cells in nodular lymphocyte predominance and in other types of Hodgkin's disease. *Am J Pathol* 1989;135:351.
52. Poppema S, Hepperle B. Restricted V gene usage in T-cell lymphomas as detected by anti-T-cell receptor variable region reagents. *Am J Pathol* 1991;138:1479.
53. Rubin B, Martin EPG, Arnaud J, et al. Expression and signal transduction of T-cell antigen receptor (TCR)/CD3 complexes on fresh or *in vitro* expanded T lymphocytes from patients with Hodgkin's and non-Hodgkin's lymphomas. *Scand J Immunol* 1997;45:715.
54. Morimoto C, Schlossman SF. CD26 a key costimulatory molecule on CD4 memory T cells. *Immunologists* 1994;2:4.
55. Fleischer B. CD26: a surface protease involved in T-cell activation. *Immunol Today* 1997;15:180.
56. Poppema S, Lai R, Visser L, Yan XJ. CD45 (leucocyte common antigen) expression in T and B lymphocyte subsets. *Leuk Lymphoma* 1995;20:217.
57. Mosmann TR Cherwinski H, Bond MW, Giedlin MA Coffman RL. Two types of helper T cell clone. I. Definition according to profiles of lymphokine activities and secreted proteins. *J Immunol* 1986;136:2348.
58. Gorschluter M, Bohlen H, Hasenclever D, Diehl V, Tesch H. Serum cytokine levels correlate with clinical parameters in Hodgkin's disease. *Ann Oncol* 1995;6:477.
59. Poppema S, Visser L, De Leij L. Reactivity of presumed anti–natural killer cell antibody Leu 7 with intrafollicular T lymphocytes. *Clin Exp Immunol* 1983;54:834.
60. Yoshimoto T, Bendelac A, Hu-Li J, Paul WE. Defective IgE production by SJL mice is linked to the absence of $CD4^+$, $NK1.1^+$ T cells that promptly produce interleukin 4. *Proc Natl Acad Sci USA* 1995;92: 11931.
61. Butch AW, Chung G, Hoffmann JW, Nahm MH. Cytokine expression by germinal center cells. *J Immunol* 1997;150:39.
62. Brinkmann V, Kristofic C. Massive production of Th2 cytokines by human $CD4^+$ effector T cells transiently expressing the natural killer cell marker CD57/HNK1. *Immunology* 1997;91:541.
63. Vollenweider L, Lazzarato M, Groscurth P. Proliferation of IL-2 activated lymphocytes preferably occurs in aggregates by cells expressing the CD57 antigen. *Scand J Immunol* 1995;42:381.
64. Fox DA, Hussey RE, Fitzgerald KA, et al. Ta_1, a novel 105 kD human T cell activation antigen defined by a monoclonal antibody. *J Immunol* 1984;133:1250.
65. Mattern T, Scholz W, Feller AC, Flad H-D, Ulmer AJ. Expression of CD26 (dipeptidyl peptidase IV) on resting and activated human T lymphocytes. *Scand J Immunol* 1991;33:737
66. Kameoka J, Tanaka T, Nojima Y, Schlossman SF, Morimoto C. Direct association of adenosine deaminase with a T cell activation antigen, CD26. *Science* 1993;261:466–469.
67. Torimoto T, Dang NH, Vivier E, Tanaka T, Schlossman SF, Morimoto C. Coassociation of CD26 (dipeptidyl peptidase IV) with CD45 on the surface of human T lymphocytes. *J Immunol* 1991;147:2514–2517.
68. Sloan-Lancaster J, Evavold BD, Allen PM. Induction of T cell anergy by altered T-cell receptor ligand on live antigen-presenting cells. *Nature* 1993;363:156.
69. Schwarz RH. Models of T cell anergy: Is there a common molecular mechanism? *J Exp Med* 1996;184:1.
70. Tsiagbe VK, Yoshimoto T, Asakawa J, Cho SY, Meruelo D, Thorbecke GJ. Linkage of superantigen-like stimulation of syngeneic T cells in a mouse model of follicular center cell B cell lymphoma to transcription of endogenous mammary tumor virus. *EMBO J* 1993;12:2313.
71. Groux H, Bigler M, de Vries JE, Roncarolo M. Interleukin-10 induces a long-term antigen-specific anergic state in human $CD4^+$ T cells. *J Exp Med* 1996;184:19.

72. Kehrl JH, Wakefield LM, Roberts AB, et al. Production of transforming growth factor beta by human T lymphocytes and its potential role in the regulation of T cell growth. *J Exp Med* 1986;163:1037.
73. Munro JM, Freedman AS, Aster JC, et al. *In vivo* expression of the B7 costimulatory molecule by subsets of antigen-presenting cells and the malignant cells of Hodgkin's disease. *Blood* 1994;83:793.
74. Hsu S, Waldron JW, Hsu P, Hough J. Cytokines in malignant lymphomas: Review and prospective evaluation. *Hum Pathol* 1993;24: 1040.
75. Kadin ME, Agnarsson BA, Ellingsworth LR, Newcom SR. Immunohistochemical evidence of a role for transforming growth factor beta in the pathogenesis of nodular sclerosing Hodgkin's disease. *Am J Pathol* 1990;136:1209.
76. Bargou RC, Emmerich F, Krappmann D, et al. Constitutive nuclear factor-κB-RelA activation is required for proliferation and survival of Hodgkin's disease tumor cells. *J Clin Invest* 1997;100:2961.
77. Ohshima K, Suzumiya J, Akamatu M, Takeshita M, Kikuchi M. Human and viral interleukin-10 in Hodgkin's disease, and its influence on $CD4^+$ and $CD8^+$ T lymphocytes. *Int J Cancer* 1995;62:5.
78. Hsu S-M, Lin J, Xie S-S, Hsu P-L, Rich S. Abundant expression of transforming growth factor-β1 and -β2 by Hodgkin's Reed-Sternberg cells and by reactive T lymphocytes in Hodgkin's disease. *Hum Pathol* 1993;24:249.
79. Newcom SR, Kadin ME, Ansari AA. Production of transforming growth factor-beta activity by Ki-1 positive lymphoma cells and analysis of its role in the regulation of Ki-1 positive lymphoma growth. *Am J Pathol* 1988;131:569.
80. Reinhold D, Bank U, Bühling F, et al. Transforming growth factor-β1 (TGF-β1) inhibits DNA synthesis of PMW-stimulated PBMC via suppression of IL-2 and IL-6 production. *Cytokine* 1994;6:382.
81. Potters M, Diepstra A, Meulenaar R, Visser L, Poppema S. The absence of effective T-cell activation in Hodgkin's disease may be the result of TGF-β production by Reed-Sternberg cells (abstract). *Blood* 1997;10:265b.
82. Newcom SR, Kadin ME, Ansari AA, Diehl V. L-428 nodular sclerosing Hodgkin's cell secrete a unique transforming growth factor-beta active at physiologic pH. *J Clin Invest* 1988;82:1915.
83. Lawrence DA. Transforming growth factor-β: a general review. *Eur Cytokine Netw* 1996;7:363.
84. Newcom SR, Tagra KK. High molecular weight transforming growth factor β is excreted in the urine in active nodular sclerosing Hodgkin's disease. *Cancer Res* 1992;52:6768.
85. Schwab U, Stein H, Gerdes J, et al. Production of a monoclonal antibody specific for Hodgkin and Sternberg-Reed cells of Hodgkin's disease and a subset of normal lymphoid cells. *Nature* 1982;299:65.
86. Pinto A, Aldinucci D, Gloghini A, et al. The role of eosinophils in the pathobiology of Hodgkin's disease. *Ann Oncol* 1997;8(Suppl 2):89.
87. Smith CA, Farrah T, Goodwin RG. The TNF receptor superfamily of cellular and viral proteins: activation, costimulation, and death. *Cell* 1994;76:959.
88. Gruss H-J, Pinto A, Gloghini A, et al. CD30 ligand expression in nonmalignant and Hodgkin's disease-involved lymphoid tissues. *Am J Pathol* 1996;149:469.
89. Carbone A, Gloghini A, Gruss H, Pinto A. CD40 ligand is constitutively expressed in a subset of T cell lymphomas and on the microenvironmental reactive T cells of follicular lymphomas and Hodgkin's disease. *Am J Pathol* 1995;147:912.
90. Grewal I, Flavell RA. A central role of CD40 ligand in the regulation of $CD4^+$ T-cell responses. *Immunol Today* 1996;17:410.
91. Abbas AK. Die and let live: eliminating dangerous lymphocytes. *Cell* 1996;84:655.
92. Zhang X, Brunner T, Carter L, et al. Unequal death in T helper cell (Th)1 and Th2 effectors: Th1, but not Th2, effectors undergo rapid Fas/FasL-mediated apoptosis. *J Exp Med* 1997;185:1837.
93. Varadhachary AS, Perdow SN, Hu C, Ramanarayanan M, Salgame P. Differential ability of T cell subsets to undergo activation-induced cell death. *Proc Natl Acad Sci USA* 1997;94:5778.
94. Walker PS, Saas P, Dietrich PY. Role of Fas ligand (CD95L) in immune escape: the tumor cell strikes back. *J Immunol* 1997;158:4521.
95. Poppema S, Potters M, Visser L, van den Berg JS. Immune escape mechanisms in Hodgkin's disease. *Ann Oncol* (in press).
96. Baba M, Imai T, Yoshida T, Yoshie O. Constitutive expression of various chemokine genes in human T-cell lines infected with human T-cell leukemia virus type 1: role of the viral transactivator Tax. *Int J Cancer* 1996;66:124.
97. Imai T, Yoshida T, Baba M, Nishimura M, Kakizaki M, Yoshie O. Molecular cloning of a novel T-cell directed CC chemokine expressed in thymus by signal sequence trap using Epstein-Barr virus vector. *J Biol Chem* 1996;271:21514.
98. Imai T, Baba M, Nishimura M, Kazizaki M, Takagi S, Yoshie O. The T-cell directed CC-chemokine TARC is a highly specific ligand for CC chemokine receptor 4. *J Biol Chem* 1997;272:15036.
99. Bonecchi R, Bianchi G, Bordignon PP, et al. Differential expression of chemokine receptors and chemotactic responsiveness of type 1 T helper cells (Th1s) and Th2s. *J Exp Med* 1998;187:129.
100. Sallusto F, Lenig D,Mackay CR, Lanzavecchia A. Flexible programs of chemokine receptor expression on human polarized T helper 1 and 2 lymphocytes. *J Exp Med* 1998;187:875.
101. Loetscher P, Uguccioni M, Bordoli L, Baggiolini M, Moser B. CCR5 is characteristic of TH1 lymphocytes. *Nature* 1998;391:344.

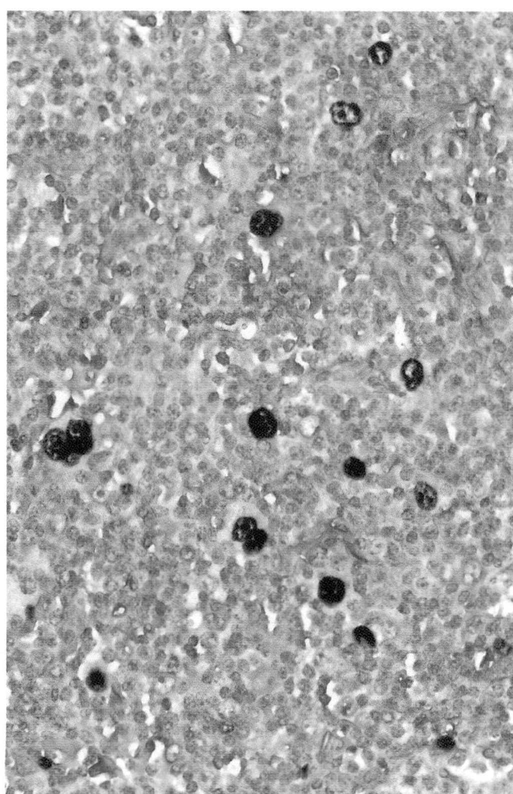

PLATE 1. Epstein-Barr viral (EBV) gene expression in Reed-Sternberg cells. Polymerase III transcript (EBER) in situ hybridization. (This plate is printed in black and white as Figure 6-5A.)

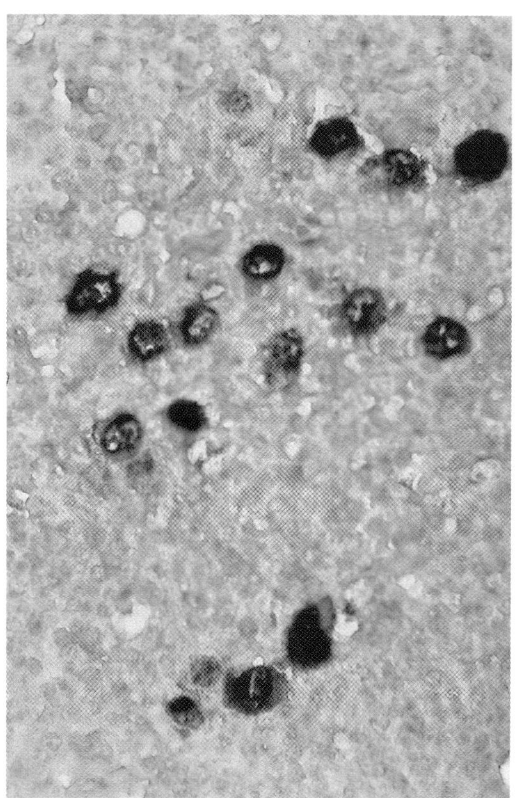

PLATE 2. Epstein-Barr viral (EBV) gene expression in Reed-Sternberg cells. EBER *in situ* hybridization with CD15 labeling of Hodgkin's cells. (This plate is printed in black and white as Figure 6-5B.)

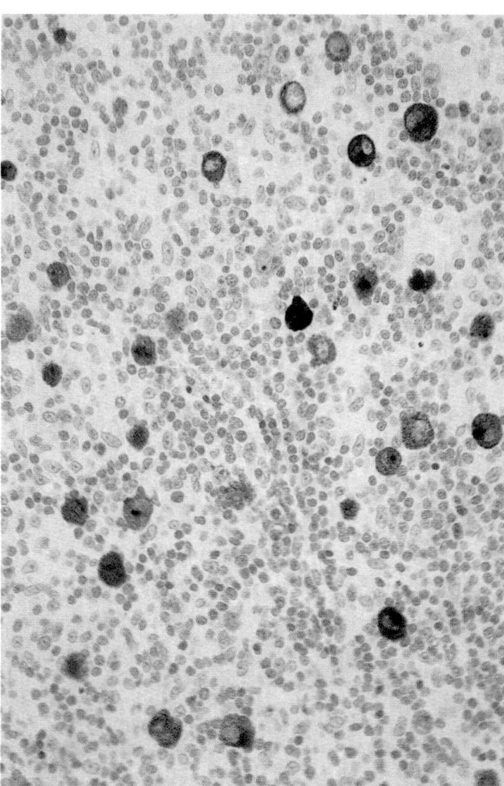

PLATE 3. Epstein-Barr viral (EBV) gene expression in Reed-Sternberg cells. Latent membrane protein 1 (LMP1) immunohistochemistry. (This plate is printed in black and white as Figure 6-5C.)

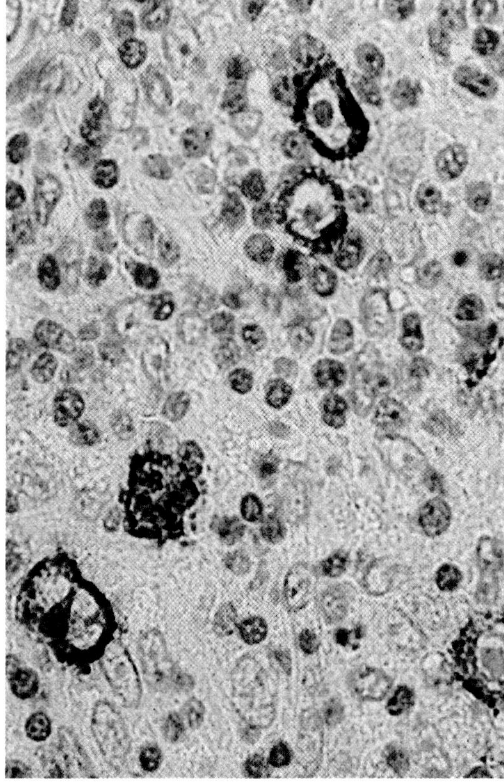

PLATE 4. Epstein-Barr viral (EBV) gene expression in Reed-Sternberg cells. Latent membrane protein 2 (LMP2) immunohistochemistry. (This plate is printed in black and white as Figure 6-5D.)

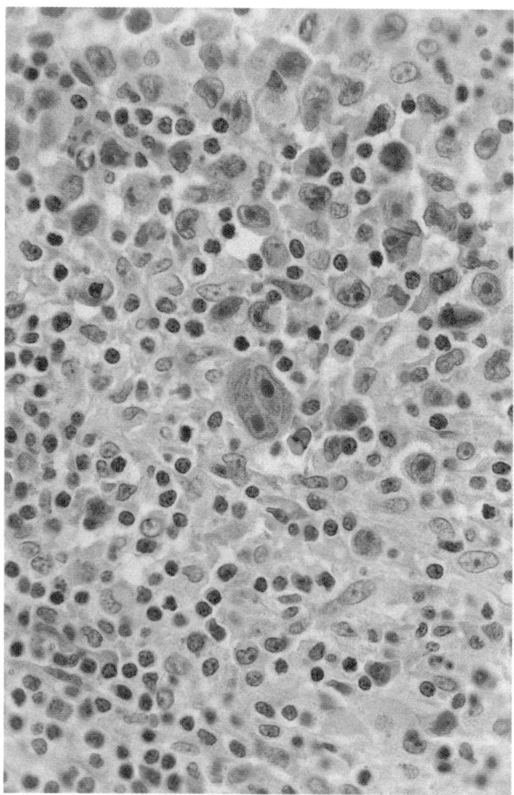

PLATE 5. A diagnostic Reed-Sternberg cell with two nuclei is seen in the center, with a prominent eosinophilic nucleolus present in each nucleus. There is some chromatin clearing around each nucleolus. Several mononuclear Reed-Sternberg variants are also present in the bottom half of the field. (This plate is printed in black and white as Figure 7-1.)

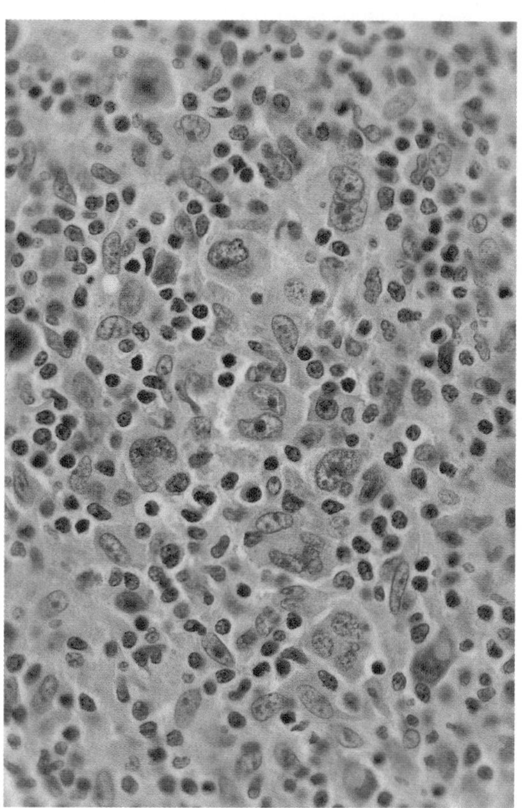

PLATE 6. A diagnostic Reed-Sternberg cell is seen in the center, and many mononucleated and multinucleated Reed-Sternberg variants are seen throughout the field. (This plate is printed in black and white as Figure 7-2.)

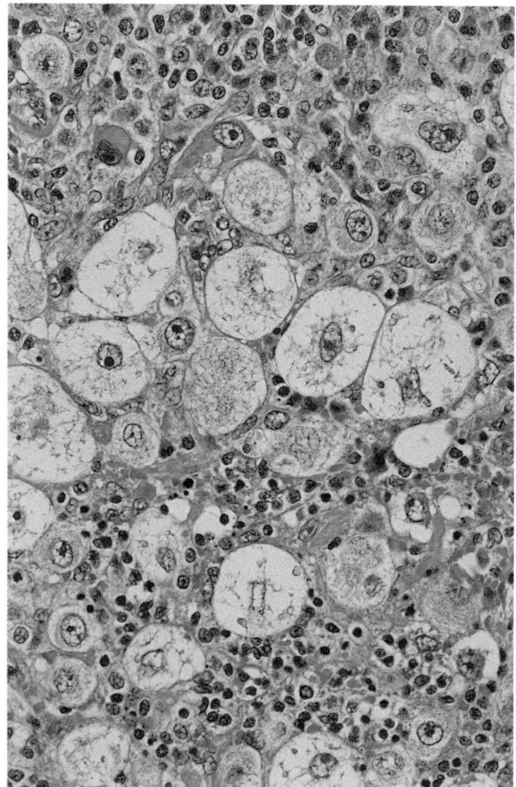

PLATE 7. Several lacunar cells are present. A "mummified" Reed-Sternberg cell is in the upper left corner. (This plate is printed in black and white as Figure 7-3.)

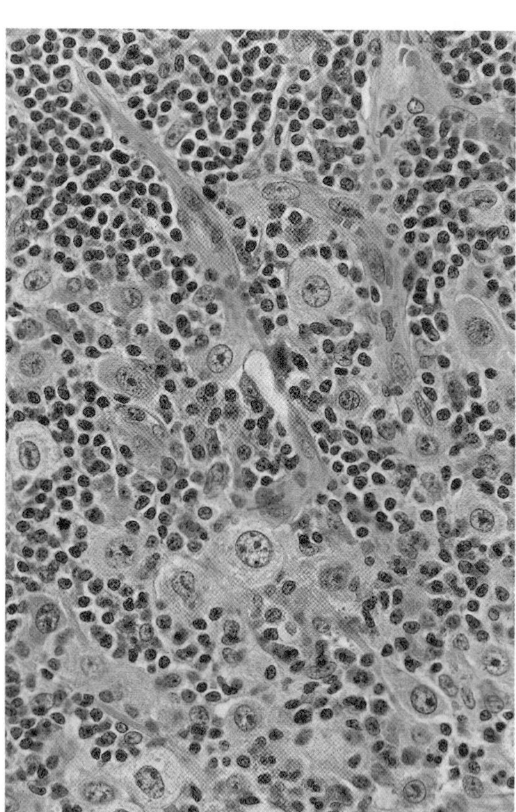

PLATE 8. The background cells consist predominantly of small lymphocytes, along with scattered eosinophils, histiocytes, and plasma cells. (This plate is printed in black and white as Figure 7-4.)

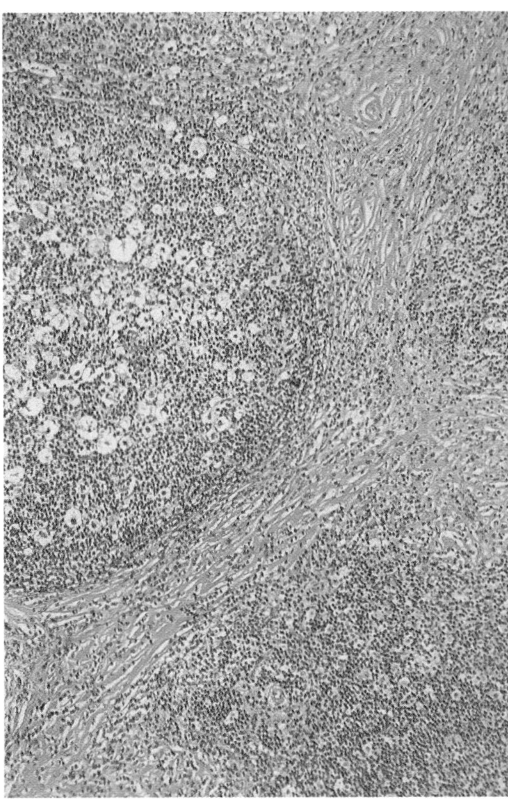

PLATE 9. Nodular sclerosis Hodgkin's disease. Broad bands of fibrosis separate several nodules. (This plate is printed in black and white as Figure 7-5.)

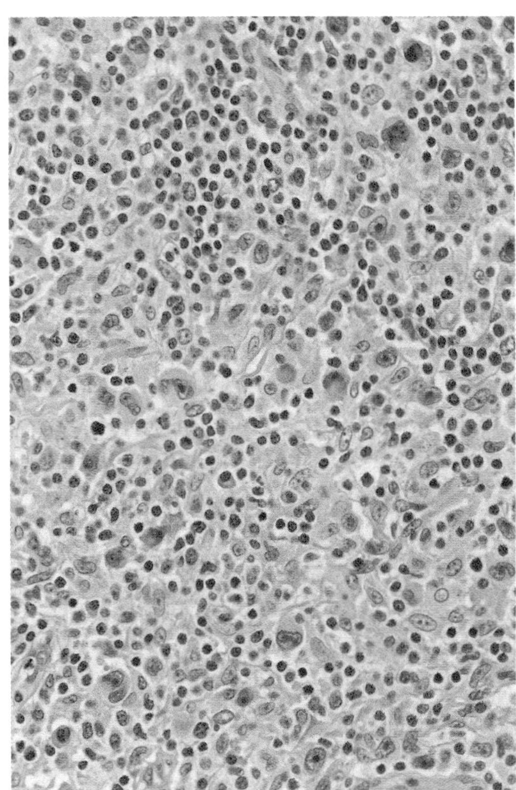

PLATE 10. Mixed cellularity Hodgkin's disease. There is an absence of fibrous bands. (This plate is printed in black and white as Figure 7-6.)

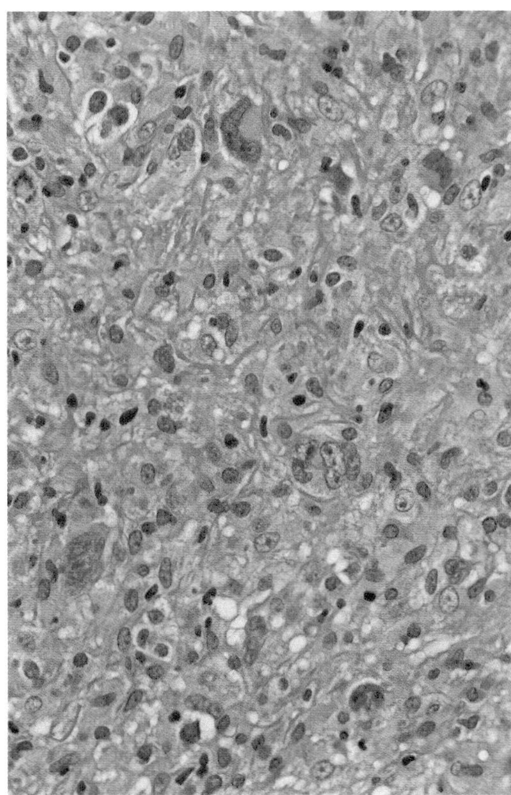

PLATE 11. Lymphocyte depletion, diffuse fibrosis type. There is a reticulin collagen fibrosis around single cells. Although the Hodgkin's cells appear atypical, results of immunophenotyping studies were characteristic of Hodgkin's disease in this case. (This plate is printed in black and white as Figure 7-7.)

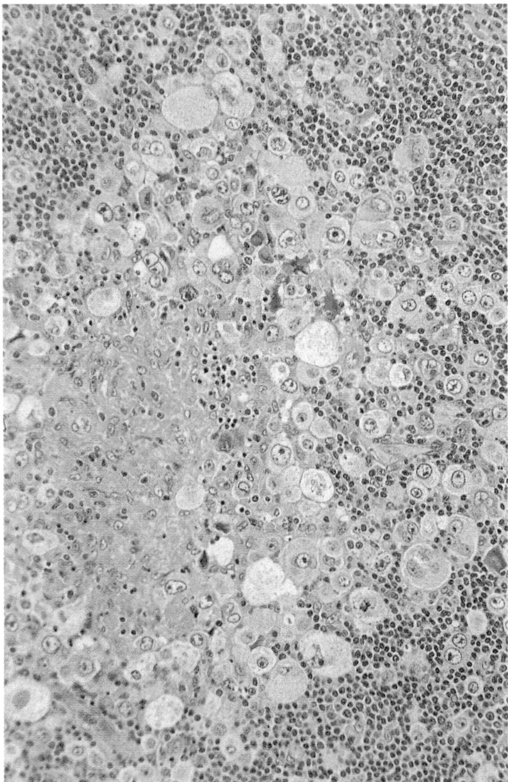

PLATE 12. Syncytial form of nodular sclerosis Hodgkin's disease; sheets of lacunar cells are clustered around a central area of necrosis. (This plate is printed in black and white as Figure 7-8.)

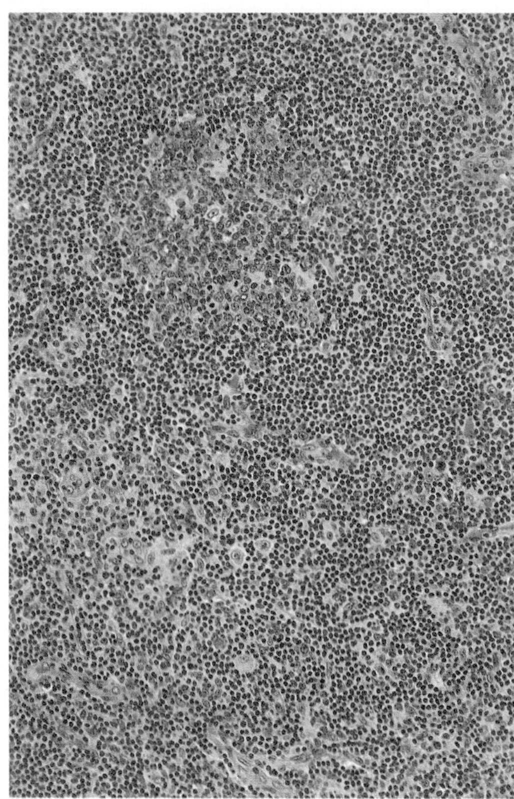

PLATE 13. Interfollicular Hodgkin's disease. At the top is a reactive follicle. Several Hodgkin's cells are seen in the interfollicular region in the bottom half of the field. (This plate is printed in black and white as Figure 7-9.)

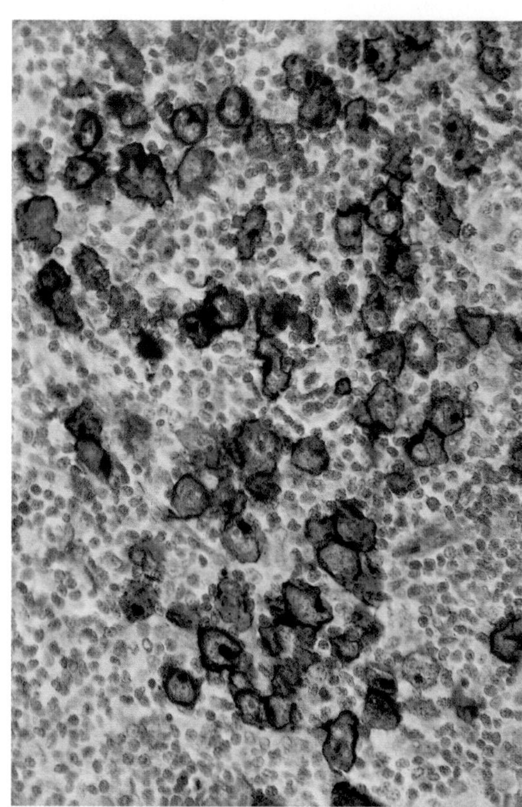

PLATE 14. Immunostaining for CD30. There is strong membrane and paranuclear staining, and weaker cytoplasmic staining, of the Hodgkin's cells. (This plate is printed in black and white as Figure 7-10.)

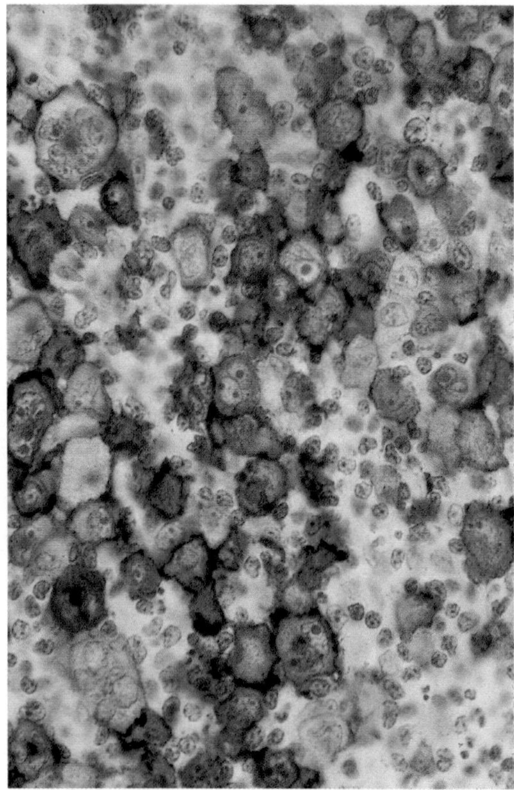

PLATE 15. Immunostaining for CD15. There is strong membrane and paranuclear staining of the Hodgkin's cells. (This plate is printed in black and white as Figure 7-11.)

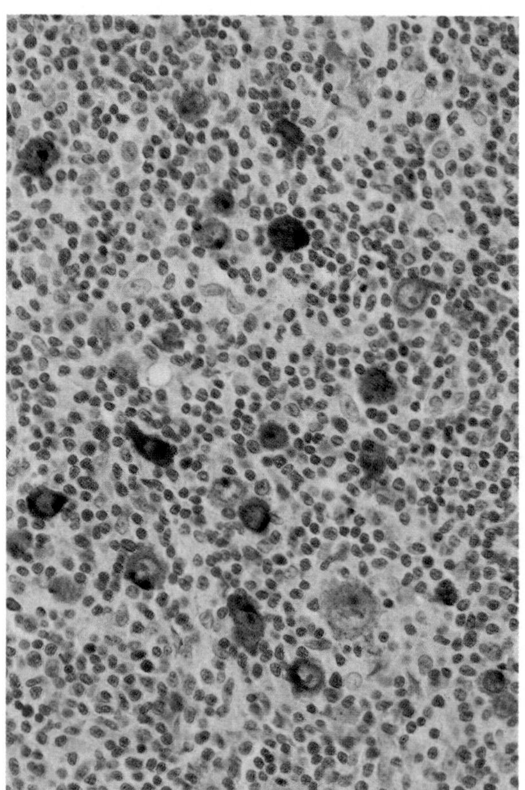

PLATE 16. Immunostaining for Epstein-Barr virus (EBV) latent membrane protein (LMP) in a case of EBV-associated Hodgkin's disease. There is strong cytoplasmic staining, with paranuclear accentuation in the Hodgkin's cells. EBV- small lymphocytes do not stain for LMP in Hodgkin's disease. (This plate is printed in black and white as Figure 7-12.)

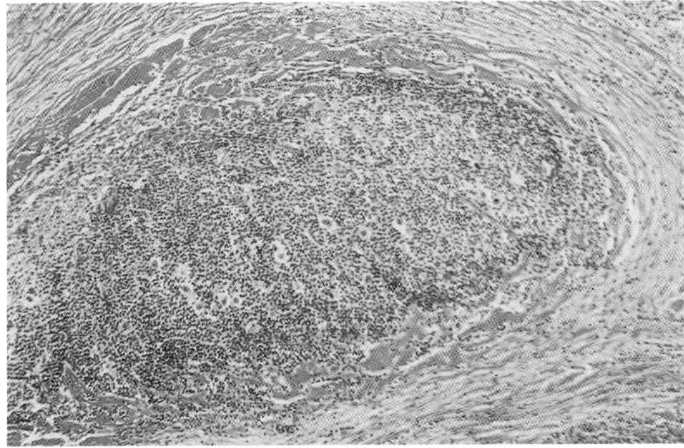

PLATE 17. Cytokine expression in Hodgkin's disease, nodular sclerosing type. Nodule containing Hodgkin–Reed-Sternberg cells surrounded by dense collagen bands (H&E stain). (This plate is printed in black and white as Figure 9-2A.)

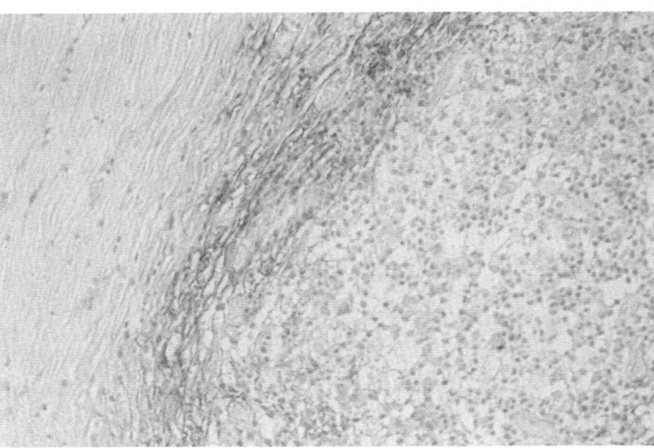

PLATE 18. Cytokine expression in Hodgkin's disease, nodular sclerosing type. Immunohistochemical stain for TGF-β1 decorating collagen fibers surrounding lymphoid nodule. (This plate is printed in black and white as Figure 9-2B.)

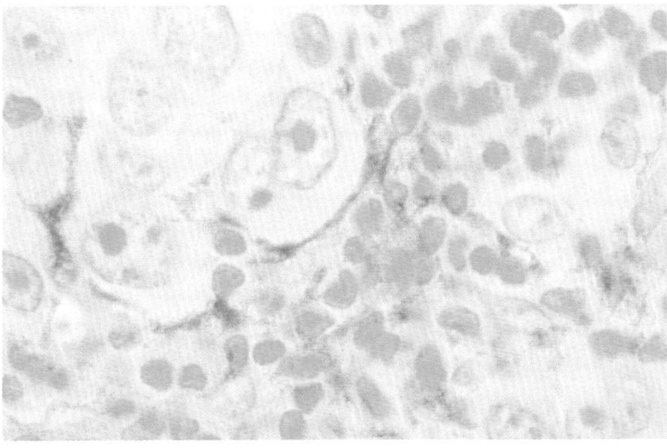

PLATE 19. Cytokine expression in Hodgkin's disease, nodular sclerosing type. TGF-β1 on surface of Hodgkin–Reed-Sternberg cells. (This plate is printed in black and white as Figure 9-2C.)

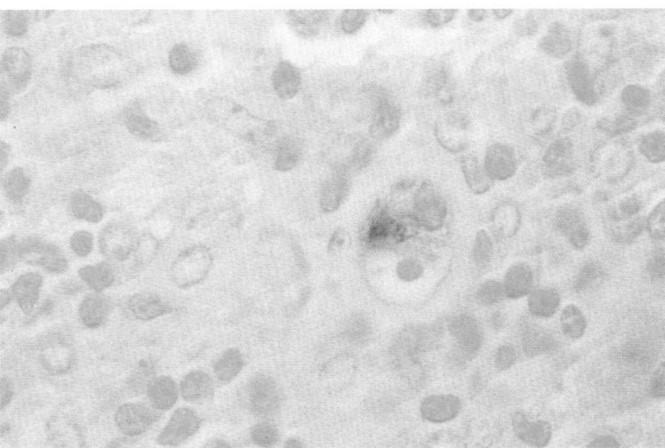

PLATE 20. Cytokine expression in Hodgkin's disease, nodular sclerosing type. within cytoplasm of Reed-Sternberg cell. (This plate is printed in black and white as Figure 9-2D.)

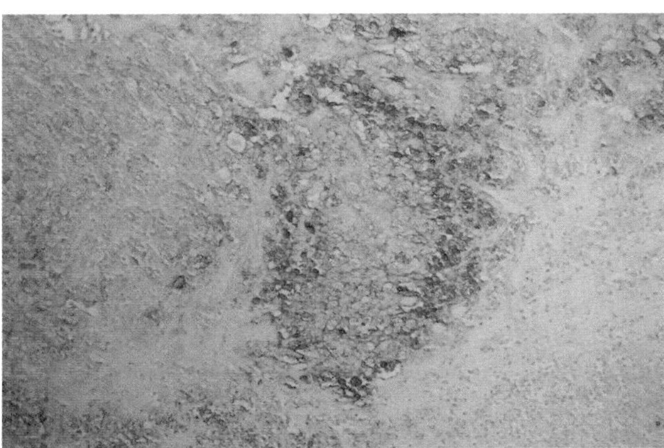

PLATE 21. Cytokine expression in Hodgkin's disease, nodular sclerosing type. CD40 expressed on surface of Hodgkin–Reed-Sternberg cells concentrated at the periphery of abnormal lymphoid nodule. (This plate is printed in black and white as Figure 9-2E.)

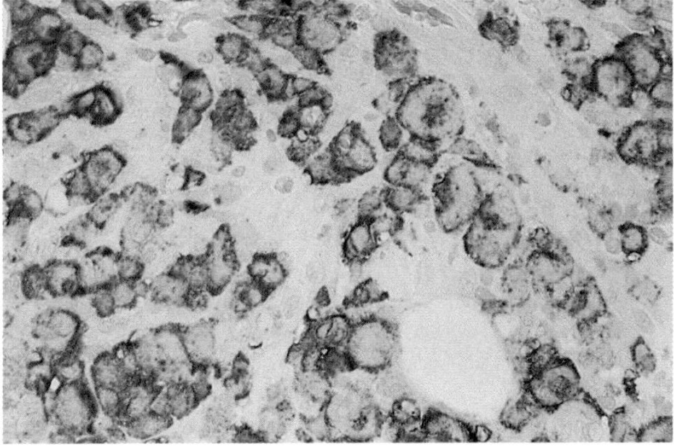

PLATE 22. Immunohistochemical demonstration of a subunit of IL-2 receptor (IL-2Rα) in CD30- cutaneous anaplastic large-cell lymphoma (ALCL). Virtually all tumor cells stain for IL-2Rα in ALCL. Reproduced with permission from ref. 25. (This plate is printed in black and white as Figure 9-3A.)

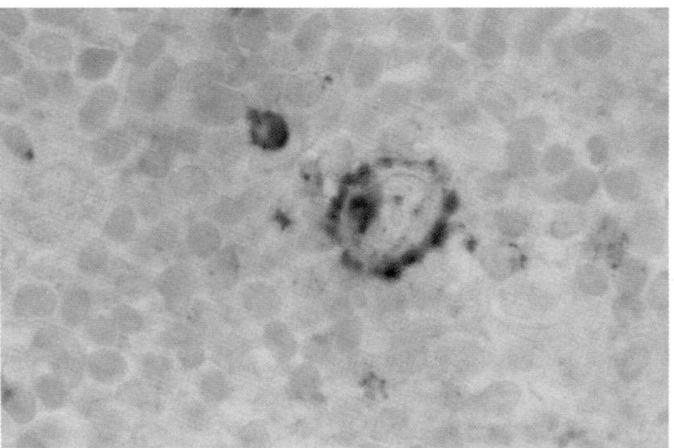

PLATE 23. Immunohistochemical demonstration of a subunit of IL-2 receptor (IL-2Rα) in Hodgkin's disease. A large Reed-Sternberg cell shows cytoplasmic and surface staining. Reproduced with permission from ref. 25. (This plate is printed in black and white as Figure 9-3B.)

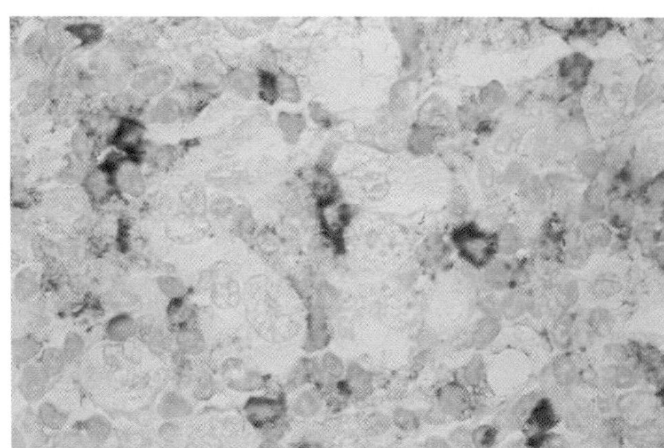

PLATE 24. Immunohistochemical demonstration of a subunit of IL-2 receptor (IL-2Rα) in Hodgkin's disease. Only small lymphocytes around Hodgkin–Reed-Sternberg cells are stained for IL-2Rα. Reproduced with permission from ref. 25. (This plate is printed in black and white as Figure 9-3C.)

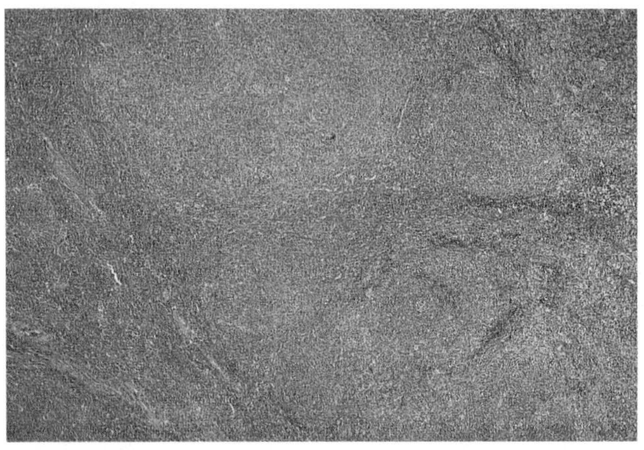

PLATE 25. Nodular lymphocyte predominance Hodgkin's disease showing large irregular nodules, which are closely packed (hematoxylin and eosin). (This plate is printed in black and white as Figure 11-1A.)

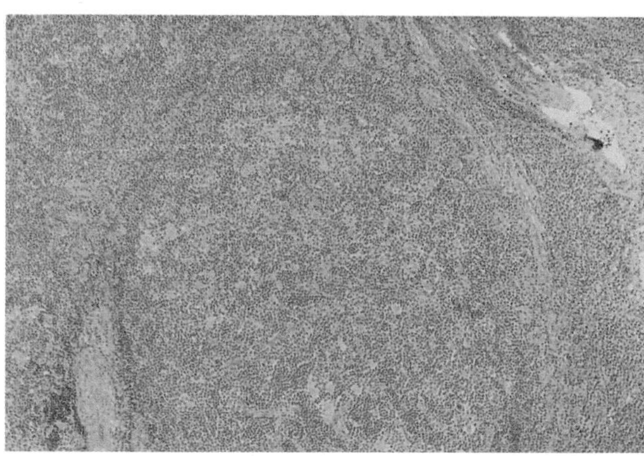

PLATE 26. A nodule of nodular lymphocyte predominance Hodgkin's disease is shown, composed mostly of small lymphocytes with scattered epithelioid histiocytes (hematoxylin and eosin). (This plate is printed in black and white as Figure 11-1B.)

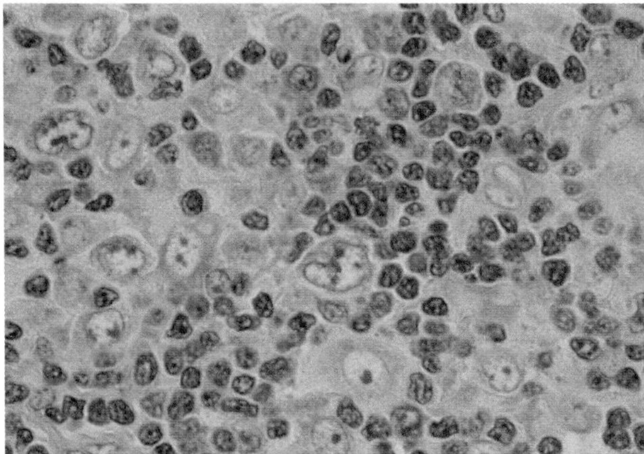

PLATE 27. High magnification, showing characteristic L&H or "popcorn" cells (Giemsa stain). (This plate is printed in black and white as Figure 11-2.)

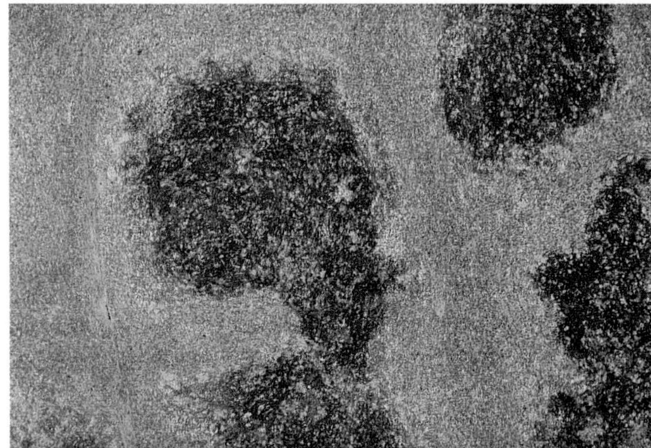

PLATE 28. Follicular dendritic cells form large networks in nodular lymphocyte predominance Hodgkin's disease (immuno–alkaline phosphatase, CD21). (This plate is printed in black and white as Figure 11-3.)

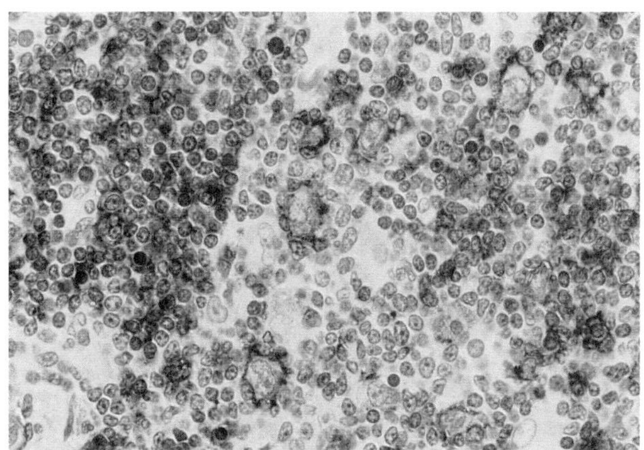

PLATE 29. In addition to small lymphocytes, several L&H cells show a membrane-bound immunoreaction for CD20 (immuno–alkaline phosphatase). (This plate is printed in black and white as Figure 11-4.)

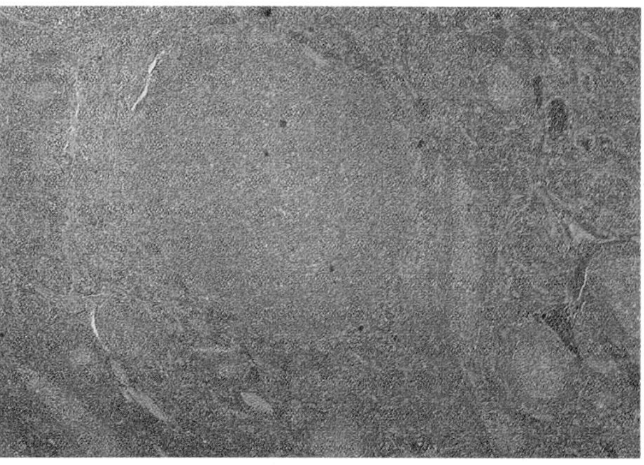

PLATE 30. A large progressively transformed germinal center is surrounded by several small germinal centers (Giemsa stain). (This plate is printed in black and white as Figure 11-5A.)

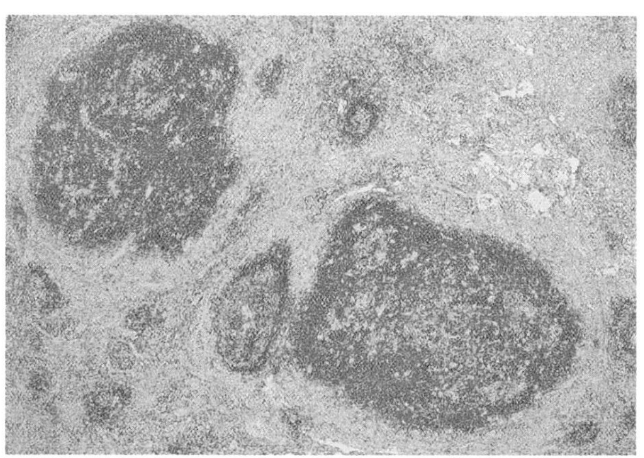

PLATE 31. The progressively transformed germinal centers are composed mainly of B cells, similar to the surrounding reactive follicles (immuno–alkaline phosphatase, CD20). (This plate is printed in black and white as Figure 11-5B.)

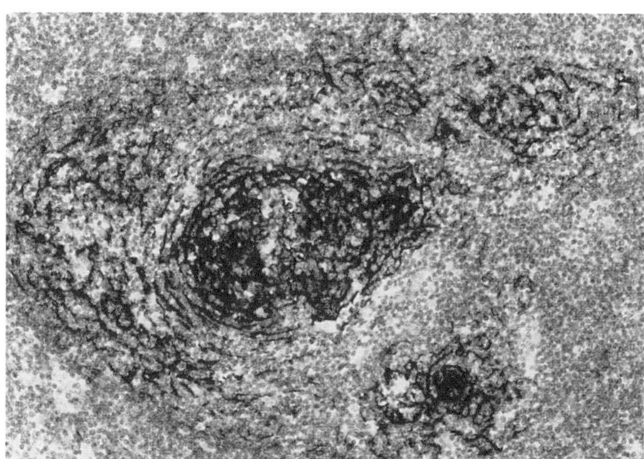

PLATE 32. Nodular infiltrate of lymphocyte-rich classical Hodgkin's disease. Eccentrically localized remnants of germinal centers are visualized by immunostaining for follicular dendritic cells (immuno–alkaline phosphatase, CD21). (This plate is printed in black and white as Figure 11-6.)

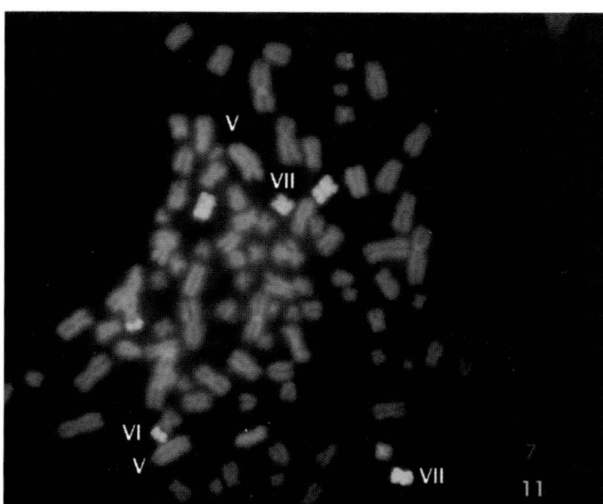

PLATE 33. Fluorescence in situ hybridization (FISH) with painting probes for chromosomes 7 *(red)* and 11 *(green)* in L-428. Markers V: duplication within the long arm of chromosome 7: dup(7)(q22q36); markers VII: deletion of the long arm of chromosome 11—del(11)(q14~21); marker VI: chromosome 11 material attached to the short arm of chromosome 9. (This plate is printed in black and white as Figure 14-4A.)

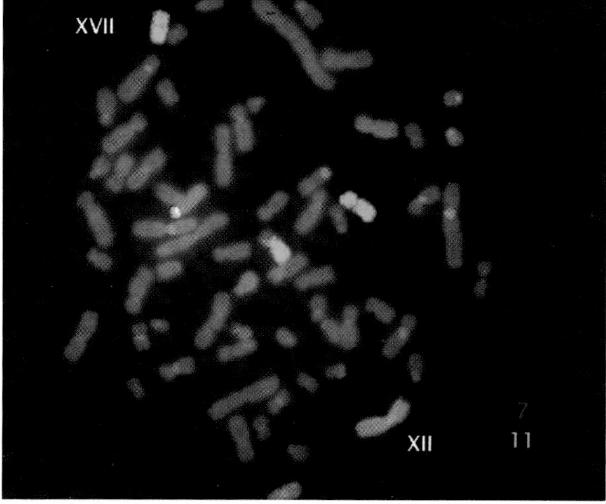

PLATE 34. Fluorescence in situ hybridization (FISH) with painting probes for chromosomes 7 *(red)* and 11 *(green)* in L-1236. Marker XII: attachment of 7q22-q36 to 7p22, leading to a duplication of this chromosome segment within marker XII; marker XVII: deletion of the long arm of chromosome 11—del(11)(q14~21). (This plate is printed in black and white as Figure 14-4B.)

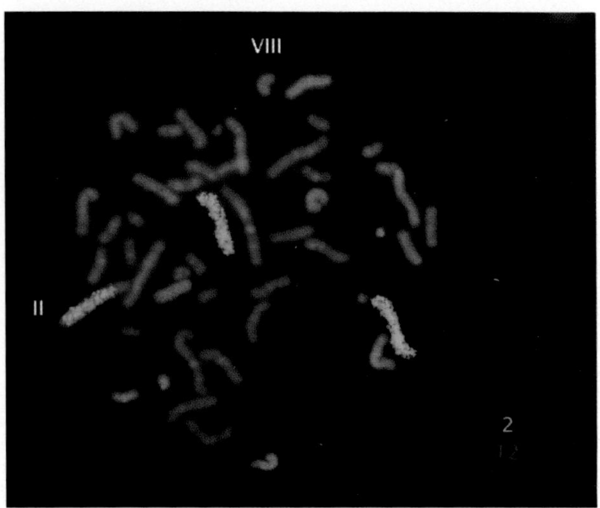

PLATE 35. FISH with painting probes for chromosomes 2 *(green)* and 12 *(red)* in L-428. Marker II: involvement of 2p23~25 in a chromosomal rearrangement, leading to elongation of 2p; marker VIII: deletion of the long arm of chromosome 12—del(12)(q15). (This plate is printed in black and white as Figure 14-5A.)

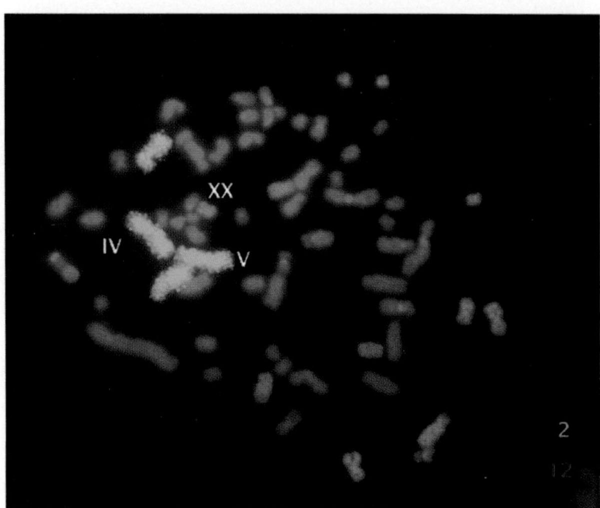

PLATE 36. FISH with painting probes for chromosomes 2 *(green)* and 12 *(red)* in L-1236. Markers IV and V: duplications within the short arm (p15 to p23) and the long arm (q33 to q37) of chromosome 2; marker XX: deletion of the long arm of chromosome 12—del(12)(q15). (This plate is printed in black and white as Figure 14-5B.)

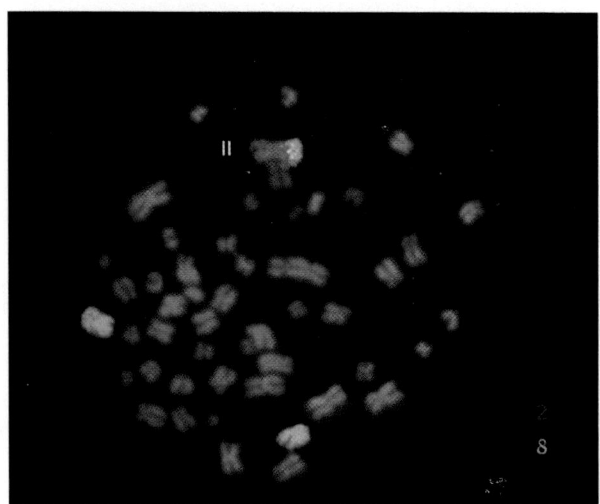

PLATE 37. FISH with painting probes for chromosomes 2 *(red)* and 8 *(green)* in L-428. Marker II: rearrangement between 2p23~25 and 8q13~21. (This plate is printed in black and white as Figure 14-6A.)

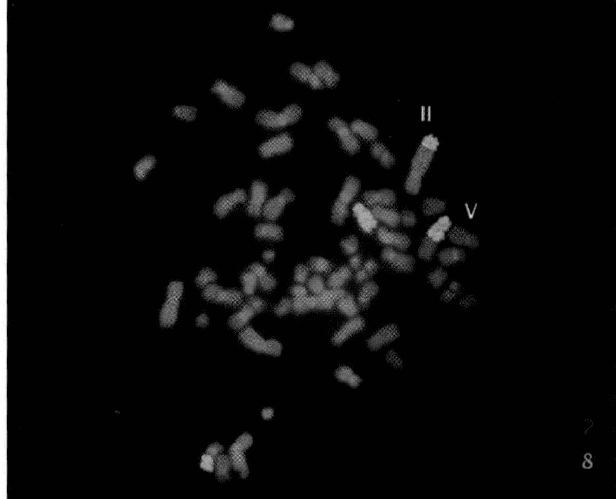

PLATE 38. FISH with painting probes for chromosomes 2 *(red)* and 8 *(green)* in L-540. Marker II: rearrangement between 2q37 and 8q13~21; marker V: involvement of 8q24 in a chromosomal rearrangement leading to elongation of 8q. (This plate is printed in black and white as Figure 14-6B.)

Hodgkin's Disease, edited by P. M. Mauch,
J. O. Armitage, V. Diehl, R. T. Hoppe, and L. M. Weiss.
Published by Lippincott Williams & Wilkins, Philadephia 1999.

CHAPTER 11

Pathology of Lymphocyte Predominance Hodgkin's Disease

Martin-Leo Hansmann, Lawrence M. Weiss, Harald Stein, Nancy Lee Harris, and Elaine S. Jaffe

HISTORICAL ASPECTS AND CURRENT CLASSIFICATION SYSTEMS

Rosenthal was the perhaps the first to call attention to the inverse relationship between the number of mature lymphocytes and the number of Reed-Sternberg cells in Hodgkin's disease (referred to as lymphogranulomatosis), suggesting that the lymphocyte-rich and Reed-Sternberg cell–poor forms of the disease responded well to radiotherapy and had the best survival (1). The earliest clear recognition of what we now call lymphocyte predominance Hodgkin's disease was by Jackson and Parker, who divided Hodgkin's disease into three subtypes: paragranuloma, granuloma, and sarcoma (2). Paragranuloma was originally termed early Hodgkin's disease by Jackson (3) but was renamed when it was recognized that this form of the disease could persist for many years. Paragranuloma characteristically showed only a few or no Hodgkin or Reed-Sternberg cells, many lymphocytes, and only a few or no eosinophilic granulocytes and plasma cells without fibrosis or necrosis; a nodular growth pattern was not specifically noted. Jackson and Parker described cases of paragranuloma that did not convert into granuloma during the clinical course and considered these cases to be a completely different disease from the other types of Hodgkin's disease (2). Similar findings were reported by other investigators, who used terms such as lymphoreticular medullary reticulosis (4), benign Hodgkin's disease (5), Hodgkin's disease grade I (6), reticular lymphoma (7), and indolent Hodgkin's disease (8). Meanwhile, Rappaport, in a study of follicular lymphoma, first called attention to a nodular variant of this disease (9).

In the Lukes and Butler classification, paragranuloma was divided into two types: lymphocytic and/or histiocytic (L&H), nodular and lymphocytic and/or histiocytic (L&H), diffuse (10,11). Lukes and Butler provided the most accurate and comprehensive descriptions yet, recognizing a Reed-Sternberg variant, the L&H cell, that differed in morphology from those of the other types of Hodgkin's disease. However, it was decided at Rye that the six-tiered classification of Lukes and Butler was too complex for clinical use, and it was simplified (12). In the Rye classification, four types of Hodgkin's disease were distinguished: lymphocyte predominance, nodular sclerosis, mixed cellularity, and lymphocyte depletion; lymphocyte predominance encompassed both types of L&H Hodgkin's disease.

Several years later, Lennert and Mohri pointed out that, in fact, lymphocyte predominance Hodgkin's disease was heterogeneous and could be subdivided into four subtypes: (a) nodular paragranuloma, (b) diffuse paragranuloma, (c) lymphocyte predominant other than paragranuloma (lymphocyte-rich mixed type), and (d) Hodgkin's disease showing partial involvement of lymph nodes (13). The nodular and diffuse forms of paragranuloma corresponded to the nodular and diffuse L&H forms of the Lukes and Butler classification, whereas subtype c (lymphocyte-rich mixed type) and subtype d (partial involve-

M.-L. Hansmann: Department of Pathology, University of Frankfurt, Frankfurt, Germany.

L. M. Weiss: Department of Pathology, City of Hope National Medical Center, Duarte, California.

H. Stein: Institute of Pathology, Universitätsklinikum Freier Universität Berlin, Berlin, Germany.

N. L. Harris: Department of Pathology, Harvard Medical School and Massachusetts General Hospital, Boston, Massachusetts.

E. S. Jaffe: Hematopathology Section, Department of Pathology, National Cancer Institute, National Institutes of Health, Bethesda, Maryland.

ment) seemed to be variants of classical Hodgkin's disease. These two variants contained a paucity of Hodgkin's and Reed-Sternberg cells, lacked L&H cells, and showed a high proportion of lymphocytes.

In the following years, numerous investigations focused on the nature of nodular and diffuse paragranuloma, providing overwhelming evidence that paragranuloma is a distinct entity, differing from all other types of Hodgkin's disease (14–17). Clinical, morphologic, and immunohistochemical findings gave support to this point of view. Patients with paragranuloma usually presented with an early stage at diagnosis and a relatively indolent course (16,18–20). Morphologic investigations, including ultrastructural studies, pointed out that paragranuloma showed features of B-cell neoplasia. The L&H cells had similar ultrastructural features to the centroblasts of germinal centers (17). In addition, follicular dendritic cells, characteristic of lymphoid follicles, could be detected in the neighborhood of L&H cells by electron microscopy. Immunohistochemical studies showed strong support for a B-cell lineage for L&H cells (Table 1) (17,21–23). Its frequent association with progressive transformation of germinal centers also suggested an association with lymphoid follicles (17).

The evolution of the concept that the nodular variant of lymphocyte predominance Hodgkin's disease represents a distinct clinicopathologic entity culminated in 1994 when a new classification of lymphoid neoplasia, called the Revised European-American Classification of Lymphoid Neoplasms (REAL classification), was proposed (24). In the REAL classification, Hodgkin's disease is subdivided into lymphocyte predominance, nodular with or without diffuse areas, and the forms of classical Hodgkin's disease: nodular sclerosis, mixed cellularity and lymphocyte-depletion types. In addition, a provisional entity termed lymphocyte rich classical Hodgkin's disease was included. Lymphocyte rich classical Hodgkin's disease encompasses the lymphocyte predominant mixed cellularity of Lennert and Mohri as well as "follicular" Hodgkin's disease as subsequently described by Ashton-Key et al. (13,25). Similarly, in the newly proposed WHO classification, there are separate categories for nodular lymphocyte predominance Hodgkin's disease (with or without diffuse areas) and lymphocyte-rich classical Hodgkin's disease, which may be nodular or diffuse.

In 1996, the European Task Force on Lymphoma *(publication in preparation)* performed a study of lymphocyte predominance Hodgkin's disease with the goal of clarifying the features that distinguish it from classical Hodgkin's disease, including lymphocyte-rich classical Hodgkin's disease (see Chapter 31). Immunohistochemical studies were shown to be of particular value in distinguishing true lymphocyte predominance Hodgkin's disease from other forms of Hodgkin's disease rich in small lymphocytes.

TABLE 1. *Morphologic, immunophenotypic, and genetic features of L&H cells vs. classical Hodgkin's cells*

	L&H cells	Hodgkin's cells
Nuclei	Polylobated	Mono- or binucleate
Nucleoli	Small to medium	Large
Classic Reed-Sternberg	Rare	Common
CD20	>95%	24% (97)
CD45	>95%	7% (98)
CD30	<5%	89% (99)
CD15	<5%	87% (100)
Epithelial membrane antigen	25–50%	5%
EBV-LMP	<1%	40–50%
In situ hybridization for light chains	Monotypic	—
Immunoglobulin genes rearranged	Clonal	Clonal
V region mutations	+	+
Productive rearrangements	+	–

HISTOPATHOLOGY

Nodular Lymphocyte Predominance Hodgkin's Disease, With or Without Diffuse Areas

At low magnification, the lymph node shows complete or subtotal effacement of the architecture. The capsule is usually intact without pericapsular infiltration, and there may be a rim of uneffaced lymphoid tissue, which may be normal or hyperplastic or may show progressive transformation of germinal centers. Fibrosis is uncommon but may be present and may be band-like; mimicking nodular sclerosis. In most cases, a nodular or a nodular and partly diffuse infiltration pattern is found in the effaced areas (Fig. 1a). The nodules are typically large and relatively numerous, sometimes resembling progressively transformed germinal centers (Fig. 1); they are typically closely packed, but in some cases the nodules are poorly demarcated and difficult to discern, and a diffuse architecture may be focally present. The existence of a purely diffuse form of nodular lymphocyte predominance is debated because, typically, some degree of nodularity is found when the entire lymph node is carefully examined. If a large number of well-prepared sections shows no evidence of nodularity, the possibility of either lymphocyte-rich classical Hodgkin's disease or T-cell–rich large B-cell lymphoma should be seriously considered. The diagnosis of diffuse lymphocyte predominance Hodgkin's disease should not be made on the basis of small biopsy specimens or without immunophenotyping.

A mixture of lymphocytes and histiocytes, particularly epithelioid histiocytes, is characteristic of nodular lymphocyte predominance Hodgkin's disease. Epithelioid

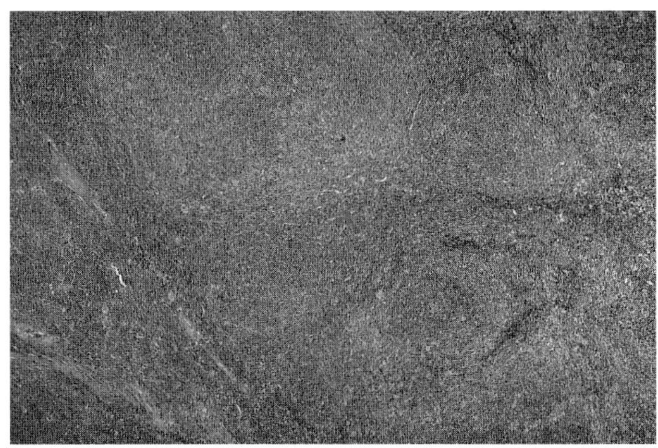
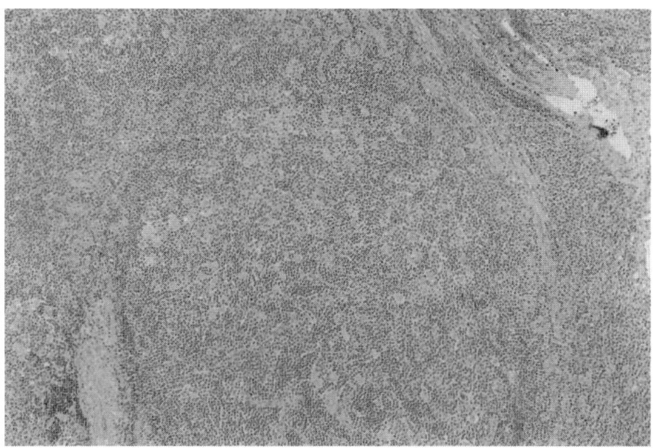

FIG. 1. A: Nodular lymphocyte predominance Hodgkin's disease showing large irregular nodules, which are closely packed (hematoxylin and eosin). **B:** A nodule of nodular lymphocyte predominance Hodgkin's disease is shown, composed mostly of small lymphocytes with scattered epithelioid histiocytes (hematoxylin and eosin). (These figures are printed in color as Plates 25 and 26.)

histiocytes are preferentially found in the outer rim of nodular infiltrates. They are arranged in small groups or clusters, and well-formed granulomas may be present in rare cases. Eosinophils and neutrophils are rare. Plasma cells are not common and are seen only between follicles.

The neoplastic cells of nodular lymphocyte predominance are the L&H cells (popcorn cells), usually found in and around the nodules (Fig. 2). In diffuse areas, the L&H cells are still often arranged in a vaguely nodular pattern. Characteristically, L&H cells resemble centroblasts but are larger and have lobulated nuclei and small to moderate-sized basophilic nucleoli, often present adjacent to the nuclear membrane (Fig. 2). The cytoplasm is broad and only slightly basophilic. Ultrastructural studies demonstrate that L&H cells have the appearance of centroblasts of germinal centers. In addition, follicular dendritic cells characteristic of the B-cell follicle can be found in the vicinity of the L&H cells (17,27). Classical Hodgkin and Reed-Sternberg cells are few in number or completely lacking. If classic Hodgkin cells and Reed-Sternberg cells are easily detected, a diagnosis of lymphocyte-rich classical Hodgkin's disease should be suspected. In some cases, L&H cells may resemble lacunar cells because both cell types show irregularly shaped or lobulated nuclei, small nucleoli, and broad pale to slightly basophilic cytoplasm. Although, in rare cases, it may be difficult to distinguish between L&H cells and lacunar cells by routine histology, lacunar cells are usually larger, with more abundant cytoplasm than L&H cells.

The number of L&H cells varies considerably from case to case. When they are numerous, the distinction between nodular lymphocyte predominance Hodgkin's disease and nodular lymphocyte predominance Hodgkin's disease with transition to large B-cell lymphoma may be difficult. However, large cell lymphoma should be diagnosed only when large areas of lymph nodes contain confluent L&H cells or centroblasts, particularly when they form sheets outside the nodules.

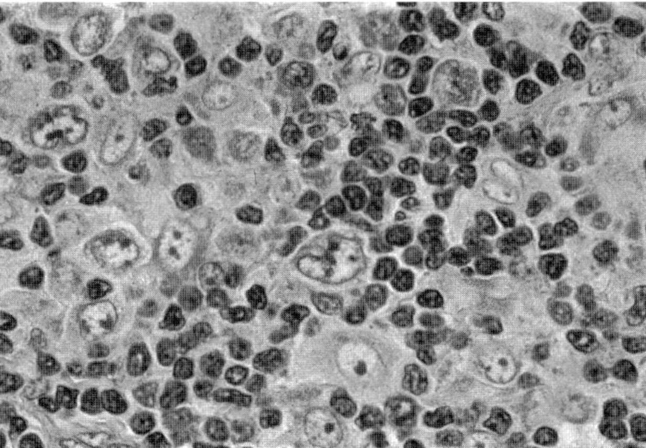

FIG. 2. High magnification, showing characteristic L&H or "popcorn" cells (Giemsa stain). (This figure is printed in color as Plate 27.)

Lymphocyte-Rich Classical Hodgkin's Disease, Nodular or Diffuse

Cases of lymphocyte-rich classical Hodgkin's disease may resemble either mixed cellularity, nodular sclerosis, or nodular lymphocyte predominance Hodgkin's disease and may be either nodular or diffuse. Many cases of lymphocyte-rich classical Hodgkin's disease have a close resemblance to mixed cellularity Hodgkin's disease, with a diffuse or vaguely nodular low-magnification appearance. Hodgkin and Reed-Sternberg cells are relatively rare, and the background is dominated by small mature lymphocytes. Eosinophils and neutrophils are usually restricted to blood vessels. Reed-Sternberg cells and variants are not easy to find but, when encountered, have identical features to the Hodgkin cells of mixed cellularity. Some cases of lymphocyte-rich classical Hodgkin's disease may show a distinctly nodular appearance that may closely mimic nodular lymphocyte predominance Hodgkin's disease. The nodules of lymphocyte-rich classical Hodgkin's disease often contain small reactive germinal centers, with Hodgkin and Reed-Sternberg cells present in and near the mantle zones, a pattern that has been called follicular Hodgkin's disease (25).

IMMUNOHISTOCHEMICAL FINDINGS

Nodular Lymphocyte Predominance Hodgkin's Disease

In typical cases, the nodules of nodular lymphocyte predominance Hodgkin's disease demonstrate large numbers of small polyclonal B lymphocytes in addition to L&H cells when stained with CD20 or CD79a (27,28). The interfollicular areas are dominated by T lymphocytes that are CD3-positive, and there may be only rare B cells (29). However, there is a wide variation in the number of T cells in the nodules; T cells tend to increase in numbers over time, and in some cases, the T cells may outnumber B cells, either in the entire section or in selected nodules. In all cases, individual L&H cells tend to be surrounded by T cells. Often, one or more of the T cells forming rings around L&H cells are CD57 positive (30). T cells expressing CD57 are usually numerous in the nodules and are found to a lesser extent in the diffuse parts of nodular lymphocyte predominance Hodgkin's disease (28,31,32). The nodules are associated with large nodular meshworks of follicular dendritic cells staining positively with anti-CD21 (Fig. 3); follicular dendritic cells are absent in diffuse areas (29,33,34).

The neoplastic cells in nodular lymphocyte predominance Hodgkin's disease show a characteristic immunohistochemical profile (22,35–37). The L&H cells are positive for leukocyte common antigen (CD45) and for B-cell antigens (CD20, CD45RA, CD79a) (Fig. 4), usually negative for CD30, and almost always negative for CD15. CD15 will become positive with a neuraminidase predigestion (38). This marker profile has proved to be a consistent finding in nearly all cases that were examined by a panel of pathologists in the study of the European Task Force on Lymphoma *(publication in preparation)*. Occasionally, a few CD30-positive blasts can be found. However, a careful evaluation of the morphology of these cells reveals that they lie either outside the nodules or in their outer rim, are smaller than L&H cells, show round to oval nuclei, and are most probably reactive immunoblasts, frequently found in the parafollicular regions of normal lymph nodes. The L&H cells are usually positive for J chain, a feature of B cells (39,40). In about 25% to 50% of cases, the L&H cells express epithelial membrane antigen (40). This antigen is more easily detected in Bouin's-fixed sections. They are also usually positive for BCL6 but are negative for BCL2 (41,42). The L&H cells always lack positivity for T-cell markers such as CD3 and CD45RO and are virtually always negative for Epstein-Barr virus (EBV) latent membrane protein (43).

The detection of immunoglobulins in L&H cells by immunohistochemistry is variable. Using conventional immunohistochemical techniques, most observers have found no good evidence of immunoglobulin expression in L&H cells (22,44,45). Others have found L&H cells to express one or the other light chain in the same case (17, 30,40). However, there have been cases reported in which light chain restriction could be demonstrated (46,47). Notably, nearly all such cases have expressed κ light chains.

When proliferation markers such as Ki-67 are stained, most L&H cells show positivity, whereas only a few bystander lymphocytes are in cycle (48,49). If immunohistochemical double staining techniques are used, the

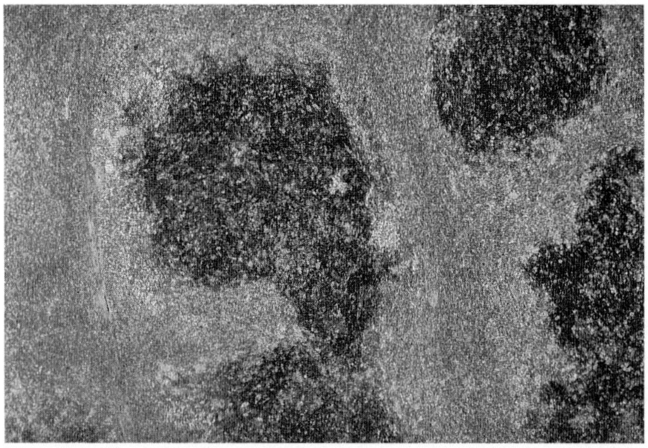

FIG. 3. Follicular dendritic cells form large networks in nodular lymphocyte predominance Hodgkin's disease (immuno–alkaline phosphatase, CD21). (This figure is printed in color as Plate 28.)

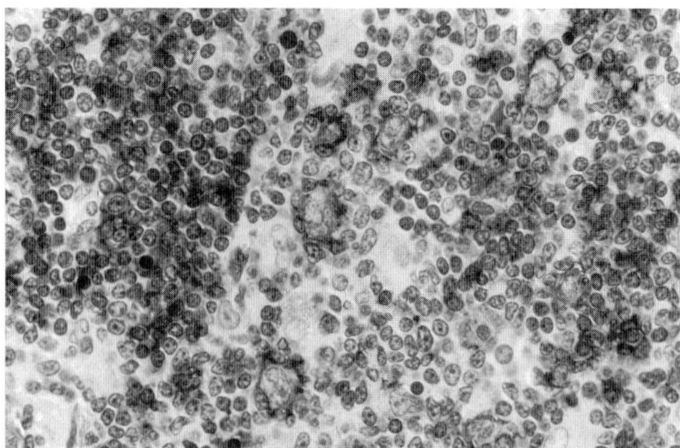

FIG. 4. In addition to small lymphocytes, several L&H cells show a membrane-bound immunoreaction for CD20 (immuno–alkaline phosphatase). (This figure is printed in color as Plate 29.)

proliferating background lymphocytes are mainly T cells, with infrequent B cells showing evidence of proliferative activity (48).

Lymphocyte-Rich Classical Hodgkin's Disease, Nodular and Diffuse

The immunophenotype of the neoplastic cells in lymphocyte-rich classical Hodgkin's disease, nodular and diffuse, is identical to that of classical Hodgkin's disease, as described in Chapter 7. There are, however, differences in the background infiltrate, as many cases of lymphocyte-rich classical Hodgkin's disease, particularly those with a nodular architecture, have a B-cell–rich infiltrate, in contrast to the marked T-cell predominance usually found in other types of classical Hodgkin's disease. Networks of follicular dendritic cells can be found in the nodules, representing the framework of follicles.

MOLECULAR BIOLOGICAL STUDIES

Considering the various technical problems and possibilities of misinterpretation of immunohistochemical staining for immunoglobulin in L&H and Hodgkin and Reed-Sternberg cells, *in situ* hybridization studies have been used to visualize light-chain mRNA in neoplastic cells (44,50–52). However, *in situ* hybridization techniques are limited by the sensitivity of the probes and the limitation in the identification of cells showing a positive signal. Probably as a consequence of the low copy numbers of mRNA and the relative low sensitivity of the method applied, the earliest studies could not identify mRNA for immunoglobulin light chains in L&H cells (44,50). In subsequent studies, which enhanced the sensitivity by using special cocktails of digoxigenin-labeled probes or using radioactively labeled ribonucleic probes, it was possible to demonstrate monotypic light-chain mRNA expression in L&H cells; these studies detected nearly exclusively mRNA for κ light chain (51, 52). In one of the studies, there was also evidence for light-chain restriction in a subset of the small B cells in some cases (52).

The detection of EBV in different forms of Hodgkin's disease by *in situ* hybridization has become important in the understanding of the development of classical Hodgkin's disease. Epstein-Barr virus can be identified in the Hodgkin's cells in 40% to 50% of cases of classical Hodgkin's disease, a finding that has been suggested to be important in the transformation from B cells to neoplastic Hodgkin's cells. However, EBV is rarely detectable in the L&H cells of nodular lymphocyte predominance Hodgkin's disease (52–56); however, one well-documented case of EBV-positive nodular lymphocyte predominance has recently been reported (57).

There is only scant information on the cytogenetics of nodular lymphocyte predominance Hodgkin's disease. In one reported case, a variety of chromosomal aberrations were found, including hyperdiploid, 6q-, and +21 (58).

Using Southern blot hybridization techniques, investigators studying nodular lymphocyte predominance Hodgkin's disease did not provide evidence of clonal rearrangements of the immunoglobulin gene locus, T-cell receptor genes, or the rearrangement of the *bcl-2* gene (59,60). Given the small number of neoplastic cells, any clone present might be below the level of detection. Polymerase chain reaction investigations require only short segments of DNA and can be carried out on partially degraded DNA from formalin-fixed and paraffin-embedded tissue, and smaller amounts of DNA are needed than for Southern blots, allowing application to single cells. A seminested polymerase chain reaction method was used by Tamaru et al. on whole tissue sections of nodular lymphocyte predominance Hodgkin's disease (67). Clonal bands were detected in many cases; however, this technique leaves doubt whether the clonal signals found were derived from the rare L&H and Reed-Sternberg cells or from clones of bystander B cells (61).

The technique of single-cell polymerase chain reaction, which permits investigations of single L&H cells micromanipulated from frozen sections, seems to have answered the question of clonality and derivation of the neoplastic cells in nodular lymphocyte predominance Hodgkin's disease (62–66). This technique was first used to analyze VH rearrangements in single cells picked from reactive follicles, including mantle cells, centrocytes, and centroblasts (65). It was found that mantle cells were clonally unrelated to one another and had rearranged but nonmutated immunoglobulin V region genes like naive B cells. Germinal centers were dominated by a few B-cell clones exhibiting somatic hypermutations and intraclonal diversity, showing ongoing somatic mutations of the immunoglobulin V region genes. In the first reported study of nodular lymphocyte predominance Hodgkin's disease, a single case was investigated (66). The results showed that L&H cells had rearranged immunoglobulin genes and were therefore B cells; the L&H cells showed bands of the same size, suggesting that they were derived from the same clone. The comparison of the VH sequences of rearrangements with the most homologous germline genes showed nucleotide differences indicating somatic point mutations and intraclonal diversity of the L&H cells. These findings showed that L&H cells were clonal B cells at the germinal center stage of differentiation.

Initially, other studies using similar techniques sometimes yielded conflicting results. In the approach of Delabie and colleagues, cell suspensions from formalin-fixed and paraffin-embedded tissue were used (67). Single L&H cells immunostained for epithelial membrane antigen were selected by a micropipette and investigated by a seminested polymerase chain reaction for immunoglobulin V region rearrangements. The cells examined showed immunoglobulin V region gene rearrangements indicating a B-cell derivation but showed no clonal relationship. However, more recent studies by the same group and two other groups using another micromanipulation technique showed clonality of L&H cells in all 21 patients investigated (68–70). In addition, clonal V gene rearrangements harboring somatic mutations were detected in each case. Braeuninger et al. and Marafioti et al. also gave evidence for intraclonal diversity by sequencing rearranged immunoglobulin genes of CD 20-positive L&H cells (69,70). The vast majority of L&H cells studied appeared to have potentially functional immunoglobulin gene rearrangements. This is in agreement with the ability to express immunoglobulin mRNA or protein on the cell surface, which has been detected by *in situ* hybridization or immunohistochemistry in a proportion of cases.

The molecular biological findings in cases of lymphocyte-rich classical Hodgkin's disease have not been studied by these techniques.

DIFFERENTIAL DIAGNOSIS

Progressive Transformation of Germinal Centers

Progressively transformed germinal centers are enlarged germinal centers composed of increased numbers of mantle cells and decreased numbers of germinal center cells (71–73). Single or clustered epithelioid histiocytes may occasionally be found but are less common than in nodular lymphocyte predominance Hodgkin's disease. The progressively transformed germinal centers are typically round and widely spaced, and normal reactive lymphoid follicles are seen between them. Low magnification can provide important information for the differential diagnostic decision between progressive transformation of germinal centers and nodular lymphocyte predominance Hodgkin's disease. In cases of reactive hyperplasia showing progressive transformation of germinal centers, germinal centers are characteristically numerous, and only a few progressively transformed germinal centers are found (Fig. 5a) (73). In contrast, in nodular lymphocyte predominance Hodgkin's disease, the nodules are closely packed, and germinal centers are almost never seen in involved areas of the lymph node. However, a peripheral rim of reactive lymphoid tissue may show well-preserved germinal centers.

In comparison with the centroblasts observed in progressive transformation of germinal centers, L&H cells are usually larger and show more lobulated nuclei. Moreover, L&H cells are often found at the periphery of or outside the nodules, in contrast to centroblasts, which are confined to follicles. The immunophenotype of progressively transformed germinal centers and nodular lymphocyte predominance Hodgkin's disease are similar. However, some features are useful for differential diagnosis (74). In progressive transformation of germinal centers, staining for CD20 reveals well-circumscribed nodules of B cells, predominantly small, that occupy the entire nodule (Fig. 5b). In contrast, in nodular lymphocyte predominance Hodgkin's disease, staining for CD20 reveals irregular nodules showing a moth-eaten appearance, with frequent unstained T cells surrounding large CD20-positive tumor cells. Staining for T-cell antigens may show many T cells in both conditions; however, their distribution is distinctive. In progressive transformation of germinal centers, as in normal germinal centers, T cells are scattered singly and are only rarely found rosetting around large B cells. In contrast, in nodular lymphocyte predominance, the T cells form irregular aggregates and clumps, with rosettes formed around the large B cells. Staining for follicular dendritic cells or CD57 is not particularly helpful because the patterns may be similar unless there is distinct rosetting of CD57-positive cells

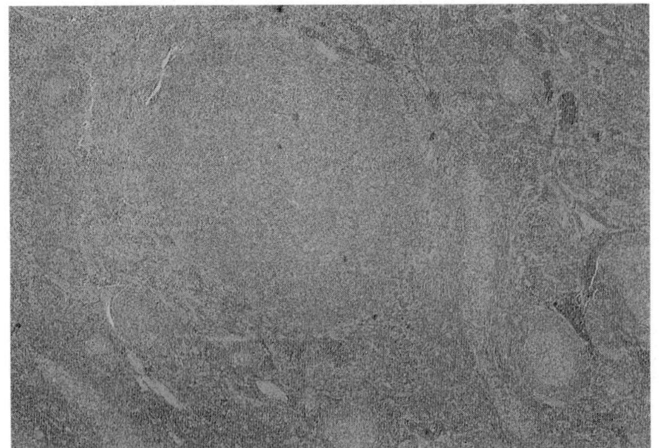
A

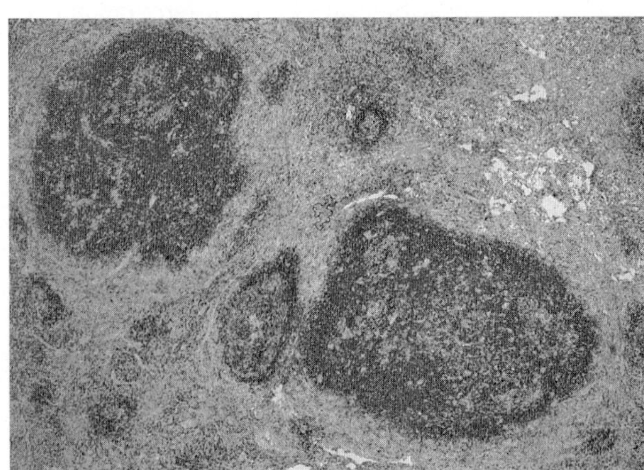
B

FIG. 5. A: A large progressively transformed germinal center is surrounded by several small germinal centers (Giemsa stain). **B:** The progressively transformed germinal centers are composed mainly of B cells, similar to the surrounding reactive follicles (immuno–alkaline phosphatase, CD20). (These figures are printed in color as Plates 30 and 31.)

around the large B cells. In Bouin's-fixed tissue, most cases of nodular lymphocyte predominance express epithelial membrane antigen on large cells; this reaction pattern is absent in progressive transformation of germinal centers.

Follicular Lymphoma

The differentiation between nodular lymphocyte predominance Hodgkin's disease and follicular lymphoma is usually not difficult. The follicles of follicular lymphoma are usually smaller than the nodules of nodular lymphocyte predominance Hodgkin's disease and often show extension outside of the capsule, a phenomenon that never occurs in nodular lymphocyte predominance Hodgkin's disease. The follicles of follicular lymphomas are composed of centrocytes intermingled with a few up to moderate or large numbers of centroblasts. The latter may be large and can show features of L&H cells. In cases in which the centrocytes are relatively small and resemble lymphocytes, the differential diagnosis between follicular lymphoma and nodular lymphocyte predominance Hodgkin's disease may become difficult. In these cases, immunostaining for CD20, CD3, CD57, J-chain, κ/λ-immunoglobulin light chain, and IgM heavy chain may help in establishing the diagnosis (Table 2) (64). The CD20-positive L&H cells in nodular lymphocyte predominance Hodgkin's disease are easily detected not only in the nodular but also in the interfollicular areas of the involved tissue. If T-cell antibodies (CD3, CD57) are used, in many cases of nodular lymphocyte predominance Hodgkin's disease complete or incomplete rosettes around the L&H cells are detected, whereas in follicular lymphoma, rosetting T cells are never found. The expression of one immunoglobulin light chain in small lymphoid cells and centroblasts can be found by immunohistochemistry in most cases of follicular lymphomas in frozen sections and in some cases in paraffin sections but not in nodular lymphocyte predominance Hodgkin's disease. In contrast to follicular lymphoma, nodular lymphocyte predominance Hodgkin's disease does not have detectable immunoglobulin heavy chain gene rearrangements by Southern blotting and does not show the t(14;18) (59,60).

Nodular Lymphocyte Predominance Hodgkin's Disease Versus Lymphocyte-Rich Classical Hodgkin's Disease

As in nodular lymphocyte predominance Hodgkin's disease, small lymphocytes comprise the majority of the cells in lymphocyte-rich classical Hodgkin's disease. Eosinophils and plasma cells may or may not be admixed. This type of Hodgkin's disease may also show a nodular or follicular growth pattern, further mimicking nodular lymphocyte predominance Hodgkin's disease, as described by Ashton-Key (25). However, in contrast to nodular lymphocyte predominance Hodgkin's disease, the nodules, when present, appear to represent expanded mantle zones. In typical cases, the neoplastic cells of lymphocyte-rich classical Hodgkin's disease have the characteristic features of similar cells described in other types of classical Hodgkin and Reed-Sternberg cells. When a nodular architecture is present, the Hodgkin and Reed-Sternberg cells are typically found in the outer areas of the nodules, which seem to be expanded mantle zones, interfollicular areas, or adjacent monocytoid B-cell proliferations. Residual intact germinal centers are also frequently identified within the nodules, in contrast with nodular lymphocyte predominance Hodgkin's disease. In cases with many classical Hodgkin and Reed-Sternberg cells, the diagnosis of lymphocyte-rich classical Hodgkin's disease may not be difficult. However, there are cases in which cells resembling L&H cells with occasional Hodgkin and Reed-Sternberg cells occur in a nodular lymphocytic background. These cases may be impossible to distinguish from nodular lymphocyte predominance Hodgkin's disease on morphologic grounds and may require immunohistochemical studies. Some cases of lymphocyte-rich classical Hodgkin's disease may show a diffuse growth pattern. In such cases, the differential diagnosis with nodular lymphocyte predominance Hodgkin's disease is less problematic. The presence of

TABLE 2. *Immunohistochemical and molecular biological studies in the differential diagnosis between nodular lymphocyte predominance Hodgkin's disease and follicular lymphoma*

	Nodular lymphocyte predominance Hodgkin's disease	Follicular lymphoma
CD20	L&H cells in nodules and interfollicular areas	Centroblasts/centrocytes within follicular structures
CD3, CD4, CD57	Aggregates of T cells; T-cell rosettes around L&H cells	Scattered T cells; no T-cell rosettes
Ig:Kλ IgM	Polyclonal lymphocytes; L&H cells negative or rarely κ-positive	Clonal in centroblasts/centrocytes
bcl-2 protein	L&H cells negative	Centroblasts/centrocytes usually x positive
Immunoglobulin heavy-chain gene	No clonal band detected by Southern blot	Rearranged by Southern blot
t(14;18)	Absent	85%

admixed eosinophils or plasma cells also argues against nodular lymphocyte predominance Hodgkin's disease.

The immunohistochemical staining pattern of lymphocytes and follicular dendritic cells of lymphocyte-rich classical Hodgkin's disease is similar to that of nodular lymphocyte predominance Hodgkin's disease in that the nodules are composed predominantly of B cells with nodular meshworks of follicular dendritic cells. However, in lymphocyte-rich classical Hodgkin's disease, the B-cell–rich nodules sometimes show concentric rings of follicular dendritic cells with a central accumulation of follicular dendritic cells, similar to the pattern seen in Castleman's disease (Fig. 6). The Hodgkin and Reed-Sternberg cells of classical Hodgkin's disease are positive for CD30 and CD15 and negative for CD45 and may or may not express B-cell markers, whereas those of nodular lymphocyte predominance Hodgkin's disease are CD20 positive and lack CD15 and CD30 (Table 1). *In situ* hybridization for EBV or immunohistochemical studies for EBV latent membrane protein may show positivity in the tumor cells of lymphocyte-rich classical Hodgkin's disease but not in nodular lymphocyte predominance Hodgkin's disease.

T-Cell–Rich Large B-Cell Lymphoma

The distinction between the diffuse variants of lymphocyte predominance and lymphocyte-rich classical Hodgkin's disease and T-cell–rich large B-cell lymphoma may be extremely difficult and in some cases even impossible on morphologic and immunohistochemical grounds. The term T-cell–rich B-cell lymphoma was introduced by Ramsay et al.; it has been used to refer to B-cell lymphomas in which an unusually prominent reactive T-cell infiltrate is found (75). The term has been used heterogeneously for cases with over 50% T cells and for cases with over 90% T cells (76–78). Many reported cases probably represent "usual" diffuse large B-cell lymphomas or even low-grade lymphomas with many T cells. However, Delabie et al. and Chittal et al. have described an unusual form of large B-cell lymphoma with a background of T cells and histiocytes resembling diffuse lymphocyte predominance Hodgkin's disease (79,80). McBride et al. reported similar cases misdiagnosed as mixed cellularity Hodgkin's disease; in that study, the atypical cells very closely resembled classical Reed-Sternberg cells and variants (81). These cases appear to represent a distinct entity with an aggressive clinical course, often involving liver, spleen, and bone marrow. T-cell/histiocyte–rich large B-cell lymphoma is characterized by a diffuse infiltrate consisting mainly of T lymphocytes and histiocytes that are not neoplastic and a minority of medium-sized to large neoplastic B cells comprising 5% or less of the total cellular population (75, 79,80,82). The large B cells may resemble L&H cells of nodular lymphocyte predominance or may resemble centroblasts or immunoblasts. This histologic picture may be extremely difficult to differentiate from nodular lymphocyte predominance Hodgkin's disease with a diffuse pattern. Indeed, it has been debated whether T-cell–rich large B-cell lymphoma is a distinct entity or is rather an aggressive variant of nodular lymphocyte predominance Hodgkin's disease (83,84). In the REAL and WHO classifications, T-cell–rich large B-cell lymphoma is included as a subtype of diffuse large cell B-cell lymphoma.

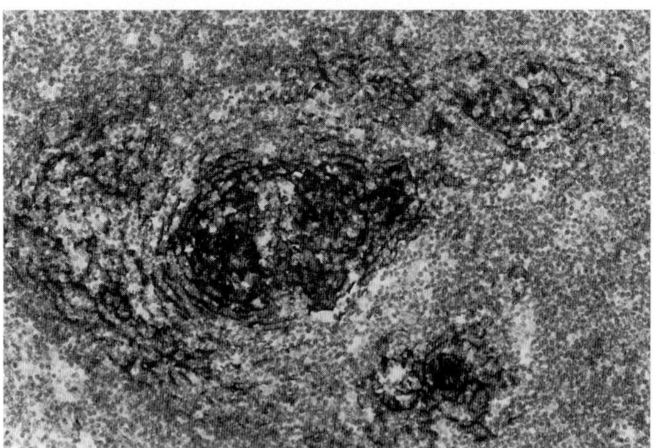

FIG. 6. Nodular infiltrate of lymphocyte-rich classical Hodgkin's disease. Eccentrically localized remnants of germinal centers are visualized by immunostaining for follicular dendritic cells (immuno–alkaline phosphatase, CD21). (This figure is printed in color as Plate 32.)

Criteria for the differential diagnosis between T-cell–rich large B-cell lymphoma and nodular lymphocyte predominance are listed in Table 3. The immunophenotype of the neoplastic cells in T-cell/histiocyte–rich large B-cell lymphoma may be identical to that of lymphocyte predominance Hodgkin's disease. The neoplastic cells of T-cell/histiocyte–rich large B-cell lymphoma express CD45, CD20, and CD79a and are often epithelial membrane antigen positive (85). They may have cytoplasmic immunoglobulin and are CD15 and CD30 negative. Thus, the differential diagnosis rests on the background infiltrate. The presence of nodular meshworks of follicular dendritic cells, numerous small B lymphocytes, and CD57-positive cells favors lymphocyte predominance Hodgkin's disease, whereas their absence favors T-cell/histiocyte–rich large B-cell lymphoma. The presence of clear-cut immunoglobulin light-chain restriction by immunohistochemistry or clonal immunoglobulin gene rearrangements by Southern blot would favor T-cell/histiocyte–rich large B-cell lymphoma. Finally, clinical features may provide a clue to the diagnosis because lymphocyte predominance Hodgkin's disease only rarely presents with disease involving the liver, spleen, and bone marrow, although these organs are commonly involved in T-cell/histiocyte–rich large B-cell lymphoma.

Some cases of T-cell–rich large B-cell lymphoma may contain neoplastic cells resembling classic Hodgkin or

TABLE 3. *Criteria for the differential diagnosis between nodular lymphocyte predominance Hodgkin's disease, including its diffuse variant, and T-cell-rich large B-cell lymphoma*

	Nodular lymphocyte predominance	T-cell-rich large B-cell lymphoma
Architecture	Nodular pattern (nearly always) Sometimes bands of fibrosis	Diffuse pattern Occasional nodularity Sometimes diffuse fibrosis
Neoplastic component		
Distribution	Found in "nodules"	Scattered
Popcorn appearance	+/–	–/+
Centroblast-like	–/+	+/–
RS/RS-like cells	–/+	–/+
CD45	+	+
CD20	+	+
CD30	–	–
CD15	–	–
EMA	–/+	–/+
J-chain	+	–
Monotypic Ig	–/+	+/–
MIB-1/Ki-67 index	High	High
EBV	–	–
Ig gene rearrangement studies on whole tissue sections	–	+/–
Reactive component		
T cells	++ (CD4+)	++++ (CD4, CD8+)
B or mixed B&T	+	–
T-cell rosettes	+	–
CD57+ cells	Varying, occasional rosettes	Rare
Histiocytes	Few to many (epithelioid)	Few to many
FDC-meshworks	+	–
Clinical Findings		
Stage	I or II	III or IV
Bone marrow involvement	–	Frequently +

Table modified from the E.A.H.P. Workshop, Toledo, October 1994.

Reed-Sternberg cells, making the differential diagnosis with classical Hodgkin's disease is more problematic (81,85,86). Distinction between classical Hodgkin's disease and T-cell/histiocyte–rich large B-cell lymphoma rests on the detection of CD15 and CD30 and the absence of CD45 on the neoplastic cells in classical Hodgkin's disease, as a significant subset of cases of classical Hodgkin's disease may express CD20. The identification of EBV in the Hodgkin and Reed-Sternberg cells of classical Hodgkin's disease may also be of benefit, as cases of T-cell/histiocyte–rich large B-cell lymphoma are rarely EBV positive.

The analysis of the rearranged V genes in the neoplastic cells of T-cell–rich large B-cell lymphoma reveals mutations indicating a germinal center cell origin of these lymphomas (87). The evaluation of the mutation pattern speaks in favor of the involvement of the tumor cells of an antigen-driven selection process.

TRANSFORMATION OF NODULAR LYMPHOCYTE PREDOMINANCE HODGKIN'S DISEASE TO LARGE B-CELL LYMPHOMA

About 2% to 3% of patients with nodular lymphocyte predominance develop large-cell lymphoma of the B type (88,89). Large cell lymphoma may be found in the same lymph node that is involved by nodular lymphocyte predominance, in another lymph node at a distant site, or rarely at an extranodal localization. The occurrence of large cell lymphoma in patients with nodular lymphocyte predominance Hodgkin's disease may be simultaneous or subsequent, or in rare cases large cell lymphoma may be seen before nodular lymphocyte predominance Hodgkin's disease (45,88–92).

The large cell lymphomas are morphologically variable. Some are composed of cells resembling L&H cells. Others may span the spectrum of all subtypes of diffuse large cell lymphomas of B type—centroblastic (monomorphic, polymorphic, or multilobated), immunoblastic, or anaplastic. Burkitt-like lymphomas may rarely develop. The large cell lymphomas arising in nodular lymphocyte predominance Hodgkin's disease characteristically express a B-cell phenotype (CD19- and CD20-positive) as well as immunoglobulin light-chain restriction. In lymph nodes containing both nodular lymphocyte predominance Hodgkin's disease and large cell lymphoma, the large cell lymphoma is typically demarcated from the nodular lymphocyte predominance Hodgkin's disease. However, in some cases, transitional areas containing numerous L&H cells may exist between the large cell lymphoma and nodular lymphocyte predominance Hodgkin's disease. It may occasionally be difficult to differentiate between nodular lymphocyte predominance Hodgkin's disease with clusters of L&H cells and nodular lymphocyte predominance Hodgkin's disease with transition to large cell lymphoma. However, transformation to large cell lymphoma should be diagnosed only when large areas of the lymph node are effaced by L&H cells (36,88).

In situ hybridization studies have shown the same immunoglobulin light-chain mRNA in the L&H cells of nodular lymphocyte predominance Hodgkin's disease and in large cell lymphoma in some of the cases investigated, indicating the presence of the same tumor clone (93). In several studies, polymerase chain reaction techniques using tissue sections have been applied to examine cases of nodular lymphocyte predominance associated with large cell lymphoma (94–96). In these studies, consensus primers to the VH and JH regions were used to identify clonal B-cell populations. In the vast majority of cases of large cell lymphoma associated with nodular lymphocyte predominance Hodgkin's disease, clonal rearrangements could be found in the large cell component. However, clonal B-cell proliferations in nodular lymphocyte predominance Hodgkin's disease were found in only a few cases. Identical sequences of rearranged V genes in two cases, both in the nodular lymphocyte predominance Hodgkin's disease infiltrate and the large cell lymphoma, were detected by Greiner et al. (94).

Use of clonospecific oligonucleotides to detect rearranged V-gene sequences in large cell lymphoma allowed Wickert et al. to identify a corresponding clonal B-cell proliferation in the associated nodular lymphocyte predominance Hodgkin's disease in only a few cases (96). No clonal immunoglobulin gene rearrangement was identified in any case of nodular lymphocyte predominance Hodgkin's disease using polymerase chain reaction on whole sections or on enriched L&H cells by microdissection in another study (95). In this study, clone-specific primers designed for the recognition of V-gene rearrangements of nodular lymphocyte predominance Hodgkin's disease–associated large cell lymphoma were not successful in detecting the corresponding clone in nodular lymphocyte predominance Hodgkin's disease. In the above studies, the failure to detect clonal populations in nodular lymphocyte predominance Hodgkin's disease may be related to the sensitivity of the methods used, as whole section polymerase chain reaction usually does not detect monoclonality in nodular lymphocyte predominance Hodgkin's disease.

CONCLUSIONS

In summary, the past decades have provided a wealth of new information regarding the entity known as nodular lymphocyte predominance Hodgkin's disease. The morphologic definition and criteria for distinguishing it from other forms of Hodgkin's disease and from reactive conditions and other lymphomas have been clarified. It has a distinctive immunophenotype, which distinguishes it from other forms of Hodgkin's disease. Through immunophenotyping and molecular genetic studies, nodular lymphocyte predominance Hodgkin's disease is clearly established as a clonal proliferation of B cells of germinal center origin. Similar studies have led to the recognition that classical Hodgkin's disease may also be a clonal outgrowth of B cells at the germinal center stage. Although the neoplastic cells of nodular lymphocyte predominance Hodgkin's disease appear to be capable of synthesizing and expressing immunoglobulins and their precursors able to undergo antigen-driven selection, the neoplastic cells of classical Hodgkin's disease appear to be unable to produce immunoglobulin.

What is it, then, that distinguishes classical Hodgkin's disease from large–B-cell lymphoma and nodular lymphocyte predominance from classical Hodgkin's disease? The background of nonneoplastic lymphoid cells and the distinctive clinical features still separate Hodgkin's disease from most non-Hodgkin's lymphomas. Although both nodular lymphocyte predominance and classical Hodgkin's disease are B-cell disorders, their distinct genetic and immunophenotypic features suggest important differences in pathogenesis. Thus, although we have learned a great deal, we are in a sense not much ahead of Jackson and Parker, who in 1944 recognized that paragranuloma was a distinct entity, different from both classical Hodgkin's disease and other malignant lymphomas.

REFERENCES

1. Rosenthal SR. Significance of tissue lymphocytes in the prognosis of lymphogranulomatosis. *Arch Pathol* 1936;21:628.
2. Jackson H Jr, Parker F Jr. Hodgkin's disease. II. Pathology. *N Engl J Med* 1944;231:35.
3. Jackson H Jr. Classification and prognosis of Hodgkin's disease and allied disorders. *Surg Gynecol Obstet* 1937;64:465.
4. Robb-Smith AHG. The lymph node biopsy. *Recent Adv Clin Pathol* 1947:350.
5. Harrison CV. Benign Hodgkin's disease (Hodgkin's paragranuloma). *J Pathol Bacteriol* 1952;64:513.
6. Thomson AD. The thymic origin of Hodgkin's disease. *Br J Cancer* 1955;9:37.
7. Lumb G. *Tumours of lymphoid tissue.* Edinburgh: Livingston, 1954.
8. Symmers WSC. The lymphoreticular system. In: Raven RW, ed. *Cancer,* vol 2. London: Butterworth, 1958:478.
9. Rappaport H, Winter WJ, Hicks EB. Follicular lymphoma: A re-evaluation of its position in the scheme of malignant lymphoma, based on a survey of 253 cases. *Cancer* 1956;9:792.
10. Lukes RJ, Butler JJ. The pathology and nomenclature of Hodgkin's disease. *Cancer Res* 1966;26:1063.
11. Lukes RJ. Relationship of histologic features to clinical stages in Hodgkin's disease. *Am J Roentgenol* 1963;90:944.
12. Lukes RJ, Craver LF, Hall TC, Rappaport H, Rubin T. Report of the nomenclature committee. *Cancer Res* 1966;26:1311.
13. Lennert K, Mohri N. Histologische Klassifizierung and Vorkommen des Morbus Hodgkin. *Internist (Berl)* 1974;15:57.
14. Mason DY, Banks PM, Chan J, et al. Nodular lymphocyte predominance Hodgkin's disease. A distinct clinicopathological entity. *Am J Surg Pathol* 1994;18:526.
15. Poppema S, Kaiserling E, Lennert K. Hodgkin's disease with lymphocyte predominance, nodular type (nodular paragranuloma) and progressively transformed germinal centers—a cytohistological study. *Histopathology* 1979;3:295.
16. Poppema S, Kaiserling E, Lennert K. Epidemiology of nodular paragranuloma (Hodgkin's disease with lymphocytic predominance, nodular). *J Cancer Res Clin Oncol* 1979;95:57.
17. Poppema S, Kaiserling E, Lennert K. Nodular paragranuloma and progressively transformed germinal centers. Ultrastructural and immunohistologic findings. *Virchows Arch [Cell Pathol]* 1979;31:211.
18. Hansmann ML, Zwingers T, Boske A, Loffler H, Lennert K. Clinical features of nodular paragranuloma (Hodgkin's disease, lymphocyte predominance type, nodular). *J Cancer Res Clin Oncol* 1984;108:321.
19. Miettinen M, Franssila KO, Saxen E. Hodgkin's disease, lymphocytic predominance nodular: increased risk for subsequent non-Hodgkin's lymphomas. *Cancer* 1983;51:2293.
20. Regula DP, Hoppe RT, Weiss LM. Nodular and diffuse types of lymphocyte predominance Hodgkin's disease. *N Engl J Med* 1988;318:214.
21. Regula DP, Weiss LM, Warnke RA, Dorfman RF. Lymphocyte predominance Hodgkin's disease: a reappraisal based upon histological and immunophenotypical findings in relapsing cases. *Histopathology* 1987;11:1107.
22. Pinkus GS, Said JW. Hodgkin's disease, lymphocyte predominance

type, nodular—a distinct entity? Unique staining profile of L&H variants of Reed-Sternberg cells defined by monoclonal antibodies to leukocyte common antigen, granulocyte specific antigen, and B-cell specific antigen. *Am J Pathol* 1985;116:1.
23. Pinkus GS, Said JW. Hodgkin's disease, lymphocyte predominance type, nodular- further evidence for a B cell derivation: L&H variants of Reed-Sternberg cells express L26, a pan B cell marker. *Am J Pathol* 1988;133:211.
24. Harris NL, Jaffe ES, Stein H, et al. A revised European-American classification of lymphoid neoplasms. A proposal from the International Lymphoma Study Group. *Blood* 1994;84:1361.
25. Ashton-Key M, Thorpe PA, Allen JP, Isaacson PG. Follicular Hodgkin's disease. *Am J Surg Pathol* 1995;19:1294.
26. Stein H, Gerdes J, Schwab U, et al. Identification of Hodgkin and Sternberg-Reed cells as a unique cell type derived from a newly-detected small-cell population. *Int J Cancer* 1982;30:445.
27. Hansmann ML, Wacker HH, Radzun HJ. Paragranuloma is a variant of Hodgkin's disease with predominance of B-cells. *Virchows Arch [Pathol Anat Histopathol]* 1986;409:171.
28. Poppema S. The nature of the lymphocytes surrounding Reed-Sternberg cells in nodular lymphocyte predominance and in other types of Hodgkin's disease. *Am J Pathol* 1989;135:351.
29. Hansmann ML, Stein H, Dallenbach F, Fellbaum C. Diffuse lymphocyte-predominant Hodgkin's disease (diffuse paragranuloma): a variant of the B-cell-derived nodular type. *Am J Pathol* 1991;138:29.
30. Timens W, Visser L, Poppema S. Nodular lymphocyte predominance type of Hodgkin's disease is a germinal center lymphoma. *Lab Invest* 1986;54:457.
31. Hansmann ML, Fellbaum C, Hui PK, Zwingers T. Correlation of content of B cells and Leu 7-positive cells with sybtype and stage in lymphocyte predominance type Hodgkin's disease. *Cancer Res Clin Oncol* 1988;114:405.
32. Kamel OW, Gelb AB, Shibuya RB, Warnke RA. Leu7 (CD57) reactivity distinguishes nodular lymphocyte predominance Hodgkin's disease, T cell rich B cell lymphoma and follicular lymphoma. *Am J Pathol* 1993;142:541.
33. Alavaikko JF, Hansmann ML, Nebendahl C, Parwaresch MR, Lennert K. Follicular dendritic cells in Hodgkin's disease. *Am J Clin Pathol* 1991;95:194.
34. Alavaikko MJ, Blanco G, Aine R. Follicular dendritic cells have prognostic relevance in Hodgkin's disease. *Am J Clin Pathol* 1994;101: 761.
35. Pinkus GS, Said JW. Hodgkin's disease, lymphocyte predominance type, nodular—further evidence for a B cell derivation. L & H variants of Reed-Sternberg cells express L26, a pan B cell marker. *Am J Pathol* 1988;133:211.
36. Chittal SM, Alard C, Rossi JF, et al. Further phenotypic evidence that nodular, lymphocyte-predominant Hodgkin's disease is a large B-cell lymphoma in evolution. *Am J Surg Pathol* 1990;14:1024.
37. Chittal SM, Caveriviere P, Schwarting R, et al. Monoclonal antibodies in the diagnosis of Hodgkin's disease: the search for a rational panel. *Am J Surg Pathol* 1988;12:9.
38. Hsu SM, Ho YS, Li PJ, et al. L&H variants of Reed-Sternberg cells express sialylated Leu M1 antigen. *Am J Pathol* 1986;122:199.
39. Stein H, Hansmann ML, Lennert K, Brandtzaeg P, Gatter KC, Mason DY. Reed-Sternberg and Hodgkin's cells in lymphocyte-predominant Hodgkin's disease of nodular subtype contain J chain. *Am J Clin Pathol* 1986;86:292.
40. Poppema S. The diversity of the immunohistological staining pattern of Sternberg-Reed cells. *J Histochem Cytochem* 1980;28:788.
41. Falini B, Bigerna B, Pasqualucci L, et al. Distinctive expression pattern of the BCL-6 protein in nodular lymphocyte prodominance Hodgkin's disease. *Blood* 1996;87:465.
42. Algara P, Martinez P, Sanchez L, et al. Lymphocyte predominance Hodgkin's disease (nodular paragranuloma)-A bcl-2 negative germinal centre lymphoma. *Histopathology* 1991;19:69.
43. Weiss LM, Chang KL. Association of the Epstein-Barr virus with hematolymphoid neoplasia. *Adv Anat Pathol* 1996;3:1.
44. Momose H, Chen Y-Y, Ben-Ezra J, Weiss LM. Nodular, lymphocyte predominant Hodgkin's disease: study of immunoglobulin light chain protein and mRNA expression. *Hum Pathol* 1992;23:1115.
45. Sundeen JT, Cossman J, Jaffe ES. Lymphocyte predominant Hodgkin's disease nodular subtype with coexistent "large cell lymphoma." Histological progression or composite malignancy? [see comments]. *Am J Surg Pathol* 1988;12:599.
46. Li G, Hansmann M. Lymphocyte predominant Hodgkin's disease of nodular subtype combined with pulmonary lymphoid infiltration and hypogammaglobulinemia. *Virchows Arch [Pathol Anat Histopathol]* 1989;145:481.
47. Schmid C, Pan L, Diss T, Isaacson PG. Expression of B-cell antigens by Hodgkin's and Reed-Sternberg cells. *Am J Pathol* 1991;139:701.
48. Hell K, Lorenzen J, Hansmann ML, Fellbaum C, Busch R, Fischer R. Expression of the proliferating cell nuclear antigen in the different types of Hodgkin's disease. *Am J Clin Pathol* 1993;99:598.
49. Gerdes J, van Baarlen J, Pileri S, Schwarting R, van Unnik JAM, Stein H. Tumor cell growth fraction in Hodgkin's disease. *Am J Pathol* 1987;128:390.
50. Ruprai AK, Pringle JH, Angel CA, Kind CN, Lauder I. Localization of immunoglobulin light chain mRNA expression in Hodgkin's disease by *in situ* hybridization. *J Pathol* 1991;164:37.
51. Hell K, Pringle JH, Hansmann ML, et al. Demonstration of light chain mRNA in Hodgkin's disease. *J Pathol* 1993;171:137.
52. Stoler MH, Nichols GE, Symbula M, Weiss LM. Nodular L&H lymphocyte predominance Hodgkin's disease: evidence for a kappa light chain-restricted monotypic B cell neoplasm. *Am J Pathol* 1995;146:812.
53. Weiss LM, Chen YY, Liu X, Shibata DM. A correlative *in situ* hybridization and polymerase chain reaction study. *Am J Pathol* 1991; 139:1259.
54. Brousset P, Chittal S, Schlaifer D, et al. Detection of Epstein-Barr virus messenger RNA in Reed-Sternberg cells of Hodgkin's disease by *in situ* hybridization with biotinylated probes on specially processed modified acetone methyl benzoate xylene (ModAMeX) sections. *Blood* 1991;77:1781.
55. Shibata D, Hansmann ML, Weiss LM, Nathwani BN. Epstein-Barr virus infection and Hodgkin's disease: a study of fixed tissues using the polymerase chain reaction. *Hum Pathol* 1991;22:1262.
56. Hansmann ML, Shibata D, Lorenzen J, Hell K, Nathwani BN, Fischer R. Incidence of Epstein-Barr virus, bcl-2 expression and chromosomal translocation t(14;18) in large cell lymphoma associated with paragranuloma (lymphocyte-predominant Hodgkin's disease). *Hum Pathol* 1994;25:240.
57. Khalidi H, Lones MA, Zhou Y, Weiss LM, Medeiros LJ. Detection of Epstein-Bar virus in the L&H cells of nodular lymphocytic predominance Hodgkin's disease. Report of a case documented by immunohistochemical, *in situ* hybridization, and polymerase chain reaction methods. *Am J Clin Pathol* 1997;108:687.
58. Hansmann M-L, Gödde-Salz E, Hui PK, Müller-Hermelink HK, Lennert K. Cytogenetic findings in nodular paragranuloma (Hodgkin's disease with lymphocytic predominance; nodular) and in progressively transformed germinal centers. *Cancer Genet Cytogenet* 1986;21:319.
59. Lorenzen J, Hansmann ML, Pezzella F, et al. Expression of the bcl-2 oncogene product and chromosomal translocation t(14;18) in Hodgkin's disease. *Hum Pathol* 1992;23:1205.
60. Said JW, Sassoon AF, Shintaku IP, Kurtin PJ, Pinkus GS. Absence of bcl-2 major breakpoint region and J_H gene rearrangement in lymphocyte predominance Hodgkin's disease: results of Southern blot analysis and polymerase chain reaction. *Am J Pathol* 1991;138:261.
61. Tamaru J, Hummel M, Zemlin M, Kalvelage B, Stein H. Hodgkin's disease with a B-cell phenotype often shows a VDJ rearrangement and somatic mutations in the V_H genes. *Blood* 1994;84:708.
62. Küppers R, Rajewsky K. The origin of Hodgkin and Reed-Sternberg cells in Hodgkin's disease. *Annu Rev Immunol* 1998;16:471.
63. Küppers R, Hansmann M-L, Rajewsky K. Micromanipulation and PCR analysis of single cells from tissue sections. In: Weiss D, Blackwell K, Herzenberg LA, Herzenberg LA, eds. *Weir's handbook of experimental immunology.* London: Blackwell Scientific, 1996:31.
64. Hansmann ML, Küppers R. Pathology and "molecular histology" of Hodgkin's disease and the border to non-Hodgkin's lymphomas. *Baillieres Clin Haematol* 1996;9:459.
65. Küppers R, Zhao M, Hansmann ML, Rajewsky K. Tracing B cell development in human germinal centres by molecular analysis of single cells picked from histological sections. *EMBO* 1993;12:4955.
66. Küppers R, Rajewsky K, Zhao M, et al. Hodgkin disease: Hodgkin and Reed-Sternberg cells picked from histological sections show clonal immunoglobulin gene rearrangements and appear to be derived from B cells at various stages of development. *Proc Natl Acad Sci USA* 1994;91:10962.
67. Delabie J, Tierens A, Wu G, Weisenburger DD, Chan WC. Lymphocyte predominance Hodgkin's disease: lineage and clonality determination using a single-cell assay. *Blood* 1994;84:3291.

68. Ohno T, Striblem JA, Wu G, Hinrichs SH, Weisenburger DD, Chan WC. Clonality in nodular lymhocyte-predominant Hodgkin's disease. *N Engl J Med* 1997;65:337.
69. Marafioti T, Hummel M, Anagnostopoulos I, et al. Origin of nodular lymphocyte-predominant Hodgkin's disease from a clonal expansion of highly mutated germinal-center B cells. *N Engl J Med* 1997;337:453.
70. Braeuninger A, Küppers R, Strickler JG, Wacker HH, Rajewsky K, Hansmann ML. Hodgkin and Reed-Sternberg cells in lymphocyte predominant Hodgkin disease represent clonal populations of germinal center-derived tumor B cells. *Proc Natl Acad Sci USA* 1997;94:9337.
71. Burns BF, Colby TV, Dorfman RF. Differential diagnostic features of nodular L&H Hodgkin's disease, including progressive transformation of germinal centers. *Am J Surg Pathol* 1984;8:253.
72. Osborne BM, Butler JJ. Clinical implications of progressive transformation of germinal centers. *Am J Surg Pathol* 1984;8:725.
73. Hansmann ML, Fellbaum C, Hui PK, Moubayed P. Progressive transformation of germinal centers with and without association to Hodgkin's disease. *Am J Clin Pathol* 1990;93:219.
74. Nguyen P, Ferry J, Harris NL. Progressive transformation of germinal centers and nodular lymphocyte predominance Hodgkin's disease: a comparative immunohistochemical study. *Am J Surg Pathol* 1999;23:27–33.
75. Ramsay AP, Smith WJ, Isaacson PG. T-cell-rich B-cell lymphoma. *Am J Surg Pathol* 1988;12:433.
76. Macon WR, Williams ME, Greer JP, Stein RS, Collins RD, Cousar JB. T-Cell-rich B-cell lymphomas. A clinicopathologic study of 19 cases. *Am J Surg Pathol* 1992;16:351.
77. Ng C, Chan J, Hui P, Lau W. Large B-cell lymphomas with a high content of reactive T-cells. *Hum Pathol* 1989;20:1145.
78. Scarpa A, Bonetti F, Zamboni G, Menestrina F, Chilosi M. T-cell-rich B-cell lymphoma [letter to editor]. *Am J Surg Pathol* 1989;13:335.
79. Chittal SM, Brousset P, Voigt JJ, Delsol G. Large B-cell lymphoma rich in T-cells and simulating Hodgkin's disease. *Histopathology* 1991;19:211.
80. Delabie J, Vandenberghe E, Kennes C, et al. Histiocyte-rich B-cell lymphoma. A distinct clinicopathologic entity possibly related to lymphocyte predominant Hodgkin's disease, paragranuloma subtype. *Am J Surg Pathol* 1992;16:37.
81. McBride JA, Rodriguez J, Luthra R, Ordonez NG, Cabinillas F, Pugh WC. T-cell-rich B large cell lymphoma simulating lymphocyte-rich Hodgkin's disease. *Am J Surg Pathol* 1996;20:193.
82. Chan A. T-cell-Rich B-Cell Lymphoma. What is new? What is cool? *Am Clin Pathol* 1997;108:489.
83. De Jong D, Van Gorp J, Sie-Go D, Van Heerde P. T-cell-rich B-cell non-Hodgkin's lymphoma: a progressed form of follicle center cell lymphoma and lymphocyte predominance Hodgkin's disease. *Histopathology* 1996;28:15.
84. Skinnider B, Connors J, Gascoyne R. Bone marrow involvement in T-cell-rich-B-cell lymphoma. *Am J Clin Pathol* 1997;108:570.
85. Osborne BM, Buttler JJ, Pugh WC. The value of immunophenotyping on paraffin sections in the identification of T-cell rich B-cell large cell lymphomas. *Am J Surg Pathol* 1990;14:933.
86. Osborne BM, Butler JJ, Pugh WC. The value of immunophenotyping on paraffin sections in the identification of T-cell rich B-cell large cell lymphoma: lineage confirmed by J_H rearrangement. *Am J Surg Pathol* 1990;14:933.
87. Küppers R, Rajewsky K, Hansmann ML. Diffuse large cell lymphomas are derived from mature B-cells carrying V region genes with a high load of somatic mutations and evidence of selection for antibody expression. *Eur J Immunol* 1997;27:1398.
88. Hansmann ML, Stein H, Fellbaum C, Hui PK, Parwaresch MR, Lennert K. Nodular paragranuloma can transform into high-grade malignant lymphoma of B type. *Hum Pathol* 1989;20:1169.
89. Miettinen M, Franssila KO, Saxen E. Hodgkin's disease, lymphocyte predominance nodular: increased risk for subsequent non-Hodgkin's lymphomas. *Cancer* 1983;51:2293.
90. Gonzalez CL, Medeiros LJ, Jaffe ES. Composite lymphoma. A clinicopathologic analysis of nine patients with Hodgkin's disease and B-cell non-Hodgkin's lymphoma. *Am J Clin Pathol* 1991;96:81.
91. Grossman DM, Hanson CA, Schnitzer B. Simultaneous lymphocyte predominant Hodgkin's disease and large cell lymphoma. *Am J Surg Pathol* 1991;15:668.
92. Jaffe ES, Zarate-Osorno A, Kingma DW, Raffeld M, Medeiros LJ. The interrelationship between Hodgkin's disease and non-Hodgkin's lymphoma. *Ann Oncol* 1994;5(Suppl 1):S7.
93. Hell K, Hansmann ML, Pringle JH, Lauder I, Fischer R. Combination of Hodgkin's disease and diffuse large cell lymphoma: an *in situ* hybridization study for immunoglobulin light chain messenger RNA. *Histopathology* 1995;27:491.
94. Greiner TC, Gascoyne RD, Anderson ME, et al. Nodular lymphocyte-predominant Hodgkin's disease associated with large cell lymphoma: Analysis of Ig gene rearrangements by V-J polymerase chain reaction. *Blood* 1996;88:657.
95. Pan LX, Diss TC, Peng HZ, Norton AJ, Isaacson PG. Nodular lymphocyte predominance Hodgkin's disease: a monoclonal or polyclonal B-cell disorder? *Blood* 1996;87:2428.
96. Wickert RS, Weisenburger DD, Tierens A, Greiner TC, Chan WC. Clonal relationship between lymphocyte predominance Hodgkin's disease and concurrent or subsequent large cell lymphoma of B lineage. *Blood* 1995;86:2312.
97. Chang KL, Arber DA, Weiss LM. CD20: A review. *Appl Immunohistochem* 1996;4:1.
98. Weiss LM, Arber DA, Chang KL. CD45: a review. *Appl Immunohistochem* 1993;1:166.
99. Chang KL, Arber DA, Weiss LM. CD30: a review. *Appl Immunohistochem* 1993;1:244.
100. Arber DA, Weiss LM. CD15: a review. *Appl Immunohistochem* 1993; 1:17.

Hodgkin's Disease, edited by P. M. Mauch,
J. O. Armitage, V. Diehl, R. T. Hoppe, and L. M. Weiss.
Published by Lippincott Williams & Wilkins, Philadephia 1999.

CHAPTER 12

Relationship between Hodgkin's Disease and Non-Hodgkin's Lymphomas

Elaine S. Jaffe and Konrad Mueller-Hermelink

Hodgkin's disease and non-Hodgkin's lymphomas have long been regarded as distinct disease entities based on differences in pathology, immunophenotype, clinical features, and response to therapy. However, recent observations suggest that these disorders may be more closely related than previously thought. Whereas non-Hodgkin's lymphomas have been recognized for many years to be derived from B and T lymphocytes, the origin of the malignant cell in Hodgkin's disease has been more controversial. At various times, the neoplastic cells in Hodgkin's disease, the Reed-Sternberg cells and variants, have been postulated to be lymphocytes, histiocytes, interdigitating dendritic cells, or even granulocytes (1).

Considerable progress has been made regarding the origin of the neoplastic cell in Hodgkin's disease (see Chapter 8). Recent data suggest that the malignant cell of Hodgkin's disease is a B cell in all, or nearly all, cases (2–5). The existence of a T-cell form of Hodgkin's disease is not totally excluded, but if it exists, it is relatively uncommon. If Hodgkin's disease is derived from an altered B lymphocyte, it is not surprising that areas of overlap with B-cell non-Hodgkin's lymphomas should occur both biologically and clinically (Fig. 1) (6). This chapter reviews the synchronous or metachronous appearance of classical Hodgkin's disease and non-Hodgkin's lymphoma as well as other areas of biological overlap (Table 1). If the Reed-Sternberg cell is viewed as a crippled B cell, the biological and molecular events leading to this state are complex. These events may occur in the context of a normal immune system, in the setting of non-Hodgkin's lymphoma, or in the setting of immunodeficiency, such as the acquired immune deficiency syndrome or iatrogenic immune suppression following solid organ transplantation. Cells resembling Reed-Sternberg cells and variants may be observed in these diverse clinical settings and may represent early steps in the transformation to Hodgkin's disease. Studies of these cases at the interface of Hodgkin's disease and non-Hodgkin's lymphoma may also provide insight into the pathogenesis of *de novo* Hodgkin's disease.

E. S. Jaffe: Hematopathology Section, Department of Pathology, National Cancer Institute, National Institutes of Health, Bethesda, Maryland.

K. Mueller-Hermelink: Institute for Pathology, University of Wurzburg, Wurzburg, Germany.

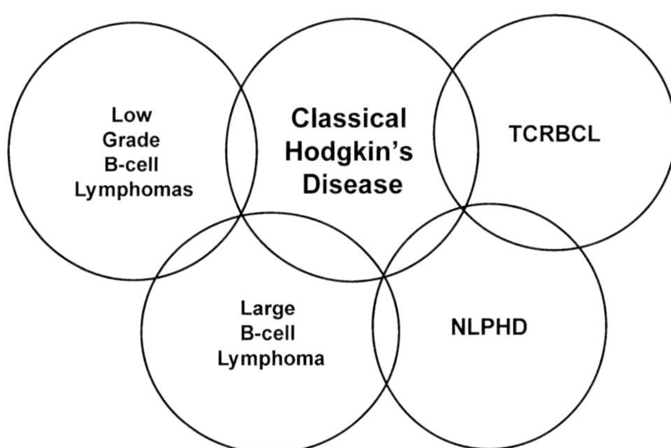

FIG. 1. Hodgkin's disease and non-Hodgkin's lymphomas: biological interfaces. Hodgkin's disease is derived from an altered B lymphocyte. The precise molecular events that result in the Reed-Sternberg cell are not fully elucidated. However, it is likely that these events can occur *de novo* in a normal B cell or secondarily in a neoplastic B cell. Therefore, biological interfaces are identified between Hodgkin's disease and diverse subtypes of B-cell lymphoma. Abbreviations: TCRBCL, T-cell–rich B-cell lymphoma; NLPHD, nodular lymphocyte predominance Hodgkin's disease.

TABLE 1. *Interrelationship between classical Hodgkin's disease and non-Hodgkin's lymphomas*[a]

	NHL subtypes (%)[b]	Association with EBV
NHL following cHD	Large B-cell (45%)	14% of all B-cell subtypes: (mainly in high grade subtypes)
	Burkitt/Burkitt-like (45%)	
	Other B-cell (10%)	
Composite cHD/NHL	Follicular (45%)	No
	Large B-cell (45%)	50% (in both HD and NHL)
	Other B-cell (10%)	No
cHD following NHL[c]	CLL	90% (in HD)
	Follicular lymphoma	No
	Large B-cell	No
	Mycosis fungoides	ND
	Other PTL (rare)	Yes

[a]Abbreviations: NHL, non-Hodgkin's lymphoma; cHD, classical Hodgkin's disease; CLL, chronic lymphocytic leukemia; EBV, Epstein-Barr virus; ND, not determined; PTL, peripheral T-cell lymphomas.

[b](%) Approximate distribution of associated lymphomas and lymphocytic leukemias based on published data.

[c]Accurate relative incidence figures for cHD following NHL are not available; only most common associations are shown.

Other benign and malignant conditions contain Reed-Sternberg–like cells that may mimic Hodgkin's disease. Examples of such conditions include peripheral T-cell lymphomas, anaplastic large-cell lymphomas, and even poorly differentiated carcinomas. These disorders represent examples of morphologic overlap with Hodgkin's disease but, for the most part, lack evidence of a biological relationship to Hodgkin's disease (Fig. 2). These conditions are best discussed in the context of differential diagnosis and are not covered here. However, there are some disorders for which a biological overlap has been postulated, such as anaplastic large-cell lymphoma and lymphomatoid papulosis. A true biological relationship with Hodgkin's disease is controversial for these proliferations and probably not supported by most recent data. However, it is appropriate to review the data and discuss their implications.

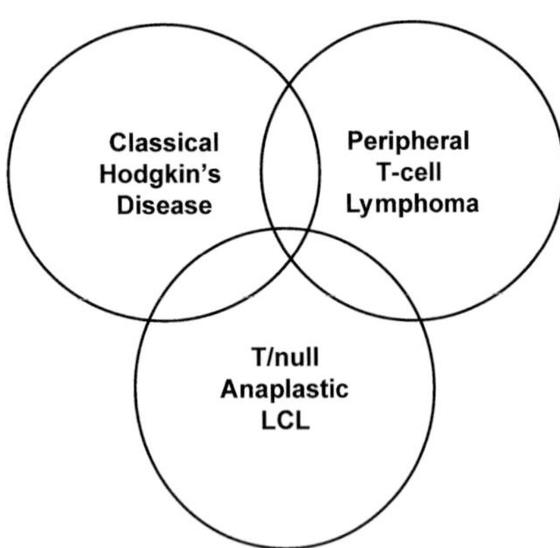

FIG. 2. Hodgkin's disease and non-Hodgkin's lymphomas: morphologic interfaces. In contrast to true biological interfaces, morphologic interfaces occur between Hodgkin's disease and other non-Hodgkin's lymphomas. These morphologic interfaces may provide problems in differential diagnosis but do not reflect an underlying biological relationship. Abbreviations: LCL, large cell lymphoma.

COMPOSITE LYMPHOMA: HODGKIN'S DISEASE AND B-CELL NON-HODGKIN'S LYMPHOMA

Composite lymphoma may be defined as the simultaneous occurrence of Hodgkin's disease and non-Hodgkin's lymphoma in the same anatomic site or biopsy specimen (7,8). The definition of composite lymphoma historically also has been applied to two variants of non-Hodgkin's lymphoma. However, in such cases, phenotypic and genotypic studies have indicated that the two histologic types of non-Hodgkin's lymphoma are clonally related in most instances. For example, large B-cell lymphomas that occur with follicular lymphomas are considered evidence of histologic progression within the same B-cell clone (9). As such, in recent years the term composite lymphoma has been more narrowly defined to situations in which the clonal relationship of the two neoplasms is more ambiguous. As with the B-cell non-Hodgkin's lymphomas, an analysis of composite Hodgkin's disease and non-Hodgkin's lymphoma may shed light on the nature of the malignant cell in Hodgkin's disease and may provide insight into the pathogenesis of this tumor.

Composite Hodgkin's disease and non-Hodgkin's lymphoma most often represents a B-cell non-Hodgkin's lymphoma in association with classical Hodgkin's disease, usually of the nodular sclerosis or mixed cellularity subtype. The type of B-cell non-Hodgkin's lymphoma involved reflects the incidence of B-cell lymphoma subtypes in the population. Therefore, most composite lymphomas involve follicular lymphomas and diffuse large B-cell lymphomas (10–13). Uncommonly, other types of B-cell lymphoma may be seen in association with classical Hodgkin's disease, including marginal zone B-cell lymphomas and mantle-cell lymphomas (14). The association of chronic lymphocytic leukemia with Hodgkin's disease has some distinctive features and is discussed separately.

Biopsy specimens usually show a segregation of the two histologic patterns within the lymph node. However, in some instances, the Hodgkin's disease and non-Hodgkin's lymphoma may be more intertwined. For example, in some cases of follicular lymphoma with coexistent Hodgkin's disease, the Hodgkin's disease may be found in the interfollicular paracortical regions.

Immunohistochemical studies are usually required for the diagnosis of a composite lymphoma. The neoplastic cells of the Hodgkin's disease component should retain the classical phenotype of Hodgkin's disease: CD30-positive, CD15-positive, and negative for leukocyte common antigen and both B-cell–associated and T-cell–associated antigens. Some cases of *de novo* Hodgkin's disease express CD20, and therefore, it is not unexpected that a minority of the Reed-Sternberg cells in composite lymphoma also may be CD20 positive (15). The expression of CD20 in the Hodgkin's disease component might imply a clonal relationship, but genetic studies would be required for confirmation of an association.

Epstein-Barr virus has been implicated in the pathogenesis of many cases of Hodgkin's disease and is most often associated with the mixed cellularity and lymphocyte depletion subtypes (see Chapter 6). Epstein-Barr virus has also been investigated in composite lymphomas. In most cases studied, the expression of Epstein-Barr virus was concordant in both components; that is, the neoplastic cells of both the Hodgkin's disease and the non-Hodgkin's lymphoma were either both positive or both negative (16). Approximately 33% of composite lymphomas were positive for Epstein-Barr virus sequences in the neoplastic cells. In all positive cases, the non-Hodgkin's lymphoma component was an aggressive B-cell lymphoma, either large B-cell or Burkitt-like. Cases of composite follicular lymphoma and Hodgkin's disease were negative for Epstein-Barr virus in both components.

Only very limited molecular studies have been applied to composite lymphomas. With the advent of techniques permitting the microdissection of individual tumor cells, it is likely that future studies will shed more light on the interrelationship of Hodgkin's disease and non-Hodgkin's lymphoma occurring as composite lymphomas.

Clinically, composite lymphoma presents in an older age group. In one series the median age at presentation was 62 years (10). This clinical presentation is more typical of the underlying non-Hodgkin's lymphoma and coincides with the second peak seen in epidemiologic studies of Hodgkin's disease, in which a bimodal age distribution is seen. The prognosis for patients with composite Hodgkin's disease and non-Hodgkin's lymphoma is most dependent on the histologic subtype of the non-Hodgkin's lymphoma identified. Patients with diffuse large B-cell lymphoma and Hodgkin's disease should be treated for the most "aggressive histology," in this instance the non-Hodgkin's lymphoma. The clinical course of patients with composite follicular lymphoma and Hodgkin's disease is more indolent. Relapses of either non-Hodgkin's lymphoma, Hodgkin's disease, or composite lymphoma may be seen following therapy.

A situation closely related to composite lymphoma is the simultaneous presentation of Hodgkin's disease and non-Hodgkin's lymphoma in different anatomic sites (17). Only a small number of cases have been identified, perhaps because in a patient undergoing diagnostic biopsy, if a biopsy does lead to a definite diagnosis, a second biopsy of another anatomic site is rarely performed. Although the true frequency of simultaneous Hodgkin's disease and non-Hodgkin's lymphoma is difficult to assess, it seems to be a rare phenomenon. The distribution of the non-Hodgkin's lymphoma subtypes encountered is similar to that of composite lymphoma, with follicular lymphomas and diffuse large B-cell lymphomas being the most frequent.

The coexistence of classical Hodgkin's disease with nodular lymphocyte predominance Hodgkin's disease can be considered a type of composite lymphoma. In recent years nodular lymphocyte predominance Hodgkin's disease has been considered a distinct entity, separable from classical Hodgkin's disease in virtually all cases on morphologic, immunophenotypic, and clinical grounds (18). Nodular lymphocyte predominance Hodgkin's disease has a mature B-cell phenotype and contains functional rather than crippled immunoglobulin genes (19,20). Just as classical Hodgkin's disease may occur in the setting of a non-Hodgkin's lymphoma of B-cell phenotype, classical Hodgkin's disease has also been reported in association with rare cases of nodular lymphocyte predominance Hodgkin's disease (21–23). This association has been reported as composite lymphoma as well as metachronous events involving biopsy specimens at different points in time.

NON-HODGKIN'S LYMPHOMAS FOLLOWING HODGKIN'S DISEASE

An increased risk of non-Hodgkin's lymphoma in patients successfully treated for Hodgkin's disease was first reported by Krikorian et al. (24). All patients had been treated with both radiation and chemotherapy and had been in complete remission for 4 to 10 years. The actuarial risk of developing non-Hodgkin's lymphoma was estimated at 4.4%, and it was postulated that the non-Hodgkin's lymphomas represented a complication from a persistent immunologic deficit. It is known that patients with Hodgkin's disease have underlying defects in cell-mediated immunity and that these defects persist following therapy (25,26). The most common subtypes of non-Hodgkin's lymphoma have been diffuse large B-cell lymphoma or other high-grade B-cell lymphomas classified as Burkitt-like or small noncleaved, non-Burkitt's in the Working Formulation (27,28). However, rare cases of low-grade non-Hodgkin's lymphoma also have been reported (29).

Subsequent series have confirmed the previous findings. The time to non-Hodgkin's lymphoma following a diagnosis of Hodgkin's disease has ranged from 1 to 26 years. The risk of secondary non-Hodgkin's lymphoma is approximately 5%. The risk of non-Hodgkin's lymphoma appears greater in patients showing evidence of underlying immunodeficiency or immune suppression, such as low peripheral blood lymphocyte counts, advanced clinical stage, or systemic symptoms (28).

The histologic subtype of non-Hodgkin's lymphoma does not appear related to the subtype of Hodgkin's disease or the treatment received. All of the non-Hodgkin's lymphomas have been of B-cell phenotype, and most patients have presented with intraabdominal disease. The pathologic and clinical features are similar to those of the aggressive B-cell non-Hodgkin's lymphomas reported in association with other immunodeficiency states, such as the acquired immune deficiency syndrome. Thus, although these findings are of interest, they do not necessarily shed light on the nature of the malignant cell in Hodgkin's disease or point to a clonal relationship between the two tumors. One recent study of a single case provided evidence for distinct B-cell clones in the two tumors using a single-cell microdissection assay and PCR amplification (30). A "small noncleaved" Burkitt-like lymphoma presented as an abdominal mass involving the cecum 41 months after the initial presentation with nodular sclerosis Hodgkin's disease. As has been the case in previous reports, the patient was in remission for Hodgkin's disease at the time of presentation with the non-Hodgkin's lymphoma. Epstein-Barr viral sequences were not studied in this case.

Based on the similarities of these lymphomas to those seen in immunodeficiency states, and the underlying immunologic deficits in patients with Hodgkin's disease, one might expect these lymphomas to be positive for Epstein-Barr virus. However, Epstein-Barr virus was identified uncommonly in non-Hodgkin's lymphoma associated with Hodgkin's disease. Only two of 14 (14%) non-Hodgkin's lymphomas that followed Hodgkin's disease contained Epstein-Barr virus when studied by *in situ* hybridization for EBER1 mRNA (16). Additionally, two cases of simultaneous Hodgkin's disease and large-cell lymphoma of B-cell type were also Epstein-Barr virus-negative.

Although the pathogenesis of most non-Hodgkin's lymphomas following Hodgkin's disease remains uncertain, it still may be related to the underlying immunodeficiency of Hodgkin's disease. Parallels may be drawn with many of the non-Hodgkin's lymphomas associated with human immunodeficiency virus infection (HIV). Most such Epstein-Barr virus-negative non-Hodgkin's lymphomas are Burkitt's lymphomas with rearrangements of the *c-myc* oncogene (31). A common pathogenesis may be operative in non-Hodgkin's lymphoma following Hodgkin's disease and HIV-associated non-Hodgkin's lymphoma. In support of this possibility, a number of the non-Hodgkin's lymphomas following Hodgkin's disease have been small noncleaved or Burkitt-like. In addition, patients with Hodgkin's disease often exhibit evidence of polyclonal B-cell hyperplasia and plasmacytosis, as is commonly seen in HIV-positive patients, perhaps suggesting that similar immunologic stimuli may be involved in both groups of patients.

MEDIASTINAL LARGE B-CELL LYMPHOMA AND NODULAR SCLEROSIS HODGKIN'S DISEASE

One of the more common occurrences in patients with composite lymphoma, or non-Hodgkin's lymphoma following Hodgkin's disease, is the association of mediastinal or thymic B-cell lymphoma with nodular sclerosis Hodgkin's disease (10,27,32). Nodular sclerosis Hodgkin's disease and mediastinal large B-cell lymphoma share a number of common clinical features. They both show a female predominance and present in young adults, with the median age of presentation for thymic B-cell lymphoma being slightly older than that of nodular sclerosis Hodgkin's disease (33–35). Both lymphomas present with an anterior mediastinal mass with involvement of the thymus gland and frequent involvement of supraclavicular lymph nodes.

Mediastinal large B-cell lymphomas have been reported following treatment for Hodgkin's disease, but in contrast to most non-Hodgkin's lymphomas, which usually present more than 10 years after primary diagnosis and treatment, the mediastinal lymphomas have presented early in the course of disease, frequently within 1 year of diagnosis. This close association suggests a different pathogenesis for these non-Hodgkin's lymphomas than for other secondary late-occurring B-cell non-Hodgkin's lymphomas. Because the malignant cell of Hodgkin's disease is thought to be a crippled or altered B lymphocyte, both mediastinal large B-cell lymphoma and nodular sclerosis Hodgkin's disease might be derived from a common cell of origin, possibly a thymic B cell (36).

At a recent workshop held in Wurzburg, Germany exploring the interrelationship of Hodgkin's disease and non-Hodgkin's lymphoma, several cases were encountered that relate to a possible association of mediastinal large B-cell lymphoma and nodular sclerosis Hodgkin's disease. Five cases were encountered with a transitional histologic appearance, showing features of both Hodgkin's disease and mediastinal large B-cell lymphoma. The histology in these cases most closely resembled a large B-cell lymphoma, with sheeting out of malignant cells, a sparse inflammatory background, and infiltration of adjacent soft tissue. Fibrous bands were either absent (three cases) or focal (two cases). Necrosis, which is usually a prominent feature in histologically aggressive nodular sclerosis Hodgkin's disease (grade II), was either absent or focal. However, most of the cases did show some vague nodularity, reminiscent of that seen in nodular sclerosis Hodgkin's disease.

The immunohistochemical phenotype of these cases was also "transitional." Although all cases were CD30-positive, and usually CD15-positive (4/5), both CD20 and

CD79a were expressed on the neoplastic cells in the majority of cases. The neoplastic cells were frequently positive for leukocyte common antigen as well. Thus, the immunologic phenotype was intermediate between that of a B-cell non-Hodgkin's lymphoma and Hodgkin's disease. All cases were negative for Epstein-Barr virus, arguing against a role for Epstein-Barr virus in the process. These cases underscore the close relationship between Hodgkin's disease and non-Hodgkin's lymphomas of B-cell type and support a B-cell derivation for the malignant cell of Hodgkin's disease.

Clinically, patients with features of both Hodgkin's disease and thymic B-cell lymphoma should be treated for an aggressive non-Hodgkin's lymphoma. The clinical course in these patients was generally aggressive, and many had relapsed following conventional treatment for Hodgkin's disease with either radiation or chemotherapy. In addition, relapse often occurred at distant sites, such as kidneys or central nervous system. These are common sites of spread for mediastinal large B-cell lymphoma. An unexpected finding based on review of the literature and the cases presented at the Wurzburg workshop is that most of these cases presented in men (10/11). This fact is surprising because both nodular sclerosis Hodgkin's disease and mediastinal large B-cell lymphoma are more common in women than men. Whether mediastinal large B-cell lymphoma represents an unusual evolution of nodular sclerosis Hodgkin's disease in these patients is purely speculative.

HODGKIN'S DISEASE FOLLOWING NON-HODGKIN'S LYMPHOMA

Although a risk for non-Hodgkin's lymphoma following Hodgkin's disease has been known for some time, Hodgkin's disease following non-Hodgkin's lymphoma has been considered rare. Carrato and colleagues reported five cases occurring 5 to 23 years after a primary diagnosis of non-Hodgkin's lymphoma (37). Travis and colleagues reviewed the experience of the national SEER Cancer Registry (38). They found that Hodgkin's disease was the most common cancer occurring after treatment for non-Hodgkin's lymphoma, with an observed-to-expected risk ratio of 4.16:1. Hodgkin's disease was more common than acute leukemia, a malignancy often associated with the carcinogenic effects of alkylating agent chemotherapy.

In a recent study expanding on Hodgkin's disease following non-Hodgkin's lymphoma, all of the non-Hodgkin's lymphomas were of B-cell origin, with a median age at presentation of the non-Hodgkin's lymphoma of 54 years (39). The most common histologic subtypes of the underlying non-Hodgkin's lymphoma were follicular lymphoma or diffuse large B-cell lymphoma. The median interval between non-Hodgkin's lymphoma and Hodgkin's disease was 5 years. The patients had generally received chemotherapy, either alone or in combination with radiation therapy. Lymph nodes represented the site of presentation of Hodgkin's disease in all cases. Although it is difficult to draw firm conclusions in a heterogeneously treated patient population, most of the patients did respond to therapy for Hodgkin's disease. The most common histologic subtype of Hodgkin's disease was nodular sclerosis. Hodgkin's disease has also been reported in association with certain T-cell malignancies, most commonly mycosis fungoides and chronic lymphocytic leukemia (see below).

As expected, the immunologic phenotypes of the Hodgkin's disease and non-Hodgkin's lymphoma were discordant. In one study in which *bcl-2* rearrangements were investigated by polymerase chain reaction (PCR) in an unselected series of 32 cases of Hodgkin's disease, *bcl-2* rearrangements were found in only two cases, both of which arose in the setting of prior follicular lymphoma (40). In one case, identical chromosomal breakpoints were identified in the Hodgkin's disease and the follicular lymphoma. This finding would suggest a clonal relationship between the two tumors. However, given the sensitivity of the PCR technique, it is difficult to rule out the presence of small numbers of follicular lymphoma B cells in the lymph node involved by Hodgkin's disease, even if they were not detected by conventional histologic or immunohistochemical means.

In a separate study in which the role of Epstein-Barr virus was investigated in cases of Hodgkin's disease following non-Hodgkin's lymphoma, in none of the cases was Epstein-Barr virus positive in the Reed-Sternberg cells (16). This finding is perhaps unexpected because Epstein-Barr virus has been shown to play a role in the occurrence of Hodgkin's disease following chronic lymphocytic leukemia.

CHRONIC LYMPHOCYTIC LEUKEMIA AND CLASSICAL HODGKIN'S DISEASE

The development of classical Hodgkin's disease in a patient with chronic lymphocytic leukemia has been recognized for some time and has been considered a form of Richter's transformation (41,42). Early reports had described Reed-Sternberg–like cells in the setting of chronic lymphocytic leukemia or in Richter's syndrome (43). However, it was often assumed that these cases represented pleomorphic non-Hodgkin's lymphomas resembling Hodgkin's disease rather than true occurrences of Hodgkin's disease (44–46). More recently, several groups have documented both histologically and immunophenotypically the association of Hodgkin's disease and chronic lymphocytic leukemia, suggesting that the association is real (47–50).

Two histologic patterns are observed. In one, the Hodgkin's disease is histologically segregated from the chronic lymphocytic leukemia, either involving a different lymph node or anatomic site or within a single lymph node (48,51). In these cases, Reed-Sternberg cells and variants are found in the usual cellular milieu of

Hodgkin's disease, with numerous T lymphocytes, plasma cells, eosinophils, and other inflammatory cells. The Reed-Sternberg cells display the usual phenotype of classical Hodgkin's disease and are typically positive for Epstein-Barr virus sequences by *in-situ* hybridization. Expression of CD20 by at least some of the Reed-Sternberg cells is commonly observed.

A second pattern is more frequently encountered. In this instance, Reed-Sternberg cells and variants are seen in a background of otherwise typical chronic lymphocytic leukemia, without the apparent cellular background of Hodgkin's disease (11,47,52). However, on closer inspection, although the Reed-Sternberg cells are surrounded by small lymphocytes, with immunohistochemical studies they are found to be rosetted by T cells, as is typical of Hodgkin's disease (47). The surrounding B cells have the usual phenotype of chronic lymphocytic leukemia and are monoclonal with coexpression of CD5. This process can be considered a form of composite lymphoma because both diseases are present in the same anatomic site.

By immunohistochemical studies, the Reed-Sternberg cells display the usual phenotype of Hodgkin's disease: CD30-positive and CD15-positive. Expression of some B-cell–associated antigens is variable. Epstein-Barr virus appears to play a major role in the development of Hodgkin's disease in this setting (53). The Reed-Sternberg cells have been positive for Epstein-Barr virus by *in-situ* hybridization or staining for latent membrane protein (LMP-1) in more than 90% of the cases studied. Although most of the background chronic lymphocytic leukemia cells are negative for Epstein-Barr virus, a small number of Epstein-Barr virus–positive cells is often found. In one study, Epstein-Barr virus positivity was identified in a small population of the lymphocytes in the underlying chronic lymphocytic leukemia several years before the development of Hodgkin's disease. This observation suggests that a first step in this transformation may be Epstein-Barr virus infection of chronic lymphocytic leukemia B lymphocytes (50). Rare cases in which the Reed-Sternberg cells are negative for Epstein-Barr virus have been described, indicating that there may be other mechanisms involved in this transformation (54).

A recent study attempted to examine the clonal relationship between chronic lymphocytic leukemia and Hodgkin's disease using microdissection techniques and PCR amplification of immunoglobulin heavy-chain genes (IgH) (55). The IgH CDRIII sequences from the Reed-Sternberg cells were identical to those from the chronic lymphocytic leukemia cells in two cases. In one case, the clonal relationship between the two disorders could not be examined because PCR products could not be obtained from the Reed-Sternberg cells. However, these studies provide further evidence that the Reed-Sternberg cells in both chronic lymphocytic leukemia and classical Hodgkin's disease are derived from transformed B lymphocytes.

Clinically, the development of Hodgkin's disease in a patient with chronic lymphocytic leukemia usually portends an aggressive clinical course (49,53). Most of the patients have developed progressive dissemination of Hodgkin's disease, usually with a poor response to therapy. The median survival is under 2 years following the diagnosis of Hodgkin's disease. It is interesting to speculate on the role of immune deficiency in the development of Hodgkin's disease following chronic lymphocytic leukemia. Patients with chronic lymphocytic leukemia typically display defects in both cellular and humoral immunity, with an increased risk of viral infections. Perhaps an increased viral load of Epstein-Barr virus is associated with the secondary development of Hodgkin's disease. In this regard, it has been suggested that treatment with fludarabine, which leads to profound lymphocytopenia, may increase the risk of secondary Hodgkin's disease (56).

HODGKIN'S DISEASE AND T-CELL LYMPHOMAS

In general, T-cell lymphomas are less often reported in association with Hodgkin's disease than B-cell lymphomas (17). This observation may reflect the lower frequency of T-cell malignancies, with the risk of coincidence with Hodgkin's disease being equal to that for B-cell disease. Alternatively, it might indicate that patients with T-cell lymphomas are not at risk to develop Hodgkin's disease. Finally, the coincidence may be underreported because of the difficulty in distinguishing Hodgkin's disease from peripheral T-cell lymphoma. Because peripheral T-cell lymphomas are associated with a prominent inflammatory background and sometimes contain pleomorphic cells resembling Reed-Sternberg cells, the observation of Reed-Sternberg cells in this setting might be assumed to be a manifestation of the T-cell malignancy and not actually Hodgkin's disease. However, if the association of Hodgkin's disease with non-Hodgkin's lymphoma is an indication of the clonal relationship of the two disorders, as a B-cell origin is likely for most cases of Hodgkin's disease, it is not surprising that Hodgkin's disease is rarely found with T-cell lymphomas. In one well-documented case, cytogenetic studies were performed on both the Hodgkin's disease and the associated peripheral T-cell lymphoma (57). Evidence of two distinct clones was obtained.

Cells resembling Reed-Sternberg cells both morphologically and immunophenotypically have been reported in a number of T-cell malignancies including mycosis fungoides, adult T-cell leukemia/lymphoma, and peripheral T-cell lymphomas, unspecified (58–60). The most common association is that of Hodgkin's disease and mycosis fungoides. Since 1979, more than 20 well-documented reports of Hodgkin's disease in association with mycosis fungoides have appeared in the literature (61–65). In one case studied with molecular techniques, a common clonal T-cell gene rearrangement was found in tissues involved by lymphomatoid papulosis, mycosis fungoides, and Hodgkin's disease (66). However, a second report provided evidence for distinct clonal origins of mycosis fungoides and Hodgkin's disease in two patients studied with molecular techniques (65). The confirmation of an association between mycosis fungoides, lymphomatoid papulosis, and Hodgkin's disease is complicated by the existence of common morphological and even phenotypical characteristics of the neoplastic cells (58). Expression of both CD15 and CD30 has been reported in the pleomorphic tumor cells of both mycosis fungoides and lymphomatoid papulosis (67,68). Therefore, do cases of Hodgkin's disease in the setting of mycosis fungoides and lymphomatoid papulosis represent instances of true Hodgkin's disease, or are these pleomorphic T-cell malignancies simulating Hodgkin's disease (69)?

In instances of mycosis fungoides and Hodgkin's disease occurring in the same patient, the diagnosis of mycosis fungoides usually precedes that of Hodgkin's disease by months to years. This observation would further support the view that some of these cases might represent pleomorphic T-cell lymphomas simulating Hodgkin's disease. However, in some cases the diagnosis of Hodgkin's disease may precede the appearance of mycosis fungoides, or the two disorders may present simultaneously (61,70–72). An association of mycosis fungoides and Hodgkin's disease is further supported by the diagnosis of Hodgkin's disease in the relatives of patients with mycosis fungoides (73). In a large epidemiologic study, Hodgkin's disease was the most common lymphoproliferative or hematopoietic malignancy occurring in family members. Of 526 consecutive patients with mycosis fungoides or Sezary syndrome, 21 had first-degree relatives with some form of lymphoma or leukemia. Hodgkin's disease accounted for one-third of the total cases reported. These observations further support an association between mycosis fungoides and Hodgkin's disease and suggest that genetically determined immunoregulatory pathways may represent shared pathways of oncogenesis in these disorders.

A relationship between Hodgkin's disease and mycosis fungoides is further complicated by controversy as to whether a T-cell form of Hodgkin's disease exists (see Chapter 8). It is generally agreed that the vast majority of cases of Hodgkin's disease are of B-cell origin. However, cases of Hodgkin's disease expressing T-cell–associated antigens, including the relatively specific marker CD3, have been described (74). Whether such cases represent instances of aberrant antigenic expression or true T-cell forms of Hodgkin's disease is not yet resolved. In our experience, such cases usually lack clonal T-cell receptor gene rearrangements *(unpublished observations).*

The existence of a T-cell form of Hodgkin's disease is complicated by cases of anaplastic large-cell lymphoma, which may contain Reed-Sternberg–like cells. Both anaplastic large-cell lymphoma and Hodgkin's disease are CD30-positive. Recent studies for the expression of cytotoxic-associated molecules have confirmed the distinction of anaplastic large cell lymphoma from Hodgkin's disease. While most cases of anaplastic large cell lymphoma express cytotoxic molecules, the neoplastic cells of Hodgkin's disease are negative for these antigens in most cases (75,76). These features further aid in the differential diagnosis of Hodgkin's disease and anaplastic large-cell lymphoma.

Reed-Sternberg–like cells have been observed in a number of peripheral T-cell lymphomas, including angioimmunoblastic T-cell lymphoma. A Hodgkin's-like morphology has also been reported in adult T-cell leukemia/lymphoma (59,60). This histologic pattern appears to precede the development of acute adult T-cell leukemia/lymphoma in the few published cases. One report suggested that the Reed-Sternberg–like cells were Epstein-Barr virus-positive transformed B cells and not part of the neoplastic T-cell process (77). In contrast to the neoplastic T cells, the Reed-Sternberg–like cells lacked HTLV-I–associated sequences. We too have observed such Reed-Sternberg–like cells in peripheral T-cell lymphomas *(unpublished observations).* The Reed-Sternberg–like cells contained Epstein-Barr virus sequences and expressed the CD20 antigen, as distinct from the expression of T-cell antigens on the neoplastic T cells. Notably, both adult T-cell leukemia/lymphoma and angioimmunoblastic T-cell lymphoma are malignancies associated with immune suppression and an increased risk of opportunistic infections. The presence of Epstein-Barr virus-transformed B-cell blasts may represent a manifestation of the underlying immunodeficiency in these conditions.

HODGKIN'S DISEASE AND EPSTEIN-BARR VIRUS–POSITIVE LYMPHOPROLIFERATIVE DISORDERS

Recently it has been shown that patients with rheumatologic disorders receiving long-term immunosuppressive therapy with methotrexate are at increased risk to develop Epstein-Barr virus–positive lymphoproliferative disorders (78,79). These Epstein-Barr virus–positive lymphoproliferative disorders may resemble both Hodgkin's disease and non-Hodgkin's lymphoma (80). This complication has been seen in patients with both rheumatoid arthritis and dermatomyositis. It is most likely related to the immunosuppressive effects of methotrexate rather than a direct oncogenic effect because the atypical lymphoproliferations frequently regress when the immunosuppression is withdrawn (78,79). In most cases the patients have been receiving immunosuppressive therapy for at least 1 year.

The cases reported appear to represent a spectrum of Epstein-Barr virus–positive B-cell proliferations ranging from polymorphic B-cell lymphomas, as seen in solid organ transplantation, to lymphomas resembling both Hodgkin's disease and large B-cell lymphoma (80). Cases of lymphoproliferative disorder resembling Hodgkin's disease often occur in soft tissue or other nonnodal sites, whereas cases with features of more typical Hodgkin's disease tend to present in lymph nodes. Immunohistochemical studies may be of value in distinguishing typical Hodgkin's disease from other lymphoproliferative disorders because the lymphoproliferative disorders are usually negative for CD15 in the atypical cells. Virtually all cases are positive for CD30 because Epstein-Barr virus induces increased expression of the CD30 antigen in B cells and B-cell lines (81).

The clinical management of these cases is complex. Clearly, in cases resembling an Epstein-Barr virus–positive lymphoproliferative disorder in the posttransplant setting, the immunosuppression should be withdrawn, and the patient observed for spontaneous regression. The same approach might be followed even in lymph nodes resembling more typical Hodgkin's disease or even non-Hodgkin's lymphoma because some cases will spontaneously regress. However, if the lesions persist, conventional therapy for Hodgkin's disease is recommended.

It is of interest that classical Hodgkin's disease is relatively uncommon following solid organ transplantation. However, an increased risk of Hodgkin's disease following allogeneic bone marrow transplantation has been observed (82). Such cases are virtually always positive for Epstein-Barr virus.

HODGKIN'S DISEASE AND T-CELL–RICH B-CELL LYMPHOMA

In recent years several groups have reported the existence of cases histologically resembling Hodgkin's disease but having the immunophenotype of T-cell–rich B-cell lymphoma (83–85). The cases may resemble either classical Hodgkin's disease or, more often, lymphocyte predominant Hodgkin's disease. The differential diagnosis of such cases is discussed in detail in Chapters 7 and 11. We comment only briefly on the biological significance of T-cell–rich B-cell lymphomas resembling classical Hodgkin's disease.

Modern studies of the biology of Hodgkin's disease have suggested that classical Hodgkin's disease may in fact be a T-cell–rich B-cell lymphoma (2). A B-cell origin for the malignant cells of Hodgkin's disease is apparent in nearly all cases. Reed-Sternberg cells elaborate numerous cytokines, which lead to the prominent inflammatory background that is an essential component of the histologic diagnosis (86). T cells comprise the majority of the nonneoplastic lymphocytes in most cases of classical Hodgkin's disease.

The events that lead to the development of a Reed-Sternberg cell are as yet unknown. However, it is likely that this process involves multiple steps. Moreover, cases of Hodgkin's disease show significant variation from case to case in the expression of B-cell–associated antigens (15,87). By definition, if all of the neoplastic cells are CD20-positive, the diagnosis of T-cell–rich B-cell lymphoma over Hodgkin's disease is favored. However, cases of T-cell–rich B-cell lymphoma resembling classical Hodgkin's disease may be related to Hodgkin's disease. Interestingly, T-cell–rich B-cell lymphoma has a more aggressive course than Hodgkin's disease, with these patients frequently failing to respond to conventional therapy for Hodgkin's disease (83–85). Moreover, the expression of B-cell antigens by a high proportion of the malignant cells (>20%) was shown to be an adverse prognostic factor in a large series from the German Hodgkin Study Group (88).

HODGKIN'S DISEASE AND ANAPLASTIC LARGE-CELL LYMPHOMA

Classical Hodgkin's disease and anaplastic large-cell lymphoma share some morphologic and immunophenotypic features (89). CD30 antigen expression, which is the hallmark of anaplastic large-cell lymphoma, is of course also found in Reed-Sternberg cells. This common biologic feature led to early speculation that Hodgkin's disease and anaplastic large-cell lymphoma might be related (90). However, subsequent studies have suggested that these disorders are distinct and that there is no true biologic or clinical overlap.

Hodgkin's-related anaplastic large-cell lymphoma was initially described as a form of anaplastic large-cell lymphoma closely resembling Hodgkin's disease (91,92). The patients were often young boys or men with mediastinal masses who responded poorly to conventional therapy for Hodgkin's disease but appeared to respond to third-generation therapy designed for non-Hodgkin's lymphoma. It is now apparent that most such cases are in fact aggressive forms of Hodgkin's disease, probably within the spectrum of nodular sclerosis Hodgkin's disease, grade II, that histologically resemble anaplastic large-cell lymphoma (93,94). (Some of these cases may represent examples of transitional nodular sclerosis Hodgkin's disease/mediastinal large B-cell lymphoma, as described above.)

By contrast, some cases of anaplastic large-cell lymphoma may histologically resemble nodular sclerosis Hodgkin's disease, having a vaguely nodular growth pattern and areas of fibrosis. However, careful immunophenotypic evaluation will usually show an absence of CD15, expression of epithelial membrane antigen and T-cell–associated antigens, and frequent positivity for ALK-1, which detects the anaplastic large cell lymphoma kinase (93,95,96).

Recent studies have shown no biologic overlap between true anaplastic large-cell lymphoma and classical Hodgkin's disease. The neoplastic cells of anaplastic large-cell lymphoma usually express one or more T-cell–associated antigens and have a cytotoxic phenotype (75,76). By contrast, the malignant cells of most cases of Hodgkin's disease lack cytotoxic antigens such as TIA-1, granzyme B, and perforin. One early report suggested that the t(2;5)(p23;q35) characteristic of anaplastic large-cell lymphoma could be detected by a sensitive reverse transcriptase–PCR method in cases of typical Hodgkin's disease (97). However, subsequent studies have found no evidence of the t(2;5), by either molecular or cytogenetic means, in the neoplastic cells of classical Hodgkin's disease or cases classified as Hodgkin's-like anaplastic large-cell lymphoma (93,94,96,98,99).

Reevaluation of well-documented cases of anaplastic large-cell lymphoma show that most of these tumors do not contain cells resembling true Reed-Sternberg cells. The cells of anaplastic large-cell lymphoma may be lobated, but they usually lack prominent nucleoli. There is abundant slightly basophilic cytoplasm, usually with a prominent perinuclear hof or Golgi zone. There is usually a spectrum in cell size, which is generally lacking in the neoplastic cells of Hodgkin's disease (93).

DIAGNOSTIC CONSIDERATIONS

Areas of both biological and morphologic overlap with Hodgkin's disease frequently cause diagnostic difficulty to the pathologist. Although scientifically we have become aware of a close relationship between non-Hodgkin's lymphoma and Hodgkin's disease, these disorders generally are approached with different treatment modalities. For the clinician, the distinction between Hodgkin's disease and non-Hodgkin's lymphoma is important in making treatment decisions. Therefore, it is highly desirable to have consistent and reproducible diagnostic guidelines for pathologists at multiple treatment centers to employ.

An international workshop was held recently in Wurzburg, Germany to examine diagnostically challenging cases at the interface between Hodgkin's disease and non-Hodgkin's lymphoma with the goal of establishing uniform criteria by which such cases may be diagnosed and treated in the future (100). Sixty-two cases were contributed by ten expert pathologists, representing examples of the following areas of potential biological or morphologic overlap:

- Interface of anaplastic large-cell lymphoma versus classical Hodgkin's disease
- Interface of T-cell–rich B-cell lymphoma versus classical Hodgkin's disease, mixed cellularity and nodular sclerosis subtypes
- Interface of diffuse "paragranuloma type" of lymphocyte predominance Hodgkin's disease versus classical Hodgkin's disease, mixed cellularity subtype
- Classical Hodgkin's disease occurring simultaneously or in the course of any non-Hodgkin's lymphoma (composite lymphomas)
- Primary extranodal classical Hodgkin's disease—does it exist?
- T-cell type of Hodgkin's disease—does it exist?
- Lymphoproliferative disorders in the immunosuppressed host (including methotrexate-associated Epstein-Barr virus–positive lymphoproliferative disease) simulating classical Hodgkin's disease

After discussion and evaluation of immunohistochemical studies, a consensus diagnosis could be reached in all cases. As always, the diagnosis of classical Hodgkin's disease relies on the identification of classical Reed-Sternberg cells with an appropriate growth pattern (often interfollicular) in an inflammatory background that is composed of inflammatory cells including small T lymphocytes, plasma cells, histiocytes, and granulocytes. Twenty-two of 23 cases of classical Hodgkin's disease were investigated immunohistochemically; such studies proved valuable in resolving diagnostically difficult cases (Table 2).

In all cases, CD30 expression could be observed in the paranuclear Golgi region in at least some of the neoplastic cells. CD15 is expressed in 70% to 80% of unselected cases of Hodgkin's disease and was found in 68% of cases in the workshop series (87,100,101). Thirty-six percent of the workshop cases expressed CD20, a figure somewhat higher than that expected in the literature (87,102). However, the expression of CD20 was weaker on the neoplastic cells than on the surrounding B lymphocytes, and usually only a minority of the tumor cells stained. In addition, the staining intensity varied among individual tumor cells, a feature characteristic of Hodgkin's disease (102). In a minority of cases of Hodgkin's disease, the neoplastic cells expressed T-cell–associated antigens such as CD3 or CD43. Cytotoxic granules (TIA-1, granzyme B) also have been reported in a minority of cases of Hodgkin's disease (76,104). However, again, usually only a minority of the neoplastic cells express these antigens. Epithelial membrane antigen is usually negative in Reed-Sternberg cells. However, the expression of epithelial membrane antigen varies somewhat with the antibody used, the detection method, and

TABLE 2. *Workshop on gray zone lymphomas: Immunophenotypes of 22 cases classified by the panel as classical Hodgkin's disease*

CD30	CD15	CD20	Cases[a]
+	+	–	11
+	+	+	4
+	–	–	3
+	–	+	4

[a]Number of cases with indicated immunophenotype.

the fixative. Epithelial membrane antigen is much more readily detected in Bouin's-fixed tissues.

The differential diagnosis of nodular lymphocyte predominance Hodgkin's disease versus T-cell–rich B-cell lymphoma is discussed in Chapter 11 and is not covered here. However, the distinction of T-cell–rich B-cell lymphoma from classical Hodgkin's disease is sometimes problematic because of potential biological overlap between these conditions. As in classical Hodgkin's disease, in T-cell–rich B-cell lymphoma, the tumor cells form a minority of the infiltrate. Reed-Sternberg–like cells are sometimes observed. However, in contrast to the often perifollicular pattern of mixed cellularity Hodgkin's disease, the tumor cells in T-cell–rich B-cell lymphoma do not shown any relationship to preserved follicles. In addition, small T cells, although they are extremely abundant, do not show rosetting of individual tumor cells. The T cells frequently show nuclear irregularities and in the past have been misconstrued as part of the neoplastic process, considered "diffuse mixed lymphoma" (104) in the Working Formulation (106).

Immunohistochemically, the tumor cells of T-cell–rich B-cell lymphoma strongly express CD20 and are often positive for CD79a (Table 3). Light-chain restriction and immunoglobulin heavy-chain gene rearrangement are often shown but are not considered essential for the diagnosis (107–109). Additionally, the tumor cells are negative for vimentin, in contrast to classical Hodgkin's disease (103). The inflammatory infiltrate differs from that of both nodular lymphocyte predominance Hodgkin's disease and classical Hodgkin's disease. Small B cells and CD57-positive T cells are virtually absent in T-cell–rich B-cell lymphoma. Plasma cells and granulocytes are also infrequent, with the inflammatory background composed almost entirely of T lymphocytes and histiocytes.

Anaplastic large-cell lymphoma is admittedly heterogeneous from a morphologic standpoint. The tumor cells may be monomorphic or pleomorphic. Pleomorphic tumor cells include kidney-shaped hallmark cells and show a strong tendency to infiltrate lymph node sinuses. In some cases morphologic similarities to Hodgkin's disease with typical lacunar cells and Reed-Sternberg–like cells may be observed. In contrast to one early report (97), the presence of the translocation t(2;5)(p23;q35) in the neoplastic cells or immunohistochemical detection of the NMP-ALK fusion protein rules out Hodgkin's disease as a differential diagnosis (93,96,98,110).

In ALK1-negative cases, expression of antigens related to T cells (CD3, CD43, CD45R0), epithelial membrane antigen, or CD45 supports the diagnosis of anaplastic large-cell lymphoma. The significance of expression of cytotoxic granules ($TIA1^+$ and/or granzyme B^+) has not yet been decisively established. Cases with strong expression of CD30, CD15, and cytotoxic granules are problematic but in all likelihood are more closely related to Hodgkin's disease than to anaplastic large-cell lymphoma. The presence of CD15, CD20, or Epstein-Barr virus latent membrane protein all are strong arguments toward the diagnosis of classical Hodgkin's disease. Most cases with a B-cell phenotype and anaplastic large-cell morphology represent a tumor-cell–rich form of lymphocyte depletion or nodular sclerosis, type II Hodgkin's disease (111). As discussed above, there are rare cases that appear to be transitional between classical Hodgkin's disease and a mediastinal large B-cell lymphoma. These cases may contain Reed-Sternberg–like cells, a paucity of inflammatory cells, and express CD30, CD15, CD20 and/or CD79a, and CD45. The clinical behavior in the small number of cases studied appears very aggressive, with failure of treatment approaches generally effective for Hodgkin's disease. Therefore, treatment for aggressive non-Hodgkin's lymphoma may be more efficacious in such cases.

CONCLUSION

From the above observations, we may draw the following conclusions: (a) Hodgkin's disease and non-Hodgkin's lymphoma occur together with greater frequency than would be expected by chance alone; (b) the association favors a lymphoid origin for the malignant cell of Hodgkin's disease and, given the predominance of B-cell non-Hodgkin's lymphoma, would be consistent with a B-cell origin in the majority of cases; (c) a clonal relationship may exist between certain forms of classical Hodgkin's disease and non-Hodgkin's lymphoma, most likely follicular lymphoma, large B-cell lymphoma, and chronic lymphocytic leukemia; (d) the data support the concept that usual Hodgkin's disease may be an altered lymphoid malignancy, with secondary transformation by

TABLE 3. *Summary of antigen expression in classical Hodgkin's disease, T-cell-rich B-cell lymphoma, and nodular lymphocyte predominance Hodgkin's disease*

	Tumor cells					Background cells	
	CD30	CD20	CD79a	J chain	Vimentin	TIA1/CD57 ratio	B cells
Classical HD	+	−/+	−	−	+	↑	↓
TCRBCL	−	+	+/−	−/+	−	↑	↓↓
NLPHD	−/+	+	−/+	+/−	−	↓	↑

a virus such as Epstein-Barr virus and/or other candidates yet to be identified; and (e) the late-occurring non-Hodgkin's lymphoma in patients in remission for Hodgkin's disease are rarely Epstein-Barr virus positive and may have a similar pathogenesis to the Burkitt-like lymphomas seen in association with HIV infection.

Clearly, the cases of Hodgkin's disease occurring in association with non-Hodgkin's lymphoma, either as composite lymphomas or as secondary Hodgkin's disease, differ clinically from usual Hodgkin's disease. The patients are elderly, and the clinical behavior of the Hodgkin's disease is usually aggressive, especially in the context of chronic lymphocytic leukemia. The question may be posed: Are such cases truly Hodgkin's disease, or do they represent a Hodgkin's disease–like transformation induced by Epstein-Barr virus or other unknown causes? Until the molecular events that cause classical Hodgkin's disease are fully elucidated, this question cannot be addressed. However, it is important for both the pathologist and the clinician to be aware of these transformations, as they do impact on the clinical management of the patient. The study of such cases also may yield clues to the pathogenesis of usual Hodgkin's disease.

REFERENCES

1. Jaffe ES. The elusive Reed-Sternberg cell (editorial). *N Engl J Med* 1989;320:529.
2. Stewards RS. Hodgkin's disease—time for a change (editorial; comment]. *N Engl J Med* 1997;337:495.
3. Kanzler H, Kuppers R, Hansmann ML, Rajewsky K. Hodgkin and Reed-Sternberg cells in Hodgkin's disease represent the outgrowth of a dominant tumor clone derived from (crippled) germinal center B cells. *J Exp Med* 1996;184:1495.
4. Tamaru J, Hummel M, Zemlin M, Kalvelage B, Stein H. Hodgkin's disease with a B-cell phenotype often shows a VDJ rearrangement and somatic mutations in the VH genes. *Blood* 1994;84:708.
5. Küppers R, Rajewsky K, Zhao M, et al. Hodgkin's disease: Hodgkin and Reed Sternberg cells picked from histological sections show clonal immunoglobulin gene rearrangements and appear to be derived from B cells at various stages of development. *Proc Natl Acad Sci USA* 1994;91:1092.
6. Jaffe ES, Zarate-Osorno A, Medeiros LJ. The interrelationship of Hodgkin's disease and non-Hodgkin's lymphomas—lessons learned from composite and sequential malignancies. *Semin Diagn Pathol* 1992;9:297.
7. Custer R, Bernard W. The interrelationship of Hodgkin's disease and other lymphatic tumors. *Am J Med Sci* 1948;216:625.
8. Kim H, Hendrickson M, Dorfman R. Composite lymphoma. *Cancer* 1977;40:959.
9. Sander CA, Yano T, Clark HM, et al. p53 mutation is associated with progression in follicular lymphomas. *Blood* 1993;82:1994.
10. Gonzalez CL, Medeiros LJ, Jaffe ES. Composite lymphoma. A clinicopathologic analysis of nine patients with Hodgkin's disease and B-cell non-Hodgkin's lymphoma. *Am J Clin Pathol* 1991;96:81.
11. Hansmann ML, Fellbaum C, Hui PK, Lennert K. Morphological and immunohistochemical investigation of non-Hodgkin's lymphoma combined with Hodgkin's disease. *Histopathology* 1989;15:35.
12. Paulli M, Rosso R, Kindl S, et al. Nodular sclerosing Hodgkin's disease and large cell lymphoma. Immunophenotypic characterization of a composite case. *Virchows Arch Pathol Anat Histopathol* 1992;421:271.
13. Guarner J, del Rio C, Hendrix L, Unger ER. Composite Hodgkin's and non-Hodgkin's lymphoma in a patient with acquired immune deficiency syndrome. *In-situ* demonstration of Epstein-Barr virus. *Cancer* 1990;66:796.
14. Aguilera NS, Howard LN, Brissette MD, Abbondanzo SL. Hodgkin's disease and an extranodal marginal zone B-cell lymphoma in the small intestine: an unusual composite lymphoma. *Mod Pathol* 1996;9: 1020.
15. Schmid C, Pan L, Diss T, Isaacson P. Expression of B-cell antigens by Hodgkin's and Reed-Sternberg cells. *Am J Pathol* 1991;139:701.
16. Kingma DW, Medeiros LJ, Barletta J, et al. Epstein-Barr virus is infrequently identified in non-Hodgkin's lymphomas associated with Hodgkin's disease. *Am J Surg Pathol* 1994;18:48.
17. Jaffe ES, Zarate-Osorno A, Kingma DW, Raffeld M, Medeiros LJ. The interrelationship between Hodgkin's disease and non-Hodgkin's lymphomas. *Ann Oncol* 1994;5(suppl 1):s7.
18. Mason D, Banks P, Chan J, et al. Nodular lymphocyte predominance Hodgkin's disease: a distinct clinico-pathological entity. *Am J Surg Pathol* 1994;18:528.
19. Marafioti T, Hummel. M, Anagnostopoulos I, et al. Origin of nodular lymphocyte-predominant Hodgkin's disease from a clonal expansion of highly mutated germinal-center B cells. *N Engl J Med* 1997;337: 453.
20. Ohno T, Stribley JA, Wu G, Hinrichs SH, Weisenburger DD, Chan WC. Clonality in nodular lymphocyte-predominant Hodgkin's disease. *N Engl J Med* 1997;337:459.
21. Gelb AB, Dorfman RF, Warnke RA. Coexistence of nodular lymphocyte predominance Hodgkin's disease and Hodgkin's disease of the usual type. *Am J Surg Pathol* 1993;17:364.
22. Hansmann M, Stein H, Fellbaum C, Hui P, Parwaresch M, Lennert K. Nodular paragranuloma can transform into high-grade malignant lymphoma of B type. *Hum Pathol* 1989;20:1169.
23. Miettinen M, Franssila KO, Saxen E. Hodgkin's disease, lymphocytic predominance nodular. Increased risk for subsequent non-Hodgkin's lymphomas. *Cancer* 1983;51:2293.
24. Krikorian JG, Burke JS, Rosenberg SA, Kaplan HS. Occurrence of non-Hodgkin's lymphoma after therapy for Hodgkin's disease. *N Engl J Med* 1979;300:452.
25. Levy R, Kaplan HS. Impaired lymphocyte function in untreated Hodgkin's disease. *N Engl J Med* 1974;290:181.
26. Fisher RI, DeVita VT Jr, Bostick F, et al. Persistent immunologic abnormalities in long-term survivors of advanced Hodgkin's disease. *Ann Intern Med* 1980;92:595.
27. Zarate-Osorno A, Medeiros LJ, Longo DL, Jaffe ES. Non-Hodgkin's lymphomas arising in patients successfully treated for Hodgkin's disease. A clinical, histologic, and immunophenotypic study of 14 cases. *Am J Surg Pathol* 1992;16:885.
28. Bennett M, MacLennan K, Hudson G, Hudson B. Non-Hodgkin's lymphoma arising in patients treated for Hodgkin's disease in the BNLI: a 20-year experience. *Ann Oncol* 1991;2(Suppl 2):83.
29. Shimizu K, Hara K, Kunii A. Non-Hodgkin's lymphoma following Hodgkin's disease. A case report and immunohistochemical corroboration. *Am J Clin Pathol* 1986;86:370.
30. Ohno T, Trenn G, Wu G, Abou-Elella A, Reis HR, Chan WC. The clonal relationship between nodular sclerosis Hodgkin's disease with a clonal Reed-Sternber cell population and a subsequent B-cell small non-cleaved cell lymphoma. *Mod Pathol* 1998;11:485.
31. Gaidano G, Carbone A, Dalla-Favera R. Pathogenesis of AIDS-related lymphomas: molecular and histogenetic heterogeneity. *Am J Pathol* 1998;152:623.
32. Perrone T, Frizzera G, Rosai J. Mediastinal diffuse large-cell lymphoma with sclerosis. A clinicopathologic study of 60 cases. *Am J Surg Pathol* 1986;10:176.
33. A clinical evaluation of the International Lymphoma Study Group classification of non-Hodgkin's lymphoma. *Blood* 1997;89:3909.
34. Moller P, Moldenhauer G, Momburg F, et al. Mediastinal lymphoma of clear cell type is a tumor corresponding to terminal steps of B cell differentiation. *Blood* 1987;69:1087.
35. Lamarre L, Jacobson J, Aisenberg A, Harris N. Primary large cell lymphoma of the mediastinum. *Am J Surg Pathol* 1989;13:730.
36. Addis B, Isaacson P. Large cell lymphoma of the mediastinum: a B-cell tumor of probable thymic origin. *Histopathology* 1986;10:379.
37. Carrato A, Filippa D, Koziner B. Hodgkin's disease after treatment of non-Hodgkin's lymphoma. *Cancer* 1987;60:887.
38. Travis LB, Gonzalez CL, Hankey BF, Jaffe ES. Hodgkin's disease following non-Hodgkin's lymphoma. *Cancer* 1992;69:2337.
39. Zarate-Osorno A, Medeiros J, Jaffe ES. Hodgkin's disease coexistent with plasma cell dyscrasia. *Arch Pathol Lab Med* 1992;116:969.

40. LeBrun DP, Ngan BY, Weiss LM, Huie P, Warnke RA, Cleary ML. The bcl-2 oncogene in Hodgkin's disease arising in the setting of follicular non-Hodgkin's lymphoma. *Blood* 1994;83:223.
41. Richter M. Generalized reticular cell sarcoma of lymph nodes associated with lymphocytic leukemia. *Am J Pathol* 1928;4:285.
42. Choi H, Keller RH. Coexistence of chronic lymphocytic leukemia and Hodgkin's disease. *Cancer* 1981;48:48.
43. Han T. Chronic lymphocytic leukemia in Hodgkin's disease. Report of a case and review of the literature. *Cancer* 1971;28:300.
44. Dick F, Maca R. The lymph node in chronic lymphocytic leukemia. *Cancer* 1978;41:283.
45. Foucar K, Rydell RE. Richter's syndrome in chronic lymphocytic leukemia. *Cancer* 1980;46:118.
46. Caveriviere P, Mallem O, Al Saati T, Delsol G. Reed-Sternberg-like cells in Richter's syndrome express granulocytic- associated-antigen (Leu-M1) [letter]. *Am J Clin Pathol* 1986;85:755.
47. Williams J, Schned A, Cotelingam JD, Jaffe ES. Chronic lymphocytic leukemia with coexistent Hodgkin's disease: Implications for the origin of the Reed-Sternberg cell. *Am J Surg Pathol* 1991;15:33.
48. Brecher M, Banks P. Hodgkin's disease variant of Richter's syndrome: report of eight cases. *Am J Clin Pathol* 1990;93:333.
49. Fayad L, Robertson LE, O'Brien S, et al. Hodgkin's disease variant of Richter's syndrome: experience at a single institution. *Leuk Lymphoma* 1996;23:333.
50. Rubin D, Hudnall SD, Aisenberg A, Jacobson JO, Harris NL. Richter's transformation of chronic lymphocytic leukemia with Hodgkin's-like cells is associated with Epstein-Barr virus infection. *Mod Pathol* 1994;7:91.
51. Weisenberg E, Anastasi J, Adeyanju M, Variakojis D, Vardiman JW. Hodgkin's disease associated with chronic lymphocytic leukemia. Eight additional cases, including two of the nodular lymphocyte predominant type. *Am J Clin Pathol* 1995;103:479.
52. Chittal S, Caveriviere P, Schwarting R, et al. Monoclonal antibodies in the diagnosis of Hodgkin's disease. The search for a rational panel. *Am J Surg Pathol* 1988;12:9.
53. Momose H, Jaffe ES, Shin SS, Chen YY, Weiss LM. Chronic lymphocytic leukemia/small lymphocytic lymphoma with Reed-Sternberg-like cells and possible transformation to Hodgkin's disease. Mediation by Epstein-Barr virus. *Am J Surg Pathol* 1992;16:859.
54. Cha I, Herndier BG, Glassberg AB, Hamill TR. A case of composite Hodgkin's disease and chronic lymphocytic leukemia in bone marrow. Lack of Epstein-Barr virus. *Arch Pathol Lab Med* 1996;120:386.
55. Ohno T, Smir BN, Weisenburger DD, Gascoyne RD, Hinrichs SD, Chan WC. Origin of the Hodgkin/Reed-Sternberg cells in chronic lymphocytic leukemia with "Hodgkin's transformation." *Blood* 1998; 91:1757.
56. Giles FJ, O'Brien SM, Keating MJ. Chronic lymphocytic leukemia in (Richter's) transformation. *Semin Oncol* 1998;25:117.
57. Wlodarska I, Delabie J, De Wolf-Peeters C, et al. T-cell lymphoma developing in Hodgkin's disease: evidence for two clones. *J Pathol* 1993;170:239.
58. van der Putte SC, Toonstra J, Go DM, van Unnik JA. Mycosis fungoides. Demonstration of a variant simulating Hodgkin's disease. A report of a case with a cytomorphological analysis. *Virchows Arch B Cell Pathol Incl Mol Pathol* 1982;40:231.
59. Picard F, Dreyfus F, Le Guern M, et al. Acute T-cell leukemia/lymphoma mimicking Hodgkin's disease with secondary HTLV I seroconversion. *Cancer* 1990;66:1524.
60. Ohshima K, Kikuchi M, Yoshida T, Masuda Y, Kimura N. Lymph nodes in incipient adult T-cell leukemia-lymphoma with Hodgkin's disease-like histologic features. *Cancer* 1991;67:1622.
61. Simrell CR, Boccia RV, Longo DL, Jaffe ES. Coexisting Hodgkin's disease and mycosis fungoides. Immunohistochemical proof of its existence. *Arch Pathol Lab Med* 1986;110:1029.
62. Hawkins KA, Schinella R, Schwartz M, et al. Simultaneous occurrence of mycosis fungoides and Hodgkin disease: clinical and histologic correlations in three cases with ultrastructural studies in two. *Am J Hematol* 1983;14:355.
63. Clement M, Bhakri H, Monk B, Pettingale KW, Pembroke AC, du Vivier A. Mycosis fungoides and Hodgkin's disease. *J R Soc Med* 1984;77:1037.
64. Kaufman D, Gordon LI, Variakojis D, et al. Successfully treated Hodgkin's disease followed by mycosis fungoides: case report and review of the literature. *Cutis* 1987;39:291.
65. Brousset P, Lamant L, Viraben R, et al. Hodgkin's disease following mycosis fungoides: phenotypic and molecular evidence for different tumour cell clones. *J Clin Pathol* 1996;49:504.
66. Davis T, Morton C, Miller-Cassman R, Balk S, Kadin M. Hodgkin's disease, lymphomatoid papulosis, and cutaneous T-cell lymphoma derived from a common T-cell clone. *N Engl J Med* 1992;326:1115.
67. Ralfkiaer E, Bosq J, Gatter KC, et al. Expression of a Hodgkin and Reed-Sternberg cell associated antigen (Ki-1) in cutaneous lymphoid infiltrates. *Arch Dermatol Res* 1987;279:285.
68. Wieczorek R, Suhrland M, Ramsay D, Reed ML, Knowles DM. Leu-M1 antigen expression in advanced (tumor) stage mycosis fungoides. *Am J Clin Pathol* 1986;86:25.
69. Scheen SRd, Banks PM, Winkelmann RK. Morphologic heterogeneity of malignant lymphomas developing in mycosis fungoides. *Mayo Clin Proc* 1984;59:95.
70. Caya JG, Choi H, Tieu TM, Wollenberg NJ, Almagro UA. Hodgkin's disease followed by mycosis fungoides in the same patient. Case report and literature review. *Cancer* 1984;53:463.
71. Park CS, Chung HC, Lim HY, et al. Coexisting mycosis fungoides and Hodgkin's disease as a composite lymphoma: a case report. *Yonsei Med J* 1991;32:362.
72. Lipa M, Kunynetz R, Pawlowski D, Kerbel G, Haberman H. The occurrence of mycosis fungoides in two patients with preexisting Hodgkin's disease. *Arch Dermatol* 1982;118:563.
73. Greene MH, Pinto HA, Kant JA, et al. Lymphomas and leukemias in the relatives of patients with mycosis fungoides. *Cancer* 1982;49: 737.
74. Kadin ME, Muramoto L, Said J. Expression of T-cell antigens on Reed-Sternberg cells in a subset of patients with nodular sclerosing and mixed cellularity Hodgkin's disease. *Am J Pathol* 1988;130:345.
75. Foss HD, Anagnostopoulos I, Araujo I, et al. Anaplastic large-cell lymphomas of T-cell and null-cell phenotype express cytotoxic molecules. *Blood* 1996;88:4005.
76. Krenacs L, Wellmann A, Sorbara L, et al. Cytotoxic cell antigen expression in anaplastic large cell lymphomas of T- and null-cell type and Hodgkin's disease: evidence for distinct cellular origin. *Blood* 1997;89:980.
77. Ohshima K, Suzumiya J, Kato A, Tashiro K, Kikuchi M. Clonal HTLV-I-infected CD4- T-lymphocytes and non-clonal non-HTLV-I-infected giant cells in incipient ATLL with Hodgkin-like histologic features. *Int J Cancer* 1997;72:592.
78. Georgescu L, Quinn GC, Schwartzman S, Paget SA. Lymphoma in patients with rheumatoid arthritis: association with the disease state or methotrexate treatment [see comments]. *Semin Arthritis Rheum* 1997;26:794.
79. Kamel OW, van de Rijn M, Weiss, LM, et al. Brief report: reversible lymphomas associated with Epstein-Barr virus occurring during methotrexate therapy for rheumatoid arthritis and dermatomyositis [see comments]. *N Engl J Med* 1993;328:1317.
80. Kamel OW, Weiss LM, van de Rijn M, Colby TV, Kingma DW, Jaffe ES. Hodgkin's disease and lymphoproliferations resembling Hodgkin's disease in patients receiving long-term low-dose methotrexate therapy. *Am J Surg Pathol* 1996;20:1279.
81. Andreesen R, Osterholz J, Lohr G, Bross K. A Hodgkin cell-specific antigen is expressed on a subset of auto- and alloactivated T (helper) lymphoblasts. *Blood* 1984;6:1299.
82. Rowlings PA, Curtis RE, Kingma DW, et al. Hodgkin disease following allogeneic bone marrow transplantation: Long latency and association with Epstein-Barr virus (abstract). Blood 1997;90(suppl 1): 379a.
83. Chittal S, Brousset P, Voigt J, Delsol G. Large B-cell lymphoma rich in T-cells and simulating Hodgkin's disease. *Histopathology* 1991;19: 211.
84. Delabie J, Vandenberghe E, Kennes C, et al. Histiocyte-rich B-cell lymphoma. A distinct clinicopathologic entity possibly related to lymphocyte predominant Hodgkin's disease, paragranuloma subtype. *Am J Surg Pathol* 1992;16:37.
85. McBride JA, Rodriguez J, Luthra R, Ordonez NG, Cabanilas F, Pugh WC. T-cell–rich B large-cell lymphoma simulating lymphocyte rich Hodgkin's disease. *Am J Surg Pathol* 1996;20:193.
86. Gruss HJ, Pinto A, Duyster J, Poppema S, Herrmann F. Hodgkin's disease: a tumor with disturbed immunological pathways. *Immunol Today* 1997;18:156.
87. Zukerberg L, Collins A, Ferry J, Harris N. Coexpression of CD15 and

CD20 by Reed-Sternberg cells in Hodgkin's disease. *Am J Pathol* 1991;139:475.

88. von Wasielewski R, Mengel M, Fischer R, et al. Classical Hodgkin's disease. Clinical impact of the immunophenotype. *Am J Pathol* 1997; 151:1123.
89. Leoncini L, Del Vecchio M, Kraft R, et al. Hodgkin's disease and CD30-positive anaplastic large cell lymphomas—a continuous spectrum of malignant disorders. *Am J Pathol* 1990;137:1047.
90. Stein H, Mason D, Gerdes J, et al. The expression of the Hodgkin's disease associated antigen Ki-1 in reactive and neoplastic lymphoid tissue: evidence that Reed-Sternberg cells and histiocytic malignancies are derived from activated lymphoid cells. *Blood* 1985;66:848.
91. Zinzani PL, Bendandi M, Martelli M, et al. Anaplastic large-cell lymphoma: clinical and prognostic evaluation of 90 adult patients. *J Clin Oncol* 1996;14:955.
92. Pileri S, Bocchia M, Baroni C, et al. Anaplastic large cell lymphoma ($CD30^+$/$Ki\text{-}1^+$): results of a prospective clinicopathologic study of 69 cases. *Br J Haematol* 1994;86:513.
93. Benharroch D, Meguerian-Bedoyan Z, Lamant L, et al. ALK-positive lymphoma: a single disease with a broad spectrum of morphology. *Blood* 1998;91:2076.
94. Nakamura S, Shiota M, Nakagawa A, et al. Anaplastic large cell lymphoma: a distinct molecular pathologic entity: a reappraisal with special reference to p80(NPM/ALK) expression. *Am J Surg Pathol* 1997; 21:1420.
95. Chittal SM, Delsol G. The interface of Hodgkin's disease and anaplastic large cell lymphoma. *Cancer Surv* 1997;30:87.
96. Pittaluga S, Wiodarska I, Pulford K, et al. The monoclonal antibody ALK1 identifies a distinct morphological subtype of anaplastic large cell lymphoma associated with 2p23/ALK rearrangements. *Am J Pathol* 1997;151:343.
97. Orscheschek K, Merz H, Hell J, Binder T, Bartels H, Feller AC. Large-cell anaplastic lymphoma-specific translocation (t[2;5] [p23;q35]) in Hodgkin's disease: indication of a common pathogenesis? *Lancet* 1995;345:87.
98. Wellman A, Otsuki T, Vogelbruch M, Clark HM, Jaffe ES, Raffeld M. Analysis of the t(2;5) (p23;q35) translocation by reverse trasnscription-polymerase chain reaction in $CD30^+$ anaplastic large-cell lymphomas, in other non-Hodgkin's of T-cell phenotype, and in Hodgkin's disease. *Blood* 1995;86:2321.
99. Weber-Matthiesen K, Deerberg-Wittram J, Rosenwald A, Poetsch M, Grote W, Schlegelberger B. Translocation t(2;5) is not a primary event in Hodgkin's disease. Simultaneous immunophenotyping and interphase cytogenetics. *Am J Pathol* 1996;149:463.
100. Rudiger T, Jaffe ES, Delsol G, et al. Workshop report on Hodgkin's lymphoma and related diseases. *Ann Oncol* 1998;9:S31–S38.
101. Warnke RA, Weiss LM, Chan JKC, Cleary ML, Dorfman RF. Tumors of lymph nodes and spleen. In: Rosai J, Sobin LH, eds. *Atlas of tumor pathology,* vol 14. Washington, DC: American Registry of Pathology, 1995:277.
102. Chu WS, Abbondanzo SL, Frizzera G. Inconsistency of the immunophenotype of Reed-Sternberg cells in simultaneous and consecutive specimens from the same patients. A paraffin section evaluation in 56 patients. *Am J Pathol* 1992;141:11.
103. Rüdiger T, Ott G, Ott MM, Müller-Deubert SM, Müller-Hermelink HK. Differential diagnosis between classical Hodgkin's lymphoma, T-cell–rich B-cell lymphoma and paragranuloma by paraffin immunohistochemistry. *Am J Surg Pathol* 1998;22:1184.
104. Oudejans JJ, Kummer JA, Jiwa M, et al. Granzyme B expression in Reed-Sternberg cells of Hodgkin's disease. *Am J Pathol* 1996; 148:233.
105. Non-Hodgkin's Lymphoma Pathologic Classification Project. National Cancer Institute sponsored study of classifications of non-Hodgkin's lymphomas: summary and description of a Working Formulation for clinical usage. *Cancer* 1982;49:2112.
106. Jaffe ES. Post-thymic T-cell lymphomas. In: Jaffe ES, ed. *Surgical pathology of the lymph nodes and related organs.* Philadelphia: WB Saunders, 1995:344.
107. Osborne B, Butler J, Pugh W. The value of immunophenotyping on paraffin sections in the identification of T-cell–rich B-cell large-cell lymphomas. *Am J Surg Pathol* 1990;14:933.
108. Macon W, Williams M, Greer J, Stein R, Collins R, Cousar J. T-Cell–Rich B-Cell Lymphomas. A clinicopathologic study of 19 cases. *Am J Surg Pathol* 1992;16:351.
109. Baddoura FK, Chan WC, Masih AS, Mitchell D, Sun NC, Weisenburger DD. T-cell–rich B-cell lymphoma. A clinicopathologic study of eight cases [see comments]. *Am J Clin Pathol* 1995;103:65.
110. Pulford K, Lamant L, Morris SW, et al. Detection of anaplastic lymphoma kinase (ALK) and nucleolar protein nucleophosmin (NPM)-ALK proteins in normal and neoplastic cells with the monoclonal antibody ALK1. *Blood* 1997;89:1394.
111. MacLennan K, Bennett M, Tu A, et al. Relationship of histopathologic features to survival and relapse in nodular sclerosing Hodgkin's disease. *Cancer* 1989;64:1686.

Hodgkin's Disease, edited by P. M. Mauch,
J. O. Armitage, V. Diehl, R. T. Hoppe, and L. M. Weiss.
Lippincott Williams & Wilkins, Philadephia ©1999.

CHAPTER 13

Cytogenetics of Hodgkin's Disease

Andreas H. Sarris, Suresh C. Jhanwar, and Fernando Cabanillas

The frequency and types of chromosomal aberrations observed in Hodgkin's disease can contribute to the understanding of this disorder. One of the major controversies in the biology of Hodgkin's disease is the identity of the normal cells that give rise to the Reed-Sternberg cells and their variants. Single-cell analysis of Reed-Sternberg cells from biopsies of Hodgkin's disease reveal the presence of rearranged immunoglobulin genes, suggesting derivation from germinal center-derived B-lymphocytes (see Chapter 8). In contrast to normal follicular center cells or follicular center-cell lymphomas, the Reed-Sternberg cells of nodular sclerosis or mixed cellularity Hodgkin's disease show no evidence of somatic hypermutations. Instead they carry clonal mutations in the immunoglobulin locus that cripple the immunoglobulin receptor, and would be expected to cause apoptosis. The Reed-Sternberg cells are rescued from apoptosis, but the nature of the salvaging signal(s) remains undefined. By comparing the most common break points observed in Hodgkin's disease and the non-Hodgkin's lymphomas, tumors known to be derived from lymphocytes, one can support the derivation of Reed-Sternberg cells from lymphocytes. One can also use this information to identify candidate genes that may protect Reed-Sternberg cells from apoptosis.

Another controversy is the clonality of Reed-Sternberg cells and their variants. Some investigators have argued in the past that Hodgkin's disease was not a malignancy, but an inflammatory or infectious disorder since most of the cells in Hodgkin's disease tissues are reactive mononuclear cells. Clonality of Reed-Sternberg cells is directly supported by single-cell sequencing of the immunoglobulin receptor, and by the results of classic cytogenetic analysis. Although clonality by itself is not proof of malignancy, it can add weight to the hypothesis that Hodgkin's disease is a malignant lymphoid disorder. This is supported by the ability of Reed-Sternberg cells to invade viscera, and by the presence of clonal chromosomal abnormalities, including numerical chromosomal gains or losses, translocations, inversions, or deletions. Many of the altered chromosomal bands are known to contain oncogenes, tumor suppressor genes, protein kinases, or proteins involved in the regulation of apoptosis. It is possible that the clonal deregulation of these loci may protect the Reed-Sternberg cells from apoptosis, and may contribute to the multistep progression to malignancy.

The relationship between Hodgkin's disease and some types of non-Hodgkin's lymphomas has been another source of controversy. The genetic evidence previously mentioned revealed that the Reed-Sternberg cells are derived from B cells and that they have rearranged immunoglobulin genes. Those of nodular sclerosis and mixed cellularity histology carry clonal crippling mutations of the immunoglobulin receptor without evidence of somatic hypermutation. By contrast, cases of lymphocyte predominance have clonal rearrangements of the immunoglobulin locus and evidence of ongoing somatic hypermutation, suggesting ongoing antigen selection as seen with follicular center-cell lymphomas. Therefore, Hodgkin's disease has molecular similarities to germinal center B-cell–derived lymphomas. Some non-Hodgkin's lymphomas such as cutaneous T-cell lymphoma and anaplastic large-cell lymphoma may contain Reed-Sternberg–like cells, and can thus be histologically confused with Hodgkin's disease. This distinction is especially problematic for the newly described anaplastic large-cell lymphoma—Hodgkin's-like—which can be extremely difficult to differentiate from Hodgkin's disease. Some non-Hodgkin's lymphomas have characteristic cytogenetic aberrations, including the t(2;5) in CD30-positive anaplastic large-cell lymphoma, and the t(14;18) in fol-

A. H. Sarris and F. Cabanillas: Department of Lymphoma-Myeloma, University of Texas M. D. Anderson Cancer Center, Houston, Texas.

S. C. Jhanwar: Cytogenetics Service, Memorial Sloan-Kettering Cancer Center, New York, New York.

licular center-cell lymphoma. Therefore, determination of the global karyotype, particularly the presence of t(14; 18) and t(2;5), can help to elucidate the relationship, and possibly the differential diagnosis between Hodgkin's disease and these other lymphomas.

Familial Hodgkin's disease represents only 2% to 5% of all cases of Hodgkin's disease, but there is neither a strong association of Epstein-Barr virus (EBV) infection of Reed-Sternberg cells among members of these families nor differences in EBV seropositivity nor germline mutations of p53 between them and controls. The association of familial Hodgkin's disease with certain human leukocyte antigen (HLA) haplotypes suggests that an environmental factor, possibly infectious, may be responsible for causing disease in individuals with the appropriate genetic predisposition.

CLASSICAL CYTOGENETICS

Established cytogenetic guidelines accept clonality if the same chromosomal abnormality is seen in at least two metaphases for structural aberrations or chromosome gains, or in three metaphases for chromosome loss. Abnormal chromosomes that cannot be identified as a result of complex rearrangements between specific chromosomes are called marker chromosomes (1). It then should not be surprising that karyotypic analysis of Hodgkin's disease has been frustrating, and that some of the observed abnormalities do not meet these strict clonality criteria. Probable reasons include the paucity of the Reed-Sternberg cells or their variants in Hodgkin's disease tissues, the lack of knowledge about their growth requirements *in vitro,* and the practical limitation of obtaining and analyzing only a limited number of metaphases with routine classic banding cytogenetic techniques. Therefore, it is possible that some of the single abnormal metaphases that do not satisfy the previously mentioned criteria of clonality do represent malignant Reed-Sternberg clones in Hodgkin's disease. It may be possible to bypass some of these problems by transplanting Hodgkin's disease tissues in mice with severe combined immunodeficiency, and thus enriching for the malignant cells, but this will not be a practical approach to routine clinical cytogenetics. Fluorescence immunophenotyping and interphase cytogenetics as a tool for investigations of neoplasms (FICTION) and other molecular techniques may be useful at the investigational level, but they are limited to analysis of specific abnormalities, and they cannot obtain global karyotypes that are essential to establish prognostically significant chromosomal abnormalities, and to identify genes that may be responsible for the malignant transformation in this disease.

The reported karyotypes of Hodgkin's disease are extremely complex, and polyploidy is very common. Most abnormal karyotypes are characterized by multiple chromosome gains or losses, translocations, inversions, and deletions (2–12). A typical karyotype, previously unreported, of a patient with Hodgkin's disease from M. D. Anderson Cancer Center is shown in Figure 1. It includes 77 chromosomes with multiple structural abnormalities, t(11; 14)(q22;q32), and 9 unidentifiable marker chromosomes (4). This break point on chromosome 11q22 is different from the break point observed in mantle cell lymphoma which involves 11q13, the locus of the bcl-1 gene (13).

The published cytogenetic experience in Hodgkin's disease is summarized in Table 1. Material from 391 patients with Hodgkin's disease was reviewed and included 294 analyzable metaphases. Overall, normal diploid karyotypes were seen in 142 patients or 48% of those with analyzable metaphases (2–12). This observation has fueled the controversy about whether these normal karyotypes arise from the reactive mononuclear infiltrate, or whether the Reed-Sternberg cells may have normal karyotypes in some patients. Abnormal metaphases, defined as those with either numerical or structural chromosomal abnormalities, were seen in 152 patients or 52% of those with analyzable metaphases. However, in individual series the frequency of abnormal metaphases ranged from 13% to 92%. This extreme variability probably reflects methodologic differences, including the analysis of samples that have variable cellularity or contain different numbers of malignant cells. In addition, differences in elapsed time from biopsy to placing the cells in culture, the exact culture conditions used to generate metaphases, and the exact banding techniques can all affect the number of abnormal metaphases observed.

Most abnormal karyotypes are hyperdiploid with several extra chromosomes. There is a broad distribution of chromosome numbers, and the highest reported chromosome number is 119, which corresponds to a hyperpentaploid cell (Fig. 2). These data are consistent with results obtained with Feulgen staining of tissue sections that demonstrated aneuploid Reed-Sternberg cells, but diploid infiltrating mononuclear cells (14).

When gains or losses of individual chromosomes are analyzed (Fig. 3), the gains exceed losses for most chromosomes. The exception is chromosomes 13, 15, 22, and Y, which are lost more often than they are gained. One might speculate that selective loss of chromosome 13, occurring in 35% of analyzable metaphases, might be occurring in individuals who already carry a germline mutation inactivating the other allele of the retinoblastoma gene. Since heterozygous inactivation of retinoblastoma gene is relatively common in the general population, it is possible that Hodgkin's disease is more likely to develop in patients who already carry a germline mutation in the retinoblastoma gene. This may provide a basis for future investigations of factors affecting the development of second tumors, which frequently occur after curative therapy in patients with Hodgkin's disease. Similarly, the high frequency of chromosome 9 gain seen in Fig. 3, might reflect the presence of tumor promoter or apoptosis protection

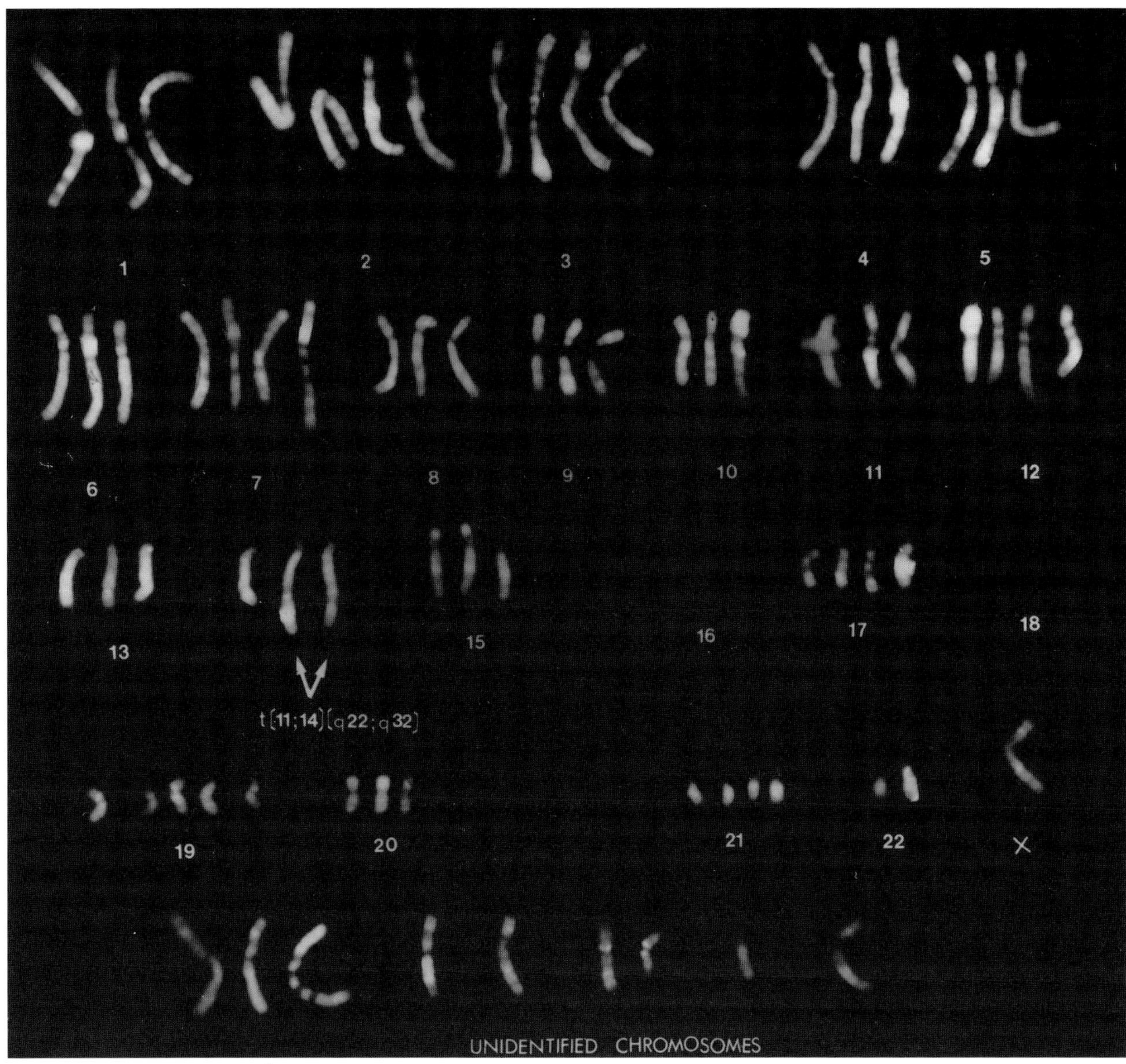

FIG. 1. Karyotype of a patient with mixed cellularity Hodgkin's disease. [From previously unpublished karyotypes that formed the basis of a published report (4).]

genes in this chromosome, whose overexpression may rescue Reed-Sternberg cells from apoptosis.

The reported structural abnormalities include translocations, inversions, deletions, or duplications, and their distribution among the different arms of each chromosome is summarized in Figure 4. It is obvious that 2p, 3q, 4q, 6q, 8q, 7q, 9p, 13p, 14q, 17q, 19p, 20q, 21q, 22q, and Xp are involved more frequently than the contralateral arm of the same chromosome. When the relative size of the p and q arms of each chromosome is taken into consideration, these data suggest that 2p, 3q, 6q, 7q, 9p, 13p, 14p, and 17q are altered much more than expected from their sizes, relative to the contralateral arm of the same chromosome. This is particularly striking when chromosomes 9p and 13p are considered, because the p arms are much smaller than the q arms in these two chromosomes. These data are consistent with the presence of tumor suppressor genes that are inactivated, and/or tumor promoter genes that are activated by these complex chromosomal alterations. The numerous unidentifiable marker chromosomes resulting from complex rearrangements involving several chromosomes are commonly seen, and these may mask other important genes.

A more detailed attempt to identify candidate genes for oncogenesis in Hodgkin's disease is to determine how often specific chromosomal bands are involved among the 128 metaphases that have been reported in detail. Table 2 summarizes the frequencies of the most commonly involved loci (translocations, deletions, or duplications).

TABLE 1. *Cytogenetic analysis in Hodgkin's disease*

Author	Patients	Patients with analyzable metaphase	Patients with abnormal metaphases		95% CI
			All	%[a]	
Reeves and Pickup (210)	5	5	4	80	28–99
Hossfeld et al. (2)	6	6	6	100	54–100
Kristoffersson et al. (3)	20	18	11	61	36–83
Cabanillas et al. (4)	49	29	18	62[b]	42–79
Dennis et al. (5)	12	12	9	75	43–95
Koduru et al. (6)	51	39	5	13	4–27
Schouten et al. (7)	37	29	13	45	26–64
Banks et al. (8)	7	5	3	60	15–95
Ladanyi et al. (9)	95	57	13	23	13–36
Tilly et al. (10)	60	49	33	67	53–80
Poppema et al. (11)	28	25	23	89	72–98
Schlegelberger et al. (12)	21	20	14	70	46–88
Total 391	294	152	52	46–58	

Series are listed in chronological order with respect to publication date. Only series reporting banded chromosomes from Hodgkin's disease tissue are shown here.
[a]Percentage of those with analyzable metaphases.
[b]Unpublished individual karyotypes.
CI, confidence intervals.

Band 14q32, which contains the immunoglobulin heavy chain locus (15), is altered in 14% of all reported cases, consistent with the B-cell origin of Hodgkin's disease. Other rearranged bands contain genes that are involved in lymphocyte activation, such as CD47 (16) and CD86 (17) on 3q11, B7 (18) on 3q26-29, interleukin-2 (IL-2) (19,20) on 4q28, and CD27 (21) on 12p (11–13). The genes for the immunomodulatory proteins interferon-α (IFN-α) and -β (IFN-β) are located on 9 p21-24, (22–24) and the gene for the α chain of the IFN-γ receptor is also located on 6q24-25 (18,25). It is possible that activation of these genes will rescue Reed-Sternberg cells from apoptosis, either by direct action on them or indirectly by affecting other accessory cells.

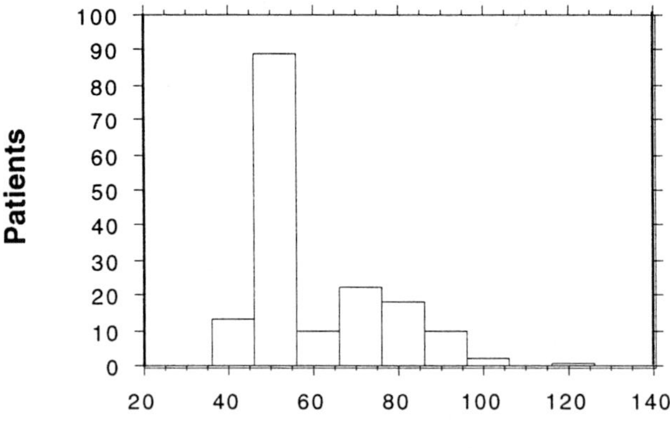

FIG. 2. Histogram of chromosome numbers in Hodgkin's disease. Prepared from the 165 reported karyotypes of the series listed in Table 1. These include aneuploid karyotypes, normal karyotypes, karyotypes with 46 chromosomes and balanced translocation(s), or abnormal karyotypes with 46 chromosomes resulting from balanced chromosome loss and gain.

Another set of bands includes various oncogenes including the *ski* (26) on 3q26-29, c-*myc* (27) on 8q24, *all-1* (28) and c-*cbl* (29) on 11q21-23, *tel* (30) on 12p11-13, TCL-1 (31–33) on 14q 32, *bcl*-8 (34) on 15p11-13, *axl* (35,36) on 19p12-13, and *src* (37,38) on 20q12-13. It is conceivable that translocations, deletions, insertions, or duplications in these chromosomal bands would constitutively activate these proteins or increase their level of expression. The resulting increase in their activity may thus contribute to salvage from apoptosis, and may even play a direct role in the multistep evolution toward the malignant phenotype the Reed-Sternberg cells.

Another set of bands contains the genes for a variety of transcription factors, such as binding regulatory factor 1q41 (39), which is responsible for the major histocompatibility complex (MHC) class II deficiency that is seen in the bare lymphocyte syndrome. The genes for a DNA-binding protein (40) are located on 3q26-29, a zinc finger protein (41) on 7q21-22, the DNA-binding protein RFX-3 (42) on 9p21-24, the interferon-responsive transcriptional regulator ISGF3 (43) on 14 p77, zinc finger protein HZF-4 (44) on 19p 12-13, and B-*myb* (45) on 20q12-13. Alterations of these bands might contribute to the malignant nature of Reed-Sternberg cells by altering the transcription of blocks of genes that either affect the cell cycle, or rescue cells from apoptosis, or contribute to the multistep progression to malignancy.

Protein kinases, cyclins, and their regulators are also known to directly affect the growth and differentiation of cells. Alterations of their activity has been implicated as the causative agent of the malignant transformation of

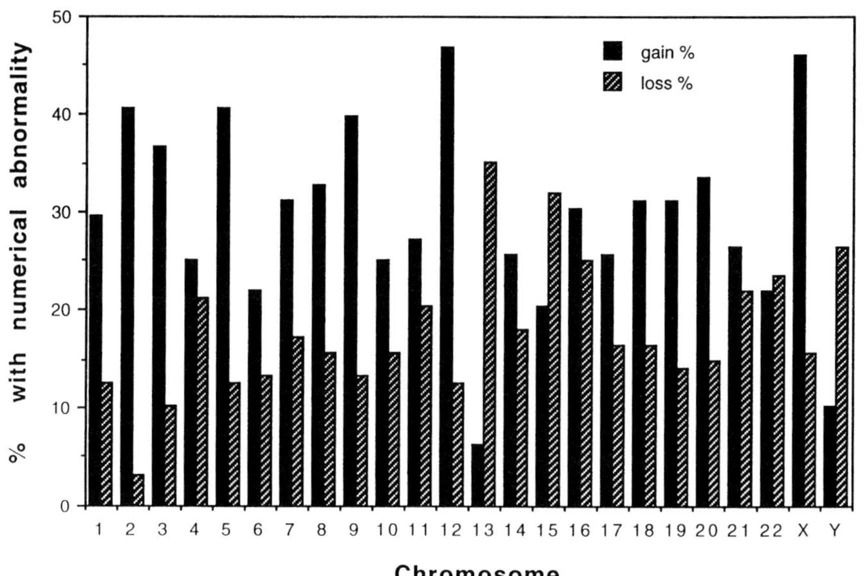

FIG. 3. Numerical gains or losses of individual chromosomes in Hodgkin's disease. Compiled from the 128 abnormal karyotypes of series of Table 1 that were reported in detail.

many tumors. Several protein kinases are encoded in chromosomal loci that are frequently affected in Hodgkin's disease. These include the genes for the iota isoform of protein kinase C (46) on 3q11-13, the tyrosine protein kinase atk/bpk (47) on 4q28, the serine kinase transforming growth factor-β (TGF-β) signaling protein (48) on 4q28, the tyrosine protein kinase HEK (49) on 6q15-16, a tyrosine kinase belonging to the EPH kinase family (50,51) on 7q21-22, an ephrin-like protein kinase (52) on 7q31-35, and MST-1 kinase (53,54) on 20q12-13. In addition, *src*, the human homologue of the transforming gene of the Rous sarcoma virus (37,38), is a protein kinase gene that has been localized to 20q12-13. The genes for cyclin E (55) and cyclin H (56) are localized on 19 p12-13 and 4q32-34, respectively. The cyclin-dependent protein kinase-4 inhibitors p15 (57) and p16 (58), which act as physiologic tumor suppressor genes and whose inactivation has been implicated as a factor in the pathogenesis of many tumors, are localized on chromosome 9p21. The gene for a third member of the family of inhibitors of cyclin-dependent protein kinases, p19 (59), is located on band p19p13, which is altered in 9% of Hodgkin's disease. Rearrangement or deletions of the p16 gene have been associated with poor prognosis in B-cell non-Hodgkin's lymphoma (60,61), but their role in the prognosis of Hodgkin's disease remains undefined.

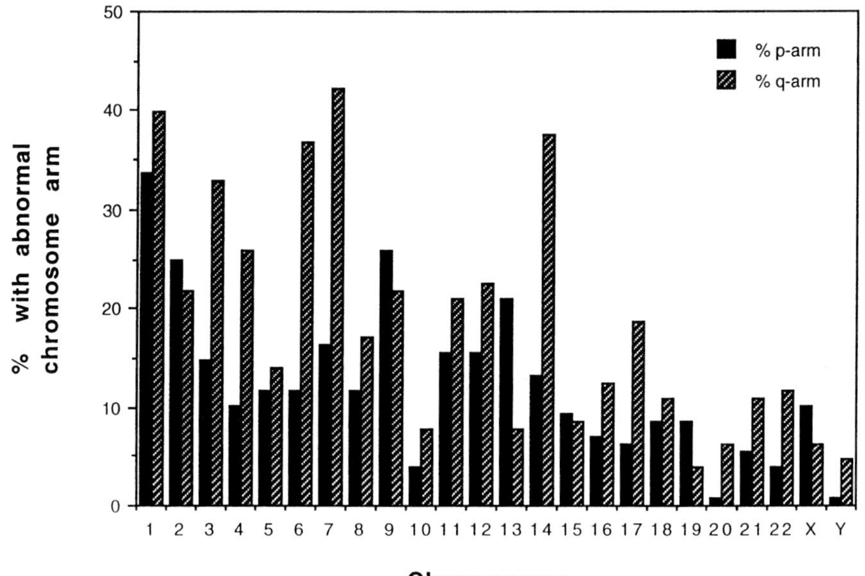

FIG. 4. Alterations of specific chromosome arms in Hodgkin's disease. Compiled from the 128 abnormal karyotypes from the series of Table 1 that were reported in detail.

TABLE 2. *Chromosomal regions that are altered in 3 or more patients with Hodgkin's disease*

Band	Number involved	% of all	95% CI	Genetic loci mapping in area
1q41	7	6	2–11	Binding regulatory factor (mutated in primary MHC class II deficiency (39); TGF-β2 (76)
2p25	7	6	2–11	Calcium-binding protein (211)
3p11	6	5	2–10	
3q11-13	4	3	1–8	Retrovirus-related reverse transcriptase (212); CD47 (16); CD86 (17)
3q26-29	19	15	9–22	DNA-binding protein (40); macrophage stimulating protein (78); proto-oncogene *ski* (26); protein kinase C-iota (46) ERS transcription factor (213); transferrin receptor (79); lymphocyte activation antigen B7 (18) Thrombopoietin (100)
4q28	6	5	2–10	TGF-β signaling protein (48); tyrosine protein kinase ATK/BPK (47); IL-2 (19,20)
4q32-34	5	4	1–9	Vascular endothelial growth factor (80); cyclin-H (56)
6q15-16	12	9	5–16	Protein tyrosine kinase HEK (49)
6q24-25	9	7	3–13	α-chain of IFN-α receptor (25)
7q21-22	19	14	9–22	*mdr*-I (99); protein kinase C; EPH tyrosine kinase (50, 51); zinc finger protein (41); type I collagen α-2 chain (98)
7q31-35	14	11	6–18	Caspase 2 (62); ephrin-like protein kinase (52)
8p22-23	7	6	2–11	
8q24	8	6	3–12	C-*myc* proto-oncogene (27)
9p21-24	11	9	4–15	IFN-α and IFN-β (22–24, 214); p15 (57), p16 (58); DNA-binding protein RFX-3 (42)
11q21-23	17	13	8–20	Inhibitor of apoptosis protein-1 (63, 64); IL-10 receptor (81) *all*-1 (28); c-*cbl* proto-oncogene (29)
12p11-13	18	14	9–210	Lactate dehydrogenase H-chain (93); parathyroid hormone-related protein (97); CD27 (21); *tel* proto-oncogene (30) Tumor necrosis factor receptor-1 (215)
12q21-24	17	13	8–20	Insulin-like growth factor-1 (82); variant platelet factor-4 (67); stem cell factor (83)
13p11	15	12	7–19	
14p11	12	9	5–16	α-subunit of interferon-responsive transcriptional regulator ISGF3 (43)
14q32	18	14	9–21	Heavy chain of the immunoglobulin locus (15); IL-8 (68); *tcl*-1 proto-oncogene (31, 32)
15p11-13	7	6	2–11	*bcl*-8 (34)
19p12-13	10	8	4–14	*Ax1* proto-oncogene (35, 36); zinc-finger protein HZF-4 (44); TGF-β1 (77); p19 (59)
20q12-13	7	6	2–11	Cyclin-E (55); MST-1 kinase (53, 54); *b-myb* (45); human *src* (37, 38); CD40 (66)

These data are based on the 128 reported abnormal karyotypes by Tilly et al. (10) (*n*=31), Schouten et al. (7) (*n*=13), Kristoffersson et al. (3) (*n*=4); Ladanyi et al. (9) (*n*=10), Dennis et al. (5) (*n*=9), Banks et al. (8) (*n*=3), Koduru et al. (6) (*n*=5), Cabanillas et al. (4) (*n*=18), Hossfeld and Schmidt (2) (*n*=6), Schlegelberger et al. (12) (*n*=12), Reeves and Pickup (210) (*n*=4), and Poppema et al. (11) (*n*=13). These authors reported 152 abnormal metaphases, but only 128 abnormal metaphases were reported in detail. The genes contained in these chromosomal loci were identified by online search of the human genome transcript map at the National Center for Biotechnology Information (www.ncbi.nlm.nih.gov/gene/map/) and of a published map of the human genome (216, 217). Only genes considered likely to contribute to the malignant transformation of the Reed-Sternberg cells are shown here.

CI, confidence interval; IFN, interferon; IL, interleukin; MHC, major histocompatibility complex; TGF, transforming growth factor.

Members of the apoptotic cascade are also good candidates for salvaging Reed-Sternberg cells from apoptosis. Inactivation of caspase-2 (62), which is coded in 7q31-35, could block apoptosis of Reed-Sternberg cells by inactivating or by reducing the activity of this essential intermediary enzyme. The same effect could be caused by any alterations of 11q21-23 that increase the activity of the inhibitor of apoptosis protein-1 (63,64). The gene for co-stimulatory molecule CD40, which is known to protect germinal-center B-cells from apoptosis (65), has been mapped to 20q12-13 (66), which is altered in 6% of Hodgkin's disease. Therefore, alterations of this chromosomal locus may rescue Reed-Sternberg cells from apoptosis, if they cause increased expression or cause the constitutive activation of CD40.

Bands 12q21-24 and 19q32 contain genes encode for two chemokines: variant platelet factor-4 (67) and IL-8 (68). The superfamily of chemokines contains many small basic proteins that are secreted from lymphocytes, monocytes macrophages, or bone marrow stromal cells in response to interferons, tumor necrosis factor, interleukins, or bacterial lipopolysaccharide (69). Chemokines have diverse functions, including chemotaxis, lymphocyte activation, inhibition of early hemopoietic progenitor proliferation, (70) and inhibition of the *in vitro* replication of human immunodeficiency virus strains (71). Both IL-8 and platelet factor-4 can suppress the proliferation of certain subsets of early human hemopoietic progenitors (72–74). Therefore, their overexpression by Reed-Sternberg cells may contribute to the anemia seen in Hodgkin's disease. In addition, overexpression of IL-8 by the Reed-Sternberg cells may account for the leukocyte chemotaxis and for the mononuclear reactive infiltrate seen in tumors by releasing other chemoattractants from T cells (75). The role of other known or unknown chemokines in the chemotaxis of the reactive infiltrate in Hodgkin's disease remains undefined, but would be an attractive subject of future investigation.

Another group of structural abnormalities involves chromosomal bands that contain loci coding for various growth factors, or their receptors. These include the genes for TGF-β_2 (76) on 1q41, TGF-β_1 (77) on 19p12-13, macrophage-stimulating protein (78) on 3q26-29, transferrin receptor (79) on 3q26-29, TGF-β signaling protein and 48 IL-219 on 4q28, vascular endothelial growth factor (80) on 4q32-34, erythropoietin on 7q22, the receptor for IL-10 (81) on 11 q21-23, and insulin-like growth factor-I (82) or stem cell factor (83) on 12 q21-24. It is possible that overexpression of these growth factors, alterations of their receptors, or constitute activation of their signaling proteins will contribute to the salvation of Reed-Sternberg cells from apoptosis. Overexpression of the stem cell factor may cause a paracrine loop since its receptor, C-KIT, is frequently expressed by Reed-Sternberg cells (84). Similarly, it is possible that rearrangements of the 11q21-23 would result in constitutive expression or activation of the receptor for IL-10. This could result in an autocrine loop, because IL-10 is known to be secreted by Reed-Sternberg cells (85,86) and its levels are significantly elevated in the serum of a significant fraction of patients with Hodgkin's disease (87). IL-10 is known to protect T cells (88–90), B cells (91), and normal hemopoietic progenitors (92) from apoptosis. Therefore, activation of this autocrine loop could contribute to the rescue of Reed-Sternberg cells from either spontaneous or chemotherapy-induced apoptosis. It is possible that activation of this loop in some patients is the underlying basis for the poor prognosis associated with elevation of serum IL-10 levels in Hodgkin's disease (87).

Several other bands encode various genes whose activation might explain other features of Hodgkin's disease. Note should be made of the location of the heavy chain of lactate dehydrogenase in chromosomal band 12p12, which is altered in 14% of the cases (93). Serum lactate dehydrogenase is elevated in 33% of patients with Hodgkin's disease (Sarris, unpublished observations on 787 untreated Hodgkin's disease patients), and is associated with inferior failure-free survival (87,94–96). Even though it is difficult to imagine how elevation serum lactate dehydrogenase might alter the prognosis of this disease, it is possible to speculate that chromosomal changes around 12q12 dysregulate both the lactate dehydrogenase locus and another unknown loci whose alteration confers poor prognosis. The same area (12p11-13) contains the gene for parathyroid hormone-related protein (97), whose overexpression may underlie the hypercalcemia observed in some cases of Hodgkin's disease. Alteration of 7q21-22 may affect the synthesis the α-2 chain of type I collagen (98), and contribute to the sclerosis seen in Hodgkin's disease. Alteration of 7q21-22 may cause overexpression of the human transport protein MDR-1 (99), which actively extrudes many drugs from cells, and may thus contribute to chemotherapy resistance in some cases of Hodgkin's disease. Alterations of 3q26-29 may cause oversecretion of thrombopoietin (100) and may thus be responsible for the thrombocytosis occasionally seen in Hodgkin's disease.

It should be emphasized that these observations do not prove that expression of the genes contained in these chromosomal loci have been altered. They may, however, form the basis of future research to define with molecular means if these genes are altered in Reed-Sternberg cells, or to identify candidate genes that may rescue Reed-Sternberg cells from apoptosis. Thus we may gain insight in the pathogenesis of Hodgkin's disease.

SPECIAL TECHNIQUES OF CYTOGENETIC ANALYSIS: "FICTION"

Classic cytogenetic analysis is limited by the small number of metaphases that can be routinely analyzed, and by the inability to determine the nature of the cells giving rise to these metaphases. These are not significant problems in most non-Hodgkin's lymphomas, because the malignant lymphocytes compose the bulk of the tumor, and they often divide in culture. However, it is a significant problem in Hodgkin's disease, where the malignant cells often represent <1% of the cellular elements in the tumor, and cannot be grown easily in culture. This has led to arguments that the observed karyotypes represent the reactive infiltrate of mononuclear cells. This argument may be plausible for those cases of Hodgkin's disease exhibiting only normal metaphases, but appears unlikely for those with extremely complex karyotypes. If the reactive lymphoid infiltrate was the source, these complex karyotypes should have been germline, and should have been detectable in the peripheral blood of the patient or relatives at the time of diagnosis or even after remission. Such karyotypes have not been observed in familial Hodgkin's disease, making this argument unlikely.

Recently FICTION has been developed to focus on the cytogenetic analysis of the malignant cells. This technique takes advantage of the frequent expression of various antigens, such as CD30, on the malignant Reed-Sternberg and Hodgkin's disease cells. This specific staining coupled with the size and number of nuclei allows the identification of Reed-Sternberg cells by immunocytochemistry, since CD30 is rarely expressed by the reactive mononuclear cell infiltrate. The cytogenetic composition of these cells can then be determined with fluorescent *in situ* DNA hybridization using probes specific for either a chromosomal centromere (numerical abnormalities) or for a specific DNA rearrangement (structural abnormalities). Therefore, by its design, FICTION is limited to those cases where the Reed-Sternberg cells bear a selectable cytochemical marker, but it cannot determine a global karyotype since it can only probe for aberrations in a specific chromosome number, or for deletions or translocations for which there are available fluorescent probes.

Even with these limitations, FICTION has contributed to our understanding of Hodgkin's disease. Recent studies examined Hodgkin's disease tissue with antibodies to CD30 and with centromeric probes for chromosomes 1, 2, 4, 8, 12, 15, 17, X, and Y. With this technique it was established that all Reed-Sternberg cells in a given case contained numerical chromosome abnormalities. By contrast, the reactive cells were diploid in all but one of the 34 cases that have been reported. In cases with complex and hyperdiploid karyotypes, the cytogenetic results agreed with chromosome abnormalities detected by FICTION. These data support the clonality of the Reed-Sternberg cells and their variants in Hodgkin's disease, and suggest that the extreme karyotypic abnormalities represent multiple subclones that exist *in vivo* within the tumor, and are not generated as tissue culture artifacts during cytogenetic preparation (101–103).

The numerical alterations (gains or losses) that were detected by FICTION in all reported cases are graphically demonstrated in Figure 5, and are grossly consistent with the reported numerical changes by classic cytogenetics that are shown in Figure 3. In addition, they provide additional evidence that the abnormal karyotypes are derived from the malignant Reed-Sternberg cells, and not from the bystander reactive mononuclear infiltrates. The FICTION data coupled with the data from the classic cytogenetics argue strongly that the Reed-Sternberg cells and their variants are the source of the cytogenetic abnormalities in Hodgkin's disease, and that they are clonal, as has already been proved by the direct DNA sequencing of the rearranged immunoglobulin locus in individual cells. Even though clonality is not always equivalent with malignancy, the clonal involvement of specific loci, and the ability of Reed-Sternberg cells to invade viscera, or to be serially transplanted in mice with severe combined immunodeficiency (Richard Ford, personal communication), prove that Hodgkin's disease is a malignant tumor of clonal Reed-Sternberg cells, and is consistent with its derivation from germinal center B-cells as has been suggested by polymerase chain reaction (PCR) of single Reed-Sternberg cells.

The t(2;5)(p23;q35).

In the years since its initial description, anaplastic large-cell lymphoma (104) has been recognized as a distinct clinicopathologic entity and has been included in both the revised Kiel (105) and in the revised European-American lymphoma (106) classifications. Pathologically, in anaplastic large-cell lymphoma the lymph node sinuses are infiltrated by anaplastic large cells with pleomorphic nuclei, prominent nucleoli, and abundant basophilic cytoplasm that is often vacuolated in cytologic smears (107). Since its initial description, many pathologic variants have been described, including the monomorphic (108,109), the small cell (110), the lymphohistiocytic (111), the sarcomatoid (112), the microvil-

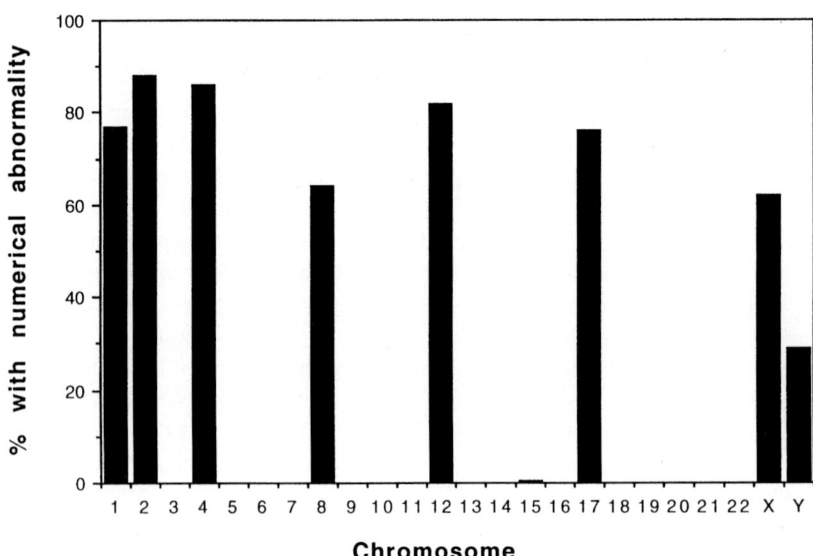

FIG. 5. Numerical chromosome changes (gains or losses) detected by fluorescence immunophenotyping and interphase cytogenetics as a tool for investigations of neoplasms (FICTION). The data are expressed for each chromosome as the percent of the 34 patients reported.

lous (113), and the Hodgkin's-like variant (114,115). The latter has been included in the revised European-American lymphoma classification as a provisional entity, but criteria for its diagnosis and its distinction from Hodgkin's disease are not yet universally accepted (106).

Immunocytochemical investigations (see Chapters 7 and 12) reveal that both anaplastic large-cell lymphoma and Hodgkin's disease express CD30 (116,117). This is a transmembrane protein belonging to the tumor necrosis factor receptor gene family that is also expressed by nonneoplastic activated T lymphocytes (118). Among malignant lymphomas, only anaplastic large-cell lymphoma and Hodgkin's disease express C-KIT, the cellular receptor for stem cell growth factor (84). The presence of CD30, C-KIT, and sclerosis in both anaplastic large-cell lymphoma and in Hodgkin's disease has made the distinction between those disorders difficult, and has led some pathologists to consider them extremes on a continuum of malignant lymphoid neoplasms (119). The clinical and morphologic similarity between lymphomatoid papulosis and anaplastic large-cell lymphoma, especially the primary cutaneous form, and the detection of a common T-cell clone in cutaneous T-cell lymphoma, Hodgkin's disease, and lymphomatoid papulosis that developed over time in one patient (120), have suggested the existence of a biologic relationship between these disorders.

By classic cytogenetics the t(2;5)(p23;q35) has been often deleted in anaplastic large-cell lymphoma (121–125), but neither 2p23 nor 5q35 alterations have been reported in Hodgkin's disease karyotypes with any frequency (Table 2). The t(2;5) fuses sequences from the nucleophosmin gene that is located on chromosome 5q35, to a novel gene, designated anaplastic lymphoma kinase, on chromosome 2p23 (126). The nucleophosmin locus is highly conserved and codes for a nuclear phosphoprotein that is involved in the late stages of ribosomal assembly (127,128). The anaplastic lymphoma kinase (*alk*) locus codes for a novel transmembrane protein kinase that has sequence homology to the β chain of the insulin receptor, the β chain of the insulin-like growth factor-1 receptor, the leukocyte tyrosine kinase, and the *Drosophila* homologue Sevenless. The fusion protein generated by the t(2;5)(p23;q35) consists of nucleophosism amino-terminal sequences fused to ALK carboxy-terminal cytoplasmic sequences, which include the consensus protein tyrosine kinase residues. Gene transduction experiments have demonstrated that this fusion protein is sufficient for malignant transformation (129).

As predicted by the break-point locations, the t(2:5) fusion protein is soluble (126) and has in fact been isolated (130) as a hyperphosphorylated phosphotyrosine-containing protein of 80,000 daltons from t(2;5)-positive cell lines (131). Antibodies raised against the kinase domain of the ALK stained both nucleus and cytoplasm of the malignant cells from biopsies of patients with anaplastic large-cell lymphomas that bear a t(2;5) translocation (131).

The presence of t(2;5) rearrangement in anaplastic large-cell lymphoma has been determined by various methods, including reverse-transcriptase PCR (RT-PCR), long-range genomic DNA PCR, fluorescent *in situ* hybridization (FISH), and immunocytochemistry based on polyclonal or monoclonal antibodies. The frequency of t(2;5) has ranged from 12% to 80%, and was 37% for all the 537 patients reported so far (131–143). One study of patients with anaplastic large-cell lymphoma has reported a frequency of 80% for t(2;5) using RT-PCR (139). This frequency is much higher than the frequency reported in pediatric or adult anaplastic large-cell lymphoma by either cytogenetics or by molecular methods. However, because of the small number of patients examined, the 95% confidence intervals ranged from 28% to 99%. It is therefore not clear whether this frequency is statistically higher than most published results. The t(2;5) was also detected by long-range genomic DNA PCR in 6 of 38 anaplastic large-cell lymphomas for an overall frequency of 16% and 95% confidence intervals of 6% to 31% (Fig. 6) (143). The t(2;5)-specific amplicon sizes generated by long-range genomic DNA PCR were different for all anaplastic large-cell lymphomas analyzed, suggesting unique genomic DNA break points (142–144). This was confirmed by DNA sequencing (142,145) and provides an additional internal control against sample cross-contamination in the laboratory. This is a distinct advantage over RT-PCR, which generates amplicons of the same size in essentially all patients, because the break points occur in the same nucleophosmin and anaplastic kinase

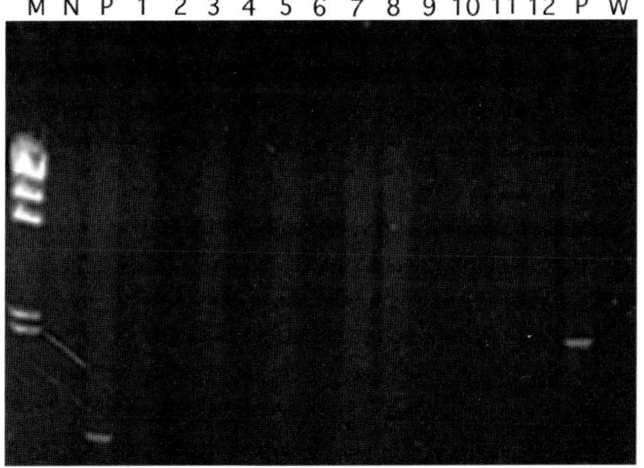

FIG. 6 The t(2;5) is not detectable by long-range genomic DNA polymerase chain reaction (PCR) in Hodgkin's disease. The conditions of the long-range genomic DNA PCR have been previously reported (150). M: The Hind III digest of the bacteriophage l DNA used as molecular weigh markers. P: Two different anaplastic large cell lymphoma tumors known to be t(2;5)-positive. N: Negative control with normal genomic DNA. W: Negative control obtained by omitting DNA from the PCR reaction. Lanes 1–12: Genomic DNA extracted from 12 different primary Hodgkin's disease tumors.

introns in the vast majority of patients. Among all published series the t(2;5) was present only in lymphomas with T-cell or null-cell histology, but was absent from B-cell lymphomas with anaplastic morphology. However, the latter are not considered as anaplastic large-cell lymphomas in the revised European-American lymphoma classification (106).

The overall frequency of t(2;5) among all 592 screened cases of Hodgkin's disease is 4%, with 95% confidence intervals extending from 2% to 6%, and is much lower than the frequency of 37% for all the previously reported 537 patients with anaplastic large-cell lymphoma (Table 3) (131,132,135–137,139–141,143,146–151). More detailed analysis shows that the t(2;5) has not been detected in 11 of 15 series that include 505 patients (131,136,140,141, 143,146–151) (Fig. 6). However, the t(2;5) has been detected in four of 15 series that include 87 patients (132, 135,137,139). Among these series the frequency of t(2;5) positivity ranges from 5% to 85% (Table 2). Orscheschek and co-workers (139) using RT-PCR reported the highest frequency of 85% for t(2;5) in 13 cases of Hodgkin's disease. This frequency was similar to the frequency of 80% reported by them in unselected cases of anaplastic large-cell lymphoma (139). It remains unclear why these investigators have reported similarly high frequencies of t(2;5) in both anaplastic large-cell lymphoma and in Hodgkin's disease, but contamination remains a distinct possibility.

There are several possibilities that either singly or in combination may contribute to the variable detection of t(2;5) in Hodgkin's disease. A major problem is the difficulty of the differential diagnosis between Hodgkin's disease and anaplastic large-cell lymphoma, especially the Hodgkin's-like variant (106,114,119,152). It is not clear if all patients in the four series that detected the t(2;5) in Hodgkin's disease in fact had this diagnosis, because no slide review was performed. Another source of uncertainty for the PCR-based results is the ever-present danger of sample cross-contamination in the laboratory. Even though most series report satisfactory positive and negative controls, this problem is in practice almost impossible to exclude. This is particularly true for RT-PCR, which gives rise to identical amplicons for the vast majority of patients, because the genomic break points involve the same *alk* and nucleophosmin introns. The generation of identical PCR amplicons can be avoided by long-range genomic DNA PCR, which generates unique amplicons for each patient. This would make sample cross-contamination obvious by the generation of identical-size amplicons (138,142,143, 151,153). Immunocytochemistry, in addition to avoiding the issue of sample cross-contamination, also allows one to directly determine that the sample examined contains either anaplastic large-cell lymphoma or Reed-Sternberg cells. The absence of t(2;5) by immunocytochemistry is in agreement with the genomic DNA-PCR studies in Hodgkin's disease (Table 3).

The detection of t(2;5) only in T-cell or null-cell but not in B-cell anaplastic large-cell lymphomas, the derivation of the Reed-Sternberg cells from germinal center B-cells,

TABLE 3. *Frequency of t(2;5) in Hodgkin's disease*

Author	Method	Patients	% Positive	95% CI
Bullrich et al. (132)	Southern	9	22	3–60
Shiota et al. (131)	IM, RT-PCR	20	0	0–17
Ladanyi et al. (146)	RT-PCR	41	0	0–9
Weiss et al. (147)	RT-PCR	34	0	0–10
Ngan (135)	RT-PCR	24	21	7–42
Yee et al. (137)	RT-PCR	41	5	1–17
Orsheschek et al. (139)	RT-PCR	13	85	55–98
Herbst et al. (148)	ISH, IM	82	0	0–4
Wellmann et al. (136)	RT-PCR	34	0	0–10
Elmberger et al. (140)	RT-PCR	21	0	0–16
Lamant et al. (141)	C,IM, RT-PCR	23	0	0–15
Weber-Matthiesen et al. (149)	FICTION	12[a]	0	0–25
Sarris et al. (142, 143) (updated)	DNA-PCR, IM	142[b]	0	0–2.6
Pulford et al. (218)	IM	50	0	0–7
Waggott et al. (151)	DNA-PCR	46	0	0–8
Total		592	4	2–6

Series are listed in chronological order with respect to publication date.

RT-PCR reverse-transcriptase polymerase chain reaction; ISH, *in-situ* hybridization; IM, immunocytochemistry; C, classic cytogenetics; FICTION, fluorescence immunocytochemistry and interphase cytogenetics; CI, confidence intervals.

[a]These authors report only one positive patient; however, by their own discussion this patient is either unevaluable or negative for t(2;5). For this reason this series is quoted as showing no evidence of t(2;5).

[b]These data are updated by the addition of patients with Hodgkin's disease whose biopsies were stained with either polyclonal or monoclonal antibodies against the cytoplasmic domain of anaplastic lymphoma kinase.

the negative results by classic cytogenetics, the predominantly negative results with molecular genetics, and the negative results with immunocytochemical methods suggest that t(2;5) is not a primary event in Hodgkin's disease.

The t(14;18)(q32;q21)

The t(14;18)(q32;q21) was characterized initially in follicular center-cell lymphomas, where it was shown to result in the dysregulation of BCL-2 production by juxtaposing the immunoglobulin heavy-chain locus on 14q32 with the *bcl-2* locus on 18q21. The *bcl-2* locus encodes a mitochondrial protein whose overexpression protects lymphoid or nonlymphoid cells from apoptosis (154). Extensive studies have documented the presence of t(14;18) in most follicular center-cell lymphomas (155–162), and the frequency appears to be higher when large DNA fragments were analyzed by pulse-field electrophoresis (163). Since Reed-Sternberg cells are derived from B cells with rearranged immunoglobulin genes, it is reasonable to probe for the presence of t(14;18) in Hodgkin's disease.

Examination of Hodgkin's disease for t(14;18) is limited by the paucity of the malignant Reed-Sternberg and Hodgkin's cells in the nodal tissues. By classic cytogenetic analysis the 18q arm containing the *bcl-2* locus is structurally altered only in 12% of the reported Hodgkin's disease karyotypes (Fig. 4). However, chromosomal alterations involving the *bcl-2* locus itself on 18q21 are rare, and have been reported in only two patients: one with lymphocyte-depleted Hodgkin's disease whose karyotype has not been reported in detail, (11) and in another with mixed cellularity Hodgkin's disease whose karyotype is also complex (4). Therefore, by classic cytogenetics the detection of t(14;18) is 2/128 among fully described karyotypes, or 1.6% (Table 2).

Investigation by restriction enzyme analysis of genomic DNA extracted from Hodgkin's disease tissue has been reported in three series (164–166) that included in 55 patients. There were no detectable *bcl-2* locus rearrangements among these patients (0%; 95% confidence intervals 0%–7%, Table 4). However, since the sensitivity of the technique requires at least 1% to 5% of clonal cells to allow detection of the rearranged bands, and since the malignant cells in Hodgkin's disease are often <1% of the cell number, a negative result by restriction enzyme analysis is not particularly compelling.

Several assays based on consensus primers and PCR amplification have been developed that amplify both the major break-point region and the minor cluster region of the *bcl-2* locus with sensitivities as low as 10^{-5} and 10^{-6} (167). The importance of both positive and negative controls for the amplification reaction has been emphasized by all investigators, as well as the need for stringent precautions to avoid contamination of patient samples with rearranged DNA that bears the t(14;18) and is often ubiquitous in research laboratories.

With the use of sensitive PCR it was established that apparently healthy blood donors and normal human vol-

TABLE 4. *Frequency of t(14;18) in Hodgkin's disease*

Author	Method	Patients	% Positive	95% CI
Weiss et al. (219)	Restriction	10	0	0–31
Shibata et al. (173)	PCR	6	0[a]	0–46
Stetler-Stevenson et al. (164)	PCR	53	32	20–46
Louie et al. (174)	PCR	26	0	0–13
Algara et al. (165)	Restriction, PCR	11	7	0–28
Masih et al. (178)	PCR	49	29	34–64
Athan et al. (166)	Restriction, PCR	34	0	0–10
LeBrun et al. (179)	PCR	38	11	3–25
Gupta et al. (181, 184)	PCR	52	27	16–41
Lorenzen et al. (175, 180)	PCR	7	0	0–41
Poppema et al. (11)	PCR	28	39	22–59
Reid et al. (182)	PCR	74	9	4–19
Corbally et al. (185)	PCR	60	12[b]	5–23
Mitani et al. (183)	PCR	44	7	1–19
Kneba et al. (186)	PCR	140	2[c]	0–6
Hell et al. (177)	PCR	16	0	0–21
Segal et al. (176)	PCR	14	0	0–23
Gravel et al. (187)	PCR	115	50	41–60
Total		800	18[d]	15–21

Series are listed in chronological order with respect to publication date.
[a]Reactive nodes were positive 0/11.
[b]Reactive nodes were positive in 3/34.
[c]Reactive nodes were positive in 0/30.
[d]This frequency calculation is based on the sum of 144 positive cases reported.
CI, confidence intervals.

unteers often carry in their peripheral blood B cells with the t(14;18) (168–170) and that the frequency of this observation increases with age. The same clone(s) persist in a given subject over time, but with the limited reported follow-up time no follicular center-cell lymphomas have yet developed in these subjects. Similarly, PCR has detected the t(14;18) in hyperplastic nodes without any evidence of follicular center-cell lymphoma (171,172).

The detection of t(14;18) by PCR amplification of genomic DNA of Hodgkin's disease has yielded conflicting results. No amplicons for t(14;18) were detected in 10 of 17 series (166,173–177). However, 7 of 17 series reported PCR amplicons consistent with the presence of t(14;18) (11,164,165,178–187), with frequencies that ranged from 2% to 39%. One investigator reported both negative and positive results (175,180). Overall, positive results were reported in 86 of 630 cases analyzed by PCR, or in 86 of 685 cases that have been analyzed either by PCR or by restriction enzyme analysis. The overall frequency is 13%, with 95% confidence intervals ranging from 9% to 14% (Table 4).

Several reasons may account for the variable detection of t(14;18) in Hodgkin's disease. It is not clear whether all PCR assays used were equally sensitive, and spurious laboratory contamination has been shown to be common in PCR for t(14;18) (188). In one series (181) sequencing of the t(14;18) amplicons revealed unique break points for each patient and thus eliminated cross-contamination as a source of the positive results. Other investigators (164) minimized the possibility of contamination by analyzing multiple samples from each patient and by verifying that the t(14;18) amplicons varied in size from one patient to the other. Even if contamination is excluded as a source for the t(14;18) amplicon in some series, it remains a possibility in most PCR series. Another series that reported a frequency of 11% by PCR noted that all the patients with Hodgkin's disease who were positive for t(14;18) had a previous or concurrent diagnosis of follicular center-cell lymphoma (179). The follicular lymphoma was the most likely cause of the positive results in this instance, because the t(14;18) PCR reaction frequently can be positive in blood or marrow in patients with this disease, even if it is of limited clinical stage or is in apparent clinical complete remission (162,189–192). Three series (173,185,186) have analyzed tissues from both Hodgkin's disease and from reactive follicular hyperplasia by PCR, and detected t(14;18)-specific amplicons in 3 of 75 reactive lesions, for an overall frequency of 4% and 95% CI of 1 to 11% (Table 4). These data raise the possibility that the t(14;18) is not present in the malignant Reed-Sternberg cells, but rather in the reactive lymphoid infiltrate. Analysis of Hodgkin's tumor tissues with fluorescent *in situ* hybridizations or with PCR of single Reed-Sternberg cells supports this interpretation (11,187).

Some investigators have used BCL-2 protein expression by immunocytochemistry as a means to infer the presence of t(14;18) in Hodgkin's disease. However, bcl-2 protein expression was highly variable without any obvious correlation with the detection of t(14;18) by PCR (174,177,180,186). The level of expression of BCL-2 can be affected by factors other than t(14;18), including IL-10 (92) and especially by the Latent Membrane Protein-1 (LMP-1) protein of EBV (193,194). Since IL-10 is often elevated in the sera of patients with Hodgkin's disease, and the expression of LMP-1 in the Reed-Sternberg cells can vary depending on patient age and geographic location, (195) studies of BCL-2 expression cannot be used to infer the presence of t(14;18) in Hodgkin's disease.

The absence of t(14;18) from the vast majority of patients by classic cytogenetics, combined with the low frequency of t(14;18) amplicons by PCR in both Hodgkin's disease and reactive lymph nodes, and the results of fluorescent *in situ* hybridization or the PCR analysis of single cells, all suggest that the t(14;18)(q32;q21) is not a primary event in the molecular pathogenesis of Hodgkin's disease.

FAMILIAL HODGKIN'S DISEASE

Although the cytogenetic aberrations seen in Hodgkin's disease are not germline, familial cases are estimated to represent between 2% and 5% of all cases of Hodgkin's disease (196,197). The predisposition to have the same histology within a given kindred (198,199) may be explained by environmental factors, such as EBV or other unknown viruses, or by genetic predisposition. In two studies that evaluated the role of EBV in Hodgkin's disease, there was no strong association with EBER-1 expression in Reed-Sternberg cells, and no difference in EBV seroprevalence between patients with Hodgkin's disease and controls (200,201). Other factors such as gene mutations could also play a role, but p53 mutations do not appear to play a critical role in familial Hodgkin's disease (202–204).

The hypothesis of a genetic predisposition to develop Hodgkin's disease has been explored by determining the HLA genotypes of several kindreds with familial Hodgkin's disease. Several HLA types have been observed repeatedly in these kindreds including HLA DR5 (205), B27 (205), B18 (206,207), Bw35 and Bw37 (208), B7,198 and B5 (209). Since it is known that the immune response is genetically determined by the HLA type, it is possible that uncommon genetic susceptibilities allow the development of Hodgkin's disease as an uncommon consequence of a common event, such as EBV infection.

CONCLUSION

Cytogenetic studies in Hodgkin's disease are limited when compared to those in non-Hodgkin's lymphoma.

However, the available data show that clonal chromosomal observations are common in this disorder and support its malignant nature. These data are consistent with the results of single-cell PCR analysis of Reed-Sternberg cells that suggest that most Reed-Sternberg cells are derived from germinal center B cells with rearranged immunoglobulin genes. The absence of t(2;5) in Hodgkin's disease is consistent with its derivation from B cells and supports the notion that it is different from anaplastic large-cell lymphoma, which is likely derived from cytotoxic T cells. The paucity of cases of Hodgkin's disease with t(14;18) suggests a lack of relationship between Hodgkin's disease and follicular center-cell lymphomas. This is consistent with the molecular evidence that reveals the presence of clonal crippling mutations in the immunoglobulin receptor in Reed-Sternberg cells, compared with somatic hypermutation in follicular center-cell lymphomas.

Analysis of familial Hodgkin's disease kindreds fails to reveal a germline mutation frequently associated with Hodgkin's disease. However, the association of certain HLA types with familial Hodgkin's disease suggests that genetic predisposition, possibly an altered immune response to one or more common infectious agents, may be a pathogenic factor in some patients. The cytogenetics of Hodgkin's disease and the derivation of Reed-Sternberg cells from germinal center B cells that are destined to undergo apoptosis suggest that multiple mechanisms may be involved in the immortalization of these cells. These may involve growth factors, cell cycle–related proteins, oncogenes, protein kinases, or tumor suppressor genes. It therefore may not be entirely coincidental that Hodgkin's disease and most solid tumors have no single cytogenetic abnormality. Most epithelial malignancies are also derived from cells that are committed, and are thus destined to undergo terminal differentiation and apoptosis. Thus in both solid tumors and Hodgkin's disease a multistep process may be responsible for the initiation and the establishment of the malignant phenotype. Molecular investigation of the loci depicted in Table 2 may shed light in these steps and uncover additional genes involved in them.

ACKNOWLEDGMENT

We thank Ms. Joyce Palmer for assistance with the manuscript.

REFERENCES

1. Mitelman F. ISCN (1991): Guidelines for Cancer Cytogenetics. Supplement to an International System for Human Cytogenetic Nomenclature. Basel, Switzerland: Karger, 1991:1–54.
2. Hossfeld DK, Schmidt CG. Chromosome findings in effusions from patients with Hodgkin's disease. *Int J Cancer* 1978;21:147–156.
3. Kristoffersson U, Heim S, Mandahl N, Olsson H, Akerman M, Mitelman F. Cytogenetic studies in Hodgkin's disease. *Acta Pathol Microbiol Immunol Scand [A]* 1987;95:289–295.
4. Cabanillas F, Pathak S, Trujillo J, et al. Cytogenetic features of Hodgkin's disease suggest possible origin from a lymphocyte. *Blood* 1988;71:1615–1617.
5. Dennis TR, Stock AD, Winberg CD, Sheibani K, Rappaport H. Cytogenetic studies of Hodgkin's disease. Analysis of involved lymph nodes from 12 patients. *Cancer Genet Cytogenet* 1989;37:201–208.
6. Koduru PR, Offit K, Filippa DA, Lieberman PH, Jhanwar SC. Cytogenetic and molecular genetic analysis of abnormal cells in Hodgkin's disease. *Cancer Genet Cytogenet* 1989;43:109–118.
7. Schouten HC, Sanger WG, Duggan M, Weisenburger DD, MacLennan KA, Armitage JO. Chromosomal abnormalities in Hodgkin's disease. *Blood* 1989;73:2149–2154.
8. Banks RE, Gledhill S, Ross FM, Krajewski A, Dewar AE, Weir-Thompson EM. Karyotypic abnormalities and immunoglobulin gene rearrangements in Hodgkin's disease. *Cancer Genet Cytogenet* 1991; 51:103–111.
9. Ladanyi M, Parsa NZ, Offit K, Wachtel MS, Filippa DA, Jhanwar SC. Clonal cytogenetic abnormalities in Hodgkin's disease. *Genes Chromosomes Cancer* 1991;3:294–299.
10. Tilly H, Bastard C, Delastre T, et al. Cytogenetic studies in untreated Hodgkin's disease. *Blood* 1991;77:1298–1304.
11. Poppema S, Kaleta J, Hepperle B. Chromosomal abnormalities in patients with Hodgkin's disease: evidence for frequent involvement of the 14q chromosomal region but infrequent bcl-2 gene rearrangement in Reed-Sternberg cells. *J Natl Cancer Inst* 1992;84:1789–1793.
12. Schlegelberger B, Weber-Matthiesen K, Himmler A, et al. Cytogenetic findings and results of combined immunophenotyping and karyotyping in Hodgkin's disease. *Leukemia* 1994;8:72–80.
13. Raffeld M, Jaffe ES. bcl-1, t(11,14), and mantle cell-derived lymphomas. *Blood* 1991;78:259–263.
14. Haber MM, Knowles DM, Inghirami G. Image analysis of the Reed-Sternberg cells of Hodgkin's disease. *Mod Pathol* 1992;5:78A.
15. Balazs I, Purrello M, Rubinstein P, Alhadeff B, Siniscalco M. Highly polymorphic DNA site D14S1 maps to the region of Burkitt lymphoma translocation and is closely linked to the heavy chain gamma 1 immunoglobulin locus. *Proc Natl Acad Sci USA* 1982;79:7395–7399.
16. Lindberg FP, Gresham HD, Schwarz E, Brown EJ. Molecular cloning of integrin-associated protein: an immunoglobulin family member with multiple membrane-spanning domains implicated in alpha v beta 3-dependent ligand binding. *J Cell Biol* 1993;123:485–496.
17. Freeman GJ, Gribben JG, Boussiotis VA, et al. Cloning of B7-2: a CTLA-4 counter-receptor that costimulates human T cell proliferation. *Science* 1993;262:909–911.
18. Selvakumar A, White PC, Dupont B. Genomic organization of the mouse B-lymphocyte activation antigen B7. *Immunogenetics* 1993;38: 292–295.
19. Seigel LJ, Harper ME, Wong-Staal F, Gallo RC, Nash WG, O'Brien SJ. Gene for T-cell growth factor: location on human chromosome 4q and feline chromosome B1. *Science* 1984;223:175–178.
20. Shows T, Eddy R, Haley L, et al. Interleukin 2 (IL2) is assigned to human chromosome 4. *Somat Cell Mol Genet* 1984;10:315–318.
21. Camerini D, Walz G, Loenen WA, Borst J, Seed B. The T cell activation antigen CD27 is a member of the nerve growth factor/tumor necrosis factor receptor gene family. *J Immunol* 1991;147:3165–3169.
22. Capon DJ, Shepard HM, Goeddel DV. Two distinct families of human and bovine interferon-alpha genes are coordinately expressed and encode functional polypeptides. *Mol Cell Biol* 1985;5:768–779.
23. Shows TB, Sakaguchi AY, Naylor SL, Goedell DV, Lawn RM. Clustering of leukocyte and fibroblast interferon genes of human chromosome 9. *Science* 1982;218:373–374.
24. Trent JM, Olson S, Lawn RM. Chromosomal localization of human leukocyte, fibroblast, and immune interferon genes by means of in situ hybridization. *Proc Natl Acad Sci USA* 1982;79:7809–7813.
25. Aguet M, Dembic Z, Merlin G. Molecular cloning and expression of the human interferon-gamma receptor. *Cell* 1988;55:273–280.
26. Nomura N, Sasamoto S, Ishii S, Date T, Matsui M, Ishizaki R. Isolation of human cDNA clones of ski and the ski-related gene, sno. *Nucleic Acids Res* 1989;17:5489–5500.
27. Colby WW, Chen EY, Smith DH, Levinson AD. Identification and nucleotide sequence of a human locus homologous to the v-myc oncogene of avian myelocytomatosis virus MC29. *Nature* 1983;301: 722–725.
28. Gu Y, Nakamura T, Alder H, et al. The t(4;11) chromosome transloca-

tion of human acute leukemias fuses the ALL-1 gene, related to Drosophila trithorax, to the AF-4 gene. *Cell* 1992;71:701–708.
29. Langdon WY, Blake TJ. The human CBL oncogene. *Curr Top Microbiol Immunol* 1990;166:159–164.
30. Golub TR, Barker GF, Bohlander SK, et al. Fusion of the TEL gene on 12p13 to the AML1 gene on 21q22 in acute lymphoblastic leukemia. *Proc Natl Acad Sci USA* 1995;92:4917–4921.
31. Virgilio L, Isobe M, Narducci MG, et al. Chromosome walking on the TCL1 locus involved in T-cell neoplasia. *Proc Natl Acad Sci USA* 1993;90:9275–9279.
32. Virgilio L, Narducci MG, Isobe M, et al. Identification of the TCL1 gene involved in T-cell malignancies. *Proc Natl Acad Sci USA* 1994; 91:12530–12534.
33. Fu TB, Virgilio L, Narducci MG, Facchiano A, Russo G, Croce CM. Characterization and localization of the TCL-1 oncogene product. *Cancer Res* 1994;54:6297–6301.
34. Dyomin VG, Rao PH, Dalla-Favera R, Chaganti RSK. BCL8, a novel gene involved in translocations affecting band 15q11–13 in diffuse large-cell lymphoma. *Proc Natl Acad Sci USA* 1997;94:5728–5732.
35. Neubauer A, Fiebeler A, Graham DK, et al. Expression of axl, a transforming receptor tyrosine kinase, in normal and malignant hematopoiesis. *Blood* 1994;84:1931–1941.
36. O'Bryan JP, Fridell YW, Koski R, Varnum B, Liu ET. The transforming receptor tyrosine kinase, Axl, is post-translationally regulated by proteolytic cleavage. *J Biol Chem* 1995;270:551–557.
37. Le Beau MM, Westbrook CA, Diaz MO, Rowley JD. Evidence for two distinct c-src loci on human chromosomes 1 and 20. *Nature* 1984;312: 70–71.
38. Parker RC, Mardon G, Lebo RV, Varmus HE, Bishop JM. Isolation of duplicated human c-src genes located on chromosomes 1 and 20. *Mol Cell Biol* 1985;5:831–838.
39. Steimle V, Durand B, Barras E, et al. A novel DNA-binding regulatory factor is mutated in primary MHC class II deficiency (bare lymphocyte syndrome). *Genes Dev* 1995;9:1021–1032.
40. Dickinson LA, Joh T, Kohwi Y, Kohwi-Shigematsu T. A tissue-specific MAR/SAR DNA-binding protein with unusual binding site recognition. *Cell* 1992;70:631–645.
41. Tommerup N, Vissing H. Isolation and fine mapping of 16 novel human zinc finger-encoding cDNAs identify putative candidate genes for developmental and malignant disorders. *Genomics* 1995;27:259–264.
42. Reith W, Ucla C, Barras E, et al. RFX1, a transactivator of hepatitis B virus enhancer I, belongs to a novel family of homodimeric and heterodimeric DNA-binding proteins. *Mol Cell Biol* 1994;14:1230–1244.
43. Veals SA, Schindler C, Leonard D, et al. Subunit of an alpha-interferon-responsive transcription factor is related to interferon regulatory factor and Myb families of DNA-binding proteins. *Mol Cell Biol* 1992;12:3315–3324.
44. Abrink M, Aveskogh M, Hellman L. Isolation of cDNA clones for 42 different Kruppel-related zinc finger proteins expressed in the human monoblast cell line U-937. *DNA Cell Biol* 1995;14:125–136.
45. Nomura N, Takahashi M, Matsui M, et al. Isolation of human cDNA clones of myb-related genes, A-myb and B-myb [published erratum appears in *Nucleic Acids Res* 1989;17(3):1282]. *Nucleic Acids Res* 1988;16:11075–11089.
46. Selbie LA, Schmitz-Peiffer C, Sheng Y, Biden TJ. Molecular cloning and characterization of PKC iota, an atypical isoform of protein kinase C derived from insulin-secreting cells. *J Biol Chem* 1993;268: 24296–24302.
47. Tanaka N, Asao H, Ohtani K, Nakamura M, Sugamura K. A novel human tyrosine kinase gene inducible in T cells by interleukin 2. *FEBS Lett* 1993;324:1–5.
48. Lechleider RJ, de Caestecker MP, Dehejia A, Polymeropoulos MH, Roberts AB. Serine phosphorylation, chromosomal localization, and transforming growth factor-beta signal transduction by human bsp-1. *J Biol Chem* 1996;271:17617–17620.
49. Wicks IP, Wilkinson D, Salvaris E, Boyd AW. Molecular cloning of HEK, the gene encoding a receptor tyrosine kinase expressed by human lymphoid tumor cell lines. *Proc Natl Acad Sci USA* 1992;89: 1611–1615.
50. Bennett BD, Wang Z, Kuang WJ, et al. Cloning and characterization of HTK, a novel transmembrane tyrosine kinase of the EPH subfamily. *J Biol Chem* 1994;269:14211–14218.
51. Bennett BD, Zeigler FC, Gu Q, et al. Molecular cloning of a ligand for the EPH-related receptor protein-tyrosine kinase Htk. *Proc Natl Acad Sci USA* 1995;92:1866–1870.
52. Hirai H, Maru Y, Hagiwara K, Nishida J, Takaku F. A novel putative tyrosine kinase receptor encoded by the eph gene. *Science* 1987;238: 1717–1720.
53. Creasy CL, Chernoff J. Cloning and characterization of a member of the MST subfamily of Ste20-like kinases. *Gene* 1995;167:303–306.
54. Creasy CL, Chernoff J. Cloning and characterization of a human protein kinase with homology to Ste20. *J Biol Chem* 1995;270:21695–21700.
55. Demetrick DJ, Matsumoto S, Hannon GJ, et al. Chromosomal mapping of the genes for the human cell cycle proteins cyclin C (CCNC), cyclin E (CCNE), p21 (CDKN1) and KAP (CDKN3). *Cytogenet Cell Genet* 1995;69:190–192.
56. Makela TP, Tassan JP, Nigg EA, Frutiger S, Hughes GJ, Weinberg RA. A cyclin associated with the CDK-activating kinase MO15. *Nature* 1994;371:254–257.
57. Hannon GJ, Beach D. p15INK4B is a potential effector of TGF-beta-induced cell cycle arrest. *Nature* 1994;371:257–261.
58. Serrano M, Hannon GJ, Beach D. A new regulatory motif in cell-cycle control causing specific inhibition of cyclin D/CDK4. *Nature* 1993; 366:704–707.
59. Okuda T, Hirai H, Valentine VA, et al. Molecular cloning, expression pattern, and chromosomal localization of human CDKN2D/INK4d, an inhibitor of cyclin D-dependent kinases. *Genomics* 1995;29:623–630.
60. Garcia-Sanz R, Gonzalez M, Vargas M, et al. Deletions and rearrangements of cyclin-dependent kinase 4 inhibitor gene p16 are associated with poor prognosis in B cell non-Hodgkin's lymphomas. *Leukemia* 1997;11:1915–1920.
61. Garcia-Sanz R, Gonzalez M, Chillon MC, et al. Deletions and rearrangements of cyclin-dependent kinase 4 inhibitor gene p16 are associated with poor prognosis in B-cell non-Hodgkin's lymphomas. *Br J Haematol* 1998;102:145.
62. Wang L, Miura M, Bergeron L, Zhu H, Yuan J. Ich-1, an Ice/ced-3-related gene, encodes both positive and negative regulators of programmed cell death. *Cell* 1994;78:739–750.
63. Rajcan-Separovic E, Liston P, Lefebvre C, Korneluk RG. Assignment of human inhibitor of apoptosis protein (IAP) genes xiap, hiap-1, and hiap-2 to chromosomes Xq25 and 11q22-q23 by fluorescence in situ hybridization. *Genomics* 1996;37:404–406.
64. Liston P, Roy N, Tamai K, et al. Suppression of apoptosis in mammalian cells by NAIP and a related family of IAP genes. *Nature* 1996; 379:349–353.
65. Liu YJ, Joshua DE, Williams GT, Smith CA, Gordon J, MacLennan IC. Mechanism of antigen-driven selection in germinal centres. *Nature* 1989;342:929–931.
66. Lafage-Pochitaloff M, Herman P, Birg F, et al. Localization of the human CD40 gene to chromosome 20, bands q12-q13.2. *Leukemia* 1994;8:1172–1175.
67. Eisman R, Surrey S, Ramachandran B, Schwartz E, Poncz M. Structural and functional comparison of the genes for human platelet factor 4 and PF4alt. *Blood* 1990;76:336–344.
68. Mukaida N, Shiroo M, Matsushima K. Genomic structure of the human monocyte-derived neutrophil chemotactic factor IL-8. *J Immunol* 1989;143:1366–1371.
69. Oppenheim JJ, Zachariae CO, Mukaida N, Matsushima K. Properties of the novel proinflammatory supergene "intercrine" cytokine family. *Annu Rev Immunol* 1991;9:617–648.
70. Broxmeyer HE, Sherry B, Cooper S, et al. Comparative analysis of the human macrophage inflammatory protein family of cytokines (chemokines) on proliferation of human myeloid progenitor cells. Interacting effects involving suppression, synergistic suppression, and blocking of suppression. *J Immunol* 1993;150:3448–3458.
71. Cocchi F, DeVico AL, Garzino-Demo A, Arya SK, Gallo RC, Lusso P. Identification of RANTES, MIP-1a and MIP-1b as the Major HIV-Suppressive Factors produced by CD8+ T cells. *Science* 1995;270: 1811–1815.
72. Broxmeyer HE. Suppressor cytokines and regulation of myelopoiesis. Biology and possible clinical uses. *Am J Pediatr Hematol Oncol* 1992; 14:22–30.
73. Broxmeyer HE, Benninger L, Hague N, et al. Suppressive effects of the chemokine (macrophage inflammatory protein) family of cytokines on proliferation of normal and leukemia myeloid cell proliferation. In: Guigon M, Lemoine FM, Dainiak N, Schechter A, Najman A,

eds. *The negative regulation of hematopoiesis; from fundamental concepts to clinical applications,* vol 229. Paris: Colloque INSERM/John Libbey Eurotext, 1993:141–154.

74. Sarris AH, Broxmeyer HE, Wirthmueller U, et al. Human interferon-inducible protein 10: expression and purification of recombinant protein demonstrate inhibition of early human hematopoietic progenitors. *J Exp Med* 1993;178:1127–1132.
75. Taub DD, Anver M, Oppenheim JJ, Longo DL, Murphy WJ. T lymphocyte recruitment by interleukin-8 (IL-8). IL-8-induced degranulation of neutrophils releases potent chemoattractants for human T lymphocytes both in vitro and in vivo. *J Clin Invest* 1996;97:1931–1941.
76. Barton DE, Foellmer BE, Du J, Tamm J, Derynck R, Francke U. Chromosomal mapping of genes for transforming growth factors beta 2 and beta 3 in man and mouse: dispersion of TGF-beta gene family. *Oncogene Res* 1988;3:323–331.
77. Fujii D, Brissenden JE, Derynck R, Francke U. Transforming growth factor beta gene maps to human chromosome 19 long arm and to mouse chromosome 7. *Somat Cell Mol Genet* 1986;12:281–288.
78. Han S, Stuart LA, Degen SJ. Characterization of the DNF15S2 locus on human chromosome 3: identification of a gene coding for four kringle domains with homology to hepatocyte growth factor. *Biochemistry* 1991;30:9768–9780.
79. Schneider C, Owen MJ, Banville D, Williams JG. Primary structure of human transferrin receptor deduced from the mRNA sequence. *Nature* 1984;311:675–678.
80. Lee J, Gray A, Yuan J, Luoh SM, Avraham H, Wood WI. Vascular endothelial growth factor-related protein: a ligand and specific activator of the tyrosine kinase receptor Flt4. *Proc Natl Acad Sci USA* 1996; 93:1988–1992.
81. Liu Y, Wei SH, Ho AS, de Waal Malefyt R, Moore KW. Expression cloning and characterization of a human IL-10 receptor. *J Immunol* 1994;152:1821–1829.
82. Rotwein P, Pollock KM, Didier DK, Krivi GG. Organization and sequence of the human insulin-like growth factor I gene. Alternative RNA processing produces two insulin-like growth factor I precursor peptides. *J Biol Chem* 1986;261:4828–4832.
83. Martin FH, Suggs SV, Langley KE, et al. Primary structure and functional expression of rat and human stem cell factor DNAs. *Cell* 1990; 63:203–211.
84. Pinto A, Gloghini A, Gattei V, Aldinucci D, Zagonel V, Carbone A. Expression of the c-kit receptor in human lymphomas is restricted to Hodgkin's disease and CD30+ anaplastic large cell lymphomas. *Blood* 1994;83:785–792.
85. Ohshima K, Suzumiya J, Akamatu M, Takeshita M, Kikuchi M. Human and viral interleukin-10 in Hodgkin's disease, and its influence on CD4+ and CD8+ T lymphocytes. *Int J Cancer* 1995;62:5–10.
86. Herbst H, Foss H-D, Samol J, et al. Frequent expression of interleukin-10 by Epstein-Barr virus-harboring tumor cells of Hodgkin's disease. *Blood* 1996;87:2918–2929.
87. Sarris AH, Kliche KO, Peethambaram PP, Witzig T, Andreeff M, Cabanillas F. Interleukin-10 as a prognostic factor for Hodgkin's disease (HD) treated with ABVD: results from MD Anderson (MDA) and Mayo Clinic (MC). *Blood* 1997;90(suppl 1):335a.
88. Taga K, Cherney B, Tosato G. IL-10 inhibits apoptotic cell death in human T cells starved of IL-2. *Int Immunol* 1993;5:1599–1608.
89. Taga K, Chretien J, Cherney B, Diaz L, Brown M, Tosato G. Interleukin-10 inhibits apoptotic cell death in infectious mononucleosis T cells. *J Clin Invest* 1994;94:251–260.
90. Brunetti M, Martelli N, Colasante A, Piantelli M, Musiani P, Aiello FB. Spontaneous and glucocorticoid induced apoptosis in human mature T lymphocytes. *Blood* 1995;86:4199.
91. Koury MJ. Programmed cell death (apoptosis) in hematopoiesis. *Exp Hematol* 1992;20:391.
92. Weber-Nordt RM, Henschler R, Schott E, et al. Interleukin-10 increases Bcl-2 expression and survival in primary human CD34+ hematopietic progenitor cells. *Blood* 1996;88:2549–2558.
93. Sakai I, Sharief FS, Pan YC, Li SS. The cDNA and protein sequences of human lactate dehydrogenase B. *Biochem J* 1987;248:933–936.
94. Straus DJ, Gaynor JJ, Myers J, et al. Prognostic factors among 185 adults with newly diagnosed advanced Hodgkin's disease treated with alternating potentially noncross-resistant chemotherapy and intermediate-dose radiation therapy. *J Clin Oncol* 1990;8:1173–1186.
95. Sarris AH, Straus D, Preti A, et al. A Prognostic Model For Advanced Hodgkin's Disease at M.D. Anderson validated with an independent set of patients treated at Memorial Sloan-Kettering. *Blood* 1996;88 (suppl 1):893a.
96. Desalbens B, Garidi R, Tabuteau S, Legrand S, Dutel JL. Prognostic value of seric LDH among 150 homogeneously treated Hodgkin's diseases. *Br J Haematol* 1998;102:116.
97. Suva LJ, Winslow GA, Wettenhall RE, et al. A parathyroid hormone-related protein implicated in malignant hypercalcemia: cloning and expression. *Science* 1987;237:893–896.
98. Tromp G, Kuivaniemi H, Stacey A, et al. Structure of a full-length cDNA clone for the prepro alpha 1(I) chain of human type I procollagen. *Biochem J* 1988;253:919–922.
99. Chen CJ, Chin JE, Ueda K, et al. Internal duplication and homology with bacterial transport proteins in the mdr1 (P-glycoprotein) gene from multidrug-resistant human cells. *Cell* 1986;47:381–389.
100. Sohma Y, Akahori H, Seki N, et al. Molecular cloning and chromosomal localization of the human thrombopoietin gene. *FEBS Lett* 1994; 353:57–61.
101. Weber-Matthiesen K, Deerberg J, Poetsch M, Grote W, Schlegelberger B. Clarification of dubious karyotypes in Hodgkin's disease by simultaneous fluorescence immunophenotyping and interphase cytogenetics (FICTION). *Cytogenet Cell Genet* 1995;70:243–245.
102. Weber-Matthiesen K, Deerberg J, Poetsch M, Grote W, Schlegelberger B. Numerical chromosome aberrations are present within the CD30+ Hodgkin and Reed-Sternberg cells in 100% of analyzed cases of Hodgkin's disease. *Blood* 1995;86:1464–1468.
103. Nolte M, Werner M, von Wasielewski R, Nietgen G, Wilkens L, Georgii A. Detection of numerical karyotype changes in the giant cells of Hodgkin's lymphomas by a combination of FISH and immunocytochemistry applied to paraffin sections. *Histochem Cell Biol* 1996; 105:401–404.
104. Stein H, Mason DY, Gerdes J, et al. The expression of the Hodgkin's disease associated antigen Ki-1 in reactive and neoplastic lymphoid tissue: evidence that Reed-Sternberg cells and histiocytic malignancies are derived from activated lymphoid cells. *Blood* 1985;66: 848–858.
105. Stansfeld AG, Diebold J, Noel H, et al. Updated Kiel classification for lymphomas. *Lancet* 1988;1:292–293.
106. Harris NL, Jaffe ES, Stein H, et al. A revised European-American classification of lymphoid neoplasms: a proposal from the International Lymphoma Study Group. *Blood* 1994;84:1361–1392.
107. Greer JP, Kinney MC, Collins RD, et al. Clinical features of 31 patients with Ki-1 anaplastic large-cell lymphoma. *J Clin Oncol* 1991; 9:539–547.
108. Chott A, Kaserer K, Augustin I, et al. Ki-1-positive large cell lymphoma. A clinicopathologic study of 41 cases. *Am J Surg Pathol* 1990; 14:439–448.
109. Chan JK, Ng CS, Hui PK, et al. Anaplastic large cell Ki-1 lymphoma. Delineation of two morphological types. *Histopathology* 1989;15: 11–34.
110. Kinney MC, Collins RD, Greer JP, Whitlock JA, Sioutos N, Kadin ME. A small-cell-predominant variant of primary Ki-1 (CD30)+ T-cell lymphoma. *Am J Surg Pathol* 1993;17:859–868.
111. Pileri S, Falini B, Delsol G, et al. Lymphohistiocytic T-cell lymphoma (anaplastic large cell lymphoma CD30+/Ki-1 + with a high content of reactive histiocytes). *Histopathology* 1990;16:383–391.
112. Chan JK, Buchanan R, Fletcher CD. Sarcomatoid variant of anaplastic large-cell Ki-1 lymphoma. *Am J Surg Pathol* 1990;14:983–988.
113. Kinney MC, Glick AD, Stein H, Collins RD. Comparison of anaplastic large cell Ki-1 lymphomas and microvillous lymphomas in their immunologic and ultrastructural features. *Am J Surg Pathol* 1990;14: 1047–1060.
114. Pileri S, Bocchia M, Baroni CD, et al. Anaplastic large cell lymphoma (CD30+/Ki-1+): results of a prospective clinico-pathological study of 69 cases. *Br J Haematol* 1994;86:513–523.
115. Stein H, Herbst H, Anagnostopoulos I, Niedobitek G, Dallenbach F, Kratzsch HC. The nature of Hodgkin and Reed-Sternberg cells, their association with EBV, and their relationship to anaplastic large-cell lymphoma. *Ann Oncol* 1991;2:33–38.
116. Schwab U, Stein H, Gerdes J, et al. Production of a monoclonal antibody specific for Hodgkin and Sternberg-Reed cells of Hodgkin's disease and a subset of normal lymphoid cells. *Nature* 1982;299:65–67.
117. Stein H, Dallenbach F. Diffuse large cell lymphomas of B and T cell

type. In: Knowles DM, ed. *Neoplastic hematopathology.* Baltimore: Williams and Wilkins, 1992:675–714.

118. Durkop H, Latza U, Hummel M, Eitelbach F, Seed B, Stein H. Molecular cloning and expression of a new member of the nerve growth factor receptor family that is characteristic for Hodgkin's disease. *Cell* 1992;68:421–427.
119. Leoncini L, Del Vecchio MT, Kraft R, et al. Hodgkin's disease and CD30-positive anaplastic large cell lymphomas—a continuous spectrum of malignant disorders. A quantitative morphometric and immunohistologic study. *Am J Pathol* 1990;137:1047–1057.
120. Davis TH, Morton CC, Miller-Cassman R, Balk SP, Kadin ME. Hodgkin's disease, lymphomatoid papulosis, and cutaneous T-cell lymphoma derived from a common T-cell clone. *N Engl J Med* 1992; 326:1115–1122.
121. Le Beau MM, Bitter MA, Larson RA, et al. The t(2;5)(p23;q35): a recurring chromosomal abnormality in Ki-1-positive anaplastic large cell lymphoma. *Leukemia* 1989;3:866–870.
122. Bitter MA, Franklin WA, Larson RA, et al. Morphology in Ki-1(CD30)-positive non-Hodgkin's lymphoma is correlated with clinical features and the presence of a unique chromosomal abnormality, t(2;5)(p23;q35). *Am J Surg Pathol* 1990;14:305–316.
123. Mason DY, Bastard C, Rimokh R, et al. CD30-positive large cell lymphomas ("Ki-1 lymphoma") are associated with a chromosomal translocation involving 5q35 [see comments]. *Br J Haematol* 1990; 74:161–168.
124. Offit K, Ladanyi M, Gangi MD, Ebrahim SA, Filippa D, Chaganti RS. Ki-1 antigen expression defines a favorable clinical subset of non-B cell non-Hodgkin's lymphoma. *Leukemia* 1990;4:625–630.
125. Sandlund JT, Pui CH, Roberts WM, et al. Clinicopathologic features and treatment outcome of children with large-cell lymphoma and the t(2;5)(p23;q35). *Blood* 1994;84:2467–2471.
126. Morris SW, Kirstein MN, Valentine MB, et al. Fusion of a kinase gene, ALK, to a nucleolar protein gene, NPM, in non-Hodgkin's lymphoma. *Science* 1994;263:1281–1284.
127. Borer RA, Lehner CF, Eppenberger HM, Nigg EA. Major nucleolar proteins shuttle between nucleus and cytoplasm. *Cell* 1989;56:379–390.
128. Chan WY, Liu QR, Borjigin J, et al. Characterization of the cDNA encoding human nucleophosmin and studies of its role in normal and abnormal growth. *Biochemistry* 1989;28:1033–1039.
129. Kuefer MU, Look AT, Pulford K, et al. Retrovirus-mediated gene transfer of NMP-ALK causes lymphoid malignancy in mice. *Blood* 1997;90:2901–2910.
130. Shiota M, Fujimoto J, Semba T, Satoh H, Yamamoto T, Mori S. Hyperphosphorylation of a novel 80 kDa protein-tyrosine kinase similar to Ltk in a human Ki-1 lymphoma cell line, AMS3. *Oncogene* 1994;9: 1567–1574.
131. Shiota M, Fujimoto J, Takenaga M, et al. Diagnosis of t(2;5)(p23;q35)-associated Ki-1 lymphoma with immunohistochemistry. *Blood* 1994; 84:3648–3652.
132. Bullrich F, Morris SW, Hummel M, Pileri S, Stein H, Croce CM. Nucleophosmin (NPM) gene rearrangements in Ki-1-positive lymphomas. *Cancer Res* 1994;54:2873–2877.
133. Downing JR, Shurtleff SA, Zielenska M, et al. Molecular detection of the (2;5) translocation of non-Hodgkin's lymphoma by reverse transcriptase-polymerase chain reaction. *Blood* 1995;85:3416–3422.
134. Lopetagui JR, Sun LH, Chan KC, et al. Association of t(2;5) in CD30-positive anaplastic large cell lymphoma vs Hodgkin's disease. *Mod Pathol* 1995;8:115A.
135. Ngan B. The presence of transcripts of the fusion of kinase gene ALK to nucleophosmin gene NPM in the t(2;5) (p23;q35) translocation defines subsets of non-Hodgkin's lymphoma with or without CD30 (Ki-1) expression and Hodgkin's disease. *Mod Pathol* 1995;8:118A.
136. Wellmann A, Otsuki T, Vogelbruch M, Clark HM, Jaffe ES, Raffeld M. Analysis of the t(2;5)(p23;q35) translocation by reverse transcription-polymerase chain reaction in CD30+ anaplastic large-cell lymphomas, in other non-Hodgkin's lymphomas of T-cell phenotype, and in Hodgkin's disease. *Blood* 1995;86:2321–2328.
137. Yee HT, Ponzoni M, Merson A, et al. Chimeric NPM-ALK transcripts of t(2;5) in anaplastic large cell lymphoma (ALCL) and Hodgkin's disease (HD). *Mod Pathol* 1995;8:124A.
138. Waggott W, Lo Y-MD, Bastard C, et al. Detection of NPM-ALK DNA rearrangement in CD30 positive anaplastic large cell lymphoma. *Br J Haematol* 1995;89:905–907.
139. Orscheschek K, Merz H, Hell J, Binder T, Bartels H, Feller AF. Large-cell anaplastic lymphoma-specific translocation (t[2;5] p23;q35]) in Hodgkin's disease: indication of a common pathogenesis? *Lancet* 1995;345:87–90.
140. Elmberger PG, Lozano MD, Weisenburger DD, Sanger W, Chan WC. Transcripts of the npm-alk fusion gene in anaplastic large cell lymphoma, Hodgkin's disease, and reactive lymphoid lesions. *Blood* 1995; 86:3517–3521.
141. Lamant L, Meggetto F, al Saati T, et al. High incidence of the t(2;5) (p23;q35) translocation in anaplastic large cell lymphoma and its lack of detection in Hodgkin's disease. Comparison of cytogenetic analysis, reverse transcriptase-polymerase chain reaction, and P-80 immunostaining. *Blood* 1996;87:284–291.
142. Sarris AH, Luthra R, Waasdorp M, et al. Genomic DNA PCR Defines unique t(2;5) breakpoints in anaplastic large cell lymphoma (ALCL). *Blood* 1996;88(suppl 1, part 2):143b.
143. Sarris AH, Luthra R, Padimitracopoulou V, et al. Rapid amplification of genomic DNA detects the t(2;5)(p23;q35) in anaplastic large-cell lymphoma, but not in other non-Hodgkin's lymphomas, Hodgkin's disease, or lymphomatoid papulosis. *Ann Oncol* 1997;8(suppl 2):59–63.
144. Sarris AH, Luthra R, Cabanillas F, Morris SW, Pugh WC. Genomic DNA amplification and the detection of t(2;5)(p23;q35) in lymphoid neoplasms. *Leukemia Lymphoma* 1998;29:507–514.
145. Luthra R, Pugh WC, Waasdorp M, et al. Mapping of genomic t(2;5) (p23;q35) breakpoints in patients with anaplastic large cell lymphoma by sequencing long-range PCR products. *Hematopathol Mol Hematol* 1998;11:173–183.
146. Ladanyi M, Cavalchire G, Morris SW, Downing J, Filippa DA. Reverse transcriptase polymerase chain reaction for the Ki-1 anaplastic large cell lymphoma-associated t(2;5) translocation in Hodgkin's disease. *Am J Pathol* 1994;145:1296–1300.
147. Weiss LM, Lopategui JR, Sun L-H, Kamel OW, Koo CH, Glackin G. Absence of the t(2;5) in Hodgkin's disease. *Blood* 1995;85:2845–2847.
148. Herbst H, Anagnostopoulos J, Heinze B, Dürkop H, Hummel M, Stein H. ALK gene products in anaplastic large cell lymphomas and Hodgkin's disease. *Blood* 1995;86:1694–1700.
149. Weber-Matthiesen K, Deerberg-Wittram J, Rosenwald A, Poetsch M, Grote W, Schlegelberger B. Translocation t(2;5) is not a primary event in Hodgkin's disease. Simultaneous immunophenotyping and interphase cytogenetics. *Am J Pathol* 1996;149:463–468.
150. Sarris AH, Luthra R, Papadimitracopoulou V, et al. Amplification of genomic DNA demonstrates the presence of the t(2;5)(p23;q35) in anaplastic large cell lymphoma, but not on other non-Hodgkin's lymphomas, Hodgkin's disease, or lymphomatoid papulosis. *Blood* 1996; 88:1771–1779.
151. Waggott W, Delsol G, Jarret RF, et al. NPM-ALK gene fusion and Hodgkin's disease [letter]. *Blood* 1997;90:1712–1713.
152. Pileri SA, Piccaluga A, Poggi S, et al. Anaplastic large cell lymphoma: update of findings. *Leukemia Lymphoma* 1995;18:17–25.
153. Wellman A, Thieblemont C, Fest T, Laszlo K, Jaffe E, Raffeld M. Detection of NMP-ALK rearrangements using an XL (extra large)-PCR assay and an analysis of genomic breakpoint sequences. *Blood* 1996;88(suppl 1, part 1):552a.
154. Miyashita T, Reed JC. Bcl-2 oncoprotein blocks chemotherapy-induced apoptosis in a human leukemia cell line. *Blood* 1993;81:151–157.
155. Yunis JJ, Oken MM, Kaplan ME, Ensrud KM, Howe RR, Theologides A. Distinctive chromosomal abnormalities in histologic subtypes of non-Hodgkin's lymphoma. *N Engl J Med* 1982;307:1231–1236.
156. Tsujimoto Y, Finger LR, Yunis J, Nowell PC, Croce CM. Cloning of the chromosome breakpoint of neoplastic B cells with the t(14;18) chromosome translocation. *Science* 1984;226:1097–1099.
157. Tsujimoto Y, Gorham J, Cossman J, Jaffe E, Croce CM. The t(14;18) chromosome translocations involved in B-cell neoplasms result from mistakes in VDJ joining. *Science* 1985;229:1390–1393.
158. Tsujimoto Y, Croce CM. Analysis of the structure, transcripts, and protein products of bcl-2, the gene involved in human follicular lymphoma. *Proc Natl Acad Sci USA* 1986;83:5214–5218.
159. Graninger WB, Seto M, Boutain B, Goldman P, Korsmeyer SJ. Expression of Bcl-2 and Bcl-2-Ig fusion transcripts in normal and neoplastic cells. *J Clin Invest* 1987;80:1512–1515.
160. Cleary ML, Sklar J. Nucleotide sequence of a t(14;18) chromosomal breakpoint in follicular lymphoma and demonstration of a breakpoint-cluster region near a transcriptionally active locus on chromosome 18. *Proc Natl Acad Sci USA* 1985;82:7439–7443.
161. Cleary ML, Galili N, Sklar J. Detection of a second t(14;18) break-

point cluster region in human follicular lymphomas. *J Exp Med* 1986; 164:315–320.

162. Gribben JG, Freedman A, Woo SD, et al. All advanced stage non-Hodgkin's lymphomas with a polymerase chain reaction amplifiable breakpoint of bcl-2 have residual cells containing the bcl-2 rearrangement at evaluation and after treatment. *Blood* 1991;78:3275–3280.
163. Zelenetz AD, Chu G, Galili N, et al. Enhanced detection of the t(14;18) translocation in malignant lymphoma using pulsed-field gel electrophoresis. *Blood* 1991;78:1552–1560.
164. Stetler-Stevenson M, Crush-Stanton S, Cossman J. Involvement of the bcl-2 gene in Hodgkin's disease. *J Natl Cancer Inst* 1990;82:855–858.
165. Algara P, Martinez P, Sanchez L, et al. Lymphocyte predominance Hodgkin's disease (nodular paragranuloma)—a bcl-2 negative germinal centre lymphoma. *Histopathology* 1991;19:69–75.
166. Athan E, Chadburn A, Knowles DM. The bcl-2 gene translocation is undetectable in Hodgkin's disease by Southern blot hybridization and polymerase chain reaction. *Am J Pathol* 1992;141:193–201.
167. Lee MS, Chang KS, Cabanillas F, Freireich EJ, Trujillo JM, Stass SA. Detection of minimal residual cells carrying the t(14;18) by DNA sequence amplification. *Science* 1987;237:175–178.
168. Dolken G, Illerhaus G, Hirt C, Mertelsmann R. BCL-2/JH rearrangements in circulating B cells of healthy blood donors and patients with nonmalignant diseases. *J Clin Oncol* 1996;14:1333–1344.
169. Limpens J, Stad R, Vos C, et al. Lymphoma-associated translocation t(14;18) in blood B cells of normal individuals. *Blood* 1995;85: 2528–2536.
170. Liu Y, Hernandez AM, Shibata D, Cortopassi GA. Bcl-2 translocation frequency rises with age in humans. *Proc Natl Acad Sci USA* 1994; 199491:8910–8914.
171. Limpens J, de Jong D, van Krieken JH, et al. Bcl-2/JH rearrangements in benign lymphoid tissues with follicular hyperplasia. *Oncogene* 1991; 6:2271–2276.
172. Aster JC, Kobayashi Y, Shiota M, Mori S, Sklar J. Detection of the t(14;18) at similar frequencies in hyperplastic lymphoid tissues from American and Japanese patients. *Am J Pathol* 1992;141:291–299.
173. Shibata D, Hu E, Weiss LM, Brynes RK, Nathwani BN. Detection of specific t(14;18) chromosomal translocations in fixed tissues. *Hum Pathol* 1990;21:199–203.
174. Louie DC, Kant JA, Brooks JJ, Reed JC. Absence of t(14;18) major and minor breakpoints and of Bcl-2 protein overproduction in Reed-Sternberg cells of Hodgkin's disease. *Am J Pathol* 1991;139:1231–1237.
175. Lorenzen J, Hansmann ML, Shibata D, et al. Bcl-2 in potential precursors of nodular paragranuloma and its dedifferentiated variant (large cell B-lymphoma). *Verh Dtsch Ges Pathol* 1992;76:169–172.
176. Segal GH, Scott M, Braylan RC. Semi-automated ELISA-based detection system for verifying the authenticity of amplified t(14;18)-containing products. *Diagn Mol Pathol* 1996;5:114–120.
177. Hell K, Lorenzen J, Fischer R, Hansmann ML. Hodgkin cells accumulate mRNA for bcl-2. *Lab Invest* 1995;73:492–496.
178. Masih A, Sun J, Strobach S, Mitchell D, Wu K. Detection of t(14;18) in Hodgkin's disease by the polymerase chain reaction: correlation with EBV genome and histologic subtype. *Lab Invest* 1991;64:77a.
179. LeBrun D, Ngan BY, Warnke R, Cleary M. *Bcl*-2 in Hodgkin's disease: a correlative study of t(14:18) and *bcl*-2 oncogenic protein expression. *Lab Invest* 1992;66:81a.
180. Lorenzen J, Hansmann ML, Pezzella F, et al. Expression of the bcl-2 oncogene product and chromosomal translocation t(14;18) in Hodgkin's disease. *Hum Pathol* 1992;23:1205–1209.
181. Gupta RK, Whelan JS, Lister TA, Young BD, Bodmer JG. Direct sequence analysis of the t(14;18) chromosomal translocation in Hodgkin's disease. *Blood* 1992;79:2084–2088.
182. Reid AH, Cunningham RE, Frizzera G, O'Leary TJ. bcl-2 rearrangement in Hodgkin's disease. Results of polymerase chain reaction, flow cytometry, and sequencing on formalin-fixed, paraffin-embedded tissue. *Am J Pathol* 1993;142:395–402.
183. Mitani S, Oka N, Aoki N, Hojo I, Ota U, Mori S. Rearrangement of *bcl*-2 is detectable in Hodgkin's disease by polymerase chain reaction. *Jpn J Cancer Res* 1994;85:1229–1232.
184. Gupta RK, Lister TA, Bodmer JG. The t(14;18) chromosomal translocation and Bcl-2 protein expression in Hodgkin's disease. *Leukemia* 1994;8:1337–1341.
185. Corbally N, Grogan L, Keane MM, Devaney DM, Dervan PA, Carney DN. *Bcl*-2 rearrangement in Hodgkin's disease and lymph nodes. *Hematol Pathol* 1994;101:756–760.
186. Kneba M, Eick S, Herbst H, et al. Low incidence of mbr *bcl*-2/JH fusion genes in Hodgkin's disease. *J Pathol* 1995;175:381–389.
187. Gravel S, Delsol G, Al Saati T. Single-cell analysis of the t(14;18) (q32;q21) chromosomal translocation in Hodgkin's disease demonstrates the absence of this translocation in neoplastic Hodgkin and Reed-Sternberg cells. *Blood* 1998;91:2866–2874.
188. Johnson PWM, Cotter FE, Swinbank K, Selby PJ. International variability in the molecular detection of lymphoma. *Proc Am Soc Clin Oncol* 1998;17:16a.
189. Price CG, Meerabux J, Murtagh S, et al. The significance of circulating cells carrying t(14;18) in long remission from follicular lymphoma. *J Clin Oncol* 1991;9:1527–1532.
190. Finke J, Slanina J, Lange W, Dolken G. Persistence of circulating t(14; 18)-positive cells in long-term remission after radiation therapy for localized-stage follicular lymphoma. *J Clin Oncol* 1993;11: 1668–1673.
191. Lambrechts AC, Hupkes PE, Dorssers LC, van't Veer MB. Translocation (14;18)-positive cells are present in the circulation of the majority of patients with localized (stage I and II) follicular non-Hodgkin's lymphoma. *Blood* 1993;82:2510–2516.
192. Soubeyran P, Cabanillas F, Lee MS. Analysis of the expression of the hybrid gene bcl-2/IgH in follicular lymphomas. *Blood* 1993;81: 122–127.
193. Henderson S, Rowe M, Gregory C, et al. Induction of bcl-2 expression by Epstein-Barr virus latent membrane protein 1 protects infected B cells from programmed cell death. *Cell* 1991;65:1107–1115.
194. Rowe M, Peng-Pilon M, Huen DS, et al. Upregulation of bcl-2 by the Epstein-Barr virus latent membrane protein LMP1: a B-cell-specific response that is delayed relative to NF-kappa B activation and to induction of cell surface markers. *J Virol* 1994;68:5602–5612.
195. Glaser SL, Lin RJ, Stewart SL, et al. Epstein-Barr virus-associated Hodgkin's disease: epidemiologic characteristics in international data. *Int J Cancer* 1997;70:375–382.
196. Ferraris AM, Racchi O, Rapezzi D, Gaetani GF, Boffetta P. Familial Hodgkin's disease: a disease of young adulthood? *Ann Hematol* 1997; 74:131–134.
197. Kerzin-Storrar L, Faed MJ, MacGillivray JB, Smith PG. Incidence of familial Hodgkin's disease. *Br J Cancer* 1983;47:707–712.
198. Bowers TK, Moldow CF, Bloomfield CD, Yunis EJ. Familial Hodgkin's disease and the major histocompatibility complex. *Vox Sang* 1977;33: 273–277.
199. Smakal S, Golan T, Blaha M, Dienstbier Z, Hermanska Z. [Familial occurrence of Hodgkin's disease]. *Bratisl Lek Listy* 1990;91:770–775.
200. Lin AY, Kingma DW, Lennette ET, et al. Epstein-Barr virus and familial Hodgkin's disease. *Blood* 1996;88:3160–3165.
201. Schlaifer D, Rigal-Huguet F, Robert A, et al. Epstein-Barr virus in familial Hodgkin's disease. *Br J Haematol* 1994;88:636–638.
202. Weintraub M, Lin AY, Franklin J, Tucker MA, Magrath IT, Bhatia KG. Absence of germline p53 mutations in familial lymphoma. *Oncogene* 1996;12:687–691.
203. Gupta RK, Norton AJ, Lister TA, Bodmer JG. p53 protein expression in Reed-Sternberg cells of Hodgkin's disease. *Leukemia* 1993;7: S31–33.
204. Gupta RK, Patel K, Bodmer WF, Bodmer JG. Mutation of p53 in primary biopsy material and cell lines from Hodgkin disease. *Proc Natl Acad Sci USA* 1993;90:2817–2821.
205. Robertson SJ, Lowman JT, Grufferman S, et al. Familial Hodgkin's disease. A clinical and laboratory investigation. *Cancer* 1987;59: 1314–1319.
206. Marshall WH, Barnard JM, Buehler SK, Crumley J, Larsen B. HLA in familial Hodgkin's disease. Results and a new hypothesis. *Int J Cancer* 1977;19:450–455.
207. Hornmark-Stenstam B, Landberg T, Low B. HLA antigens in Hodgkin's disease of very long survival. *Acta Radiol Oncol Radiat Phys Biol* 1978;17:283–288.
208. Greene MH, McKeen EA, Li FP, Blattner WA, Fraumeni JF Jr. HLA antigens in familial Hodgkin's disease. *Int J Cancer* 1979;23: 777–780.
209. Lynch HT, Saldivar VA, Guirgis HA, et al. Familial Hodgkin's disease and associated cancer. A clinical-pathologic study. *Cancer* 1976;38: 2033–2041.
210. Reeves BR, Pickup VL. The chromosome changes in non-Burkitt lymphomas. *Hum Genet* 1980;53:349–355.
211. Kobayashi M, Takamatsu K, Fujishiro M, Saitoh S, Noguchi T. Mole-

cular cloning of a novel calcium-binding protein structurally related to hippocalcin from human brain and chromosomal mapping of its gene. *Biochim Biophys Acta* 1994;1222:515–518.
212. Ono M, Yasunaga T, Miyata T, Ushikubo H. Nucleotide sequence of human endogenous retrovirus genome related to the mouse mammary tumor virus genome. *J Virol* 1986;60:589–598.
213. Monte D, Coutte L, Dewitte F, et al. Genomic organization of the human ERM (ETV5) gene, a PEA3 group member of ETS transcription factors. *Genomics* 1996;35:236–240.
214. Owerbach D, Rutter WJ, Shows TB, Gray P, Goeddel DV, Lawn RM. Leukocyte and fibroblast interferon genes are located on human chromosome 9. *Proc Natl Acad Sci USA* 1981;78:3123–3127.
215. Derre J, Kemper O, Cherif D, Nophar Y, Berger R, Wallach D. The gene for the type 1 tumor necrosis factor receptor (TNF-R1) is localized on band 12p13. *Hum Genet* 1991;87:231–233.
216. Schuler GD, Boguski MS, Stewart EA, et al. A gene map of the human genome. *Science* 1996;274:540–546.
217. Schuler GD, Boguski MS, Hudson TJ, et al. Genome maps 7. The human transcript map. Wall chart. *Science* 1996;274:547–562.
218. Pulford K, Lamant L, Morris SW, et al. Detection of anaplastic lymphoma kinase (ALK) and nucleolar protein nucleophosmin (NPM)-ALK proteins in normal and neoplastic cells with the monoclonal antibody ALK1. *Blood* 1977;89:1394–1404.
219. Weiss LM, Warnke RA, Sklar J, Cleary ML. Molecular analysis of the t(14;18) chromosomal translocation in malignant lymphomas. *N Engl J Med* 1987;317:1185–1189.

Hodgkin's Disease, edited by P.M. Mauch,
J.O. Armitage, V. Diehl, R.T. Hoppe, and L.M. Weiss.
Lippincott Williams & Wilkins, Philadephia ©1999.

CHAPTER 14

Cytogenetic Findings in Hodgkin's Disease Cell Lines

Christa Fonatsch, Andrea Jox, Berthold Streubel, Jürgen Wolf, and Volker Diehl

CLASSIC CYTOGENETIC STUDIES IN HODGKIN'S DISEASE

Chromosome studies in lymph nodes from patients with Hodgkin's disease are limited by the low number of Hodgkin and Reed-Sternberg cells and their low mitotic rate. Reviewing the literature, the success in preparing metaphases from a lymph node suspension ranged from 36% to 90%. Clonal karyotype abnormalities were found in about 10% (1) to 66% (2) of the cases. In the remaining cases the prepared metaphases exhibited a normal karyotype whereby single metaphases with sporadic abnormalities were often observed.

Within the same lymph node, cytogenetically normal cells are detected at a higher rate than clonally abnormal ones. These cells are considered to be derived from contaminating normal bystander cells, which consist mostly of T lymphocytes, histiocytes, and plasma cells. They surround the neoplastic Hodgkin–Reed-Sternberg cells and compose the largest fraction of the tumor mass.

A compilation of the published cytogenetic data comprising 105 chromosomally aberrant Hodgkin's disease cases revealed the presence of a karyotype in the near-triploid to near-tetraploid range in 57 of the cases (54%). A near-diploid karyotype with complex numerical and structural aberrations was found in 30 of the cases (29%). In 18 cases (17%) a near-diploid chromosome number containing only minor numerical or structural chromosome abnormalities was observed, e.g., a gain or loss of a single chromosome or chromosome segment (1–7).

C. Fonatsch and B. Streubel: Institut für Medizinische Biologie der Universität Wien, Wien, Austria.

A. Jox, J. Wolf and V. Diehl: Department of Internal Medicine, Klinik I für Innere Medizin der Universität zu Koln, Koln, Germany.

Although near-diploid karyotypes with only minor chromosome anomalies were predominantly observed in early cytogenetic studies of Hodgkin's disease (reviewed in ref. 6), recent publications present mostly near-triploid to near-tetraploid karyotypes with many numerical and structural chromosome aberrations (2,4,7).

The occurrence of clonal abnormalities does support the concept that Hodgkin's disease is a malignant disease. However, it remains to be established whether the near-diploid cells with minor chromosome aberrations represent the same neoplastic cell population as metaphases with major complex aberrations do. It was suggested that the lymphoma cells in Hodgkin's disease may present a diploid range in early stages of cytogenetic progression. Hossfeld and Schmidt (8) described clonal anomalies in near-diploid effusion cells from six patients with Hodgkin's disease but did not detect typical Hodgkin–Reed-Sternberg cells in five of these patients. They suspected that the diploid cells could represent precursors of the polyploid Reed-Sternberg cells. The classic giant Reed-Sternberg cell is taken as as a product of at least two or three endomitotic cycles (9).

So far no specific structural or numerical chromosome abnormality has been delineated in Hodgkin's disease. Nevertheless common numerical abnormalities were observed such as gains of chromosomes 1, 2, 3, 5, 9, 11, 12, 15, 20, and 21, whereby the most frequent gains concern chromosomes 2, 5, 9, and 12. Likewise, loss of chromosomes 6, 10, 13, 15, 17, 18, 21, 22, X, and Y seems to be nonrandom, whereby chromosomes 13, 21, and 22 were most frequently lost (4,10).

In addition, specific chromosomes and chromosome arms are nonrandomly involved in structural rearrangements. In one-third of Hodgkin's disease cases, structural abnormalities of chromosome 1 are found. The changes include deletions, translocations, duplications, inversions, and isochromosome formations of 1q. Furthermore, the chromosome arms 2p, 3q, 4q, 6q, 7q, 11q, 12p, 12q, 13p, 14q, and 15p are specifically affected by rearrangements (2,4,10,11). Interestingly, the short arms of chromosomes 13 and 15 harbor genes encoding ribosomal RNA. These so-called nucleolus organizer regions of the acrocentric chromosomes are rarely involved in chromosome aberrations obtained from other malignant diseases. Their involvement in chromosomal aberrations in Hodgkin's disease might thus be a peculiarity of this disease.

CHROMOSOME BANDING AND FLUORESCENCE *IN SITU* HYBRIDIZATION STUDIES IN CONTINUOUSLY GROWING HODGKIN–REED-STERNBERG CELL LINES

Since the analysis of primary lymph node suspensions obtained from fresh lymphoma tissue is difficult to perform and since it is not possible to clarify whether the obtained chromosomal aberrations derive from Hodgkin–Reed-Sternberg cells or bystander cells, Hodgkin–Reed-Sternberg cell lines were used to analyze their chromosomal structure in detail. The recently established method of combined classical chromosome banding analysis with fluorescence *in situ* hybridization (FISH) using whole chromosome painting probes (WCP) allowed us to further clarify the derivation of the as yet unidentified chromosomal markers and rearrangements in the Hodgkin's disease–derived cell lines L-428 (Fig. 1), L-540 (Fig. 2), and L-1236 (Fig. 3). Although Hodgkin's disease–derived cell lines are characterized by a genomic instability resulting in the sporadic occurrence of random chromosomal abnormalities in single metaphases, several nearly identical chromosomal aberrations were identified in L-428 as well as in L-1236 (Table 1). A deleted chromosome 11 with breakpoint in 11q14~21 was observed in L-428 (marker VII, Figs. 1 and 4A) and in L-1236 (marker XVII, Figs. 3 and 4B). Marker VII of the cell line L-540, which was thought to be a deleted chromosome 11 after Giemsa-banding, had to be reinterpreted as a deleted chromosome 9 del(9)(q22) after FISH. Markers VIII (L-428) (Figs. 1 and 5A) and XX (L-1236) (Figs. 3 and 5B) seem to be identically deleted chromosomes 12—del(12)(q15). Marker V in L-428 represents a duplication within the long arm of chromosome 7 (7q22 to 7q36) (Figs. 1 and 4A), whereas in marker XII of L-1236 the segment 7q22 to 7q36 was attached to the short arm of chromosome 7, resulting in a duplication 7q22 to 7q36 in this cell line, too (Figs. 3 and 4B).

Furthermore, recurrent breakpoints were detected in all three cell lines (Table 1). Breaks occurred in L-428 and L-236 in 1p22, leading to a duplication in L-428 (marker I) and to a deletion in L-1236 (marker II). Marker I in L-540 resulted from a translocation of 12p to 1p13. A translocation of chromosome 8 material to 2p23~25 led to the marker II in L-428 (Figs. 1 and 6A), and a duplication from 2p15 to 2p23 was observed in markers IV and V of L-1236 (Figs. 3 and 5B). The elongation of the long arm of chromosome 2 in L-540 (marker II) is due to a translocation t(2;8)(q37;q13~21) (Figs. 2 and 6B), whereas in L-1236 markers IV and V

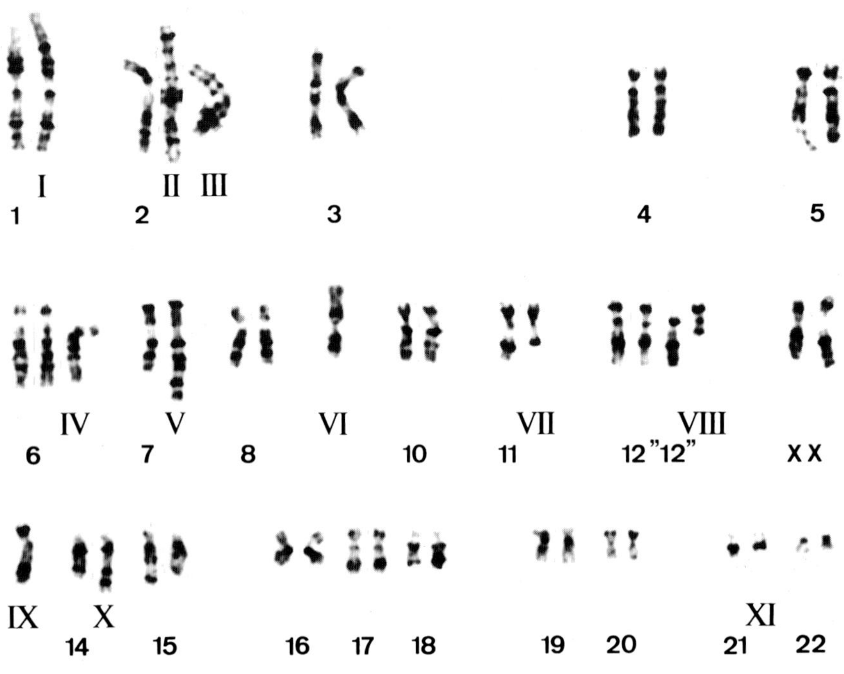

FIG. 1. L-428. Representative G-band karyogram with 12 derivative chromosomes (markers I–XI, "12"). (From ref. 12, with permission.)

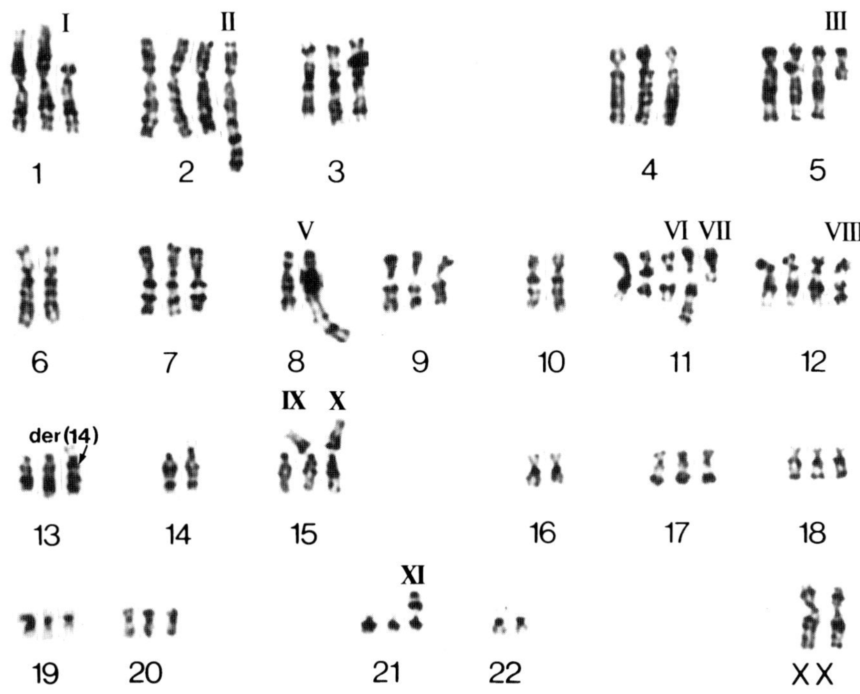

FIG. 2. L-540. Representative G-band karyogram with 12 derivative chromosomes [markers I–XI, der(14)]. (From ref. 12, with permission.)

show a duplication within the long arm—dup(2)(q33q37). Cytogenetically identical break points in 8q13~21 led to the formation of markers II in L-428 and L-540. In L-428 the segment 8q13~21-qter is translocated to the short arm of chromosome 2 (2p23~25) as described (Figs. 1 and 6A), and in L-540 the same chromosome segment 8q13~21-qter is attached to the long arm of chromosome 2 (2q37) (Figs. 2 and 6B). In L-540 as well as in L-1236, rearrangements of 8q24 are found; translocation of a part of the long arm of chromosome 6 (6q15-qter) to 8q24 led to the elongated marker V in L-540, a rearrangement of chromosome 1 and chromosome 14 material, and 8q24 made up marker XIV in L-1236.

Chromosome 14 is involved in rearrangements in all three cell lines. The elongation of the long arm of a chromosome 14 in L-428 (marker X, Fig. 1) is due to a translocation of chromosome 9 material to 14q32. In L-540 intercalation of 14q11 between chromosome 15 and chromosome 1p material was proven by *in situ* hybridization with T cell receptor-α gene probes (markers IX

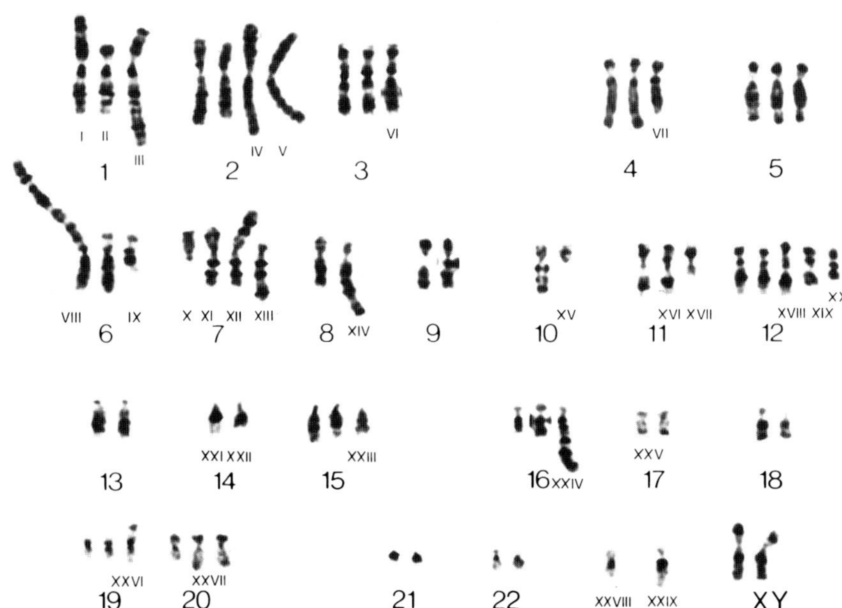

FIG. 3. L-1236. Representative G-band karyogram with 29 derivative chromosomes (markers I–XXIX) (From ref. 14, with permission.)

TABLE 1. *Identical chromosome aberrations and break points in three Hodgkin–Reed-Sternberg cell lines*

Identical aberrations	Markers involved in Hodgkin–Reed-Sternberg cell line L-428	L-540	L-1236
del(11)(q14~21)	VII		XVII
del(12)(q15)	VIII		XX
dup(7)(q22q36), der(7)t(7;7)(p22;q22)	V		XII
Identical breakpoints			
1p22	I		II
2p23~25	II		IV,V
2q37		II	IV,V
6q15		V	IX
8q13~21	II	II	
8q24		V	XIV
14q24		der(14)	XXII

and X, Fig. 2) (12). Furthermore, in the karyogram of L-540 (Fig. 2) the third chromosome 13, bearing satellites, was identified as a chromosome 14—der(14)—in which the segment 14q11-q24 was replaced by chromosome 11 material. Finally, in L-1236 markers I and XXI represent a balanced translocation t(1;14)(p34;q22) and marker XXII is a deleted chromosome 14 del(14)(q24). Chromosome 6 is rearranged in all three cell lines: in L-540 and L-1236 we found break points in 6q15 (marker V in L-540, marker IX in L-1236), and in L-428 unidentified chromosome material is attached to 6q23 (marker IV).

Rearrangements involving the short arms of acrocentric chromosomes and thus the nucleolus organizer regions were found in L-428 and L-540. In L-428 a rearrangement of an unidentified chromosome segment with the short arm of chromosome 13 builds up marker IX. Marker XII is composed of chromosome 21 and part of the long arm of an X chromosome that is translocated to 21p (Fig. 1). In L-540 the identical markers IX and X show a rearrangement of the short arm of chromosome 15 with 14q11 and 1p; marker XI is due to a translocation of 7q22-qter to 21p12 (Fig. 2).

Comparing the cytogenetic results obtained from the Hodgkin–Reed-Sternberg cell lines as well as from primary Hodgkin–Reed-Sternberg cells the following aberrations were detected in both sources: the short arm of chromosome 1, which is affected by deletions, translocations, and duplications in all three cell lines (13–15), is also described as altered in a number of cases described by Döhner et al. (4) and Schlegelberger et al. (2), and in cases published earlier (6,11). According to our studies the short arm of chromosome 2 (p23~25) is affected in the cell lines L-428 and L-1236, but this was also found in primary Hodgkin's disease cases examined by Tilly et al. (7) and by Schlegelberger et al. (2). The band q37 of the long arm of chromosome 2 shows aberrations in L-540 and L-1236 comparable to a case studied by Döhner

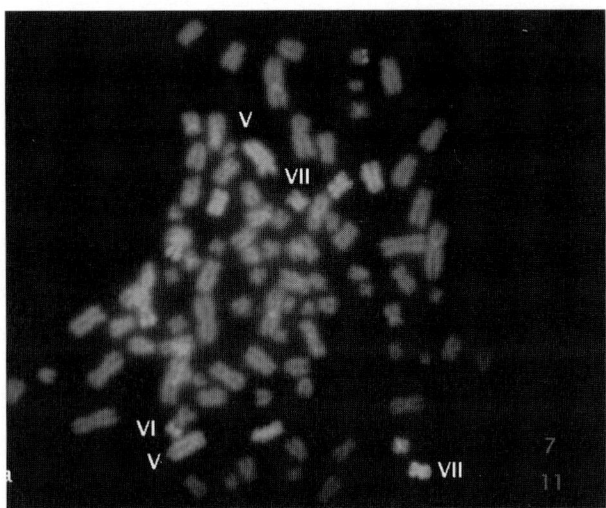

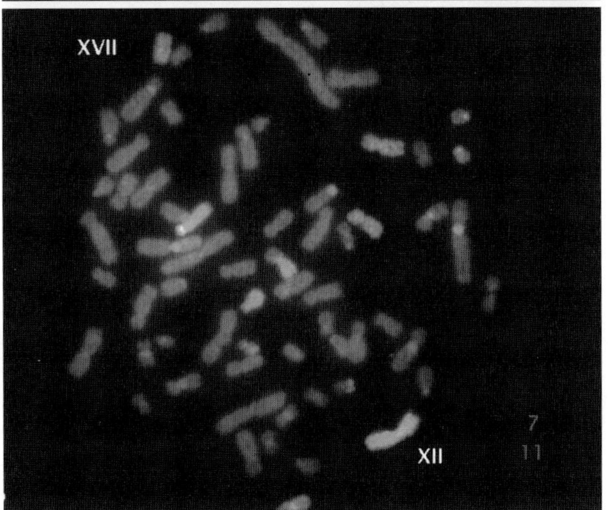

FIG. 4. Fluorescence *in situ* hybridization (FISH) with painting probes for chromosomes 7 *(red)* and 11 *(green)*. **A:** L-428. Markers V: duplication within the long arm of chromosome 7: dup(7)(q22q36); markers VII: deletion of the long arm of chromosome 11—del(11)(q14~21); marker VI: chromosome 11 material attached to the short arm of chromosome 9. **B:** L-1236. Marker XII: attachment of 7q22-q36 to 7p22, leading to a duplication of this chromosome segment within marker XII; marker XVII: deletion of the long arm of chromosome 11—del(11)(q14~21). (Fig. 4B from ref. 14, with permission. This figure is reproduced in color as Plates 33 and 34.

et al. (4). Chromosome 7 is affected by numerical and structural aberrations of the short and of the long arm in all three cell lines and likewise in a number of primary Hodgkin's disease cases. Especially the chromosome bands 7q22 to q35 are nonrandomly involved in aberrations in Hodgkin's disease lymphomas (2,4,7; cases reviewed in ref. 11).

The long arm of chromosome 11 has been described as being affected in a number of cases (4,6,7,16). Reeves et al. (17) published a case of Hodgkin's disease that has been analyzed repeatedly over a period of 5 years showing a deleted chromosome 11—del(11)(q13q23)—during the

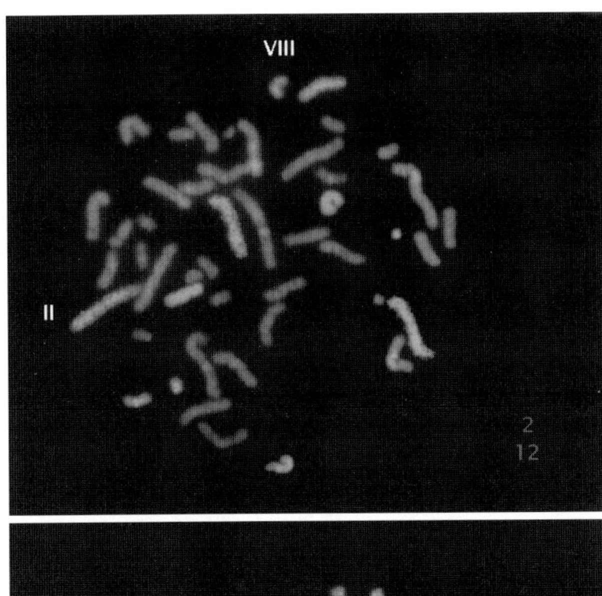

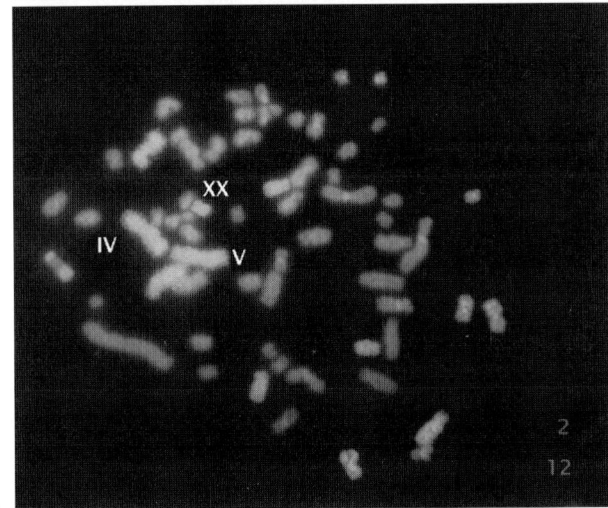

FIG. 5. FISH with painting probes for chromosomes 2 *(green)* and 12 *(red)*. **A:** L-428. Marker II: involvement of 2p23~25 in a chromosomal rearrangement, leading to elongation of 2p; marker VIII: deletion of the long arm of chromosome 12—del(12)(q15). **B:** L-1236. Markers IV and V: duplications within the short arm (p15 to p23) and the long arm (q33 to q37) of chromosome 2; marker XX: deletion of the long arm of chromosome 12—del(12)(q15). (This figure is reproduced in color as Plates 35 and 36.)

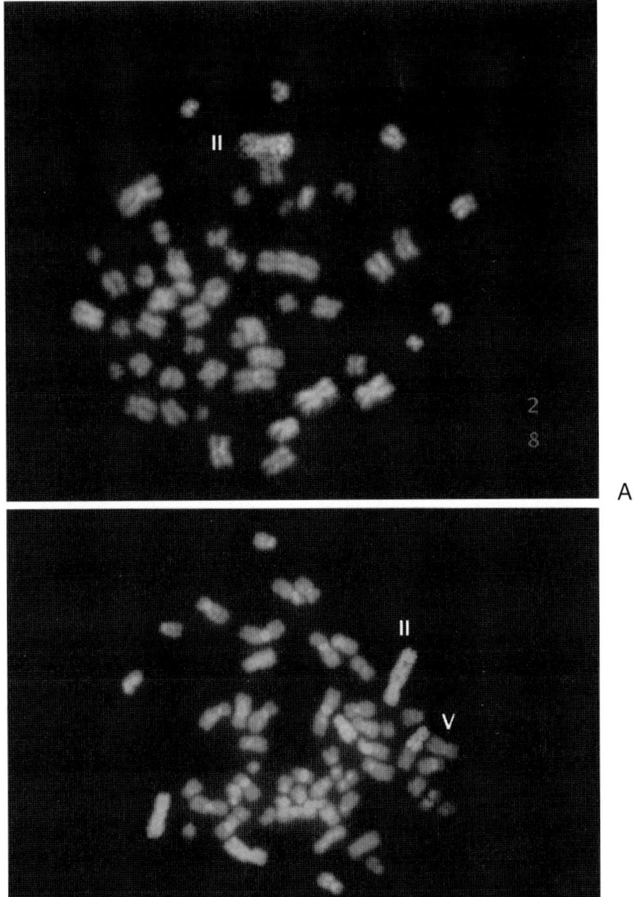

FIG. 6. FISH with painting probes for chromosomes 2 *(red)* and 8 *(green)*. **A:** L-428. Marker II: rearrangement between 2p23~25 and 8q13~21. **B:** L-540. Marker II: rearrangement between 2q37 and 8q13~21; marker V: involvement of 8q24 in a chromosomal rearrangement leading to elongation of 8q. (This figure is reproduced in color as Plates 37 and 38.)

whole time period. A nearly identical marker, a chromosome 11 with deletion in q14~21, was detected by our group in L-428 and in L-1236. Remarkably, a translocation affecting this chromosome region—t(6;11)(q21;q14~21)—in addition to supernumerary chromosomes 3 and 7 has been detected in a severe combined immunodeficient (SCID) mouse tumor, generated by inoculation of primary Hodgkin's disease tumor material (18; Fonatsch, unpublished observations). In most published cases the break point in 11q is indicated as in 11q23, but it must be mentioned that break point designation was determined after chromosome banding and not proven by, for example, FISH. Therefore FISH analysis of the chromosome 11 abnormalities could probably lead to a reinterpretation of the location of the break-points. Recently, from 11q14~21 an interesting clathrin assembly lymphoid myeloid (CALM) leukemia gene was isolated and characterized (19). This gene is found to be rearranged in the malignant cells of acute leukemias that derive from a very early precursor cell and show a translocation t(10;11)(p13;q14~21) (20).

The long arm of chromosome 12 from q15 to q24 is nonrandomly involved in structural aberrations in Hodgkin's disease cases described by Tilly et al. (7), Döhner et al. (4), and Schlegelberger et al. (2). In one of these cases a deletion in 12q15 was detected (4) that was also found in the Hodgkin–Reed-Sternberg cell lines L-428 and L-1236. Interestingly, the specific expression of restin (*Re*ed-*St*ernberg *in*termediate associated protein), a novel intermediate filament associated protein, was detected in Hodgkin–Reed-Sternberg cells (21), whereby the restin gene was assigned to the chromosome subband 12q24.3. Whether loss or translocation of this gene does play a role in the development or progression of Hodgkin's disease remains to be elucidated.

The nonrandomness of numerical as well as structural aberrations of chromosome 14 has been mentioned in a compilation of 40 cases of Hodgkin's disease by Thangavelu and Le Beau (6) and also in a later review (11). Whereas Tilly et al. (7), Döhner et al. (4), and Schlegelberger et al. (2) claim that 14q11 and 14q32 are often involved in structural aberrations in primary Hodgkin–Reed-Sternberg cells, we found, beneath these abnormalities, also breaks in 14q22 and 14q24 in the cell lines L-540 and L-1236.

DO RRNA GENES PLAY A ROLE IN HODGKIN'S DISEASE?

In primary Hodgkin–Reed-Sternberg cells as well as in Hodgkin–Reed-Sternberg cell lines, short arms of the acrocentric chromosomes 13, 14, 15, 21, and 22 harboring genes encoding ribosomal RNA were frequently involved in chromosomal rearrangements. These regions are also known as the nucleolus organizer regions. It can be speculated that the nonrandom involvement of chromosomal segments bearing the nucleolus organizer regions may contribute to the malignant transformation of the Hodgkin–Reed-Sternberg cell. The juxtaposition of transcriptionally active genes for ribosomal RNA to a specific gene (a proto-oncogene?) may alter the control of expression of this gene by its own specific promoter or enhancer sequence, and thus could lead to the enhanced expression of this gene (12). In recent publications of cytogenetic data in primary material of Hodgkin's disease, the nonrandom involvement of the short arms of acrocentric chromosomes in rearrangements was emphasized. Tilly et al. (7) described rearrangements of the short arms of chromosomes 13, 14, and 15 in 12 out of 31 chromosomal abnormal cases of Hodgkin's disease. Döhner et al. (4) described 15p11 aberrations in four out of nine cases in which clonal chromosome aberrations were detected. Schlegelberger et al. (2) registered breaks in the short arm of acrocentric chromosomes in 5 out of 12 Hodgkin's disease cases revealing clonal chromosome aberrations in their tissue preparations. It has to be further analyzed whether genes encoding ribosomal RNA or other as yet unidentified genes that are also mapped to the short arm of the acrocentric chromosomes are rearranged with another gene leading to a Hodgkin–Reed-Sternberg cell–specific chromosomal aberration.

SOURCE OF ERRORS IN CYTOGENETICS OF PERMANENT HODGKIN'S DISEASE CELL LINES AND OF PRIMARY MATERIAL

It is impossible to discriminate between disease-specific karyotype deviations, chromosomal aberrations that occur due to a previous chemo- and/or radiotherapy, and cytogenetic abnormalities occurring during culturing of Hodgkin–Reed-Sternberg cell lines. Nevertheless, Hodgkin–Reed-Sternberg cell lines are characterized by an intrinsic chromosomal instability. This genomic instability in combination with the mutagenic effect of cytostatic agents and/or radiotherapy may lead to the occurrence of complex chromosome aberrations *in vivo* and *in vitro* that are disease inherent but not disease specific. Thus, a number of complex duplications, deletions, and insertions affecting three to four chromosomes within a single marker (for example, marker XIII and XXIV in L-1236) are suggested to be induced by mutagenic agents and/or by *in vitro* culturing of cells. It cannot be excluded that a Hodgkin–-RS cell–specific rearrangement is hidden in these complex marker chromosomes.

Until now, karyotype analysis of most of the Hodgkin's disease cases was performed using conventional chromosome banding techniques. Thus, the interpretation of multiple structural aberrations was difficult to perform and sometimes not possible at all. Using the recently established method of Giemsa banding followed by FISH, most of the former described chromosomal aberrations in Hodgkin–Reed-Sternberg cell lines were confirmed. However, some marker chromosomes had to be reinterpreted as follows: Marker VII of L-540, which is similar to markers VII in L-428 and XVII in L-1236, does not correspond to a deleted chromosome 11 (as in L-428 and L-1236) but represents a deleted chromosome 9 with break point in 9q21~22. Marker XII of L-428 is composed of the long arm of an X chromosome translocated to the short arm of a chromosome 21. Regarding these results obtained from the Hodgkin–Reed-Sternberg cell lines, it cannot be excluded that some of the chromosomal aberrations described in primary Hodgkin–Reed-Sternberg cell have to be reinterpreted using FISH techniques. Thus, the application of newly established methods such as FISH using different types of DNA probes, multicolor FISH, and comparative genomic hybridization (CGH) in combination with conventional banding techniques might lead to the detection of specific candidate chromosomal break points in Hodgkin's disease. One can speculate that a Hodgkin–Reed-Sternberg cell–specific chromosomal aberration contributes to the malignant phenotype of Hodgkin–Reed-Sternberg cells.

THE CONTRIBUTION OF CHROMOSOME ANOMALIES TO THE MALIGNANT TRANSFORMATION IN HODGKIN'S DISEASE: A SCENARIO

An inherent genetically determined karyotype instability can be suspected in a number of Hodgkin's disease patients. This is underlined by the fact that nonneoplastic cells of Hodgkin's disease patients, such as phytohemagglutinin-stimulated lymphocytes, B cells from lymphoblastoid cell lines, and fibroblasts, are characterized by an increased rate of spontaneous chromosomal anomalies (22,23). Recently, microsatellite instability was demonstrated in tumors of Hodgkin's disease patients indicative of the predisposition of some Hodgkin's disease patients to genetic instability (24). Moreover, a high rate of nonclonal minor karyotype abnormalities was noted in many direct preparations of Hodgkin's disease–derived tissues. Therefore, sporadic abnormalities in Hodgkin's disease tumor tissue as well as in nonmalignant cells of Hodgkin's disease patients might be due to a generalized inherent karyotype instability.

Recently it has been demonstrated that Hodgkin–Reed-Sternberg cells clonally derive from germinal center B cells. Furthermore, somatic mutations were detected within their rearranged immunoglobulin genes, rendering potentially functionally immunoglobulin genes nonfunctional (reviewed in ref. 25). Under physiologic conditions those cells would undergo apoptosis within the germinal center. The mechanism protecting Hodgkin–Reed-Sternberg cells from this programmed cell death is unknown. In germinal center B cells the exchange of V genes within a VDJ recombination can occur and has been described as receptor editing (26). Thus, in these cells specific recombinases are expressed causing the exchange of V genes. If one assumes that the inherent chromosomal instability observed in Hodgkin's disease patients is due to the aberrant expression of repair genes or genes that cause double-strand breaks, one might speculate that chromosomal breaks and recombinations do occur, especially during the germinal center reaction of the lymphocytes leading to the expression of an antiapoptotic and/or transforming gene. Specific chromosomal rearrangements involving the V gene loci are frequently detected in follicular lymphoma cells and Burkitt's lymphoma cells, providing evidence that double-strand breaks can occur in B cells. However, the molecular mechanism associated with the numerous random and nonrandom structural chromosome aberrations in Hodgkin–Reed-Sternberg cells has to be further investigated.

REFERENCES

1. Koduru PRK, Offit K, Filippa DA, Lieberman PH, Jhanwar SC. Cytogenetic and molecular genetic analysis of abnormal cells in Hodgkin's disease. *Cancer Genet Cytogenet* 1989;43:109.
2. Schlegelberger B, Weber-Matthiesen K, Himmler A, et al. Cytogenetic findings and results of combined immunophenotyping and karyotyping in Hodgkin's disease. *Leukemia* 1994;8:72.
3. Banks RE, Gledhill S, Ross FM, Krajewski A, Dewar AE, Weir-Thompson EM. Karyotypic abnormalities and immunoglobulin gene rearrangements in Hodgkin's disease. *Cancer Genet Cytogenet* 1991;51:103.
4. Döhner H, Bloomfield CD, Frizzera G, Frestedt J, Arthur DC. Recurring chromosome abnormalities in Hodgkin's disease. *Genes Chrom Cancer* 1992;5:392.
5. Ladanyi M, Parsa NZ, Offit K, Wachtel MS, Filippa DA, Jhanwar SC. Clonal cytogenetic abnormalities in Hodgkin's disease. *Genes Chrom Cancer* 1991;3:294.
6. Thangavelu M, Le Beau MM. Chromosomal abnormalities in Hodgkin's disease. *Hematol Oncol Clin North Am* 1989;3:221.
7. Tilly H, Bastard C, Delastre T, et al. Cytogenetic studies in untreated Hodgkin's disease. *Blood* 1991:77:1298.
8. Hossfeld DK, Schmidt CG. Chromosome findings in effusions from patients with Hodgkin's disease. *Int J Cancer* 1978;21:147.
9. Anastasi J, Bauer KD, Variakojis D. DNA aneuploidy in Hodgkin's disease. A multiparameter flow cytometric analysis with cytologic correlation. *Am J Pathol* 1987;128:573.
10. Drexler HG. Recent results on the biology of Hodgkin and Reed-Sternberg cells. I. Biopsy material. *Leukemia Lymphoma* 1992;8:283.
11. Heim S, Mitelman F. *Cancer cytogenetics.* New York: Wiley-Liss, 1995.
12. Fonatsch C, Gradl G, Kolbus U, Rieder H, Tesch H. Chromosomal in situ hybridization of a Hodgkin's disease-derived cell line (L540) using DNA probes for TCRA, TCRB, MET and rRNA. *Hum Genet* 1990;84:427.
13. Fonatsch C, Diehl V, Schaadt M, Burrichter H, Kirchner HH. Cytogenetic investigations in Hodgkin's disease: I. Involvement of specific chromosomes in marker formation. *Cancer Genet Cytogenet* 1986;20:39.
14. Wolf J, Kapp U, Bohlen H, et al. Peripheral blood mononuclear cells of a patient with advanced Hodgkin's lymphoma give rise to permanently growing Hodgkin-Reed Sternberg cells. *Blood* 1996;87:3418.
15. Fonatsch C, Gradl G, Rademacher J. Genetics of Hodgkin's lymphoma. In: Diehl V, Pfreundschuh M, Löffler M, eds. *Recent results in cancer research, new aspects in the diagnosis and treatment of Hodgkin's disease.* Berlin: Springer, 1989:35.
16. Cabanillas F, Pathak S, Trujillo J, et al. Cytogenetic features of Hodgkin's disease suggest possible origin from a lymphocyte. *Blood* 1998;71:1615.
17. Reeves BR, Nash R, Lawler SD, Fisher C, Treleaven JG, Wiltshaw E. Serial cytogenetic studies showing persistence of original clone in Hodgkin's disease. *Cancer Genet Cytogenet* 1990;50:1.
18. Kapp U, Wolf J, Hummel M, et al. Hodgkin's lymphoma derived tissue serially transplanted into severe combined immunodeficient (SCID)-mice. *Blood* 1993;82:1247.
19. Dreyling MH, Martinez-Climent JA, Zheng M, Mao J, Rowley JD, Bohlander SK. The t(10;11)(p13;q14) in the U937 cell line results in the fusion of the AF10 gene and CALM, encoding a new member of the AP-3 clathrin assembly protein family. *Proc Natl Acad Sci USA* 1996;3:4804.
20. Dreyling MH, Schrader K, Fonatsch C, et al. MLL and CALM are fused to AF10 in morphologically distinct subsets of acute leukemia with translocation t(10,11):both rearrangements are associated with a poor prognosis. *Blood* 1998;91:4662–4667.
21. Hilliker C, Delabie J, Speleman F, et al. Localization of the gene (RSN) coding for restin, a marker for Reed-Sternberg cells in Hodgkin's disease, to human chromosome band 12q24.3 and YAC cloning of the locus. *Cytogenet Cell Genet* 1994;65:172.
22. Barrios L, Caballin MR, Mirò R, et al. Chromosome abnormalities in peripheral blood lymphocytes from untreated Hodgkin's patients. A possible evidence for chromosome instability. *Hum Genet* 1998;78:320.
23. Fonatsch C, Kirchner HH, Schaadt M, Günzel M, Diehl V. Sister chromatid exchange in lymphoma lines and lymphoblastoid cell lines before and after heterotransplantation into nude mice. *Int J Cancer* 1981, 28: 441.
24. Mark Z, Toren A, Amariglio N, Schiby G, Brok-Simoni F, Rechavi G. Instability of dinucleotide repeats in Hodgkin's disease. *Am J Hematol* 1998;57:148.
25. Küppers R, Rajewsky K. The origin of Hodgkin and Reed Sternberg cells in Hodgkin's disease. *Annu Rev Immunol* 1998;16:471.
26. Fanning L, Bertrand FE, Steinberg C, Wu GE. Molecular mechanisms involved in receptor editing at the Ig heavy chain locus. *Int Immunol* 1998;10:241.

SECTION IV

Staging and Initial Evaluation

Hodgkin's Disease, edited by P. M. Mauch, J. O. Armitage, V. Diehl, R. T. Hoppe, and L. M. Weiss. Lippincott Williams & Wilkins, Philadephia ©1999.

CHAPTER 15

Clinical Evaluation and Staging of Hodgkin's Disease

Rajnish K. Gupta, Mary K. Gospodarowicz, and T. Andrew Lister

A clinical stage classification serves as a guide in determining prognosis and treatment. It is also mandatory for comparison of results obtained with different types of treatment in various cancer centers. The TNM system is not applicable to lymphoma, since it is based on the concept of a primary tumor and metastasis. The prerequisite for any staging classification remains unchanged, in that it should provide a basis for the most accurate prediction possible of the pattern of the illness, and be relevant to the therapy prescribed. The goals of staging have been previously stated (1) and include (a) determining the extent of disease (staging), (b) defining the location of disease within the lymphoid system and associated prognostic factors, and (c) defining disease manifestations that can be reevaluated during and after treatment to determine the effectiveness of therapy (outcome).

HISTORICAL PERSPECTIVE

In 1825 Thomas Hodgkin, at the age of 27, was appointed lecturer in morbid anatomy and later curator of the museum of the newly created Guy's Hospital Medical School. He was a man of many parts, a Quaker, an expert morbid anatomist, physician, and philanthropist (in which role he was deeply involved in the rights of the natives of the colonies). In 1829 he provided the first description of aortic valve disease, but in 1832, in his historic paper entitled "On Some Morbid Appearances of the Absorbent Glands and Spleen" (2), read by Dr. Lee to the Medical-Chirurgical Society in London on January 10, 1832, he provided the first clear description of the disease that was later to bear his name. He briefly described the clinical histories and post mortem findings of massive enlargement of the lymph nodes and spleen in six patients and added the description of a seventh patient who had been seen by his friend Robert Carswell in 1828.

Hodgkin described the lymph nodes as unusually large and firm—different from the softer and smaller nodes seen in patients with tuberculosis. The enlarged nodes were often seen only in the neck and chest, but also in the abdomen and groin. The spleen was also massively enlarged in these patients. Hodgkin stated, "This enlargement of the glands appeared to be a primitive (i.e., primary) affection of those bodies rather than the result of an irritation propagated to them from some ulcerated surface or other inflamed texture." The gross specimens of three of these cases are still preserved in the Gordon Museum of Guy's Hospital.

Hodgkin was probably correct in noting that others had observed the same condition, although he was the first to recognize that he was dealing with a primary disease of the lymph nodes and not a response to an inflammatory condition (he does not, however, appear to have recognized its malignant nature). For example, David Craigie (2a) in 1828 stated in his book *Elements of General and Pathological Anatomy,* "Either after repeated attacks on inflammation, alternating with resolution, or with a slow and indistinct form of the disease, a gland, or a cluster of glands gradually enlarges, and resisting all means of resolution, becomes unusually hard. The great hardness, and the malignant tendency of this growth, have procured for it from most authors the ominous names of scirrhus and cancer." Craigie also mentions a case described by Cruickshank in 1786, "in which the tracheobronchial

R. K. Gupta: Department of Medical Oncology, St. Bartholomew's and The Royal London School of Medicine and Dentistry and St. Bartholomew's Hospital, London, United Kingdom.

T. A. Lister: Department of Medical Oncology, St. Bartholomew's Hospital, London, United Kingdom.

M. K. Gospodarowicz: Department of Radiation Oncology, University of Toronto and Princess Margaret Hospital, Toronto, Ontario, Canada.

lymphatic glands were affected with this morbid change to such an extent as to cause fatal suffocation."

In 1838 Richard Bright, a consultant physician at Guy's Hospital, referred to Hodgkin's original cases in a paper on abdominal tumors. However, it was due to Sir Samuel Wilks' generosity that the disease bears its present name. In 1856 Wilks described amyloidosis and included some of Hodgkin's original cases in his paper. In 1865, having collected a series of 15 cases, he chose to emphasize the separate nature of Hodgkin's original cases in a second paper, "Cases of the Enlargement of the Lymphatic Glands and Spleen (or Hodgkin's Disease) with Remarks" (3). He acknowledged Hodgkin's pioneering work, and named the condition after him. Wilks' initial descriptions give us some of our earliest understanding of Hodgkin's disease. He described the disease as a cancer that started and remained in the lymph nodes for a long time, perhaps years, before involving the spleen, and then spreading to other organs. He also noted anemia, weight loss, and fevers in some of his patients with Hodgkin's disease. Wilks clearly observed the anemia and cachexia of his patients and called attention to intermittent fever in at least one instance.

The early staging classifications for Hodgkin's disease merely reflected the natural history of the disease, since no effective therapy was available. The first recorded classification was proposed by Trousseau (4) in Paris in 1865, in an excellent descriptive essay on *l'adénie* or enlargement of lymph nodes, suggesting a new entity consisting of glandular tumors. His description of the illness may be divided into three stages: latent, progressive, and cachectic. The definitions of these stages is best provided by the following translation direct from Trousseau's paper: the latent stage "is characterized by the tendency of certain individuals to present with enlarged nodes (glands), arising from some cause.... Blood shows no appreciable abnormality." The progressive stage is "initially localized but becomes generalized over a period of 18–24 months.... Anemia becomes apparent only in the second phase of the disease.... There is loss of appetite and digestive difficulty." The final stage of cachexia is "associated with an alteration in the blood picture.... The illness results in anemia and cachexia and is not accompanied by leucocytosis."

In 1879 Gowers (5) wrote:

> Varieties may be distinguished according[ly] as the glandular affection exists alone or is associated with enlargement of the spleen, and as the latter depends upon the presence of limited growths, or of a diffused increase in the pulp tissue. The distribution of the glandular enlargement also constitutes a salient distinction between different cases. In some it is general, and uniform in degree; in others, certain glands are much more enlarged than others, and these may or may not be the glands first affected. In some cases, again, one group of glands may be the seat of great enlargement, and constitute a tumour having the characters of a local growth.

Gowers therefore proposed the following stages (varieties of distribution): 1, "local growth only"; 2, "local enlargement preponderating"; and 3, "general uniform infection." Each stage could be associated with splenic involvement and an increased white cell count. Gowers was unclear whether stage 1, local growth only, was related to the two other stages. This anatomico-clinical approach seemed appropriate at the time, reflecting the morbid macroscopic anatomic findings at post mortem examination, as described by Hodgkin (2) in 1832, Bright (6) in 1838, and Wilks (3) in 1865.

In 1902 Dorothy Reed (7) described not only the features of what are now known as Sternberg-Reed cells, but also two functional stages of Hodgkin's disease, including an initial stage of increasing lymphadenopathy during which the individual was in apparently normal physical condition and a second stage of advancing disease with progressive asthenia, cachexia, and anemia. The clinical course was further defined in 1911 by Ziegler (8), who described 11 more or less distinct patterns, which was reformulated in 1920 by Longcope and McAlpin (9), dividing Hodgkin's disease into seven distinct clinical forms: localized, mediastinal, generalized, acute, larval, splenomegalic, and osteoperiostitic. The localized form was described as mostly involving the cervical nodes, while the mediastinal form represented a variation of the localized form involving the mediastinal nodes. In the generalized form, "there is an extension of the localised process to neighboring groups of nodes and the disease becomes more or less generalized."

Both the acute and larval forms were associated with symptoms. In the acute form "death may occur within a few weeks, or at most months. In this form, the enlargement of the lymph nodes is often widespread, but not very great." In the larval form the disease appeared to be limited exclusively to the thoracic or abdominal lymph nodes with no peripheral involvement. The symptoms were varied and included abdominal symptoms and fever. In the splenomegalic form, disease was confined in the spleen and the final form was a result of extralymphatic spread to bone and bone marrow.

Possibly the simplest and most satisfactory division of cases was proposed by Jackson and Parker (10,11), who based their classification on both distinctive pathologic findings and clinical pictures. In 1951 Craver (12) published a staging classification dividing the disease into three categories: class I, localized disease; class II, regional or intermediate disease; and class III, generalized disease. Unfortunately, although this was one of the first important classification systems in the postwar era, the terms *localized* and *regional* were variously interpreted. An anatomic staging system with greater specificity and clarity was first proposed by Peters (13) with a three-stage classification: stage I involves a single site or lymph node region, stage II involves two or three proximal lymphatic regions, and stage III involves two or more distinct lymphatic regions. This system was further modified by Peters and Middlemiss (14) to take into account constitutional symptoms of generalized disease in stage II. In 1964, Kaplan and colleagues (15) proposed modification of Peters's stage III to distinguish nodal disease above and below the diaphragm as defined by lymphangiography (as being stage III) from disease that has extended to involve extralymphatic tissues (stage IV). They also proposed extending the concept of classification of constitutional symptoms from stage II to all four stages.

These changes were ratified at both the Paris meeting in February 1965 (16), and at the Rye conference in New York in September 1965 (17), and lymph node chains were designated as regions for the purpose of staging. The only difference between the conclusions of the two meetings concerned patients with two contiguous lymph node areas, who were classified as stage II in Paris, and stage I_2 at the Rye meeting. Specific guidelines were also laid down for the investigation of a patient with Hodgkin's disease. Interestingly, at that time all stages were subclassified as A or B to indicate the absence or presence, respectively, of defined systemic symptoms. Those symptoms were otherwise explained as (a) fever, (b) night sweats, or (c) pruritus. Weight loss, although important to document, did not relegate a patient to a B subgroup.

Further changes were proposed to the Rye classification by Petersen and Milham (18), Musshoff and Boutis (19), and Rosenberg and Kaplan (20) to maximize the potential of radiation therapy. Two major modifications were adopted in the Ann Arbor staging classification in 1971 (21). The first removed the ambiguity in defining stage I and stage IV. Musshoff and colleagues found in a retrospective analysis of their own patients with Hodgkin's disease a striking difference in prognosis between patients with essentially localized extralymphatic organ involvement, essentially contiguous with an involved lymph node region (designated as "p.c." type), and disseminated extralymphatic involvement (their "p.d." type). Therefore, the designation "E" emerged to distinguish extranodal contiguous extension from truly disseminated disease, that is for proximal or contiguous extranodal disease that could be encompassed within an irradiation field that would be appropriate for nodal disease of the same anatomic extent and treated with a tumoricidal dose. This presumed the equivalent prognosis of localized extranodal disease and nodal disease of the same extent treated with a tumoricidal dose to appropriately designed irradiation fields.

The second modification introduced the concept of pathologic stage. This was made possible by performing staging laparotomy with splenectomy, and liver and multiple lymph node biopsies, a technique designed to maximize accurate anatomic description of disease extent, given the limitations inherent in clinical investigation of abdominal Hodgkin's disease. It was to be undertaken if subsequent management could be influenced by findings from these procedures. It must be remembered, however, that staging laparotomy was developed as an investigational tool, for example, in the early Stanford studies and the H_2 trial of the European Organization for Research and Treatment of Cancer (EORTC), to define the extent of Hodgkin's disease in patients rather than specifically to have an impact on treatment. Its role in designing treatment plans for patients became evident later with the development of chemotherapy and the increased knowledge of the morbidity and mortality risks of the staging procedure. Thus, initially, the procedure was used to enhance our understanding of the distribution of Hodgkin's disease, while its influence on treatment occurred later.

The designations of clinical stage (CS) and pathologic stage (PS) were suggested to clarify on which basis the anatomic stage was determined (Fig. 1). Clinical stage referred to the extent of disease determined as a result of diagnostic tests following a single diagnostic biopsy. Pathologic stage was developed primarily to acknowledge the greater accuracy of disease extent determined following staging laparotomy and bone marrow biopsy, unless bone marrow biopsy is positive in the absence of staging laparotomy, which would permit the designation of stage IV disease. In practice, however, most clinicians use the designation PS to indicate stage determined after

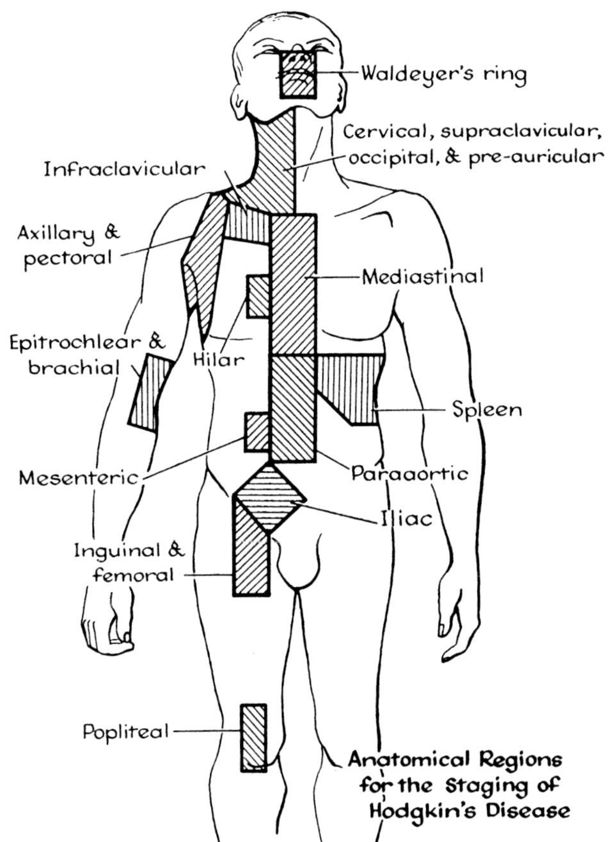

FIG. 1. The anatomic definitions of separate lymph node regions adopted for staging purposes at the Rye symposium on Hodgkin's disease. (From ref. 90, with permission.)

exploratory laparotomy with splenectomy. As this procedure is now rarely performed, most patients can be considered as clinically staged, even if a bone marrow biopsy or second lymph node biopsy has been obtained (22).

Once again, these proposed changes were agreed to at the Workshop on the Staging of Hodgkin's Disease, held at Ann Arbor, Michigan, in April 1971 and reflected the state of the art in diagnosis (Table 1) (21), assessment of prognostic factors, and treatment of the disease at that time. This is illustrated by the opening remarks of the Ann Arbor committee: "To facilitate communication and exchange information," and "To provide guidance of prognosis and to assist in therapeutic decisions" (20). All cases of Hodgkin's disease continued to be subclassified as A or B to indicate the respective absence or presence of constitutional symptoms. Interestingly, however, these were now documented as unexplained night sweats, fever, and/or loss of 10% or more of body weight during the 6 months prior to diagnosis. Pruritus was excluded, having been shown to have little or no influence on prognosis (23).

TABLE 1. *Ann Arbor recommendations for the diagnostic evaluation of patients with Hodgkin's disease*

A. Mandatory procedures
   1. Biopsy, with interpretation by a qualified pathologist
   2. History, with special attention to the presence and duration of fever, night sweats, and unexplained loss of 10% or more of body weight in the 6 months preceding admission
   3. Physical examination
   4. Laboratory tests
      a. Complete blood cell count and platelet count
      b. Erythrocyte sedimentation rate
      c. Serum alkaline phosphatase
   5. Radiographic examinations
      a. Chest (posteroanterior and lateral)
      b. Lymphangiogram
      c. Intravenous urogram
      d. Skeletal survey (spine and pelvis)
B. Contingent procedures
   1. Chest tomography (frontal or lateral), *if* pulmonary, hilar, and/or mediastinal involvement is present or suspected
   2. Bone marrow biopsy (needle or open), *if* CS III, alkaline phosphatase elevated, anemia, or at time of laparotomy
   3. Laparotomy and splenectomy, *if* decisions regarding management are likely to be influenced
   4. Inferior vena cavography, *if* lymphangiogram or urogram equivocal or unsatisfactory
   5. Liver biopsy (needle), *if* there is a strong clinical indication of hepatic involvement
C. Optional ancillary procedures
   1. Radioisotopic bone scans, in selected patients with bone pain and negative or equivocal roentgenograms
   2. Radioisotopic liver or spleen scans, in selected patients; limited value
   3. Tests of immunologic function
   4. Additional blood chemistry determinations: uric acid, calcium, copper, and so forth
D. Promising procedures for clinical investigations
   1. Radiogallium (^{67}Ga) and radioselenium (^{75}Se) scans
   2. Biologic indicators of disease activity: reduced serum Fe^{2+}, elevated Cu^{2+}

From ref. 21.

TABLE 2. *Ann Arbor staging classification*

Stage	Definitions
I	Involvement of a single lymph node region (I) or of a single extralymphatic organ or site (I_E)
II	Involvement of two or more lymph node regions on the same side of the diaphragm (II) or localized involvement of an extralymphatic organ or site and of one or more lymph node regions on the same side of the diaphragm (II_E)
III	Involvement of lymph node regions on both sides of the diaphragm (III), which may also be accompanied by involvement of the spleen (III_S) or by localized involvement of an extralymphatic organ or site (III_E) or both (III_{SE})
IV	Diffuse or disseminated involvement of one or more extralymphatic organs or tissues, with or without associated lymph node involvement

The absence or presence of fever, night sweats, and/or unexplained loss of 10% or more of body weight in the 6 months preceding admission are to be denoted in all cases by the suffix letters A or B, respectively. The clinical stage (CS) denotes the stage as determined by all diagnostic examinations and a single biopsy only. If a second biopsy of any kind has been obtained, whether negative or positive, the term *pathologic stage* (PS) is used.
From ref. 22.

In the two decades since the Ann Arbor meeting, several significant changes in the management of Hodgkin's disease took place. Important prognostic criteria were recognized, such as bulky disease and multiple sites of disease affecting the outlook adversely if such patients were treated with radiation alone. Also, computed tomography (CT) was introduced and was demonstrated to be an accurate and efficient imaging technique in staging.

The Ann Arbor staging classification (Table 2) (22) for Hodgkin's disease was formulated to provide a rational basis upon which curative treatment decisions could be made for patients at initial presentation. The classification became rapidly and widely adopted, with most investigators following the guidelines laid down by the Committee on Hodgkin's Disease Staging (21,22). Indeed, the Ann Arbor classification for Hodgkin's disease (1971) has been adopted by the Union Internationale Centre le Cancer (UICC) staging committee as an official staging system (1). During the early 1970s, patients with stages I, II, and IIIA disease were usually treated with radiotherapy following laparotomy; the remainder were mostly treated with combination chemotherapy.

SITES OF INVOLVEMENT AND PATTERNS OF PRESENTATION

It has been widely accepted, based on the work of Gilbert (24), Peters (13,25), and Kaplan (26), that Hodgkin's disease starts at a single site, usually a lymph node, and clinically progresses to adjacent lymphoid tissues before disseminating to distant nonadjacent sites and organs. It appears to begin in an area within the lymphatic system and to spread in an orderly manner to contiguous lymph nodes via lymphatic channels. Noncontiguous spread and hematologic distribution is more common with recurrent disease. However, this theory of contiguous spread did have its opponents (27).

As patients were evaluated more completely with techniques such as lymphangiography and histologic assessment with laparotomy and splenectomy, evidence supported the view that Hodgkin's disease was usually unifocal in its origin and progressed in an orderly and predictable manner (28,29). This was apparently particularly true for most patients in the younger age groups with classic histologic subtypes of disease. A study of 100 consecutive patients at Stanford, at a time when surgical staging was being performed, documented the distribution of disease (28). Figure 2 illustrates the most common anatomic patterns of Hodgkin's disease in these patients.

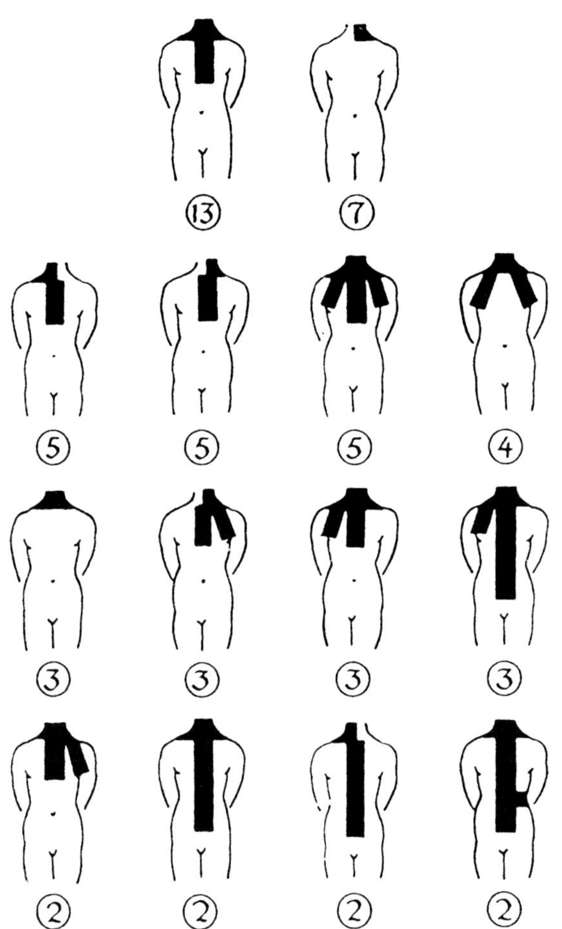

FIG. 2. Evidence of an orderly progression in the spread of Hodgkin's disease. Most common anatomic patterns of Hodgkin's disease in 100 consecutive patients who underwent staging laparotomy at Stanford (28). The number of patients are in circles. (From ref. 28, with permission.)

The pattern of disease at presentation also appears to be associated with the histologic subtype, as described by Mauch and colleagues (30) in a detailed study of 719 patients with Hodgkin's disease who underwent staging laparotomy. For example, most patients with nodular lymphocyte-predominant Hodgkin's disease present with localized peripheral disease often in the upper neck, whereas patients with the lymphocyte-depletion subtype of disease usually present with abdominal nodal involvement and often have extranodal disease. The majority of patients with nodular sclerosis histology have disease above the diaphragm and mediastinal node involvement. Disease in the liver is most frequently seen in patients with mixed-cellularity or lymphocyte-depletion Hodgkin's disease and systemic symptoms.

These patterns of spread of Hodgkin's disease have considerable therapeutic implications, particularly if extended-field radiotherapy is advocated as the treatment of choice. For example, it is rare to have Hodgkin's disease in the neck and also in the lower abdomen without disease in the upper abdomen. It is unusual to have bilateral axillary involvement without disease being present in the lower neck areas as well. It is extremely unusual to have liver involvement with Hodgkin's disease or bone marrow infiltration without having disease in the spleen. It is uncommon to have pulmonary disease at presentation without Hodgkin's disease being present within intrathoracic lymph nodes, usually on the ipsilateral side. It is also claimed that if the theory that Hodgkin's disease spreads in a pattern explained by the contiguity along lymphatic channels is correct, then it is likely that it can spread via the thoracic duct, possibly in either direction, without clinical involvement of the mediastinum.

STAGING SYSTEM—PRESENT

Adherence to the Ann Arbor guidelines gradually became less strict for three reasons: First, new features of prognostic importance were recognized. It became clear that for patients with exclusively nodal disease treated with conventional extended-field radiation, prognosis correlated not only with stage and the presence of symptoms but also with other factors such as "bulk" of disease and in some studies the number of involved nodal sites—features not defined within stage. Subsequently, chemotherapy has been introduced for patients with "unfavorable" early-stage disease, a management decision independent of pathologic definition of stage by laparotomy. Second, the need for a staging laparotomy was questioned by some investigators following the demonstration of an excellent prognosis for patients who had relapsed after initial radiotherapy and were subsequently treated with chemotherapy. Third, new techniques for determining sites of disease have been introduced. For example, CT and magnetic resonance imaging (MRI) became available and have been introduced into routine staging, replacing others recommended in the Ann Arbor report.

TABLE 3. *Cotswolds classification*

Stage	Definitions
I	Involvement of a single lymph node region or lymphoid structure (e.g., spleen, thymus, Waldeyer's ring)
II	Involvement of two or more lymph node regions on the same side of the diaphragm (the mediastinum is a single site; hilar lymph nodes are lateralized); the number of anatomic sites should be indicated by a suffix (e.g., II_3)
III	Involvement of lymph node regions or structures on both sides of the diaphragm
III_1	With or without splenic, hilar, celiac, or portal nodes
III_2	With paraaortic, iliac, mesenteric nodes
IV	Involvement of extranodal site(s) beyond that designated E

Annotation:
A, No B symptoms.
B, Fever, drenching sweats, or weight loss.
X, Bulky disease, >1/3 widening of mediastinum at T5-6, or >10 cm maximum dimension of nodal mass.
E, Involvement of a single extranodal site, contiguous or proximal to known nodal site.
CS, Clinical stage.
PS, Pathologic stage.
From ref. 31.

Thus, to update the Ann Arbor staging classification and justify the use of imaging techniques such as CT scanning, a meeting was organized in the Cotswolds, England, in 1988 (31). At this meeting it was decided to retain the general framework of the Ann Arbor classification, extending it to define the number of sites and bulky disease, and subdividing pathologic stage III disease into stages III_1 and III_2, as defined by Desser and colleagues (32) (Table 3). The clinical criteria for hepatic and splenic involvement were tightened, with the abolition of abnormal liver function findings as denoting liver involvement.

The major changes (Table 4) were as follows: (a) legitimize the use of CT scanning for the detection of intraabdominal disease, (b) redefine clinical involvement of liver and spleen, (c) formally introduce the concept of bulk of disease at a given site, and (d) draw attention to the problem of equivocal complete remission. It seemed appropriate to adopt these changes for the following reasons: (a) CT scanning was already in general use for the detection of both intraabdominal and intrathoracic disease and is regarded by many to be at least as useful as lymphangiography. (b) Laparotomy studies had demonstrated the inaccuracy of the clinical criteria for involvement of the liver and spleen in the Ann Arbor classification. The demonstration of focal filling defects with either CT or ultrasound at least increased the possibility of accurate clinical staging. It was recognized that this was still not as accurate as wedge biopsy of the liver or splenectomy. (c) Bulk disease had clearly been defined as an adverse prognostic factor. (d) It had been well documented that residual radiologic abnormalities after both radiotherapy and chemotherapy in a patient in otherwise good health and with no clinical evidence of Hodgkin's disease did not necessarily imply active disease. However, by definition, they do preclude the designation "complete remission" (CR). This situation was partly a reflection of the sensitivity of current imaging techniques, and, in the absence of pathologic confirmation, the outcome was designated as unconfirmed/uncertain complete remission—CR(u).

TABLE 4. *Cotswolds revision of the Ann Arbor staging system*

Stage	Ann Arbor system	Cotswolds revision
I	Single nodal area or structure (e.g., mediastinum = 1; left neck = 1; spleen = 1; Waldeyer's = 1; thymus = 1)	Same
II	Two or more single nodal areas on the same side of the diaphragm	Right and left hilum: one area each, independent of mediastinum; number of anatomic nodal areas to be indicated by a subscript (II_4)
III	At least one nodal area on both sides of the diaphragm	III_1 = upper abdomen (splenic, celiac, portal) III_2 = lower abdomen (including paraaortic, mesenteric
IV	Visceral involvement	Same
B symptoms	Fever >38°C or drenching sweats during the last month, weight loss >10% in 6 months	Same
A	No symptoms	Same
E	Extranodal involvement by contiguity, encompassable in the nodal radiation field	Same
X		Bulky disease, >1/3 widening of mediastinum at T5-6 level, or >10 cm maximum dimension of nodal mass
CR(u)		Unconfirmed/uncertain complete remission (residual imaging abnormality)

PROGNOSIS RELATED TO STAGE

The presenting stage as presently defined has a strong prognostic value. However, the influence of the number of involved nodal regions on both remission duration and overall survival was not initially considered in the Ann Arbor classification, which did not take into account the volume of disease. For example, the total tumor burden can be greater in some patients with stage II than in those with stage III disease. Also, as all prognostic indicators are strongly interrelated, the relevant indicators may differ as a function of the stages. Multivariate analysis has now become mandatory (33).

The prognostic significance of bulk of disease, particularly within the mediastinum, has now been well documented (34). However, the definition of bulk is rather confusing in the literature. The definition that found greatest acceptance for the mediastinum involved measuring the greatest transverse diameter of the mediastinal mass on a standard posteroanterior chest radiograph and dividing by the maximal diameter of the chest wall at its pleural surfaces, usually at the level of the diaphragm (35) (Fig. 3). A ratio exceeding one-third was considered bulky and an adverse feature, with a significantly increased incidence of relapse both in the mediastinum and in nodal sites outside the chest.

The Cotswolds committee recommended a different approach. Mediastinal bulk was defined as the ratio of the maximum transverse tumor mass diameter to the internal thoracic diameter at the level of the T5-6 interspace (Fig. 4). The Cotswolds committee used the T5-6 criteria to define a more consistent, reliable, and therefore reproducible measurement rather than using the widest diameter of the chest or thoracic cage, because they believed the later measurement could vary with the depth of inspiration, underlying lung or parenchymal disease such as emphysema, or other clinical factors. At present there are no established criteria for the definition of bulk using measurements obtained from CT scans.

Several studies describing prognostic factors have been performed (36–38). Although results were not entirely consistent, probably due to different analytical techniques, variable definitions of certain factors, and different cohorts of patients studied, there are major areas of agreement.

With reference to presenting stage, the presence of systemic symptoms has always been considered one of the main prognostic indicators. There is a strong correlation between the percentage of patients with systemic symptoms and the stage and the number of involved lymph node areas, as shown by Kaplan (38). However, when these fac-

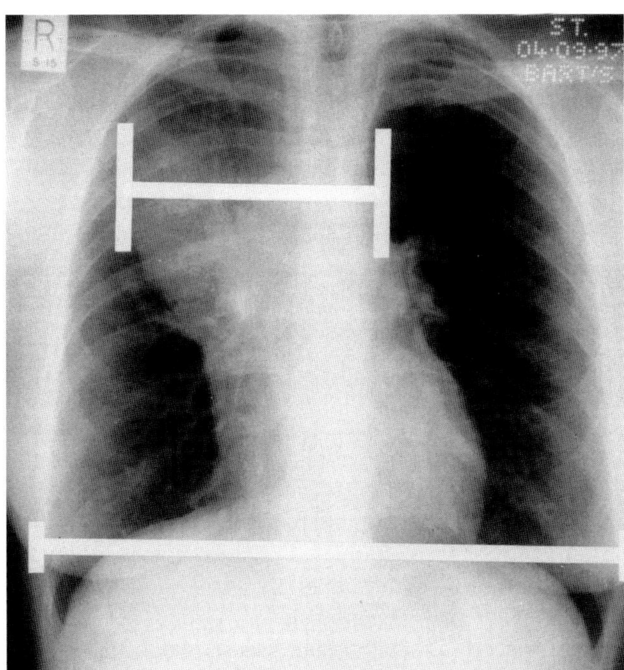

FIG. 3. A chest radiogram of a female patient with mediastinal involvement of Hodgkin's disease at presentation. The maximum transverse diameter of the mass (11.5 cm) is divided by the maximal diameter of the chest (26.5 cm), as described by Mauch et al. (35), to yield a ratio of 0.43. (Note that the internal thoracic diameter at the T5-6 interspace is 22.5 cm—a ratio of 0.51.)

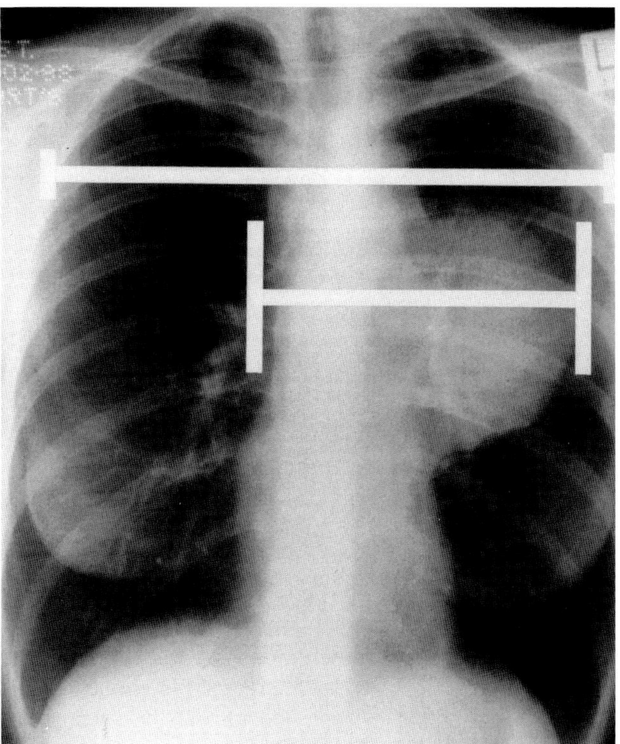

FIG. 4. A chest radiogram of another female patient with mediastinal involvement of Hodgkin's disease at presentation. The maximum transverse diameter of the mass (14.0 cm) is divided by the internal thoracic diameter at the T5-6 interspace (26.0 cm) as described in the Cotswolds report (31), yielding a ratio of 0.54. (Note that the maximal diameter of the chest is 28.5 cm—a ratio of 0.49.)

tors are taken into account in multivariate analysis, systemic symptoms retain significance (36,37). Indeed, recent studies have revealed correlations between the total tumor burden and systemic symptoms—the more accurately the tumor mass is evaluated, the less the prognostic significance of these systemic symptoms (33).

There is also a strong correlation between erythrocyte sedimentation rate (ESR) and the number of involved sites (16), and ESR also relates to the bulk of disease (33). Systemic symptoms and ESR are correlated with each other, but have independent significant prognostic impact. It has been suggested that a combination of ESR and systemic symptoms might be the simplest way to define favorable and unfavorable groups (36).

CLINICAL EVALUATION BEFORE THERAPY

History and Physical Examination

A detailed history should be obtained and the following recorded: (a) age; (b) gender; (c) presence or absence of unexplained fever and its duration; (d) unexplained sweating, especially at night, and its severity; (e) unexplained loss of weight as a percentage of usual body weight and rapidity of loss; and (f) unexplained pruritus, its extent, and severity. Note should also be made of performance status; alcohol-induced pain; a family history of Hodgkin's disease; other lymphoproliferative, myeloproliferative, or tissue malignancies; previous immunosuppressive illness (e.g., acquired immune deficiency syndrome); a history of previous malignancy including other lymphomas; and prior treatment with chemotherapy or radiotherapy.

A careful and complete physical examination must be performed by a physician experienced in the management of patients with Hodgkin's disease. Special attention must be directed to the areas where lymphadenopathy commonly occurs and the number of sites noted. A measurement of the largest mass in each region must be made. Waldeyer's ring should always be examined especially in patients with high neck disease. The size of the liver and spleen in centimeters below the costal margin in the midclavicular line must be recorded.

Symptoms and Signs

Symptoms and Presenting Features

The majority of patients present with overt disease. However, the presenting symptoms and signs may be relatively nonspecific, often more compatible with infection than with malignant disease. Occult presentation of the disease is very uncommon, but the incidence of clinically occult disease has been an importance influence in the development of therapeutic strategy.

The most common characteristic clinical presentation of Hodgkin's disease is a young adult noticing an otherwise asymptomatic lump (70% of cases). The enlarged lymph gland, which is usually nontender, occurs most frequently in the lower neck, often in the supraclavicular fossa, but may be present high in the neck or axilla. Less often it is found in the inguinal-femoral region.

Another not uncommon presentation is the discovery of a mediastinal mass on routine plain chest radiograph. The mass may be fairly large without producing local symptoms. Less commonly, symptoms of retrosternal chest pain, cough, or shortness of breath may indicate an intrathoracic presentation of Hodgkin's disease. Rarely the disease may result in effusions of the pericardium or the pleura, although the presence of small amounts of pericardial and pleural fluid is not uncommon in patients with bulky mediastinal disease. The syndrome secondary to superior vena cava obstruction is rarely seen in patients with Hodgkin's disease.

A significant proportion of patients with undiagnosed Hodgkin's disease develop systemic symptoms prior to the discovery of lymphadenopathy. As mentioned above, typical symptoms of Hodgkin's disease are fever, night sweats, pruritus, fatigue, and weight loss, none of which is specific. The fever of Hodgkin's disease is much like that of an infection, being more noticeable in the evening, and becoming more severe and continuous over time. The so-called Pel-Ebstein fever (39,40) is the characteristic intermittent fever associated with Hodgkin's disease. It is uncommon and recurs at variable intervals of several days or weeks lasting for 1 to 2 weeks before waning. However, a low-grade fever and drenching night sweats are found in about 25% of all patients at presentation, and usually in those with more advanced disease, in whom the incidence increases to 50%.

Other nonspecific symptoms such as chest pain, bronchial obstruction, abdominal pain, ascites, jaundice, bone pain, spinal cord compression, and peripheral edema are all uncommon presenting features. One unusual presenting symptom of Hodgkin's disease is pain. Alcohol ingestion has a rare but intriguing and as yet unexplained association with pain in Hodgkin's disease. The pain is characteristically severe, occurring within a few minutes of the ingestion of even a small amount of alcohol, and localizing to areas involved by Hodgkin's disease. It occurs more often at sites of bony involvement, but may also occur at the site of lymphadenopathy.

Retroperitoneal lymphadenopathy may give rise to characteristic discomfort and pain felt in the paravertebral or loin regions, particularly in the supine position. Patients may also present with abdominal swelling secondary to hepatomegaly or splenomegaly or, rarely, with ascites. Very advanced intraabdominal disease may be associated with obstruction of the ureters or compression of the renal vein, and, rarely, nephrotic syndrome may occur. There is, however, a well-described paraneoplastic nephrotic syndrome in patients with early-stage Hodgkin's disease who do not have retroperitoneal disease.

Other manifestations of Hodgkin's disease include a normochromic normocytic anemia, or more rarely a

Coombs' positive hemolytic anemia. Skin lesions associated with Hodgkin's disease include ichthyosis, urticaria, erythema multiforme, erythema nodosum, necrotizing lesions, hyperpigmentation, and skin infiltration. Several paraneoplastic neurologic syndromes have been reported in association with the disease but all are very rare. Symptomatic hypercalcemia is extremely uncommon in patients presenting with Hodgkin's disease and is usually associated with involvement of bone or, rarely, abnormalities in vitamin D metabolism (see Chapter 20 for a more detailed discussion).

Pruritus, although nonspecific and currently not a defined B symptom (see below), if severe, may be an important systemic symptom of disease (41), often preceding the diagnosis for months or even a year or more. It may occur early in the course of Hodgkin's disease in 10% to 15% of all patients, and it has been reported that 85% of patients may experience pruritus at some time during the course of the disease. It is usually generalized in character, and occasionally sufficiently severe to induce intense scratching, leading to extensive excoriations.

The pathophysiologic mechanisms leading to pruritus in Hodgkin's disease are unknown. However, since itching is known to be caused by a number of cytokines including those resulting from the breakdown of tissue, it has been suggested that in Hodgkin's disease pruritus may be due to an autoimmune reaction in which such substances are activated by tumor lysis (42).

Signs and Clinical Features (30,38)

On examination there is usually a rubbery consistency to the nodes, which are nontender; 60% to 80% of patients have enlarged nodes in the cervical and supraclavicular regions, 10% to 20% in the axilla, and 6% to 12% in the inguinal region. Exclusive infradiaphragmatic lymphadenopathy is seen in at most 10% of patients. At presentation mediastinal nodes are involved in up to 60% of cases, and retroperitoneal nodes in 25% of cases. Occasionally, alcohol-induced lymph node discomfort, ranging up to sharp pain, may be noted (<10%). Splenomegaly is found in 30% of patients at presentation and hepatomegaly in less than 5%. Table 5 shows the distribution of disease and involved sites in untreated pathologically staged patients with Hodgkin's disease.

TABLE 5. *Involved sites of disease in untreated pathologically staged patients with Hodgkin's disease*

Site	Percentage involved
Waldeyer's ring	1–2
Cervical nodes	
Right side	50–60
Left side	60–70
Axillary nodes	
Right side	25–35
Left side	30–35
Mediastinal nodes	50–60
Hilar nodes	15–35
Spleen	30–35
Liver	2–6
Paraaortic nodes	30–40
Iliac nodes	15–20
Mesenteric nodes	1–4
Inguinal nodes	8–15
Bone marrow	1–4
Other extranodal sites (lung, bone, etc.)	10–12
Total extranodal	10–15

Recommended Studies for Initial Evaluation (Tables 6 and 7)

An adequate surgical biopsy should be undertaken. Where possible, a whole lymph node should be taken for pathologic examination. Inguinal nodes should not be biopsied if equally suspicious peripheral nodes are present elsewhere. When the diagnosis of Hodgkin's disease is made from biopsy of an extranodal site, a node biopsy confirmation of diagnosis is desirable unless the diagnosis is considered unequivocal. The diagnosis should always be based on representative, appropriately prepared material. Radiologic investigation should include chest radiographs (posteroanterior and lateral) and CT of the thorax, abdomen, and pelvis, with intravenous contrast if necessary and with images at 1-cm intervals. Imaging of

TABLE 6. *Cotswolds recommendations for investigation of patients with Hodgkin's disease*

Recommended
- History and examination
  - B symptoms: weight loss >10% during previous 6 months, documented fever, night sweats
- Radiology
  - Plain chest radiograph
  - Computed tomography of the thorax
  - Computed tomography of the abdomen and pelvis[a]
  - Bipedal lymphogram[a]
- Hematology
  - Full blood count[c]
  - Lymphocyte count[c]
  - Erythrocyte sedimentation rate[c]
  - Bone marrow biopsy[b]
- Biochemistry
  - Tests of liver function[c]
  - Albumin, lactate dehydrogenase, calcium levels[c]

Under special circumstances
- Ultrasonographic scanning
- Magnetic resonance imaging

Other imaging techniques
- Isotope scanning
- Gallium
- Technetium

[a]Both not usually required.
[b]Not for stage IA or IIA with favorable features.
[c]Do not determine stage; may not influence management.
From ref. 31.

TABLE 7. *Recommended studies for initial evaluation*

Mandatory for the Cotswolds classification	Histology and immunophenotyping
	Past and familial history, clinical examination as per Cotswolds recommendations
	Blood counts and routine workup: ESR, LDH, alkaline phosphatase, albumin, liver function, virology
	Chest radiograms: computed tomography of chest, abdomen, and pelvis; bone marrow aspiration and biopsy if indicated
Recommended for disease assessment	Liver and spleen ultrasonography and if doubtful percutaneous liver biopsy
	Gallium scanning/gallium SPECT
	β_2-microglobulin, interleukin-6 and interleukin-10 levels
Investigational noninvasive	Magnetic resonance imaging (bone/bone marrow), technetium bone scanning
	Immunoscintigram with antiferritin or anti-CD30 antibodies
	Histologic expression and/or serum levels of soluble CD8, CD25, CD30, IL-6, and other cytokines
Investigational invasive	Staging laparotomy, laparoscopy
Recommended for toxicity assessment	Heart: ECG, MUGA, or echocardiogram
	Pulmonary: lung function tests
	Thyroid and gonadal functions: FSH, LH, and TSH (semen analysis and sperm storage)
	Psychosocial adaptation

ECG, electrocardiogram; ESR, erythrocyte sedimentation rate; FSH, follicle stimulating hormone; LDH, lactate dehydrogenase; LH, luteinizing hormone; MUGA, multiple uptake gated acquisition; SPECT, single proton emission computed tomography; TSH, thyroid stimulating hormone.

the neck, although not absolutely necessary, is increasingly being employed. There is considerable normal variation in the size of mediastinal and hilar nodes, but those measuring >10 mm in shortest cross-section can be considered abnormal. Retrocrural lymph nodes >6 mm can be considered as abnormal. In the remaining abdomen and pelvis, lymph nodes of more than 15 mm in shortest cross section are strongly suspicious, certainly in the paraaortic region, and almost always abnormal. However, although unequivocal abnormal findings on CT scanning may represent Hodgkin's disease, there is a risk of false positives, particularly within the abdomen, when using these criteria. Therefore, when lymph nodes in the 15- to 20-mm range are seen, it is often advisable to obtain further evaluation using gallium-67 scanning or lymphangiography, or undertake a percutaneous biopsy, or in some cases a laparotomy, if it is important to determine the accuracy of staging, being that there may be a moderately high risk of false-positive results. An ultrasound of the liver and spleen should also be performed.

Gallium-67 citrate scanning was initially investigated in the 1960s and 1970s following the observation that uptake was most pronounced in viable tumor (43). The exact role of gallium-67 scanning in the staging of lymphoma has yet to be defined, although it is increasingly used in conjunction with CT (44), particularly at diagnosis. It is clearly useful in the assessment and evaluation of mediastinal disease before and after treatment (45) (see Chapter 16).

Laboratory Tests

Laboratory investigations (see Table 5) should include (a) complete blood count, including hemoglobin, platelet count, white blood cell count, and differential (including absolute lymphocyte count); (b) ESR at 1 hour; and (c) biochemical tests of liver, bone, and renal function, including serum alkaline phosphatase, aspartate aminotransferase (AST-glutamyl oxalo acetic transaminase), alanine aminotransferase (ALT-glutamyl pyruvate transaminase), γ-glutamyl transaminase, lactate dehydrogenase (LDH), albumin, and calcium. Although these investigations may not necessarily contribute directly to staging, they may influence treatment modification and guide further investigations to other potential sites of disease.

Recommendation for Bone Marrow Biopsy

It is well recognized that marrow infiltration by malignant cells occurs in up to 5% of newly-diagnosed cases of patients with Hodgkin's disease. This is closely associated with advanced clinical stage and is found in less than 1% of early-stage Hodgkin's disease (i.e., stage IA or IIA). A study of 613 cases of Hodgkin's disease reported by Macintyre and colleagues (46) found that the result of bone marrow biopsy influenced the mode of treatment in less than 1% of cases. It has also been suggested that it was only helpful in patients with B symptoms.

A survey conducted in the United Kingdom and reported in 1995 by Howard and colleagues (47) revealed a significant variation in clinical practice with respect to bone marrow biopsy of newly diagnosed patients with Hodgkin's disease. They concluded that this invasive and often painful procedure was performed more frequently in patients with Hodgkin's disease than was recommended on the basis of published studies and guidelines. In view of the result from the German Lymphoma Study

Group (48) in 1995, together with the recommendation from the Cotswolds meeting (31), it would seem that bone marrow trephine from at least one site should be advocated for patients with B symptoms, or clinical stages III and IV, or bulk disease, or abnormalities in the peripheral blood count such as anemia, leukopenia, or thrombocytopenia. Patients with recurrent disease should all undergo a bone marrow biopsy for both morphologic and cytogenetic analysis, particularly if high-dose therapy is to be considered (49).

Supplementary Investigations

Further imaging studies to confirm clinical involvement at a given site include isotope scanning (e.g., gallium for extent of nodal involvement or technetium for involvement of bone); MRI; and other imaging studies necessary to resolve the significance of symptoms or physical signs [e.g., positron emission tomography (PET)]. Biopsy of a specific site to determine pathologic involvement may include bone marrow trephine from at least one site for selected patients, as previously discussed; percutaneous or laparoscopic liver biopsy; CT-guided bone biopsy; percutaneous or open lung biopsy; selective biopsy of any other extranodal tissue site; and laparotomy (only if the findings would alter the treatment plan). Staging laparotomy should include wedge and needle biopsy of the liver to provide histologic evidence of involvement, bone marrow biopsy, splenectomy with assessment of extent of splenic involvement, and nodal biopsies from suspected areas in paraaortic, celiac, splenic hilar, and iliac regions.

Cotswolds Recommendations

The Cotswolds report (31) (Table 6) makes detailed recommendations on the clinical and laboratory investigations that should accompany a history and clinical examination for all patients.

The recommended pretreatment evaluation procedures include a number of parameters that although not directly related to staging are nevertheless of importance in terms of prognosis, and may be taken into consideration when planning treatment. These include features not considered in the Ann Arbor report, such as performance status, age, gender, assessment of mediastinal bulk, and measurements of serum LDH and albumin. Measurements of ESR, total lymphocyte count, and number of nodal sites of involvement are also of prognostic importance, and are recommended in the initial evaluation. Once these have been completed and a clinical stage determined, a treatment plan may be devised. The results of the investigations should be discussed with the patient. Treatment options should be outlined, together with potential side effects including acute toxicities and long-term morbidity. In view of the possibility of infertility secondary to systemic chemotherapy, semen analysis and sperm storage should be made available for men. For women, at present, there are no reliable methods of protecting ovarian function from systemic chemotherapy (see Chapter 36).

Chest

Chest radiography with posteroanterior and lateral views should be performed on all patients. Several studies have demonstrated that 10% to 20% of lymphoma cases are upstaged following CT scanning, compared with plain chest radiography (50,51), and the management is altered in up to 60% of patients. CT scanning is also useful in eradicating false-positive findings: in one study 25 suspected sites of disease on plain radiographs were disproved by CT scanning (51) (see Chapter 16 for more detailed discussion).

Thoracic CT is therefore now recommended for all new patients. Until recently, it was the general policy to perform CT only when plain chest radiographs were normal, to detect small nodes behind the cardiomediastinal shadow. However, the greater accuracy of CT scanning in detecting parenchymal abnormalities, pericardial involvement, chest wall involvement, and retrocardiac nodes, especially in the presence of mediastinal Hodgkin's disease, has redefined the role of CT from being a contingent procedure (38) to being a mandatory procedure. Thoracic CT scanning has been extremely valuable in recognizing and delineating disease for subsequent radiation planning (52,53).

Abdomen

The advent of CT has made it easier to detect intraabdominal disease. The procedure is easier to administer and less labor intensive than bipedal lymphangiography. It is also better at defining celiac, rectocrural, splenic, renal hilar, and porta-hepatis nodes. The overall accuracy of CT compared with bipedal lymphangiography is very similar (54), though in some cases specificity may be slightly better with bipedal lymphangiography (55), with distortion of the architecture due to replacement being a reliable sign of tumor involvement; but false-positive findings may result from benign replacement by fat, fibrosis, or reactive hyperplasia, and may be as high as 12% (56). A study of 139 patients who had laparotomy plus CT and/or lymphograms as part of their initial staging for Hodgkin's disease evaluated the relative ability of the two techniques to detect disease in the abdomen. It was concluded that lymphangiography of the lower abdomen was more sensitive and provided more information than CT, and therefore should continue to be used (57). Nevertheless, it is now rarely performed, although there may still be a role for bipedal lymphangiography in patients who present with subdiaphragmatic Hodgkin's disease and are being considered for treatment with radiotherapy. The use of lymphangiograms in this situation allows for more precise shaping of blocks and protection of normal tissues.

The CT scan also provides detailed information about the liver and spleen and may be useful in clinically defining involvement of these organs, according to the Cotswolds recommendations. However, even with the latest CT scanners, it is still difficult to reliably diagnose splenic involvement. Castellino and colleagues (55) found the overall accuracy of CT detection to be only 58% (sensitivity 33% and specificity 76%). These dismal results are the reason for performing staging laparotomy in cases in which management could be altered with this information.

Hepatic involvement occurs in approximately 5% of cases of Hodgkin's disease (58). Involvement usually appears as microscopic or small macroscopic foci. Size alone is therefore inaccurate as an indicator of the presence of disease, and liver function tests may be abnormal in the absence of histologic involvement. The current Cotswolds guidelines recommend the demonstration of multiple focal defects (not cystic or vascular) by at least two imaging techniques, such as CT, isotope scanning, ultrasonography, or MRI. Low-field-strength MRI was found by Richards and colleagues (59) to be sensitive in detecting liver lymphoma. However, others (60) found it to be inconclusive. In a group of 13 biopsy-proven hepatic lymphoma cases, it was found that T1- and T2-weighted techniques were useful in detecting focal, and T2-weighted techniques were useful in detecting mixed (focal and diffuse), hepatic involvement; diffuse infiltration was undetectable by MRI (61).

Splenic involvement has not been reliably and accurately predicted by CT, isotope scanning, ultrasound scans, or MRI. The diagnostic accuracy of abdominal ultrasound was compared with that of CT and laparotomy in 100 patients with Hodgkin's disease (62). The authors concluded that if, in the staging of patients with Hodgkin's disease, a CT scan was considered to be negative, then the splenic texture and size should be examined by ultrasound. An earlier report suggested that the accuracy of MRI may be significantly enhanced by the use of a new contrast agent, superparamagnetic iron oxide, which causes a change in splenic magnetic resonance signal intensity (63). Using this technique, splenic lymphoma could be unambiguously identified in all eight patients studied. A larger study with pathologic correlation will be needed to evaluate this technique further.

Bone

Bone disease at presentation is uncommon but may be present at some time in the course of the disease in up to 21% of patients with Hodgkin's disease (64–66). Isotope bone scans using radiolabeled technetium-99 (^{99}Tc) pyrophosphate or ^{99}Tc-methylene diphosphonate are very sensitive; specificity can be enhanced by using another imaging technique to support the isotope scan findings, such as MRI. Isotope bone scans should be undertaken in patients with bone or joint pain, with a raised alkaline phosphatase, or in whom areas of bone disease are suspected on CT or plain radiology.

Gastrointestinal Tract

The gastrointestinal tract is a common site of extranodal infiltration in non-Hodgkin's lymphoma but is rarely involved in Hodgkin's disease. If indicated, barium studies with endoscopic biopsy are the investigations of choice in confirming suspected involvement.

Central Nervous System

Central nervous system involvement in Hodgkin's disease is rare but may occur, presenting either intracranially or with spinal, extranodal deposits. If suspected, diagnosis can be readily established with plain radiography, CT, MRI, myelography, and cytology of the cerebrospinal fluid.

Pathologic Staging

Pathologic staging is dependent on histologic confirmation of involvement, not, as is often misunderstood, merely based on postlaparotomy findings. Apart from the diagnostic histology, the most common site of biopsy is the bone marrow, being involved in up to 5% of previously untreated patients (67–69); MRI or scintigraphy bone marrow guided biopsy may occasionally improve sensitivity of the procedure.

The question of exploratory laparotomy in previously untreated patients is a vexing one (see Chapters 17 and 18). None of the current imaging techniques has been accurate or reliable enough in detecting splenic involvement to dispense with this procedure in cases that would involve a major change in therapy if splenic disease were found. Use of prognostic factors has made it easier to define patients who are most and least likely to have splenic disease (70,71). However, these predictions are not absolute and some believe that staging laparotomy and splenectomy remains a relevant investigation for selected patients (72).

The UICC (1) now states specifically that the pathologic classification of Hodgkin's disease should include definition of all the four stages following the same criteria as for clinical stage, but with additional information obtained following laparotomy. Splenectomy, liver biopsy, lymph node biopsy, and bone marrow biopsy are mandatory for the establishment of pathologic stage.

Anatomic Staging Criteria

Clinical Stage

Lymph node involvement is demonstrated by (a) clinical enlargement of a node when alternative pathology may reasonably be ruled out (suspicious nodes should always be biopsied if treatment decisions are based on their involvement); and (b) enlargement on plain radiograph, CT, or lymphangiography.

Spleen involvement is demonstrated by unequivocal palpable splenomegaly alone, or equivocal palpable splenomegaly with radiologic confirmation (ultrasound or CT) of either enlargement or multiple focal defects that are neither cystic nor vascular (radiologic enlargement alone is inadequate).

Liver involvement is demonstrated by multiple focal defects that are neither cystic nor vascular and noted with at least two imaging techniques. Clinical enlargement alone with or without abnormalities of liver function tests is not adequate.

Lung involvement is demonstrated by radiologic evidence of parenchymal involvement in the absence of other likely causes especially infection.

Bone involvement is demonstrated by a history of pain or elevation of serum alkaline phosphatase, supported by plain radiologic changes or evidence from other imaging studies (isotope, CT, or MRI).

CNS involvement is demonstrated by (a) a spinal intradural deposit or spinal cord or meningeal involvement, which may be diagnosed on the basis of the clinical history and findings supported by plain radiology, myelography, CT, and/or MRI (spinal extradural deposits should be carefully assessed as they may be the result of soft tissue disease that represents extension from bone metastasis or disseminated disease); and (b) intracranial involvement, which will rarely be diagnosed clinically at presentation. It should be considered on the basis of a space-occupying lesion in the face of disease in additional extranodal sites.

Other sites of involvement: clinical involvement of other extranodal sites may only be diagnosed if the site is contiguous or proximal to a known nodal site (i.e., an E lesion).

Pathologic Stage

PS depends on histologic confirmation of specific sites of involvement such as bone, bone marrow, lung, liver, skin, and so forth.

Criteria for B Symptoms

The criteria for B symptoms are unexplained weight loss of more than 10% of the body weight during the 6 months before initial staging investigation, unexplained persistent or recurrent fever with temperatures above 38°C during the previous month, and recurrent drenching night sweats during the previous month. Although other symptoms may be associated with Hodgkin's disease, they will not be classified as B symptoms, although some (such as severe pruritus, discussed earlier) may prove to be of prognostic significance and should be recorded.

Fever and weight loss appear to have more prognostic significance than drenching night sweats, which are considered by some to be the least important of the B symptoms (34,73,74). It is of interest that, although B symptoms generally correlate with advanced stage and bulk disease, on occasions patients with early or small-volume Hodgkin's disease will have significant B symptoms—a feature that remains unexplained.

Particular Problems

Mediastinal Disease

The term *mediastinal* includes the following nodal subgroups: (a) prevascular, aortopulmonary; (b) paratracheal, pretracheal, subcarinal; and (c) posterior mediastinal. Hilar (bronchopulmonary) nodes are considered to be outside the mediastinum and should be defined and recorded separately. Disease within the chest is usually in the anterior mediastinum, often at the site of the thymus. Internal mammary nodes are part of the lymphatic system of the chest wall and they drain the diaphragm. Paravertebral nodes, although in the posterior mediastinum, also drain the chest wall and diaphragm. Where possible, all these should be documented separately. Anterior extension of a mediastinal mass into the sternum or chest wall or extension to lung or pericardium should be recorded as extranodal extension.

Criteria for Bulk

The bulk of palpable lymph nodes will be defined by the largest dimension (in centimeters) of the single largest lymph node or conglomerate node mass in each region of involvement. A node or nodal mass must be 10 cm or greater to be recorded as bulky . Abdominal nodal bulk is defined by the largest dimension of a single node or conglomerate nodal mass using CT, MRI, or ultrasonography. It should be remembered, however, that different definitions of bulk disease have been used, such as 6 cm (75,76) and 5 cm (77).

A mediastinal mass, as described before, is defined as bulky on a posteroanterior chest radiograph when the maximum width is equal to or greater than one-third of the internal transverse diameter of the thorax at the level of the T5-6 interspace (Fig. 4). The chest radiograph should be taken with maximal inspiration in the upright position at a source–skin distance of 2 m.

Criteria for Extranodal Spread

Involvement of extralymphatic tissue on one side of the diaphragm by limited direct extension from an adjacent nodal site will be classified as extranodal extension (E) with the implicit expectation of a prognosis equivalent to that for treatment of nodal disease of the same anatomic extent. The E category may also include an apparently discrete single extranodal deposit consistent with extension from a regionally involved node. Multiple extranodal deposits will not be included. A single extralymphatic site as the only site of disease should be classified as IE, but this is extremely uncommon in Hodgkin's disease.

Staging Notation (31)

For CS and PS, symptomatic disease should be noted as B, and asymptomatic as A .

Nodal Disease (I–III)

Stage I: involvement of a single lymph node region (e.g., cervical, axillary, inguinal, mediastinal) or lymphoid structure such as spleen, thymus, or Waldeyer's Ring.

Stage II: involvement of two or more lymph node regions or lymph node structures on the same side of the diaphragm. Hilar nodes should be considered to be lateralized, and when involved on both sides they constitute stage II disease. The number of anatomic regions should be indicated by a subscript (e.g., II_3). For the purpose of defining the number of anatomic regions, all nodal disease within the mediastinum is considered to be a single lymph node region, and hilar involvement constitutes an additional site of involvement.

Stage III: involvement of lymph node regions or lymphoid structures on both sides of the diaphragm. This may be subdivided stage III1 or III2, stage III1 being used for patients with spleen or splenic hilar, celiac, or portal node involvement, and stage III2 for those with paraaortic, iliac, inguinal, or mesenteric node involvement.

Bulky Disease

The subscript X will be used if bulky disease is present. No subscripts will be used in the absence of bulk.

Extranodal Disease

The subscript E is used if limited extranodal extension as described above is documented. More extensive extranodal disease will be designated as stage IV.

Pathologic Stage

PS at a given site will be denoted by a subscript (e.g., M, bone marrow; H, liver; L, lung; O, bone; P, pleura; D, skin).

All the necessary information should be available prior to assigning the stage. For example, a 63-year-old man who presents with bilateral cervical nodes, night sweats, weight loss of 15 kg, with a mediastinal mass on the chest radiogram (>1/3), and involvement of right hilum, with abdominal CT showing paraaortic and pelvic adenopathy with no definite involvement of the liver and with negative bone marrow, should be staged as CS $IIIB_X$. A patient who is asymptomatic but has bilateral cervical and right axillary lymph nodes with a small mediastinal mass is staged as CS II_4A.

CLINICAL EVALUATION DURING THERAPY

During treatment, whether with radiotherapy or combination chemotherapy, clinical evaluation must be made at regular intervals, e.g., prior to each cycle of treatment, and should include a physical examination (with particular emphasis on documenting the reduction in previous sites of lymphadenopathy, and checking that those sites not involved at presentation remain unaffected). Imaging is used as guide to therapeutic response, and this is particularly true with cyclical chemotherapy, which should be discontinued or changed if the patient fails to show objective evidence of response. Radiologic examination should be performed in all patients in whom an abnormality was detectable at presentation, to ensure continuing response to therapy and that no new lesions have arisen. Chest radiographs are also useful to ensure that lung fields are clear of any occult infection and the possible effects of treatment, for example with bleomycin. However, patients with disease visible only on an initial CT scan should have a repeat scan after every two cycles of chemotherapy.

Should all physical abnormalities seen at presentation and any abnormalities visible on plain radiology resolve during treatment (for example, after three courses of chemotherapy), a CT scan to document response at that point may be useful for evaluating the rate of response and the number of cycles of treatment received as "consolidation." Constitutional symptoms should be assessed as well as those related to treatment toxicity, and performance status recorded. Abnormal laboratory results, such as a raised ESR and/or LDH, must also be monitored with every cycle of therapy. Gallium scans and/or PET scans may also be performed during active treatment and may have prognostic significance (78).

Definition of Treatment Outcome

One month following the completion of planned therapy (or sooner if the outcome is unfavorable), response should be documented on the basis of the clinical situation and the results of repeated imaging investigations that were abnormal at presentation, supplemented by bone marrow and tissue biopsy where appropriate. Following mantle-field irradiation, a reassessment CT scan of the chest should be postponed for 1 to 3 months. It is worthwhile noting that after radiation therapy, the regression of disease may be slow and that residual fibrotic mass may still be visible on a chest radiograph or CT images. Further investigations may be necessary to define the nature of any residual abnormality. These include the use of gallium scanning (79,80), MRI, or, in unusual or highly suspicious lesions, a possible rebiopsy.

MRI also gives excellent anatomic details, but has not been demonstrated to be superior to CT. It may be possible to predict response and size of residual mediastinal mass by measuring sequential T2 signal intensity following commencement of therapy (81). Whole-body PET scanning with fluorine-18-deoxyglucose is a promising tool in evaluating disease regression (80,82), although longer follow-up of these of studies is necessary to confirm the early impressions (see chapter by Castellino and Podoloff).

The criteria for reporting response to therapy are as follows:

Complete Remission

The patient has no clinical, radiologic, or other evidence of Hodgkin's disease. Changes consistent with the effects of previous therapy (i.e., radiation fibrosis) may be present.

Complete Remission (Unconfirmed/Uncertain)

This category [CR(u)] of response has been included to denote patients in whom remission status is unclear, as the patient is otherwise in good health with no clinical evidence of Hodgkin's disease, but some radiologic abnormality, not absolutely consistent with the effects of therapy, persists at a site of previous disease (Table 8). Implicit in this designation is considerable uncertainty about the significance of such abnormalities, it being well known that abnormal widening of the mediastinum or architectural distortion of lymphographic studies may persist for many years without therapy and without evidence of recurrent Hodgkin's disease (83,84).

Attempts to resolve the dilemma of persistent disease versus residual anatomic distortion not indicative of Hodgkin's disease should include investigations such as radiologic imaging, MRI, and gallium scanning. Within the bounds of acceptable morbidity, pathologic examination may be appropriate, although the difficulties of sampling artifacts are acknowledged. Unusual or highly suspicious lesions should be rebiopsied. Persistent elevation of the ESR, while not diagnostic of active Hodgkin's disease, is an indication for very close surveillance (85,86). Guidelines for criteria used to assign response category based on measurements of residual abnormalities on posttreatment CT scans have been published (87) (see Table 8).

TABLE 8. *Criteria used to assign CR, CR(u), and PR Categories from posttreatment computed tomography scan*

Anatomic site	CR	CR(u)	PR[a]
Thorax (cm)	<1.0	1.1–2.0	>2.1
Retrocrural (cm)	<0.6	0.7–1.6	>1.7
Abdomen (cm)	<1.5	1.6–2.5	>2.6

[a]Less than 50% of original nodal mass.

CR, complete remission; CR(u), unconfirmed/uncertain complete remission; PR, partial remission.

From ref. 87.

Partial Remission

Partial remission is defined as a decrease by at least 50% in the sum of the products of the largest perpendicular diameters of all measurable lesions. There should also be an objective improvement in nonevaluable but clinically evident malignant disease, resolution of B symptoms, and no new lesions.

Progressive Disease

Progressive disease is defined as a 25% or more increase in the size of a least one measurable lesion, or the appearance of a new lesion, or recurrence of B symptoms that cannot otherwise be explained.

RECOMMENDATIONS FOR FOLLOW-UP AFTER TREATMENT

Following completion of therapy, restaging, and documentation of response, it is recommended that patients be seen at 3-month intervals during the first and second year of therapy, 4-month intervals in the third year, 6-month intervals in the fourth and fifth years, and annually thereafter. The frequency and type of radiologic studies should reflect the initial sites of disease. Appropriate investigation should accompany any concern about symptoms or signs of possible recurrent disease. A full blood count, ESR, biochemical profile, and chest radiograph should be performed at each visit. The use and frequency of complicated and expensive imaging studies such as CT scanning and gallium scanning is variable, and perhaps controversial, and is the subject of ongoing studies. An assessment of long-term complications of therapy should be undertaken at regular intervals and their presence or absence documented.

Although the Cotswolds committee stated the follow-up arrangements as outlined, a retrospective study of hospital notes to examine the effectiveness of routine clinical review in detecting relapse after treatment for Hodgkin's disease questioned such arrangements (88). The cohort consisted of 210 patients with Hodgkin's disease recruited to a chemotherapy protocol between 1984 and 1990 who had achieved a complete or partial remission following treatment. The 210 patients generated 2,512 outpatient reviews, and 37 relapses were detected. Thirty relapses were diagnosed in patients who described symptoms which in 15 cases had resulted in an earlier appointment being arranged. In only four cases was relapse detected as a result of routine physical examination or investigation of a patient who showed no symptoms. The report concluded that relapse of Hodgkin's disease after treatment is usually detected as a result of the investigation of symptoms, rather than by routine screening of asymptomatic patients. It was therefore proposed that the frequency of routine follow-up visits should be reduced, and greater emphasis placed on patient education. This should underline the importance of symptoms and encourage patients to arrange an earlier appointment should these develop.

Another retrospective study examined the cost and benefit of routine follow-up evaluation in 709 patients treated with radiotherapy for early-stage Hodgkin's disease (89). The authors concluded that the majority of relapses occurred within 5 years of treatment, and were usually identified by the patient's history and routine physical examination. Chest radiographs were useful, particularly during the first 3 years of follow-up, but routine abdominal radiograms, full blood counts, and other laboratory tests rarely led to the detection of recurrence.

Routine follow-up, however, is also important for assessment of long-term complications of therapy, as well as for screening for possible recurrence. It is therefore possible to suggest that a full blood count would be useful in revealing abnormalities consistent with bone marrow dysfunction, for example. Chest radiograph should be considered at each annual visit after 5 years, and annual mammography could be undertaken at 8 to 10 years after treatment. Women are also advised to undergo annual cervical smears. It would also be appropriate to consider routine testing of thyroid function, with a total thyroxine (T_4) and thyroid-stimulating hormone (TSH) level, again at least on an annual basis, and particularly for those patients who received mantle-field irradiation or any other field involving the neck.

RECOMMENDATIONS FOR STAGING OF RECURRENT DISEASE

All staging classification systems both past and present refer only to the extent of disease at the first presentation of the illness. Patients with possible recurrent disease should be evaluated in much the same way. A detailed history, with particular emphasis on symptoms, previous symptoms, the stage of illness, and past treatment, should be recorded in detail, with particular reference to doses of chemotherapy received and dates of delivery. This is especially important for anthracycline-based combinations. Special note should be made of any toxicities experienced during treatment, and residual effects that may have persisted. A thorough clinical examination should be performed, again recording (with measurements) sites of nodal involvement.

Investigations should be undertaken in line with those recommended by the Cotswolds committee (31) (see Table 6), together with review of previous radiology and previous histology (including lymph node and bone marrow biopsies). A cardiac assessment may also be required in those patients who have previously received anthracycline-based chemotherapy and/or mantle-field irradiation. Although the Cotswolds staging notation (and indeed the Ann Arbor) applies only to presenting stage, it is often used at recurrence as a shorthand to document the extent of recurrent disease. The UICC TNM system (1) suggests the use of the prefix *r* for this purpose when patients are staged after a disease-free interval.

REFERENCES

1. Sobin LH, Wittekind CH, eds. *UICC TNM classification of malignant tumours,* 5th ed. New York: Wiley-Liss, 1997.
2. Hodgkin T. On some morbid appearances of the absorbent glands and spleen. *Med Chir Trans* 1832;17:68.

2a. Craigie D. *Elements of general and pathological anatomy.* Edinburgh: Adam Black, 1928.

3. Wilks S. Cases of enlargement of the lymphatic glands and spleen (or Hodgkin's disease), with remarks. *Guy's Hosp Rep* 1865;11:56.
4. Trousseau A. De l'adénie. *Clin Med L'Hôtel Dieu Paris* 1865;3:555.
5. Gowers WR. Hodgkin's disease. In: Reynolds JR, ed. *A system of medicine.* London: Macmillan, 1879:306.
6. Bright R. Observations on abdominal tumours and intumescence. *Guy's Hosp Rep* 1838;3:401.
7. Reed DM. On the pathological changes in Hodgkin's disease, with especial reference to tuberculosis. *Johns Hopkins Hosp Rep* 1902;10:133.
8. Ziegler K. *Die hodgkinsche krankheit.* Jena: Gustav Fischer, 1911.
9. Longcope WT, McAlpin KR. Hodgkin's disease. *Oxford Med* 1920;4 (1):1.
10. Jackson H Jr, Parker F Jr. Hodgkin's disease. I. General considerations. *N Engl J Med* 1944;230:1.
11. Jackson H. Jr, Parker F. Jr. Hodgkin's disease. II. Pathology. *N Engl J Med* 1944;231:35.
12. Craver LF. Hodgkin's disease. In: Tice F, ed. *Practice of medicine*, vol 5. Hagerstown, MD: WF Pryor, 1951:152.
13. Peters MV. A study of survivals in Hodgkin's disease treated radiologically. *Am J Roentgenol* 1950;63:299.
14. Peters MV, Middlemiss KCH. A study of Hodgkin's disease treated by irradiation. *Am J Roentgenol* 1958;79:114.
15. Kaplan HS, Bagshaw MA, Rosenberg SA. Présentation de protocoles d'essai radiothérapeutiques des lymphomes malins de l'Université de Stanford. *Nouv Rev Fr Hematol* 1964;4:95.
16. Tubiana M. Hodgkin's disease: historical perspective and clinical presentation. *Baillieres Clin Haematol* 1996;9(3):503.
17. Rosenberg SA. Report of the committee on the staging of Hodgkin's disease. *Cancer Res* 1966;26:1310.
18. Petersen GR, Milham S Jr. Hodgkin's disease mortality and occupational exposure to wood. *J Natl Cancer Inst* 1974;53:957.
19. Musshoff K, Renemann H, Boutis L, Afkham J. Extranodular lymphogranulomatosis—diagnosis, therapy and prognosis in two different types of organ involvement. Contribution to the phase classification of Hodgkin's disease. *Fortschr Geb Rontgentstr Nuklearmed* 1968;109: 776–786.
20. Rosenberg SA, Kaplan HS. Hodgkin's disease and other malignant lymphomas. *Calif Med* 1970;113:23.
21. Rosenberg SA, Boiron M, DeVita VT Jr, et al. Report of the committee on Hodgkin's disease staging procedures. *Cancer Res* 1971;31:1862.
22. Carbone PP, Kaplan HS, Musshoff K, et al. Report of the Committee on Hodgkin's Disease Staging Classification. *Cancer Res* 1971;31:1860.
23. Tubiana M, Attié E, Flamant R, Gerard-Marchant R, Hayat M. Prognostic factors in 454 cases of Hodgkin's disease. *Cancer Res* 1971;31:1801.

24. Gilbert R. Radiotherapy in Hodgkin's disease (malignant granulomatosis): anatomic and clinical foundations; governing principles; results. *Am J Roentgenol* 1939;41:198.
25. Peters MV, Alison RE, Bush RS. Natural history of Hodgkin's disease as related to staging. *Cancer* 1966;19:308.
26. Kaplan HS. The radical radiotherapy of regionally localized Hodgkin's disease. *Radiology* 1962;78:553.
27. Smithers DW, Lillicrap SC, Barnes A. Patterns of lymph node involvement in relation to hypotheses about the modes of spread of Hodgkin's disease. *Cancer* 1974;34:1179.
28. Rosenberg SA, Kaplan HS. Evidence for an orderly progression in the spread of Hodgkin's disease. *Cancer Res* 1966;26:1225.
29. Kaplan HS. On the natural history, treatment and prognosis of Hodgkin's disease. In: *Harvey Lectures 1968–69*. New York: Academic Press, 1970:215.
30. Mauch PM, Kalish LA, Kadin M, Coleman CN, Osteen R, Hellman S. Patterns of presentation of Hodgkin disease. *Cancer* 1993;71:2062.
31. Lister TA, Crowther D, Sutcliffe SB, et al. Report of a committee convened to discuss the evaluation and staging of patients with Hodgkin's disease: Cotswolds Meeting. *J Clin Oncol* 1989;7:1630.
32. Desser RK, Golomb HM, Ultmann JE, et al. Prognostic classification of Hodgkin' disease in pathological stage III, based on anatomic considerations. *Blood* 1977;49:883.
33. Specht L. Prognostic factors in Hodgkin's disease. *Cancer Treat Rev* 1991;18:21.
34. Specht L. Prognostic factors in Hodgkin's disease. *Semin Radiat Oncol* 1996;6:146.
35. Mauch P, Goodman R, Hellman S. The significance of mediastinal involvement in early stage Hodgkin's disease. *Cancer* 1978;42:1039.
36. Tubiana M, Henry-Amar M, van der Werf-Messing B, et al. A multivariate analysis of prognostic factors in early stage Hodgkin's disease. *Int J Radiat Oncol Biol Phys* 1985;11:23.
37. Henry-Amar M, Somers R. Survival outcome after Hodgkin's disease: a report from the international data base on Hodgkin's disease. *Semin Oncol* 1991;17:758.
38. Kaplan HS. *Hodgkin's disease,* 2nd ed. Cambridge, MA: Harvard University Press, 1980.
39. Pel PK. Zur Symptomatologie der sorgenannten Pseudoleukämie. II. Pseudoleukämie oder chronisches Rückfallsfieber? *Berl Klin Wehnschr* 1887;24:644.
40. Ebstein W von. Das chronische Rückfallsfieber, eine neu Infectionskrankheit. *Berl Klin Wehnschr* 1887;24:565.
41. Gobbi PG, Cavalli C, Gendarini A, et al. Reevaluation of prognostic significance of symptoms in Hodgkin's disease. *Cancer* 1985;56:2874.
42. Newbold PCH. Skin markers of malignancy. *Arch Dermatol* 1970;102: 680.
43. Edwards CL, Hayes RL. Tumor scanning with 67Ga citrate. *J Nucl Med* 1969;10:103.
44. Devizzi L, Maffioli L, Bonfante V, et al. Comparison of gallium scan, computed tomography, and magnetic resonance in patients with mediastinal Hodgkin's disease. *Ann Oncol* 1997;8(suppl 1):53.
45. Bogart JA, Chung CT, Mariados NF, et al. The value of gallium imaging after therapy for Hodgkin's disease. *Cancer* 1998;82:754.
46. Macintyre EA, Vaughan Hudson B, Linch DC, Vaughan Hudson G, Jelliffe AM. The value of staging bone marrow trephine biopsy in Hodgkin's disease. *Eur J Haematol* 1987;39:66.
47. Howard MR, Taylor PRA, Lucraft HH, Taylor MJ, Proctor SJ. Bone marrow examination in newly-diagnosed Hodgkin's disease: current practice in the United Kingdom. *Br J Cancer* 1995;71:210.
48. Munker R, Hasenclever D, Brosteanu O, Hiller E, Diehl V. Bone marrow involvement in Hodgkin's disease: an analysis of 135 consecutive cases. *J Clin Oncol* 1995;13:403.
49. Chao NJ, Nademanee AP, Long GD, et al. Importance of bone marrow cytogenetic evaluation before autologous bone marrow transplantation for Hodgkin's disease. *J Clin Oncol* 1991;9:1575.
50. Gallagher CJ, White FE, Tucker AE, et al. The role of computerised tomography in the diagnosis of intrathoracic lymphoma. *Br J Cancer* 1984;49:621.
51. Hopper KD, Diehl LF, Lesar M, Barnes M, Granger E, Baumann J. Hodgkin's disease: clinical utility of CT in initial staging and treatment. *Radiology* 1988;169:17.
52. Rostock RA, Giangreco A, Wharam MD, Lenhard R, Siegelman SS, Order SE. CT scan modification in the treatment of mediastinal Hodgkin's disease. *Cancer* 1982;49:2267.
53. Rostock RA, Siegelman SS, Lenhard RE, Wharam MD, Order SE. Thoracic CT scanning for mediastinal Hodgkin's disease: results and therapeutic implications. *Int J Radiat Oncol Biol Phys* 1983;9:1451.
54. Blackledge G, Best JJ, Crowther D, Isherwood I. Computed tomography (CT) in the staging of patients with Hodgkin's disease: a report on 136 patients. *Clin Radiol* 1980;31:143.
55. Castellino R, Hoppe RT, Blank N. Computed tomography, lymphangiography and staging laparotomy: correlation in initial staging of Hodgkin's disease. *Am J Radiol* 1984;143:37.
56. Castellino RA, Billingham M, Dorfman RF. Lymphographic accuracy in Hodgkin's disease and malignant lymphoma with a note on the "reactive" lymph node as a cause of most false-positive lymphograms. *Invest Radiol* 1974;9:155.
57. Mansfield CM, Fabian C, Jones S, et al. Comparison of lymphangiography and computed tomographic scanning in evaluating abdominal disease in stages III and IV Hodgkin's disease. *Cancer* 1990; 66:2295.
58. Kaplan HS, Dorfman RF, Nelsen TS, Rosenberg SA. Staging laparotomy and splenectomy in Hodgkin's disease: analysis of indications and patterns of involvement in 285 consecutive, unselected patients. *Natl Cancer Inst Monogr* 1973;36:291.
59. Richards MA, Webb JAW, Reznek RH, et al. Detection of spread of malignant lymphoma to the liver by low field strength magnetic resonance imaging. *Br Med J* 1986;293:1126.
60. Weinreb JC, Brateman L, Maravilla KR. Magnetic resonance imaging of hepatic lymphoma. *Am J Roentgenol* 1984;143:1211.
61. Weissleder R, Stark DD, Elizondo G, et al. MRI of hepatic lymphoma. *Magn Reson Imaging* 1988;6:675.
62. Munker R, Stengel A, Stäbler A, Hiller E, Brehm G. Diagnostic accuracy of ultrasound and computed tomography in the staging of Hodgkin's disease. *Cancer* 1995;76:1460.
63. Weissleder R, Elizondo E, Stark DD, et al. The diagnosis of splenic lymphoma by MR imaging: value of superparamagnetic iron oxide. *Am J Roentgenol* 1989;152:175.
64. Sweet DL Jr, Kinnealey A, Ultmann JE. Hodgkin's disease: problems of staging. *Cancer* 1978;42:957.
65. Braunstein EM. Hodgkin's disease of bone: radiographic correlation with the histological classification. *Radiology* 1980;137:643.
66. Braunstein EM, White SJ. Non-Hodgkin lymphoma of bone. *Radiology* 1980;135:59.
67. Grann V, Pool JL, Mayer K. Comparative study of bone marrow aspiration and biopsy in patients with neoplastic disease. *Cancer* 1966;19: 1898.
68. Rosenberg SA. Hodgkin's disease of the bone marrow. *Cancer Res* 1971;31:1733.
69. O'Carroll DL, McKenna RW, Brunning RD. Bone marrow manifestations of Hodgkin's disease. *Cancer* 1976;38:1717.
70. Leibenhaut M, Hoppe R, Efron B, et al. Prognostic indicators of laparotomy findings in clinical stage I–II supradiaphragmatic Hodgkin's disease. *J Clin Oncol* 1989;7:81.
71. Mauch P, Larson D, Osteen R, et al. Prognostic factors for positive surgical staging in patients with Hodgkin's disease. *J Clin Oncol* 1990;8:257.
72. Sombeck MD, Mendenhall NP, Kaude JV, Torres GM, Million RR. Correlation of lymphangiography, computed tomography, and laparotomy in the staging of Hodgkin's disease. *Int J Radiat Oncol Biol Phys* 1993; 15:567.
73. Crnkovich MJ, Hoppe RT, Rosenberg SA. Stage IIB Hodgkin's disease: the Stanford experience. *J Clin Oncol* 1986;4:472.
74. Crnkovich MJ, Leopold K, Hoppe RT, Mauch PM. Stage I to IIB Hodgkin's disease: the combined experience at Stanford University and the Joint Center for Radiation Therapy. *J Clin Oncol* 1987;5:1041.
75. Thar TL, Million RR, Hausner RJ, McKetty MHB. Hodgkin's disease, Stages I and II. *Cancer* 1979;43:1101.
76. Fabian C, Mansfield C, Dahlberg S, et al. Low-dose involved field radiation after chemotherapy in advanced Hodgkin's disease. *Ann Intern Med* 1994;120:903.
77. Bartlett NL, Rosenberg SA, Hoppe RT, Hancock SL, Horning SJ. Brief chemotherapy, Stanford V, and adjuvant radiotherapy for bulky or advanced-stage Hodgkin's disease: a preliminary report. *J Clin Oncol* 1995;13:1080.
78. Hagemeister FB, Purugganan R, Podoloff DA, et al. The gallium scan predicts relapse in patients with Hodgkin's disease treated with combined modality therapy. *Ann Oncol* 1994;5(suppl 2):59.

79. Salloum E, Brandt DS, Caride VJ, et al. Gallium scans in the management of patients with Hodgkin's disease: a study of 101 patients. *J Clin Oncol* 1997;15:518.
80. Bangerter M, Griesshammer M, Binder T, et al. New diagnostic imaging procedures in Hodgkin's disease. *Ann Oncol* 1996;7(suppl 4):55.
81. Nyman RS, Rehn SM, Glimelius BL, Hagberg HE, Hemmingsson AL, Sundstrom CJ. Residual mediastinal masses in Hodgkin disease: prediction of size with MR imaging. *Radiology* 1989;170:435.
82. Hoh CK, Glaspy J, Rosen P, et al. Whole-body FDG-PET imaging for staging of Hodgkin's disease and lymphoma. *J Nucl Med* 1997; 38:343.
83. Jochelson M, Mauch P, Balikian J, et al. The significance of the residual mediastinal mass in treated Hodgkin's disease. *J Clin Oncol* 1985; 3:637.
84. Radford JA, Cowan RA, Flanagan M, et al. The significance of residual mediastinal abnormality on the chest radiograph following treatment for Hodgkin's disease. *J Clin Oncol* 1988;6:940.
85. Friedman S, Henry-Amar M, Cosset JM, et al. Evolution of erythrocyte sedimentation rate as predictor of early relapse in post therapy early-stage Hodgkin's disease. *J Clin Oncol* 1988;6:596.
86. Henry-Amar M, Friedman S, Hayat M, et al. Erythrocyte sedimentation rate predicts early relapse and survival in early-stage Hodgkin's disease. The EORTC Lymphoma Cooperative Group. *Ann Intern Med* 1991; 114:361.
87. Radford JA, Crowther D Rohatiner AZS, et al. Results of a randomized trial comparing MVPP chemotherapy with a hybrid regime, ChlVPP/EVA, in the initial treatment of Hodgkin's disease. *J Clin Oncol* 1995;13:2379.
88. Radford JA, Eardley A, Woodman C, Crowther D. Follow up policy after treatment for Hodgkin's disease: too many clinic visits and routine tests? A review of hospital records. *Br Med J* 1997;314:343.
89. Torrey MJ, Poen JC, Hoppe RT. Detection of relapse in early-stage Hodgkin's disease: role of routine follow-up studies. *J Clin Oncol* 1997;15:1123.
90. Kaplan HS, Rosenberg SA. The treatment of Hodgkin's disease. *Med Clin North Am* 1966;50:1591.

Hodgkin's Disease, edited by P. M. Mauch,
J. O. Armitage, V. Diehl, R. T. Hoppe, and L. M. Weiss.
Lippincott Williams & Wilkins, Philadephia ©1999.

CHAPTER 16

Diagnostic Radiology and Nuclear Medicine Imaging in Hodgkin's Disease

Ronald A. Castellino and Donald A. Podoloff

Diagnostic radiology (including interventional radiology) and nuclear medicine studies play a major and at times pivotal role in the management of patients with Hodgkin's disease. These studies provide information that leads to a more precise staging of disease at the time of initial diagnosis, thereby influencing decisions about treatment planning, periodic monitoring of sites of known disease during treatment to judge efficacy of therapy, surveillance of the patient following treatment to detect relapse, and restaging should a relapse be detected. Medical and radiation oncologists, while well acquainted with these various imaging modalities, should keep the following points in mind when ordering diagnostic imaging tests:

1. Detection versus delineation of disease: Frequently, the simple detection of disease site(s) in various anatomic regions, or nodal versus extranodal locations, is sufficient for determining stage and therefore treatment. At other times, however, a more precise delineation of the extent of disease at specific anatomic sites is needed, as for example radiation therapy treatment planning and determination of bulky disease.
2. Impact on management: In general, an imaging test should provide information that contributes to the clarity of management decisions, be it at the initial staging or subsequently. This is equally true if the result is positive (disease is found) or negative (no evidence of disease), either because it provides new information or is simply confirmatory. Since the oncologist has in-depth knowledge about known patterns of disease at presentation as well as patterns of relapse, imaging studies are most useful when directed at sites that have a high probability of involvement, or at sites where the detection of disease would affect management.
3. Baseline imaging studies. Comparison to prior studies, whether obtained at the time of initial staging or following treatment, can be most helpful when interpreting a subsequent study. This not only facilitates the detection of an interval change but also provides information about possible etiology.
4. Accuracy of the imaging study. Determining the accuracy of imaging tests, as well as other clinical assessments, requires comparison with some type of gold standard, ideally histopathologic evaluation of the anatomic site/structure being evaluated. When staging laparotomies were routinely performed in newly diagnosed Hodgkin's disease, the derived information was useful in assessing the accuracy of the clinical examination as well as imaging studies for disease below the diaphragm. However, staging laparotomies have not been routinely performed for almost two decades, so that currently the gold standard is some type of indirect assessment, such as comparison with other clinical or imaging information, or clinical follow-up. The following terms, illustrated in Figure 1, are used to define accuracy (1):
   a. *Sensitivity* is the ability of a test to correctly identify disease when present.
   b. *Specificity* is the ability of a test to correctly identify the absence of disease when no disease is present.
   c. *Positive predictive value* is how often the test is correct when interpreted as positive.
   d. *Negative predictive value* is how often the test is correct when interpreted as negative.
   e. *Overall accuracy* is the proportion of correct test results in the total number of tests.
5. Because imaging studies are subjectively interpreted, and because the findings and therefore interpreta-

R. A. Castellino: Department of Radiology, Cornell University Medical College and Memorial Sloan-Kettering Cancer Center, New York, New York.

D. A. Podoloff: Department of Nuclear Medicine, Division of Diagnostic Imaging, M. D. Anderson Cancer Center, University of Texas, Houston, Texas.

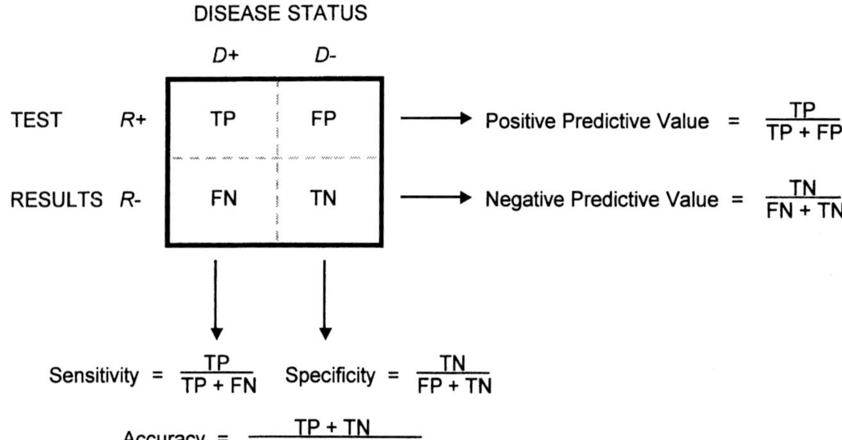

FIG. 1. Bayesian 2 × 2 classification table of test results compared with a gold standard of diagnosis. TP, true positive; FP, false positive; FN, false negative; TN, true negative; D, disease status; R, test result. (From ref. 47.)

tions are not always clearly negative or positive, results are appropriately stated/implied as positive, probably positive, indeterminate, probably negative, or negative. For this reason, receiver operator characteristic (ROC) curves (1) have been developed to evaluate imaging studies, which plot sensitivity and specificity pairs (Fig. 2).

6. Just as there are variations in access to technology and therapeutic expertise in the oncology community, there likewise are variations in the diagnostic radiology and nuclear medicine community regarding access to state-of-the-art imaging equipment and, importantly, the level of expertise of the radiologists and nuclear medicine physicians who perform, supervise, and interpret these studies. When interpreting the literature that addresses accuracy of imaging studies, care must be taken to ensure that the comparative studies are performed with the same level of equipment and imaging expertise for each modality and that the clinical design ensures an unbiased, objective result. Finally, similar to other aspects of medicine, diagnostic imaging is continually evolving, not only in refinements of existing technologies, but also in the introduction of new forms of image acquisition.

IMAGING MODALITIES

Diagnostic radiology and nuclear medicine images are generated by the interaction of different forms of energy with the patient, with capture of this energy by some sort of detector to enable viewing. The most common form of energy used in this setting is the x-ray, which describes the ionizing electromagnetic radiations (photons) that are emitted when electrons interact with matter. X-ray–gen-

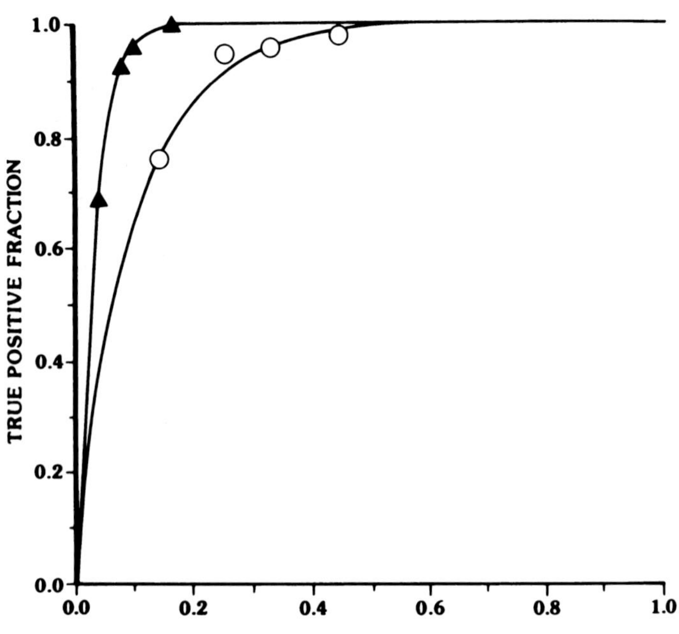

FIG. 2. Receiver operator characteristic (ROC) curves for comparing two imaging tests. The more accurate test is shown by the curve with the higher sensitivity and lower false-positive ratio (i.e., the curve closest to the left horizontal and upper vertical axes). (From ref. 47.)

erated medical images rely on differences in absorption (attenuation coefficients) of the photons caused by interactions with matter of different atomic number and the detection of the transmitted photons. The detection devices include radiographic films (for general plain film radiography), fluorescent intensifying screens (fluoroscopy), and electronic detection devices (computed tomography [CT] and digital radiography).

Nuclear medicine studies depend on the detection of the spontaneous decay of unstable elements, which produces photons called alpha, beta, or gamma rays. Medical ultrasound images are produced by pulsing a high-frequency sound wave into the body and detecting the reflected sound waves, based on differences in acoustical impedance between various tissues and tissue interfaces. Magnetic resonance (MR) images are generated by detection of radio-frequency signals from within the body, as described in more detail below. These imaging modalities share the common characteristic of detection of energy emitted from within the body, as compared to x-ray–generated medical images, which are formed by detection of energy transmitted through the body.

X-ray Imaging

General radiography (plain films) continues to represent the majority of all types of medical imaging, in large part due to the lower cost of equipment and short procedure time (with the exception of positive contrast studies such as barium gastrointestinal tract examinations and excretory urograms). Although not as highly operator dependent as more complex cross-section imaging studies, nonetheless the diagnostic content of these examinations is critically dependent on obtaining a technically optimal study. Attention to radiographic factors, patient positioning, and film processing cannot be overemphasized.

X-ray CT scanning has had a major impact on the entire field of oncologic imaging, including evaluating patients with Hodgkin's disease. Substantial improvements in technology over the past decade have produced superior diagnostic images. The recent introduction of helical/spiral CT scanning permits image acquisition during shorter periods of time, which minimizes artifacts or misregistrations from physiologic motion, and ensures that the entire volume is imaged, avoiding potential loss of information by differences in slice sampling and/or motion between acquisition of adjacent images. Careful selection by the technologists and radiologists of the scanning parameters, slice thickness and intervals, and other radiographic factors is necessary for an optimized CT scan.

Administration of IV contrast media during CT scanning is commonly performed, primarily to increase the ability to detect abnormalities within solid organs, such as the liver and spleen. It is also used to further investigate the etiology of mass lesions based on an assessment of vascular supply as determined by contrast enhancement. The correct method of IV contrast media administration must be used in the diagnostic study, which should be performed with a bolus technique (preferentially with a power-assisted injector) with rapid scanning during the early phase of arterial contrast enhancement. Images obtained during a phase of contrast equilibrium can frequently mask the presence of space-occupying lesions (Fig. 3). A reasonable guide to whether the imaging study was performed during the optimal phase is the presence

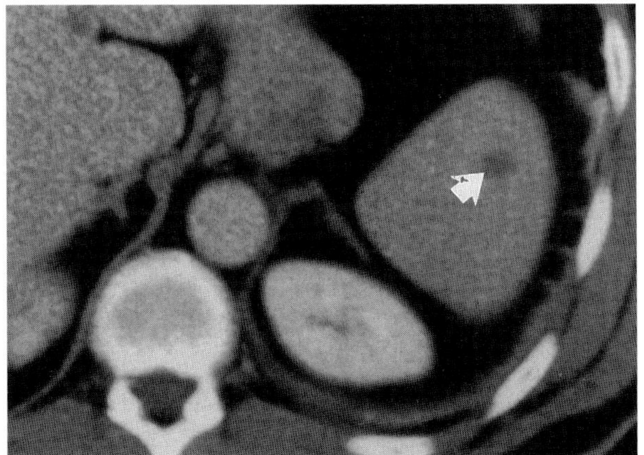

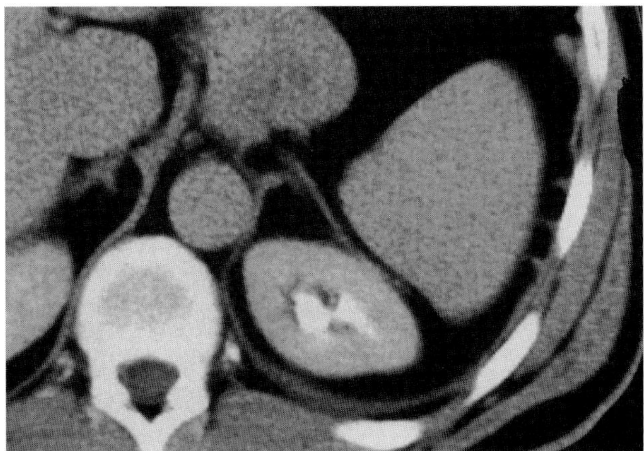

FIG. 3. A 60-year-old man with newly diagnosed Hodgkin's disease. Contrast-enhanced computed tomography (CT) scan **(A)** through the spleen demonstrates a focal, poorly defined filling defect *(arrow)* that, upon repeat scanning seven minutes later **(B)**, is no longer apparent. This is an example of a splenic lesion that becomes isointense on images performed after the bolus phase of i.v. contrast media administration. Note the early nephrogram **(A)** compared to the excretion of contrast media in the renal collecting system **(B)**, which can indicate that the scan was performed early during the vascular opacification phase.

of obvious vascular enhancement (e.g., intense demarcation of the intrahepatic, portal, and hepatic veins). If the images are obtained when there is contrast media within the renal pelvis and ureters, this suggests that the imaging was performed several minutes later than optimal.

Finally, with particular regard to patients with Hodgkin's disease, the early contrast media enhancement of the spleen is characteristically patchy, so that the spleen normally demonstrates a mottled parenchyma that could erroneously be interpreted as involvement by Hodgkin's disease. This is due to the early arterial opacification of splenic parenchyma prior to opacification of the larger venous vascular spaces within this organ. This applies not only to x-ray contrast media but also to contrast media enhancement with magnetic resonance imaging (MRI) studies utilizing gadolinium (Fig. 4).

Ultrasound

The interaction of high-frequency sound waves with tissues is complex, and can be described in terms of transmission, reflection, refraction, defraction, scattering, and absorption. These interactions in turn are influenced by the characteristics of the tissues that interact with the propagated ultrasound wave, the frequency and wavelength of the ultrasound, and the specific acoustic impedance of the various tissues. The anatomic image that is provided has unique characteristics that are often useful to further define areas of known or suspected abnormality detected on other imaging studies. Also, the real-time capabilities of ultrasound often lead to its use as the initial diagnostic imaging examination for nononcologic applications (e.g., echocardiography, static and Doppler studies of the venous system for thrombus).

Sound waves are poorly propagated through air and bone, which markedly limits application of this modality in evaluating intrathoracic structures (with the exception of the heart) and portions of the abdomen and pelvis. Furthermore, the generation of optimal diagnostic images is highly operator dependent. For this reason, ultrasound is infrequently used as the initial imaging modality in the oncologic patient population in the United States. However, in European and other countries ultrasound is used more frequently, and with relatively good results, perhaps in part related to lack of access to CT scanning.

Magnetic Resonance Imaging (MRI)

This cross-sectional and three-dimensional imaging technique is based on principles of nuclear magnetic resonance (NMR), which has long been used for chemical analysis purposes. The methodology employed for image formation is quite complex, and the various pulse sequences available to more precisely define anatomic structure and/or function contribute greatly to the power of this imaging technology. Fortunately, hydrogen not only has the greatest sensitivity to NMR compared to other biologically relevant nuclei, but it is also the most abundant atom in the body, and thus is used most frequently in developing clinical MR images. Because the

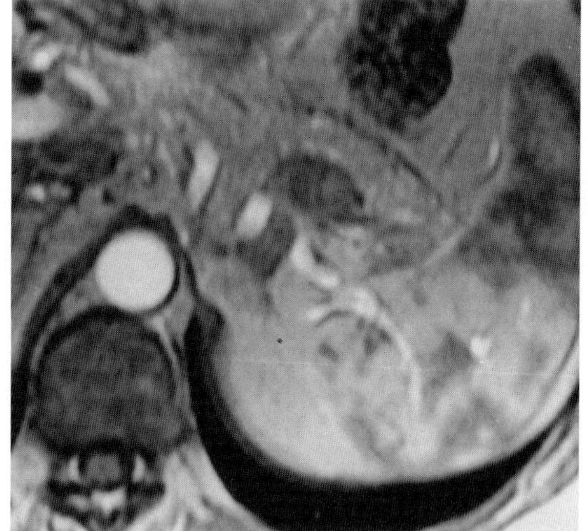

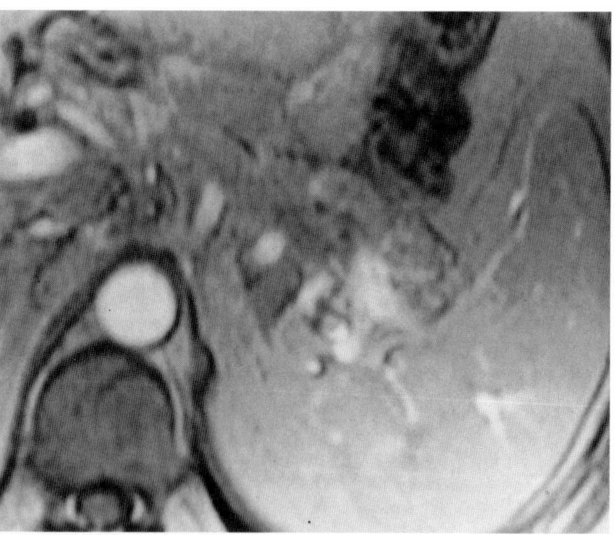

FIG. 4. A 50-year-old man with nodular sclerosing Hodgkin's disease. Magnetic resonance (MR) scan during early phase of i.v. gadolinium administration **(A)** demonstrates a markedly mottled splenic parenchyma. Repeat MR scan minutes later **(B)** demonstrates a uniformly homogeneous splenic parenchyma, due to vascular enhancement by the gadolinium of the intrasplenic vascular lakes, with a persistent single focus of decreased signal intensity *(arrow)* compatible with involvement by Hodgkin's disease. The earlier vascular phase of contrast enhancement, whether with iodinated contrast on CT studies or gadolinium on MR studies, can produce marked inhomogeneity in the splenic parenchyma due to vascular lakes, which must be differentiated from pathologic entities.

relaxation characteristics of the hydrogen proton are affected by its immediate chemical milieu, MRI is able to clearly differentiate tissues primarily composed of the hydrogen proton in water (HOH) from that in fat ($-CH_2-$), as well as from nuclei in other tissues. These differences can be manipulated by choosing the appropriate RF pulse sequence.

The resultant MR images demonstrate cross-sectional anatomic detail similar to that encountered with x-ray CT (with the exception that MRI can also display slices in coronal and sagittal planes, as well as the axial plane generated with x-ray CT). However, whereas x-ray CT consistently depicts anatomic and pathologic information in the same patient with identical levels of brightness due to the constant x-ray attenuation coefficients of these tissues, the relative brightness (ranging from black, or signal void, to white) of the identical structure on MRI can greatly vary depending on the applied RF pulse signal. This leads to MR's increased capability of tissue characterization as compared to x-ray CT, a significant advantage that leads to MRI's particular adaptation in oncologic imaging as a problem solver.

Nuclear Medicine

Ever since its introduction in 1969, gallium citrate 67 (Ga 67) has generated considerable interest in evaluating patients with Hodgkin's disease (2). The reason for gallium's localization in tumors include increased permeability of tumor vessels, the large extracellular fluid space in some tumors, and binding by intracellular protein such as lactoglobulin. In the past two decades, there has been significant improvement in instrumentation and technique. At this time, Ga 67 citrate imaging with single photon emission computed tomography (SPECT) has been shown to be more sensitive than gallium planar imaging, especially in the middle and anterior mediastinum (3). Whole body images must be acquired with the camera as close to the patient as possible at a speed that is sufficient to achieve 3 to 4 million counts in the total image. Often this will take 20 to 30 minutes. Although not generally used to up- or downstage patients with Hodgkin's disease, there are anecdotal reports in the literature indicating that Ga 67 citrate imaging may be useful. More importantly, a baseline gallium scan prior to therapy is necessary in order to judge response once therapy is initiated.

One must be alert to potential pitfalls in gallium scan interpretation. There is a high proportion of patients with bilateral submandibular, bilateral hilar, and diffuse pulmonary uptake during and after therapy. The necessity for anatomic correlation of the gallium scan cannot be overemphasized. As an example, the position of loops of bowel, whether or not an anatomic abnormality is seen on CT, and the presence or absence of hilar adenopathy are of critical importance in interpreting gallium scans. False-positive gallium scans with bilateral hilar activity are always associated with negative chest x-rays and normal CT scans. Nonspecific uptake also occurs in infection and inflammation; additionally, false-positive results have been reported in sarcoidosis, thymic hyperplasia, thyrotoxicosis, and salidanitis. Posttherapy findings include bilateral hilar, submandibular, and diffuse pulmonary uptake (4,5).

Thallium-201 chloride, Tc-99m methoxyisobutylisonitrile, and somatostatin receptor agents have all been tried in the low-grade non–gallium-avid lymphomas. These agents must be considered investigational presently and their exact role in Hodgkin's disease is not known (6,7).

Positron emission tomography (PET) imaging with 18-F-dioxyglucose (FDG) is based on detection of regional FDG uptake, which correlates with glucose metabolism, which in turn is increased in malignant tumors. The role of PET scanning in Hodgkin's disease would seem to be similar to that of gallium, although the information concerning prognosis has not yet been rigorously developed in the literature. Newman et al. (8) studied 16 patients with non-Hodgkin's lymphoma and five patients with Hodgkin's disease. Blinded, independent interpretation of PET and CT studies were followed by a direct comparison of the images. Measurement of tumor uptake of FDG was performed on positive PET scans. Fifty-four foci of abnormal uptake were detected with PET in 13 patients, and 49 corresponding sites of lymphadenopathy and/or masses were detected with CT. All sites of adenopathy seen at CT were detected at PET. Three patients with Hodgkin's disease had negative findings at abdominal PET, CT, and subsequent staging laparotomy.

INITIAL STAGING

Chest

Frontal posteroanterior (PA) and lateral chest radiographs are performed in virtually all patients with newly diagnosed Hodgkin's disease. Careful evaluation of well-performed studies provides substantial information about involvement of various lymph node sites within the thorax, as well as of lung parenchyma, detection of pleural fluid and at times the involvement of the chest wall. Numerous studies, however, have shown that CT scans of the thorax clearly detect disease at sites that, even in retrospect, cannot be seen on conventional chest radiographs, and that the precise anatomic delineation of disease is greatly enhanced (Fig. 5). Furthermore, several of these studies have indicated that such incremental information derived from routinely performed CT studies has a direct impact on patient management. Therefore, the current standard of practice is the routine performance of CT studies of the chest.

A representative study is that reported from Stanford Medical Center (9), in which data from 203 consecutive,

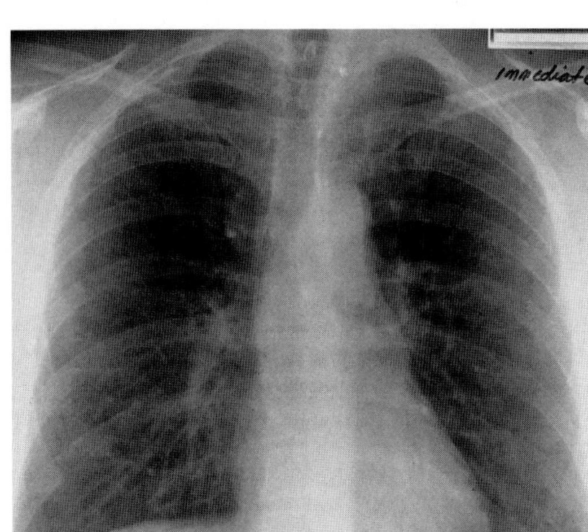

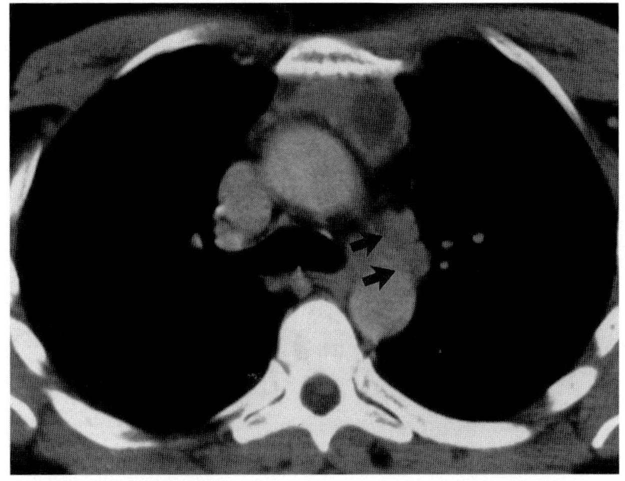

FIG. 5. A 36-year-old man with newly diagnosed nodular sclerosing Hodgkin's disease. PA chest x-ray **(A)** is unremarkable without evidence of mediastinal lymphadenopathy. Thoracic CT scan **(B)** demonstrates a prevascular nonhomogeneous mass and aortopulmonary window adenopathy *(arrows)* that, even in retrospect, was not visible on the PA chest radiograph **(A)**.

newly diagnosed patients with Hodgkin's disease underwent chest CT studies and chest radiography. Not surprisingly, CT scans demonstrated disease at specific anatomic sites that were unremarkable on chest radiography in as many as 15% of cases (Table 1). Importantly, based on this incremental information provided by the CT scans, patient management was modified in 9.4% of all patients (13.8% of those undergoing radiotherapy alone and 8.2% of those receiving combined modality therapy). Hopper and colleagues (10) performed a similar analysis of 107 cases to determine incremental data from CT studies, and then applied their findings to evaluate how patient management might be modified based on treatment protocols at other medical centers. Their analysis demonstrated an impact on management ranging from 6.5 to 62.7% of cases.

Although Ga 67 citrate imaging has been found to be most useful in the chest (specifically in the mediastinum), most feel that gallium imaging is of no benefit in initial staging in the vast majority of Hodgkin's disease patients (11). Hagemeister et al. (12) reported an overall sensitivity of only 64%, although the specificity was high at 98%, with older, single-channel gamma cameras and low-dose gallium imaging.

Devizzi et al. (13) studied 125 patients with previously untreated Hodgkin's disease in two different prospective trials. Staging procedures included Ga 67, chest and abdominal CT, and/or MRI. All three tests were performed in 53 patients at staging and in 47 at restaging. Gallium imaging at staging showed lower sensitivity than CT and MRI (90% vs. 96% and 100%, respectively). Nevertheless, by using CT and gallium scan together, the sensitivity is

TABLE 1. *Location of thoracic Hodgkin's disease at initial presentation (%) (n=203)*

	CX− CT−	CX+ CT+	CX− CT+	Change in treatment[a]
Lymph nodes				
Superior mediastinal	16	77	7	0.5
Hilar	72	21	7	1.0
Subcarinal	78	7	15	3.5
Internal mammary	95	1	4	0
Posterior mediastinal	95	2	3	1.0
Cardiophrenic angle	92	1	7	1.5
Lung parenchyma	92	8	0	0
Pleura	87	10	3	0
Pericardium	94	2	4	1.0
Chest wall	94	1	6	2.5
Any site	13	78	8	9.4

CT, computed tomography; CX, chest radiography; −, negative findings; +, positive findings.
[a]Incidence of treatment modification based on incremental CT data in total patient study (*n*=203).
From ref. 9.

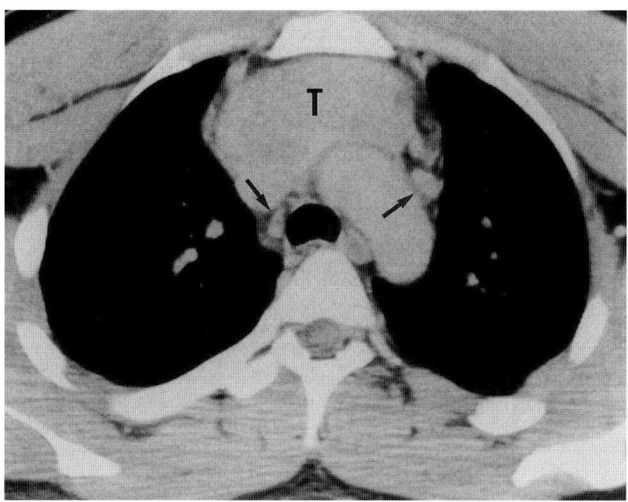

FIG. 6. A 29-year-old man with newly diagnosed nodular sclerosing Hodgkin's disease. CT scan demonstrates a prevascular mediastinal mass, with configuration and location compatible with thymus (T), as well as focal prevascular and paratracheal lymphadenopathy *(arrows)*. (Biopsy proven.)

equal to that observed with MRI (100%). They concluded that as a single technique Ga 67 imaging cannot substitute for CT or MRI in staging patients with Hodgkin's disease.

Lymph Nodes

Approximately 85% of patients with newly diagnosed Hodgkin's disease show radiographic evidence of intrathoracic lymphadenopathy at the time of initial presentation (9). When this is noted, almost invariably the superior mediastinal lymph nodes (paratracheal and/or prevascular) and/or thymus will be involved (Figs. 5B and 6). Rarely is there evidence of intrathoracic disease at other sites (lung, pleura, pericardium) without concomitant radiographic evidence of intrathoracic lymphadenopathy. Thus, from the imaging point of view, the superior mediastinal lymph nodes (and thymus) appear to be the gateway for Hodgkin's disease involving the thorax.

Lymph node sites that are particularly difficult to evaluate on chest radiography, but that are readily demonstrated on CT studies, include the subcarinal, cardiophrenic angle (14) (also called paracardiac or diaphragmatic) and internal mammary lymph node groups (Fig. 7). In addition, CT scans can evaluate lymph node groups that are external to the bony thorax, such as those in the axilla and subpectoral spaces (Fig. 8). Although enlarged axillary lymph nodes are amenable to palpation, in patients with a large body habitus CT studies can reveal enlarged axillary lymph nodes that even on repalpation are not discernible. Enlarged lymph nodes in the subpectoral region also are difficult to detect on physical examination, unless massively enlarged. Presence of disease at these sites can have implication for radiotherapy treatment planning.

Although calcification within intrathoracic lymph nodes occasionally occurs following therapy, the detection of calcification at the time of initial diagnosis prior to treatment has also been reported.

Lung

The pulmonary parenchyma and bronchial tree can become involved by direct extension from adjacent lymph node masses that infiltrate these structures (which is compatible with an E designation) or by the presence of separate, more distant foci (Fig. 7B) (compatible with stage IV disease). Mediastinal masses that demonstrate sharp interfaces between the mass and adjacent aerated lung do not involve the adjacent lung on imaging studies.

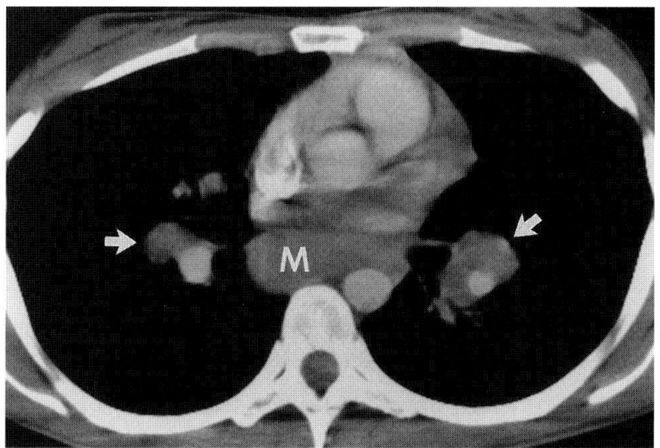

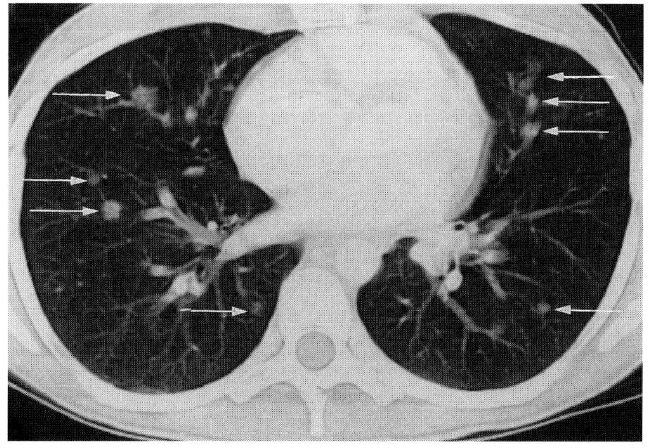

FIG. 7. A 24-year-old woman with nodular sclerosing Hodgkin's disease, stage IIB. CT scan, mediastinal window **(A)**, demonstrates a large subcarinal mass (*M*) as well as bilateral hilar lymphadenopathy *(arrows)*. Lung window **(B)** demonstrates multiple pulmonary nodules *(arrows)*, some relatively sharply defined, whereas others have ill-defined margins, which are often seen with lymphomatous involvement of pulmonary parenchyma *(arrows)*.

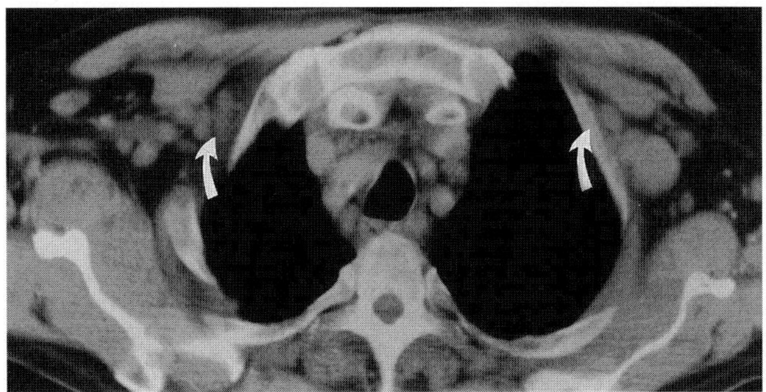

FIG. 8. A 69-year-old man with bulky axillary and mediastinal lymphadenopathy. Note also the enlarged subpectoral lymph nodes *(arrows)*.

When this interface becomes poorly defined, the differential diagnosis must consider nonspecific, subsegmental compressive atelectasis adjacent to the enlarging mass as well as local invasion (Fig. 9B).

Pulmonary parenchymal involvement can range from one or more isolated nodules to apparent complete consolidation of a segment or lobe. In general, nodular deposits have poorly defined margins as compared to the typically sharply marginated coin lesion seen in metastases from carcinomas and sarcomas. The presence of an air bronchogram within the pulmonary mass further suggests the etiology of Hodgkin's disease (Fig. 10).

Pleura and Pericardium

The presence of a pleural effusion, as noted above, is almost invariably associated with mediastinal lymphadenopathy. Since such effusions often resolve following mediastinal radiation, a reasonable assumption is that the pleural fluid is the result of lymphatic and/or venous compromise rather than intrinsic pleural disease. However, at times pleural masses are identified on imaging studies, and often have an extrapleural appearance suggesting that they may represent enlargement of intercostal lymph nodes rather than intrinsic involvement of the pleura itself. The radiographic detection of an intrinsic pleural mass is uncommon.

The presence of pericardial fluid is also almost invariably associated with mediastinal lymphadenopathy. Although such fluid could also simply be related to lymphatic and/or venous compromise, its presence is generally considered a manifestation of E disease. The rare instance when focal, nodular thickening of the pericardium is detected presumably represents true intrinsic involvement, but this is a very uncommon finding in Hodgkin's disease.

Chest Wall

Bulky mediastinal lymphadenopathy frequently abuts, and appears contiguous with, the adjacent chest wall. As long as there is no focal anatomic distortion and the intervening fascial planes appear intact, this does not imply local invasion. However, when the converse is present, intrinsic involvement of the chest wall can be diagnosed (Fig. 9A). MRI may be particularly useful in this situation, since differences in signal intensity on certain pulse sequences can identify areas of tumor infiltration independent of anatomic distortion (15). Less commonly, patients may demonstrate apparent isolated foci of chest wall involvement distant from the ever-present mediastinal mass. Whether this represents distant metastases or simply involvement of intercostal lymph nodes that have

A

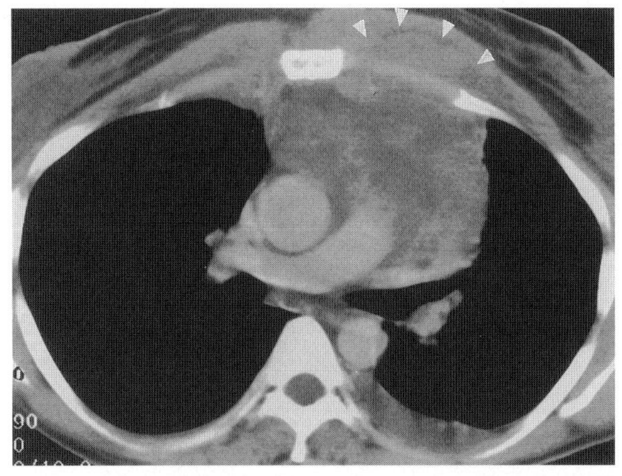

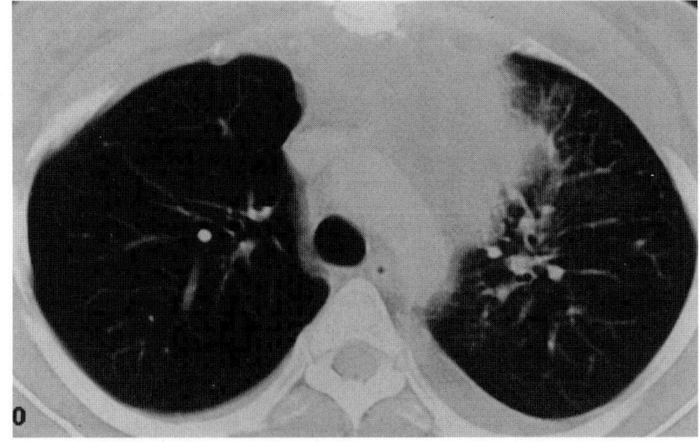

B

FIG. 9. A 37-year-old woman with newly diagnosed nodular sclerosing Hodgkin's disease. CT scan, mediastinal window **(A)**, demonstrates a large prevascular mediastinal mass that invades through the left parasternal anterior chest wall *(arrows)* and a left pleural effusion. Lung window **(B)** several centimeters cephalad demonstrates an indistinct margin between the left superior mediastinal mass and adjacent lung parenchyma, compatible with adjacent compressive subsegmental atelectasis or infiltration by tumor (compare with the sharp margin between lung and right superior mediastinal mass).

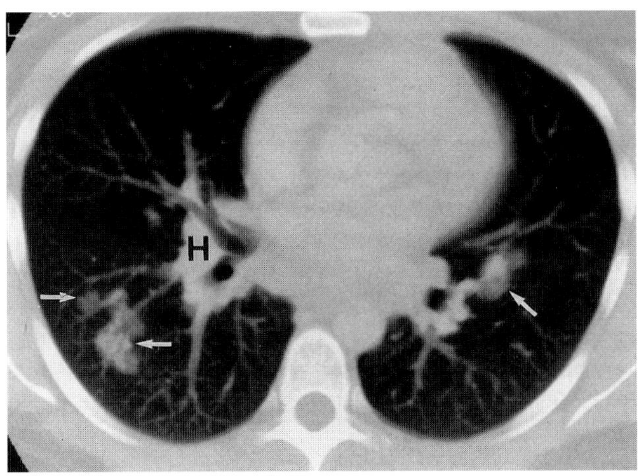

FIG. 10. A 27-year-old woman with newly diagnosed nodular sclerosing Hodgkin's disease. CT scan shows bilateral, poorly defined, pulmonary parenchymal lesions (*arrows*), with associated right hilar (H) and superior mediastinal (not shown) adenopathy. Note the air bronchograms in the right lung mass (From ref. 48.)

become enlarged and locally invaded adjacent chest wall tissues is unclear.

Comment

Numerous studies have concluded that the presence of bulky disease within the mediastinum carries a poorer prognosis, which has led to incorporation of more aggressive treatment strategies in this patient population. The determination of bulk has been based on various measurements on PA chest radiographs, although at least 27 different definitions have been proposed to make this assessment; and, it is clear that measurements derived from PA chest radiographs, from which the boundaries of the mediastinal mass can only be inferred, are imprecise when compared to the three-dimensional data available from chest CT scans (16). Nonetheless, current clinical practice relies on the definition of mediastinal bulky disease as representing a mediastinal width at the level of maximum disease divided by the maximal thoracic width (to the inside of the rib cage) of 33% or greater.

Not surprisingly, the presence of bulky mediastinal lymphadenopathy places other intrathoracic sites at greater risk for involvement. Diehl et al. (17) reported their experience in 108 consecutive, previously untreated patients with Hodgkin's disease in whom intrathoracic disease was present in 77 (71%). Although the 45 patients with bulk disease represented 58% (45/77) of all patients with intrathoracic involvement, this group of patients accounted for the majority of cases with pleural (22/26, or 85%), pericardial (24/26, or 92%), and/or chest wall (8/10, or 80%) disease.

CT scanning represents the standard for chest imaging in patients with Hodgkin's disease. Early experience (18,19) with MRI for this purpose is limited and, in general, MR scanning provides little incremental information compared to carefully performed CT studies at the time of initial staging to warrant its routine use or replacement of CT. As a problem solver, or in specific situations such as assessment of chest wall invasion (15), it appears to be useful.

Abdomen and Pelvis

Virtually all patients with newly diagnosed Hodgkin's disease undergo CT scanning of the abdomen and pelvis. Prior to the introduction of CT, lymphography was the single most reliable method to determine the presence of subdiaphragmatic disease. In experienced hands, lymphography demonstrates slightly improved sensitivity and specificity as compared to CT when evaluating the retroperitoneal lymph nodes (20). However, CT scanning has the distinct advantage of being able to evaluate lymph node sites not opacified with lymphography as well as other organs (such as the spleen and liver) (Figs. 11 and 12A). In addition, most radiologists are very comfortable in the performance and interpretation of CT studies, whereas similar skills regarding lymphography, which were never widespread, currently reside in only a few major cancer centers and other practice settings.

Information derived from the era when staging laparotomy was routinely performed on newly diagnosed patients with Hodgkin's disease was very useful in assessing the accuracy of imaging studies, specifically lymphography. Such confirmatory data has not been available since the early 1980s, so that there is limited similar experience on the accuracy of CT studies based on histopathologic confirmation. Similar data for MRI is almost not available.

There are less rigorous Ga 67 citrate studies available concerning Hodgkin's disease in the abdomen and pelvis. Because of the excretion of Ga 67 in the feces, it would be anticipated not to perform as well in the abdomen as it does in the chest or mediastinum.

Lymph Nodes

Based on laparotomy data, approximately 35% of patients with newly diagnosed Hodgkin's disease have involvement of the subdiaphragmatic lymph nodes. The orderly progression of Hodgkin's disease establishes that in patients with supradiaphragmatic presentation of disease the upper retroperitoneal lymph nodes are at highest risk for involvement; whereas, in those unusual instances of disease presentation in the inguinal nodes, the contiguous lymph node groups, i.e., those in the external and common iliac regions, are at greatest risk for involvement.

Based on staging laparotomy data, the sensitivity and specificity of lymphography when performed and interpreted by experienced radiologists are very high, with

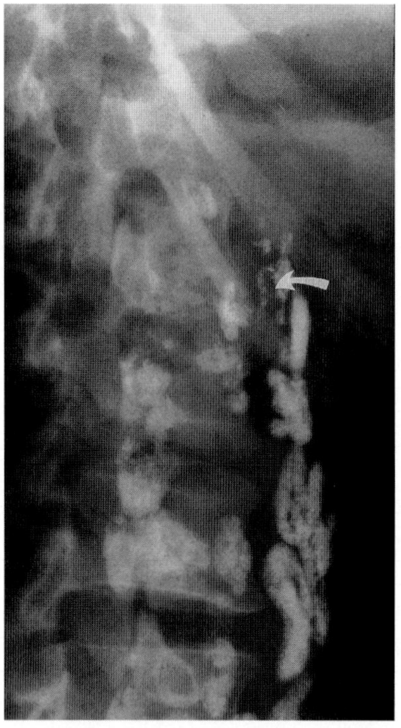

A

FIG. 11. A 22-year-old woman with newly diagnosed Hodgkin's disease. Lymphogram **(A)** is normal, except for one lymph node with irregular opacification *(arrow)* of questionable significance. CT scan through the upper abdomen **(B)** demonstrates a focal defect within splenic parenchyma, which resolved following therapy, compatible with Hodgkin's disease. CT scan in the mid-abdomen **(C)** demonstrates several focally enlarged lymph nodes *(arrows)*. Note the absence of opacification of these lymph nodes by lymphographic contrast media *(open arrow)*.

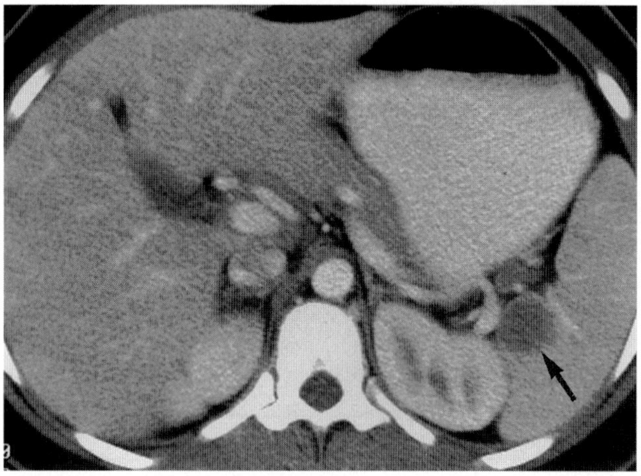

B

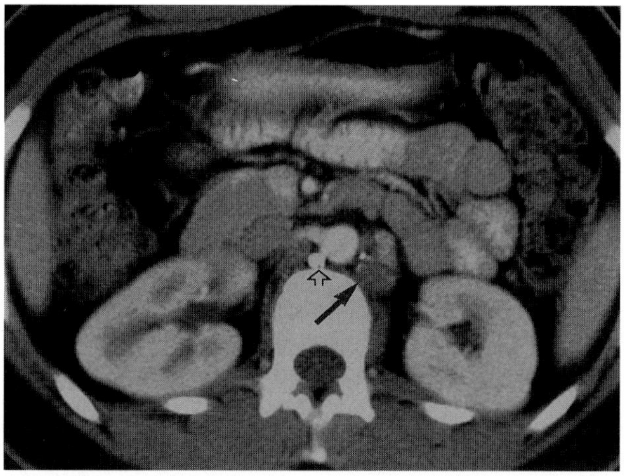

C

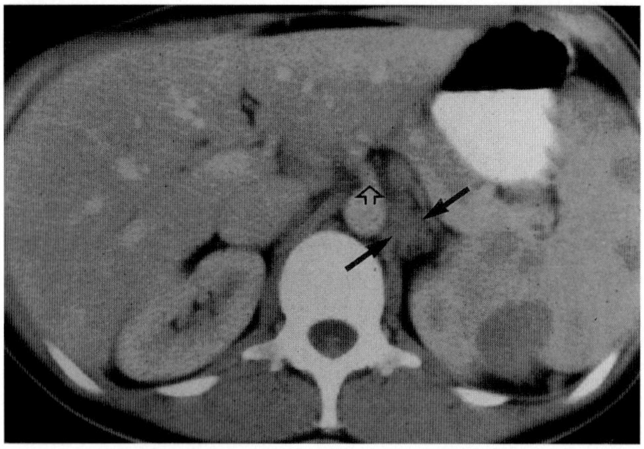

A

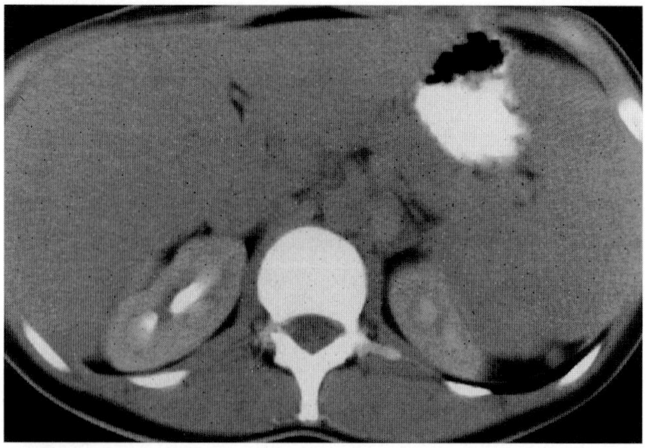

B

FIG. 12. A 30-year-old woman with newly diagnosed Hodgkin's disease. Contrast-enhanced CT scans of the upper abdomen **(A)** demonstrate focal lymphadenopathy *(arrows)* adjacent to the origin of the celiac artery *(open arrow)* and focal defects within a modestly enlarged spleen **(B)**. A repeat scan **(B)** minutes later no longer demonstrates the intrasplenic defects, which are now isointense with the adjacent normal splenic parenchyma. Note good vascular opacification and absence of contrast media in the renal collecting system during the optimal bolus phase of IV contrast media administration **(A)** as compared to **(B)**.

TABLE 2. *Accuracy of lymphography in 632 patients with newly diagnosed malignant lymphoma, based on staging laparotomy findings*

	Hodgkin's disease (n=416)	Non-Hodgkin's lymphoma (n=216)
Sensitivity	93% (100/107)	89% (101/114)
Specificity	92% (284/309)	86% (88/102)
Overall accuracy	92% (384/416)	88% (189/216)
Positive predictive value	80% (100/125)	88% (101/115)
Negative predictive value	98% (284/291)	87% (88/101)

From ref. 21.

reported data frequently in the low to middle 90 percentile range (21) (Table 2). The fact that lymphography does not opacify mesenteric lymph nodes is of little import in this patient population, since this nodal site is infrequently involved in newly diagnosed patients, and, when involved, these nodes are usually normal in size, so even CT studies that evaluate this lymph node site cannot reliably assess mesenteric nodal involvement.

Lymph nodes in the upper retroperitoneum, i.e., at sites not routinely opacified by lymphography such as those above the renal vascular pedicle, including at the base of the celiac axis, can be identified on CT studies as being involved when enlarged (Fig. 12). Likewise, enlarged lymph nodes extending into the porta hepatis and along the splenic vascular pedicle to the splenic hilus, and those at the posterior iliac crest (22) are readily displayed on CT (and MR) studies (Fig. 13).

Accuracy data on CT evaluation of subdiaphragmatic lymph nodes is limited (20) (Table 3). The available data was generated with the CT scanners that were used in the late 1970s and early 1980s, and comparable data on more advanced CT scanners that provide higher spatial resolution are not available.

CT has clearly replaced lymphography as the imaging method of choice in evaluating the subdiaphragmatic lymph nodes (23,24). Lymphography continues to have a potential role when the CT scan is equivocal, i.e., when scattered clusters of lymph nodes <1 cm in size raise concern about possible involvement, although the nodes are not enlarged by CT size criteria. The lymphogram's ability to display the internal architecture of the opacified lymph nodes can either provide reassurance that these nodes are normal or depict the presence of disease in nodes that are still normal in size (Fig. 14).

CT interpretation of lymphadenopathy is typically based on detection of lymph nodes >1 cm in short-axis measurement (Fig. 15). Although subcentimeter lymph nodes are normally seen in the retroperitoneal fat, when there are clusters of subcentimeter lymph nodes at sites with high probability of initial involvement below the diaphragm, then these CT features also warrant consideration for early involvement by Hodgkin's disease.

The other cross-sectional imaging techniques of ultrasound and MRI similarly rely on depiction of metastases based on lymph node size criteria (25). The presence of intervening gas and bony structures, which impairs complete evaluation of subdiaphragmatic lymph nodes, has led to ultrasound not being employed in the United States. In European and other countries, however, ultrasound is utilized more frequently, in part perhaps due to the less widespread availability of newer generation CT scanners. There are only limited data regarding MRI in lymph node assessment. However, since MRI also depends on the same size criteria as CT (>1 cm in short axis measurement) for an interpretation

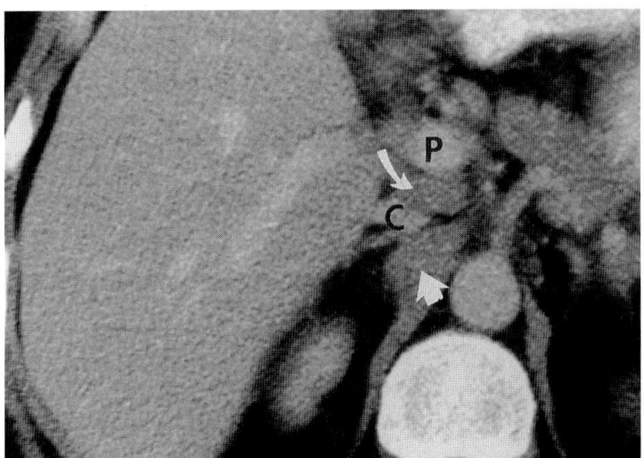

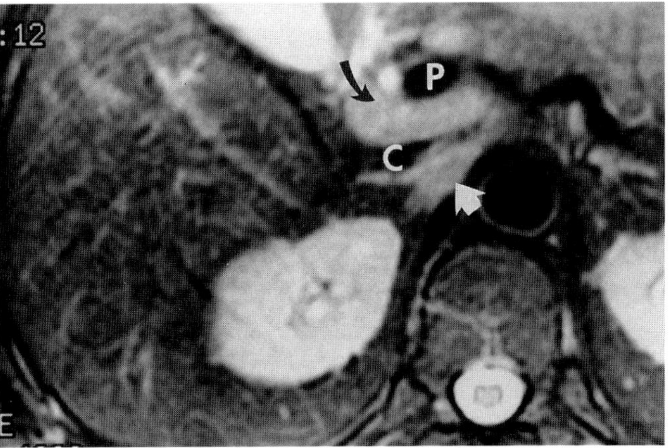

FIG. 13. A 50-year-old man with Hodgkin's disease. CT scan **(A)** demonstrates an enlarged portacaval lymph node *(curved arrow)*, as well as added soft tissue *(broad arrow)* adjacent to the anterior aspect of the right diaphragmatic crus, also compatible with lymphadenopathy. MR scan **(B)** at approximately the same level demonstrates increased signal from the soft tissue in the portacaval *(curved arrow)* and right retrocrural *(broad arrow)* spaces, supporting the presence of lymphadenopathy. P, portal vein; C, inferior vena cava.

TABLE 3. *Histopathologic correlations of CT and LAG in newly diagnosed, previously untreated patients with Hodgkin's disease based on staging laparotomy findings (n = 121)*

	Paraaortic nodes		Mesenteric nodes	Spleen	Liver
	LAG	CT	CT	CT	CT
Sensitivity	17/20 (85)	13/20 (65)	0/1 (0)	17/51 (33)	1/4 (25)
Specificity	85/87 (98)	80/87 (92)	90/91 (99)	53/70 (76)	117/117 (100)
Accuracy					
Overall	102/107 (95)	93/107 (87)	90/92 (98)	70/121 (58)	118/121 (98)
Positive report	17/19 (89)	13/20 (65)	0/1 (0)	17/34 (50)	1/1 (100)
Negative report	85/88 (97)	80/87 (92)	90/91 (99)	53/87 (61)	117/120 (98)

Numbers in parentheses are percentages.

In seven patients, no retroperitoneal nodes were biopsied, and in an additional seven patients the lymphographically positive nodes were not biopsied, leaving 107 cases for analysis.

CT, computed tomography; LAG, lymphography.

From ref. 20.

of lymphadenopathy, there is little reason to suggest that this technology would be significantly superior to CT.

Spleen and Liver

Staging laparotomy data have demonstrated that organ size is a poor criterion for involvement, unless the spleen or liver is markedly enlarged (which is readily detected by physical examination). Further, focal deposits of Hodgkin's disease frequently reside in normal-sized organs. Thus, efforts to use organ size based on CT volume measurements to assess disease status have not been useful (26). Properly performed contrast-enhanced CT (20) and MRI (27) studies can clearly demonstrate focal deposits of tumor that are 1.0 cm in size or larger (Figs. 3A, 11B, 12A, and 16A). Ultrasound appears to have similar sensitivity and specificity. However, not infrequently, involvement of the spleen and liver occurs as one or more subcentimeter deposits of tumor that are difficult if not impossible to detect with confidence with current cross-sectional imaging techniques. Thus, when focal defects within the spleen or liver are detected, and other etiologies (Fig. 16) can be confidently excluded (28), such information is useful for staging purposes. However, the absence of such findings should not provide confidence that these organs are free of disease.

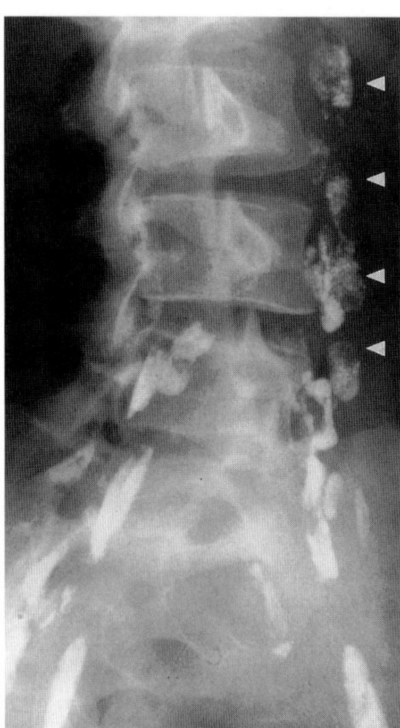

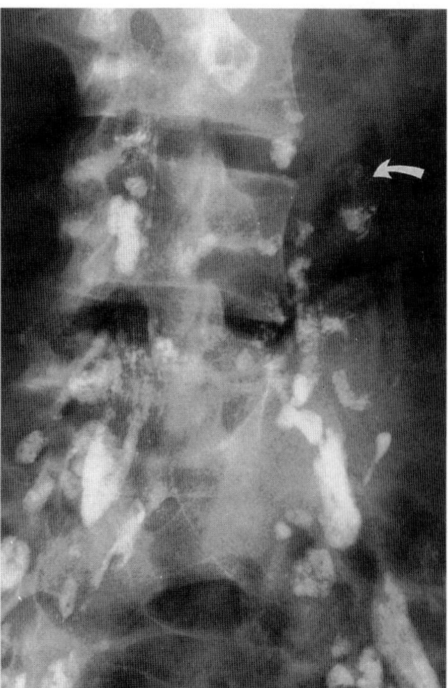

A,B

FIG. 14. A: A 14-year-old girl with newly diagnosed Hodgkin's disease. Lymphogram, left posterior oblique projection, demonstrates marked internal architectural distortion of multiple left paraaortic lymph nodes *(arrowheads)*, which are not enlarged, compatible with involvement by Hodgkin's disease (biopsy proven at staging laparotomy). **B:** An 18-year-old man with newly diagnosed Hodgkin's disease. Lymphogram, LPO projection, demonstrates uneven opacification of the lower paraaortic and upper common iliac lymph nodes, which are normal in size (compare with the homogeneously opacified lymph nodes more caudally). Note in particular the focally replaced lymph node to the left of L4 *(arrow)*.

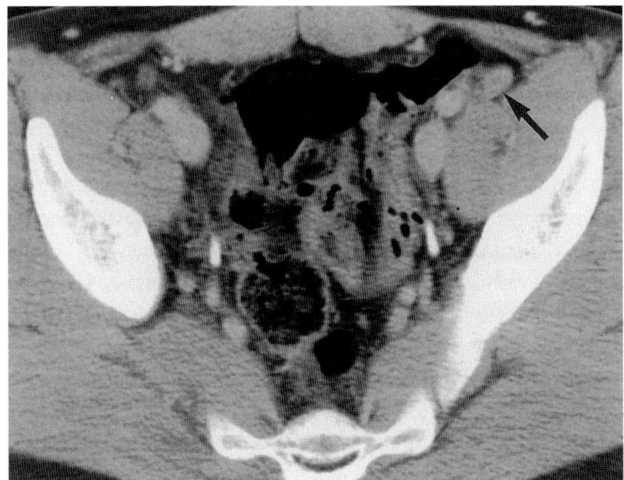

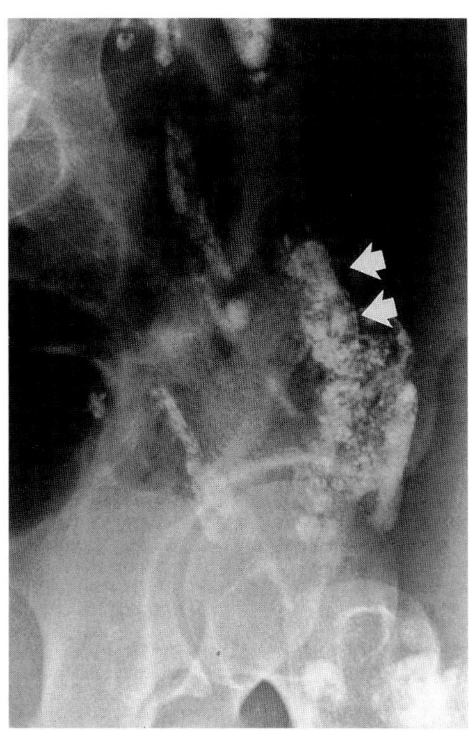

FIG. 15. A 21-year-old man with newly diagnosed lymphocyte-predominance Hodgkin's disease. CT scan through the low pelvis **(A)** demonstrates focally enlarged left external iliac lymph nodes *(arrow)*, whereas nodes more cephalad were unremarkable by CT size criteria. Lymphogram, LPO projection **(B)**, confirms lower left external iliac lymphadenopathy with modest enlargement but marked internal architectural distortion. Nodes more cephalad were also normal. This noncontiguous pattern can be seen with lymphocyte-predominance Hodgkin's disease, whereas it is extremely rare with other histologic subtypes, at the time of presentation.

Gastrointestinal and Genitourinary Systems

For all practical purposes, and unlike the non-Hodgkin's lymphomas, Hodgkin's disease does not intrinsically involve these organ systems. However, these organ systems can be impinged on by adjacent lymphadenopathy as well as become infiltrated by adjacent tumor. In such situations, cross-sectional CT studies as well as positive contrast radiography of these organ systems (barium studies of the gastrointestinal tract and excretory urography, respectively) can demonstrate such findings with ease. Imaging evidence suggesting intrinsic involvement of these organs systems should prompt suspicion of another etiology, such as a concomitant non-Hodgkin's lymphoma or an incidental epithelial tumor, as well as inflammatory or infectious etiologies.

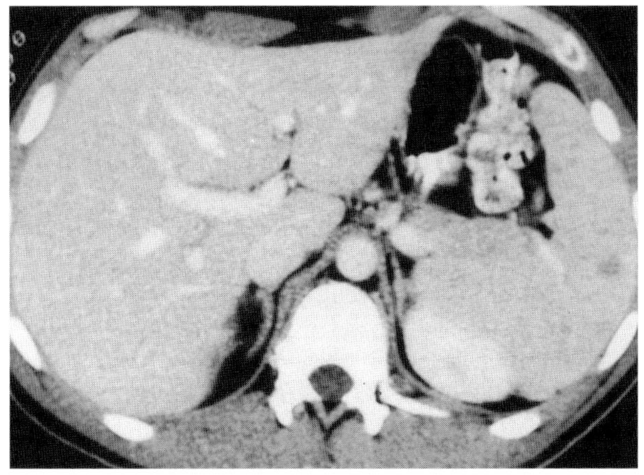

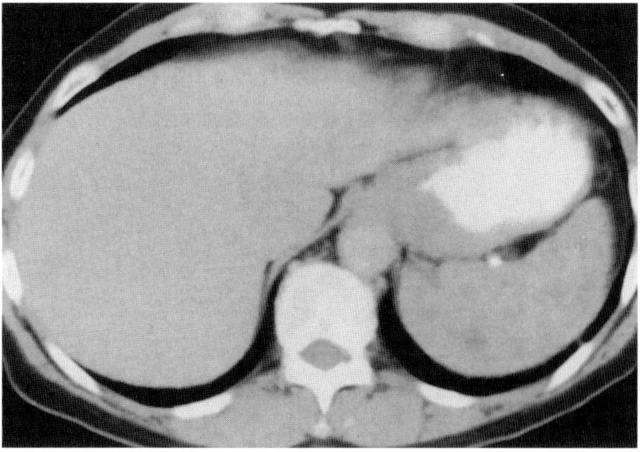

FIG. 16. A: A 23-year-old man with newly diagnosed Hodgkin's disease, stage IVB. CT scan demonstrates poorly defined filling defects within the spleen due to Hodgkin's disease. **B:** In a 56-year-old woman, CT scan through the upper abdomen demonstrates multiple poorly defined filling defects within splenic parenchyma, raising concern for involvement by Hodgkin's disease. Splenectomy specimen, however, demonstrated multiple lymphangiomas without evidence of Hodgkin's disease. (Courtesy of B. Nixon, M.D.)

Miscellaneous

Bone Marrow

When positive, bone marrow biopsies provide useful information for staging. However, negative bone marrow biopsies are of limited value since only a small fraction of bone marrow is evaluated with this technique. MRI has the potential to be useful in the assessment of bone marrow involvement, based on its ability to distinguish marrow that has undergone normal fatty replacement from that which maintains active hematopoiesis (29,30). Thus, when tumor deposits are present in the normal fat-containing marrow, their presence can be identified on conventional MRI (Fig. 17). Spotty involvement of marrow, such as typically seen with Hodgkin's disease, is more likely to be identified than when the marrow is diffusely, homogeneously involved. Abnormal areas on such MR images could then be percutaneously sampled to obtain histologic verification (Fig. 17). Bone marrow involvement is difficult to appreciate on Ga 67 imaging because gallium accumulates in normal bone marrow. A discrete cutoff of bone marrow is often seen on gallium studies in the thoracic spine after radiation therapy to the mediastinum (Fig. 18).

Skeletal System

Involvement of cortical bone is unusual at initial presentation. When caused by metastatic disease, the deposits are usually lytic or mixed lytic and blastic, presumably as a result of hematogenous spread of disease or involvement of cortical bone underlying bone marrow involvement. The characteristic ivory vertebrae that are often associated with Hodgkin's disease usually are a result of an adjacent lymph node mass that locally invades the adjacent bony structures, and this can occur in other portions of the bony skeleton as well (Fig. 19). Local invasion of bone from an adjacent lymph node mass results in frank bone destruction, with the creation of a lytic defect. Radioisotope bone scanning is

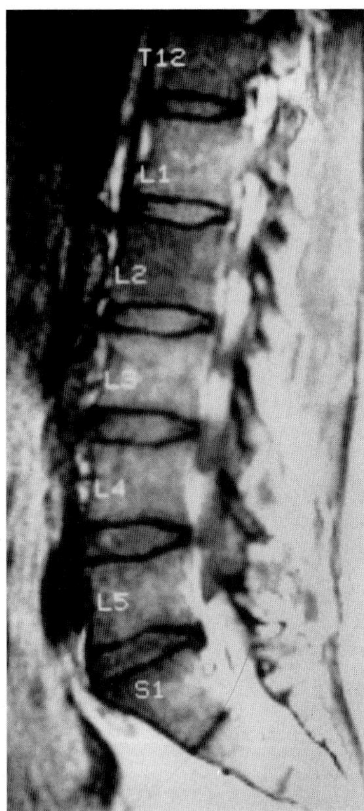

FIG. 17. A 28-year-old man with newly diagnosed Hodgkin's disease with complaints of back pain. Conventional spine radiographs and radionuclide studies were negative. Magnetic resonance imaging (MRI) demonstrated abnormally low signal at T12 and L2 on T1-weighted images, suggesting infiltration of the marrow. Conventional iliac crest bone marrow biopsy results were negative; however, image-guided percutaneous biopsy of L2 was positive for marrow involvement by Hodgkin's disease. (From ref. 49.)

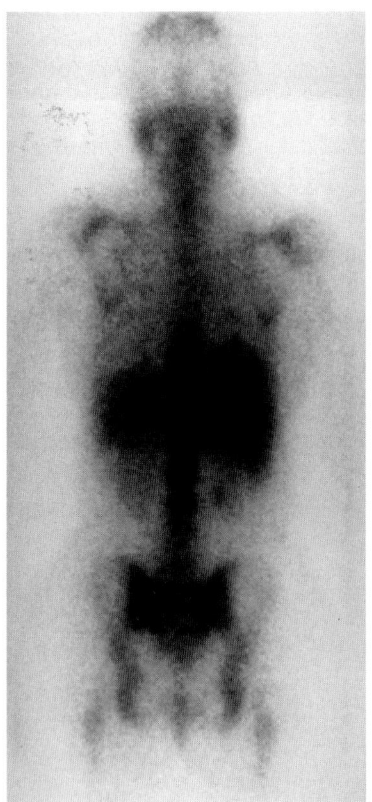

FIG. 18. A posterior whole-body scan of a patient who had previously received mediastinal radiation and chemotherapy. Note the normal distribution of gallium with visualization of the parotid glands, the bone marrow, liver, and spleen. Also note the abrupt cutoff of normal bone marrow in the lower thoracic spine just above the liver. The abrupt change from normal marrow distribution to absence of marrow in upper thoracic spine is characteristic of postradiation changes. The fact that the kidneys are faintly visualized below the spleen and the liver is an indication that the patient has had prior chemotherapy. The examination was performed using 8 to 10 mCi of Ga 67 Citrate and the scans were done 72 hours after the intravenous administration of the radiopharmaceutical.

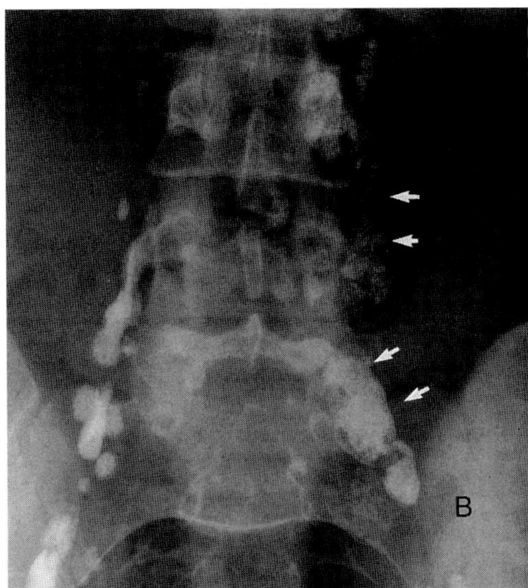

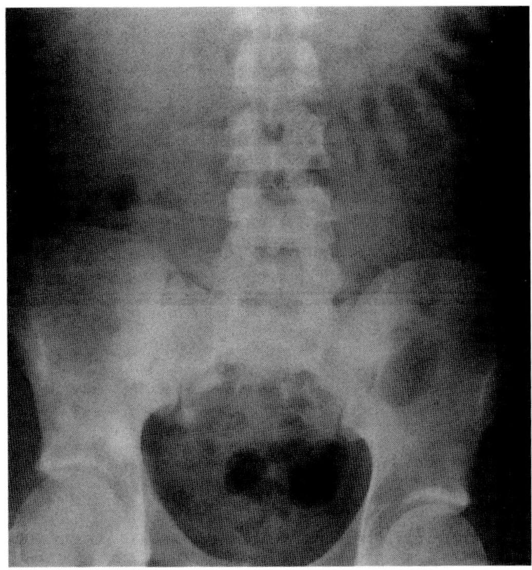

FIG. 19. A: A 20-year-old woman with newly diagnosed Hodgkin's disease. The lymphogram is positive, with modestly enlarged left paraaortic and common iliac lymph nodes with internal architectural distortion *(arrows)*. The increased density in the adjacent left iliac bone *(B)* is due to cortical bone involvement from the adjacent lymphadenopathy. **B:** A 30-year-old man with previously treated Hodgkin's disease. Abdominal radiograph demonstrates multiple blastic metastases, predominantly involving the right iliac bone. (Autopsy proven.)

very sensitive in the early detection of skeletal involvement; however, since this is an uncommon if not rare manifestation at the time of initial presentation, the routine use of radionuclide bone scans has long been abandoned.

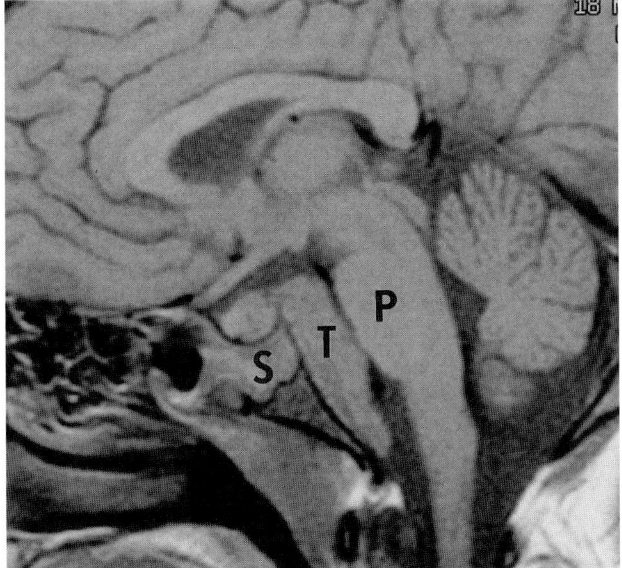

FIG. 20. An 18-year-old man presented with diplopia and left fifth and sixth cranial nerve involvement. Sagittal MR scan through the midline demonstrates a lobular soft tissue mass (*T*) in the prepontine cistern, which displaces the pons (*P*) posteriorly and locally invades the sella (*S*) and left cavernous sinus. Other imaging studies demonstrated axillary, abdominal, and pelvic lymphadenopathy, biopsy of which revealed nodular sclerosing Hodgkin's disease. All sites of disease regressed following chemotherapy.

Central Nervous System

As with the gastrointestinal and genitourinary systems, for all practical purposes, and unlike the non-Hodgkin's lymphomas, Hodgkin's disease does not intrinsically involve the central nervous system. However, the central nervous system can become secondarily involved by extension of disease from adjacent lymphadenopathy or infiltration of the leptomeninges by tumor (Fig. 20). Appropriate symptoms or signs should prompt performance of MRI, often with gadolinium enhancement, which is highly successful in demonstrating such involvement.

INTRATREATMENT SURVEILLANCE STUDIES

At times, diagnostic radiographic studies of sites of known disease are performed to evaluate response during treatment. Usually, such intratreatment imaging studies will readily demonstrate a decrease in size of these disease sites, although the presence of abundant sclerosis in the untreated tumor can mask the true tumor response. Although such information is useful, to date there is no information that rate of response as determined by shrinkage of the initial mass, or masses, is necessarily predictive of eventual relapse or survival.

However, Ga 67 imaging using high-activity (8–10 mCi) techniques with SPECT has been shown to provide prognostic information of clinical value. During and after therapy, the disease-free interval is longer in gallium-negative than in gallium-positive individuals with treated Hodgkin's disease. Further, mid-cycle review after three or four courses of therapy is an excellent prognostic indicator of eventual outcome. In a study performed by Hagemeister and colleagues (31) in 37 patients with Hodgkin's disease, all patients who were judged to be Ga 67 negative after chemotherapy survived. The only deaths that occurred were in patients who were gallium positive at the conclusion of therapy. More recently Front et al. (32) have reported that after just one therapy cycle important prognostic information can be obtained in patients with Hodgkin's disease. This work supports changing therapy after one cycle if the gallium image is positive (Fig. 21).

The real value of gallium imaging lies in its ability to lead to earlier interventions; i.e., in patients whose gallium scan remains positive at early or mid-cycle treatment review, there is a high likelihood of subsequent treatment failure (Fig. 22).

The importance of gallium imaging in Hodgkin's disease is that a persistently positive study mid-cycle or at completion of therapy carries a poor prognosis. In our

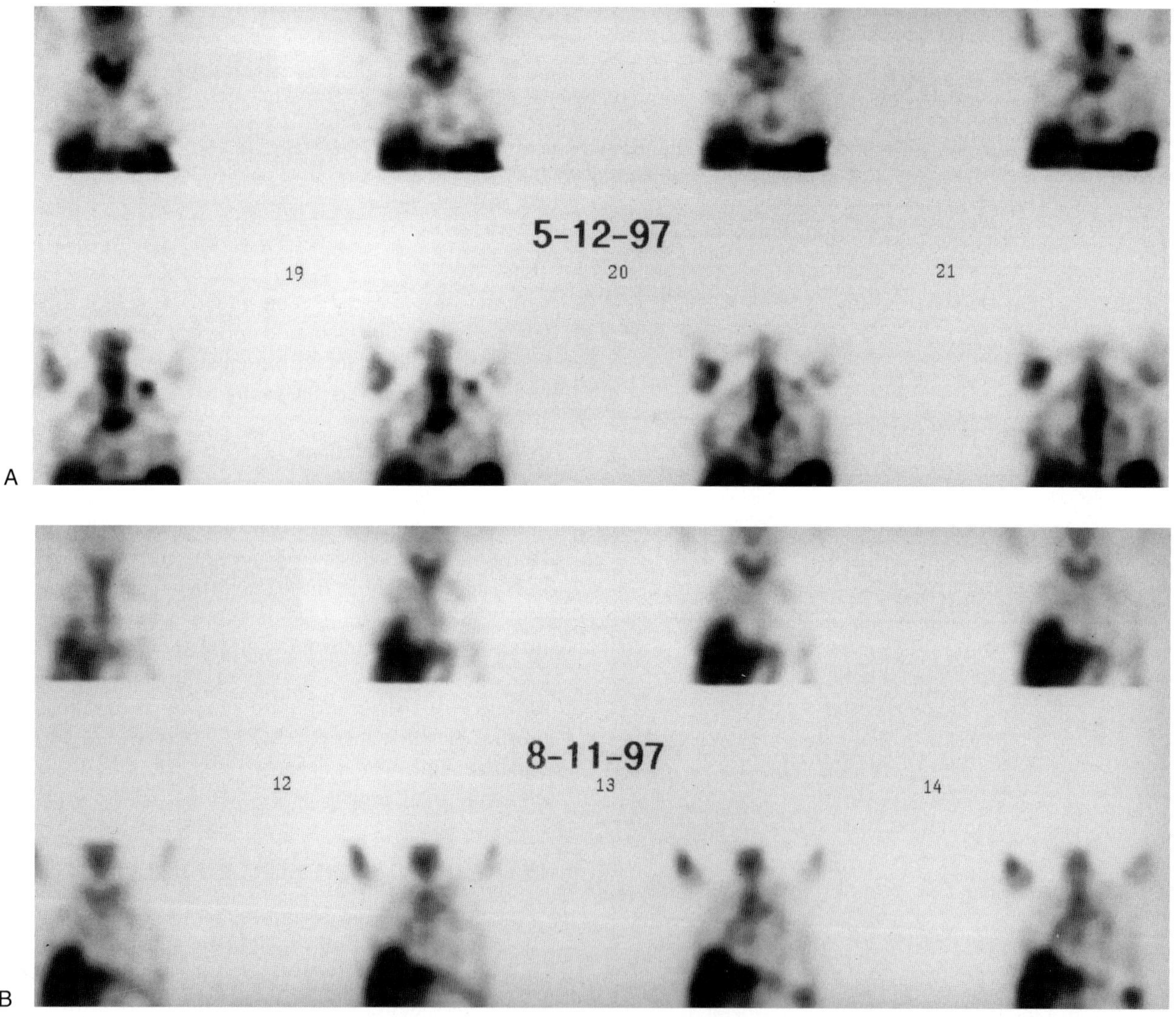

FIG. 21. A: A 36-year-old man with stage IIA Hodgkin's disease. A single photon emission computed tomography (SPECT) examination of the chest reveals left supraclavicular and anterior mediastinal adenopathy that is gallium avid. **B:** The same patient after two cycles of therapy. Note the absence of activity in the mediastinum and left supraclavicular region, and the faint bilateral hilar uptake, which is a manifestation of prior therapy. It is characteristic for such patients to have normal chest x-rays and CT scans when the gallium scan is positive in the hilar regions. Both these SPECT studies were performed 72 hours after intravenous injection of 10 mCi of Ga 67 citrate.

study (31) we noted that gallium scan predicted relapse in patients with Hodgkin's disease treated with combined modality therapy. The major rationale for pretherapy gallium studies is to determine the state of gallium avidity prior to the introduction of therapy. The positive posttherapy mid-cycle scan would appear to be of value in identifying early treatment failures.

The conversion of a pretreatment positive gallium scan to a negative scan has been suggested to reflect long-term favorable response, whereas persistence of gallium positivity would indicate incomplete response. Recently, Salloum et al. (33) presented their data on 101 newly diagnosed patients whose gallium scans were positive, of which all but four reverted to negative following therapy. Although the four patients with persistently positive scans died from progressive disease or relapsed, 16 of 97 patients with negative posttreatment gallium scans also relapsed. The negative predictive value for all patients was 83.5%; however, when stratified by stage (I–II vs. III–IV) it was 94.2% and 64.5%, respectively. The authors emphasize that "a good outcome in a group of patients with an excellent prognosis does not prove the predictive value of negative posttreatment Ga^{67} scans as much as it confirms the favorable prognosis of patients with early-stage disease."

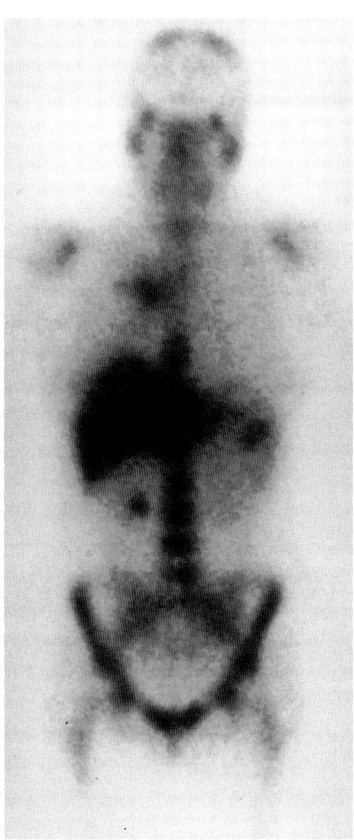

FIG. 22. Anterior whole-body gallium image performed 72 hours after the intravenous injection of approximately 10 mCi of Ga 67 citrate. The fact that there is visualization of the submandibular glands and parotid glands as well as intense activity in the lacrimal glands indicates that the patient has previously been treated. Despite the fact that this patient had undergone several courses of therapy, there is a residual gallium-avid lesion noted in the right suprahilar region. The irregular borders of this region suggest that it represents residual active Hodgkin's disease. Additionally, the patient has a focal area of abnormal gallium accumulation in an enlarged, poorly functioning spleen. This patient later succumbed to his disease.

It is known that patients with early-stage Hodgkin's disease who require only radiotherapy have a good prognosis. The salvage rates in these patients are high and the data would suggest that the more limited the relapse, the better the prognosis (34). Such patients do not appear to benefit from gallium imaging.

POSTTREATMENT SURVEILLANCE STUDIES

Following completion of therapy, current practice is to monitor patients with periodic clinical, laboratory, and imaging studies (35,36) to evaluate for evidence of disease relapse or treatment-related complications. Most would agree that a set of baseline studies is useful to have following treatment, which can then be compared with follow-up surveillance studies.

There is little information, about the optimal frequency of such periodic surveillance or about the impact of detecting relapse one or several months earlier than would have occurred if the surveillance program (clinical and imaging) were done at longer intervals. Most oncologists have adopted surveillance schedules based on the likelihood of relapse related to the patient's initial histology and stage, and, in general, imaging studies are ordered to coincide with the clinic visit. However, the frequency with which such studies should be performed is not clearly known, although statistical models (37) exist that can be used to guide clinical practice.

Posttreatment Residual Mass

A common problem confronting the oncologist and diagnostic radiologist is the persistence of a mass at a site that was originally involved following completion of therapy. The persistent mass raises the question of whether there is residual viable tumor, which would lead to further treatment considerations, or whether this persistent mass simply represents the residua of successfully treated disease.

Such assessment can be made based on surveillance over time, since the residua of successfully treated disease would remain stable or perhaps slightly decrease over time, whereas persistent disease would at some point demonstrate interval tumor growth. However, in this clinical setting this information is preferably obtained when the residual mass is first noted, so that if there is persistent viable tumor, therapeutic options could be initiated when the likelihood of salvage was greatest. CT images usually contain no information that is useful in this assessment. If no enhancement of the residual mass following IV contrast media is clearly documented (determined by comparison with a noncontrast set of CT images), a conclusion can be made that the mass contains no blood supply, and thus no viable tissue. However, this result is rarely seen, in part due to the frequent coexistence of an inflammatory component that has a blood supply.

MRI has the potential to make this differentiation, as different pulse sequences can satisfactorily discriminate between non–water-containing masses (such as fibrous tissue) and cellular masses (such as residual tumor) (38,39). However, following successful treatment of tumor masses, these residual masses commonly contain an inflammatory component for several months that in itself is cellular (40,41). Thus, such assessment by MRI is more reliable only months after completion of therapy, not at the time when potentially more effective therapeutic interventions could be made.

Image-guided percutaneous biopsy of such masses (42) can be readily accomplished, and if the result demonstrates persistent viable tumor, then such information is useful. However, the simple recovery of necrotic tissue does not imply that the entire mass is made up of similar material, as foci of viable tumor simply may not have been sampled.

Gallium tends to underestimate early recurrence and small deposits of disease (Fig. 22). The greatest interest in gallium scanning today is in the prediction of early treatment failure in patients with residual abnormality in the chest. In a retrospective study by Cooper et al. (43), 48 patients were noted to have pretherapy gallium-avid mediastinal Hodgkin's disease. At the completion of chemotherapy, 44 patients had normal findings on gallium scans but relapse occurred in 12 of the 44, and nine of these relapses occurred in the mediastinum.

Bogart et al. (44) retrospectively reviewed gallium imaging and treatment outcome in 60 patients with Hodgkin's disease. Based on the gallium scan, 46 patients were in complete remission after initial treatment, 10 were in partial remission, and four had persistent or progressive disease. Ten of 29 patients (34%) with gallium complete remission after chemotherapy subsequently had recurrences compared with no recurrences in 17 patients receiving initial radiotherapy or combined chemoradiation. Eight of 10 patients received further therapy after gallium partial remission and nine patients remained disease free. The survival did not differ in patients achieving a gallium complete remission or a partial remission. The authors conclude that Ga 67 imaging may help confirm the presence of active Hodgkin's disease but is unreliable in defining disease remission after chemotherapy. The results of this study are not unexpected since once again false negatives due to small deposits are not expected to be imaged by nuclear techniques.

Thymic Hyperplasia

Although the emergence of a mediastinal mass following therapy is usually due to disease relapse, at times a similar appearance can be caused by an increase in size of the thymus. This entity has become well established over the past decade, is more frequently seen in teenagers and young adults (although it can be seen in other ages), and appears to be some type of rebound phenomenon following therapy. Histologically, the thymus will demonstrate evidence of nonspecific hyperplasia and/or development of cysts (45). The findings, although readily apparent on imaging studies, are nonspecific, and currently CT, MRI, and gallium (which can also be positive with thymic hyperplasia) cannot distinguish between thymic hyperplasia and recurrent disease (Fig. 23).

Posttreatment Complications

Posttherapy complications, such as radiation fibrosis or drug toxicity, can be manifested on imaging studies, particularly chest radiography and chest CT exams. The ability to distinguish the effects of therapy (Fig. 24) from persistent or recurrent tumor is important. The increasingly effective treatment of Hodgkin's disease has resulted in the well-established increased incidence of secondary tumors and acceleration of degenerative vascular disease, both situations which can be identified on imaging studies. These situations are addressed in more detail in Chapter 33. Gallium distribution is affected by therapy. Bilateral hilar, salivary gland, and diffuse lung uptake can all be manifestations of posttherapy effects (4,5) (Fig. 25).

Miscellaneous

In addition to being at risk for disease relapse or illness related to therapy, previously treated patients with Hodgkin's disease are susceptible to the variety of illnesses that affect the general population. It is therefore important to keep this in mind and not assume that newly developing abnormalities on imaging (as well as clinical or laboratory findings) necessarily relate to the patient's underlying disease and prior therapy. Although the imaging findings often will suggest an etiology not related to the patient's underlying disease or treatment, which can then be further pursued clinically, at times such findings are nonspecific and may require obtaining tissue for a definitive diagnosis. Particularly vexing are entities that closely mimic Hodgkin's disease relapse, such as can be seen in sarcoid-like reactions in patients who have a history of malignant disease (46). The development of intrathoracic lymphadenopathy and pulmonary parenchymal disease, which is typical for sarcoid, can, in a patient

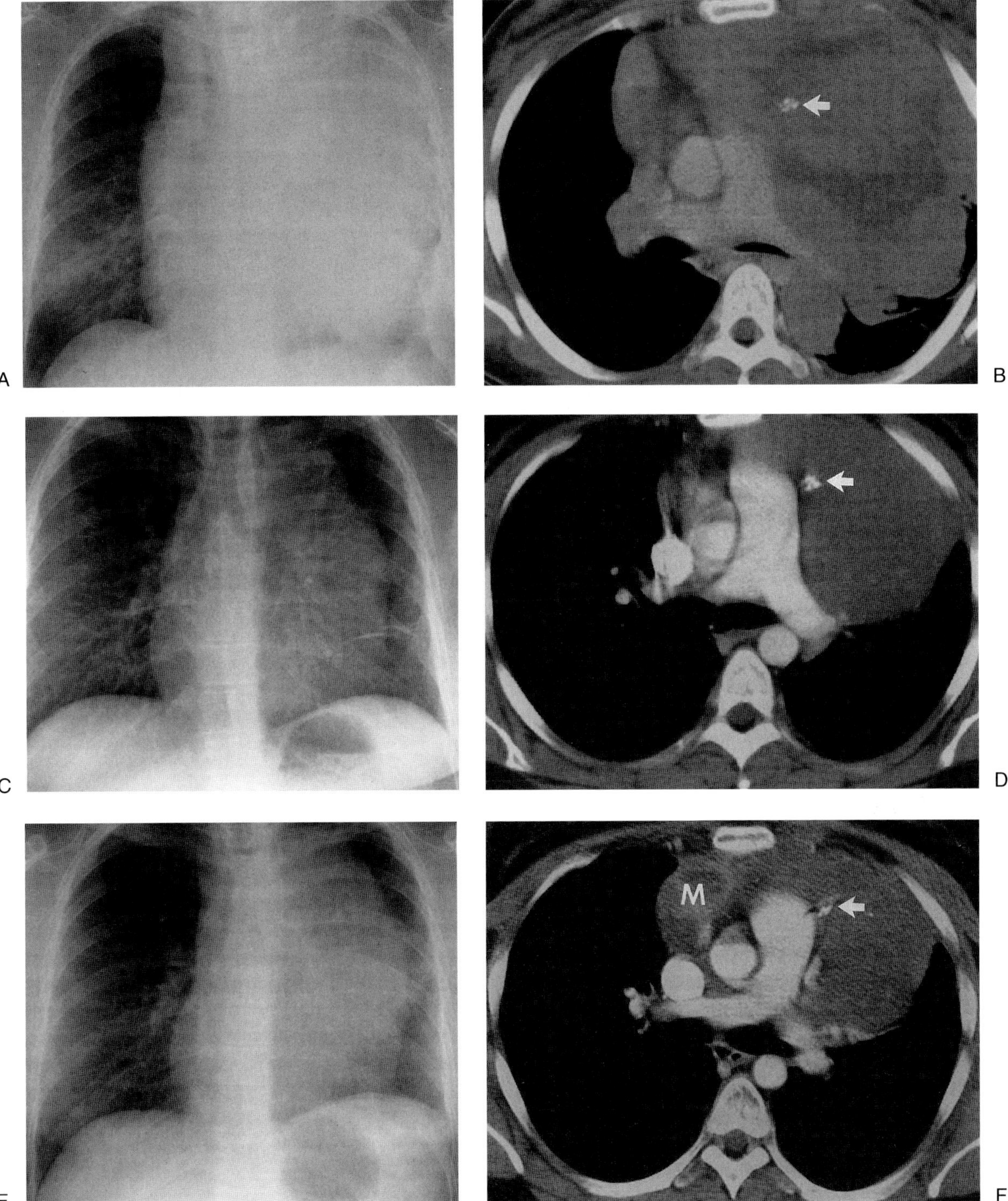

FIG. 23. A 29-year-old woman with newly diagnosed Hodgkin's disease (mediastinal biopsy). Pretreatment chest radiograph **(A)** and CT scan **(B)** demonstrate a large, nonhomogeneous, predominantly left-sided anterior mediastinal mass that abuts (although not clearly invades) the left anterior chest wall. Focal calcification is seen within the mass *(arrow)*. Frontal chest radiograph **(C)** and CT scan **(D)** 7 months later, postchemotherapy, demonstrate reduction of the mediastinal mass, although a significant residual mass persists. Interval resolution of the prior left pleural effusion is seen as well as a decrease in size of the right mediastinal component. Frontal chest radiograph **(E)** and CT scan **(F)** 5 months later demonstrate minimal interval decrease in size of the predominant left mediastinal mass. However, the CT scan shows interval increase in the right superior mediastinal mass (M), which is heterogeneous, compatible with disease progression (although the left-sided mediastinal mass has continued to regress), thymic hyperplasia/cyst, or emergence of a new disease entity. Surgical biopsy revealed diffuse large-cell lymphoma.

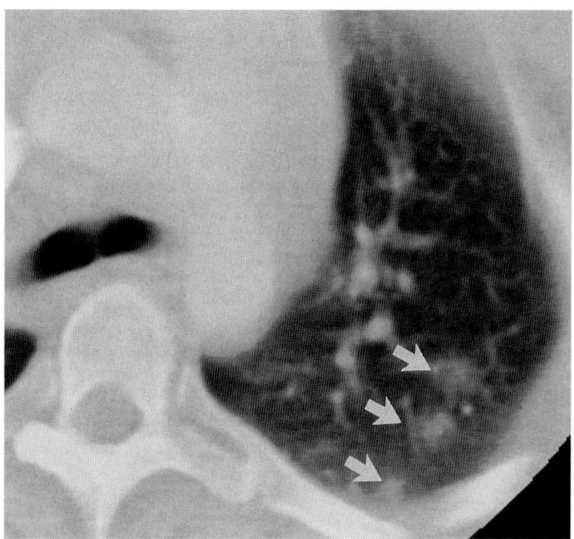

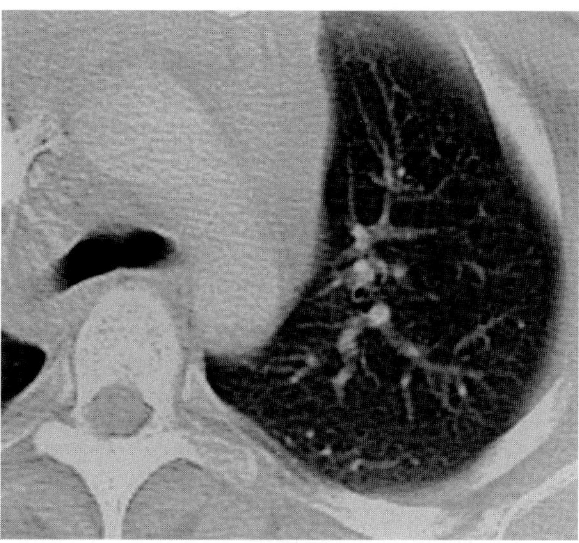

FIG. 24. A 21-year-old woman with newly diagnosed nodular sclerosing Hodgkin's disease presenting with extensive mediastinal lymphadenopathy (not shown). Mid-therapy scan **(A)** demonstrates a persistent although decreased mediastinal mass, with interval appearance of poorly defined pulmonary nodules *(arrows)*, raising the possibility of progressive Hodgkin's disease, intercurrent infection, or drug toxicity (the patient was on bleomycin). Two months later, CT scan **(B)** demonstrates resolution of the pulmonary nodules following withdrawal of bleomycin, suggesting that the pulmonary nodules were simply a manifestation of bleomycin drug toxicity.

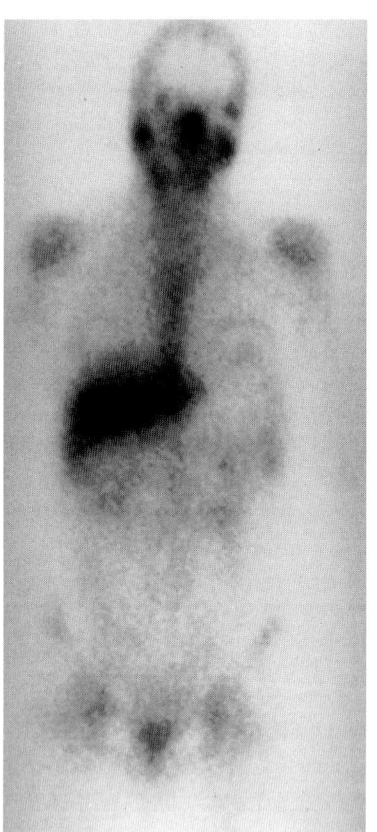

FIG. 25. This patient with Hodgkin's disease underwent treatment and subsequently had a complete remission. Whole body scan performed 72 hours after the intravenous injection of 10 mCi of Ga 67 citrate reveals normal gallium distribution to the central bone marrow, the liver, and nasopharynx. The activity seen in the parotid glands and submandibular glands and lacrimal glands indicates that the patient has had prior therapy. Note that this patient underwent a splenectomy.

with a history of Hodgkin's disease, readily be mistaken for evidence of disease relapse.

REFERENCES

1. Begg CB, McNeil BJ. Assessment of radiologic tests: control of bias and other design considerations. *Radiology* 1988;167:565.
2. Edwards CL, Hy RL. Tumor scanning with Ga-67 citrate. *Nucl Med* 1969;10:103–105.
3. Tuhma SS, Rosenthal DS, Kaplan W, English RJ, Holman BL. Lymphoma evaluation with Ga-67 SPECT. *Radiology* 1987;164:111–114.
4. Podoloff DA. Diffuse lung uptake of Ga-67 in treated lymphoma: Another milestone on the road to understanding. *Radiology* 1996;199: 318–320.
5. Bar-Shalom R, Israel O, Harim N, et al. Diffuse lung uptake of Ga-67 after treatment of lymphoma: Is it of clinical importance? *Radiology* 1996;199:473–476.
6. Ziegles P, Noucadie N, Huglo D, et al. Comparison of Tc-99m methoxyisobutylisonitrile and Ga-67: what's scanning in the assessment of lymphomas. *Eur J Nucl Med* 1995;22:126–131.
7. Krenning EP, Kwekheboom DJ, Bakker WH, et al. Somatostatin receptor scintigraphy with [In-111 DTPA-dphe] and [I-123-Tyr-3]-Octreotide in the Rotterdam experience with more than 1,000 patients. *Eur J Nucl Med* 1993;20(8):716–731.
8. Newman JS, Francis JR, Kaminski MS, et al. Imaging of lymphoma with PET with 2-[F-18]-fluoro-2-deoxy D-glucose: Correlation with CT. *Radiology* 1994;190:111–116.
9. Castellino RA, Blank N, Hoppe RT, Cho C. Hodgkin's disease: contributions of chest CT in the initial staging evaluation. *Radiology* 1986; 106:603–605.
10. Hopper KD, Diehl LF, Lesar M, et al. Hodgkin's disease: Clinical utility of CT in initial staging and treatment. *Radiology* 1988;169:17.
11. Larcos G, Farlow DC, Antico VF, et al. The role of high dose Ga-67 scintigraphy in staging untreated patients with lymphomas. *Aust NZ J Med* 1994;24:5–8.
12. Hagemeister FB, Fesus SM, Lamki LM, et al. Role of the gallium scan in Hodgkin's disease. *Cancer* 1990;65:1090–1096.
13. Devizzi L, Maffioli L, Bonfante V, et al. Comparison of gallium scan, computed tomography, and magnetic resonance in patients with mediastinal Hodgkin's disease. *Ann Oncol* 1997;1(8):53–56.
14. Cho CS, Blank N, Castellino RA. CT evaluation of cardiophrenic angle lymph nodes in patients with malignant lymphoma. *AJR* 1984;143: 719–721.
15. Bergin CJ, Healy MV, Zincone GE, Castellino RA. MRI evaluation of chest wall involvement in malignant lymphoma. *J Comput Assist Tomogr* 1990;14:926–932.
16. Hopper KD, Diehl LF, Lynch JD, et al. Mediastinal bulk in Hodgkin disease: Method of measurement versus prognosis. *Invest Radiol* 1991; 26:1101–1109.
17. Diehl LF, Hooper KD, Giguere J, et al. The pattern of intrathoracic Hodgkin's disease assessed by computed tomography. *J Clin Oncol* 1991;9:438–443.
18. Tesoro-Tess JD, Balzarini I, Ceglia E, et al. Magnetic resonance imaging in the initial staging of Hodgkin's disease and non-Hodgkin's lymphoma. *Eur J Radiol* 1991;12:81–90.
19. Skillings JR, Bramwell V, Nicholson RL, et al. Magnetic resonance imaging in the initial staging of Hodgkin's disease and non-Hodgkin's lymphoma. *Cancer* 1991;67:1838–1843.
20. Castellino RA, Hoppe RT, Blank N, Young SW, Rosenberg SA, Kaplan HS. Computed tomography, lymphography, and staging laparotomy: correlations in initial staging of Hodgkin's disease. *AJR* 1984;143: 37–41.
21. Marglin S, Castellino RA. Lymphographic accuracy in 632 consecutive, previously untreated cases of Hodgkin's disease and non-Hodgkin's lymphoma. *Radiology* 1981;140:351–353.
22. Castellino RA. Lymph nodes of the posterior iliac crest: CT and lymphographic observations. *Radiology* 1990;175:687–689.
23. North LB, Wallace S, Lindell MM, et al. Lymphography for staging lymphomas: Is it still a useful procedure? *AJR* 1993;161:867–869.
24. Libson E, Polliack A, Bloom RA. Value of lymphangiography in the staging of Hodgkin's disease. *Radiology* 1994;193:757–759.
25. Hanna SL, Fletcher BD, Boulden TF, et al. MR imaging of infradiaphragmatic lymphadenopathy in children and adolescents with Hodgkin's disease: Comparison with lymphography and CT. *J Magn Reson Imaging* 1993;3:461.
26. Hancock SLI, Scidmore NS, Hopkins KL, et al. Computed tomography assessment of splenic size as a predictor of splenic weight and disease involvement in laparotomy staged Hodgkin's disease. *Int J Radiat Oncol Biol Phys* 1994;28:93–99.
27. Weissleder R, Elizondo G, Stark DD, et al. The diagnosis of splenic lymphoma by MR imaging. *AJR* 1989;152:175.
28. Warshauer DM, Molina PL, Worawattanakul S. The spotted spleen: CT and clinical correlation in a tertiary care center. *J Comput Assist Tomogr* 1998;22(5):694–702.
29. Altehoefer C, Blum U, Bathmann J, et al. Comparative diagnostic accuracy of magnetic resonance imaging and immunoscintigraphy for detection of bone marrow involvement in patients with malignant lymphoma. *J Clin Oncol* 1997;15:1754–1760.
30. Hoane BR, Shields AF, Porter BA, Borrow JW. Comparison of initial lymphoma staging using computed tomography (CT) and magnetic resonance (MR) imaging. *Am J Hematol* 1994;47:100–105.
31. Hagemeister FB, Purugganan R, Podoloff DA, et al. The gallium scan predicts relapse in patients with Hodgkin's disease treated with combined modality therapy. *Ann Oncol* 1994;5(suppl 2):S59–S63.
32. Front D, Bar-Shalom R, Mor M, et al. Prediction of outcome of patients with Hodgkin's disease (HD) by Ga-67 scintigraphy after one cycle of chemotherapy. *J Nucl Med* 1998;39(5):101–118.
33. Salloum E, Schwab Brandt D, Caride VJ, et al. Gallium scans in the management of patients with Hodgkin's disease: a study of 101 patients. *J Clin Oncol* 1997;15:518–527.
34. Roach M III, Brophy N, Cox R, et al. Prognostic factors for patients relapsing after radiotherapy for early stage Hodgkin's disease. *J Clin Oncol* 1990;8:623–629.
35. Castellino RA, Cassady JR, Blank N, Kaplan HS. Roentgenologic aspects of Hodgkin's disease. II. Role of routine radiographs in detecting initial relapse. *Cancer* 1973;31:316–323.
36. Heron CW, Husband JE, Williams MP, Cherryman GR. The value of thoracic computed tomography in the detection of recurrent Hodgkin's disease. *Br J Radiol* 1988;61:567.
37. Chang PJ, Parker BR, Donaldson SS, Thompson EI. Dynamic probabilistic model for determination of optimal timing of surveillance chest radiography in pediatric Hodgkin disease. *Radiology* 1989;173:71.
38. Nyman R, Forsgren G, Glimelius B. Long-term follow-up of residual mediastinal masses in treated Hodgkin's disease using MR imaging. *Acta Radiol* 1996;37:323–326.
39. Rahmouni A, Tempany C, Jones R, et al. Lymphoma: Monitoring tumor size and signal intensity with MR imaging. *Radiology* 1993;188:445.
40. Lee JKT, Glazer HS. Controversy in the MR imaging appearance of fibrosis. *Radiology* 1990;177:21.
41. Webb R. MR imaging of treated mediastinal Hodgkin disease. *Radiology* 1989;170:315.
42. Wittich GR, Nowels KW, Korn RL, et al. Coaxial transthoracic fineneedle biopsy in patients with a history of malignant lymphoma. *Radiology* 1992;183:175.
43. Cooper DL, Caride VJ, Zloty M, et al. Gallium scans in patients with mediastinal Hodgkin's disease treated with chemotherapy. *J Clin Oncol* 1993;11:1092–1098.
44. Bogart JA, Chung CT, Mariados NF, et al. The value of gallium imaging after therapy for Hodgkin's disease. *Cancer* 1998;82(4):754–759.
45. Wong-You-Cheong J, Radford JA. Case report: Enlargement of a mediastinal mass during treatment of Hodgkin's disease may be due to accumulation of fluid within thymic cysts. *Clin Radiol* 1995;50:61–62.
46. Hunsaker AR, Munden RF, Pugatch RD, et al. Sarcoid-like reaction in patients with malignancy. *Radiology* 1996;200:255–261.
47. Castellino RA, DeLaPaz RL, Larson SM. Imaging techniques in cancer. In: DeVita V, Hellman S, Rosenberg SA, eds. *Principles and practice of oncology.* Philadelphia: JB Lippincott, 1993:507–531.
48. Castellino RA. Diagnostic radiology. In: Canellos GP, Lister TA, Sklar JL, eds. *The lymphomas.* Philadelphia: WB Saunders, 1998:187–206.
49. Castellino RA. Malignant lymphoma in adults. In: Bragg DG, Thompson WM, eds. *Categorical course on imaging of cancers: diagnosis, staging and follow-up challenges.* American College of Radiology, 1992:127–136.

SUGGESTED READINGS

Au V, Leung AN. Radiologic manifestations of lymphoma in the thorax. *AJR* 1997;168:93–98.

Castellino RA. Hodgkin disease: Practical concepts for the diagnostic radiologist. *Radiology* 1986;159:305.

Libshitz HJ, ed. Imaging the lymphomas. *Radiol Clin North Am* 1990;28. 669–899.

Musumeci R, Tesoro-Tess JD. New imaging techniques in staging lymphomas. *Curr Opin Oncol* 1994;6:464.

Stomper PC, Cholewinski SP, Park J, et al. Abdominal staging of thoracic Hodgkin disease: CT-lymphangiography-Ga-67 scanning correlation. *Radiology* 1993;187:381.

Hodgkin's Disease, edited by P. M. Mauch,
J. O. Armitage, V. Diehl, R. T. Hoppe, and L. M. Weiss.
Lippincott Williams & Wilkins, Philadephia ©1999.

CHAPTER 17

Surgical Procedures in Hodgkin's Disease

Samuel Singer and Robert T. Osteen

HISTORY OF SURGERY IN HODGKIN'S DISEASE

The therapy of Hodgkin's disease throughout the 19th century was largely symptomatic. From 1920 to 1950 there was some interest in the use of radical surgery for the treatment of localized Hodgkin's lymphoma. During this period there were reports of isolated Hodgkin's lesions that were treated with surgery and in a few instances long survival resulted (over 5 years) (1). These largely anecdotal studies were among the first to suggest that Hodgkin's disease can be cured, and that the disease in some patients may be localized and is not always disseminated from the onset. Stimulated by these early studies together with the limitations of kilovoltage radiotherapy techniques available during this time period, an increasing number of surgeons began to report favorable outcomes in selected, apparently localized cases of Hodgkin's disease. In 1947 Hellwig (2) reported that 25% of his series of 130 patients had survived for 5 years or more and that of 21 patients with a single primary focus in which radical surgery alone was performed, 12 were long-term survivors with no evidence of recurrence for periods of 5 to 20 years. Subsequent selected series of patients with localized disease treated by radical surgery achieved surprisingly high 5-year survival rates (3,4). From these studies it was documented that only a fraction of the lymph nodes in a radical node dissection specimen are likely to contain Hodgkin's disease and that other nodes immediately adjacent to them may be uninvolved. However, in most of the series that reported good results with radical surgery, radiotherapy had been given postoperatively and may have been responsible for the favorable outcome. With the advent of megavoltage radiotherapy, tumoricidal doses of radiotherapy could be delivered to entire chains of deep or superficial lymph nodes with little or no skin reaction or cosmetic deformity. This consideration along with the fact that radical surgery often produced cosmetic disfigurement end results and significant functional disability led most surgeons to accept that radical surgery was not indicated in the primary management of Hodgkin's disease.

Historical Review of Surgical Staging

Hodgkin's disease is characterized by an axial distribution of nodal disease and a contiguous, predictable pattern of spread. Staging systems and anatomic descriptions of the sites of tumor involvement in relation to the diaphragm were developed to differentiate patients who would benefit from treatment with radiation therapy alone from those who would require systemic therapy. The first useful staging classification for Hodgkin's disease relative to potentially curative therapy was proposed by Peters et al. (5), based on survival data of patients treated with radiation therapy. This three-stage Peters classification formed the basis of our current staging system. In 1965, the Rye classification improved the staging of Hodgkin's disease by providing a separate stage for disseminated disease outside the lymph node system and specifying guidelines for the pretreatment evaluation of patients (6,7). The Ann Arbor classification of 1971 (8) allowed for the definition of direct extralymphatic extension of a focal nature and the important distinction between clinically staged and pathologically staged disease. Based on data that localized extension of disease did not alter prognosis, patients whose disease spread from lymph nodes to adjacent organs were not considered to have diffuse dissemination. These patients were classified by the extent of lymph node involvement and labeled with the subscript E to represent direct extension (9). If there was splenic involvement, the patient's stage was

S. Singer and R. T. Osteen: Division of Surgical Oncology, Harvard Medical School and Brigham and Women's Hospital, Boston, Massachusetts.

labeled with the subscript S. Constitutional symptoms such as temperature greater than 38°C, night sweats, or weight loss of >10% body weight over a 6-month period were considered to confer a worse prognosis and were classified as B. Patients without these symptoms were staged in the A category. Data presented at the Ann Arbor conference determined that the available radiologic tests could not accurately predict splenic involvement. The exploratory laparotomy was therefore introduced to stage patients whose treatment would be altered by the presence or absence of subdiaphragmatic involvement. Staging laparotomy was originally developed by the Stanford University group to provide information about the patterns of involvement for subdiaphragmatic Hodgkin's disease (10,11).

As the patterns of subdiaphragmatic tumor involvement were surgically defined and correlated with clinical prognostic factors, changes to the Ann Arbor staging classification were considered. A new international staging classification based on a modification of the Ann Arbor staging system was proposed during a meeting held in Cotswold, England in 1989 (12). This new system recommended accounting for the presence of bulky disease [size greater than 10 cm maximum dimension or a mediastinal mass greater than one-third the transthoracic diameter at T5-T6 on an upright posteroanterior (PA) chest film] using the subscript X.

Clinical Presentation

The majority of patients with Hodgkin's lymphoma present with superficial adenopathy. The lymph node enlargement may be detected by the patient or on physical examination by a physician for unrelated symptoms. Often patients give a history of waxing and waning adenopathy over a period of months to years prior to diagnosis. Lymph node enlargement is usually manifested in the neck region as a painless, rubbery mass, with isolated axillary and inguinal lymph node presentations much less common. The involved solitary or multiple lymph nodes tend to be situated in an axial location, and contiguous nodal involvement is common. Fifty to sixty percent of patients with Hodgkin's disease present with mediastinal involvement (13). Thoracic adenopathy or a mediastinal mass may be detected on a routine chest radiography. Most patients who present with a mediastinal mass experience some degree of chest heaviness or discomfort and a cough. Some may have shortness of breath as a result of airway or lung compression. Such symptoms are almost always present when the chest disease is bulky (more than one-third the lateral chest wall diameter). Bulky disease that may result in an superior vena cava syndrome may also be seen at presentation (14,15). Abdominal nodal involvement is uncommon in asymptomatic patients, but it is more common in older patients or when a systemic symptom such as fever, night sweats, or weight loss is present. Epitrochlear nodes, Waldeyer's ring, the testes, and the intestine are rarely presenting sites for Hodgkin's disease. It is important to examine all peripheral lymph node sites and the spleen for evidence of disease.

Indications for Biopsy

The indications for peripheral lymph node biopsy depend on the size, shape, texture and location of the adenopathy. Soft, flat and elliptical nodes about 0.5 to 1 cm in size are commonly found in the submental and submandibular locations of normal patients. Similarly, soft elliptical 0.5-cm nodes are frequently palpated in the jugular or cervical chain, particularly in thin normal patients. Acute oral/pharyngeal infections are the most frequent cause of head and neck adenopathy in young patients. Posterior cervical nodes commonly enlarge secondary to scalp irritation and are rarely involved by Hodgkin's disease. Adenopathy secondary to infection may result in firm, spherical, enlarged lymph nodes that are often nontender and may be difficult on exam to distinguish from a lymph node involved by Hodgkin's disease. A patient with a suspected underlying infectious process and a firm, spherical lymph node greater than 1 cm in size may be followed clinically for a 4- to 8-week period. If the enlarged lymph node persists after treatment and resolution of the presumed infectious process, then a biopsy of the node should be performed. The majority of patients referred to the surgeon for biopsy of suspected Hodgkin's disease have had enlarged lymph nodes that have not responded to prior antibiotic treatment. Discrete, hard, and firm lymph nodes in older patients should be biopsied for diagnosis without delay. In an older patient with a hard mass in the upper or middle neck, a careful oral/pharyngeal and laryngeal exam for a primary tumor involving these sites should be performed. Similarly, primary tumors of the nasopharynx may present with posterior cervical adenopathy. Supraclavicular adenopathy is a common site for lymphoma, tumor, or infectious processes that arise from the lung or retroperitoneal space. Soft inguinal and axillary nodes are commonly felt in patients without cancer or Hodgkin's disease. In the absence of an infection or trauma in the extremity of a patient with an enlarged, solitary axillary mass, the most likely diagnoses are lymphoma, melanoma, and breast cancer. Thus, any firm, enlarging, greater than 1 cm peripheral lymph node in the absence of infection/trauma should undergo biopsy for histologic diagnosis.

Peripheral Lymph Node Biopsy

There are four different methods of biopsy available to the surgeon to establish a tissue diagnosis: fine-needle aspiration, core biopsy, open incisional biopsy, and open excisional biopsy. In a fine-needle aspiration the tip of the needle is guided into the tumor mass, with two or three passes of the needle often required to ensure adequate sampling of the mass. The specimen is then evaluated by the cytopathologist for evidence of malignancy. Fine-needle aspiration is particularly useful for patients suspected of having a primary cancer of the head and neck (nonlymphomatous) or thyroid, as it avoids contamination of surrounding tissue planes prior to definitive therapy. However, if a lymphoma is suspected based on the needle aspiration or it is nondiagnostic, then an open lymph node biopsy is necessary to establish tissue architecture and subtyping. If the node is 1 to 3 cm in size, a carefully performed excisional biopsy is the procedure of choice for a peripheral node. For nodes larger than 3 cm or nodes fixed to underlying structures, an incisional biopsy is often the most prudent approach with an aim of sampling 1 to 2 cm^3 of nodal tissue. Although, a 3-mm core biopsy theoretically could be used for peripheral nodes, it still provides relatively small fragments of tissue for the pathologist and is often more traumatic and less controlled than an open biopsy. The importance of adequate tissue sampling cannot be overemphasized, since most of the suspicious node may contain normal lymphocytes, plasma cells, and fibrous stroma and only a scattering of the malignant Reed-Sternberg cells and their mononuclear variants characteristic of Hodgkin's disease. Sufficient tissue is also essential for the accurate histologic classification of Hodgkin's into lymphocyte-predominance, nodular sclerosis, mixed-cellularity, and lymphocyte-depletion subtypes. In about 10% to 15% of cases it may be difficult to establish a diagnosis of Hodgkin's disease and distinguish it from other benign and malignant lymphoproliferative conditions (see Chapter 12). Occasionally multiple biopsies are needed to obtain diagnostic tissue or sufficient tissue for classification. Thus, an open biopsy is the preferred approach in most situations since it is more likely to yield sufficient pathologic information compared to core biopsy or fine-needle aspiration. See Table 1 for a summary of the advantages and disadvantages of each type of biopsy. In difficult or atypical cases, consultative review of biopsy material by another hematopathologist is recommended prior to initiation of therapy.

Mediastinoscopy

An anterosuperior mediastinal mass in the absence of peripheral adenopathy requires an accurate tissue diagnosis. Although these lesions may be reached by fine-needle biopsy, this approach is not recommended because it yields nondiagnostic cells or, when diagnostic for lymphoma, it is inadequate for subclassification of the lymphoma (16). To obtain sufficient diagnostic tissue, one of several surgical approaches may be selected depending on the anatomic location of the mass. Mediastinoscopy (cervical or anterior), anterior mediastinotomy, median sternotomy, thoracotomy, or thoracoscopy can usually be used to evaluate, perform a biopsy, and obtain sufficient nodal tissue for definitive diagnosis. These procedures are performed under general anesthesia and allow a minimally invasive surgical approach to biopsy. Median sternotomy or thoracotomy is rarely required since complete surgical removal of the mass is not indicated in the treatment of Hodgkin's disease, and the morbidity of these open procedures is excessive compared to the minimally invasive procedures available to establish a tissue diagnosis.

The choice of cervical or anterior mediastinoscopy depends on the anatomic location of the mass. Both are preferable to thoracoscopy because they can be performed on an outpatient basis (17). Cervical mediastinoscopy provides biopsy capability under direct

TABLE 1. *Type of biopsy technique: advantages and disadvantages*

Type of biopsy	Advantages	Disadvantages
Fine-needle aspiration	Minimally invasive, often may be performed in outpatient or office setting with minimal risk; often useful for diagnosing recurrent disease or if open biopsy is difficult or hazardous	Grading and subtyping may be extremely difficult if not impossible since such small samples of malignant cells are obtained; requires considerable expertise in cytopathology
Core needle biopsy	Minimal contamination of tissue planes and the availability of tissue architecture; this technique is especially useful for large, deep-seated tumors in the pelvis or paraspinal area, which then avoids an open surgical biopsy	The small sample size may not be representative of the entire tumor and may miss high-grade areas of the tumor that are not sampled with a core biopsy; often requires radiologic guidance with potential risk of bleeding and injury to surrounding normal structures
Open incisional biopsy	Provides a small (1 cm × 1 cm × 1 cm) yet representative piece of tissue with minimal violation of normal surrounding tissues	For deep-seated pelvic or abdominal lymph nodes requires general anesthesia with abdominal wall incision
Open excisional biopsy	Used for lymph nodes <3 cm in size that are not fixed to surrounding structures; no sampling error, provides sufficient tissue for special studies, allows for meticulous homeostasis	Most invasive technique for deep-seated pelvic or abdominal lymph nodes requires general anesthesia with abdominal wall incision

vision in the paratracheal middle mediastinum, behind the aortic arch and innominate veins. This approach is of no benefit when tumors are in the anterior or posterior paravertebral mediastinum. Thus, cervical mediastinoscopy is the procedure of choice for the diagnosis of midmediastinal lymphomas. Limited thoracotomy is very useful for the diagnosis of mediastinal lymphomas, particularly in the anterior mediastinum. The procedure may be accomplished with parasternal mediastinotomy via removal of a costal cartilage, or via a more extensive anterior thoracotomy. Both cervical and anterior mediastinoscopy can be performed on an outpatient basis. Video thoracoscopy is used to approach inaccessible posterior lesions, suspicious lung nodules, or for the restaging of anterior lesions on which previous biopsies have already been performed (18). Peripheral lung lesions may be excised by performing wedge resections using visually guided thoracoscopy with minimal morbidity. With the advent of cross-sectional imaging and the judicious use of mediastinoscopy and video thoracoscopy, an accurate diagnosis should be obtained for any mediastinal mass. Thus, sternotomy or thoracotomy with their associated morbidity are rarely required to establish a diagnosis of mediastinal Hodgkin's. Although a frozen section may be obtained to assure adequate sampling of lesional tissue at the time of biopsy, a definitive diagnosis of lymphoma is usually not possible on frozen-section material.

Biopsy of Deep Retroperitoneal Adenopathy

Hodgkin's rarely involves retroperitoneal lymph nodes without significant neck or mediastinal lymph node involvement, so isolated biopsy of a retroperitoneal lymph node is usually not required to establish a diagnosis of Hodgkin's disease. Fine-needle aspiration is the least invasive approach to an enlarged retroperitoneal lymph node. With sufficient sampling a diagnosis may be made in 80% of cases; however, fine-needle aspiration has been unsuccessful in establishing the histologic subtype of Hodgkin's disease. Rarely, fine-needle aspiration may be indicated to prove involvement of retroperitoneal nodes in a patient with an established diagnosis. Tissue cores of 1.5 mm by 2 cm in size can be obtained with a 14-gauge core biopsy needle. With the core biopsy approach, sufficient tissue for both diagnosis and subtype is possible. Both the core biopsy and fine-needle aspiration technique are more often of use in the patient with a previously established diagnosis of Hodgkin's disease where the presence of recurrent retroperitoneal or abdominal disease needs to be documented.

Another minimally invasive approach for assessment of retroperitoneal adenopathy is laparoscopic lymph node biopsy. This has been a well-recognized procedure for sampling pelvic lymph nodes by gynecologists and urologists, but has not been widely reported for hematologic disease, which commonly involves less accessible periaortic nodes. Although this approach does require a general anesthetic, a recent series suggests a high diagnostic yield (90%) and a relatively short hospital stay (19). With this technique a more complete sampling of the diseased lymph node is possible compared to percutaneous computed tomography (CT)-guided approaches to diagnosis. A significant disadvantage to the laparoscopic approach is the inability to directly palpate the nodal disease so as to determine the best and safest node to biopsy for diagnosis. Significant retroperitoneal fibrosis may make definitive diagnosis without open biopsy extremely difficult. For retroperitoneal nodes below the pelvic brim, a transverse incision 2 cm above the inguinal ligament provides access for open biopsy of iliac lymph nodes. For superficial external iliac nodes, this approach can be performed under a local anesthetic and does not require a hospital stay. For retroperitoneal adenopathy above the pelvic brim, a midline incision usually provides the best exposure for biopsy. During the open biopsy it is usually advisable for the hematopathologist to perform a touch prep or frozen section on a small piece of the biopsied lymph node to verify that sufficient diagnostic tissue has been obtained. This approach avoids the problem of having to repeat an open biopsy.

Biopsy of Extranodal Sites

When the diagnosis of Hodgkin's disease is made from biopsy of an extranodal site, a concomitant nodal biopsy for confirmation of diagnosis is usually needed unless the diagnosis is considered unequivocal. Extranodal sites include liver, bone, or lung. Percutaneous or open Tru-cut core biopsies of liver may be accomplished with minimal risk. Wedge liver biopsies may also provide sufficient tissue for diagnosis and may be performed by laparoscopy or laparotomy. Bone biopsies of symptomatic bone lesions may be radiologically directed or marked by radionuclide scan for open biopsy. Marrow involvement in Hodgkin's disease is often spotty and associated with fibrosis. Magnetic resonance imaging may be a potentially valuable tool in investigating bone marrow involvement and can help in directing image-guided biopsies (20). In patients with clinical stage IIIA through IVB disease, systemic symptoms, bone lesions, bone pain, or elevated serum alkaline phosphatase bilateral posterior iliac crest bone marrow core biopsies should be obtained. Fewer than 1% of patients with clinical stage IA and IIA disease will have bone marrow involvement, so bone marrow biopsy may be omitted in these patients. Occasionally, biopsy of extranodal pulmonary parenchymal involvement is required for complete staging. This is probably best approached through thoracoscopic wedge excision of the suspicious pulmonary nodule as a negative needle biopsy is not helpful. Cutaneous lesions are easily biopsied under local anesthesia to document skin involvement.

Processing of Fresh Biopsy Tissue for Immunohistochemistry and Molecular Genetic Studies

The most important aspect of evaluating a lymph node for possible lymphoma is to have an experienced hematopathologist process, prepare, and evaluate the tissue. Improperly fixed or prepared tissue may be nondiagnostic or uninterpretable. If accessible peripheral adenopathy for biopsy is limited, it may be prudent to have the biopsy performed at a center where an experienced hematopathologist can prepare the specimen to optimize the diagnostic yield and avoid the problem of having the patient undergo a second biopsy procedure to establish a definitive diagnosis. The surgeon performing a lymph node biopsy should notify the hematopathologist of the patient's history and send the nodal tissue to the pathologist in an empty container (if processed immediately) or in sterile saline (never in fixative). Typically a portion of tissue is separately fixed in formalin, B5 media, snap frozen, and a portion sent in sterile culture media for cytogenetics. The B5-fixed portion of nodal tissue allows for optimal preservation of cellular and nuclear features, which are often critical for appropriate lymphoma diagnosis. The B5 fixative is a mercury-based solution that requires the implementation of costly procedures for proper disposal and is often not available at many community hospitals. Reliable interpretation of the immunohistochemistry is dependent on the careful application of specific monoclonal antibody protocols to unstained 5-m paraffin-embedded sections. The surgeon performing a diagnostic biopsy for lymphoma should be sure an experienced hematopathologist is available prior to initiating the procedure and should deliver the fresh tissue to the pathologist for both routine and special studies.

SURGICAL STAGING

Current Indications for Staging Laparotomy

The routine use of staging laparotomy remains controversial and the procedure has acceptable but significant morbidity and rare mortality (21,22). Several studies have failed to show a survival advantage for patients undergoing pathologic staging with laparotomy compared to those undergoing clinical staging only (23,24). Since the purpose of staging laparotomy is to improve staging and limit therapy, one would not expect survival to be affected. Thus, the decision to perform a staging laparotomy depends on institutional treatment policies and operative morbidity.

Currently, staging laparotomy primarily serves to identify those patients whose Hodgkin's disease may be treated with radiation therapy alone and possibly to limit the radiotherapy treatment volume and thus the potential long-term side effects. The procedure is justified only if its results will alter therapy and permit the treating physician to customize the radiation therapy fields to the individual patient. Recent reviews of surgically staged patients presenting with supradiaphragmatic Hodgkin's disease suggest that 20% to 30% of clinical stage IA to IIA and 35% of clinical stage IB to IIB patients will have occult splenic or upper abdominal node involvement not detected by routine radiographic staging (25,26). The studies have selected favorable prognostic factors that help identify those patients unlikely to have subdiaphragmatic involvement. Selected subgroups such as clinical stage IA females, clinical stage IIA females younger than 26 years of age with limited nodal disease, and clinical stage IA males with lymphocyte-predominant Hodgkin's disease on histology have a low risk of occult abdominal involvement (6% to 9%). Given this low risk, these subgroups of patients may be candidates for radiation therapy alone without staging laparotomy. The remainder of clinical stage I and II patients (about 80%) remain at considerable risk for tumor involvement in the spleen or abdominal nodes (24% to 36%) that will be outside the field of radiotherapy unless radiation fields are extended or if the patients are treated by chemotherapy (26,27).

Preoperative Staging Studies of Importance to the Surgeon

Preoperatively the surgeon should carefully review the patient's history for constitutional symptoms and perform a complete clinical nodal and abdominal exam. Routine blood work, including complete blood count, platelet count, prothrombin time, and liver function tests, should be reviewed (Table 2), because abnormalities may indicate advanced Hodgkin's disease or a concurrent medical problem that may pose an anesthesia or surgery risk. The surgeon should review the abdominal pelvic CT scan and

TABLE 2. *Recommended preoperative staging studies*

History	Detailed history with special attention to presence or absence of systemic symptoms
Physical exam	Detailed physical exam with special attention to nodal chains, size of liver and spleen, and bony tenderness
Routine laboratory tests	Complete blood count, prothrombin time, liver function tests
Chest radiograph	
Chest CT scan	
Abdominal/pelvic CT scan	
Gallium scan	
Core needle biopsy of bone marrow	Biopsy may be omitted in patients with clinical stage IA and IIA disease

CT, computed tomography.

gallium scan, since any suspicious areas on these studies should be targeted for complete and careful examination during the laparotomy. Bipedal lymphangiography may provide complementary information to the CT scan with regard to abdominal node involvement and is particularly sensitive for identifying small changes in nodal architecture. However, most centers are now using CT scans alone, since lymphangiography has been felt to be tedious, difficult to perform, and of limited value. Bone marrow biopsy of specimens at least 2 cm in length should be performed and reviewed prior to laparotomy unless the patient presents with clinical stage IA or IIA disease (because this subgroup of patients has a less than 1% chance of bone marrow involvement).

Contraindications for Staging Laparotomy

A staging laparotomy should not be performed unless information obtained from the laparotomy will be used to determine the therapeutic approach. Although in the past laparotomy was used as a research tool to determine the patterns of involvement of Hodgkin's and the accuracy of clinical/radiologic staging, these reasons no longer justify its application. Thus, laparotomy should be performed only if the knowledge obtained from the procedure will influence the type and scope of therapy recommended for the individual patient. It should be carried out by surgeons and pathologists experienced in performing a complete staging procedure. Significant cardiac, respiratory, or renal risk factors are relative contraindications to laparotomy. Obesity (greater than 20% over ideal body weight) adds considerable morbidity to laparotomy and increases the difficulty of complete nodal assessment and therefore serves as a relative contraindication to staging laparotomy. Complications seen with any type of surgery in obese patients include wound infection, wound dehiscence, incisional hernia, thrombophlebitis and pulmonary embolus. Obesity may also be predictive of increased postoperative pulmonary morbidity, since obesity leads to decreased lung volumes and an increase work of breathing. Thus, postoperative problems related to ineffective cough, atelectasis, hypoxemia, and infections all occur with greater frequency in obese patients.

Age is a relative contraindication to staging laparotomy because of an increasing morbidity noted for patients over 60 years of age. These patients are at some increased risk because their physiologic reserve is compromised, and they require careful assessment of the individual organ systems including cardiovascular, respiratory, renal, cerebrovascular, hepatic, and endocrine before considering laparotomy. Patients 40 to 60 years of age should be seriously considered for staging laparotomy since they have a higher risk of mortality from treatment-related complications and poorer survival after relapse; staging laparotomy may allow for delivery of minimal treatment with a high disease-free survival. Thus, for each patient the potential risks must be weighed carefully against the impact the staging information will have on planning subsequent therapy.

Preoperative Surgical Preparation

Because of the small but finite risk of postsplenectomy sepsis, all patients should undergo immunization at least 1 week prior to the planned staging laparotomy. Patients should be routinely given the new polysaccharide-conjugate vaccines against pneumococcus, *Haemophilus influenzae* type B, and meningococcus type C if feasible. The patient should also be told that if symptoms of a significant infection develop such as fever or stiff neck, medical attention and antibiotic therapy should be sought immediately because of the potential fulminate nature of these capsular bacterial infections. Children are particularly susceptible to postsplenectomy sepsis, and in addition to vaccination they should receive oral prophylactic penicillin until age 18. All patients should undergo revaccination at 5- to 6-year intervals.

Operative Technique for Open Staging Laparotomy

A complete staging laparotomy begins with a detailed inspection and palpation of the abdomen, including all nodal groups. This exploration is performed through an upper midline incision made from xiphoid to umbilicus. A left upper quadrant incision is not advisable since this provides poor exposure for the staging part of the procedure. The spleen is removed and sectioned into 0.3-cm slices and if disease is present the total number of nodules recorded. Routine wedge biopsy of the right lobe of the liver and Tru-cut needle biopsy of the left lobe of the liver should be performed. Grossly abnormal areas of liver should be biopsied as well. Biopsy of right and left paraaortic and iliac nodes should be performed. Palpation by an experienced surgeon is probably the most reliable way to identify involved nodes since they often feel rubbery/firm even if they are only 1.5 cm in size. If there are no suspicious nodes, then several normal-feeling nodes are biopsied. Splenic hilar, porta-hepatic, and celiac nodes are assessed and biopsied in a similar fashion.

Particular attention should be paid to the palpation of the paraaortic area just underneath the diaphragm, and any suspicious node biopsied. Iliac nodes may be assessed by direct palpation through the upper midline incision, and it is rarely necessary to extend the incision below the umbilicus. A bone marrow biopsy should be performed through the anterior iliac crest if a marrow biopsy was not previously performed preoperatively. Radiopaque titanium clips should be placed on the splenic pedicle so that the radiotherapist can minimize the lateral extent of the radiation field and thus minimize radiation to the left lower lobe of the lung, the kidney, and the colon.

Currently, oophoropexy (the placement of ovaries out of their normal position) is not indicated unless a pelvic radiation field is anticipated. Thus, the need to perform oophoropexy should be discussed with the radiation oncologist prior to planned laparotomy. The main indications for oophoropexy are for patients who present with primary subdiaphragmatic disease or for patients receiving pelvic radiotherapy for recurrent disease. The ovaries are usually very mobile and may be moved from their usual lateral location near the iliac lymph nodes to a position as close to the midsagittal plane as possible, either behind or in front of the uterus, where they are sutured in place with synthetic absorbable sutures. The lateral extent of each ovary is marked with double clips so as to assist the radiotherapist in the radiographic visualization of the ovaries to allow for appropriate placement of lead shields. In the Stanford series more than 70% of the patients who underwent midline oophoropexy and pelvic radiotherapy with midpelvic shielding have continued to have normal menstrual periods, with a substantial number of patients going on to conceive full-term infants. The failure of return of menstrual function in the remaining 30% of patients was attributed to the difficulty of placing the ovaries exactly in the midline. Even a 1-cm shift of the ovary lateral to midline was felt to result in a appreciably larger scatter dose to the ovary. A recent study suggests that a greater percentage of patients treated with pelvic radiotherapy had preserved ovarian function with laterally transposed ovaries compared to medial transposed ovaries (28). However, there have been no reported pregnancies among women who have been treated with pelvic radiotherapy after oophoropexy by the lateral ovarian transposition technique.

The frequency of key anatomical subdiaphragmatic regions involved with Hodgkin's disease in 285 consecutive cases has been published by the Stanford group (Table 3) (13). Liver involvement is extremely rare in the absence of an involved spleen. Bone marrow involvement is usually associated with constitutional symptoms and otherwise extensive disease. Skin, subcutaneous fat, gastrointestinal tract, and breast involvement rarely occur in Hodgkin's disease.

The concept of partial splenectomy as part of a staging laparotomy was initially introduced as a means of preserving splenic function and preventing overwhelming postsplenectomy sepsis. In a series of partial splenectomy for ten children with Hodgkin's disease, it was reported that all ten had one-third to one-fourth of their spleen removed, and only one spleen had histologic evidence of Hodgkin's disease (29). There were no reported deaths, episodes of sepsis, or evidence of Hodgkin's recurrence. An analysis of the risk of disease understaging by partial splenectomy was performed by Dearth et al. (30) by examining the spleens of 112 patients staged with laparotomy; 13 patients (11.6%) were found to have limited splenic involvement, with five or fewer nodules localized to a single pole of the spleen and with no visible subcapsular involvement. In another study of 180 patients by Sterchi et al. (31), a 6.2% risk of understaging with partial splenectomy was found. Thus, from both these studies it was felt that partial splenectomy could not exclude occult splenic involvement, and that these patients would be consistently undertreated. In addition to underestimating the stage of disease, the other risk of partial splenectomy would be an increased recurrence in the area of the splenic remnant if the patient is understaged and this area is not treated. A recent series suggests that many of these relapses may occur after 3 years and thus stresses the importance of continued close follow-up for recurrence beyond 3 years (32). The spleen remains the most frequently involved intraabdominal organ and is the only site involved in 50% of cases with a positive laparotomy result (21).

Postoperative management and recovery after staging laparotomy typically involves early ambulation postoperatively with pneumatic compression boots applied prior to induction of anesthesia. The nasogastric tube is typically removed on postoperative day 1, with clear liquids instituted on postoperative day 2. A majority of patients are advanced to regular diet by postoperative day 3 and may be discharged on oral pain medication.

TABLE 3. *Subdiaphragmatic anatomic distribution of Hodgkin's disease in 285 consecutive unselected and untreated cases*

Site of involvement	Number of cases involved	% of 285 consecutive cases
Spleen	99	35
Paraaortic	90	32
Splenic hilar/celiac	36	13
Left iliac	36	13
Right iliac	31	11
Left groin	27	9
Right groin	22	8
Liver	9	3
Mesenteric	3	1
Bone marrow	9	3

From ref. 13.

Most patients are off all pain medication by the 2nd or 3rd week postsurgery and may begin treatment with either radiotherapy or chemotherapy depending on the results of their laparotomy.

Laparoscopic Splenectomy and Lymph Node Staging

Recently laparoscopic techniques for splenectomy have been developed with the intent of reducing morbidity and improving lengths of stay compared to those with conventional open techniques. The series involving laparoscopic splenectomy have largely been confined to removing normal-sized spleens in patients with Hodgkin's, idiopathic thrombocytic purpura, and hemolytic anemia. In fact an enlarged spleen is a relative contraindication to the laparoscopic approach. The first laparoscopic splenectomy for Hodgkin's was performed in 1992 (33). Since then there have been several case reports and small series that have detailed the technique of laparoscopic splenectomy together with laparoscopic lymph node biopsy (34–37). This minimally invasive technique is performed using a five-puncture technique, with the patient under general anesthesia and in the supine position. After producing a pneumoperitoneum, a 10-mm trocar is placed in the umbilical area. A 30-degree viewing laparoscope is placed through the umbilical trocar and a general abdominal inspection is carried out. Four other 10-mm trocars are then placed as shown in Figure 1. Lymph node biopsies are taken from the iliac, paraaortic, hepatic, celiac, and mesenteric areas. Wedge and Tru-cut liver biopies are performed via the laparoscope. The spleen is then removed by ligating the main splenic artery through the lesser sac. The splenocolic ligament is cut with an electrocautery scissors. The spleen is then elevated and the segmental splenic arteries and veins are dissected close to the splenic capsule and serially ligated and divided. The short gastric vessels are ligated and divided using extracorporeal techniques. Finally, the retroperitoneal attachments to the spleen are divided and the spleen is placed in a heavy plastic bag. For Hodgkin's patients, the spleen must be delivered intact, since if it is morcellated in the bag it would be impossible for the pathologist to reliably identify small focal nodules of Hodgkin's disease. Typically, the bag containing the spleen is brought through to the umbilical trocar site and the incision is enlarged 3 to 5 cm to permit removal of the bag with the intact spleen. The need for delivering the entire spleen intact remains an important reason for not using a laparoscopic approach for Hodgkin's staging.

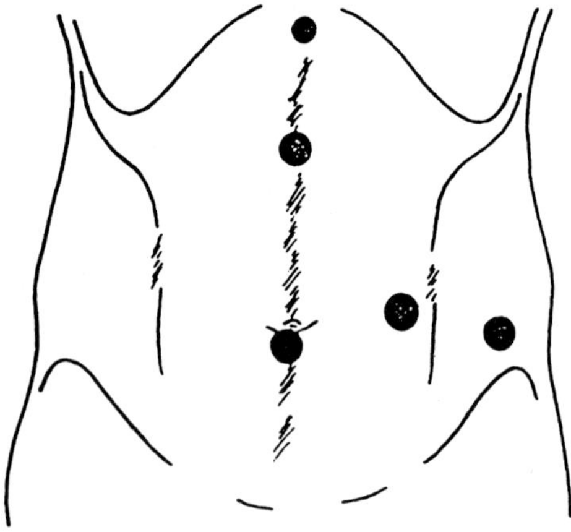

FIG. 1. Location of trocar sites for laparoscopic splenectomy.

The technique of laparoscopic staging laparotomy is still evolving, and series combining laparoscopic splenectomy with lymph node biopsy remain small (34,37). This new technique has not been directly compared to open staging laparotomy in terms of accuracy of pathologic staging. Even preliminary studies comparing the morbidity, length of hospital stay, and hospital cost are inconclusive and include many patients with a diagnosis other than Hodgkin's disease (19,38–40). Even in these series the shorter hospital stays of the laparoscopic approach (3 days versus 5 days) are largely offset by the twofold longer operative times in laparoscopic compared to open approaches. The main disadvantages of the laparoscopic approach are the surgeon's loss of tactile sensation and loss of depth perception, the longer operative times, and the higher cost of instruments. Additionally, should bleeding occur, it is more difficult to control with the laparoscopic approach. The inability of the surgeon to palpate a firm, involved, often small lymph node with the laparoscopic technique may lead the operating surgeon to overlook a node that would have been easily identified by an experienced surgeon using the open technique. Before this new technique is widely applied to Hodgkin's patients, well-designed trials should be developed to test its accuracy in pathologic staging, and prospective randomized trials should clearly demonstrate a reduction in morbidity and cost compared to open laparotomy.

Complications of Surgical Staging

The major complications that may occur following staging laparotomy include cardiopulmonary arrest, wound infection, dehiscence, postoperative surgical bleeding, gastrointestinal bleeding, gastric stress ulceration, pulmonary embolism, pneumonia, sepsis, small bowel obstruction, pancreatitis, pancreatic pseudocyst, and subphrenic abscess. Minor complications include pleural effusions, prolonged ileus, atelectasis, and urinary tract infections. The morbidity and mortality of the procedure vary among institutions; however, the major complication rate ranges from 5% to 13%, and the minor complication rate from 2% to 22%. The complication rates are dependent on patient age and comorbid disease as well as on the experience of the operating surgeon. Mortality has ranged from 0% to 1% depending on the series (21,22,41).

The late complications that may develop after staging laparotomy include postsplenectomy sepsis, adhesions, hernia, and small bowel obstruction. Postsplenectomy sepsis is a significant problem in children, particularly in those under 10 years of age. Splenectomized children appear to be at significantly increased risk of fulminant bacterial sepsis due to streptococcus and hemophilus. A study of 1,170 splenectomized Hodgkin's patients revealed 16 instances of serious infection; six of these patients went on to die—a 0.5% late mortality rate (42). A retrospective national survey by the children's cancer study group showed 20 episodes of severe sepsis in 18 of 200 children splenectomized for Hodgkin's disease, with ten deaths (43). From these studies it was difficult to determine if treatment with radiotherapy/chemotherapy rather than splenectomy may have contributed to a substantial proportion of these infections. Sudden severe infections have an incidence of 5% to 10% in children postsplenectomy (44). The use of prophylactic antibiotics and capsular vaccine prophylaxis in this high-risk group has reduced the incidence of postsplenectomy sepsis and death dramatically (45). In adult patients who are appropriately vaccinated and informed of the risks of postsplenectomy sepsis, there has been a marked reduction in the incidence of overwhelming sepsis. These adult splenectomized patients have a sepsis incidence no different from nonsplenectomized patients with Hodgkin's disease (46).

Surgical Evaluation of Recurrent Disease

For new, recurrent, superficial peripheral adenopathy in the patient who has been treated in the past for Hodgkin's disease, an open or excision biopsy under local anesthesia is the procedure of choice. For deep abdominal or retroperitoneal adenopathy, a CT-guided core biopsy and/or aspiration is often sufficient to confirm a diagnosis of recurrent Hodgkin's disease. This approach has the advantage of not requiring an anesthetic and is minimally invasive. If the node is not accessible to CT-guided biopsy or there is insufficient tissue, then a laparoscopic or open biopsy under general anesthesia may be performed. While the patient is under the general anesthetic, a frozen section or touch prep should be performed to see if sufficient diagnostic tissue has been obtained. If not, a more representative biopsy can often be obtained while the patient is still anesthetized.

REFERENCES

1. Slaughter D, Craver L. Hodgkin's disease: five year survival rate; value of early surgical treatment; notes on four cases of long duration. *Am J Roentgen* 1942;47:596.
2. Hellwig C. Malignant lymphoma; the value of radical surgery in selected cases. *Surg Gynecol Obstet* 1947;84:950–958.
3. Slaughter D, Economou S, Southwick H. Surgical management of Hodgkin's disease. *Ann Surg* 1958;148:705.
4. Pack G, Molander D. The surgical treatment of Hodgkin's disease. *Cancer Res* 1966;26:1254.
5. Peters M, Hasselbach R, Brown T. The natural history of lymphomas related to the clinical classification. In: Zarafonetis C, ed. *Proceedings of the International Conference on Leukemia-lymphoma.* Philadelphia: Lea & Febiger, 1968:357.
6. Lukes R, Butler J, Hicks E. Natural history of Hodgkin's disease as related to its pathologic picture. *Cancer* 1966;19:317.
7. Keller AR, Kaplan HS, Lukes RJ, Rappaport H. Correlation of histopathology with other prognostic indicators in Hodgkin's disease. *Cancer* 1968;22(3):487–499.
8. Carbone PP, Kaplan HS, Musshoff K. Report of the Committee on Hodgkin's Disease Staging Classification. *Cancer Res* 1971;31(11): 1860–1861.
9. Musshoff K. Prognostic and therapeutic implications of staging in extranodal Hodgkin's disease. *Cancer Res* 1971;31:1814–1827.
10. Glatstein E, Guernsey JM, Rosenberg SA, Kaplan HS. The value of laparotomy and splenectomy in the staging of Hodgkin's disease. *Cancer* 1969;24(4):709–718.
11. Glatstein E, Trueblood HW, Enright LP, et al. Surgical staging of abdominal involvement in unselected patients with Hodgkin's disease. *Radiology* 1970;97:425.
12. Lister TA, Crowther D, Sutcliffe SB, et al. Report of a committee convened to discuss the evaluation and staging of patients with Hodgkin's disease: Cotswolds meeting. *J Clin Oncol* 1989;7(11):1630–1636.
13. Kaplan HS, Dorfman RF, Nelsen TS, Rosenberg SA. Staging laparotomy and splenectomy in Hodgkin's disease: analysis of indications and patterns of involvement in 285 consecutive, unselected patients. *Natl Cancer Inst Monogr* 1973;36:291–301.
14. Yellin A, Rosen A, Reichert N, Lieberman Y. Superior vena cava syndrome. The myth—the facts. *Am Rev Respir Dis* 1990;141(5 pt 1): 1114–1118.
15. Yellin A, Mandel M, Rechavi G, et al. Superior vena cava syndrome associated with lymphoma. *Am J Dis Child* 1992;146(9):1060–1063.
16. Bonfiglio TA, Dvoretsky PM, Piscioli F, et al. Fine needle aspiration biopsy in the evaluation of lymphoreticular tumors of the thorax. *Acta Cytol* 1985;29(4):548–553.
17. Rendina EA, Venuta F, De Giacomo T, et al. Comparative merits of thoracoscopy, mediastinoscopy, and mediastinotomy for mediastinal biopsy. *Ann Thorac Surg* 1994;57(4):992–995.
18. Bonadies J, D'Agostino RS, Ruskis AF, Ponn RB. Outpatient mediastinoscopy. *J Thorac Cardiovasc Surg* 1993;106(4):686–688.
19. Rhodes M, Rudd M, O'Rourke N, et al. Laparoscopic splenectomy and lymph node biopsy for hematologic disorders. *Ann Surg* 1995;222(1): 43–46.
20. Smith SR, Roberts N, Percy DF, Edwards RH. Detection of bone marrow abnormalities in patients with Hodgkin's disease by T1 mapping of MR images of lumbar vertebral bone marrow. *Br J Cancer* 1992;65(2): 246–251.
21. Taylor MA, Kaplan HS, Nelsen TS. Staging laparotomy with splenectomy for Hodgkin's disease: the Stanford experience. *World J Surg* 1985; 9(3):449–460.
22. Muskat PC, Johnson RA, Bowers GJ. Staging laparotomy in Hodgkin's lymphoma: 1979 to 1988. *Am J Surg* 1991;162(6):603–606; discussion 606–607.
23. Tubiana M, Henry-Amar M, Carde P, et al. Toward comprehensive management tailored to prognostic factors of patients with clinical stages I and II in Hodgkin's disease. The EORTC Lymphoma Group controlled clinical trials: 1964–1987. *Blood* 1989;73(1):47–56.
24. Carde P, Hagenbeek A, Hayat M, et al. Clinical staging versus laparotomy and combined modality with MOPP versus ABVD in early-stage Hodgkin's disease: the H6 twin randomized trials from the European Organization for Research and Treatment of Cancer Lymphoma Cooperative Group. *J Clin Oncol* 1993;11(11):2258–2272.
25. Leibenhaut MH, Hoppe RT, Efron B, et al. Prognostic indicators of laparotomy findings in clinical stage I–II supradiaphragmatic Hodgkin's disease. *J Clin Oncol* 1989;7(1):81–91.
26. Mauch P, Larson D, Osteen R, et al. Prognostic factors for positive surgical staging in patients with Hodgkin's disease [see comments]. *J Clin Oncol* 1990;8(2):257–265.
27. Mauch P, Somers R. Controversies in the use of diagnostic staging laparotomy and splenectomy in the management of Hodgkin's disease. *Ann Oncol* 1992;3(suppl 4):41–43.
28. Hadar H, Loven D, Herskovitz P, et al. An evaluation of lateral and medial transposition of the ovaries out of radiation fields. *Cancer* 1994; 74(2):774–779.
29. Boles ET Jr, Haase GM, Hamoudi AB. Partial splenectomy in staging

laparotomy for Hodgkin's disease: an alternative approach. *J Pediatr Surg* 1978;13(6D):581–586.
30. Dearth JC, Gilchrist GS, Telander RL, et al. Partial splenectomy for staging Hodgkin's disease: risk of false-negative results. *N Engl J Med* 1978;299(7):345–346.
31. Sterchi JM, Buss DH, Beyer FC. The risk of improperly staging Hodgkin's disease with partial splenectomy. *Am Surg* 1984;50(1):20–22.
32. Duchesne G, Crow J, Ashley S, et al. Changing patterns of relapse in Hodgkin's disease. *Br J Cancer* 1989;60(2):227–230.
33. Carroll BJ, Phillips EH, Semel CJ, et al. Laparoscopic splenectomy. *Surg Endosc* 1992;6:183–185.
34. Lefor AT, Flowers JL, Heyman MR. Laparoscopic staging of Hodgkin's disease. *Surg Oncol* 1993;2(3):217–220.
35. Lefor AT, Flowers JL, Judmaier G, et al. Laparoscopic wedge biopsy of the liver: a combined biopsy-plugging device based on the Menghini- or Trucut needle for percutaneous liver biopsy: clinical experience. *J Am Coll Surg* 1994;178(3):307–308.
36. Greene FL, Brown PA. Laparoscopic approaches to abdominal malignancy. *Semin Surg Oncol* 1994;10(6):386–390.
37. Carroll BJ, Decker RW, Chandra M, Phillips EH. Laparoscopic staging of Hodgkin's disease (meeting abstract). *Proc Annu Meet Am Soc Clin Oncol* 1995;14:A1284.
38. Moores DC, McKee MA, Wang H, et al. Pediatric laparoscopic splenectomy. *J Pediatr Surg* 1995;30(8):1201–1205.
39. Beanes S, Emil S, Kosi M, et al. A comparison of laparoscopic versus open splenectomy in children. *Am Surg* 1995;61(10):908–910.
40. Smith CD, Meyer TA, Goretsky MJ, et al. Laparoscopic splenectomy by the lateral approach: a safe and effective alternative to open splenectomy for hematologic diseases. *Surgery* 1996;120(5):789–794.
41. Sterchi JM, Myers RT. Staging laparotomy in Hodgkin's disease. *Ann Surg* 1980;191(5):570–575.
42. Dresser R, Ultmann J. Risk of severe infection in patients with Hodgkin's disease or lymphoma after diagnostic laparotomy and spleenectomy. *Ann Intern Med* 1972;77:143–146.
43. Chilcote R, Baehner R, Hammond D. Septicemia and meningitis in children splenectomized for Hodgkin's disease. *N Engl J Med* 1976; 295:798–800.
44. Schneeberger AL, Girvan DP. Staging laparotomy for Hodgkin's disease in children. *J Pediatr Surg* 1988;23(8):714–717.
45. Hays DM, Ternberg JL, Chen TT, et al. Postsplenectomy sepsis and other complications following staging laparotomy for Hodgkin's disease in childhood. *J Pediatr Surg* 1986;21(7):628–632.
46. Abrahamsen AF, Borge L, Holte H. Infection after splenectomy for Hodgkin's disease. *Acta Oncol* 1990;29(2):167–170.

Hodgkin's Disease, edited by P. M. Mauch,
J. O. Armitage, V. Diehl, R. T. Hoppe, and L. M. Weiss.
Lippincott Williams & Wilkins, Philadephia ©1999.

CHAPTER 18

Role of Staging Laparotomy in Hodgkin's Disease

Patrice Carde and Eli Glatstein

Claude Bernard observed that "when a physician performs an autopsy and observes some anomalies . . ., he feels satisfied. However, this just tells nothing about the cause of the disease, the activity of the drugs, or the cause of death. The pathological examination does not teach more, . . . because the microscopic lesions found after the death were present before, often for a long time, and cannot explain the death itself." Bernard predicted that "modern experimental medicine would be founded in the first place on the knowledge of the internal environment where normal and morbid influences, as well as medicinal influences, take place." He added, ". . . how to know about the environment of such a complex organism as in man and in superior animals except by plunging into it and penetrating it through experimental methods applied to living beings? This means that, in order to analyze the characteristics of life, one must necessarily enter the living organisms using the vivisection procedures" (1). What else inspired Dr. Saul A. Rosenberg, in the early 1960s, when he first asked a surgeon to perform an exploratory laparotomy? This bold step was the logical extension of the first data supporting the concept that Hodgkin's disease was "curable" (2–4). As observed by Bernard nearly a century earlier, autopsy findings in patients with Hodgkin's disease did not explain its evolution. The success of radiation therapy, in practice, was hindered by occult abdominal involvement. Yet it was quite a leap to conclude that patients would benefit from such an invasive procedure. How did this elective procedure (exploratory laparotomy) evolve into a routine diagnostic procedure (staging laparotomy)? What have been the side effects? Have these side effects contributed to the abandonment of laparotomy as a standard diagnostic procedure? Are there circumstances in which staging laparotomy remains justified? Beyond being of historical interest, the subject of abdominal surgery provides essential knowledge about the natural history of the disease, and its prognosis and treatment.

P. Carde: Department of Medical Oncology/Hematology, Institut Gustave-Roussy, Villejuif, France.

E. Glatstein: Department of Radiation Oncology, Hospital of the University of Pennsylvania, Philadelphia, Pennsylvania.

à Saul A. Rosenberg, notre maître bien-aimé, et à nos petit(e)s camarades des samedis matins de Stanford. (This chapter is dedicated to Saul A. Rosenberg, our beloved teacher, and to our "Saturday-morning friends" at Stanford.)

1960S: LAPAROTOMY AS EXPLORATION BY WESTERN PIONEERS

By Dr. Rosenberg's account, the first laparotomy was performed by the surgeon Thomas Nelsen because it was impossible to design radiation fields in a patient with Hodgkin's disease who had equivocal findings on a lymphangiogram. The "unclear" lymphangiogram prevented physicians from administering portals of radiation therapy appropriate for the extent of the disease. Surgical exploration and biopsy were required to resolve the particular conundrum. This patient recovered from surgery and is still without recurrence more than 30 years later.

The story of this first patient illustrates the delicate relationship between proposed treatment and diagnostic workup. In the 1960s, a transition had occurred in the therapeutic strategy that was facilitated by the availability of megavoltage irradiation. Aggressive treatment approaches were based on the emerging technique of "extended fields." This technique was developed by Drs. Kaplan and Rosenberg at Stanford University to prevent "a recurrence developing in the immediate vicinity of a field too narrowly irradiated" (5). The technique of irradiation did matter, as survival rates were higher in patients with localized

Hodgkin's disease when high doses rather than lower palliative doses were applied (6). Although initially advocated by Peters and Middlemiss (4), the benefit of administering "prophylactic" irradiation to clinically uninvolved neighboring nodal regions thought to contain subclinical or "occult" disease was ignored by most treating physicians in the mid-1960s. Moreover, the trial that eventually demonstrated a benefit from large anterior and posterior radiation fields intended to encompass both involved nodal areas and areas at risk for involvement commenced only in 1962, and the results were not yet available when the first exploratory laparotomies were performed (7,8).

Among physicians who practiced prophylactic treatment of uninvolved sites, the prevalent opinion of the time was that prophylactic irradiation of uninvolved nodal regions was of value only in supradiaphragmatic sites. Infradiaphragmatic nodal and visceral involvement, recognized through autopsies, was considered to occur at the end stage of disease. Lymphangiography suggested that infradiaphragmatic involvement was more frequent than initially thought, but it was the report of this first series of patients who underwent exploratory laparotomy that revealed such a high frequency of paraaortic and splenic involvement (9). In this first series, laparotomy was performed in selected patients who needed an exploratory diagnostic procedure because standard staging procedures had failed to provide a reliable determination of the extent of disease. These patients had either (a) equivocal or unsatisfactory findings on lymphangiogram, (b) splenomegaly and negative or equivocal findings on lymphangiogram, or (c) hepatomegaly or abnormal liver function test results. During laparotomy, splenectomy, biopsy of selected paraaortic nodes and of the liver, and sampling of the iliac crest bone marrow were performed. The diagnostic laparotomy, which proved to be superior to radiologic evaluation and physical examination, showed "...the all-too-frequent presence of spleen involvement" (10). Indeed, in this first study, laparotomy revealed splenic involvement in 62% of patients, almost twice as many as had been thought to have splenic involvement clinically (Table 1).

This study allowed two important observations to be made. First, the clinical or radiologic size of the spleen proved to be a poor indicator of histologic involvement. Second, the newly introduced technique of lymphangiography had no absolute value, not because the technique did not show splenic disease or disease above L-2, but because the results proved to be wrong in 18% of the patients whether they were interpreted as negative or positive. Conversely, an equivocal result on lymphangiogram proved to be negative in 77% of cases (Table 2).

Concept of a Therapeutic Impact of Exploratory Laparotomy

During the same period (1960s), physicians from Stanford University and the European Organization for Research and Treatment of Cancer (EORTC) were assessing the value of extended-field radiation through randomized studies. Both groups were frustrated by the same obstacle: comparison of the involved field versus the extended field was restricted to the supradiaphragmatic region, where physicians could rely on their physical examination findings. Relapse rates remained high, even in the extended-field arm, when radiation was limited to nodal groups above the diaphragm (8,11,12). In the EORTC series, almost 50% of relapses occurred transdiaphragmatically. Exploratory laparotomy data provided the explanation: the diaphragm was not an anatomic "barrier" but merely a muscle traversed by the lymphatics and thoracic duct. Infradiaphragmatic recurrences began to be explained by the growth of microscopic (subclinical) disease, which could have been present early in the course of the disease but was initially overlooked and thus not irradiated. During the 1960s and early 1970s, exploratory laparotomy was not part of any preestablished therapeutic strategy. Laparotomy had some impact *a posteriori* on treatment in that it could be used to identify and correct erroneous evaluations of extent of disease. Laparotomy was considered an optimal investigation because physicians were persuaded that in patients with localized disease, any relapse of Hodgkin's disease would eventually be a fatal event. As no other procedure could better ensure that all abdominal disease would be recognized, the laparotomy was soon advocated as the optimal safeguard, not only to optimize abdominal treatment but also to tailor abdominal irradiation to the extent of each patient's disease.

The Institut Gustave-Roussy, in parallel with Stanford University, had adopted a policy of routinely recommending staging laparotomy. An evaluation of 135 patients treated between 1966 and 1971 at the Institut Gustave-Roussy confirmed the diagnostic value of laparotomy but questioned its therapeutic impact and called for a random-

TABLE 1. *Splenic histologic findings as a function of preoperative splenic clinical assessment in 65 selected patients submitted to laparotomy (37 of 65 previously untreated)*

	Clinically negative (n = 27)	Clinically positive (n = 38)	All patients (n = 65)
Pathologically positive	11 (41%)	14 (37%)	25 (38%)
Pathologically negative	16 (59%)	24 (63%)	40 (62%)

Exploratory laparotomy is superior to clinical examination (Stanford series 1961–1968).
Adapted from ref. 9.

TABLE 2. *Paraaortic nodes: histologic findings as a function of prior lymphangiogram results in 65 selected patients submitted to laparotomy*

	Results of lymphangiography		
	Negative (n = 17)	Equivocal (n = 13)	Positive (n = 28)
Pathologically negative	14 (82%)	10 (72%)	5 (18%)
Pathologically positive	3 (18%)	3 (23%)	23 (82%)

Exploratory laparotomy is superior to lymphangiogram (Stanford series 1961–1968).
Adapted from ref. 9.

ized trial (13). This question was first evaluated in the EORTC H_2 trial (1972–1976) (14).

Exploratory Laparotomy: Insight into the Pathophysiology of Hodgkin's Disease

For a long time, it was questioned whether some lymphatic areas were more at risk for involvement with Hodgkin's disease than others. The observation of a *nonrandom distribution* could be explained only by a unique manner of lymphatic spread from one site to another contiguous area. A *random distribution* could be explained by a greater susceptibility of certain sites to the blind hit of a blood-borne, yet unknown, causal agent. In brief, these theories illustrated two opposing concepts concerning the natural history of Hodgkin's disease: a unifocal versus a multifocal origin.

The use of lymphangiography, which visualized paraaortic and iliac involvement, helped to demonstrate that "involvement of the paraaortic and iliac lymph node chains is the silent link between the upper trunk and the groin" (10). Lymphangiographic data illustrated why nodal recurrences occurred more frequently in certain sites (15–17). However, the interpretation of lymphangiography was often equivocal. In laparotomy series, the documentation of anatomic distribution by pathologic review of splenic, nodal, liver, and bone marrow samples supported the hypothesis that Hodgkin's disease spread in an orderly manner. This was best expressed by Kaplan (10), who stated, "The frequencies with which two (or more) specific sites are involved at time of diagnosis and the frequencies with which extension to specific sites occurs after local treatment of any given primary site or sites provide the basis for the hypothesis that, in the great majority of instances, Hodgkin's disease spreads nonrandomly and predictably via lymphatic channels to contiguous lymph node chains or other lymphatic structures." These hypotheses and observations (10) provided the rationale in the 1970s and 1980s for administering prophylactic nodal irradiation with large fields and routinely using staging laparotomy in radiotherapy-based treatment. For instance, following local irradiation, further spread involved a contiguous nodal area in 22 of 26 instances in an early report (15). With the advent of laparotomy, it could be understood why, in patients with stage IIIA disease, extended-field irradiation provided higher survival in comparison with involved-field irradiation (7), and why, in patients with clinical stage (CS) I–II disease, paraaortic and spleen irradiation reduced by 30% to 50% the risk for recurrence and death in two consecutive EORTC trials (14).

Contrary to the theory of contiguity, a random distribution of the disease, to noncontiguous nodal areas, would have supported the concept of a multifocal origin, with some areas eventually rendered more susceptible by an unknown causative (presumably viral) agent. Data supporting the spread of disease in a noncontiguous pattern that could involve any area of the entire lymphatic system had been reported (18). In stage II, the frequency of involvement for a particular site was in accord with expectations of the contiguity theory when two or three sites were involved. However, when four or more sites were involved, the distribution was more random, suggesting the existence of "other pathways of dissemination" (19–21). Moreover, random distribution was reported in patients with mixed-cellularity histology (17,19).

Interest in these competing theories declined when total nodal plus visceral irradiation and adjuvant chemotherapy came into common use. The issue of mechanism of spread became less important when the potential to cure Hodgkin's disease at presentation improved. For the last 20 years, however, late complications have jeopardized treatment results, and physicians have gradually been obliged to reduce the intensity of both radiation and chemotherapy. Thus, the question of aggressiveness of treatment, in which the risk for late complications is weighed against the potential for cure, has again emerged. Involvement by Hodgkin's disease in 236 patients with cervical presentation who had undergone a staging laparotomy was recently reported to follow an orderly progression via "functionally" (but not anatomically) contiguous lymphatic areas. Retrograde flow of contaminated lymphatic fluid in the lymphatic canals may result from their intrinsic low pressure and susceptibility to changes in lymphatic pressure. Spread differed according to the side of initial cervical involvement; for example, in left cervical presentations, the mediastinal nodes were often bypassed (Fig. 1) (22).

Thus, the claim by Kaplan (10) that based on its mode of spread, Hodgkin's disease had "to be a monoclonal neoplasm of unifocal origin which spreads secondarily by metastasis of pre-existing tumor cells, much like other

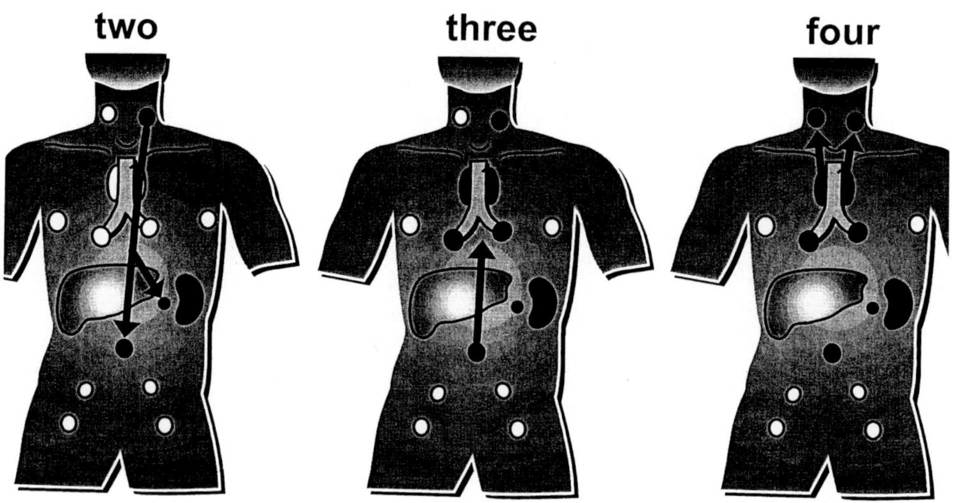

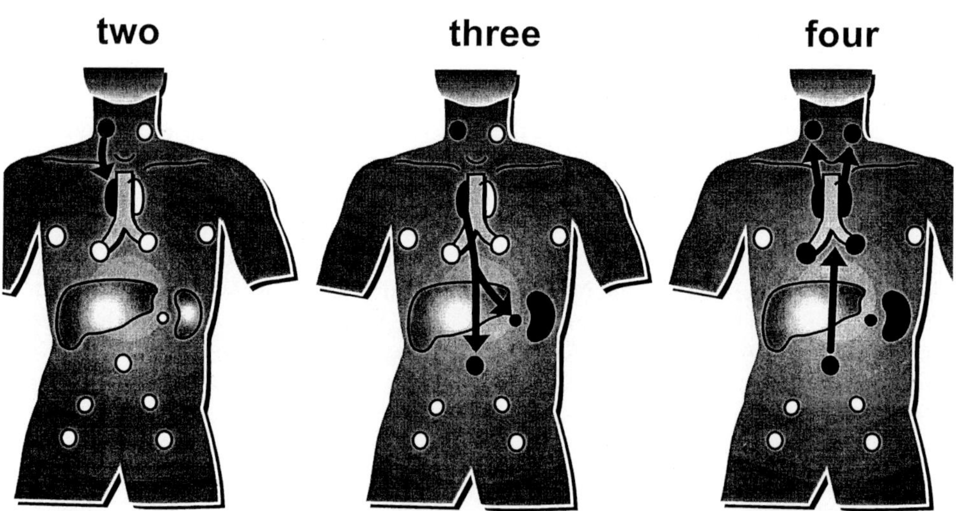

FIG. 1. Hodgkin's disease spreads in an orderly fashion. Spread differs according to the side of initial cervical involvement; in left presentations, for instance, disease bypasses the mediastinal nodes (22). In the past, prediction of spread allowed for the prophylactic treatment of even remote regions at high risk for involvement. In the future, it may help to avoid irradiation of even close regions at low risk (25).

neoplasms, except that spread is predominantly via lymphatic rather than hematogenous pathways" continues to be supported by recent findings from staging laparotomies. Indeed, unifocality can be considered not only from a topographic but also from a molecular biologic point of view. The same monoclonal Epstein-Barr viral strain was demonstrated in Reed-Sternberg cells associated with relapses scattered over 8 years (23). Similarly, monoclonal Reed-Sternberg cells were reported in three successive manifestations of Hodgkin's disease spread over 4 years (initial cervical presentation in 1971, nodal relapse in 1973, disseminated relapse in 1974); in all three manifestations, the Reed-Sternberg cells showed the same rearrangement of the immunoglobulin gene (24).

At a time when treatment intensity is being restricted, how important is the contiguity theory from a therapeutic point of view? The susceptibility (random distribution) theory called for the constitutive presence of either a causal agent or an immune defect that would induce multifocal and repeated emergence of new malignant clones, each of them responsible for a new relapse or emergence of new disease. The corresponding treatment strategy would be to deliver treatments gradually to spare host resistance in the long run. Conversely, if clonal Hodgkin's disease presents in a unique location at one point in time, spreads by contiguity, and is potentially responsible for all subsequent relapses (as now appears to be the case), then optimal initial strategy should be started at once, no matter what the intensity of treatment, to eradicate all Hodgkin's disease from the initial site(s) (25).

1970S: LAPAROTOMY AS A ROUTINE STAGING PROCEDURE

Laparotomy as an Indispensable Staging Procedure

The absence of major complications or death in the first reports rendered staging laparotomy an extremely attractive procedure, and it was recommended as a "contingent" procedure in the report on the Ann Arbor classification. Since the first stratification into "latent," "progressive," and "cachectic" states of Hodgkin's disease by Trousseau in Paris in 1865 (26), the aim of subsequent clinical staging classifications had been to assess prognosis and guide treatment. The proposal for the curability of Hodgkin's disease by Easson and Russell (2) in 1963 integrated the possibility for cure with the classification of localized disease amenable to radiation in one undivided volume. The need for a refined staging classification based on lymphangiography was proposed as early as February 1965 at the Paris meeting (27). This classification was the basis of subsequent classifications in which four stages were defined: involvement of one nodal area (I), several areas on the same side of the diaphragm (II), both sides (III), or extranodal involvement (IV). At a subsequent meeting in Rye in September 1965 (15), it was proposed to classify contiguous stage II disease as stage I2, a confusing step that was later modified at the Ann Arbor conference (28,29).

The Ann Arbor classification was directly based on two findings from early reports of the results of staging laparotomies: (a) Splenic involvement was much more frequent than expected and could not be predicted by clinical or radiographic findings (Table 1), and (b) equivocal lymphangiographic findings were usually associated with negative findings in paraaortic node specimens obtained at laparotomy (Table 2). The Ann Arbor classification established a dual staging system, the first component being a "mandatory" clinical staging and the second a "contingent" pathologic staging in which specific symbols were used to identify pathologic splenic and abdominal nodal involvement detected at laparotomy. The results of both clinical and pathologic staging were to be noted. In pathologic staging, use of the initial letters of the names of sampled sites (i.e., hepatic, nodal, marrow, abbreviated by the symbols H+/-, N+/-, M+/-, respectively) indicated that additional biopsies of these organs had been performed beyond those of clinical staging, and the status of involvement was noted. Mention of the initial letter of the word spleen (S+/-) along with the symbols for pathologic stage indicated that the information had been obtained through laparotomy. Such a subtle notation probably led to a slight ambiguity in the abbreviation "PS" between the meaning "pathologic stage," as initially intended, and "postsurgical stage," as many believed to be correct. The statement of Kaplan (10), "The newer Ann arbor classification . . . has the added virtue of distinguishing between the clinical stage, based solely on the original tissue biopsy, history, physical examination, and radiographic findings, and the pathological stage, based in addition on histological findings in tissues obtained at laparotomy or supplemental biopsies," emphasizes the evolution of thinking about staging laparotomy in the 1970s. In 1973, the National Practice Survey in Hodgkin's Disease assigned staging laparotomy a weight of 21% to 29% of the total scores for workup, follow-up, and treatment planning (30). This emphasis on laparotomy can be understood only when one considers the possibilities that meticulous staging offers in regard to patient stratification, prognosis, treatment planning, and comparison of results among many academic centers (31–33).

Results of Laparotomy Staging

The value of routine staging laparotomy and splenectomy was initially reported from the Stanford University study of a series of 50 consecutive unselected patients (34), which was later updated (Table 3). This early series called attention to the frequency of splenic and paraaortic involvement, the association of B symptoms and splenic involvement, and the rarity of liver involvement, especially in the absence of B symptoms. Moreover, staging laparotomy data demonstrated that equivocal lymphangiogram

TABLE 3. *Nodal and visceral findings in 100 unselected patients submitted to laparotomy at Stanford University*

Sites examined	Preoperative assessment	Patients without symptoms: bx-positive at laparotomy	Patients with symptoms: bx-positive at laparotomy	All patients with abdominal disease at laparotomy (%)
Spleen	84 negative	11/51	9/33	20/84 (24)
	16 positive	2/6	6/10	8/16 (50)
Paraaortic nodes	57 negative	5/33	2/24	7/57 (12)
	20 equivocal	3/13	1/7	4/20 (20)
	23 positive	8/11	10/12	18/23 (78)
Liver	85 negative	1/53	1/32	2/85 (2)
	15 positive	0/4	1/11	1/15 (7)

Routine exploratory laparotomy in 100 consecutive patients yields high numbers of cases with unsuspected abdominal disease, primarily splenic (Stanford series).
Adapted from ref. 10, update of ref. 34.
bx, biopsy.

findings overstated the probability of abdominal involvement. From 1968 to 1977, 814 patients underwent laparotomy in the Stanford series, and overall, the clinical stage (CS) was altered in 32%. In patients with CS IIA and IIB, the results were upstaged 29% and 27%, respectively. Interestingly, there was a 35% incidence of downstaging in CS IIIA patients and a 19% incidence in CS IIIB patients (10), a finding also noted in other series (35,36).

Additional data have been reported from the EORTC trials. The EORTC conducted three successive trials from 1972 to 1988 in which 527 patients with supradiaphragmatic CS I–II Hodgkin's disease underwent a staging laparotomy (H_2, n = 144; H_5 favorable, n = 237; H_6 favorable, n = 126). Entry criteria included a negative lymphangiogram (or abdominal and pelvic computed tomogram in the H_{6F} trial) and a Jamshidi bone marrow biopsy. Percutaneous liver biopsy was performed in case of suspected liver involvement. Overall, 22% of patients (n = 116) were found to have pathologic stage (PS) III (21%) or stage IV (1%) disease. The great majority of patients had splenic involvement; the spleen was the only involved abdominal site in 40% of patients with positive findings at laparotomy. Iliac and isolated paraaortic involvement was rarely seen (Carde, *unpublished data*). Similar rarity of lower infradiaphragmatic involvement alone has been observed in other series (36,37).

The International Database on Hodgkin's Disease (IDHD) has gathered the largest series of patients for analysis of the results of staging laparotomy. A total of 14,315 patients, treated at major centers from the early 1960s to 1987, were entered into the IDHD database (38). Based on the numbers provided in the statistical report, it is possible to recalculate the proportion of these patients who were recorded by clinical and pathologic staging, respectively (Table 4). For the whole cohort, there were 21% of patients with CS I, 43% with CS II, 23% with CS III, and 13% of patients with CS IV Hodgkin's disease. Forty-three percent of patients underwent a staging laparotomy (n = 6,093). This percentage varied with time. For example, before 1970, 14% of patients with CS II disease had a staging laparotomy compared with 63% in the 1970s and 40% after 1980. In the subset of patients who underwent laparotomy, the distribution of pathologic stages was 18% for PS I, 39% for PS II, 36% for PS III, and 8% for PS IV Hodgkin's disease.

Based on these data, 29% of patients presenting with supradiaphragmatic CS I–II Hodgkin's disease were upstaged to PS III or (rarely) PS IV. In this series of patients undergoing a staging laparotomy, primary infradiaphragmatic presentations of Hodgkin's disease were rare (4%, n = 240).

Guidelines for Staging Laparotomy

Laparotomy has never been considered a trivial surgical procedure. It has always been classified as major

TABLE 4. *Findings in 6,108 selected patients submitted to staging laparotomy (International Database on Hodgkin's Disease)*

Clinical stage	No. pts	Pathological stage postlaparotomy (%)				Change of stage (%)	
		I	II	III	IV	Up	Down
I	1,386	73	—	25	2	27	—
II	3,077	—	69	29	2	31	—
III	1,318	4	17	68	11	11	21
IV	327	0	5	14	80	—	19

From ref. 38; data recalculated from Tables III3–III6, pp 197–200.

abdominal surgery. Although the surgical aspects of staging laparotomy are detailed in another chapter (see Chapter 17), four features of staging laparotomy are briefly mentioned below.

1. The surgery includes splenectomy; sampling of splenic hilar nodes; placement of a radiopaque clip at the splenic pedicle; mandatory sampling of celiac, hepatic portal, and paraaortic nodes; biopsy of any suspected palpable nodes; liver wedge and deep-needle biopsies; and bone marrow biopsy (13,37,39).
2. Metallic clips are placed at the site of biopsy of the retroperitoneal nodes for later comparison with the lymphangiogram to assess for adequate biopsy of suspected nodes; some advocate intraoperative radiographs to verify whether suspected nodes were sampled (13). Iliac nodal areas are palpated but not routinely sampled in most centers.
3. Oophoropexy, a procedure to move the ovaries outside the radiation field, thereby preserving hormonal function and fertility, is recommended for patients who are anticipated to need pelvic irradiation. Techniques include moving the ovaries laterally (40) or to the midline posterior and anterior to the uterus (41).
4. Finally, there may be an anesthesia risk in staging laparotomy for patients with Hodgkin's disease who present with bulky mediastinal involvement; five acute, life-threatening complications occurred in 74 such patients in one report (42). Superior vena cava and/or bronchial occlusion during intubation makes extubation impossible or dangerous; presurgical irradiation of the mediastinum and hila prevents this complication (39,42).

Comparison of Diagnostic Value of Laparotomy, Lymphangiography, and Other Procedures

No radiographic technique has been shown to match the information obtained with staging laparotomy. However, it is not clear which factors (reliability, current availability, expertise, ease, cost, or patient acceptability) have made both lymphangiography and staging laparotomy less popular. However, in the 1980s, several reports noted a decrease in the use of lymphangiography (43–45), or a decrease in the use of both lymphangiography and diagnostic laparotomy (46).

Lymphangiography versus Laparotomy

One problem with lymphangiography is that it is not intended to provide information above L-2 (celiac, hepatic portal, and splenic hilar nodes, or the spleen) (10,14,47). Table 5 reports the comparative findings of lymphangiography and laparotomy in one large study (36).

Computed Axial Tomography versus Laparotomy

Computed tomography (CT) scans may be better at assessing upper abdominal involvement than lymphography, which better visualizes a small degree of paraaortic involvement. The specificity of CT (true negatives) appears generally good. However, direct comparisons of lymphangiography and CT demonstrated that although the specificity of CT nearly matched that of lymphangiography, its sensitivity was much lower (Table 6) (48–50).

The value of CT has somewhat increased with technical improvements in diagnostic radiology (36,51). For instance, in a series of 114 patients undergoing a staging laparotomy who had negative findings on abdominal-pelvic CT, 29 (25%) had a positive result on laparotomy. Only 13 of the 29 patients had extrasplenic involvement (36). In a more sophisticated analysis of 94 patients comparing CT, splenic size, splenic weight at laparotomy, and disease involvement, splenic weight was the strongest independent risk factor for involvement with Hodgkin's disease below the diaphragm, but it depended heavily on other prognostic factors, especially histology. One-dimensional CT splenic measurement correlated poorly with histologic involvement, whereas three-dimensional measurements correlated well. However, neither splenic weight nor other parameters, such as CT-estimated splenic weight or volume, were sensitive predictors of splenic involvement (52). CT detection of lower abdominal nodal involvement (paraaortic, iliac, mesenteric nodes) is particularly deficient (49,53). Indeed, the sensitivity of CT for paraaortic or pelvic disease was found to be 20%, and it increased only to 23% when combined with lymphangiogram, suggesting that the yield of positive cases is not much improved when both lymphangiography and CT are performed (53).

TABLE 5. *Findings at laparotomy or lymphangiography in 571 patients (examinations 1969–1986)*

Laparotomy results	Lymphangiogram negative (n = 465; 81%)	Lymphangiogram positive (n = 106; 19%)
Negative	347 (75%)	44 (42%)
Positive	118 (25%)[a]	62 (58%)[b]

Twenty-five percent of patients with negative lymphangiogram have abdominal disease.
Adapted from ref. 36.
[a]Positive laparotomy in lymphangiogram negative patients mostly splenic disease, only 12 positive in paraaortic or pelvic nodes.
[b]43 positive in paraaortic or pelvic nodes.

TABLE 6. *Findings at laparotomy by computed tomographic analysis*

		Laparotomy negative		Laparotomy positive	
Series (ref.)	No. patients	True negatives (%)	False positives (%)	True positives (%)	False negatives (%)
1981 (48)	105	92	8	26	74
1993 (50)	69	84	12	63	37

Validation of New Diagnostic Procedures with Staging Laparotomy

A study comparing gallium 67 scanning with lymphangiography in 94 patients with localized Hodgkin's disease was aided by data from the 51 patients who underwent a staging laparotomy. Compared with CT and lymphangiography, scanning with gallium 67 for abdominal nodal involvement is of suboptimal sensitivity (54). Unfortunately, with the diminished use of laparotomy, none of these new procedures, including immunoscintigraphy with radiolabeled anti-CD30 antibodies, positive emission tomography (PET), and magnetic resonance imaging (MRI), can be compared extensively with lymphangiography or CT (55). The failure of newer techniques to identify occult abdominal Hodgkin's disease may be the reason why the role of laparotomy has been preserved in the Cotswolds classification (56).

Impact of Laparotomy on Treatment Decisions

Standardization of Extended-field Irradiation to Reduce Risk for Relapse

In the early 1970s, many oncologists believed that all patients with stage I–III Hodgkin's disease should receive total nodal irradiation (including splenic irradiation in clinically staged patients) to be certain that all macroscopic and microscopic disease would be treated (29). The early results of staging laparotomy provided evidence for the orderly spread of Hodgkin's disease to adjacent lymphatic sites. As the hazards of such extended irradiation became better understood, arguments were made to use more restricted irradiation ("extended-mantle" or subtotal nodal irradiation), provided that a staging laparotomy had proved the patient to be PS I or II. A similar strategy was applied between 1972 and 1976 in the H_2 trial conducted by the EORTC. Although in the previous H_1 trial (1964–1971) the relapse rates below the diaphragm after mantle irradiation alone in clinically staged patients were 11%, and 40% for patients with nodular sclerosis and MC histology, respectively, the recurrence rates below the diaphragm in the H_2 trial, in which staging laparotomies and subtotal nodal irradiation were used, did not exceed 10% (14). In parallel, splenic irradiation, which had been questioned in regard to efficacy (13), proved to be as effective as splenectomy, with limited long-term renal toxicity (57,58). Similarly, centers that utilized subtotal nodal irradiation in PS I–IIA supradiaphragmatic patients reported 10-year rates of freedom from progression in excess of 80% and recurrence rates below the diaphragm of only approximately 5% (59–62).

Oophoropexy

Oophoropexy was successful at preserving the potential for normal hormonal function and fertility in patients receiving pelvic irradiation (41,63,64). Some have argued that lateral oophoropexy (above the iliac crest) may be wiser than oophoropexy to the midline, as the central positioning is associated with more scattered radiation and possible displacement from the uterus. The lateralization technique preserved the gonadal function in 14 of 22 women treated with the inverted-Y technique (40). However, the maneuver by itself may be harmful (65,66), and some authors have recommended unilateral rather than bilateral oophoropexy. Forty-two percent of women in the EORTC H_5 trial had an oophoropexy; a unilateral procedure was performed 40% of the time (67). As few patients now receive pelvic irradiation, this procedure is rarely performed today.

Increased Hematologic Tolerance after Splenectomy

Significant differences in platelet and white blood cell counts favoring splenectomized patients have been observed during the first 4 courses of MOPP (mechlorethamine, vincristine, procarbazine, prednisone) chemotherapy (68). This was not totally unexpected, as splenectomy is used as a treatment for peripheral anemia, thrombocytopenia, and "hypersplenism." Similarly, higher platelet and white blood cell counts as well as fewer treatment interruptions were observed during total lymphoid irradiation (69). However, in a multivariate analysis of 48 patients differing only by splenectomy, age was the only significant factor for chemotherapy tolerance: age-matched dose intensity was 87% for nonsplenectomized patients versus 84% for splenectomized patients (70).

Restaging Laparotomy

As many as 40% to 50% of patients treated with chemotherapy alone for advanced Hodgkin's disease relapse. In a series of 26 patients who underwent a laparotomy and splenectomy within 2 months of the end of chemotherapy, 23% were found to have Hodgkin's disease below the diaphragm, mostly involving the spleen (71). In a study of 46 patients, 13% were found to have splenic involvement (72). However, in two reports, only 2% to 4% of patients with negative findings at clinical restaging had residual disease at restaging laparotomy after three to six cycles of MOPP chemotherapy (45,73). Today, with rare exception, diagnostic laparotomy is not recommended for restaging of patients with recurrent Hodgkin's disease.

Prognostic Value of Positive Laparotomy Findings in Supradiaphragmatic Hodgkin's Disease

The statement that "the basic observation of Peters that the anatomic extent is the single most important factor influencing survival . . . still holds true today" is supported by the 10-year relapse-free and overall survival rates of 923 patients staged by laparotomy at Stanford University: 81% and 91%, respectively, for PS I; 71% and 82% for PS II; 64% and 57% for PS III; 41% and 40% for PS IV. Moreover, prognosis depends "upon the anatomic involvement within a single stage, as defined for instance by the involvement of two or more nodal sites" (10,74).

A large number of investigators have reported that findings at laparotomy are of prognostic value and in many instances result in modification of treatment. A number of these observations and their potential impact on prognosis are set forth below. Most of these observations were made when radiation therapy alone was utilized as initial treatment. Kaplan (10) reported that nodal involvement in addition to splenic involvement, and diffuse involvement of the spleen, both had a negative impact on freedom from progression. Vascular invasion of the spleen has been reported to be associated with an increased risk for liver and bone marrow involvement, early relapse, and death (75). The fact that the liver is almost never involved in the absence of splenic involvement, and that liver involvement at relapse is almost exclusively observed in association with splenic involvement (76), ultimately led to recommendations for prophylactic liver irradiation in patients with splenic involvement (77). Similarly, the presence of Reed-Sternberg cells in the venous blood of the involved spleen during splenectomy suggested that hematogenous spread, in addition to lymphatic spread, had already taken place beyond the spleen (78).

In PS IIIA patients, a poor freedom from progression was observed if more than four splenic nodules were identified (79). Desser and colleagues (80) reported that patients with Hodgkin's disease limited to the upper abdomen had a better prognosis than patients with disease in the paraaortic or pelvic nodes. This distinction, III1 (*vide supra*) versus III2, was adopted by the Cotswolds classification (56).

To investigate further the prognostic importance of the presence and extent of abdominal involvement, the EORTC performed prospective trials that took into account prospectively registered disease-related and patient-related prognostic factors in patients treated in a homogeneous manner. The EORTC also investigated the strong correlation between the identification of prognostic factors in a specific group of patients and the treatment they received. This is best illustrated by the example of the H_2 trial (Fig. 2), in which 300 CS I–II patients with Hodgkin's disease were studied (14). In this trial, the aims were to assess (a) the prognostic value of positive findings at laparotomy and (b) the therapeutic efficacy and toxicity of splenic irradiation compared with splenectomy. Thus, laparotomy and splenectomy were randomized against clinical staging. In both arms, treatment was not modified by the findings at surgery; indeed, patients in both arms received the same treatment (subtotal nodal irradiation). The 7-year freedom from progression (68% vs. 76%) and overall survival rates (77% vs. 79%) were similar for patients with clinical staging and laparotomy staging, respectively (21).

Because treatments were not modified by the findings at laparotomy, the trial also allowed assessment of the impact of disease below the diaphragm when treatment designed for CS I–II patients was used. A total of 42% of patients with splenic involvement relapsed, compared with 17% of patients without splenic involvement. The additional recurrences in patients with splenic involvement were more likely to be in non-irradiated nodal sites

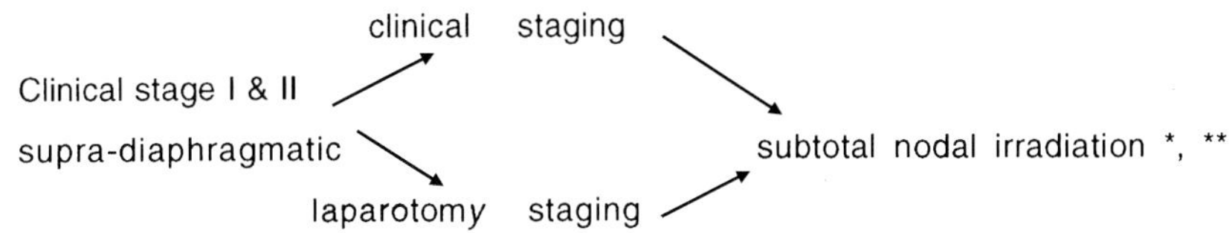

** In clinically staged patients spleen irradiation was given in addition to subtotal nodal irradiation*

*** chemotherapy given only for liver or bone marrow involvement*

FIG. 2. Design of the randomized EORTC H_2 trial in supradiaphragmatic clinical stage (CS) I–II patients (n = 300; 1972–1976).

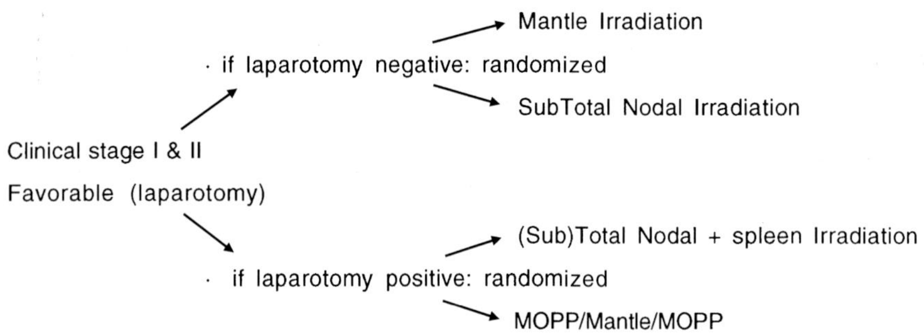

FIG. 3. Design of the randomized EORTC H5 favorable trial in supradiaphragmatic clinical stage (CS) I–II patients (n = 237; 1977–1982).

than in extranodal sites (14). After longer follow-up of the patients treated with radiation therapy alone in the H_2 trial, other prognostic factors, including the number of initial clinically involved areas and the combination of systemic symptoms and an elevated erythrocyte sedimentation rate (ESR), were seen to be strong adverse predictive factors, so that a positive laparotomy result had a pejorative significance only in the best prognostic group. Adverse factors affected only freedom from progression, not overall survival, because of successful combination chemotherapy in patients who relapsed (21).

Use of Staging Laparotomy to Tailor Treatment to Prognosis

One of the most rewarding uses of staging laparotomy has been in designing strategies to avoid adjuvant chemotherapy or restrict the extent of irradiation. One strategy was aimed at the avoidance of chemotherapy in early-stage Hodgkin's disease. Even before 1970, chemotherapy had been utilized as adjuvant treatment to increase tumor control. The first adjuvant chemotherapy trial, launched in 1964 (EORTC H_1 trial), demonstrated a freedom-from-progression advantage for single-agent chemotherapy and radiation therapy compared with radiation therapy alone (81); this still holds true 25 years later (21). However, survival differences were not noted in this trial or other trials in which adjuvant chemotherapy was added to radiation therapy (82,83). Because of concern regarding the potential hazards of chemotherapy (84), many groups decided to restrict the use of chemotherapy to patients with positive findings at laparotomy. This was the case, for instance, in the H_5 favorable trial (Fig. 3) (67). In this trial, only 18% of patients initially received chemotherapy. Treatment with radiation therapy alone based on a negative laparotomy was a strategy that resulted in a 9-year freedom from progression rate of 70% and an overall survival rate in excess of 92% (21).

Not everybody agreed that splenic involvement indicated a need for chemotherapy, and some centers reported reasonable disease-free survival rates when total nodal irradiation was combined with low-dose irradiation to the lungs and liver (10). However, in the H_5 unfavorable EORTC trial (Fig. 4), patients with positive laparotomy findings who were randomized to MOPP and mantle irradiation did better than those given subtotal or total nodal irradiation in regard to both freedom from progression and overall survival (67).

Strategies aimed at restricting radiotherapy fields after a negative laparotomy have also been explored. Frequently, patients with CS III Hodgkin's disease do not have pathologic evidence of Hodgkin's disease below the

Stratification on 4 prognostic factors : age >40, erythrocyte sedimentation rate > 70, mixed cellularity histology, absence of mediastinal involvement in clinical stage II.

H5 Favorable : no adverse feature; these patients (48% of total) required laparotomy to permit treatment adaptation. The judicious choice of characteristics for prognostic stratification led to 16% of laparotomies being positive

H5 Unfavorable trial if one factor present (52% of total):

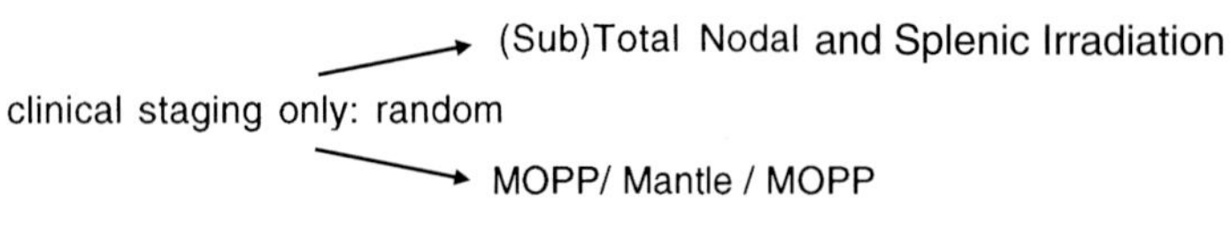

FIG. 4. H_5 trials: prognostic stratification in supradiaphragmatic clinical stage (CS) I–II patients (n = 494; 1977–1982).

diaphragm (36%) in a study by Desser et al., allowing for a reduction of radiation therapy (and in some cases chemotherapy) (37). In addition, splenectomy allows the volume of radiation to be reduced in the thorax and abdomen, so that the pleurae, lung bases, apical and diaphragmatic heart surfaces, and some of the left kidney are spared the radiation exposure to which they are subjected during splenic irradiation (37,58). In a further attempt to reduce radiation volumes, the EORTC explored the possibility of eliminating infradiaphragmatic irradiation and chemotherapy in PS I–II patients (Fig. 3). When patients were randomized to mantle irradiation or subtotal nodal irradiation, absolutely no differences were seen in freedom from progression or overall survival rates (67), and abdominal irradiation was eliminated for selected pathologically staged patients in the subsequent H_6 favorable trial. Mantle irradiation alone for laparotomy-staged I–II patients to reduce the risk for second solid tumors and for gastrointestinal and renal toxicity has also been recommended by others (85–88).

COMPLICATIONS AND LONG-TERM HAZARDS OF LAPAROTOMY

In early reports, patients undergoing laparotomy and splenectomy by skilled surgeons were spared operative mortality (9,34). Operative mortality observed after splenectomy under other circumstances was attributed to the type of hematologic disease, such as anemia and hypersplenism (10). However, the hope that patients with Hodgkin's disease could be spared surgical complications did not last for long.

Treatment Delay

Staging laparotomy does result in a delay in treatment of at least several weeks. In the randomized H_{6F} trial, patients in the laparotomy arm had a treatment delay of 28 days in comparison with the patients not undergoing laparotomy staging (89).

Immediate Complications

Although no major complications or deaths were reported in the first 65 patients at Stanford University, major complications were reported in subsequent reviews of larger numbers of patients undergoing staging laparotomy from the same institution (9,90,91). Death was also reported in one of 135 patients treated between 1966 and 1971 at the Institut Gustave-Roussy (13). The causes of perioperative mortality in different studies included complications of subphrenic abscesses and embolism (13,36,61,67). In large series or reviews, the associated operative mortality has been approximately 0.5% to 1% (36,37,92,93). Miscellaneous late postsurgical complications have been described, including cardiac arrest, pneumonia, pleural effusions, prolonged ileus, urinary infection, septicemia, deep-venous thrombosis and pulmonary embolism, gastric hemorrhage, intraperitoneal hemorrhage, and subdiaphragmatic abscess (35, 89,93–96). However, careful patient selection (i.e., avoidance of elderly patients with large mediastinal masses or patients with poor performance status) and modern surgical techniques have minimized the risks. Recent series have reported 0.3% fatal and 2.9% major nonfatal complications in 692 patients (36), and no casualty in 915 patients treated between 1968 and 1986 (97).

Myocardial infarction, an extremely rare complication, is not usually attributed to splenectomy. Splenectomy had been performed in three young patients with Hodgkin's disease later admitted for acute myocardial infarction (98). One patient, who had a myocardial infarction after administration of vinblastine, had normal coronary arteries. Another patient, who had undergone neither mediastinal irradiation nor chemotherapy before myocardial infarction, demonstrated a marked increase in platelet counts following splenectomy. The role of splenectomy and subsequent thrombocytosis as a possible pathogenic factor for development of myocardial infarction has been reviewed (98). It is unclear how this observation is linked with the functional expression of monocyte tissue factor on peripheral blood monocytes, which were found to be more numerous in patients with Hodgkin's disease who had not undergone splenectomy (99).

Late Gastrointestinal Complications of Surgery

Small-bowel obstructions were reported in nearly 10% of 133 patients undergoing staging laparotomy and splenectomy in one study. In some of these patients, repeated laparotomies had been performed (94). However, the risk is much lower (1% to 1.5%) in most other series (36). In one recent series, one of 692 patients died of multiple bowel obstructions (36). The incidence of small-bowel obstruction may be higher in younger patients, possibly because of more aggressive staging (94,100). Other complications have been described, including gastroduodenal ulcer and small-bowel perforation (101). The delivery of radiation and surgical staging both contribute to the risk for small-bowel obstruction. Doses of radiation therapy greater than 200 cGy daily may result in an especially high risk for small-bowel obstruction (Table 7) (101). Higher daily fraction sizes should not be used in the modern practice of radiation therapy for Hodgkin's disease.

TABLE 7. *Gastrointestinal complications by treatment for patients in the EORTC 42nd H_5 trials ($n = 134$; 1972–1982)*

H_2	Radiation fractionation	
	3×3.3 Gy/wk	4×2.5 Gy/wk
No laparotomy	11%	5%
Laparotomy	42%	11%

Institut Gustave Roussy series. Adapted from ref. 101.

Impairment of Immune Function

Hodgkin's disease-related immune impairment and treatment-induced immunosuppression are confounding factors in the causation of splenectomy-induced immunosuppression (10). A high serum CD8 soluble antigen level has been associated with suppressor T-cell activity and decreased concanavalin A-induced blood lymphocyte DNA synthesis (102). Moreover, constitutive immune deficiency has been observed in family members of patients with Hodgkin's disease (103). All these factors confound the role of splenectomy in immune suppression and the occurrence of cytomegalovirus and herpes-zoster infections. Conversely, it has been shown that functionally active lymphocyte populations can be removed by a spleen affected with Hodgkin's disease (104). Enhanced elimination of autologous CD4 lymphocytes labeled with indium 111 also may be a general property of tissue affected by Hodgkin's disease (105). Splenectomy has been reported in a small number of patient to protect from treatment-induced lymphopenia. Conversely, impairment of both humoral and cellular immunity has been associated more closely with treatment than with laparotomy and splenectomy (106–108).

Bacterial Sepsis Following Splenectomy

"Although the problem of bacterial sepsis in splenectomized patients is real, it is important to place it in proper perspective—the gains far outweigh the risks (which are by no mean negligible)" (10). Bacterial sepsis after splenectomy, first reported in 1919 and 1929 (109, 110), is caused most frequently by encapsulated organisms and results in infections, pneumonia, septicemia, and overwhelming postsplenectomy infection (111). In a review of 12 series (a total of 1,170 cases), 16 infections were reported, with a mortality rate of 50% (112). Overwhelming post splenectomy infection is more frequent in children where it has a high incidence and mortality rate. Overwhelming post splenectomy infection is more likely to occur within the first 5 years of Hodgkin's disease and in younger patients, but cases after 15 years have been reported (94,113,114). Bacterial infections were found more frequently in patients with advanced-stage Hodgkin's disease, in those with active disease, and in patients under treatment (95). Overwhelming post splenectomy infection occurs less frequently with less intensive treatment (114). The risk is higher when chemotherapy is given than with radiotherapy (114). Similarly, aggressive combinations of irradiation, prednisone, and chemotherapy appear to increase risk (Table 8) (115).

Whereas the phagocytic activity of the reticuloendothelial system has been found to be enhanced, possibly through the release of stimulatory factors like interleukin-5 (IL-5), the phagocytic mass is reduced to one-fifth of normal in splenectomized patients, leading to a proportional decrease in the clearance capacity for encapsulated organisms (116). Curative measures for overwhelming post splenectomy infection, generally in the presence of disseminated intravascular coagulopathy, require immediate administration of antibiotics and admission to an intensive care unit. Prophylactic measures against *Streptococcus pneumoniae* and *Haemophilus influenzae* must rely on both oral antibiotics and vaccination. Daily lifelong oral administration of penicillin is efficient (110,117), but its feasibility has been questioned (94), and antibiotic prophylaxis is not routinely recommended in adults because of poor compliance and the decreased overall risk in adults (118). However, fatal sepsis has been reported weeks to months after the all-too-frequent discontinuation of penicillin (119).

A program of prophylactic vaccination with polyvalent pneumococcal polysaccharide vaccines against the most widely prevalent types of *S. pneumoniae* is the logical and most efficient strategy to prevent postsplenectomy sepsis (120,121), although there are no guidelines for the levels of immunoglobulin G (IgG) that guarantee protection. Vaccination is advised before splenectomy rather than afterward (94) because results may be improved with the presence of spleen at vaccination. Because pneumococcal and meningococcal infections have occurred 5 to 14 years after treatment in patients who had benefited from serotype-specific pretreatment vaccinations, repeated vaccination at regular intervals after the appearance of Hodgkin's disease is recommended (122). The increase in antibody titers after administration of polyvalent pneumococcal polysaccharide vaccines against the most widely prevalent types of *S. pneumoniae* has been studied (123). In one report, the response to vaccination, assessed by monitoring responses to certain pneumococcal antigens, did not differ according to whether or not patients with Hodgkin's disease had been splenectomized (124). In another study, the response in patients with Hodgkin's disease was similar to that of patients who had undergone splenectomy for trauma and was not significantly improved when vaccination was performed before splenectomy (108). In the Boston study (122), the only factor that predicted for a better antibody response was younger age, in which case the levels matched those of normal patients. Actually, immunosuppressive treatments rather than splenectomy appear to be responsible for the reduced antibody response after vaccination (125). Moreover, data generated in Boston demonstrated the close inverse relationship between antibody titers and intensity of chemotherapy and irradiation (Table 9) (124).

In conclusion, a vaccination program against the pneumococcus, *Haemophilus*, and the meningococcus should be undertaken after splenectomy (94,108,122). Vaccination should also be carried out in patients whose spleen has been (or is to be) irradiated, as infectious casualties do occur in this population (126,127). The antibody levels for revaccination and re-revaccination are currently

TABLE 8. *Late non-postoperative bacterial sepsis following splenectomy (literature in chronologic order)*

Author (center), year (ref.)	No. patients	Age	No. serious infections (%)	No. deaths (%)
Desser and Vetmann (review), 1972 (112)	1,170	All	16 (1)	6 (0.5)
Donaldson et al. (SUH), 1972 (113)	238	All	10 (4)	3 (1.3)
Rosenstock et al., 1974 (169)	374	Children	—	2 (0.5)
Schimpff et al. (NCI), 1975 (95)	92	All	6 (6)	3 (3)
Chilcote et al. (CCSG), 1976 (170)	200	Children	18 (9)	8 (4)
Ertel et al. (Columbus), 1977 (118)	20	Children	4 (20)	3 (15)
Donaldson et al. (SUH), 1978 (114) Control group (no laparotomy) = no event (n = 60)	121	Children	14 pneumonia and meningitis (11.6%; 2.8% if radiotherapy and 18% if chemotherapy)	1 (0.8)
Weitzman and Aisenberg (Boston), 1977 (115)	119	All	3 (3)	2 (2)
Askergren et al. (Stockholm), 1980 (143)	31	Adults	2 (6)	0
Scott et al. (ESNLG), 1980 (35)	225	All	0	0
Tubiana et al. (EORTC), 1981 (14)	144	Adults	0	0
Hoppe et al. (SUH), 1982 (60)	230	Adults	—	2 (1)
Hays et al. (Intergroup), 1984 (65)	234	Children	4 (1.7)	0 (0)
Baccarani et al. (Bologna), 1986 (171)	342	Adult	5 (1.8) (more at relapse)	3 (1) (2/3 at relapse)
Leibenhaut et al. (SUH), 1987 (168)	49	Adults	—	1 (2)
Carde et al. (EORTC), 1988 (67)	237	Adults	0	0
Mauch et al. (JCRT), 1988 (62)	315	All	8 (2.5)	2 (0.6)
Donaldson et al. (SUH), 1990 (142)	100	Children	1 (1)	1 (1)
Mauch et al. (JCRT), 1990 (36)	692	All	0	0
Frezzato et al., 1993 (172)	226	All	6 (3)	4 (2)
Carde et al. (EORTC), 1993 (89)	134	Adults	—	2 (1.5)
Jockovich et al. (Florida), 1994 (94)	133	All	9 (6.8)	1 (0.8)
Breuer et al. (Harvard), 1994 (100)	247	Children	1 (0.4)	0
Zanini et al. (Milan), 1994 (173)	147	Adults	1 (0.7)	1 (0.7)

Type of infection, interval from last treatment, occurrence of a relapse, and type of treatment at time of event are important parameters that are lacking in most reports.

SUH, Stanford University Hospital; NCI, National Cancer Institute; CCSG, Children's Cancer Study Group; ESNLG, East of Scotland and New Castle Lymphoma Group; EORTC, European Organization for Research and Treatment of Cancer; JCRT, Joint Center for Radiation Therapy.

being investigated as a national service in Sweden (M. Björkholm, Karolinska Institute, Stockholm *personal communication*). Current data suggest that vaccinations should be repeated 2 to 6 years after splenectomy and treatment, and at 6-year intervals thereafter (128). Vaccines should cover all 23 pneumococcal serotypes, the meningococcus, and *Haemophilus*.

Second Cancers as a Complication of Splenectomy

Several studies have indicted staging laparotomy in the emergence of second cancers (particularly myelodysplasia and leukemia, but not solid tumors) after Hodgkin's disease (129–131). An increased relative risk (RR) for leukemia of 1.6 (95% CI, 1.1–1.8) was associated with splenectomy, but only for the first 4 years after surgery (132). In another study, the adjusted RR per unit time was 4.26-fold greater in splenectomized patients than in patients with an intact spleen (133). At the Institut Gustave-Roussy, in 892 adult patients treated between 1960 and 1984 and continuously free of Hodgkin's disease, the RR for second cancer was 2.80 (95% CI, 1.63–4.48; $p < .001$) in patients whose spleen was not treated or removed, compared with 6.87 (95% CI, 4.81–9.51; $p < .001$) in splenectomized patients or in patients whose spleen was irradiated. Multivariate regression analysis

TABLE 9. *Antibacterial vaccination in splenectomized patients: relation between antibody titers, intensity of chemotherapy, and irradiation*

Mean antibody antibacterial titers at 3 wk	Controls (n = 10)	Laparotomy + subtotal nodal irradiation (n = 15)	Laparotomy + MOPP (n = 4)	Laparotomy + subtotal nodal irradiation + MOPP (n = 10)	Laparotomy + total nodal irradiation + MOPP (n = 12)
Protein (ng)	1,566	963	658	377	283
p value		$p < .05$	$p < .05$	$p < .01$	$p < .001$

MOPP, mechlorethamine, Oncovin, procarbazine, prednisone.
Adapted from ref. 124.

that controlled for confounding variables (age, sex, clinical stage, extent of radiation therapy, and chemotherapy regimen) showed that splenic irradiation (RR = 3.67; p = .003) and splenectomy (RR = 2.54; p = .018) were also significantly correlated with an increased risk for second cancers (134). Are the prognostic characteristics and treatments of patients undergoing a laparotomy acting as confounding variables? The follow-up of patients with equivalent characteristics, treated without chemotherapy, with or without splenectomy, such as in the EORTC H_2 trial, needs careful investigation.

In addition, some large studies do not find an impact of laparotomy on risk for second cancer. In 2,846 patients with Hodgkin's disease treated within the British National Lymphoma Investigation (BNLI) during 1970–1987, the RR for second cancers (lung, all other solid tumors, non-Hodgkin's lymphoma, and particularly leukemia) did not vary significantly according to whether or not splenectomy had been performed (135). The same observation was made in 1,410 patients treated for Hodgkin's disease from 1970 to 1990 in Florence (136) and in 1,152 Norwegian patients (137). Furthermore, in 6,315 patients who underwent splenectomy for reasons other than hematologic disorders, no increase in the incidence of cancer was detected after a mean follow-up of 6.8 years (138).

THE 1980S AND 1990S: CAN LAPAROTOMY BE REPLACED? CURRENT INDICATIONS AND NEW TECHNIQUES

In recent years, the role of staging laparotomy in the diagnosis and treatment of Hodgkin's disease has decreased markedly. The increasing role of chemotherapy in patients with localized disease has made precise abdominal staging less important. In parallel, new prognostic factors have been perfected, making laparotomy less valuable than previously thought. Both chemotherapy and prognostic stratification for treatment have greatly reduced the role of staging laparotomy.

Replacement of Laparotomy by More Extended Irradiation or Systematic Use of Chemotherapy

In the 1980 edition of his book, Kaplan (10) wrote that, "the indications for routine diagnostic laparotomy would extend to virtually all patients with Hodgkin's disease, with the exception of the elderly or severely debilitated, or those with positive findings on bone marrow or liver needle biopsy or other evidence of stage IV disease." A mathematical model taking into account the risks and benefits of each procedure and using 5-year disease-free survival as an end point had shown that staging laparotomy and stage-specific treatment would almost always provide better results than combined-modality therapy, although a quite high (2%) risk for fatal sepsis had to be selected to make the model work (139). Recent work based on more sophisticated modeling and recent data have confirmed a small but significant theoretical survival advantage for staging laparotomy and splenectomy (140).

Yet, because of concerns about the morbidity and delays in treatment associated with staging laparotomy, and because of increases in freedom from recurrence with strategies combining chemotherapy and radiation therapy, programs of more extensive irradiation or chemotherapy were pursued in Toronto and France. The Toronto group compared its series of clinically staged patients with an inferior event-free survival (48.9% at 10 years) with series generated in Stanford of laparotomy-staged patients (66.8%) (141). However, the overall survivals were similar, leading to the claim that "the conclusion must be that the prevention of relapse by the use of more extensive radiation fields and/or the use of chemotherapy plus locoregional irradiation during the later period has resulted in improved relapse-free survival. Overall survival increased from 80% (1968–1972) to 92% (1973–1977)" (141).

In children, the same debate opposed maximal staging and adopted treatment that favored clinical staging and limited irradiation fields. The latter option provided lower event-free survival rates in a combined analysis of patients from St. Bartholomew's Hospital and Stanford University Medical Center but identical overall survival rates (142). In another study, no event-free survival or overall survival differences were observed in patients treated in Stockholm with total nodal irradiation, whether they were randomized to clinical or laparotomy staging (143). In a trial at the Roswell Park Memorial Institute, the workup between clinical staging and staging laparotomy was randomized; results suggested a disadvantage for surgery, but randomization allocation errors cast doubts on the results (144). Finally, results have been published for a significant number of patients successfully treated between 1972 and 1976 with three cycles of MOPP and mantle or mini-mantle irradiation (145).

Factors that Predict for Positive Laparotomy Findings

Positive laparotomy findings are correlated with patient and disease-related factors. The most common characteristics have been older age (10) and MC histology (10,12). Another predictor for disease below the diaphragm was the absence of mediastinal involvement in CS I–II patients (10,12,146). A few models have been developed to anticipate the proportion of PS III–IV patients in a defined population. A model based on age, sex, and site and size of nodal involvement in CS I of the neck has been used at the Royal Marsden Hospital to predict for abdominal disease. This model allowed laparotomy to be avoided in both high-risk patients (>50%) and low-risk patients (<15%) (147). The number of nodal areas was not assessed, although the number of sites has been identified as a major factor in one previous (148) and two later studies (36,146).

Two models have been based on large series. These have identified the population of patients who would have their stage or treatment changed following laparotomy. In the Stanford University study (97), only CS I–II patients were enrolled (n = 915). Sex was the main predicting parameter, whereas B symptoms were not. A small group of patients were identified who were at low risk for having a change in stage or treatment following laparotomy; these patients included CS I women, all CS I patients with involvement of the mediastinum, CS I men with lymphocyte-predominant histology, and CS II women younger than 27 years of age and with three or fewer sites involved. Overall, 131 of 363 (36%) CS II women were identified who had very low risk for abdominal involvement (97). In the Boston study of 692 patients, including 552 CS I–II patients (36), 21% of the study population had a low probability (<10%) of having their stage or treatment changed following laparotomy; this was the case for CS IA female patients and CS IA male patients with lymphocyte predominance histology or high-neck presentations. Patients with CS IIIB–IV disease also were at low risk for stage or treatment change. Still, laparotomy was thought to result in valuable information for treatment decisions in the majority of CS I–II patients. Overall, laparotomy was recommended for 79% of the patients. The recommendations encompassed patients with B symptoms (.001), mixed cellularity/lymphocyte depletion histology (.017), two or more supradiaphragmatic sites (.001), male sex (.034), age above 40 (.004), and CS III–IV disease (<.001). The study emphasized the case for downstaging of CS III–IV patients, especially those without B symptoms (Table 10).

Pediatric studies reached similar conclusions. One model including sex, age, B symptoms, number of involved sites above the diaphragm, and histology defined a cohort of 24% of all the patients whose risk for abdominal disease was less than 10%(100). In a Pediatric Oncology Group series of 216 children that used many of the same factors, prediction of abdominal involvement was not improved by the addition of radiologic parameters (149).

Within the EORTC, treatment policies have been based on prognostic factors identified during clinical trials. For the unfavorable subgroup of CS I–II patients in the EORTC H_2 trial, staging laparotomy did not help to identify a group for which adjuvant chemotherapy provided a freedom from progression or overall survival advantage (14,21,150). The EORTC H_2 trial (Fig. 2) was designed to evaluate the prognostic value of laparotomy findings (treatment was identical whether patients underwent laparotomy or not). In parallel, the therapeutic value and complications of splenic irradiation were assessed (14,58). The prognostic factors identified during the first two trials (12,14,17,151) were used to devise a strategy for the subsequent EORTC H_5 trial (Fig. 4). The goal was to separate, beyond classic Ann Arbor staging, patients who would require from the outset extensive irradiation (subtotal or total nodal irradiation) or combined-modality treatment with six cycles of MOPP and mantle irradiation.

Initially, only 33% of patients received chemotherapy in the H_5 trial (67); 43% received it when treatment of recurrences was included (21). A few other groups reported similar results. In the BNLI, no relapse-free survival or overall survival differences were noted in matched-pair analyses of patients with or without laparotomy (152). In the H_{5U} trial, event-free survival was better in the combined-modality arm; this arm served as a standard arm in the subsequent H_{6U} trial, which also omitted staging laparotomy (89).

TABLE 10. *Laparotomy downstaging in clinical stage III–IV*

Subgroup with clinical stage III–IV		No. patients	Pathologic stage I–II (%)	*p* value
Symptoms	A	86	47 (55)	<.001
	B	54	12 (22)	
Histology	LP/nodular sclerosis	73	40 (55)	.005
	MC/LD	67	19 (28)	
Age	≤39	111	53 (48)	.009
	≥40	29	6 (21)	
Sex	M	93	40 (43)	NS
	F	47	19 (40)	
No. sites	1	29	15 (52)	NS
	≥2	111	44 (40)	

Predictive model for positive laparotomy in clinical stage III–IV.

LP, lymphocyte predominance; MC, mixed cellularity; LD, lymphocyte depletion; NS, not significant.

Adapted from ref. 36.

Trials of Staging Laparotomy in Favorable Prognosis CS I–II Patients (EORTC H_{6F} Trial)

With the increasing use of chemotherapy as part of the treatment of CS I–II patients with poor prognostic features, the H_{6F} EORTC trial (Figs. 5 and 6) studied the value of laparotomy only in favorable prognosis patients with localized supradiaphragmatic Hodgkin's disease. This group of favorable prognosis patients was chosen to represent the population of patients who would most benefit from treatment adaptation in terms of optimizing initial control and minimizing late effects. The trial was not designed to select patients who would be at low risk for infradiaphragmatic involvement (as in the H_{5F} trial; 16% positive at laparotomy). Rather, it was designed to identify and modify treatment in patients with a positive laparotomy who were at high risk for relapse after radiation therapy alone. The incidence of positive laparotomies in the H_{6F} trial exceeded 30%. Half of the patients underwent classic staging, with laparotomy results lead-

H6F selection by exclusion from the Unfavorable group : age <50, no B symptoms & erythrocyte sedimentation rate <50 or B symptoms & erythrocyte sedimentation rate <30, not more than 3 nodal areas involved, no bulky mediastinum (M/T ratio > 0.35)

→ clinical staging & subtotal nodal + spleen irradiation

Clinical stage I & II
supra-diaphragmatic

→ laparotomy staging

if negative : Mantle field (favorable histologies) or subtotal irradiation (unfavorable histologies)

if positive : MOPP or ABVD + Mantle irradiation

(randomized as in unfavorable H6U patients)

FIG. 5. Design of the randomized EORTC H6F trial in favorable supradiaphragmatic clinical stage (CS) I–II patients: role of staging laparotomy (n = 262; 1982–1988).

ing to treatment adaptation: irradiation alone in case of negative laparotomy or addition of six cycles of chemotherapy in case of positive laparotomy. The other half of the patients were staged without laparotomy and received a standard treatment, subtotal nodal and splenic irradiation without adjuvant chemotherapy (89).

The 6-year rates for freedom from progression were 83% for the laparotomy arm and 78% in the clinical staging arm (p = NS). Overall, survival was 89% and 93%, respectively (p = NS), with the slightly higher mortality in the surgery arm attributed to laparotomy-related deaths (89). The data suggest that laparotomy can be deleted as a routine staging strategy in adult patients with favorable localized supradiaphragmatic Hodgkin's disease, at no cost in disease-free or overall survival.

The EORTC group omitted staging laparotomy from its subsequent trials of favorable CS I–II patients with supradiaphragmatic Hodgkin's disease, utilizing subtotal nodal and splenic irradiation as the standard control arm in the H_7 (1988–1993) and H_8 (1993–1998) trials. In this same group of patients, the combination of the abbreviated EBVP chemotherapy regimen (six monthly injections of epirubicin, bleomycin, vinblastine, and prednisone over 4 months) and involved-field irradiation achieved a freedom from progression superior to that attained with subtotal nodal and splenic irradiation (153,154), opening the way to explore the means to reduce further the extent of radiation therapy.

New Techniques and Procedures, and Current Indications for Laparotomy

Laparoscopic staging has been in use at the Milan Cancer Institute since the mid-1970s (33). It must be stressed that most patients who underwent laparoscopic staging were given adjuvant chemotherapy. Reports of the tech-

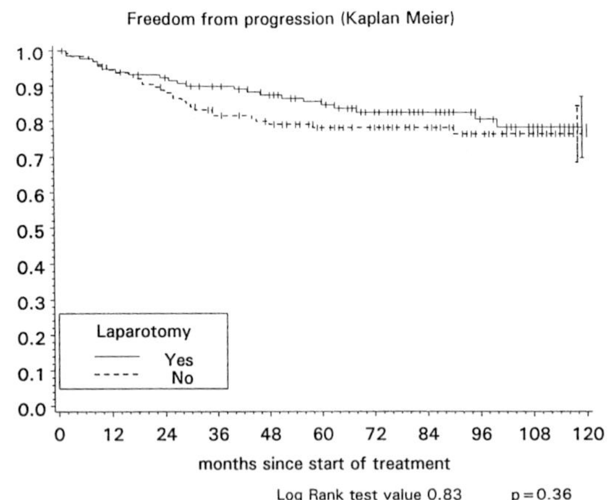

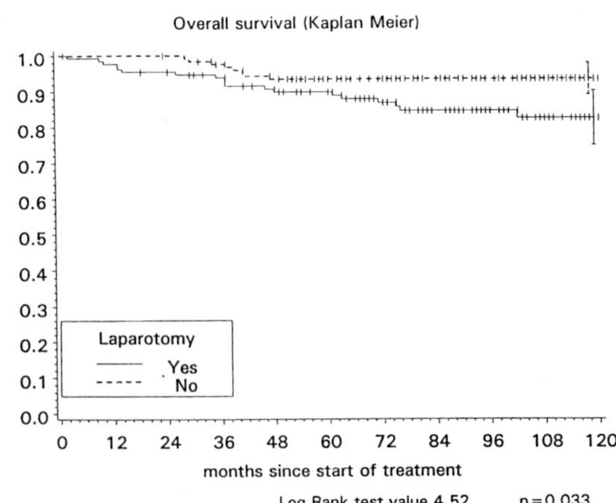

FIG. 6. Results of the EORTC H6F trial in favorable supradiaphragmatic clinical stage (CS) I–II patients randomized to clinical staging and standard irradiation versus staging laparotomy and adjusted treatment (n = 262; 1982–1988). The staging laparotomy arm demonstrated a nonsignificant higher 6-year freedom from progression, hampered by lethal laparotomy-related deaths (89).

nique have focused mainly on safety and ease of the procedure (hospitalization of approximately 3 days), but not on yield of the procedure compared with laparotomy (155–161). Complications of bleeding led to an open procedure in one of 170 cases in one study (162) and in three of 19 cases in another (163). In addition, the Milan series pointed out that in 74 patients who underwent both a laparoscopy and a laparotomy, the yield for splenic involvement was 12% and 42%, respectively, and for hepatic involvement 1% and 7%, respectively (162), which raised concerns about the diagnostic value of the laparoscopic procedure. Still, laparoscopic staging may be advantageous in selected cases. It should be noted that laparoscopic ovarian transposition has been a successful technique and may be preferred to an open procedure when diagnostic information is not needed (164).

Partial splenectomy has been performed in children in an attempt (with some success) to avoid late overwhelming post splenectomy infection, again without major complications, except an occasional need for repeated laparotomy (165). Nevertheless, laparoscopic laparotomy and hemisplenectomy are not appropriate because splenic disease may be focal or not visible when the surface is examined.

Current indications for laparotomy are restricted to selected circumstances such as planning radiation therapy alone. Most major institutions have discontinued the routine use of staging laparotomies (166). For example, the Princess Margaret Hospital discontinued laparotomy in 1977, the EORTC in 1986, and the German Hodgkin Study Group and the M. D. Anderson Cancer Center in 1988. At Stanford, laparotomy was still recommended for children in 1985 (167) but was reserved for "favorable patients" in the 1980 protocols; it also was pursued in patients with infradiaphragmatic presentations until 1989 (168), in IIIB patients until 1984, and in IIIA patients until 1990. In Milan, staging laparotomy was discontinued in 1976 for CS I–II supradiaphragmatic patients and in 1988 for CS III and for CS I–II infradiaphragmatic patients. At the Joint Center for Radiation Therapy in Boston, the only persons still submitted to laparotomy are favorable CS I–II supradiaphragmatic patients. At the Institut Gustave-Roussy, a handful of laparotomies have been performed in the last 3 years, mostly for restaging or suspected relapses; in some cases, second cancers have been discovered instead of relapse.

CONCLUSION

The staging laparotomy has greatly contributed to the understanding and management of Hodgkin's disease. None of the standard or new radiographic modalities has been able to replace laparotomy for accurate determination of Hodgkin's disease below the diaphragm. The major failing of these studies has been their inability to detect Hodgkin's disease in the spleen. A combination of modern imaging techniques and prognostic factors may be substituted for laparotomy, but because these tests do not accurately determine the anatomic extent of disease in individual patients, omission of laparotomy eliminates the strategy of tailoring treatment to the extent of disease. Most CS I–II patients, including patients with favorable prognostic features, in the absence of laparotomy staging, should be managed with combinations of radiation therapy and chemotherapy. Subtotal nodal and splenic radiation fields continues to be an alternative to combined chemotherapy and radiotherapy. The long-term success of radiation therapy and combination chemotherapy (without laparotomy) for favorable prognosis CS I–II patients will depend on the design of combinations of adjuvant chemotherapy and limited radiation therapy that will maintain a high freedom from recurrence but will allow reduction of the late effects of prior standard treatment regimens. Without laparotomy, the current practice is to use both modalities of treatment but in attenuated forms to minimize morbidity. Who knows if new modalities of combined chemotherapy and lessons learned from the laparotomy era (22) will compensate for the loss of routine laparotomy (25)? This is why, to paraphrase a prior definition of lymphangiography (44), laparotomy should be called "the Mohican who lasts."

ACKNOWLEDGMENTS

We are grateful to Professor Stephan Roth (Heinrich Heine University, Düsseldof), who provided Fig. 1 illustrating the contiguity theory; to Professor Magnus Björkholm (Karolinska Institute, Stockholm), who generously provided results of recent longitudinal studies on the immune status of Hodgkin's patients; and to Professor Saul A. Rosenberg (Stanford University), who was kind enough to track the chart of the first patient who underwent a laparotomy.

REFERENCES

1. Bernard C. *Introduction à l'étude de la médecine expérimentale*, Chapter II, Sections II and III. Paris, 1865.
2. Easson E, Russell M. The cure of Hodgkin's disease. *Br Med J* 1963; 1:1704–1707.
3. Peters M. A study in survivals in Hodgkin's disease treated radiologically. *Am J Roentgenol* 1950;63:299–311.
4. Peters M, Middlemiss K. A study of Hodgkin's disease treated by irradiation. *Am J Roentgenol* 1958;79:114–121.
5. Gilbert R. Radiotherapy in Hodgkin's disease (malignant granulomatosis); anatomic and clinical foundations; governing principles, results. *Am J Roentgenol* 1939;41:198–241.
6. Kaplan H. The radical radiotherapy of Hodgkin's disease. *Radiology* 1962;78:553–561.
7. Kaplan H. Long-term results of palliative and radical radiotherapy of Hodgkin's disease. *Cancer Res* 1966;26:1250–1252.
8. Kaplan HS, Rosenberg SA. Extended-field radical radiotherapy in advanced Hodgkin's disease: short-term results of 2 randomized clinical trials. *Cancer Res* 1966;26:1268–1276.
9. Glatstein E, Guernsey J, Rosenberg S, Kaplan H. The value of laparotomy and splenectomy in the staging of Hodgkin's disease. *Cancer* 1969;24:709–718.

10. Kaplan H. *Hodgkin's disease*, vol 2. Cambridge, MA: Harvard University Press, 1980.
11. Kaplan H. Clinical evaluation and radiotherapeutic management of Hodgkin's disease and the malignant lymphomas. *N Engl J Med* 1968; 278:892–899.
12. Tubiana M, Henry-Amar M, Hayat M, Breur K, Van Der Werf-Messing B, Burgers M. Long-term results of the E.O.R.T.C. randomized study of irradiation and vinblastine in clinical stages I and II of Hodgkin's disease. *Eur J Cancer* 1979;13:643–657.
13. Amiel JL, Lacour J, Gerard-Marchant R, et al. 135 laparotomies et splénectomies pour maladies de Hodgkin. *Bull Cancer (Paris)* 1971; 58:167–90.
14. Tubiana M, Hayat M, Henry-Amar M, et al. Five-year results of the E.O.R.T.C. randomized study of splenectomy and spleen irradiation in clinical stages I and II of Hodgkin's disease. *Eur J Cancer* 1981;17: 355–363.
15. Rosenberg S, Kaplan H. Evidence for an orderly progression in the spread of Hodgkin's disease. *Cancer Res* 1966;26:1225–1231.
16. Banfi A, Bonadonna G, Carnevali G, Oldini C, Salvini E. Preferential sites of involvement and spread in malignant lymphomas. *Eur J Cancer* 1968;4:319–324.
17. Tubiana M, Vanderwerf-Messing Bvd, Laugier A, et al. Survival after recurrence: prognostic factors and spread patterns in clinical stages I and II of Hodgkin's disease. *Natl Cancer Inst Monogr* 1973;36: 513–530.
18. Smithers D. Spread of Hodgkin's disease. *Lancet* 1970;1:1262–1267.
19. Hutchison GB. Anatomic patterns by histologic type of localized Hodgkin's disease of the upper torso. *Lymphology* 1972;5:1–14.
20. Lillicrap SC. Modes of spread of Hodgkin's disease. *Br J Radiol* 1973; 46:18–23.
21. Tubiana M, Henry-Amar M, Carde P, et al. Toward comprehensive management tailored to prognostic factors of patients with clinical stages I and II in Hodgkin's disease. The EORTC Lymphoma Group controlled clinical trials: 1964–1987. *Blood* 1989;73:47–56.
22. Roth S, Sack H, Havemann K, Willers R, Kocsis B, Schumacher V. Contiguous pattern spreading in patients with Hodgkin's disease. *Radiother Oncol* 1998;47:7–16.
23. Brousset P, Schlaifer D, Meggetto F, et al. Persistence of the same viral strain in early and late relapses of Epstein-Barr virus-associated Hodgkin's disease. *Blood* 1994;84:2447–2451.
24. Jox A, Zander T, Kornacker M, et al. Detection of identical Hodgkin-Reed Sternberg cell specific immunoglobulin gene rearrangements in a patient with Hodgkin's disease of mixed cellularity subtype at primary diagnosis and in relapse two and a half years later. *Ann Oncol* 1998;9:283–287.
25. Carde P, Noordijk EM. Studying spreading pattern in Hodgkin's disease: is it relevant to modern cancer treatment? [Editorial; Comment]. *Radiother Oncol* 1998;47:3–5.
26. Trousseau A. De l'adénie. *Cliniques médicales de l'hôtel-dieu*, vol 3. Paris, 1865:551–581.
27. La radiothérapie dans la maladie de Hodgkin. Société Francaise d'Hématologie et Société Française d'Électroradiologie Médicale, Symposium du 15 Février 1965 (Présidents J. Bernard et M. Tubiana). *Nouv Rev Fr Hematol* 1965–66;6:7–175
28. Carbone P, Kaplan H, Musshoff K, Smithers D, Tubiana M. Report of the Committee on Hodgkin's Disease Staging Classification. *Cancer Res* 1971;31:1860–1861.
29. Rosenberg SA, Boiron M, DeVita VT Jr, et al. Report of the Committee on Hodgkin's Disease Staging Procedures. *Cancer Res* 1971;31: 1862–1863.
30. Hanks G, Kinzie J, White R, Herring D, Kramer S. Patterns of care outcome studies: results of the National Practice Survey in Hodgkin's Disease. *Cancer* 1983;51:569–573.
31. Worthy T. Evaluation of diagnostic laparotomy and splenectomy in Hodgkin's disease (report no 12). *Clin Radiol* 1981;32:523–526.
32. Le Bourgeois J-P, Chauvel C, Schlienger M, Parmentier C, Tubiana M. La laparotomie dans la maladie de Hodgkin. Bilan des résultats. *Nouv Presse Med* 1974;3:2563–2567.
33. Bonadonna G, Beretta G, Castellino R, et al. Current views on surgical staging in planning the treatment of malignant lymphomas. In: Tagnon H, Staquet M, eds. *Recent advances in cancer treatment*, vol 55. New York: Raven Press, 1977:55–67.
34. Glatstein E, Trueblood W, Enright L, Rosenberg S, Kaplan H. Surgical staging of abdominal involvement in unselected patients with Hodgkin's disease. *Radiology* 1970;97:425–432.
35. Scott J, Dawson A, Proctor S, Allan N. The place of staging laparotomy in the management of Hodgkin's disease. *Clin Radiol* 1984;35: 261–263.
36. Mauch P, Larson D, Osteen R, et al. Prognostic factors for positive surgical staging in patients with Hodgkin's disease. *J Clin Oncol* 1990;8:257–265.
37. Desser RK, Moran EM, Ultmann JE. Staging of Hodgkin's disease and lymphoma. Diagnostic procedures including staging laparotomy and splenectomy. *Med Clin North Am* 1973;57:479–498.
38. Somers R, Henry-Amar M, Meerwaldt J, Carde P, eds. *Treatment strategy in Hodgkin's disease*. Colloque INSERM no 196. London: INSERM/John Libbey Eurotext, 1990.
39. Cannon WB, Nelsen TS. Staging of Hodgkin's disease: a surgical perspective. *Am J Surg* 1976;132:224–230.
40. Michel G, Lasser P, Castaigne D, Apelbaum H, Genin J, Lacour J. Transposition ovarienne. Technique, indications, résultats. *Chirurgie* 1983;109:55–60.
41. Trueblood H, Enright L, Roy G, et al. Preservation of ovarian function in pelvic irradiation for Hodgkin's disease. *Arch Surg* 1970;100: 236–237.
42. Piro A, Hellman S, Moloney W. The influence of laparotomy on management decisions in Hodgkin's disease. *Arch Intern Med* 1972;130: 844–848.
43. Jones S, Haut A, Weick J, et al. Comparison of adriamycin-containing chemotherapy (MOP-BAP) with MOPP-bleomycin in the management of advanced Hodgkin's disease. *Cancer* 1983;51:1339–1347.
44. Glatstein E. The vanishing lymphangiogram in Hodgkin's disease: the last of the Mohicans? [Editorial; Comment]. *Int J Radiat Oncol Biol Phys* 1993;25:567–568.
45. Jones SE. The staging of Hodgkin's disease revisited. *Med Oncol Tumor Pharmacother* 1984;1:15–17.
46. Moskovic E, Fernando I, Blake P, Parsons C. Lymphography—current role in oncology. *Br J Radiol* 1991;64:422–427.
47. Castellino R, Dunnick N, Goffinet D, Rosenberg S, Kaplan H. Predictive value of lymphography for sites of subdiaphragmatic disease encountered at staging laparotomy in newly diagnosed Hodgkin's disease and non-Hodgkin's lymphoma. *J Clin Oncol* 1983;1:532–536.
48. Blackledge G. A comparison of computed tomography and laparotomy in staging lymphomas. *Nouv Rev Fr Hematol* 1981;23:9–12.
49. Mansfield C, Fabian G, Jener S, et al. Comparison of lymphography and computer tomography scanning in evaluating abdominal disease in stages III and IV Hodgkin's disease. *Cancer* 1990;66:2295–2299.
50. Pluzanska A, Chmielowska E, Chmielowski M, Pasz S, Berner J, Wozniak L. Comparison of computed tomography results and pathological findings after laparotomy with splenectomy in Hodgkin's disease [in Polish]. *Acta Haematol Pol* 1993;24:27–34.
51. Hoppe R, Horning S, Hancock S, Rosenberg S. *Current Stanford clinical trials for Hodgkin's disease. Recent results in cancer research.* Berlin-Heidelberg: Springer-Verlag, 1989:182–190.
52. Hancock SL, Scidmore NS, Hopkins KL, Cox RS, Bergin CJ. Computed tomography assessment of splenic size as a predictor of splenic weight and disease involvement in laparotomy staged Hodgkin's disease. *Int J Radiat Oncol Biol Phys* 1994;28:93–99.
53. Sombeck MD, Mendenhall NP, Kaude JV, Torres GM, Million RR. Correlation of lymphangiography, computed tomography, and laparotomy in the staging of Hodgkin's disease. *Int J Radiat Oncol Biol Phys* 1993;25:425–429 (*see comments*).
54. Stomper PC, Cholewinski SP, Park J, Bakshi SP, Barcos MP. Abdominal staging of thoracic Hodgkin disease: CT-lymphangiography-Ga-67 scanning correlation. *Radiology* 1993;187:381–386.
55. Carde P, Da Costa L, Manil L, et al. Immunoscintigraphy of Hodgkin's disease: *in vivo* use of radiolabelled monoclonal antibodies derived from Hodgkin cell lines. *Eur J Cancer* 1990;26:474–479.
56. Lister TA, Crowther D. Staging for Hodgkin's disease. *Semin Oncol* 1990;17:696–703.
57. Hayat M, Carde P. Comparison of initial splenectomy and spleen irradiation in clinical stages I and II Hodgkin's disease. In: Cavalli F, Bonadonna G, Rozencweig M, eds. *Malignant lymphomas and Hodgkin's disease: experimental and therapeutic advances*. Boston: Martinus Nijhoff Publishers, 1985:379–384.
58. Le Bourgeois J, Meignan M, Parmentier C, Tubiana M. Renal conse-

quences of irradiation of the spleen in lymphoma patients. *Br J Radiol* 1979;52:56–60.

59. Farah J, Ultmann J, Griem M, Golomb H, Kalokhe U. Extended mantle radiation therapy for pathologic stage I and II Hodgkin's disease. *J Clin Oncol* 1988;6:1047–1052.
60. Hoppe R, Coleman C, Cox R, Rosenberg S, Kaplan H. The management of stage I–II Hodgkin's disease with irradiation alone or combined modality therapy: the Stanford experience. *Blood* 1982;59: 455–465.
61. Cornbleet M, Vitolo U, Ultmann J, et al. Pathologic stages IA and IIA Hodgkin's disease: results of treatment with radiotherapy alone (1968–1980). *J Clin Oncol* 1985;3:758–768.
62. Mauch P, Tarbell N, Weinstein H, et al. Stage IA and IIA supradiaphragmatic Hodgkin's disease: prognostic factors in surgically staged patients treated with mantle and paraaortic irradiation. *J Clin Oncol* 1988;6:1576–1583.
63. Le Floch O, Donaldson S, Kaplan H. Pregnancy following oophoropexy and total nodal irradiation in women with Hodgkin's disease. *Cancer* 1976;38:2263–2268.
64. Horning S. Female reproductive potential after treatment for Hodgkin's disease. *N Engl J Med* 1981;304:1377–1382.
65. Hays D, Ternberg J, Chen T, et al. Complications related to 234 staging laparotomies performed in the Intergroup Hodgkin's Disease in Childhood Study. *Surgery* 1984;96:471–478.
66. Gabriel DA, Bernard SA, Lambert J, Croom RD III. Oophoropexy and the management of Hodgkin's disease. A reevaluation of the risks and benefits. *Arch Surg* 1986;121:1083–1085.
67. Carde P, Burgers J, Henry-Amar M, et al. Clinical stages I and II Hodgkin's disease: a specifically tailored therapy according to prognostic factors. *J Clin Oncol* 1988;6:239–252.
68. Panettiere R, Coltman C. Splenectomy effects on chemotherapy in Hodgkin's disease. *Arch Intern Med* 1973;27:471–478.
69. Salzman J, Kaplan H. Effect of splenectomy on hematological tolerance during total lymphoid radiotherapy of patients with Hodgkin's disease. *Cancer* 1971;27:471–478.
70. Offner F, Piens R, Gobert AM, Coppens N, Noens L, Van Hove W. Splenectomy does not influence dose intensity of chemotherapy in advanced Hodgkin's disease regimen. *Proceedings of the Third International Symposium on Hodgkin's Lymphoma*, Cologne, Germany, September 18–23, 1995 (vol 114).
71. Goodman G, Jones S, Villar H, Silverstein M, Dabich L, Newcombe S. Surgical restaging of Hodgkin's disease. *Cancer Treat Rep* 1982;66: 751–757.
72. Sutcliffe S, Wrigley P, Timothy A, et al. Posttreatment laparotomy as a guide to management in patients with Hodgkin's disease. *Cancer Treat Rep* 1982;66:759–765.
73. Kostraba N, Peterson B, Kennedy B, Grage T, Bloomfield C. Laparotomy in the re-evaluation of patients with advanced Hodgkin's disease. *Cancer Treat Rep* 1981;65:685–687.
74. Peckham MJ, Ford HT, McElwain TJ, Harmer CL, Atkinson K, Austin DE. The results of radiotherapy for Hodgkin's disease. *Br J Cancer* 1975;32:391–400.
75. Kirschner RH, Abt AB, O'Connell MJ, Sklansky BD, Greene WH, Wiernik PH. Vascular invasion and hematogenous dissemination of Hodgkin's disease. *Cancer* 1974;34:1159–1162.
76. Shipley WU, Piro AJ, Hellman S. Radiation therapy of Hodgkin's disease: significance of splenic involvement. *Cancer* 1974;34:223–229.
77. Schultz HP, Glatstein E, Kaplan HS. Management of presumptive or proven Hodgkin's disease of the liver: a new radiotherapy technique. *Int J Radiat Oncol Biol Phys* 1975;1:1–8.
78. Bouroncle BA. Sternberg-Reed cells in the peripheral blood of patients with Hodgkin's disease. *Blood* 1966;27:544–556.
79. Hoppe R, Rosenberg S, Kaplan H, Cox R. Prognostic factors in pathological stage IIIA Hodgkin's disease. *Cancer* 1980;46:1240–1246.
80. Desser R, Golomb H, Ultmann J, et al. Prognostic classification of Hodgkin disease in pathologic stage III, based on anatomic considerations. *Blood* 1977;49:883–893.
81. Van Der Werf-Messing B. Morbus Hodgkin's disease, stages I and II: trial of the European Organization for Research on Treatment of Cancer. *Natl Cancer Inst Monogr* 1973;36:331–386.
82. Rosenberg S, Kaplan H. The evolution and summary results of the Stanford randomized clinical trials of the management of Hodgkin's disease: 1962–1984. *Int J Radiat Oncol Biol Phys* 1985;11:5–22.
83. Specht L, Gray R, Clarke M, Peto R. The influence of more extensive radiotherapy and adjuvant chemotherapy on long-term outcome of early stage Hodgkin's disease: a meta-analysis of 23 randomized trials involving 3888 patients. *J Clin Oncol* 1998;16:830–843.
84. Belpomme D, Carde P, Oldham R, et al. Malignancies possibly secondary to anticancer therapy. *Recent Results Cancer Res* 1974;49: 115–123.
85. Sutcliffe S, Gospodarowicz M, Bergsagel D, et al. Prognostic groups for management of localized Hodgkin's disease. *J Clin Oncol* 1985;3: 393–401.
86. Mandelli F, Anselmo A, Cartoni C, Cimino G, Enrici R, Biagini C. Evaluation of therapeutic modalities in the control of Hodgkin's disease. *Int J Radiat Oncol Biol Phys* 1986;12:1617–1620.
87. Ganesan T, Wrigley P, Murray P, et al. Radiotherapy for stage I Hodgkin's disease: 20 years of experience at St. Bartholomew's Hospital. *Br J Cancer* 1990;62:314–318.
88. Mauch P, Canellos G, Shulman L, et al. Mantle irradiation alone for selected patients with laparotomy-staged IA to IIA Hodgkin's disease: preliminary results of a prospective trial. *J Clin Oncol* 1995;13: 947–952.
89. Carde P, Hagenbeek A, Hayat M, et al. Clinical staging versus laparotomy and combined modality with MOPP versus ABVD in early-stage Hodgkin's disease: the H6 twin randomized trials from the European Organization for Research and Treatment of Cancer Lymphoma Cooperative Group. *J Clin Oncol* 1993;11:2258–2272.
90. Enright LP, Trueblood HW, Nelsen TS. The surgical diagnosis of abdominal Hodgkin's disease. *Surg Gynecol Obstet* 1970;130: 853–858.
91. Slavin R, Nelson T. Complications of staging laparotomy for Hodgkin's disease. *Natl Cancer Inst Monogr* 1973;36:457–459.
92. Gazet JC. Laparotomy and splenectomy. In: Smithers DW, ed. *Hodgkin's disease*. Edinburgh: Churchill Livingstone, 1973:190–200.
93. Mauch P, Kalish L, Marcus K, et al. Long-term survival in Hodgkin's disease: relative impact of mortality, infection, second tumors, and cardiovascular disease. *Cancer J Sci Am* 1995;1:33–42.
94. Jockovich M, Mendenhall NP, Sombeck MD, Talbert JL, Copeland EM III, Bland KI. Long-term complications of laparotomy in Hodgkin's disease. *Ann Surg* 1994;219:615–621; discussion 621–624.
95. Schimpff S, O'Connell M, Greene W, Wiernik P. Infections in 92 splenectomized patients with Hodgkin's disease. A clinical review. *Am J Med* 1975;59:695–701.
96. Sutcliffe S, Wrigley P, Smyth J, et al. Intensive investigation in management of Hodgkin's disease. *Br Med J* 1976;2:1343–1347.
97. Leibenhaut M, Hoppe R, Efron B, Halpern J, Nelsen T, Rosenberg S. Prognostic indicators of laparotomy findings in clinical stage I–II supradiaphragmatic Hodgkin's disease. *J Clin Oncol* 1989;7:81–91.
98. Scholz KH, Herrmann C, Tebbe U, Chemnitius JM, Helmchen U, Kreuzer H. Myocardial infarction in young patients with Hodgkin's disease—potential pathogenic role of radiotherapy, chemotherapy, and splenectomy. *Clin Invest* 1993;71:57–64.
99. Haire WD, Pirruccello SJ, Carson SD. Monocyte tissue factor in treated Hodgkin's disease. *Leuk Lymphoma* 1994;12:259–263.
100. Breuer CK, Tarbell NJ, Mauch PM, et al. The importance of staging laparotomy in pediatric Hodgkin's disease. *J Pediatr Surg* 1994;29: 1085–1089.
101. Gallez-Marchal D, Fayolle M, Henry-Amar M, LeBourgeois J, Rougier P, Cosset JM. Radiation injuries of the gastrointestinal tract in Hodgkin's disease: the role of exploratory laparotomy and fractionation. *Radiother Oncol* 1984;2:93–99.
102. Grimfors G, Andersson B, Tullgren O, et al. Increased serum CD8 soluble antigen level is associated with blood lymphocyte abnormalities and other established indicators of a poor prognosis in adult Hodgkin's disease. *Br J Haematol* 1992;80:166–171.
103. Merk K, Björkholm M, Tullgren O, Mellstedt H, Holm G. Immune deficiency in family members of patients with Hodgkin's disease. *Cancer* 1990;66:1938–1943.
104. Björkholm M, Holm G, Askergren J, Mellstedt H. Lymphocyte counts and functions in arterial and venous splenic blood of patients with Hodgkin's disease. Evidence for elimination of spontaneously DNA synthesizing cells in the spleen. *Clin Exp Immunol* 1983;52:485–492.
105. Grimfors G, Soderqvist M, Holm G, Lefvert AK, Björkholm M. A longitudinal study of class and subclass antibody response to pneumococcal vaccination in splenectomized individuals with special ref-

erence to patients with Hodgkin's disease. *Eur J Haematol* 1990;45: 101–108.
106. Björkholm M, Askergren J, Holm G, Mellstedt H. Long-term influence of splenectomy on immune functions in patients with Hodgkin's disease. *Scand J Haematol* 1980;24:87–94.
107. Björkholm M, Wedelin C, Holm G, Johansson B, Mellstedt H. Longitudinal studies of blood lymphocyte capacity in Hodgkin's disease. *Cancer* 1981;48:2010–2015.
108. Grimfors G, Holm G, Mellstedt H, Schnell PO, Tullgren O, Björkholm M. Increased blood clearance rate of indium-111 oxine-labeled autologous CD4+ blood cells in untreated patients with Hodgkin's disease. *Blood* 1990;76:583–589.
109. Morris DH, Bullock FD. The importance of spleen in the resistance to infection. *Am Surg* 1919;70:513.
110. Crosby WH. Splenectomy. In and out of fashion [Editorial]. *Arch Intern Med* 1985;145:225–227.
111. Singer DB. Postsplenectomy sepsis. *Perspect Pediatr Pathol* 1973;1: 285–311.
112. Desser RK, Ultmann JE. Risk of severe infection in patients with Hodgkin's disease or lymphoma after diagnostic laparotomy and splenectomy. *Ann Intern Med* 1972;77:143–146.
113. Donaldson S, Moore M, Rosenberg S, Vosti K. Characterization of postsplenectomy bacteremia among patients with and without lymphoma. *N Engl J Med* 1972;287:69–71.
114. Donaldson S, Glatstein E, Vosti K. Bacterial infections in pediatric Hodgkin's disease. *Cancer* 1978;41:1949–1958.
115. Weitzman S, Aisenberg A. Fulminant sepsis after successful treatment of Hodgkin's disease. *Am J Med* 1977;62:47–50.
116. Tullgren O, Giscombe R, Holm G, Johansson B, Mellstedt H, Björkholm M. Increased luminol-enhanced chemiluminescence of blood monocytes and granulocytes in Hodgkin's disease. *Clin Exp Immunol* 1991;85:436–440.
117. Krivit W, Giebink GS, Leonard A. Overwhelming postsplenectomy infection. *Surg Clin North Am* 1979;59:223–233.
118. Ertel IJ, Boles ET Jr, Newton WA Jr. Infection after splenectomy [Letter]. *N Engl J Med* 1977;296:1174.
119. Lanzkowsky P, Shende A, Karayalcin G, Aral I. Staging laparotomy and splenectomy: treatment and complications of Hodgkin's disease in children. *Am J Hematol* 1976;1:393–404.
120. LaForce FM, Eickhoff TC. Pneumococcal vaccine: the evidence mounts. *Ann Intern Med* 1986;104:110–112.
121. Shapiro ED, Berg AT, Austrian R, et al. The protective efficacy of polyvalent pneumococcal polysaccharide vaccine. *N Engl J Med* 1991;325:1453–1460 (*see comments*).
122. Molrine D, George S, Tarbell N, et al. Antibody responses to polysaccharide and polysaccharide-conjugate vaccines following treatment for Hodgkin's disease. *Ann Intern Med* 1995;123:824–828.
123. Hosea S, Burch C, Brown E, Berg R, Frank M. Impaired immune response of splenectomized patients to polyvalent pneumococcal vaccine. *Lancet* 1981;1:804–807.
124. Siber G, Weitzman S, Aisenberg A, Weinstein H, Schiffman G. Impaired antibody response to pneumococcal vaccine after treatment for Hodgkin's disease. *N Engl J Med* 1978;299:442–448.
125. Grimfors G, Björkholm M, Hammarstrom L, Askergren J, Smith CI, Holm G. Type-specific anti-pneumococcal antibody subclass response to vaccination after splenectomy with special reference to lymphoma patients. *Eur J Haematol* 1989;43:404–410.
126. Notter D, Grossman P, Rosenberg S, Remington J. Infections in patients with Hodgkin's disease: a clinical study of 300 consecutive adult patients. *Rev Infect Dis* 1980;2:761–800.
127. Coleman C, McDougall I, Dailey M, Ager P, Bush S, Kaplan H. Functional hyposplenia after splenic irradiation for Hodgkin's disease. *Ann Intern Med* 1982;96:44–47.
128. Centers for Disease Control. Update on adult immunization. Recommendations of the Immunization Practices Advisory Committee (ACIP). *MMWR Morb Mortal Wkly Rep* 1991;40:1–94.
129. van Leeuwen F, Somers R, Hart A. Splenectomy in Hodgkin's disease and second leukemias. *Lancet* 1987;2:210–212.
130. Meadows A, Obringer A, Marrero O, et al. Second malignant neoplasms following childhood Hodgkin's disease: treatment and splenectomy as risk factors. *Med Pediatr Oncol* 1989;17:477–484.
131. van Leeuwen F, Somers R, Taal B, et al. Increased risk of lung cancer, non-Hodgkin's lymphoma and leukemia following Hodgkin's disease. *J Clin Oncol* 1989;7:1046–1058.
132. Boivin JF, Hutchison GB, Zauber AG, et al. Incidence of second cancers in patients treated for Hodgkin's disease. *J Natl Cancer Inst* 1995; 87:732–741 (*see comments*).
133. Tura S, Fiacchini M, Zinzani P, Brusamolino E, Gobbi P. Splenectomy and the increasing risk of secondary acute leukemia in Hodgkin's disease. *J Clin Oncol* 1993;11:925–930.
134. Dietrich PY, Henry-Amar M, Cosset JM, Bodis S, Bosq J, Hayat M. Second primary cancers in patients continuously disease-free from Hodgkin's disease: a protective role for the spleen? *Blood* 1994;84: 1209–1215.
135. Swerdlow AJ, Douglas AJ, Vaughan Hudson G, Vaughan Hudson B, MacLennan KA. Risk of second primary cancer after Hodgkin's disease in patients in the British National Lymphoma Investigation: relationships to host factors, histology and stage of Hodgkin's disease, and splenectomy. *Br J Cancer* 1993;68:1006–1011.
136. Salvagno L, Simonato L, Soraru M, et al. Secondary leukemia following treatment for Hodgkin's disease. *Tumori* 1993;79:103–107.
137. Abrahamsen JF, Andersen A, Hannisdal E, et al. Second malignancies after treatment of Hodgkin's disease: the influence of treatment, follow-up time, and age. *J Clin Oncol* 1993;11:255–261 (*see comments*).
138. Mellemkjoer L, Olsen JH, Linet MS, Gridley G, McLaughlin JK. Cancer risk after splenectomy. *Cancer* 1995;75:577–583.
139. Rutherford C, Desforges J, Barnett A, Safran C, Davies B. The decision betwen single- and combined-modality therapy in Hodgkin's disease. *Am J Med* 1982;72:63–70.
140. Ng A, Weeks J, Mauch P, Kuntz K. Laparotomy versus no laparotomy in the management of early stage, favorable prognosis Hodgkin's disease: a decision analysis. *J Clin Oncol* 1999;17:241–252.
141. Bergsagel D, Alison R, Bean H, et al. Results of treating Hodgkin's disease without a policy of laparotomy staging. *Cancer Treat Rep* 1982;66:717–731.
142. Donaldson S, Whitaker S, Plowman P, Link M, Malpas J. Stage I–II pediatric Hodgkin's disease: long-term follow-up demonstrates equivalent survival rates following different management schemes. *J Clin Oncol* 1990;8:1128–1137.
143. Askergren J, Björkholm M, Holm G, et al. Prognostic effect of early diagnostic splenectomy in Hodgkin's disease: a randomized trial. *Br J Cancer* 1980;42:284–291.
144. Gomez GA, Reese PA, Nava H, et al. Staging laparotomy and splenectomy in early Hodgkin's disease. No therapeutic benefit. *Am J Med* 1984;77:205–210.
145. Andrieu JM, Montagnon B, Asselain B, et al. Chemotherapy-radiotherapy association in Hodgkin's disease, clinical stages IA, IIA: results of a prospective clinical trial with 166 patients. *Cancer* 1980;46:2126–2130.
146. Aragon de la Cruz G, Cardenes H, Otero J, et al. Individual risk of abdominal disease in patients with stages I and II supradiaphragmatic Hodgkin's disease. *Cancer* 1989;63:1799–1803.
147. Brada M, Easton DF, Horwich A, Peckham MJ. Clinical presentation as a predictor of laparotomy findings in supradiaphragmatic stage I and II Hodgkin's disease. *Radiother Oncol* 1986;5:15–22.
148. Peters MV, Brown TC, Rideout DF. Updated Hodgkin's disease: B. Curability of localized disease. Prognostic influences and radiation therapy according to pattern of disease. *JAMA* 1973;223:53–59.
149. Mendenhall NP, Cantor AB, Williams JL, et al. With modern imaging techniques, is staging laparotomy necessary in pediatric Hodgkin's disease? A Pediatric Oncology Group study. *J Clin Oncol* 1993;11: 2218–2225.
150. Tubiana M, Henry-Amar M, Hayat M, et al. Prognostic significance of the number of involved areas in the early stages of Hodgkin's disease. *Cancer* 1984;54:885–894.
151. Tubiana M, Attié E, Flamant R, Gérard-Marchant R, Hayat M. Prognostic factors in 454 cases of Hodgkin's disease. *Cancer Res* 1971;31: 1801–1810.
152. Haybittle J, Easterling M, Bennett M, et al. Review of British National Lymphoma Investigation studies of Hodgkin's disease and development of prognostic index. *Lancet* 1985;1:967–972.
153. Noordijk E, Carde P, Mandard A, et al. Preliminary results of the EORTC-GPMC controlled clinical trial H7 in early stage Hodgkin's disease. *Ann Oncol* 1994;5:107–112.
154. Carde P, Noordijk E, Hagenbeek A, et al. Superiority of EBVP chemotherapy in combination with involved field irradiation over subtotal nodal irradiation in favorable clinical stage I–II Hodgkin's disease: the EORTC-GPMC H7F randomized trial. *Proc Am Soc Clin Oncol* 1997;16:13.

155. Lefor AT, Flowers JL, Heyman MR. Laparoscopic staging of Hodgkin's disease. *Surg Oncol* 1993;2:217–220.
156. Childers JM, Balserak JC, Kent T, Surwit EA. Laparoscopic staging of Hodgkin's lymphoma. *J Laparoendosc Surg* 1993;3:495–499.
157. Zornig C, Emmermann A, von Waldenfels HA, Felixmuller C. Colpotomy for specimen removal in laparoscopic surgery [in German]. *Chirurg* 1994;65:883–885.
158. Tulman S, Holcomb GWd, Karamanoukian HL, Reynhout J. Pediatric laparoscopic splenectomy. *J Pediatr Surg* 1993;28:689–692.
159. Kusminsky RE, Tiley EH, Lucente FC, Boland JP. Laparoscopic staging laparotomy with intra-abdominal manipulation. *Surg Laparosc Endosc* 1994;4:103–105.
160. Silvestri F, Barillari G, Fanin R, et al. Laparoscopic splenectomy in the management of Hodgkin's disease. *Proceedings of the Third International Symposium on Hodgkin's Lymphoma*, Cologne, Germany, September 18–23, 1995 (vol 176).
161. Mann GB, Conlon KC, LaQuaglia M, Dougherty E, Moskowitz CH, Zelenetz AD. Emerging role of laparoscopy in the diagnosis of lymphoma. *J Clin Oncol* 1998;16:1909–1915.
162. Veronesi U, Spinelli P, Bonadonna G, et al. Laparoscopy and laparotomy in staging Hodgkin's and non-Hodgkin's lymphoma. *Am J Roentgenol* 1976;127:501–503.
163. Phillips EH, Carroll BJ, Fallas MJ. Laparoscopic splenectomy. *Surg Endosc* 1994;8:931–933.
164. Morice P, Castaigne D, Haie-Meder C, et al. Laparoscopic ovarian transposition for pelvic malignancies: indications and functional outcomes. *Fertil Steril* 1998;70:956–960.
165. Hoekstra HJ, Tamminga RY, Timens W. Partial splenectomy in children: an alternative for splenectomy in the pathological staging of Hodgkin's disease. *Ann Surg Oncol* 1994;1:480–486.
166. Kluin-Nelemans HC, Noordijk EM. Staging of patients with Hodgkin's disease: what should be done? *Leukemia* 1990;4:132–135.
167. Rosenberg SA. Laparotomy and splenectomy in Hodgkin's disease: a reappraisal after twenty years. *Scand J Haematol* 1985;34:289–292.
168. Leibenhaut M, Hoppe R, Varghese A, Rosenberg S. Subdiaphragmatic Hodgkin's disease: laparotomy and treatment results in 49 patients. *J Clin Oncol* 1987;5:1050–1055.
169. Rosenstock JG, D'Angio GJ, Kiesewetter WB. Proceedings: the incidence of complications following staging laparotomy for Hodgkin's disease in children. *Am J Roentgenol Radium Ther Nucl Med* 1974;120:531–535.
170. Chilcote R, Baehner R, Hammond D. Septicemia and meningitis in children splenectomized for Hodgkin's disease. *N Engl J Med* 1976;294:798–800.
171. Baccarani M, Fiacchini M, Galieni P, et al. Meningitis and septicaemia in adults splenectomized for Hodgkin's disease. *Scand J Haematol* 1986;36:492–498.
172. Frezzato M, Castaman G, Rodeghiero F. Fulminant sepsis in adults splenectomized for Hodgkin's disease. *Haematologica* 1993;78:73–77.
173. Zanini M, Viviani S, Santoro A, et al. Extended-field radiotherapy in favorable stage IA–IIA Hodgkin's disease (prognostic role of stage). *Int J Radiat Oncol Biol Phys* 1994;30:813–819.

Hodgkin's Disease, edited by P. M. Mauch,
J. O. Armitage, V. Diehl, R. T. Hoppe, and L. M. Weiss.
Lippincott Williams & Wilkins, Philadephia ©1999.

CHAPTER 19

Prognostic Factors of Hodgkin's Disease

Lena K. Specht and Dirk Hasenclever

HISTORICAL PERSPECTIVE

Early descriptions of the natural history of untreated or palliatively treated patients with Hodgkin's disease showed a disease with a highly variable clinical course, although the disease eventually proved fatal in virtually all cases (1–5). The disease might remain localized in one lymph node region for many years without causing any deterioration in the patient's physical condition. Some uncured patients have been reported to have survived more than 20 years. At the other end of the spectrum, the disease might disseminate rapidly to other lymph node regions and internal organs and cause progressive asthenia, cachexia, and death. This highly variable course prompted and continues to prompt numerous clinical studies designed to identify new prognostic factors or improve already-established prognostic factors, so that clinicians can predict outcome more accurately in individual patients.

As early as the beginning of this century, the concept had developed that Hodgkin's disease passes through successive clinical stages with an increasing spread of the disease and progressive worsening of prognosis (1). The validity of this concept has been repeatedly confirmed, and different staging classifications have been proposed over the years based on the anatomic extent of disease (6–25). A consensus was reached at the Workshop on the Staging of Hodgkin's disease at Ann Arbor in 1971 (26), and the Ann Arbor staging classification has since been universally adopted. Its prognostic significance has been amply demonstrated (27–40). The Ann Arbor staging classification remains the basis for the evaluation of patients with Hodgkin's disease. Survival curves according to clinical Ann Arbor stage for more than 14,000 patients in the International Database on Hodgkin's Disease (33) are shown in Figure 1.

Through the years, however, it became increasingly clear that the Ann Arbor staging system could not be relied on as the only prognostic tool in Hodgkin's disease. New features of prognostic importance became recognized, many of them related to the extent and volume of disease. The extent of disease may vary considerably in stages other than stage I, and the volume of disease in individual regions is not taken into account at all in the Ann Arbor classification. At a meeting in the Cotswolds region of England in 1988, a modification of the Ann Arbor staging system was devised to incorporate a designation for number of sites and bulk (41). However, the recommendations of the Cotswolds meeting have still not been universally adopted. A multitude of other prognostic factors for different Ann Arbor stages, presentations, treatments, and outcomes have been examined, and varying combinations of some of these factors are presently being employed by different centers and groups worldwide. Thus, there is a need for a general consensus on the use of prognostic factors in Hodgkin's disease.

DIFFERENT PROGNOSTIC FACTORS AND END POINTS, AND THEIR INTERRELATION

Definition and Use of Prognostic Factors

Prognostic factors are variables measured in individual patients that offer a partial explanation of the heterogeneity observed in the outcome of a given disease—in this case, Hodgkin's disease (42). There are many reasons for studying prognostic factors in Hodgkin's disease. Prognostic factors may be used to predict the outcome of a disease. However, we cannot predict exactly for individual patients. We can offer only statements of probability, and even these will be more accurate for groups of patients than for individual patients (43).

L. K. Specht: Department of Oncology, Herlev Hospital, University of Copenhagen, Herlev, Denmark.

D. Hasenclever: Institut für Medizinische Informatik, Statistik und Epidemiologie, Universität Leipzig, Leipzig, Germany.

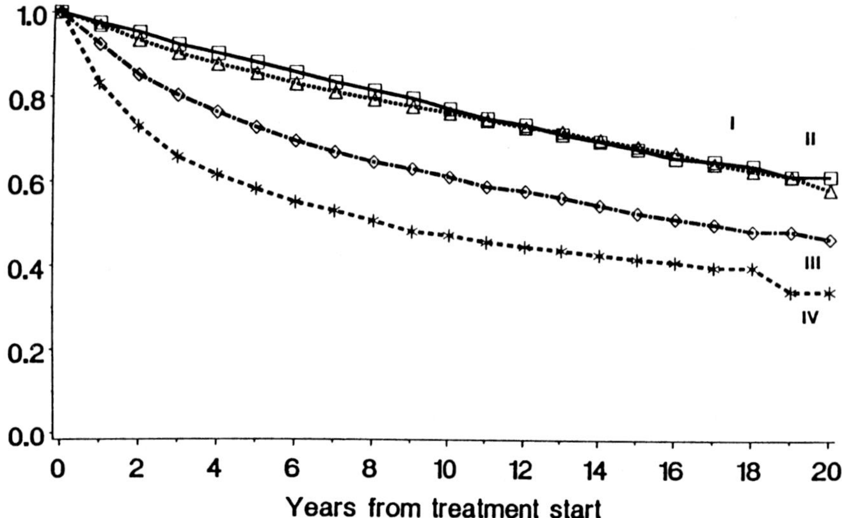

FIG. 1. Overall survival according to clinical stage for 14,037 patients in the International Database on Hodgkin's Disease treated over the past 25 years. (From ref. 33, with permission.)

On a practical level, prediction of outcome may be used to define risk groups and may thus be a determining factor in treatment selection. In the context of clinical trials, the prediction of outcome for groups of patients may be used beforehand to define eligibility and stratification criteria, and afterwards in the statistical analysis of the trial results to allow adjustments for more valid comparisons (42,43). However, it is important to realize that although known prognostic factors are important in the design and analysis of trials, they are rarely sufficiently explanatory to justify the comparison of treatments by use of nonrandomized data (44,45).

On a more theoretical level, if certain prognostic factors are found to be important, they may provide insight into a disease process and help us understand the natural history of a disease, including the effects of treatment on its course, thereby suggesting directions for future studies.

Types of Prognostic Factors

Prognostic factors can be divided into tumor-related factors and patient-related factors. Tumor-related factors reflect tumor type, extent of disease, and growth characteristics of the tumor, either directly or indirectly via surrogate measures, such as serum markers. Patient-related factors reflect the physiologic reserve of the patient (e.g., age and performance status). Both types of factors are important for outcome, but in many situations it is advisable to keep them separate, in particular if they are to form the basis for treatment selection.

Prognostic factors can also be divided according to the point in time at which they are recorded. It is generally assumed that the values of the prognostic factors are known at the point from which prognosis or time to response is measured (43). This type of prognostic factor, for which a single value is determined for each patient at the outset of the study, is called a fixed covariate. However, other prognostic variables (e.g., time to response, received dose intensity, toxicity of treatment) may be measured after the outset of a study and may even change over time. This type of prognostic factor is called a time-dependent covariate (42). Although the study of time-dependent covariates may be very interesting biologically, their use as prognostic factors is fraught with problems because the time-dependent covariates may well themselves be affected by treatment. Variables that are affected by treatment should never be used when adjusted treatment comparisons are performed (43).

Different End Points

Analyses of prognostic factors attempt to relate patient variables to an outcome variable (and to each other). In considering and comparing the results of prognostic factor analyses, it is important to define the outcome variable clearly. A simple outcome variable could be response to therapy (yes or no). However, the vast majority of patients with Hodgkin's disease respond to therapy, so a response to therapy is by no means an indication of cure or long-term survival. Disease-free survival or relapse-free survival would be a relevant outcome variable. However, strictly speaking, only patients achieving complete remission should be analyzed, and only from the time at which complete remission is achieved. It continues to be difficult to define complete remission accurately in Hodgkin's disease, particularly for disease in the mediastinum, and the exact time at which it is achieved is often uncertain. A more useful outcome variable is therefore freedom from progression or time to failure—that is, time from registration until recurrence after remission or progression or death without remission. The ultimate outcome variable remains survival. It is tempting to increase the sensitivity of analyses by analyzing cause-specific survival in Hodgkin's disease—that is, time from registration to death from Hodgkin's disease with censoring of deaths from other causes. However, it can be surprisingly difficult to be certain about the exact cause of death in particular patients, and the most certain outcome variable remains overall survival—that is, time from registration to death from any cause.

Interrelations among Different Factors

For a patient variable to qualify as a useful prognostic factor, it must be significant, independent, and clinically important (46). All patient variables are potentially of prognostic significance and many prove significant in univariate analysis. However, different variables are likely to be highly interrelated and may thus be partial substitutes for one another, and only a few in fact possess independent prognostic value. The independent prognostic information contained in a cluster of correlated variables can be equally well represented by several of the variables within the cluster. The choice of the representing variable(s) may not be entirely determined by the data but depends on medical insight, practicality considerations, and the strategy of model selection. Moreover, some factors may be prognostic for certain therapies only, some may be prognostic for certain stages only, and some may be prognostic only in the context of certain other factors. Therefore, multivariate statistical analyses, often complex, are needed to determine which factors are independently significant and which factors are merely related to well-known prognostic factors but are without independent prognostic significance. A large number of studies of prognostic factors in Hodgkin's disease in which multivariate regression techniques are used have been published. Comparisons of these studies may cause some bewilderment, as different studies seem to come up with widely differing results, both in regard to the factors found to be significant and in regard to the relative importance attributed to these factors. There are many reasons for these differences between studies, and some of the main reasons are the following (47):

- Studies vary with regard to selection criteria. Studies of highly selected patient populations may miss out important factors because patients with these factors are underrepresented in the patient population studied.
- Studies vary with regard to staging investigations. In general, if the evaluation of the anatomic extent and bulk of the disease is less accurate (e.g., no laparotomy), other factors correlated with the extent of disease (e.g., hematologic, biochemical, or immunologic indicators) will acquire greater significance.
- Studies vary with regard to treatment approach. Prognostic factors found in a particular study will predict outcome for other patients only if they are treated in a roughly similar way. Treatment may also influence studies of prognostic factors in a more subtle but no less important way. Intensive treatment is a prerequisite for cure in Hodgkin's disease. If a subgroup of patients for some reason (e.g., old age or other medical problems) receives suboptimal treatment, this subgroup will have a poorer prognosis that is at least partly explained by insufficient treatment. Statistical analysis cannot fully compensate for this type of confounding (48).
- Studies vary with regard to the range of factors analyzed. Obviously, a study cannot identify prognostic factors that were not analyzed in the study.
- Studies vary with regard to the number of patients analyzed. The number of patients analyzed determines the size of the prognostic difference that can be detected or reproduced in a given set of data. Typical analyses of about 300 patients have an 80% chance of detecting a prognostic difference in the order of 15% if the smaller subgroups are not too small. For an 80% chance of reproducing a difference of 8% to 10%, 800 to 1,200 patients must be included in a study.
- Studies vary with regard to cut points chosen for different variables (e.g., age and laboratory values). Even if cut points are chosen systematically (e.g., by the optimal P method), different studies will come up with different cut points (49,50).
- Studies vary with regard to the methods used for analysis. This issue is perhaps the one that creates the most bewilderment for clinicians. First, investigators commonly perform multivariate prognostic factor analyses by using the Cox proportional hazards regression model (51). Regression models can make more accurate predictions than other methods, such as stratification and recursive partitioning, provided they are used wisely. However, regression models make assumptions that must hold, at least approximately, for valid prognostic estimates to be obtained. For a study to be valid, model assumptions must be thoroughly examined and appropriate steps taken if assumptions are violated (52–54). Second, multivariate analyses are commonly applied to data materials in an exploratory manner, without any prior hypothesis, except that some of the variables entered are likely to possess some prognostic significance. Different studies of this kind will invariably identify differing factors and prognostic indices. From a statistical point of view, this variation is unproblematic because if one is primarily interested in prediction, the actual factors used are not important (42). Moreover, it is important to realize that the majority of factors identified by this type of analysis probably reflect the same underlying biologic characteristics. The multiple regression model will select a factor for inclusion in the model if its χ^2 value is the highest among the factors examined. However, another factor may have a χ^2 value that is only a fraction smaller. This other factor may well, simply by chance, be the one selected in another, similar study. Therefore, prognostic indices from different studies may be quite diverse sim-

ply by chance. As long as the purpose of the studies is merely predicting outcome, this is perfectly acceptable, provided the different indices are roughly equally good at predicting outcome. However, if the primary purpose of a study is to understand the biologic reasons why certain factors seem to be related to outcome, clearly it is essential that the specific range of factors be included in the model.

PROGNOSTIC FACTORS FOR PATHOLOGIC STAGE I–II HODGKIN'S DISEASE

Patients with apparently early-stage Hodgkin's disease after clinical staging were previously usually staged further with laparotomy and splenectomy. The purpose of staging these patients more accurately was to differentiate those who could be treated with radiotherapy alone from those who required additional chemotherapy (55–63). However, it is important to realize that although additional chemotherapy can prevent recurrence, a meta-analysis of all randomized trials of radiotherapy versus radiotherapy plus additional chemotherapy gave no indication of an improvement in survival in any subgroup of early-stage patients (64). The value of laparotomy and splenectomy as part of the staging procedure has therefore been challenged in later years, and the procedure is performed less frequently than before. However, the information gathered in the past from large series of patients staged with laparotomy and splenectomy has provided us with invaluable data on the intra-abdominal distribution of Hodgkin's disease.

Our knowledge of the extent and anatomic distribution of disease is more accurate in patients with pathologic stage (PS) I and II than in any other patients with Hodgkin's disease. Consequently, we would expect to be able to predict outcome for these patients with a high degree of precision.

Patients Treated with Radiotherapy Alone

The precise prediction of the risk for relapse is particularly important for patients treated with radiotherapy alone because one important use of prognostic factors is to define groups with an acceptable risk for relapse, who can be treated with radiotherapy alone, and groups with an unacceptable risk, for whom combined-modality therapy is deemed advisable (63).

The anatomic extent of disease may vary considerably in stage II, and the number of involved regions has been shown to possess independent prognostic significance. An early study from the Royal Marsden Hospital found a high relapse rate in patients with multiple nodal areas involved (65). Follow-up studies from the same institution confirmed the importance of the number of sites of nodal involvement for disease-free survival and also showed an influence of borderline significance on overall survival (66,67). Figure 2 shows relapse-free survival curves according to the number of involved sites for 131 PS I and II patients treated with radiotherapy alone at the Royal Marsden. Another early study, from the University of Florida, in which about half the patients were staged with laparotomy, found that one of the most important factors in predicting relapse is the number of sites initially involved (68). Again, this was confirmed in a follow-up study, which also showed a highly significant influence on cause-specific survival (69). In the European Organization for the Research and Treatment of Cancer (EORTC) H_2 trial, the number of involved lymph node areas proved to be a highly significant independent factor for relapse-free survival and of borderline significance for overall survival (70,71). Studies from the University of Minnesota also showed that the number of involved sites is important for relapse-free survival and overall survival (72,73). A study from the Massachusetts General Hospital, in which most patients were staged with laparotomy, showed a significantly increased risk for relapse with increasing number of sites of involvement, but no difference for survival (74). The large Australasian study on patterns of care, in which most patients were staged with laparotomy, showed an increased risk for in-field relapse with an increasing number of involved lymph node sites, whereas there was no relation to out-of-field recurrences and to overall survival (75). However, in two other large series of patients, one from Stanford University and one from Harvard University, there was no significant independent prognostic influence of the number of involved regions (76,77). In the Danish National Hodgkin Study, the number of involved regions was sig-

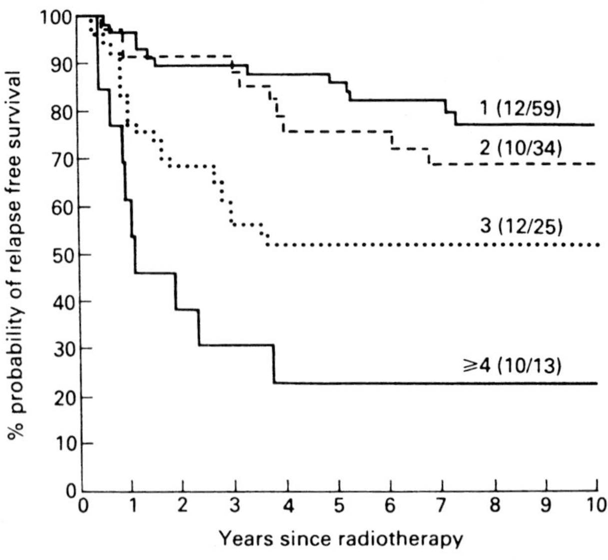

FIG. 2. Relapse-free survival according to number of involved sites for 131 patients in pathologic stage (PS) I–II treated with radiotherapy alone at the Royal Marsden Hospital. (From ref. 67, with permission.)

nificant both for relapse-free survival and overall survival (78,79). However, an estimate of the total tumor burden (*vide infra*) was an even more powerful prognostic factor, rendering the number of involved regions nonsignificant in multivariate analysis.

The volume of disease in individual regions is left out of consideration in the Ann Arbor classification. Realizing that the size of the tumor mass in single regions may be important, the Cotswolds modification of the Ann Arbor classification tried to remedy this by incorporating a designation of bulk. The extent of mediastinal involvement has attracted particular interest because mediastinal involvement, even bulky, is quite common. Measurement of mediastinal tumor mass has been carried out in different ways. Some studies have measured the maximal width of mediastinal disease in absolute terms (68,80–83). Others have used the ratios of maximum mediastinal width to maximum chest diameter (76,78,81,84–86), to chest diameter at T5-6 (87,88), to chest diameter at T6-7 (89), or to chest diameter at the carina (90). No one of these methods seems to be clearly superior to the others (91). The area of mediastinal disease on posteroanterior chest radiographs (92) and the volume of mediastinal disease on thoracic computed tomograms (93) have also been employed. Whatever method has been used, the general consensus is that disease-free survival is poorer for patients with large mediastinal masses than for patients with small or no mediastinal masses (76,77,80–83,85–90,92–100). However, the presence of a large mediastinal mass is correlated with other adverse prognostic factors, such as a large number of involved sites (84), stage II (vs. stage I) (80,87,94,97)), B symptoms (87,89), and hilar involvement (87). However, even in multivariate analyses that take other prognostic factors into account, a large mediastinal mass remains an important independent prognostic factor inversely related to disease-free survival (67,76,101). Figure 3 shows relapse-free survival curves according to mediastinal size for 315 patients in PS IA and IIA treated with radiotherapy alone at the Joint Center for Radiation Therapy. Most patients who relapse after initial radiotherapy for PS I and II are salvaged with chemotherapy. Consequently, the prognostic impact of large mediastinal adenopathy on overall survival is much smaller but still statistically significant in a number of studies (85,87,88,96). In regions other than the mediastinum, large tumor masses are uncommon in PS I and II. Most studies analyze mediastinal and peripheral bulk together, thus obscuring any independent significance of peripheral bulk (67,81,88). A study from the University of Florida did, however, show that the prognostic importance of maximum tumor dimension in any site is greater than the prognostic significance of the size of mediastinal mass alone, suggesting that bulky disease in sites other than the mediastinum is indeed prognostically significant (69).

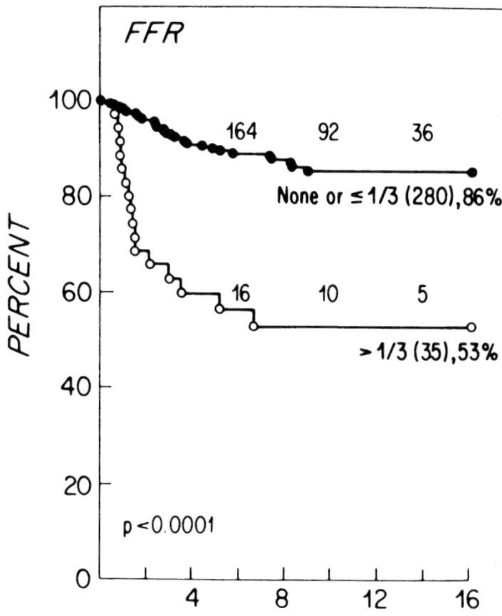

FIG. 3. Relapse-free survival according to mediastinal size for 315 patients in pathologic stages (PS) IA and IIA treated with radiotherapy alone at the Joint Center for Radiation Therapy. (From ref. 77, with permission.)

The number of involved regions and the tumor size in each region have thus been shown to be important for prognosis in PS I and II treated with radiotherapy alone. Multivariate analyses of data from the Danish National Hodgkin Study have shown that the estimated total tumor burden, combining the number of involved regions with the tumor size in each region, is by far the most important prognostic factor both for disease-free survival and overall survival (78,79,102). These findings were subsequently confirmed in a Swedish study (103). Figure 4 shows disease-free survival curves according to the estimated total tumor burden for 142 patients in PS I and II treated with radiotherapy alone in the Danish National Hodgkin Study.

The prognostic significance of different disease localizations has also been investigated. Mediastinal involvement has been associated with poorer disease-free survival (89) and overall survival (97,101). It would, however, seem to be tumor size rather than localization in the mediastinum that is important, because only bulky mediastinal involvement influences prognosis adversely, whereas nonbulky mediastinal involvement confers the same prognosis as no mediastinal involvement (67,82, 85–87,90,94,96,101,104,105). Hilar nodal involvement is rare in patients without mediastinal involvement (83,87, 89,98). A higher relapse rate was demonstrated in patients with small or no mediastinal involvement if hilar disease was present than if it was not (87), and poorer survival was demonstrated in patients with large mediastinal adenopathy if hilar disease was present (101). Other studies have not been able to demonstrate any prognostic effect of hilar adenopathy independent of mediastinal involvement (83,98). Infradiaphragmatic early-

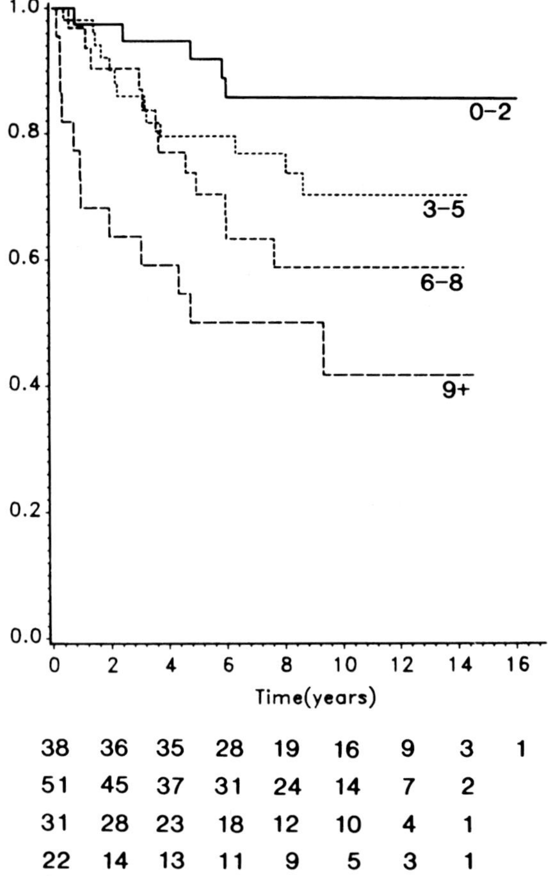

FIG. 4. Disease-free survival according to estimated total tumor burden for 142 patients in pathologic stage (PS) I–II treated with radiotherapy alone in the Danish National Hodgkin Study. (From ref. 154, with permission.)

stage disease is rare. In pathologically staged patients, infradiaphragmatic disease has not been shown to have a worse prognosis than supradiaphragmatic disease, except for patients presenting with intra-abdominal disease without peripheral adenopathy, who often have bulky disease at diagnosis and a high relapse rate (106–119). Localized extralymphatic (E) lesions were included in the Ann Arbor classification of stages I and II (26) because some studies had shown that the prognosis of patients with these lesions was no worse than that of other patients with the corresponding stages. For PS I and II patients treated with radiotherapy alone, some studies have found no prognostic influence of E lesions (76,96), whereas others have found a poorer prognosis in patients with E lesions (81,83,120). The question of whether E lesions are or are not of prognostic importance is still controversial, and it is further complicated by the fact that there is wide disagreement as to what is and what is not an E lesion (121,122). In conclusion, there seems to be no definitive evidence that particular localizations of PS I and II disease significantly affect prognosis. Prognosis seems to be determined by the bulk of disease rather than its precise anatomic localization, provided that appropriate therapy can be administered. With radiotherapy alone this may be a problem, and a number of studies suggest that patients with involvement of the pericardial nodes, extensive pericardial involvement, significant involvement of the lung or pleura, or bulky axillary disease may not be suitable for radiotherapy alone because of the toxicity associated with the large radiation volumes needed to treat these areas (63,100,123–130).

Systemic B symptoms (weight loss, unexplained fever, night sweats) have consistently been shown to influence prognosis adversely in PS I and II treated with radiotherapy alone (35,76,88,101). Repeated evaluations of the prognostic significance of B symptoms indicate that night sweats have no prognostic significance (95,131, 132) but that severe pruritus, although rarely encountered, confers a particularly ominous prognosis (131,133, 134). Fever seems to have a greater impact than weight loss, and the combination of fever and weight loss confers a significantly poorer prognosis than either symptom alone (95). Mild symptoms that do not qualify as B symptoms in the Ann Arbor definition had no prognostic influence at all (131), and symptoms that were more severe than is required to qualify as B symptoms did not further compromise prognosis (132). The presence of B symptoms is, however, correlated with the anatomic extent of disease. In studies in which the extent of disease was analyzed in greater detail, the systemic symptoms were correlated with the total tumor burden and lost their prognostic significance in multivariate analysis (78,79). This correlation of B symptoms with amount of tumor is consistent with the notion, supported by several lines of evidence, that B symptoms could be caused by aberrant production of endogenous cytokines, either by tumor cells or by reactive bystander cells (135–140).

A consensus on the histopathologic classification of Hodgkin's disease was reached in 1965 at the Rye conference (141). Slight modifications of the classification were proposed by the International Lymphoma Study Group in 1996 (142), the most important modification being the recognition of lymphocyte predominance as a distinct entity. Lymphocyte predominance is a rare subtype of Hodgkin's disease, affecting only 5% to 10% of patients with Hodgkin's disease. In cases of PS I–II treated with radiotherapy alone, patients who have lymphocyte predominance seem to have a favorable prognosis compared with patients who have other histologic subtypes, but this difference may partly be attributed to earlier stage at presentation (143–145). The precise prognostic significance of the lymphocyte predominance subtype, in particular whether the pattern of continuous late relapse found in some studies (146,147) is real, awaits further study. It is hoped that the final analyses of the multinational project on lymphocyte predominance Hodgkin's disease initiated by the European Task Force on Lymphoma will provide us with a clearer picture (148). Lymphocyte depletion is rare, very rare in early-stage disease, and its incidence is decreasing, most likely as a result of changes in diagnostic criteria (149,150).

The overwhelming majority of PS I–II patients have either the nodular sclerosis or mixed cellularity subtype, and histologic subtype usually does not provide prognostic information (76,143,151–155). One of the problems with the histopathologic classification is that in many series nodular sclerosis constitutes up to 75% of all cases (35,151,156,157). Attempts have therefore been made to subdivide the nodular sclerosis type into prognostic subgroups (158–163). The British National Lymphoma Investigation has proposed a subdivision into grades 1 and 2 of the nodular sclerosis type according to the cellular composition of the nodules of tumor tissue (156,164). In their large series of PS I–II patients, they showed that cytologic subtypes with extensive and easily recognized areas of lymphocyte depletion or numerous pleomorphic Hodgkin's cells (nodular sclerosis grade 2) were associated with a decreased survival independent of stage (152,164). The prognostic significance of nodular sclerosis grades in PS I–II was confirmed in one study (165), but not in another, larger study (166). The issue is thus still unsettled. In the Danish National Hodgkin Study of PS I and II patients, the Rye classification and the British National Lymphoma Investigation subclassification of nodular sclerosis were compared with an alternative classification based on a simple count of tumor cells in sections (154). In this study, univariate analysis showed tumor cell count to be the more significant of these classifications for prognosis. None of these histologic classifications proved independently significant in multivariate analysis. Significantly, however, a combination of the estimate of the total macroscopic tumor burden and the tumor cell count, yielding an estimate of the total tumor cell burden, was shown to be the most powerful prognostic factor of all. In conclusion, histologic subtype is not at present an important prognostic factor in PS I and II and should not play a major part in treatment decisions. However, further research, particularly in lymphocyte predominance, is in progress.

Older age has frequently been associated with poor survival in studies of prognostic factors in Hodgkin's disease (11,19,21,24,28,29,31,32,35,36,39,66,67,73,103,167–174). In many of these studies, however, deaths from all causes have been included without any correction, thus inevitably leading to a poorer prognosis for older patients. Age remained an important prognostic factor even in studies in which survival was related to that of the general population (171,172,175), in which deaths from causes other than Hodgkin's disease were excluded (36), or in which other prognostic factors were taken into account in stratified (173) or multivariate analysis (33,152,176,177). Older patients commonly have underlying medical problems that may preclude adequate staging and treatment in some cases (155,168,173,178). Adequate staging and appropriate intensive therapy is a prerequisite for cure in Hodgkin's disease, and suboptimal staging and treatment of some older patients may well explain their poorer prognosis. Significantly, in a study of patients in PS IA and IIA treated with radiotherapy alone, an increased mortality was found in older patients, but this was caused by secondary tumors rather than by recurrent Hodgkin's disease (77). In another study, older patients with early-stage disease who were staged and treated aggressively had the same potential for cure as younger patients (168). In a series from St. Bartholomew's Hospital of stage II patients treated with radiotherapy alone, age had no influence on the duration of complete remission (179). The issue regarding the prognostic importance of age *per se* is still not settled, but evidence from more recent analyses would seem to indicate that the natural history of Hodgkin's disease in older patients does not differ from that in younger patients, but that the reduced tolerance to staging and treatment may largely explain the differences seen in outcome (155).

Sex is an established prognostic factor in Hodgkin's disease, with men having a poorer prognosis than women (8,11,16,19,21,24,31,32,132,167,175). Male patients are more likely to have adverse prognostic factors (35). Nevertheless, even in multivariate analyses of PS I and II, sex often comes out as an independent prognostic factor, although not a very important one (79,132,152). Data on the prognostic influence of race are very sparse. When other prognostic factors are taken into account, prognosis seems basically the same irrespective of race, but a low socioeconomic status is highly correlated with advanced disease at diagnosis and exerts a profound influence on prognosis, especially in third world countries (180–183).

Biologic parameters (e.g., hematologic, biochemical, or immunologic indicators) are not generally very important in PS I–II, in which our knowledge of the extent and volume of tumor is quite accurate. An elevated erythrocyte sedimentation rate (ESR) is a well-established adverse prognostic factor in Hodgkin's disease (32,152,184,185). However, the ESR is correlated with other prognostic factors, such as B symptoms, age, sex, mediastinal involvement, number of involved lymph node areas, histologic subtype, stage, and total tumor burden (32,33,78,79,170,184–186). In multivariate analyses of PS I–II patients treated with radiotherapy alone, an elevated ESR had no independent prognostic significance (67,78). In a study from Manchester, a low lymphocyte count and a low albumin level were independently significant for relapse-free survival (88). Many other biologic parameters have been shown to correlate with disease activity, but their independent prognostic significance in PS I–II has not been proved (187).

The prognostic factors known to be independently significant in PS I and II treated with radiotherapy alone are summarized in Table 1.

TABLE 1. *Prognostic factors shown to be independently significant in PS I–II treated with radiotherapy alone*

Number of involved regions
Large tumor mass, particularly mediastinal
Tumor burden (combination of number of involved regions and tumor size in each region)
B symptoms (fever, weight loss, possibly severe pruritus)
(Histologic subtype)
Age
Sex

PS, pathologic stage.

Patients Receiving Combined-modality Therapy

Today, patients subjected to laparotomy and splenectomy as part of the staging procedure are given combined-modality therapy only if they turn out to be in PS III or IV (63,188). Our knowledge of prognostic factors in this group of patients therefore stems from earlier results, mostly from trials in which PS I–II patients were randomized between radiotherapy alone and combined-modality therapy. As mentioned previously, a meta-analysis in which individual patient data were used showed that the addition of chemotherapy to radiotherapy prevents recurrence but does not improve survival (64). In the meta-analysis, comparisons were made of the reduction in risk for failure with combined-modality therapy between different prognostic subgroups. The size of reduction in risk for failure seen in patients with different stages of disease, with and without B symptoms, both male and female, and of different ages was remarkably similar. Thus, there is no indication that prognostic factors for patients who receive combined-modality therapy are different from the factors for patients treated with radiotherapy alone. However, as fewer recurrences are seen with combined-modality therapy, a larger number of patients need to be analyzed for a factor to show statistical significance for relapse-free survival.

Patients Treated with Chemotherapy Alone

Chemotherapy as the sole treatment of PS I–II patients is not standard, and few data are therefore available. Two randomized trials have tested radiotherapy versus chemotherapy in these patients. In one trial, 54 patients in PS I–II were treated with chemotherapy alone; seven of them relapsed, all in previously involved sites (189). B symptoms and sex seemed to influence relapse-free survival, but the number of patients was too small for meaningful analysis of prognostic factors. In another trial, 44 patients in PS I–IIA were treated with chemotherapy alone; 12 relapsed, eight of them in previously involved areas (190). Patients with bulky disease or three or more involved areas seemed to relapse more frequently, but numbers were small (191). The precise delineation of prognostic factors in PS I–II treated with chemotherapy alone thus awaits further studies.

PROGNOSTIC FACTORS FOR LAPAROTOMY FINDINGS IN CLINICAL STAGE I–II HODGKIN'S DISEASE

Staging laparotomy with splenectomy was previously performed in large numbers of patients in clinical stage (CS) I–II, yielding a PS that differed from CS in about 30% of patients (192–196). Staging laparotomy remains the most precise way to determine the presence and extent of abdominal involvement. However, because of the associated morbidity and the fact that no survival benefit has been found in patients staged with laparotomy (197–201), the procedure is used less often today and has been largely abandoned in Europe. Instead, prognostic factors predicting the likelihood of occult disease in the abdomen are potentially useful and may aid in treatment decisions.

A number of studies have examined clinical factors for prediction of abdominal involvement in patients with supradiaphragmatic CS I or II who were subsequently staged by laparotomy. A large multivariate study from the Joint Center for Radiation Therapy showed that the number of supradiaphragmatic sites, B symptoms, and male sex were independently predictive of positive laparotomy findings (196). Female patients with CS IA and male patients with CS IA and lymphocyte predominance histology or high cervical involvement had less than a 10% risk for occult abdominal involvement. Another large multivariate study, from Stanford, found the number of involved sites, sex, histology, and age to be significant (195). In CS I disease, female patients, patients with disease limited to the mediastinum, and male patients with lymphocyte predominance histology had less than a 5% chance of positive findings at laparotomy. In CS II, women less than 27 years of age with only two or three sites of disease had less than a 10% risk for subdiaphragmatic disease. The original Stanford data also demonstrated the predictive value of histology, sex, and age (high risk in both pediatric and older adult patients) (34). The International Database on Hodgkin's Disease analyzed laparotomy findings in a total of more than 4,000 CS I–II patients and showed that male sex, mixed cellularity and lymphocyte depletion histology, and age over 50 were associated with a higher probability of positive laparotomy findings in CS IA (33). In CS IIA, the absence of mediastinal involvement, four or more involved lymph node areas, mixed cellularity and lymphocyte depletion histology, male sex, and an elevated ESR were associated with a higher probability of positive laparotomy findings. In CS IB–IIB, male sex, absence of mediastinal involvement, and extranodal localization were associated with positive laparotomy. In the EORTC studies of favorable CS I–II patients, mediastinal involvement and male sex were correlated with positive laparotomy findings (170). The investigators also found that a combination of the number of involved regions above the diaphragm, B symptoms, and ESR was predictive of subdiaphragmatic disease. Early studies from the British National Lymphoma

TABLE 2. *Prognostic factors for laparotomy findings in supradiaphragmatic CS I–II*

Number of involved regions above the diaphragm
Disease confined to upper cervical nodes
Mediastinal involvement (variable influence)
B symptoms
Age (high risk in both pediatric and older adult patients)
Sex
Histology
Erythrocyte sedimentation rate

CS, clinical stage.

Investigation and from Australia found that the presence of B symptoms increases the risk for positive laparotomy, but no relation was found between particular sites of supradiaphragmatic disease or sex and risk for intraabdominal disease (59,202). A study from the Royal Marsden found young age and male sex to be predictive of positive laparotomy findings (203). Additionally, in CS I they found that nonbulky, high cervical nodes were associated with a low risk for abdominal disease. A study from Alabama found B symptoms, histology, and sex to be independently predictive of laparotomy findings (194). A Spanish study found B symptoms, histology, and number of involved regions to be predictive of laparotomy findings, and they found increasing size of the mediastinum to be inversely correlated with the risk for abdominal disease (204). Table 2 summarizes the prognostic factors found to be significant predictors of laparotomy findings in supradiaphragmatic CS I–II disease.

In CS I–II patients with infradiaphragmatic presentation, CS IA patients had a low risk for positive findings at laparotomy if the disease was confined to inguinofemoral nodes (108–112).

PROGNOSTIC FACTORS FOR CLINICAL STAGE I–II HODGKIN'S DISEASE

Prognostic factors in CS I and II disease are to some extent similar to the ones in PS I and II. However, because our knowledge of the extent and anatomic distribution of the disease is far less accurate in patients staged without laparotomy, there is greater variation in outcome in these patients. Factors predicting positive laparotomy findings will also be predictive for outcome in these patients, because they indicate patients with more extensive disease. Additional factors, usually providing an indirect or surrogate measure of the total tumor burden and possibly also the growth characteristics of the tumor, have also proved valuable in CS patients because the direct measures in these patients are less accurate than in PS patients.

Patients Treated with Radiotherapy Alone

For a number of years, many centers treated patients with radiotherapy alone only if a staging laparotomy had been carried out to ensure that no occult abdominal disease was present. However, a number of centers have treated CS I–II patients with radiotherapy alone, and it is now clear that although the relapse rate is higher than in PS I–II, there is no difference in survival results (197–201).

In the EORTC studies of CS I–II, the number of involved regions was found to be independently significant for both disease-free survival and overall survival (70,71,170,175). In multivariate analyses of the International Database on Hodgkin's Disease, stratified for treatment and laparotomy, the number of involved regions proved significant for both disease-free survival and cause-specific survival in CS IB and IIB (33). Analyses from the Princess Margaret Hospital in Toronto, which has a large experience with radiotherapy alone in CS I–II, did not show a significant influence of the number of sites (or tumor burden), but few patients with multiple sites (or large tumor burden) were included in their material (40,205).

Patients in CS I–II with large mediastinal masses have rarely been treated with radiotherapy alone because of the high risk for relapse known from studies of PS I–II patients. Data from Toronto did, however, show a significantly higher intrathoracic relapse rate in patients with mediastinal bulk (40). The prognostic importance of a large tumor in peripheral regions has not been documented.

In regard to disease localization, CS I and II patients with disease confined to the upper cervical region have a particularly good prognosis with radiotherapy alone (35,40,170), probably because these patients are unlikely to have occult abdominal disease (*vide supra*). Subdiaphragmatic presentation in CS I–II seemed to have a decreased disease-free survival with radiotherapy alone in a couple of studies, but this was probably because it seemed to be slightly more advanced at the time of diagnosis than supradiaphragmatic disease (40,113,206). Overall, as for PS I–II, there is no clear evidence that any particular disease localization affects prognosis, except in cases in which particular localizations are associated with a particularly small or large extent of disease.

The presence of B symptoms is correlated with the extent of disease and predicts for positive laparotomy findings (33,35,176,186). Hence, B symptoms are also prognostically significant in CS I–II treated with radiotherapy alone (33,40,170,175). Figure 5 shows overall survival curves according to B symptoms for 9,087 CS I–II patients in the International Database on Hodgkin's Disease, most of whom were treated with radiotherapy alone. Histologic subtype is also prognostic for laparotomy findings and is therefore prognostically significant in some studies of CS I–II (33,40,167,170,175,205).

Older age is associated with a higher risk for occult abdominal disease. Also, as mentioned above, underlying medical problems may preclude adequate staging and

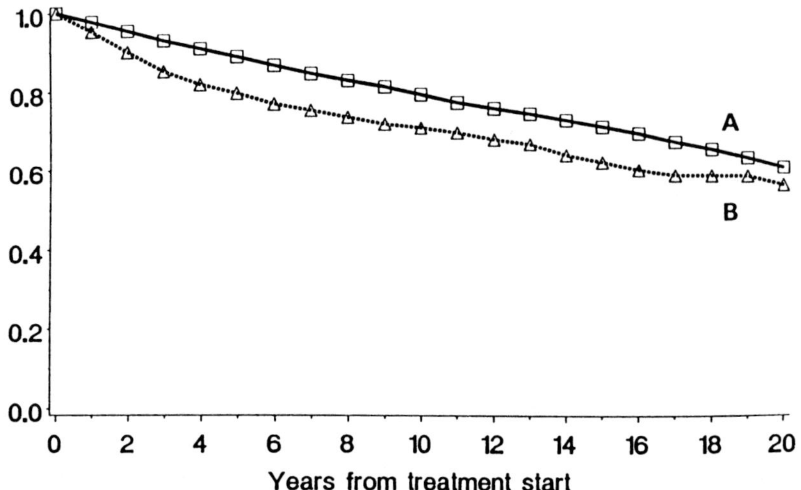

FIG. 5. Overall survival according to B symptoms for 9,087 patients in clinical stage (CS) I–II in the International Database on Hodgkin's Disease. (From ref. 33, with permission.)

treatment in some older patients. Older age was associated with poorer disease-free survival and overall survival in CS I–II patients treated with radiotherapy alone in a number of multivariate analyses (40,175,205). In the analyses of the International Database on Hodgkin's Disease, the influence of older age on disease-free survival was relatively small (33,176). Figure 6 shows disease-free survival curves according to age for 8,461 CS I–II patients achieving remission (most of them after radiotherapy alone) in the International Database on Hodgkin's Disease. The influence of age on overall survival is much greater, partly because relapse treatment seems to be less effective in older patients (*vide infra*). Sex often comes out as an independent prognostic factor in multivariate analysis, although not a very important one (33,167,170, 175,176).

Some biologic parameters (hematologic, biochemical, or immunologic) have been shown to be prognostically significant in CS I–II because they provide an indirect indication of disease extent in these patients, in whom staging was less accurate than in PS I–II (186). In the multivariate studies by the EORTC, an elevated ESR was an independent prognostic factor for both disease-free survival and overall survival in patients treated with radiotherapy alone. The EORTC has combined the ESR and B symptoms into one factor with a high prognostic significance (70,71,170,175). In the British National Lymphoma Investigation studies of CS IA and IIA and in the study from the Princess Margaret Hospital of CS I–II, an elevated ESR was also independently significant for both disease-free survival and overall survival (152,205). In the multivariate analyses of the International Database on Hodgkin's Disease, an elevated ESR had independent prognostic significance for disease-free survival in CS IA and IIA and for cause-specific survival in CS IB and IIB; most of these patients were treated initially with radiotherapy alone (33). Figure 7 shows disease-free survival curves according to ESR for 4,358 patients in CS I–II in

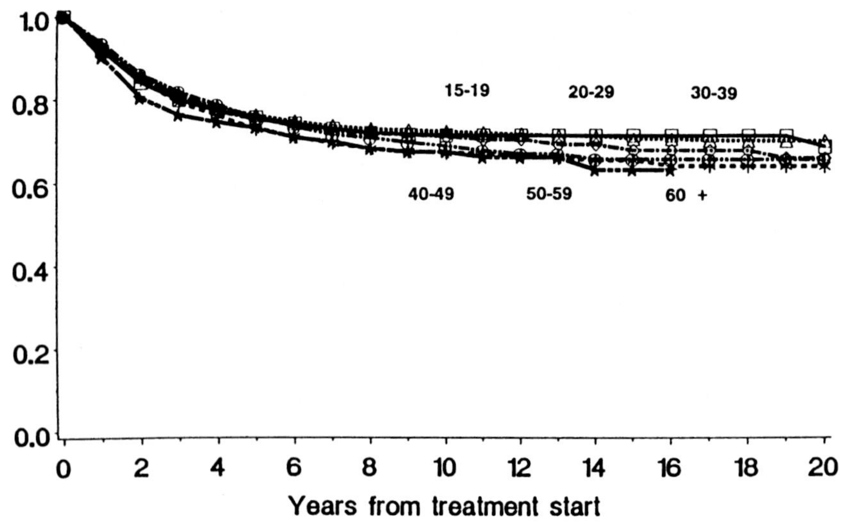

FIG. 6. Disease-free survival according to age for 8,461 patients in clinical stage (CS) I–II in the International Database on Hodgkin's Disease. (From ref. 33, with permission.)

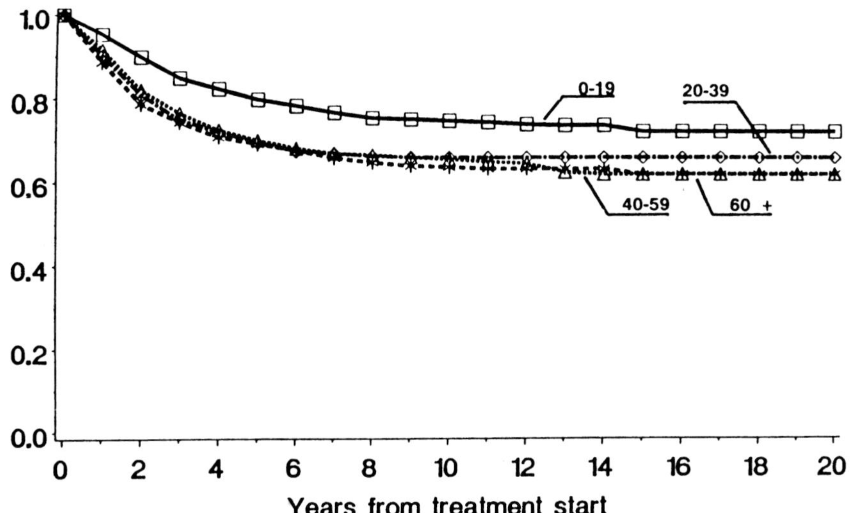

FIG. 7. Disease-free survival according to erythrocyte sedimentation rate (ESR) for 4,358 patients in clinical stage (CS) I–II in the International Database on Hodgkin's Disease. (From ref. 33, with permission.)

the International Database on Hodgkin's Disease. Anemia has been shown to be prognostically significant in several univariate analyses (24,184,185). In the multivariate analyses of the International Database on Hodgkin's Disease, anemia was independently significant for disease-free survival and cause-specific survival in CS IA, IB, and IIB (33). A decreased serum albumin level was prognostically significant in univariate analysis (184,207). In the multivariate analyses of the International Database on Hodgkin's Disease, a decreased serum albumin level was predictive of disease-free survival in CS IB and IIB (33). As mentioned previously, a host of other biologic indicators have been shown to be correlated with disease activity. However, their independent prognostic significance in CS I–II has not been proved (187).

The prognostic factors known to be independently significant in CS I–II treated with radiotherapy alone are summarized in Table 3.

Patients Treated with Combined-modality Therapy

As was the case for pathologically staged patients, a meta-analysis of individual patient data showed that combined-modality therapy reduces the risk for relapse compared with radiotherapy alone, but does not improve survival (64). The size of reduction in risk for failure in patients with different stages of disease, with and without B symptoms, both male and female, of different ages, and staged with and without laparotomy was remarkably similar. Therefore, there is also no indication in CS I–II that prognostic factors for patients treated with combined-modality therapy are different from the factors for patients treated with radiotherapy alone. Today, patients in CS I–II with adverse prognostic factors are generally given combined-modality therapy. Hence, many of the published series are selected, consisting mainly of poor-risk patients, which makes the detection of prognostic factors difficult.

TABLE 3. *Prognostic factors shown to be independently significant in CS I–II treated with radiotherapy alone*

Number of involved regions
Large mediastinal mass
Disease confined to upper cervical nodes
B symptoms
Histology
Age
Sex
Erythrocyte sedimentation rate
Anemia
Serum albumin

CS, clinical stage.

The number of involved regions was also independently significant for disease-free survival and overall survival in the EORTC studies for patients who received combined-modality therapy (175). Two other studies found the number of involved areas to be predictive for disease-free survival in patients who received combined-modality therapy (208,209). A large mediastinal mass is a highly important factor in CS I–II patients who receive combined-modality therapy (208,210–212). B symptoms, ESR, histology, age, and sex have also been shown to be prognostically significant in CS I–II patients who receive combined-modality therapy (175,209).

Patients Treated with Chemotherapy Alone

Like PS I–II patients, CS I–II patients have rarely been treated with chemotherapy alone in larger studies, and few data on prognostic factors are therefore available. In an Argentinian study in which 142 patients in CS I–II were treated with chemotherapy alone, 21 failed to achieve complete remission and 25 relapsed, 18 in previously involved areas (208). In multivariate analyses, age, number of involved areas, and tumor bulk were significant for disease-free survival, and age and tumor bulk were significant for overall survival. In another, smaller study in which 23 patients in CS I–II were treated with chemotherapy alone, three patients with bulky mediastinal disease achieved only partial remission and three relapsed, all in previously involved areas (213). However, the numbers involved were too small for any meaningful analysis of prognostic factors.

PROGNOSTIC FACTORS IN ADVANCED DISEASE

The term advanced disease is not unequivocally defined. Stages IIIB and IV certainly qualify as advanced disease, and many groups also generally include stage IIIA. Nevertheless, certain PS IIIA patients may be successfully treated with radiotherapy alone, although this has become rare in recent times. On the other hand, certain stage I or II patients with multiple adverse prognostic factors may require full systemic treatment and are included in some trials of advanced disease.

Some groups also include patients with initially localized disease who relapse after radiotherapy alone in trials of advanced disease. These patients form a biologically selected group and are reported to have a better prognosis than patients presenting in advanced stages (214–218). Prognostic factors cannot be expected to be similarly distributed in this group. Consequently, the prognosis of these patients is considered separately below.

Patients with advanced disease require systemic treatment and are typically treated with conventional chemotherapy with or without additional radiotherapy. An overview based on individual patient data of all randomized trials comparing chemotherapy alone with combined-modality therapy in Hodgkin's disease shows no general advantage of the use of radiotherapy in advanced disease (219). Thus, data with these treatment variants may be pooled for analysis of prognostic factors, although radiotherapy might play a role to control large, bulky sites.

In the vast literature on prognostic factors in advanced Hodgkin's disease, two very large sets of data have evolved from international cooperation. The International Database on Hodgkin's Disease was set up in 1989, combining individual patient data from 20 study groups in all stages (33). Besides early-stage patients, it includes 5,217 patients in stages CS III–IV, mostly treated with MOPP-type (mechlorethamine, vincristine, procarbazine, prednisone) chemotherapy. In 1995, the International Prognostic Factors Project on advanced Hodgkin's disease combined data of 5,141 advanced-stage patients mainly treated with a doxorubicin-containing regimen (220). These international efforts are particularly useful to determine the relative prognostic importance of routinely documented variables. This task requires large patient numbers for statistical analysis because the independent contributions of single prognostic factors are quantitatively small to moderate (5% to 10% in tumor control) (220).

Patients Treated with Conventional Chemotherapy with or without Additional Radiotherapy

Age is well recognized as an important patient-related prognostic factor for overall survival in advanced Hodgkin's disease (31,168,221–233). Its prognostic influence on freedom from progression is less pronounced. Besides natural mortality and a greater tendency to toxicity or reduced disease control because of a reduced, age-adapted treatment in older patients, the greater impact of age on overall survival is mainly a consequence of poor results of salvage treatment in elderly relapsed patients: 5-year survival rates after progression/relapse decrease in an ordered fashion with advancing age from about 40% in the patients up to 35 years old to less than 5% in patients between 55 and 65 years of age at diagnosis (220). Nevertheless age (e.g., above 45 years) is also an independent prognostic factor for freedom from progression in patients up to 65 years old who may be assumed to be treated homogeneously. This may be related to tumor biology, as unfavorable histologic subtypes are more frequent in these patients (33).

Sex is correlated with disease stage at presentation, as about two-thirds of advanced-stage patients are men (33,220). Male sex is an independent, although quantitatively moderate, adverse prognostic factor within advanced stages (31,33,220,224,230,234–236).

Among the tumor-related prognostic factors, histologic subtype plays a minor role as a prognostic factor in advanced Hodgkin's disease. Some studies report mixed cellularity or lymphocyte depletion subtypes as unfavorable prognostic factors (31,33,224,228,237), but several other studies do not confirm these findings (214,217,220, 221,223,229,230,234,238,239). The lymphocyte depletion subtype has rarely been diagnosed in recent times (33). As mentioned previously, the prognostic relevance of grading the nodular sclerosis subtype remains controversial (164–166,240–244). Unfavorable subtypes are moderately correlated with male sex, age, lack of mediastinal involvement, stage, systemic symptoms, and related abnormal blood parameters (33,184). Given the relatively high reclassification rate under expert pathologic review, histology subtyping does not lend itself to prognostication, at least in multicenter settings (240).

The principle that a high tumor burden correlates with an unfavorable prognosis also holds for advanced disease (229,230). However, tumor burden is much more difficult to quantify in advanced stages because pathologic staging and splenectomy have become rare. Thus, information on the number of involved areas (223,229,245), the amount of tumor in the spleen (246–251), and the subdivision of stage III (123,246–248,252–256), established as prognostic in the context of pathologic staging and radiotherapy alone, are not generally available.

Inguinal involvement may be a surrogate marker for maximal nodal spread and has been reported as independently prognostic (231). As described previously, there are various methods of measuring mediastinal bulk (257). Although very large mediastinal bulk (e.g., >0.45 of the thoracic aperture) is relatively rare, seen in fewer than 10% of cases of advanced disease (220), it has been reported as an adverse prognostic factor in some studies (231,258), but not in others (259). Large but not very large (e.g., 0.33–0.45 of the thoracic aperture) mediastinal mass is not related to prognosis in advanced Hodgkin's disease treated with modern chemotherapy (220).

Stage IV marks dissemination to extranodal sites and is independently prognostic within advanced disease (33,220,228). Bone marrow, lung or pleura, and liver involvement are each present in about 30% of cases of stage IV disease. It remains controversial whether any of these sites carries a particularly bad prognosis within stage IV. Bone marrow involvement was an adverse factor in some studies (214,230,231,260–264), but not in others (234,265,266). Pleura, lung, or liver involvement has been reported as prognostically unfavorable (238, 260,265,267), but other studies did not show a prognostic impact of any of these (214,230,231,234,245,262,268). The number of involved extranodal sites has also been reported to be independently prognostic (226,233,268), but this could not be confirmed in the International Prognostic Factors Project (220).

Several hematologic and biochemical laboratory parameters carry prognostic information in advanced Hodgkin's disease. Decreased serum levels of albumin (220,269,270) and hemoglobin (33,220,227,233,259,271) [or hematocrit (231)] as well as an elevated ESR (184, 272) or alkaline phosphatase level (232,272,273) are correlated (33,184,220,271) with one another as well as with the presence of B symptoms (33,264) and the anatomic extent of disease. These variables form a cluster of interrelated prognostic indicators that mirror both tumor burden and inflammatory processes (207). They have been variously reported as prognostic, individually or in combination. Serum albumin (220,269) and hemoglobin (220) levels show a remarkably consistent relation to prognosis over their full range of variation. Figure 8 shows freedom from progression according to serum albumin for 2,239 patients, and Figure 9 shows freedom from progression according to hemoglobin for 4,314 patients in the International Prognostic Factors Project. Moreover, hemoglobin and serum albumin levels change on a scale of weeks and are thus biometrically reliable measurements. This singles them out both as the most informative prognostic factors in advanced Hodgkin's disease and as representatives for this prognostic cluster of systemic symptoms. Given hemoglobin and serum albumin, the other members of this cluster, in particular B symptoms, lose their independent prognostic impact (220).

Leukocyte and lymphocyte counts form a second cluster of laboratory parameters. These parameters are interrelated but only weakly correlated with the first cluster mentioned above. Analysis of the joint distribution of leukocyte and lymphocyte counts in advanced Hodgkin's disease reveals a simultaneous shift away from the normal pattern toward both leukocytosis (220) and lymphocytopenia (227,230,232,233,274) that carries independent prognostic impact (220). These relatively unspecific measurements may indirectly capture dysregulation of hematopoiesis caused by cytokine release by Hodgkin's disease cells.

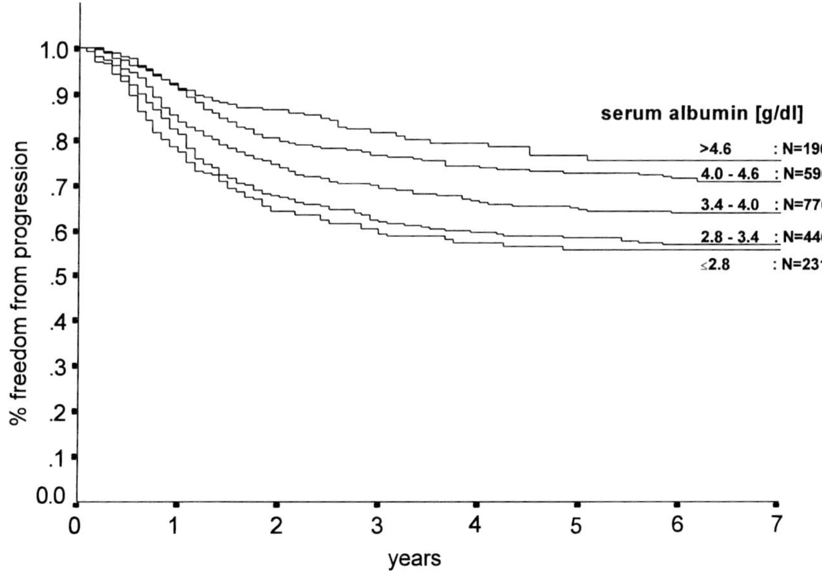

FIG. 8. Freedom from progression according to albumin levels for 2,239 patients with advanced disease in the International Prognostic Factors Project.

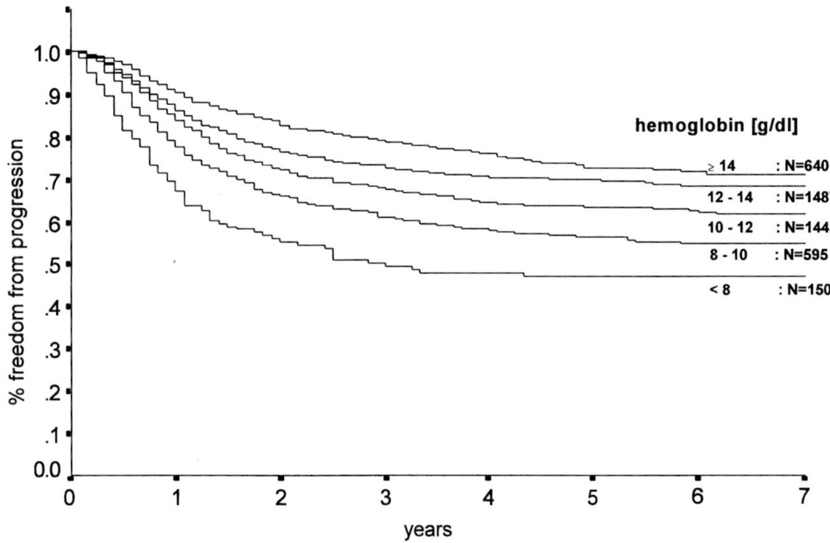

FIG. 9. Freedom from progression according to hemoglobin levels for 4,314 patients with advanced disease in the International Prognostic Factors Project.

Elevated serum lactic dehydrogenase was found to be independently prognostic by some groups (231,233), but not in the large databases of the International Database on Hodgkin's Disease and the International Prognostic Factors Project. Serum lactic dehydrogenase probably plays a lesser role in Hodgkin's disease than in high-grade non-Hodgkin's lymphoma (275). Elevated β_2-microglobulin is not generally documented but has been reported as prognostic (276). Table 4 summarizes the prognostic factors in advanced disease.

It is important to stress that the clinical features and laboratory parameters discussed so far are in biologic terms relatively nonspecific. The neoplastic cells in Hodgkin's disease are known to produce and express a number of cytokines and antigens. Increased levels of some cytokines and soluble forms of membrane-derived antigens have been detected in the serum of a majority of patients with untreated Hodgkin's disease. They are thought to correlate both with the number of tumor cells and with the activity of the Hodgkin's disease cells. Of particular interest is the CD30 surface molecule, which is consistently expressed by Hodgkin and Reed-Sternberg cells. The soluble form of the CD30 molecule is released by the cells, and with sensitive techniques it is detectable in the serum of virtually all untreated patients (135,277–279). The level of soluble CD30 is correlated with disease spread and burden. It maintains independent prognostic significance in multivariate analysis (279) and is currently one of the most promising tumor markers in Hodgkin's disease (135). It will be a task for future investigators to accumulate more extensive scientific and clinically relevant data on soluble CD30 and other specific biologic indicators, such as soluble interleukin-2 receptor (CD25) (135,138,278,280–282) and other cytokines (135–138,283,284), some of which may eventually provide the objective scientific factors needed to predict outcome more accurately for patients with advanced-stage Hodgkin's disease.

TABLE 4. *Prognostic factors in advanced disease*

Age
Sex
Histology
Stage IV disease
Tumor burden
Inguinal involvement
Very large mediastinal mass
B symptoms
Anemia
Serum albumin
Erythrocyte sedimentation rate
Serum alkaline phosphatase
Leukocytosis
Lymphocytopenia
Serum lactic dehydrogenase
Serum β_2-microglobulin

Prognostic Indices or Scores in Advanced Hodgkin's Disease

Prognostic indices or scores for advanced Hodgkin's disease may be clinically important, both for selecting patients who may be overtreated and, in particular, for identifying patients in whom standard treatment is likely to fail to eliminate disease and who may be appropriate candidates for experimental approaches.

Several groups developed prognostic indices or scores based on a few hundred cases and defined high-risk groups. Wagstaff et al. (232,285) defined risk groups based on age above 45 years, male sex, absolute lymphocyte count below 0.75×10^9/L, and stage IV disease. Straus et al. (231) proposed a five-factor score: age above 45 years, elevated serum lactic dehydrogenase, low

TABLE 5. *Adverse prognostic factors incorporated in the International Prognostic Factors Project score for freedom progression in advanced Hodgkin's disease*

Age ≥45 years
Male sex
Stage IV disease
Hemoglobin <10.5 g/dL
Serum albumin <4.0 g/dL
Leukocytosis ≥15 × 10^9/L
Lymphocytopenia <0.6 × 10^9/L or <8% of white blood cell count

hematocrit, inguinal involvement, and a mediastinal mass larger than 0.45 of the thoracic aperture. Proctor et al. (227,258) developed a numeric index to predict overall survival based on age, stage, hemoglobin level, absolute lymphocyte count, and tumor bulk (>10 cm). Gobbi et al. (31,286) set up a predictive equation based on age, sex, stage, histology, B symptoms, mediastinal mass, ESR, hemoglobin, and serum albumin.

However, none of these indices has received general acceptance. The first three of these models and the inclusion criteria used in an ongoing European Bone Marrow Transplant Group study in high-risk advanced Hodgkin's disease (287) have been compared by Fermé et al. (233). All prognostic models were reproduced, but none of the models was successful in identifying a high-risk group with a 3-year survival rate of less than 50%.

Gobbi et al. in 1994 (236) developed a parametric model to derive numeric estimates of expected survival in all stages. Seven factors were incorporated: stage, age, histology, B symptoms, serum albumin, sex, and distribution of involved areas (infradiaphragmatic disease or more than three supradiaphragmatic areas). This work was based on 5,023 patients in both early and advanced stages from the International Database on Hodgkin's Disease (33). They were treated rather heterogeneously with radiotherapy alone or mainly MOPP-type chemotherapy with or without radiotherapy. All these models used overall survival as the main end point.

The International Prognostic Factors Project on advanced Hodgkin's disease (220) was organized to develop a prognostic score to predict treatment outcome in patients with advanced-stage Hodgkin's disease treated with modern combination chemotherapy with or without radiotherapy. To focus on the effects of the first-line treatment only, the major end point was freedom from progression; deaths in remission not preceded by progression of Hodgkin's disease were censored. Data were collected from 23 centers or study groups on 5,141 patients in whom advanced-stage Hodgkin's disease had been diagnosed and who had been treated with chemotherapy with and without radiotherapy according to a defined protocol. Individual patient data on course of disease and 19 generally documented clinical features at diagnosis were collected. A prognostic score was developed from this set of data in patients up to 65 years of age. The score incorporates seven binary adverse prognostic factors (summarized in Table 5) of approximately similar prognostic impact: age of 45 years of more, male sex, stage IV disease, albumin level below 4.0 g/dL, hemoglobin level below 10.5 g/dL, leukocytosis (leukocyte count >15 x 10^9/L), and lymphocytopenia (lymphocyte count <0.6 x 10^9/L, or <8% of leukocytes, or both). The prognostic score predicts expected 5-year rates of tumor control in the range of 45% to 80%. Each additional factor reduces the prognosis by about 8%. Figure 10 shows freedom from progression according to the

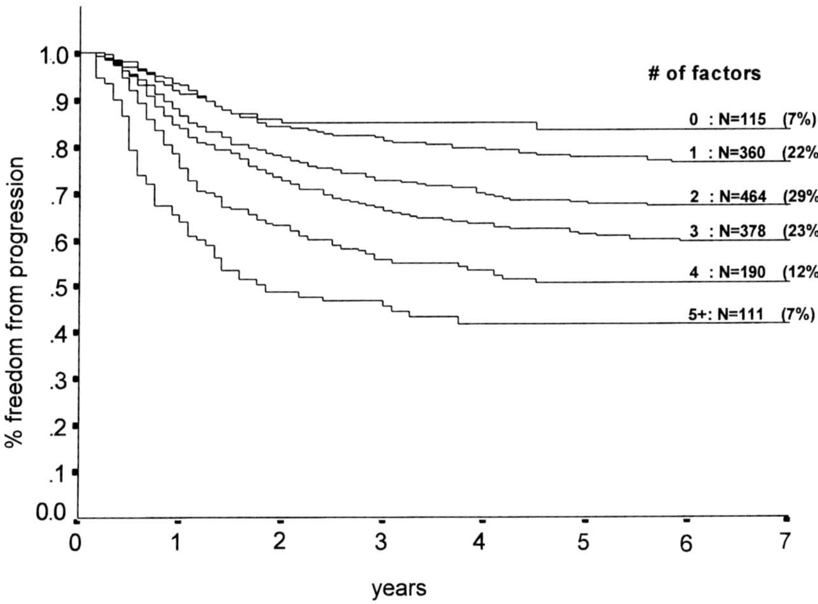

FIG. 10. Freedom from progression according to the number of adverse prognostic factors (see Table 5) for 1,618 patients with advanced disease in the International Prognostic Factors Project.

number of adverse prognostic factors for 1,618 patients with advanced disease in the International Prognostic Factors Project.

This international prognostic score was developed from the combined experience of most major study groups from the 1980s in treating advanced Hodgkin's disease mainly with doxorubicin-containing regimens. Until markers that are biologically more specific become available, the score may be useful in the design of future therapeutic trials in patients with advanced Hodgkin's disease, in the description of patient populations, and in tailoring treatment to individual patients. However, no distinct very high-risk group in advanced Hodgkin's disease can be defined in advance by routinely documented clinical features. This is particularly important to note in the context of early high-dose chemotherapy with autologous stem cell support, typically considered for consolidation in responding patients (259,270,287–290) who nevertheless remain at high risk for relapse. It should be highlighted (291,292) that the rates of tumor control at 5 years in the selected group of patients achieving a complete remission are even higher than those in all patients: 73 ± 2%, 70 ± 2%, and 65 ± 4% in the groups with at least two, at least three, and at least four adverse factors, respectively. Thus, nearly two-thirds of these patients are already cured with conventional treatment.

PROGNOSTIC FACTORS FOR OUTCOME AFTER RELAPSE

Relapses of Hodgkin's disease after radiotherapy alone are qualitatively different from relapses after chemotherapy alone or combined-modality therapy. Both freedom from second relapse and overall survival are considerably better for patients relapsing after radiotherapy alone than for the others (63,293).

Patients Relapsing after Initial Treatment with Radiotherapy Alone

About 30% of early-stage patients treated with radiotherapy alone relapse. However, most of these patients can be successfully salvaged with chemotherapy, and durable remissions are achieved in about 60% of cases (293–304).

The extent of disease at relapse has consistently been shown to be important for prognosis. In studies in which systematic restaging at relapse was carried out, relapse stage was independently significant for achievement of second complete remission (293,301), freedom from second relapse (302), and overall survival after relapse (301). Relapse site (nodal only vs. extranodal with or without nodal relapse) is highly correlated with relapse stage (293). Hence, in studies in which systematic restaging at relapse was not carried out, the importance of extent of disease at relapse was reflected in the adverse prognostic influence of extranodal relapse for achievement of second complete remission (300), freedom from second progression (305), cause-specific survival after relapse (303,304), and overall survival after relapse (295,303,304). Figure 11 shows cause-specific survival after first relapse according to type of relapse for 448 patients in the International Database on Hodgkin's Disease staged initially with laparotomy and relapsing after

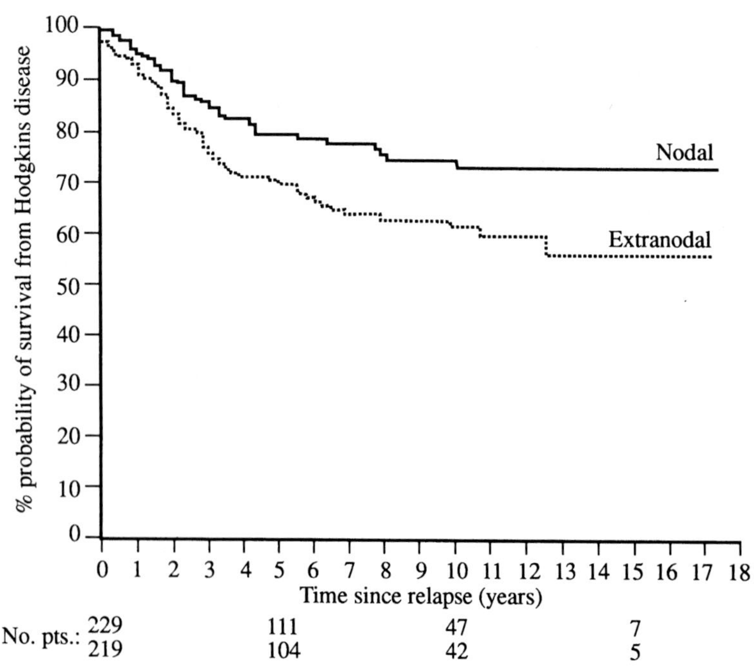

FIG. 11. Cause-specific survival from Hodgkin's disease after first relapse according to type of relapse for 448 patients in the International Database on Hodgkin's Disease who were initially staged with laparotomy and treated with irradiation alone. (From ref. 303, with permission from Elsevier Science.)

initial treatment with irradiation alone. In early studies, initial stage was important for prognosis (297,305) and a more advanced initial stage was shown to be correlated with increased risk for extranodal relapse (305). However, the prognostic significance of initial stage was not found in later studies, probably because they included fewer patients with advanced disease at presentation.

In contrast to the findings at initial treatment (*vide supra*), the histologic subtype has in many studies been found to be independently significant for achievement of second complete remission (293,299,301), freedom from second relapse (293), cause-specific survival after relapse (303,304), and overall survival after relapse (293,295,303).

Age, which had only a small effect on results of initial treatment (*vide supra*), has consistently been shown to be independently significant for prognosis after relapse, the efficacy of salvage chemotherapy being much lower in older patients (175). Older age is an independent adverse prognostic factor for achievement of second complete remission (298), freedom from second relapse (298,299,302), cause-specific survival after relapse (177,303,304), and overall survival after relapse (177,293,298,299,303,304). Whether this finding reflects a true biologic difference in the behavior of Hodgkin's disease between age groups is uncertain. It is quite possible that a significant part of the difference should be ascribed to suboptimal staging and treatment at relapse for some older patients (177). Figure 12 shows cause-specific survival after first relapse according to age (at initial treatment) for 681 patients in the International Database on Hodgkin's Disease staged initially with laparotomy and relapsing after initial treatment with irradiation alone.

The length of the initial disease-free interval has been shown in many studies not to influence prognosis after relapse, the prognosis being equally good whether relapse occurs within a year of initial radiotherapy or after many years (293,296,298,300,302–306). This is in stark contrast to the findings in patients relapsing after chemotherapy or combined-modality therapy (*vide infra*).

The prognostic factors known to be independently significant for outcome after relapse after primary treatment with radiotherapy alone are summarized in the first part of Table 6.

Patients Relapsing after Initial Treatment with Chemotherapy Alone or Combined-modality Therapy

Patients relapsing after treatment with chemotherapy or combined-modality therapy, whether for early-stage or advanced disease, have a much poorer prognosis than patients relapsing after radiotherapy alone. With second-line chemotherapy, durable remissions are obtained in only 10% to 30% of cases (190,221,293,307–329).

By far the most important prognostic factor for outcome after relapse in these patients has consistently been shown to be the extent and durability of the initial remission, irrespective of the specific initial or second-line treatment used. Patients relapsing from complete remission after more than 12 months have a much better

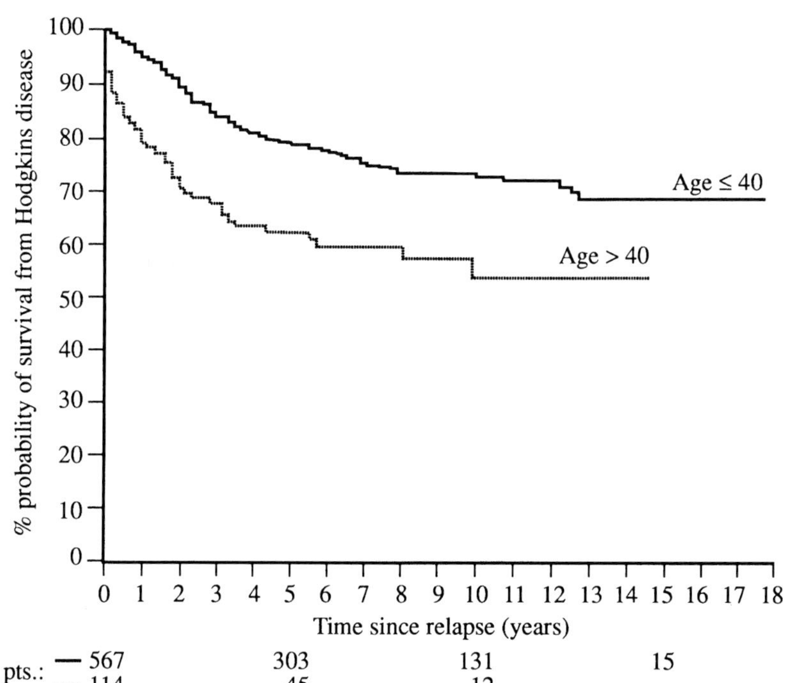

FIG. 12. Cause-specific survival from Hodgkin's disease after first relapse according to age (at initial treatment) for 681 patients in the International Database on Hodgkin's Disease who were initially staged with laparotomy and treated with irradiation alone. (From ref. 303, with permission from Elsevier Science.)

TABLE 6. *Prognostic factors shown to be independently significant for outcome after relapse*

Relapse after radiotherapy alone
Relapse stage
Extranodal relapse
Histology
Age
Relapse after chemotherapy or combined-modality therapy
Extent and duration of first remission
Relapse stage
Extranodal relapse
Number of involved sites at relapse
B symptoms at relapse
Histology
Stage IV disease at original presentation
Age
Performance status

chance of achieving a durable complete remission with second-line treatment than patients whose first remission period is less than 12 months (308,312,317–320,322, 324,328). Figure 13 shows overall survival curves from the date of relapse according to duration of initial remission for 107 patients from the National Cancer Institute relapsing after initial treatment with chemotherapy or combined-modality therapy. Patients who do not achieve complete remission even during primary treatment have the worst prognosis of all, rarely achieving durable complete remission with second-line treatment (311,312, 318,321,322,327). As would be expected, patients relapsing more than once have a dismal prognosis (323–326).

The extent of disease at relapse has also been shown to influence prognosis after relapse from chemotherapy or combined-modality therapy. Patients with advanced stage (III or IV) at relapse (320), with extranodal disease at relapse (310,322,324,326,328,329), or with more than three involved sites (328) have a significantly poorer prognosis than patients without these adverse factors. The presence of B symptoms at relapse has likewise proved significant (310,312,317,319,322,328). Histologic subtype other than nodular sclerosis (328,329), stage IV disease at original presentation (317), older age (318), and poor performance status (321) have also been shown to be associated with a poorer prognosis.

The prognostic factors known to be independently significant for outcome after relapse following primary treatment with chemotherapy or combined-modality therapy are summarized in the second part of Table 6.

A subgroup of patients relapsing after chemotherapy have anatomically limited relapse in nodal sites alone. A number of small series have shown that for selected patients in this subgroup, wide-field radiotherapy with or without additional chemotherapy offers a reasonable chance of durable disease control (317,330–340). Prognostic factor analyses in some of the larger series indicate that patients suitable for this kind of relapse treatment are those relapsing exclusively in supradiaphragmatic nodal sites, with no B symptoms at relapse, with favorable histology (lymphocyte predominance or nodular sclerosis), and after a disease-free interval of more than 12 months (334,339,340). Patients with these favorable characteristics may expect to achieve durable remission with radiotherapy in about 50% of cases.

Patients Undergoing High-dose Chemotherapy and Stem Cell Transplantation for Relapsed or Refractory Disease

High-dose chemotherapy with stem cell transplantion with or without additional radiotherapy seems to im-

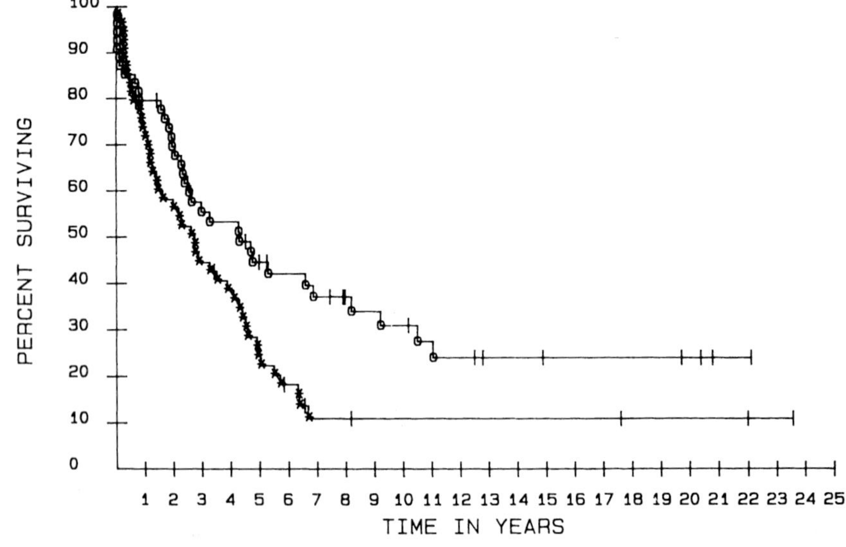

FIG. 13. Overall survival from the date of relapse for 107 patients from the National Cancer Institute relapsing after initial treatment with chemotherapy or combined-modality therapy. Patients are divided according to length of the initial remission (*upper curve*, >1 year; *lower curve*, <1 year). (From ref. 318, with permission.)

prove the prognosis for patients failing after chemotherapy or combined-modality therapy. However, randomized evidence supporting this notion is at present sparse (341), and results of phase II studies are difficult to interpret because of differences in patient selection in the various studies. Analyses of prognostic factors in several published series have demonstrated a number of independent factors affecting outcome of high-dose chemotherapy.

The chemosensitivity of the disease is a critical determinant of outcome. The response to initial therapy (342, 343), duration of initial remission (344,345), number of prior failed regimens (346–352), and response to conventional salvage therapy before transplant (347,348, 52–354) have all been shown to influence prognosis.

Disease burden before transplantation has also been shown to be important for prognosis. Stage of disease at transplantation (348), bulky disease at transplantation (348,350,355,356), extranodal relapse (344,348,351), pleural involvement or multiple pulmonary nodules at relapse (354), B symptoms at relapse (344), and an elevated serum lactic dehydrogenase level before transplantation (357) have all been shown to be prognostically important, reflecting directly or indirectly the tumor burden at the time of transplantation. As would be expected with intensive treatment, a poor performance status has proved to be an important adverse prognostic factor (346,348,349,357,358). A single study found that female patients had a significantly poorer prognosis (350). Older patients have only rarely been treated with high-dose chemotherapy and stem cell transplantation, so that the prognostic significance of older age has not been examined. Pediatric patients, however, have the same outcome as their adult counterparts (359).

The prognostic factors known to be independently significant for outcome after high-dose chemotherapy and stem cell transplantation are summarized in Table 7.

TABLE 7. *Prognostic factors shown to be independently significant for outcome after high-dose chemotherapy and stem cell transplantation*

Chemosensitivity of the disease
Response to initial therapy
Duration of initial remission
Number of prior failed regimens
Response to conventional salvage therapy
Disease burden before transplantation
Stage of disease at transplantation
Bulky disease at transplantation
Extranodal relapse
Pleural involvement or multiple pulmonary nodules at relapse
B symptoms at relapse
Elevated serum lactic dehydrogenase level at transplantation
Performance status

USE OF PROGNOSTIC FACTORS IN CLINICAL TRIALS

Rationale for Use of Prognostic Factors as Entry and Stratification Criteria

In the context of clinical trials, prognostic factors are used for three purposes: in the definition of the study population (entry and exclusion criteria), in *a priori* stratification of the study population to balance randomization within prognostic subgroups, and to describe the actual study population and adjust the analysis according to prognostic factors.

Entry and exclusion criteria are tailored specifically to a given trial. They select a study population in which the main question under study is open and in which the therapeutic difference may be expected to be clearly demonstrable if it exists and is clinically relevant.

Knowledge of prognostic factors plays a key, but not exclusive, role in the formulation of entry criteria. Ethically, only those patients may be included for whom the risks and benefits of the treatment arms are sufficiently uncertain to justify randomization. Biometrically, except in equivalence trials, patients should be excluded in whom the difference is probably negligible. On the other hand, enough cases must be retained for a meaningful trial with sufficient statistical power, and consequently entry criteria should not be overly selective so as not to preclude a result that can be generalized.

There is some debate on the adequate degree of formalization and selectivity of entry criteria (360). Some propose strictly formalized criteria designed to select a prognostically homogeneous study population because variance in the study population decreases the statistical power of the trial. Others advocate relaxation of eligibility criteria to maximize accrual and not preclude extrapolation from trial results.

In Hodgkin's disease, as in most other tumors, patient heterogeneity is pronounced and the known prognostic factors account for only a relatively small part of it. The results of a reasonably focused and powered trial may be expected not to depend markedly on a precise definition of the inclusion criteria. The treatment effect may quantitatively vary by subgroup and may be reduced or increased at the extremes of the prognostic distribution in the study population. However, the main effect will typically have the same direction in all subgroups except in rare situations (with competing risks, such as toxicity vs. treatment effectiveness). Thus, the trial outcome will typically not depend on minor variations of the eligibility criteria (361).

The decision to enter a patient in a trial eventually lies with the responsible local physician. The physician will and should decide the borderline cases that inevitably emerge. Uncontrolled selection processes at the extremes of the prognostic distribution are difficult to prevent unless a strictly consecutive entry of all qualifying patients is enforced. This is practically impossible in multicenter settings and conflicts with the imperative of informed consent.

Therefore, a certain arbitrariness in the selection of the study population is unavoidable; however, in reasonably powered trials this will not materially alter results. Nevertheless, at least in large multicenter trials with possibly less experienced participants, the decision to enter a patient in a trial should be guided by clear eligibility criteria summarizing the expert opinion of those responsible for the trial with regard to the study population in which the study question is relevant.

Randomization is the method of choice to achieve comparability in the prognostic composition of the treatment groups to be compared in a clinical trial (362,363). Proper randomization avoids not only imbalances in known prognostic factors (for which one can adjust the analysis to a certain degree by using statistical modeling) but also imbalances that are not detectable concerning unknown factors.

Randomization techniques generally work well with large numbers of patients. In small randomized trials, some imbalances by chance may occur. Stratified randomization is randomization particularly designed to balance treatment allocation within predefined subgroups. Stratification may be indicated if the study population consists of clearly different prognostic groups that are definable *a priori* by well-established prognostic factors. As it is possible to adjust the analysis statistically for moderate imbalances in known prognostic factors, stratification should be restricted to markedly different subgroups. The number of strata should remain small, as overstratification may compromise the main task of randomization, which is to balance unknown or undocumented factors.

Prognostic factors serve to describe the composition of a study population. In addition, they play a role in the final analysis. The estimate of the treatment effect in a trial may be biased and the statistical power reduced if important known or unknown prognostic factors are not accounted for (364). Thus, a trial analysis should comprise both a simple univariate test for treatment effect and one based on multivariate modeling. The trial results will be most convincing if both analyses approximately agree.

Combinations of Prognostic Factors Currently Used by Major Trial Groups

Inclusion criteria that are currently used differ by trial and study group. This is not surprising; prognosis varies on a continuum from low-risk, minimal disease to high-risk, maximally advanced disease. The population of patients with Hodgkin's disease thus does not fall into naturally defined groups that differ in prognosis and clearly require different treatment approaches. The delineation of study populations depends on prognosis, the respective therapeutic challenge, and study history. Any sharp borderline is artificial to a certain degree. Nevertheless, certain clusters of comparable selection criteria have emerged.

The classic Ann Arbor (26) or Cotswolds (41) staging systems are based on the anatomic distribution of disease. Stage correlates reasonably with prognosis, although combinations of prognostic factors in which additional information is used show better correlation. The Ann Arbor staging system is well established and universally accepted and still forms the reference system for most definitions of study entry criteria. However, most study groups currently use hybrid systems to define their study entry criteria, basically using stage and also the presence or absence of unfavorable prognostic factors (also called risk factors in this context). Prognosis of stage groups overlaps considerably; for example, a stage IIB patient with additional risk factors may have a worse prognosis than a limited IIIA patient.

Entry criteria are tailored to study questions. Combinations of prognostic factors to define entry criteria may therefore be grouped by study aims and the composition of the menu of therapeutic options. Most study groups have at least one trial in early stages and one in advanced stages. Tables 8 and 9 describe inclusion criteria currently or recently used by study groups for early-stage and advanced disease, respectively. Table 10 attempts to describe and systematize the current practice. Entry criteria may change in the future with more widespread use of prognostic scores or indices to select study populations, in particular in studies of advanced disease, as discussed below.

In early stages, patients are included from the favorable end of the prognostic distribution, in which full systemic treatment is considered overtreatment. As the prognosis in this group is excellent, study questions focus on how to cure with minimal toxicity or cost. Treatment options comprise radiotherapy alone, or reduced or less toxic chemotherapy with or without radiotherapy. Table 8 illustrates that early stages are typically defined as stage I or II without risk factors, with lists of unfavorable prognostic factors that vary by study group and have been derived mainly from radiotherapy-alone relapse data.

In addition, some groups single out for minimal treatment a small group within early stages who have minimal disease. The EORTC (365) entered a small, "very favorable" group of patients without risk factors and with a very low probability of infradiaphragmatic disease (CS IA, female sex, age under 40 years, with lymphocyte predominance or nodular sclerosis histologic subtype) in a trial of mantle-field radiotherapy alone ("minimal disease"). The British National Lymphoma Investigation (366) treated CSIA–IIA patients with lymphocyte predominance subtype, nodular sclerosis grade 1 subtype, and ESR below 10 mm/h or CS IA high cervical involvement with involved-field radiotherapy only.

TABLE 8. *Eligibility criteria of recent or current studies of early-stage disease (typically defined as stage I or II and absence of certain unfavorable prognostic factors)*

Study group	Criteria for early-stage versus intermediate-stage/advanced disease Early stage = stage I or II without any of the listed risk factors
EORTC [H_7 study (365), H_8 study]	Age >50 y 4+ involved nodal sites ESR >50 mm/h, or B symptoms and ESR >30 mm/h Bulky mediastinum (mediastinal-thoracic ratio ≥0.35) (Infradiaphragmatic disease)
BNLI (366)	Lymphocyte depletion, mixed cellularity, nodular sclerosis II, and ESR ≥60 mm/h
Manchester Lymphoma Group 1989	B symptoms Mediastinal bulk
GHSG (HD_7 study)	Large mediastinal mass (>1/3 of the thoracic aperture) Massive spleen involvement E lesions ESR >50 mm/h, or B symptoms and ESR >30 mm/h 3+ involved lymph nodal areas
Milano 1990	Stage II B symptoms Bulk
SWOG (9133 study) and CALGB (9391 study)	B symptoms Mediastinal mass ≥1/3 maximum thoracic diameter Infradiaphragmatic presentation
NCI-C (HD-6)/ECOG (IHD06)	B symptoms Mixed cellularity or lymphocyte depletion Age >40 y ESR >50 mm/h 4+ disease sites
Stanford [G_1 study (369)]	B symptoms (except night sweats only) Mediastinal mass >1/3 of maximum intrathoracic diameter 2+ E lesions

ESR, erythrocyte sedimentation rate; EORTC: European Organization for Research and Treatment of Cancer; BNLI, British National Lymphoma Group; GHSG, German Hodgkin Study Group; SWOG, Southwest Oncology Group; CALGB, Cancer and Leukemia Group B; NCI-C, National Cancer Institute of Canada; ECOG, Eastern Cooperative Oncology Group.

TABLE 9. *Eligibility criteria of recent or current studies of advanced disease*

Study group	Eligibility criteria for trials in advanced disease
EORTC [H_{34} study (370)]	III–IV
BNLI [PA(BI)OE study]	All with chemotherapy indication (i.e., IA–IIA "poor prognosis," IB–IIB, III, IV)
Manchester Lymphoma Group (VAPEC-B study)	I–II with B symptoms or bulk, III, IV
GHSG (HD_9 study)	IIB with bulk, massive spleen, or E lesion PS IIIA S PS IIIA N with bulk, E lesion, or elevated ESR CS IIIA with bulk, massive spleen, E lesions, elevated ESR or ≥3 lymph node areas IIIB–IV
Milano [MAMA study (371)]	IB, IIA bulk, IIB, III, IV
GELA [H_{89} study (233)]	IIIB, IV
NCI-US (372)	III, IV
SWOG (373)	III, IV
CALGB (221)	IIIA2, IIIB, IV
CALGB (8952 study) and SWOG (8952 study) and ECOG (5489 study) and NCI-C (HD_5 study)	III–IV + recurrent Hodgkin's disease after radiotherapy
Stanford (374)	IIB with mediastinal bulk, III, IV

PS, pathologic stage; CS, clinical stage; ESR, erythrocyte sedimentation rate; EORTC, European Organization for Research and Treatment of Cancer; BNLI, British National Lymphoma Group; GHSG, German Hodgkin Study Group; GELA, Groupe d'Etudes des Lymphomes de l'Adulte; NCI-US, National Cancer Institute of the United States; SWOG, Southwest Oncology Group; CALGB, Cancer and Leukemia Group B; ECOG, Eastern Cooperative Oncology Group; NCI-C, National Cancer Institute of Canada.

TABLE 10. *An attempt to describe and systematize current eligibility criteria (see text)*

	Typical form of entry criteria, prognostic composition	Typical study aims	Main therapeutic options
Early stage	Stages I and II without RF	Cure with minimal toxicity	Radiotherapy alone Reduced or "less toxic" chemotherapy with or without localized radiotherapy
Intermediate stage: separate study or (partially) included in early or advanced disease	± Stages I and II with RF ± Stage IIIA without RF ± Stage II with multiple RF ± Stage IIIA with RF	Overlap of aims	Overlap of treatment options
Advanced disease	IIIB–IV lower risk IIIB–IV higher risk	Improve unsatisfactory results	Full systemic treatment with or without radiotherapy required

RF, risk factors.

Studies of advanced stage include patients from the unfavorable end of the prognostic scale for whom full systemic treatment appears to be required. As the prognosis in this group is less than satisfactory, trials focus on improving results. Most study groups have patients with stage IIIB–IV as the core group for advanced disease (Table 9). Studies differ in whether they include all stage IIIA patients, none, or only selected stage IIIA patients with unfavorable prognostic factors. Some groups also include stages I and II patients with systemic risk factors.

An ongoing European Bone Marrow Transplant Group Trial (287) of the role of early high-dose therapy with autologous stem cell transplant attempts to select a higher-risk advanced-stage study population. It includes advanced-stage patients with two or more of the following factors: large mediastinal mass (>0.45 of the maximum chest diameter), bone marrow involvement, stage IV disease with more than one extranodal site, inguinal involvement, high serum levels of lactic dehydrogenase, and low hematocrit.

Stages I and II with risk factors and stage IIIA form what may be called "intermediate" stages. In these patients, the prognosis is neither excellent nor unsatisfactory. Study aims and treatment modalities therefore overlap. Study groups either have a separate trial for intermediate-stage patients or split this group, including part of it in early-stage or advanced-stage trials depending on available accrual and the particular question under study. Intermediate stage thus essentially denotes a gray zone between early and advanced disease.

Two groups [The Scotland and Newcastle Lymphoma Group (258) and Grupo Argentino de Tratamiento de la Leucemia Aguda (367)] have abandoned what was referred to above as the stage hybrid system and currently use prognostic indices or scores that cover the whole range of Hodgkin's disease to define trial entry criteria. In these approaches, stage has become one factor among others and has ceased to be the backbone of the system. Indeed, if predicting outcome is the only task, stage information is not privileged, and the best available predictor, possibly numeric, should be used. On the other hand, entry criteria do not depend on prognosis only. Stage codes the anatomic distribution of disease and may thus be particularly important to define the applicability of radiotherapy. If group-specific prognostic indices are used, intergroup comparability may be compromised. As stage is well established, at least a population description in terms of stage with and without risk factors should be provided.

The Scotland and Newcastle Lymphoma Group has challenged the classic staging system, pointing out that with their prognostic index, 10% of stage I–IIIA, 20% of stage IIB, 37% of stage IIIB, and 46% of stage IV patients belong to the high-risk category (368). Thus, the majority of stage IIIB–IV patients are predicted to do well with standard chemotherapy. The International Prognostic Factor Project (220) confirmed that prognosis within stage IIIB–IV is not homogeneous: 34%, 50%, and 81% of patients in stages IIIB, IVA, and IVB, respectively, have three or more adverse prognostic factors and may therefore be expected to demonstrate about 55% tumor control at 5 years, as opposed to 74% tumor control in patients with up to two factors. Thus, prognostic factors now make it possible to split advanced-stage patients in a lower- and a higher-risk group. Trials with aggressive experimental treatment might be restricted to the higher-risk advanced disease group. This decision depends on practical considerations, on complex toxicity-benefit trade-offs, and, in particular, on whether 74% tumor control at 5 years is considered satisfactory.

CONCLUSION AND FUTURE ASPECTS

As demonstrated in this chapter, a large number of variables have been shown to possess prognostic significance in Hodgkin's disease. Many of these factors appear to be more or less directly correlated with the total tumor mass. In current clinical practice, the move is toward tailoring treatment according to prognostic factors, decreasing treatment intensity for patients with favorable prognostic factors to reduce toxicity, and increasing treatment intensity for patients with unfavorable prognostic factors to increase the chance of cure.

In the absence of a general consensus on which factors or combinations of factors should be employed, different centers and groups worldwide currently use varying combinations of factors when allocating patients to different treatments and clinical trials. This makes it increasingly difficult to undertake large-scale analyses and comparisons between different patient series. A general consensus on which prognostic factors should be employed in clinical research and in the treatment of Hodgkin's disease in the future would be highly valuable.

REFERENCES

1. Reed DM. On the pathological changes in Hodgkin's disease, with especial reference to its relation to tuberculosis. *Johns Hopkins Hosp Rep* 1902;10:133.
2. Peters MV. The need for a new clinical classification in Hodgkin's disease: keynote address. *Cancer Res* 1971;31:1713.
3. Craft CB. Results with roentgen ray therapy in Hodgkin's disease. *Bull Staff Meet Univ Minnesota Hosp* 1940;11:391.
4. Sahyoun PF, Eisenberg SJ. Hodgkin's disease. A histopathological and clinical classification with radiotherapeutic response. *Am J Roentgenol* 1949;61:369.
5. Greco RS, Acheson RM, Foot FM. Hodgkin's disease in Connecticut from 1935 to 1962. *Arch Intern Med* 1974;134:1039.
6. Banfi A, Bonadonna G, Buraggi G, et al. Proposta di classificazione e terapia della malattia di Hodgkin. *Tumori* 1965;51:97.
7. Easson EC. Possibilities for the cure of Hodgkin's disease. *Cancer* 1966;19:345.
8. Easson EC, Russell MH. The cure of Hodgkin's disease. *Br Med J* 1963;1:1704.
9. Hilton G, Sutton PM. Malignant lymphomas: classification, prognosis, and treatment. *Lancet* 1962;1:283.
10. Hohl K, Sarasin P, Bessler W. Therapie und prognose der lymphogranulomatose Zürcher erfahrungen von 1922–1950. *Oncologia* 1951;4:1.
11. Jelliffe AM, Thomson AD. The prognosis in Hodgkin's disease. *Br J Cancer* 1955;9:21.
12. Kaplan HS. Long-term results of palliative and radical radiotherapy of Hodgkin's disease. *Cancer Res* 1966;26:1250.
13. Kaplan HS. *On the natural history, treatment, and prognosis of Hodgkin's disease*. Harvey Lectures 1968–1969. New York: Academic Press, 1970:215.
14. Kaplan HS, Bagshaw MA, Rosenberg SA. Présentation du protocole d'essai radiotherapique des lymphomes malins de l'université de Stanford. *Nouv Rev Fr Hematol* 1964;4:95.
15. Longcope WT, McAlpin KR. Hodgkin's disease. In: Christian HA, ed. *The Oxford medicine*. New York: Oxford University Press, 1920:1.
16. Meighan SS, Ramsay JD. Survival in Hodgkin's disease. *Br J Cancer* 1963;17:24.
17. Musshoff K, Boutis L. Therapy results in Hodgkin's disease Freiburg i.Br., 1948–1966. *Cancer* 1968;21:1100.
18. Musshoff K, Stamm H, Lummel G, Gössel K. Zur prognose der lymphogranulomatose. Klinisches bild und strahlentherapie. Freiburger Krankengut 1938–1958. In: Keiderling W, ed. *Beiträge zur Inneren Medizin*. Stuttgart: FK Schattauer-Verlag, 1964:549.
19. Peters MV. A study of survivals in Hodgkin's disease treated radiologically. *Am J Roentgenol* 1950;63:299.
20. Peters MV, Hasselback R, Brown TC. The natural history of the lymphomas related to the clinical classification. In: Zarafonetis CJD, ed. *Proceedings of the International Conference on Leukemia-Lymphoma*. Philadelphia: Lea & Febiger, 1968:357.
21. Peters MV, Middlemiss KCH. A study of Hodgkin's disease treated by irradiation. *Am J Roentgenol* 1958;79:114.
22. Rosenberg SA. Report of the Committee on the Staging of Hodgkin's Disease. *Cancer Res* 1966;26:1310.
23. Rosenberg SA, Kaplan HS. Hodgkin's disease and other malignant lymphomas. *Calif Med* 1970;113:23.
24. Westling P. Studies of the prognosis in Hodgkin's disease. *Acta Radiol* 1965;245(Suppl):5.
25. Ziegler K. *Die Hodgkinsche Krankheit*. Jena: Gustav Fischer Verlag, 1911.
26. Carbone PP, Kaplan HS, Musshoff K, Smithers DW, Tubiana M. Report of the Committee on Hodgkin's Disease Staging Classification. *Cancer Res* 1971;31:1860.
27. Aisenberg AC, Qazi R. Improved survival in Hodgkin's disease. *Cancer* 1976;37:2423.
28. Björkholm M, Holm G, Mellstedt H, Johansson B, Askergren J, Söderberg G. Prognostic factors in Hodgkin's disease. I. Analysis of histopathology, stage distribution and results of therapy. *Scand J Haematol* 1977;19:487.
29. Davis S, Dahlberg S, Myers MH, Chen A, Steinhorn SC. Hodgkin's disease in the United States: a comparison of patient characteristics and survival in the Centralized Cancer Patient Data System and the Surveillance, Epidemiology, and End Results Program. *J Natl Cancer Inst* 1987;78:471.
30. Fischer P, Franken T. Ein multivariates prognosemodell für den morbus Hodgkin. *Strahlenther* 1984;160:535.
31. Gobbi PG, Cavalli C, Federico M, et al. Hodgkin's disease prognosis: a directly predictive equation. *Lancet* 1988;1:675.
32. Hancock BW, Aitken M, Martin JF, et al. Hodgkin's disease in Sheffield (1971–76) (with computer analysis of variables). *Clin Oncol* 1979;5:283.
33. Henry-Amar M, Aeppli DM, Anderson J, et al. Workshop statistical report. In: Somers R, Henry-Amar M, Meerwaldt JK, Carde P, eds. *Treatment strategy in Hodgkin's disease*. Colloque INSERM no 196. London: INSERM/John Libbey Eurotext, 1990:169.
34. Kaplan HS. Survival and relapse rates in Hodgkin's disease: Stanford experience, 1961–71. *Monogr Natl Cancer Inst* 1973;36:487.
35. Kaplan HS. *Hodgkin's disease*, 2nd ed. Cambridge, MA: Harvard University Press, 1980.
36. Kennedy BJ, Loeb V, Peterson VM, Donegan WL, Natarajan N, Mettlin C. National survey of patterns of care for Hodgkin's disease. *Cancer* 1985;56:2547.
37. Musshoff K, Hartmann C, Niklaus B, Rössner R. Results of therapy in Hodgkin's disease: Freiburg i.Br. 1964–1971. In: Musshoff K, ed. *Diagnosis and therapy of malignant lymphoma*. Berlin: Springer-Verlag, 1974:206.
38. Nordentoft AM, Pedersen-Bjergaard J, Brincker H, et al. Hodgkin's disease in Denmark. *Scand J Haematol* 1980;24:321.
39. Patchefsky AS, Brodovsky H, Southard M, Menduke H, Gray S, Hoch WS. Hodgkin's disease. A clinical and pathologic study of 235 cases. *Cancer* 1973;32:150.
40. Sutcliffe SB, Gospodarowicz MK, Bergsagel DE, et al. Prognostic groups for management of localized Hodgkin's disease. *J Clin Oncol* 1985;3:393.
41. Lister TA, Crowther D, Sutcliffe SB, et al. Report of a committee convened to discuss the evaluation and staging of patients with Hodgkin's disease: Cotswolds meeting. *J Clin Oncol* 1989;7:1630.
42. George SL. Identification and assessment of prognostic factors. *Semin Oncol* 1988;15:462.
43. Byar DP. Identification of prognostic factors. In: Buyse ME, Staquet MJ, Sylvester RJ, eds. *Cancer clinical trials: methods and practice*. Oxford: Oxford University Press, 1984:423.
44. Simon R. Importance of prognostic factors in cancer clinical trials. *Cancer Treat Rep* 1984;68:185.
45. Byar DP. Problems with using observational databases to compare treatments. *Stat Med* 1991;10:663.
46. Burke HB, Henson DE. Criteria for prognostic factors and for an enhanced prognostic system. *Cancer* 1993;72:3131.
47. Specht L. Prognostic factor studies in Hodgkin's disease: problems and pitfalls. *Leukemia* 1993;7:1915.
48. Redmond C, Fisher B, Wieand HS. The methodologic dilemma in retrospectively correlating the amount of chemotherapy received in adjuvant therapy protocols with disease-free survival. *Cancer Treat Rep* 1983;67:519.
49. Altman DG, Lausen B, Sauerbrei W, Schumacher M. Dangers of using "optimal" cutpoints in the evaluation of prognostic factors. *J Natl Cancer Inst* 1994;86:829.

50. Estey E. Prognostic factors in clinical cancer trials. *Clin Cancer Res* 1997;3:2591.
51. Cox DR. Regression models and life tables. *J R Stat Soc B* 1972; 34:187.
52. Harrell FE, Lee KL, Matchar DB, Reichert TA. Regression models for prognostic prediction: advantages, problems, and suggested solutions. *Cancer Treat Rep* 1985;69:1071.
53. Marsoni S, Valsecchi MG. Prognostic factor analysis in clinical oncology: handle with care. *Ann Oncol* 1991;2:245.
54. Vollmer RT. Multivariate statistical analysis for anatomic pathology. Part II: failure time analysis. *Am J Clin Pathol* 1996;106:522.
55. Piro AJ, Hellman S, Moloney WC. The influence of laparotomy on management decisions in Hodgkin's disease. *Arch Intern Med* 1972; 130:844.
56. Kaplan HS, Dorfman RF, Nelsen TS, Rosenberg SA. Staging laparotomy and splenectomy in Hodgkin's disease: analysis of indications and patterns of involvement in 285 consecutive, unselected patients. *Natl Cancer Inst Monogr* 1973;36:291.
57. Høst H, Abrahamsen AF, Jørgensen OG, Normann T. Laparotomy and splenectomy in the management of Hodgkin's disease. *Scand J Haematol* 1973;10:327.
58. Cannon WB, Kaplan HS, Dorfman RF, Nelsen TS. Staging laparotomy with splenectomy in Hodgkin's disease. *Surg Annu* 1975;7:103.
59. British National Lymphoma Investigation. The value of laparotomy and splenectomy in the management of early Hodgkin's disease. *Clin Radiol* 1975;26:151.
60. Rutherford CJ, Desforges JF, Davies B, Barnett AI. The decision to perform staging laparotomy in symptomatic Hodgkin's disease. *Br J Haematol* 1980;44:347.
61. Kinsella TJ, Glatstein E. Staging laparotomy and splenectomy for Hodgkin's disease: current status. *Cancer Invest* 1983;1:87.
62. Rosenberg SA. Exploratory laparotomy and splenectomy for Hodgkin's disease: a commentary. *J Clin Oncol* 1988;6:574.
63. Mauch PM. Controversies in the management of early stage Hodgkin's disease. *Blood* 1994;83:318.
64. Specht L, Gray RG, Clarke MJ, Peto R, for The International Hodgkin's Disease Collaborative Group. The influence of more extensive radiotherapy and adjuvant chemotherapy on long-term outcome of early stage Hodgkin's disease: a meta-analysis of 23 randomized trials involving 3,888 patients. *J Clin Oncol* 1998;16:830.
65. Peckham MJ, Ford HT, McElwain TJ, Harmer CL, Atkinson K, Austin DE. The results of radiotherapy for Hodgkin's disease. *Br J Cancer* 1975;32:391.
66. Horwich A, Easton D, Nogueira-Costa R, Liew KH, Colman M, Peckham MJ. An analysis of prognostic factors in early stage Hodgkin's disease. *Radiother Oncol* 1986;7:95.
67. Verger E, Easton D, Brada M, Duchesne G, Horwich A. Radiotherapy results in laparotomy-staged Hodgkin's disease. *Clin Radiol* 1988;39: 428.
68. Thar TL, Million RR, Hausner RJ, McKetty MHB. Hodgkin's disease, stages I and II. Relationship of recurrence to size of disease, radiation dose, and number of sites involved. *Cancer* 1979;43:1101.
69. Mendenhall NP, Cantor AB, Barré DM, Lynch JW, Million RR. The role of prognostic factors in treatment selection for early-stage Hodgkin's disease. *Am J Clin Oncol* 1994;17:189.
70. Tubiana M, Henry-Amar M, Hayat M, et al. Prognostic significance of the number of involved areas in the early stages of Hodgkin's disease. *Cancer* 1984;54:885.
71. Tubiana M, Henry-Amar M, Hayat M, et al. The EORTC treatment of early stages of Hodgkin's disease: the role of radiotherapy. *Int J Radiat Oncol Biol Phys* 1984;10:197.
72. Lee CKK, Aeppli DM, Bloomfield CD, Levitt S. Hodgkin's disease: a reassessment of prognostic factors following modification of radiotherapy. *Int J Radiat Oncol Biol Phys* 1987;13:983.
73. Lee CKK, Aeppli DM, Bloomfield CD, Levitt SH. Curative radiotherapy for laparotomy-staged IA, IIA, IIIA Hodgkin's disease: an evaluation of the gains achieved with radical radiotherapy. *Int J Radiat Oncol Biol Phys* 1990;19:547.
74. Willett CG, Linggood RM, Meyer J, et al. Results of treatment of stage IA and IIA Hodgkin's disease. *Cancer* 1987;59:1107.
75. Barton M, Boyages J, Crennan E, et al. Radiation therapy for early stage Hodgkin's disease: Australasian patterns of care. *Int J Radiat Oncol Biol Phys* 1995;31:227.
76. Hoppe RT, Coleman CN, Cox RS, Rosenberg SA, Kaplan HS. The management of stage I–II Hodgkin's disease with irradiation alone or combined modality therapy: the Stanford experience. *Blood* 1982;59: 455.
77. Mauch P, Tarbell N, Weinstein H, et al. Stage IA and IIA supradiaphragmatic Hodgkin's disease: prognostic factors in surgically staged patients treated with mantle and paraaortic irradiation. *J Clin Oncol* 1988;6:1576.
78. Specht L, Nordentoft AM, Cold S, Clausen NT, Nissen NI. Tumour burden in early stage Hodgkin's disease: the single most important prognostic factor for outcome after radiotherapy. *Br J Cancer* 1987; 55:535.
79. Specht L, Nordentoft AM, Cold S, Clausen NT, Nissen NI. Tumor burden as the most important prognostic factor in early stage Hodgkin's disease. Relations to other prognostic factors and implications for choice of treatment. *Cancer* 1988;61:1719.
80. Fuller LM, Madoc-Jones H, Hagemeister FB, et al. Further follow-up of results of treatment in 90 laparotomy-negative stage I and II Hodgkin's disease patients: significance of mediastinal and non-mediastinal presentations. *Int J Radiat Oncol Biol Phys* 1980;6:799.
81. Liew KH, Easton D, Horwich A, Barrett A, Peckham MJ. Bulky mediastinal Hodgkin's disease management and prognosis. *Hematol Oncol* 1984;2:45.
82. Nissen NI, Nordentoft AM. Radiotherapy versus combined modality treatment of stage I and II Hodgkin's disease. *Cancer Treat Rep* 1982; 66:799.
83. Zagars G, Rubin P. Laparotomy-staged IA versus IIA Hodgkin's disease. A comparative study with evaluation of prognostic factors for stage IIA disease. *Cancer* 1985;56:864.
84. Mauch P, Goodman R, Hellman S. The significance of mediastinal involvement in early stage Hodgkin's disease. *Cancer* 1978;42:1039.
85. Mazza P, Lauria F, Sciascia R, et al. Prognostic significance of large mediastinal involvement in Hodgkin's disease. *Scand J Haematol* 1983;31:315.
86. Prosnitz LR, Curtis AM, Knowlton AH, Peters LM, Farber LR. Supradiaphragmatic Hodgkin's disease: significance of large mediastinal masses. *Int J Radiat Oncol Biol Phys* 1980;6:809.
87. Lee CKK, Bloomfield CD, Goldman AI, Levitt SH. Prognostic significance of mediastinal involvement in Hodgkin's disease treated with curative radiotherapy. *Cancer* 1980;46:2403.
88. Anderson H, Crowther D, Deakin DP, Ryder WDJ, Radford JA. A randomised study of adjuvant MVPP chemotherapy after mantle radiotherapy in pathologically staged IA–IIB Hodgkin's disease: 10-year follow-up. *Ann Oncol* 1991;2(Suppl 2):49.
89. Dorreen MS, Wrigley PFM, Laidlow JM, et al. The management of stage II supradiaphragmatic Hodgkin's disease at St. Bartholomew's Hospital. *Cancer* 1984;54:2882.
90. Schomberg PJ, Evans RG, O'Connell MJ, et al. Prognostic significance of mediastinal mass in adult Hodgkin's disease. *Cancer* 1984;53:324.
91. Erdkamp FL, Houben MJ, Breed WP, et al. The reliability and value of determining mediastinal involvement and width on chest radiographs in patients with Hodgkin's disease. *Eur J Radiol* 1993;16:143.
92. Velentjas E, Barrett A, McElwain TJ, Peckham MJ. Mediastinal involvement in early-stage Hodgkin's disease. Response to treatment and pattern of relapse. *Eur J Cancer* 1980;16:1065.
93. Willett CG, Linggood RM, Leong JC, et al. Stage IA to IIB mediastinal Hodgkin's disease: three-dimensional volumetric assessment of response to treatment. *J Clin Oncol* 1988;6:819.
94. Mauch P, Gorshein D, Cunningham J, Hellman S. Influence of mediastinal adenopathy on site and frequency of relapse in patients with Hodgkin's disease. *Cancer Treat Rep* 1982;66:809.
95. Crnkovich MJ, Leopold K, Hoppe RT, Mauch PM. Stage I to IIB Hodgkin's disease: the combined experience at Stanford University and the Joint Center for Radiation Therapy. *J Clin Oncol* 1987;5:1041.
96. Leslie NT, Mauch PM, Hellman S. Stage IA to IIB supradiaphragmatic Hodgkin's disease: long-term survival and relapse frequency. *Cancer* 1985;55:2072.
97. North LB, Fuller LM, Hagemeister FB, Rodgers RW, Butler JJ, Shullenberger CC. Importance of initial mediastinal adenopathy in Hodgkin disease. *AJR Am J Roentgenol* 1982;138:229.
98. Tarbell NJ, Thompson L, Mauch P. Thoracic irradiation in Hodgkin's disease: disease control and long-term complications. *Int J Radiat Oncol Biol Phys* 1990;18:275.
99. Mill WB, Lee FA. Prognostic parameters in early stage Hodgkin's disease. *Int J Radiat Oncol Biol Phys* 1982;8:837.

100. Hughes-Davies L, Tarbell NJ, Coleman CN, et al. Stage IA–IIB Hodgkin's disease: management and outcome of extensive thoracic involvement. *Int J Radiat Oncol Biol Phys* 1997;39:361.
101. Hagemeister FB, Fuller LM, Velasquez WS, et al. Stage I and II Hodgkin's disease: involved-field radiotherapy versus extended-field radiotherapy versus involved-field radiotherapy followed by six cycles of MOPP. *Cancer Treat Rep* 1982;66:789.
102. Specht L. Tumour burden as the main indicator of prognosis in Hodgkin's disease. *Eur J Cancer* 1992;28A:1982.
103. Enblad G. Hodgkin's disease in young and elderly patients: clinical and pathological studies. *Ups J Med Sci* 1994;99:1.
104. Anderson H, Deakin DP, Wagstaff J, et al. A randomised study of adjuvant chemotherapy after mantle radiotherapy in supradiaphragmatic Hodgkin's disease PS IA–IIB: a report from the Manchester Lymphoma Group. *Br J Cancer* 1984;49:695.
105. Hoppe RT, Horning SJ, Rosenberg SA. The concept, evolution and preliminary results of the current Stanford clinical trials for Hodgkin's disease. *Cancer Surv* 1985;4:459.
106. Krikorian JG, Portlock CS, Rosenberg SA, Kaplan HS. Hodgkin's disease, stages I and II occurring below the diaphragm. *Cancer* 1979;43:1866.
107. Barrett A, Gregor A, McElwain TJ, Peckham MJ. Infradiaphragmatic presentation of Hodgkin's disease. *Clin Radiol* 1981;32:221.
108. Cionini L, Magrini S, Mungai V, Biti GP, Ponticelli P. Stage I and II Hodgkin's disease presenting in infradiaphragmatic nodes. *Tumori* 1982;68:519.
109. Mauch P, Greenberg H, Lewin A, Cassady JR, Weichselbaum R, Hellman S. Prognostic factors in patients with subdiaphragmatic Hodgkin's disease. *Hematol Oncol* 1983;1:205.
110. Dorreen MS, Wrigley PFM, Jones AE, Shand WS, Stansfeld AG, Lister TA. The management of localized infradiaphragmatic Hodgkin's disease: experience of a rare clinical presentation at St. Bartholomew's Hospital. *Hematol Oncol* 1984;2:349.
111. Krikorian JG, Portlock CS, Mauch PM. Hodgkin's disease presenting below the diaphragm: a review. *J Clin Oncol* 1986;4:1551.
112. Leibenhaut MH, Hoppe RT, Varghese A, Rosenberg SA. Subdiaphragmatic Hodgkin's disease: laparotomy and treatment results in 49 patients. *J Clin Oncol* 1987;5:1050.
113. Specht L, Nissen NI. Hodgkin's disease stages I and II with infradiaphragmatic presentation: a rare and prognostically unfavourable combination. *Eur J Haematol* 1988;40:396.
114. Frassica DA, Schomberg PJ, Banks PM, Colgan JP, Ilstrup DM, Earle JD. Management of subdiaphragmatic early-stage Hodgkin's disease. *Int J Radiat Oncol Biol Phys* 1989;16:1459.
115. Givens SS, Fuller LM, Hagemeister FB, Gehan EA. Treatment of lower torso stages I and II Hodgkin's disease with radiation with or without adjuvant mechlorethamine, vincristine, procarbazine, and prednisone. *Cancer* 1990;66:69.
116. Mai DH-W, Peschel RE, Portlock C, Knowlton A, Farber L. Stage I and II subdiaphragmatic Hodgkin's disease. *Cancer* 1991;68:1476.
117. Roos DE, O'Brien PC, Wright J, Willson K. Treatment of subdiaphragmatic Hodgkin's disease: is radiotherapy alone appropriate only for inguino-femoral presentations? *Int J Radiat Oncol Biol Phys* 1994;28:683.
118. Enrici RM, Osti MF, Anselmo AP, et al. Hodgkin's disease stage I and II with exclusive subdiaphragmatic presentation. The experience of the departments of radiation oncology and hematology, University "La Sapienza" of Rome. *Tumori* 1996;82:48.
119. Vlachaki MT, Hagemeister FB, Fuller LM, et al. Long-term outcome of treatment for Ann Arbor stage I Hodgkin's disease: prognostic factors for survival and freedom from progression. *Int J Radiat Oncol Biol Phys* 1997;38:593.
120. Levi JA, Wiernik PH. Limited extranodal Hodgkin's disease. Unfavorable prognosis and therapeutic implications. *Am J Med* 1977;63:365.
121. Prosnitz LR. The Ann Arbor staging system for Hodgkin's disease: does E stand for error? *Int J Radiat Oncol Biol Phys* 1977;2:1039.
122. Connors JM, Klimo P. Is it an E lesion or stage IV? An unsettled issue in Hodgkin's disease staging. *J Clin Oncol* 1984;2:1421.
123. Levi JA, Wiernik PH, O'Connell MJ. Patterns of relapse in stages I, II and IIIA Hodgkin's disease: influence of initial therapy and implications for the future. *Int J Radiat Oncol Biol Phys* 1977;2:853.
124. Rostock R, Giangreco A, Wharam M, Lenhard R, Siegelman S, Order S. CT scan modification in the treatment of mediastinal Hodgkin's disease. *Cancer* 1982;49:2267.
125. Rostock RA, Siegelman SS, Lenhard RE, Wharam MD, Order SE. Thoracic CT scanning for mediastinal Hodgkin's disease: results and therapeutic implications. *Int J Radiat Oncol Biol Phys* 1983;9:1451.
126. Jochelson M, Balikian J, Mauch P, Liebman H. Peri- and paracardial involvement in lymphoma: a radiographic study of 11 cases. *Am J Roentgenol* 1983;140:483.
127. Zittoun R, Audebert A, Hoerni B, et al. Extended versus involved fields irradiation combined with MOPP chemotherapy in early clinical stages of Hodgkin's disease. *J Clin Oncol* 1985;3:207.
128. Hoppe RT. The management of stage II Hodgkin's disease with a large mediastinal mass: a prospective program emphasizing irradiation. *Int J Radiat Oncol Biol Phys* 1985;11:349.
129. Jochelson M, Herman T, Stomper P, Mauch P, Kaplan W. Planning mantle radiation therapy in patients with Hodgkin's disease: role of gallium-67 scintigraphy. *Am J Roentgenol* 1988;151:1229.
130. Leopold KA, Canellos GP, Rosenthal D, Shulman LN, Weinstein H, Mauch P. Stage IA–IIB Hodgkin's disease: staging and treatment of patients with large mediastinal adenopathy. *J Clin Oncol* 1989;7:1059.
131. Gobbi PG, Cavalli C, Gendarini A, et al. Reevaluation of prognostic significance of symptoms in Hodgkin's disease. *Cancer* 1985;56:2874.
132. Crnkovich MJ, Hoppe RT, Rosenberg SA. Stage IIB Hodgkin's disease: the Stanford experience. *J Clin Oncol* 1986;4:472.
133. Feiner AS, Mahmood T, Wallner SF. Prognostic importance of pruritus in Hodgkin's disease. *JAMA* 1978;240:2738.
134. Gobbi PG, Attardo-Parrinello G, Lattanzio G, Rizzo SC, Ascari E. Severe pruritus should be a B-symptom in Hodgkin's disease. *Cancer* 1983;51:1934.
135. Gause A, Jung W, Keymis S, et al. The clinical significance of cytokines and soluble forms of membrane-derived activation antigens in the serum of patients with Hodgkin's disease. *Leuk Lymphoma* 1992;7:439.
136. Kurzrock R, Redman J, Cabanillas F, Jones D, Rothberg J, Talpaz M. Serum interleukin 6 levels are elevated in lymphoma patients and correlate with survival in advanced Hodgkin's disease and with B symptoms. *Cancer Res* 1993;53:2118.
137. Trümper L, Jung W, Dahl G, Diehl V, Gause A, Pfreundschuh M. Interleukin-7, interleukin-8, soluble TNF receptor, and p53 protein levels are elevated in the serum of patients with Hodgkin's disease. *Ann Oncol* 1994;5(Suppl 1):93.
138. Gorschlüter M, Bohlen H, Hasenclever D, Diehl V, Tesch H. Serum cytokine levels correlate with clinical parameters in Hodgkin's disease. *Ann Oncol* 1995;6:477.
139. Foss H-D, Herbst H, Gottstein S, Demel G, Araujó I, Stein H. Interleukin-8 in Hodgkin's disease. Preferential expression by reactive cells and association with neutrophil density. *Am J Pathol* 1996;148:1229.
140. Gruss H-J, Ulrich D, Dower SK, Herrmann F, Brach MA. Activation of Hodgkin cells via the CD30 receptor induces autocrine secretion of interleukin-6 engaging the NF-κB transcription factor. *Blood* 1996;87:2443.
141. Lukes RJ, Craver LF, Hall TC, Rappaport H, Ruben P. Report of the nomenclature committee. *Cancer Res* 1966;26:1311.
142. Harris NL, Jaffe ES, Stein H, et al. A revised European-American classification of lymphoid neoplasms: a proposal from the International Lymphoma Study Group. *Blood* 1994;84:1361.
143. Russell KJ, Hoppe RT, Colby TV, Burns BF, Cox RS, Kaplan HS. Lymphocyte predominant Hodgkin's disease: clinical presentation and results of treatment, *Radiother Oncol* 1984;1:197.
144. Pappa VI, Norton AJ, Gupta RK, Wilson AM, Rohatiner AZX, Lister TA. Nodular type of lymphocyte predominant Hodgkin's disease. A clinical study of 50 cases. *Ann Oncol* 1995;6:559.
145. Bodis S, Kraus MD, Pinkus G, et al. Clinical presentation and outcome in lymphocyte-predominant Hodgkin's disease. *J Clin Oncol* 1997;15:3060.
146. Regula DP, Hoppe RT, Weiss LM. Nodular and diffuse types of lymphocyte predominance Hodgkin's disease. *N Engl J Med* 1988;318:214.
147. Orlandi E, Lazzarino M, Brusamolino E, et al. Nodular lymphocyte predominance Hodgkin's disease: long-term observation reveals a continuous pattern of recurrence. *Leuk Lymphoma* 1997;26:359.
148. Sextro M, Diehl V, Franklin J, et al., for the European Task Force on Lymphoma. Lymphocyte predominant Hodgkin's disease—a workshop report. *Ann Oncol* 1996;7(Suppl 4):61.

149. Banks PM. The pathology of Hodgkin's disease. *Semin Oncol* 1990; 17:683.
150. Medeiros LJ, Greiner TC. Hodgkin's disease. *Cancer* 1995;75:357.
151. Fuller LM, Madoc-Jones H, Gamble JF, et al. New assessment of the prognostic significance of histopathology in Hodgkin's disease for laparotomy-negative stage I and stage II patients. *Cancer* 1977;39:2174.
152. Haybittle JL, Hayhoe FGJ, Easterling MJ, et al. Review of British National Lymphoma Investigation studies of Hodgkin's disease and development of prognostic index. *Lancet* 1985;1:967.
153. Fuller LM, Hagemeister FB. Hodgkin's disease in adults: stages I and II. In: Fuller LM, Hagemeister FB, Sullivan MP, Velasquez WS, eds. *Hodgkin's disease and non-Hodgkin's lymphomas in adults and children*. New York: Raven Press, 1988:203.
154. Specht L, Lauritzen AF, Nordentoft AM, et al. Tumor cell concentration and tumor burden in relation to histopathological subtype and other prognostic factors in early stage Hodgkin's disease. *Cancer* 1990;65:2594.
155. Guinee VF, Giacco GG, Durand M, et al. The prognosis of Hodgkin's disease in older adults. *J Clin Oncol* 1991;9:947.
156. Bennett MH, MacLennan KA, Easterling MJ, Vaughan Hudson B, Vaughan Hudson G, Jelliffe AM. Analysis of histological subtypes in Hodgkin's disease in relation to prognosis and survival. In: Quaglino D, Hayhoe FGJ, eds. *The cytobiology of leukaemias and lymphomas*. Serono Symposia Publications, vol 20. New York: Raven Press, 1985: 15.
157. MacLennan KA, Bennett MH, Bosq J, et al. The histology and immunohistology of Hodgkin's disease: its relationship to prognosis and clinical behaviour. In: Somers R, Henry-Amar M, Meerwaldt JK, Carde P, eds. *Treatment strategy in Hodgkin's disease. Proceedings of the Paris International Workshop and Symposium held on June 28–30, 1989*. Colloque INSERM no 196. London: INSERM/John Libbey Eurotext, 1990:17.
158. Patchefsky AS, Brodovsky H, Southard M, Menduke H, Gray S, Hoch WS. Hodgkin's disease. A clinical and pathologic study of 235 cases. *Cancer* 1973;32:150.
159. Carbone A. Histologic subclassification of nodular sclerosis Hodgkin's disease. *Tumori* 1979;65:743.
160. Cionini L, Arganini L, Mungai V, Biti GP, Bondi R. Prognostic significance of histologic subdivision of Hodgkin's disease nodular sclerosis. *Acta Radiol Oncol* 1978;17:65.
161. Coppleson LW, Rappaport H, Strum SB, Rose J. Analysis of the Rye classification of Hodgkin's disease. The prognostic significance of cellular composition. *J Natl Cancer Inst* 1973;51:379.
162. Cross RM. A clinicopathological study of nodular sclerosing Hodgkin's disease. *J Clin Pathol* 1968;21:303.
163. Keller AR, Kaplan HS, Lukes R, Rappaport H. Correlation of histopathology with other prognostic indicators in Hodgkin's disease. *Cancer* 1968;22:487.
164. MacLennan KA, Bennett MH, Tu A, et al. Relationship of histopathologic features to survival and relapse in nodular sclerosing Hodgkin's disease. *Cancer* 1989;64:1686.
165. Ferry JA, Linggood RM, Convery KM, Efird JT, Eliseo R, Harris NL. Hodgkin disease, nodular sclerosis type. Implications of histologic subclassification. *Cancer* 1993;71:457.
166. Hess JL, Bodis S, Pinkus G, Silver B, Mauch P. Histopathologic grading of nodular sclerosis Hodgkin's disease. Lack of prognostic significance in 254 surgically staged patients. *Cancer* 1994;74:708.
167. A Collaborative Study. Radiotherapy of stage I and II Hodgkin's disease. *Cancer* 1984;54:1928.
168. Austin-Seymour MM, Hoppe RT, Cox RS, Rosenberg SA, Kaplan HS. Hodgkin's disease in patients over sixty years old. *Ann Intern Med* 1984;100:13.
169. Lokich JJ, Pinkus GS, Moloney WC. Hodgkin's disease in the elderly. *Oncology* 1974;29:484.
170. Tubiana M, Henry-Amar M, van der Werf-Messing B, et al. A multivariate analysis of prognostic factors in early stage Hodgkin's disease. *Int J Radiat Oncol Biol Phys* 1985;11:23.
171. Vaughan Hudson B, MacLennan KA, Easterling MJ, Jelliffe AM, Haybittle JL, Vaughan Hudson G. The prognostic significance of age in Hodgkin's disease: examination of 1500 patients (BNLI report no 23). *Clin Radiol* 1983;34:503.
172. Wedelin C, Björkholm M, Biberfeld P, Holm G, Johansson B, Mellstedt H. Prognostic factors in Hodgkin's disease with special reference to age. *Cancer* 1984;53:1202.
173. Walker A, Schoenfeld ER, Lowman JT, Mettlin CJ, MacMillan J, Grufferman S. Survival of the older patient compared with the younger patient with Hodgkin's disease. Influence of histologic type, staging, and treatment. *Cancer* 1990;65:1635.
174. Glimelius B, Enblad G, Kälkner M, et al. Treatment of Hodgkin's disease: the Swedish National Care Programme experience. *Leuk Lymphoma* 1996;21:71.
175. Tubiana M, Henry-Amar M, Carde P, et al. Toward comprehensive management tailored to prognostic factors of patients with clinical stages I and II in Hodgkin's disease. The EORTC Lymphoma Group controlled clinical trials: 1964–1987. *Blood* 1989;73:47.
176. Meerwaldt JH, van Glabbeke M, Vaughan Hudson B. Prognostic factors for stage I and II Hodgkin's disease. In: Somers R, Henry-Amar M, Meerwaldt JK, Carde P, eds. *Treatment strategy in Hodgkin's disease. Proceedings of the Paris International Workshop and Symposium held on June 28–30, 1989*. Colloque INSERM no 196. London: INSERM/John Libbey Eurotext, 1990:37.
177. Specht L, Nissen NI. Hodgkin's disease and age. *Eur J Haematol* 1989;43:127.
178. Enblad G, Glimelius B, Sundström C. Treatment outcome in Hodgkin's disease in patients above the age of 60: a population-based study. *Ann Oncol* 1991;2:297.
179. Ganesan TS, Oza A, Perry N, et al. Management of stage II Hodgkin's disease: 15 years of experience at St. Bartholomew's Hospital. *Ann Oncol* 1992;3:349.
180. Levy LM. Hodgkin's disease in black Zimbabweans. A study of epidemiologic, histologic, and clinical features. *Cancer* 1988;61:189.
181. Routh A, Hickman BT. Comparison of black and white patients in each stage of Hodgkin's disease during 1970–1980. *Radiat Med* 1989; 7:28.
182. Glaser SL. Hodgkin's disease in black populations: a review of the epidemiologic literature. *Semin Oncol* 1990;17:643.
183. Riyat MS. Hodgkin's disease in Kenya. *Cancer* 1992;69:1047.
184. Vaughan Hudson B, MacLennan KA, Bennett MH, Easterling MJ, Vaughan Hudson G, Jelliffe AM. Systemic disturbance in Hodgkin's disease and its relation to histopathology and prognosis (BNLI report no 30). *Clin Radiol* 1987;38:257.
185. Tubiana M, Attié E, Flamant R, Gérard-Marchant R, Hayat M. Prognostic factors in 454 cases of Hodgkin's disease. *Cancer Res* 1971;31: 1801.
186. Tubiana M. Hodgkin's disease: historical perspective and clinical presentation. *Baillieres Clin Haematol* 1996;9:503.
187. Specht L. Prognostic factors in Hodgkin's disease. *Cancer Treat Rev* 1991;18:21.
188. Specht L, Carde P, Mauch P, Magrini SM, Santarelli MT. Radiotherapy versus combined modality in early stages. *Ann Oncol* 1992;3 (Suppl 4):77.
189. Longo DL, Glatstein E, Duffey PL, et al. Radiation therapy versus combination chemotherapy in the treatment of early-stage Hodgkin's disease: seven-year results of a prospective randomized trial. *J Clin Oncol* 1991;9:906.
190. Biti GP, Cimino G, Cartoni C, et al. Extended-field radiotherapy is superior to MOPP chemotherapy for the treatment of pathologic stage I–IIA Hodgkin's disease: eight-year update of an Italian prospective randomized study. *J Clin Oncol* 1992;10:378.
191. Cimino G, Biti GP, Anselmo AP, et al. MOPP chemotherapy versus extended-field radiotherapy in the management of pathological stages I–IIA Hodgkin's disease. *J Clin Oncol* 1989;7:732.
192. Kaplan HS. Hodgkin's disease: unfolding concepts concerning its nature, management and prognosis. *Cancer* 1980;45:2439.
193. British National Lymphoma Investigation. The value of laparotomy and splenectomy in the management of early Hodgkin's disease. *Clin Radiol* 1975;26:151.
194. Trotter MC, Cloud GA, Davis M, et al. Predicting the risk of abdominal disease in Hodgkin's lymphoma. *Ann Surg* 1985;201:465.
195. Leibenhaut MH, Hoppe RT, Efron B, Halpern J, Nelsen T, Rosenberg SA. Prognostic indicators of laparotomy findings in clinical stage I–II supradiaphragmatic Hodgkin's disease. *J Clin Oncol* 1989;7:81.
196. Mauch P, Larson D, Osteen R, et al. Prognostic factors for positive surgical staging in patients with Hodgkin's disease. *J Clin Oncol* 1990;8:257.
197. Askergren J, Björkholm M, Holm G, et al. Prognostic effect of early diagnostic splenectomy in Hodgkin's disease: a randomized trial. *Br J Cancer* 1980;42:284.

198. Lacher MJ. Routine staging laparotomy for patients with Hodgkin's disease is no longer necessary. *Cancer Invest* 1983;1:93.
199. Gomez GA, Reese PA, Nava H, et al. Staging laparotomy and splenectomy in early Hodgkin's disease. No therapeutic benefit. *Am J Med* 1984;77:205.
200. Carde P, Hagenbeek A, Hayat M, et al. Clinical staging versus laparotomy and combined modality with MOPP versus ABVD in early-stage Hodgkin's disease: the H_6 twin randomized trials from the European Organization for Research and Treatment of Cancer Lymphoma Cooperative Group. *J Clin Oncol* 1993;11:2258.
201. Bergsagel DE, Alison RE, Bean HA, et al. Results of treating Hodgkin's disease without a policy of laparotomy staging. *Cancer Treat Rep* 1982;66:717.
202. Roberts SJ, Roeser HP, Kynaston B, Whitaker SV, Hocker GA, Battersby AC. Hodgkin's disease: an evaluation of staging laparotomy in 82 patients. *Aust Radiol* 1976;20:314.
203. Brada M, Easton DF, Horwich A, Peckham MJ. Clinical presentation as a predictor of laparotomy findings in supradiaphragmatic stage I and II Hodgkin's disease. *Radiother Oncol* 1986;5:15.
204. De la Cruz GA, Cardenes H, Otero J, et al. Individual risk of abdominal disease in patients with stages I and II supradiaphragmatic Hodgkin's disease. A rule index based on 341 laparotomized patients. *Cancer* 1989;63:1799.
205. Gospodarowicz MK, Sutcliffe SB, Clark RM, et al. Analysis of supradiaphragmatic clinical stage I and II Hodgkin's disease treated with radiation alone. *Int J Radiat Oncol Biol Phys* 1992;22:859.
206. Mason MD, Law M, Ashley S, et al. Infradiaphragmatic Hodgkin's disease. *Eur J Cancer* 1992;28A:1851.
207. Gobbi PG, Gendarini A, Crema A, et al. Serum albumin in Hodgkin's disease. *Cancer* 1985;55:389.
208. Pavlovsky S, Maschio M, Santarelli MT, et al. Randomized trial of chemotherapy versus chemotherapy plus radiotherapy for stage I–II Hodgkin's disease. *J Natl Cancer Inst* 1988;80:1466.
209. Lagarde P, Eghbali H, Bonichon F, de Mascarel I, Chauvergne J, Hoerni B. Brief chemotherapy associated with extended field radiotherapy in Hodgkin's disease. Long-term results in a series of 102 patients with clinical stages I–IIIA. *Eur J Cancer Clin Oncol* 1988;24: 1191.
210. Bonfante V, Santoro A, Viviani S, et al. Early stage Hodgkin's disease: ten-year results of a non-randomised study with radiotherapy alone or combined with MOPP. *Eur J Cancer* 1993;29A:24.
211. Colonna P, Jais J-P, Desablens B, et al. Mediastinal tumor size and response to chemotherapy are the only prognostic factors in supradiaphragmatic Hodgkin's disease treated by ABVD plus radiotherapy: ten-year results of the Paris-Ouest-France 81/12 Trial, including 262 patients. *J Clin Oncol* 1996;14:1928.
212. Longo DL, Glatstein E, Duffey PL, et al. Alternating MOPP and ABVD chemotherapy plus mantle-field radiation therapy in patients with massive mediastinal Hodgkin's disease. *J Clin Oncol* 1997;15: 3338.
213. Rueda A, Alba E, Ribelles N, Sevilla I, Ruiz I, Miramón J. Six cycles of ABVD in the treatment of stage I and II Hodgkin's lymphoma: a pilot study. *J Clin Oncol* 1997;15:1118.
214. Moore MR, Jones SE, Bull JM, William LA, Rosenberg SA. MOPP chemotherapy for advanced Hodgkin's disease: prognostic factors in 81 patients. *Cancer* 1973;32:52.
215. Canellos GP, Come SE, Skarin AT. Chemotherapy in the treatment of Hodgkin's disease. *Semin Hematol* 1983;20:1.
216. Cooper MR, Pajak TF, Gottlieb AJ, et al. The effects of prior radiation therapy and age on the frequency and duration of complete remission among various four-drug treatments for advanced Hodgkin's disease. *J Clin Oncol* 1984;2:748.
217. Sutcliffe SB, Wrigley PFM, Peto J, et al. MVPP chemotherapy regimen for advanced Hodgkin's disease. *Br Med J* 1978;1:679.
218. Timothy AR, Sutcliffe SBJ, Wrigley PFM, Jones AE. Hodgkin's disease: combination chemotherapy for relapse following radical radiotherapy. *Int J Radiat Oncol Biol Phys* 1979;5:165.
219. Loeffler M, Brosteanu O, Hasenclever D, et al. Meta-analysis of chemotherapy versus combined modality treatment trials in Hodgkin's disease. *J Clin Oncol* 1998;16:818.
220. Hasenclever D, Diehl V. A prognostic score for advanced Hodgkin's disease. International Prognostic Factors Project on advanced Hodgkin's disease. *N Engl J Med* 1998;339:1506–1514.
221. Canellos GP, Anderson JR, Propert KJ, et al. Chemotherapy of advanced Hodgkin's disease with MOPP, ABVD, or MOPP alternating with ABVD. *N Engl J Med* 1992;327:1478.
222. Peterson BA, Pajak TF, Cooper MR, et al. Effect of age on therapeutic response and survival in advanced Hodgkin's disease. *Cancer Treat Rep* 1982;66:889.
223. Somers R, Carde P, Henry-Amar M, et al. A randomized study in stage IIIB and IV Hodgkin's disease comparing eight courses of MOPP versus an alternation of MOPP with ABVD: a European Organization for Research and Treatment of Cancer Lymphoma Cooperative Group and Group Pierre-et-Marie-Curie controlled clinical trial. *J Clin Oncol* 1994;12:279.
224. Löffler M, Dixon DO. Swindell R. Prognostic factors of stage III and IV Hodgkin's disease. In: Somers R, Henry-Amar M, Meerwaldt JK, Carde P, eds. *Treatment strategy in Hodgkin's disease. Proceedings of the Paris International Workshop and Symposium held on June 28–30, 1989*. Colloque INSERM no 196. London: INSERM/John Libbey Eurotext, 1990:89.
225. Yelle L, Bergsagel D, Basco V, et al. Combined modality therapy of Hodgkin's disease: 10-year results of National Cancer Institute of Canada Clinical Trials Group multicenter clinical trial. *J Clin Oncol* 1991;9:1983.
226. Jaffe HS, Cadman EC, Farber LR, Bertino JR. Pretreatment hematocrit as an independent prognostic variable in Hodgkin's disease. *Blood* 1986;68:562.
227. Proctor SJ, Taylor P, Donnan P, Boys R, Lennard A, Prescott RJ. A numerical prognostic index for clinical use in identification of poor-risk patients with Hodgkin's disease at diagnosis. Scotland and Newcastle Lymphoma Group (SNLG) Therapy Working Party. *Eur J Cancer* 1991;27:624.
228. Ranson MR, Radford JA, Swindell R, et al. An analysis of prognostic factors in stage III and IV Hodgkin's disease treated at a single centre with MVPP. *Ann Oncol* 1991;2:423.
229. Specht L, Nissen NI. Prognostic factors in Hodgkin's disease stage III with special reference to tumour burden. *Eur J Haematol* 1988;41:80.
230. Specht L, Nissen NI. Prognostic factors in Hodgkin's disease stage IV. *Eur J Haematol* 1988;41:359.
231. Straus DJ, Gaynor JJ, Myers J, et al. Prognostic factors among 185 adults with newly diagnosed advanced Hodgkin's disease treated with alternating potentially noncross-resistant chemotherapy and intermediate-dose radiation therapy. *J Clin Oncol* 1990;8:1173.
232. Wagstaff J, Gregory WM, Swindell R, Crowther D, Lister TA. Prognostic factors for survival in stage IIIB and IV Hodgkin's disease: a multivariate analysis comparing two specialist centres. *Br J Cancer* 1988;58:487.
233. Fermé C, Bastion Y, Brice P, et al. Prognosis of patients with advanced Hodgkin's disease: evaluation of four prognostic models using 344 patients included in the Groupe d'Études des Lymphomes de l'Adulte Study. *Cancer* 1997;80:1124.
234. Wagstaff J, Steward W, Jones M, et al. Factors affecting remission and survival in patients with advanced Hodgkin's disease treated with MVPP. *Hematol Oncol* 1986;4:135.
235. Dienstbier Z, Chytry P, Hermanska Z, Melinova L, Penicka P, Marikova E. A multivariate analysis of prognostic factors in adult Hodgkin's disease. *Neoplasma* 1989;36:447.
236. Gobbi PG, Comelli M, Grignani GE, Pieresca C, Bertoloni D, Ascari E. Estimate of expected survival at diagnosis in Hodgkin's disease: a means of weighting prognostic factors and a tool for treatment choice and clinical research. A report from the International Database on Hodgkin's Disease (IDHD). *Haematologica* 1994;79:241.
237. Rodgers RW, Fuller LM, Hagemeister FB, et al. Reassessment of prognostic factors in stage IIIA and IIIB Hodgkin's disease treated with MOPP and radiotherapy. *Cancer* 1981;47:2196.
238. Longo DL, Young RC, Wesley M, et al. Twenty years of MOPP therapy for Hodgkin's disease. *J Clin Oncol* 1986;4:1295.
239. Hancock BW, Vaughan Hudson G, Vaughan Hudson B, et al. LOPP alternating with EVAP is superior to LOPP alone in the initial treatment of advanced Hodgkin's disease: results of a British National Lymphoma Investigation trial. *J Clin Oncol* 1992;10:1252.
240. Georgii A, Fischer R, Hubner K, Schwarze EW, Bernhards J. Classification of Hodgkin's disease biopsies by a panel of four histopathologists. Report of 1,140 patients from the German National Trial. *Leuk Lymphoma* 1993;9:365.
241. Masih AS, Weisenburger DD, Vose JM, Bast MA, Armitage JO. Histologic grade does not predict prognosis in optimally treated,

advanced-stage nodular sclerosing Hodgkin's disease. *Cancer* 1992; 69:228.

242. D'Amore ES, Lee CK, Aeppli DM, Levitt SH, Frizzera G. Lack of prognostic value of histopathologic parameters in Hodgkin's disease, nodular sclerosis type. A study of 123 patients with limited stage disease who had undergone laparotomy and were treated with radiation therapy. *Arch Pathol Lab Med* 1992;116:856.
243. Norum J, Wist E, Nordoy T, Stalsberg H. Subclassification of Hodgkin's disease, nodular sclerosis type. Prognostic value? *Anticancer Res* 1995;15:1569.
244. Van Spronsen DJ, Vrints LW, Hofstra G, Crommelin MA, Coebergh JW, Breed WP. Disappearance of prognostic significance of histopathological grading of nodular sclerosing Hodgkin's disease for unselected patients, 1972–92. *Br J Haematol* 1997;96:322.
245. Selby P, Patel P, Milan S, et al. ChlVPP combination chemotherapy for Hodgkin's disease: long term results. *Br J Cancer* 1990;62:279.
246. Stein RS, Golomb HM, Wiernik PH, et al. Anatomic substages of stage IIIA Hodgkin's disease: follow-up of a collaborative study. *Cancer Treat Rep* 1982;66:733.
247. Mauch P, Goffman T, Rosenthal DS, Canellos GP, Come SE, Hellman S. Stage III Hodgkin's disease: improved survival with combined modality therapy as compared with radiation therapy alone. *J Clin Oncol* 1985;3:1166.
248. Hoppe RT, Cox RS, Rosenberg SA, Kaplan HS. Prognostic factors in pathologic stage III Hodgkin's disease. *Cancer Treat Rep* 1982;66: 743.
249. Hoppe RT, Rosenberg SA, Kaplan HS, Cox RS. Prognostic factors in pathological stage IIIA Hodgkin's disease. *Cancer* 1980;46:1240.
250. Powlis WD, Mauch P, Goffman T, Goodman RL. Treatment of patients with "minimal" stage IIIA Hodgkin's disease. *Int J Radiat Oncol Biol Phys* 1987;13:1437.
251. Mazza P, Miniaci G, Lauria F, et al. Prognostic significance of lymphography in stage IIIs Hodgkin's disease (HD). *Eur J Cancer Clin Oncol* 1984;20:1393.
252. Desser RK, Golomb HM, Ultmann JE, et al. Prognostic classification of Hodgkin's disease in pathologic stage III, based on anatomic considerations. *Blood* 1977;49:883.
253. Farah R, Golomb HM, Hallahan DE, et al. Radiation therapy for pathologic stage III Hodgkin's disease with and without chemotherapy. *Int J Radiat Oncol Biol Phys* 1989;17:761.
254. Golomb HM, Sweet DL, Ultmann JE, Miller JB, Kinzie JJ, Gordon LI. Importance of substaging of stage III Hodgkin's disease. *Semin Oncol* 1980;7:136.
255. Levi JA, Wiernik PH. The therapeutic implications of splenic involvement in stage IIIA Hodgkin's disease. *Cancer* 1977;39:2158.
256. Brada M, Ashley S, Nicholls J, et al. Stage III Hodgkin's disease—long-term results following chemotherapy, radiotherapy and combined modality therapy. *Radiother Oncol* 1989;14:185.
257. Hopper KD, Diehl LF, Lynch JC, McCauslin MA. Mediastinal bulk in Hodgkin disease. Method of measurement versus prognosis. *Invest Radiol* 1991;26:1101.
258. Proctor SJ, Taylor P, Mackie MJ, et al. A numerical prognostic index for clinical use in identification of poor-risk patients with Hodgkin's disease at diagnosis. The Scotland and Newcastle Lymphoma Group (SNLG) Therapy Working Party. *Leuk Lymphoma* 1992;7(Suppl 7):17.
259. Hasenclever D, Schmitz N, Diehl V. Is there a rationale for high-dose chemotherapy as first line treatment of advanced Hodgkin's disease? German Hodgkin's Lymphoma Study Group (GHSG). *Leuk Lymphoma* 1995;15(Suppl 1):47.
260. Carde P, MacKintosh FR, Rosenberg SA. A dose and time response analysis of the treatment of Hodgkin's disease with MOPP chemotherapy. *J Clin Oncol* 1983;1:146.
261. Gibbs GE, Peterson BA, Kennedy BJ, Vosika G, Bloomfield CD. Long-term survival of patients with Hodgkin's disease. Treatment with cyclophosphamide, vinblastine, procarbazine and prednisone. *Arch Intern Med* 1981;141:897.
262. Höffken K, Ippisch A, Pfeiffer R, Becher R, Seeber S, Schmidt CG. Chemotherapie der fortgeschrittenen lymphogranulomatose. *Dtsch Med Wochenschr* 1985;110:618.
263. Bartl R, Frisch B, Burkhardt R, Huhn D, Pappenberger R. Assessment of bone marrow histology in Hodgkin's disease: correlation with clinical factors. *Br J Haematol* 1982;51:345.
264. Brusamolino E, Orlande E, Morra E, et al. Analysis of long-term results and prognostic factors among 138 patients with advanced Hodgkin's disease treated with the alternating MOPP/ABVD chemotherapy. *Ann Oncol* 1994;5(Suppl 2):53.
265. DeVita VT, Simon RM, Hubbard SM, et al. Curability of advanced Hodgkin's disease with chemotherapy. *Ann Intern Med* 1980;92:587.
266. Munker R, Hasenclever D, Brosteanu O, et al. Bone marrow involvement in Hodgkin's disease: an analysis of 135 consecutive cases. *J Clin Oncol* 1995;13:403.
267. Bonadonna G, Valagussa P, Santoro A. Alternating non-cross-resistant combination chemotherapy or MOPP in stage IV Hodgkin's disease. *Ann Intern Med* 1986;104:739.
268. Pillai GN, Hagemeister FB, Velasquez WS, et al. Prognostic factors for stage IV Hodgkin's disease treated with MOPP, with or without bleomycin. *Cancer* 1985;55:691.
269. Gobbi PG, Cavalli C, Gendarini A, et al. Prognostic significance of serum albumin in Hodgkin's disease. *Haematologica* 1986;71:95.
270. Straus DJ. High-risk Hodgkin's disease prognostic factors. *Leuk Lymphoma* 1995;15(Suppl 1):41.
271. MacLennan KA, Vaughan Hudson B, Easterling MJ, Jelliffe AM, Vaughan Hudson G, Haybittle JL. The presentation haemoglobin level in 1103 patients with Hodgkin's disease (BNLI report no 21). *Clin Radiol* 1983;34:491.
272. Loeffler M, Pfreundschuh M, Hasencelver D, et al. Prognostic risk factors in advanced Hodgkin's lymphoma. Report of the German Hodgkin Study Group. *Blut* 1988;56:273.
273. Aviles A, Talavera A, Garcia EL. Guzman R, Diaz-Maqueo JC. La fosfatafa alcalina como factor pronóstico en enfermedad de Hodgkin. (Alkaline phosphatase as a prognostic factor in Hodgkin's disease.) *Rev Gastroenterol Mex* 1990;55:211.
274. MacLennan KA, Vaughan Hudson B, Jelliffe AM, Haybittle JL, Vaughan Hudson G. The pretreatment peripheral blood lymphocyte count in 1100 patients with Hodgkin's disease: the prognostic significance and the relationship to the presence of systemic symptoms. *Clin Oncol* 1981;7:333.
275. The International Non-Hodgkin's Lymphoma Prognostic Factors Project. A predictive model for aggressive non-Hodgkin's lymphoma. *N Engl J Med* 1993;329:987.
276. Dimopoulos MA, Cabanillas F, Lee JJ, et al. Prognostic role of serum β_2-microglobulin in Hodgkin's disease. *J Clin Oncol* 1993;11:1108.
277. Pizzolo G, Vinante F, Chilosi M, et al. Serum levels of soluble CD30 molecule (Ki-1 antigen) in Hodgkin's disease: relationship with diseaase activity and clinical stage. *Br J Haematol* 1990;75:282.
278. Gause A, Jung W, Schmits R, et al. Soluble CD8, CD25 and CD30 antigens as prognostic markers in patients with untreated Hodgkin's lymphoma. *Ann Oncol* 1992;3(Suppl 4):49.
279. Nadali G, Vinante F, Ambrosetti A, et al. Serum levels of soluble CD30 are elevated in the majority of untreated patients with Hodgkin's disease and correlate with clinical features and prognosis. *J Clin Oncol* 1994;12:793.
280. Pui C-H, Ip SH, Thompson, et al. High serum interleukin-2 receptor levels correlate with a poor prognosis in children with Hodgkin's disease. *Leukemia* 1989;3:481.
281. Pizzolo G, Chilosi M, Vinante F, et al. Soluble interleukin-2 receptors in the serum of patients with Hodgkin's disease. *Br J Cancer* 1987; 55:427.
282. Enblad G, Sundström C, Gronowitz S, Glimelius B. Serum levels of interleukin-2 receptor (CD25) in patients with Hodgkin's disease, with special reference to age and prognosis. *Ann Oncol* 1995;6:65.
283. Pui C-H, Ip SH, Thompson E, et al. Increased serum CD8 antigen level in childhood Hodgkin's disease relates to advanced stage and poor treatment outcome. *Blood* 1989;73:209.
284. Gause A, Verpoort K, Roschansky V, et al. The clinical significance of serum CD8 antigen levels in adult patients with Hodgkin's disease. *Ann Oncol* 1991;2:579.
285. Wagstaff J, Steward W, Jones M, et al. Factors affecting remission and survival in patients with advanced Hodgkin's disease treated with MVPP. *Hematol Oncol* 1986;4:135.
286. Gobbi PG, Gobbi PG, Mazza P, Zinzani PL. Multivariate analysis of Hodgkin's disease prognosis. Fitness and use of a directly predictive equation. *Haematologica* 1989;74:29.
287. Federico M, Clo V, Carella AM. High-dose therapy autologous stem cell transplantation vs. conventional therapy: analysis of clinical characteristics of 51 patients enrolled in the HD01 protocol. EBMT/ ANZLG/Intergroup HD01 Trial. *Leukemia* 1996;10(Suppl 2):69.
288. Carella AM, Prencipe E, Pungolino E, et al. Twelve years of experi-

ence with high-dose therapy and autologous stem cell transplantation for high-risk Hodgkin's disease patients in first remission after MOPP/ABVD chemotherapy. *Leuk Lymphoma* 1996;21:63.
289. Gisselbrecht C, Fermé C. Prognostic factors in advanced Hodgkin's disease: problems and pitfalls. Towards an international prognostic index. *Leuk Lymphoma* 1995;15(Suppl 1):23.
290. Carde P. Should poor risk patients with Hodgkin's disease be sorted out for intensive treatments? *Leuk Lymphoma* 1995;15(Suppl 1):31.
291. Schmitz N, Hasenclever D, Brosteanu O, et al. Early high-dose therapy to consolidate patients with high-risk Hodgkin's disease in first remission? Results of an EBMT/GHSG matched pair analysis. *Blood* 1995;86,10(Suppl 1): ASH abst no 1742.
292. Lee SM, Radford JA, Ryder WD, Collins CD, Deakin DP, Crowther D. Prognostic factors for disease progression in advanced Hodgkin's disease: an analysis of patients aged under 60 years showing no progression in the first 6 months after starting primary chemotherapy. *Br J Cancer* 1997;75:110.
293. Healey EA, Tarbell NJ, Kalish LA, et al. Prognostic factors for patients with Hodgkin disease in first relapse. *Cancer* 1993;71:2613.
294. Canellos GP, Young RC, DeVita VT. Combination chemotherapy for advanced Hodgkin's disease in relapse following extensive radiotherapy. *Clin Pharmacol Ther* 1972;13:750.
295. Tubiana M, van der Werf-Messing B, Laugier A, et al. Survival after recurrence: prognostic factors and spread patterns in clinical stages I and II of Hodgkin's disease. *Natl Cancer Inst Monogr* 1973;36:513.
296. Timothy AR, Sutcliffe SBJ, Wrigley PFM, Jones AE. Hodgkin's disease: combination chemotherapy for relapse following radical radiotherapy. *Int J Radiat Oncol Biol Phys* 1979;5:165.
297. Mauch P, Ryback ME, Rosenthal D, Weichselbaum R, Hellman S. The influence of initial pathologic stage on the survival of patients who relapse from Hodgkin's disease. *Blood* 1980;56:892.
298. Cooper MR, Pajak TF, Gottlieb AJ, et al. The effects of prior radiation therapy and age on the frequency and duration of complete remission among various four-drug treatments for advanced Hodgkin's disease. *J Clin Oncol* 1984;2:748.
299. Vinciguerra V, Propert KJ, Coleman M, et al. Alternating cycles of combination chemotherapy for patients with recurrent Hodgkin's disease following radiotherapy. A prospectively randomized study by the Cancer and Leukemia Group B. *J Clin Oncol* 1986;4:838.
300. Santoro A, Viviani S, Villarreal CJR, et al. Salvage chemotherapy in Hodgkin's disease irradiation failures: superiority of doxorubicin-containing regimens over MOPP. *Cancer Treat Rep* 1986;70:343.
301. Olver IN, Wolf MM, Cruickshank D, et al. Nitrogen mustard, vincristine, procarbazine, and prednisolone for relapse after radiation in Hodgkin's disease. An analysis of long-term follow-up. *Cancer* 1988;62:233.
302. Roach M, Brophy N, Cox R, Varghese A, Hoppe RT. Prognostic factors for patients relapsing after radiotherapy for early-stage Hodgkin's disease. *J Clin Oncol* 1990;8:623.
303. Specht L, Horwich A, Ashley S. Salvage of relapse of patients with Hodgkin's disease in clinical stages I or II who were staged with laparotomy and initially treated with radiotherapy alone. A report from the International Database on Hodgkin's Disease. *Int J Radiat Oncol Biol Phys* 1994;30:805.
304. Horwich A, Specht L, Ashley S. Survival analysis of patients with clinical stages I or II Hodgkin's disease who have relapsed after initial treatment with radiotherapy alone. *Eur J Cancer* 1997;33:848.
305. Portlock CS, Rosenberg SA, Glatstein E, Kaplan HS. Impact of salvage treatment on initial relapses in patients with Hodgkin disease, stages I–III. *Blood* 1978;51:825.
306. Herman TS, Hoppe RT, Donaldson SS, Cox RS, Rosenberg SA, Kaplan HS. Late relapse among patients treated for Hodgkin's disease. *Ann Intern Med* 1985;102:292.
307. Krikorian JG, Portlock CS, Rosenberg SA. Treatment of advanced Hodgkin's disease with Adriamycin, bleomycin, vinblastine, and imidazole carboxamide (ABVD) after failure of MOPP therapy. *Cancer* 1978;41:2107.
308. Fisher RI, DeVita VT, Hubbard SP, Simon R, Young RC. Prolonged disease-free survival in Hodgkin's disease with MOPP reinduction after first relapse. *Ann Intern Med* 1979;90:761.
309. Sutcliffe SB, Wrigley PFM, Stansfeld AG, Malpas JS. Adriamycin, bleomycin, vinblastine and imidazole carboxamide (ABVD) therapy for advanced Hodgkin's disease resistant to mustine, vinblastine, procarbazine and prednisolone (MVPP). *Cancer Chemother Pharmacol* 1979;2:209.
310. Santoro A, Bonfante V, Bonadonna G. Salvage chemotherapy with ABVD in MOPP-resistant Hodgkin's disease. *Ann Intern Med* 1982; 96:139.
311. Tannir N, Hagemeister F, Velasquez W, Cabanillas F. Long-term follow-up with ABDIC salvage chemotherapy of MOPP-resistant Hodgkin's disease. *J Clin Oncol* 1983;1:432.
312. Harker WG, Kushlan P, Rosenberg SA. Combination chemotherapy for advanced Hodgkin's disease after failure of MOPP: ABVD and B-CAVe. *Ann Intern Med* 1984;101:440.
313. Richards MA, Waxman JH, Man T, et al. EVA treatment for recurrent or unresponsive Hodgkin's disease. *Cancer Chemother Pharmacol* 1986;18:51.
314. Pfreundschuh MG, Schoppe WD, Fuchs R, Pflüger KH, Loeffler M, Diehl V. Lomustine, etoposide, vindesine, and dexamethasone (CEVD) in Hodgkin's lymphoma refractory to cyclophosphamide, vincristine, procarbazine, and prednisone (COPP) and doxorubicin, bleomycin, vinblastine, and dacarbazine (ABVD): a multicenter trial of the German Hodgkin Study Group. *Cancer Treat Rep* 1987;71:1203.
315. Schulman P, McCarroll K, Cooper MR, Norton L, Barcos M, Gottlieb AJ. Phase II study of MOPLACE chemotherapy for patients with previously treated Hodgkin's disease: a CALGB study. *Med Pediatr Oncol* 1990;18:482.
316. Enblad G, Glimelius B, Hagberg H, Lindemalm C. Methyl-GAG, ifosfamide, methotrexate and etoposide (MIME) as salvage therapy for Hodgkin's disease and non-Hodgkin's lymphoma. *Acta Oncol* 1990; 29:297.
317. Lohri A, Barnett M, Fairey RN, et al. Outcome of treatment of first relapse of Hodgkin's disease after primary chemotherapy: identification of risk factors from the British Columbia experience 1970 to 1988. *Blood* 1991;77:2292.
318. Longo DL, Duffey PL, Young RC, et al. Conventional-dose salvage combination chemotherapy in patients relapsing with Hodgkin's disease after combination chemotherapy: the low probability for cure. *J Clin Oncol* 1992;10:210.
319. Canellos GP, Petroni GR, Barcos M, Duggan DB, Peterson BA for the Cancer and Leukemia Group B. Etoposide, vinblastine, and doxorubicin: an active regimen for the treatment of Hodgkin's disease in relapse following MOPP. *J Clin Oncol* 1995;13:2005.
320. Brice P, Bastion Y, Divine M, et al. Analysis of prognostic factors after the first relapse of Hodgkin's disease in 187 patients. *Cancer* 1996;78: 1293.
321. Fermé C, Bastion Y, Lepage E, et al. The MINE regimen as intensive salvage chemotherapy for relapsed and refractory Hodgkin's disease. *Ann Oncol* 1995;6:543.
322. Bonfante V, Santoro A, Viviani S, et al. Outcome of patients with Hodgkin's disease failing after primary MOPP-ABVD. *J Clin Oncol* 1997;15:528.
323. Straus DJ, Passe S, Koziner B, Lee BJ, Young CW, Clarkson BD. Combination chemotherapy salvage of heavily pretreated patients with Hodgkin's disease: an analysis of prognostic factors in two chemotherapy trials and the literature. *Cancer Treat Rep* 1981;65:207.
324. Straus DJ, Myers J, Koziner B, Lee BJ, Clarkson BD. Combination chemotherapy for the treatment of Hodgkin's disease in relapse. Results with lomustine (CCNU), melphalan (Alkeran), and vindesine (DVA) alone (CAD) and in alternation with MOPP and doxorubicin (Adriamycin), bleomycin, and vinblastine (ABV). *Cancer Chemother Pharmacol* 1983;11:80.
325. Perren TJ, Selby PJ, Milan S, Meldrum M, McElwain TJ. Etoposide and Adriamycin containing combination chemotherapy (HOPE-Bleo) for relapsed Hodgkin's disease. *Br J Cancer* 1990;61:919.
326. Hagemeister FB, Tannir N, McLaughlin P, et al. MIME chemotherapy (methyl-GAG, ifosfamide, methotrexate, etoposide) as treatment for recurrent Hodgkin's disease. *J Clin Oncol* 1987;5:556.
327. Fairey AF, Mead GM, Jones HW, Sweetenham JW, Whitehouse JMA. CAPE/PALE salvage chemotherapy for Hodgkin's disease patients relapsing within 1 year of ChlVPP chemotherapy. *Ann Oncol* 1993;4: 857.
328. Viviani S, Santoro A, Negretti E, Bonfante V, Valagussa P, Bonadonna G. Salvage chemotherapy in Hodgkin's disease. Results in patients relapsing more than twelve months after first complete remission. *Ann Oncol* 1990;1:123.
329. Salvagno L, Soraru M, Aversa SML, et al. Late relapses in Hodgkin's disease: outcome of patients relapsing more than twelve months after primary chemotherapy. *Ann Oncol* 1993;4:657.

330. Mauch P, Tarbell N, Skarin A, Rosenthal D, Weinstein H. Wide-field radiation therapy alone or with chemotherapy for Hodgkin's disease in relapse from combination chemotherapy. *J Clin Oncol* 1987;5:544.
331. Roach M, Kapp DS, Rosenberg SA, Hoppe RT. Radiotherapy with curative intent: an option in selected patients relapsing after chemotherapy for advanced Hodgkin's disease. *J Clin Oncol* 1987; 5:550.
332. Fox KA, Lippman SM, Cassady JR, Heusinkveld RS, Miller TP. Radiation therapy salvage of Hodgkin's disease following chemotherapy failure. *J Clin Oncol* 1987;5:38.
333. Kirkove C, Timothy AR. Radiotherapy as salvage treatment in patients with Hodgkin's disease or non-Hodgkin's lymphoma relapsing after initial chemotherapy. *Hematol Oncol* 1991;9:163.
334. Brada M, Eeles R, Ashley S, Nichols J, Horwich A. Salvage radiotherapy in recurrent Hodgkin's disease. *Ann Oncol* 1992;3:131.
335. Uematsu M, Tarbell NJ, Silver B, et al. Wide-field radiation therapy with or without chemotherapy for patients with Hodgkin disease in relapse after initial combination chemotherapy. *Cancer* 1993;72:207.
336. Leigh BR, Fox KA, Mack CF, Baier M, Miller TP, Cassady JR. Radiation salvage of Hodgkin's disease following chemotherapy failure. *Int J Radiat Oncol Biol Phys* 1993;27:855.
337. Pezner RD, Lipsett JA, Vora N, Forman SJ. Radical radiotherapy as salvage treatment for relapse of Hodgkin's disease initially treated by chemotherapy alone: prognostic significance of the disease-free interval. *Int J Radiat Oncol Biol Phys* 1994;30:965.
338. MacMillan CH, Bessell EM. The effectiveness of radiotherapy for localized relapse in patients with Hodgkin's disease (IIB–IVB) who obtained a complete response with chemotherapy alone as initial treatment. *Clin Oncol* 1994;6:147.
339. O'Brien PC, Parnis FX. Salvage radiotherapy following chemotherapy failure in Hodgkin's disease—what is its role? *Acta Oncol* 1995; 34:99.
340. Wirth A, Corry J, Laidlaw C, Matthews J, Liew KH. Salvage radiotherapy for Hodgkin's disease following chemotherapy failure. *Int J Radiat Oncol Biol Phys* 1997;39:599.
341. Linch DC, Winfield D, Goldstone AH, et al. Dose intensification with autologous bone-marrow transplantation in relapsed and resistant Hodgkin's disease: results of a BNLI randomised trial. *Lancet* 1993; 341:1051.
342. Yahalom J, Gulati SC, Toia M, et al. Accelerated hyperfractionated total-lymphoid irradiation, high-dose chemotherapy, and autologous bone marrow transplantation for refractory and relapsing patients with Hodgkin's disease. *J Clin Oncol* 1993;11:1062.
343. Ager S, Wimperis JZ, Tolliday B, et al. Autologous bone marrow transplantation for Hodgkin's disease—a five-year single centre experience. *Leuk Lymphoma* 1994;13:263.
344. Reece DE, Phillips GL. Intensive therapy and autologous stem cell transplantation for Hodgkin's disease in first relapse after combination chemotherapy. *Leuk Lymphoma* 1996;21:245.
345. Bierman PJ, Anderson JR, Freeman MB, et al. High-dose chemotherapy followed by autologous hematopoietic rescue for Hodgkin's disease patients following first relapse after chemotherapy. *Ann Oncol* 1996;7:151.
346. Jagannath S, Armitage JO, Dicke KA, et al. Prognostic factors for response and survival after high-dose cyclophosphamide, carmustine, and etoposide with autologous bone marrow transplantation for relapsed Hodgkin's disease. *J Clin Oncol* 1989;7:179.
347. Jones RJ, Piantadosi S, Mann RB, et al. High-dose cytotoxic therapy and bone marrow transplantation for relapsed Hodgkin's disease. *J Clin Oncol* 1990;8:527.
348. Anderson JE, Litzow MR, Appelbaum FR, et al. Allogeneic, syngeneic, and autologous marrow transplantation for Hodgkin's disease: the 21-year Seattle experience. *J Clin Oncol* 1993;11:2342.
349. Bierman PJ, Bagin RG, Jagannath S, et al. High dose chemotherapy followed by autologous hematopoietic rescue in Hodgkin's disease: long term follow-up in 128 patients. *Ann Oncol* 1993;4:767.
350. Chopra R, McMillan AK, Linch DC, et al. The place of high-dose BEAM therapy and autologous bone marrow transplantation in poor-risk Hodgkin's disease. A single-center eight-year study of 155 patients. *Blood* 1993;81:1137.
351. Nademanee A, O'Donnell MR, Snyder DS, et al. High-dose chemotherapy with or without total body irradiation followed by autologous bone marrow and/or peripheral blood stem cell transplantation for patients with relapsed and refractory Hodgkin's disease: results in 85 patients with analysis of prognostic factors. *Blood* 1995; 85:1381.
352. O'Brien MER, Milan S, Cunningham D, et al. High-dose chemotherapy and autologous bone marrow transplant in relapsed Hodgkin's disease—a pragmatic prognostic index. *Br J Cancer* 1996;73:1272.
353. Harding M, Selby P, Gore M, et al. High-dose chemotherapy and autologous bone marrow transplantation for relapsed and refractory Hodgkin's disease. *Eur J Cancer* 1992;28A,1396.
354. Poen JC, Hoppe RT, Horning SJ. High-dose therapy and autologous bone marrow transplantation for relapsed/refractory Hodgkin's disease: the impact of involved field radiotherapy on patterns of failure and survival. *Int J Radiat Oncol Biol Phys* 1996;36:3.
355. Crump M, Smith AM, Brandwein J, et al. High-dose etoposide and melphalan, and autologous bone marrow transplantation for patients with advanced Hodgkin's disease: importance of disease status at transplant. *J Clin Oncol* 1993;11:704.
356. Rapoport AP, Rowe JM, Kouides PA, et al. One hundred autotransplants for relapsed or refractory Hodgkin's disease and lymphoma: value of pretransplant disease status for predicting outcome. *J Clin Oncol* 1993;11:2351.
357. Lumley MA, Milligan DW, Knechtli CJC, Long SG, Billingham LJ, McDonald DF. High lactate dehydrogenase level is associated with an adverse outlook in autografting for Hodgkin's disease. *Bone Marrow Transplant* 1996;17:383.
358. Reece DE, Barnett MJ, Connors JM, et al. Intensive chemotherapy with cyclophosphamide, carmustine, and etoposide followed by autologous bone marrow transplantation for relapsed Hodgkin's disease. *J Clin Oncol* 1991;9:1871.
359. Williams CD, Goldstone AH, Pearce R, et al. Autologous bone marrow transplantation for pediatric Hodgkin's disease: a case-matched comparison with adult patients by the European Bone Marrow Transplant Group Lymphoma Registry. *J Clin Oncol* 1993;11:2243.
360. Begg CB. Selection of patients for clinical trials. *Semin Oncol* 1988; 15:434.
361. Peto R. Clinical trial methodology. *Biomedicine* 1978;28:24.
362. Peto R, Pike MC, Armitage P, et al. Design and analysis of randomized clinical trials requiring prolonged observation of each patient. I. Introduction and design. *Br J Cancer* 1976;34:585.
363. Peto R, Pike MC, Armitage P, et al. Design and analysis of randomized clinical trials requiring prolonged observation of each patient. II. Analysis and examples. *Br J Cancer* 1977;35:1.
364. Schmoor C, Schumacher M. Effects of covariate omission and categorization when analysing randomized trials with the Cox model. *Stat Med* 1997;16:225.
365. Noordijk EM, Carde P, Mandard AM, et al. Preliminary results of the EORTC-GPMC controlled clinical trial H_7 in early-stage Hodgkin's disease. EORTC Lymphoma Cooperative Group. Groupe Pierre-et-Marie-Curie. *Ann Oncol* 1994;5(Suppl 2):107.
366. Bates NP, Williams MV, Bessell EM, Vaughan Hudson G, Vaughan Hudson B. Efficacy and toxicity of vinblastine, bleomycin, and methotrexate with involved-field radiotherapy in clinical stage IA and IIA Hodgkin's disease: a British National Lymphoma Investigation pilot study. *J Clin Oncol* 1994;12:288.
367. Pavlovsky S, Schvartzman E, Lastiri F, et al. Randomized trial of CVPP for three versus six cycles in favorable-prognosis and CVPP versus AOPE plus radiotherapy in intermediate-prognosis untreated Hodgkin's disease. *J Clin Oncol* 1997;15:2652.
368. Proctor SJ, Taylor PR. Classical staging of Hodgkin's disease is inappropriate for selecting patients for clinical trials of intensive therapy: the case for the objective use of prognostic factor information in addition to classical staging. *Leukemia* 1993;7:1911.
369. Horning SJ, Hoppe RT, Mason J, et al. Stanford-Kaiser Permanente G1 study for clinical stage I to IIA Hodgkin's disease: subtotal lymphoid irradiation versus vinblastine, methotrexate, and bleomycin chemotherapy and regional irradiation. *J Clin Oncol* 1997;15:1736.
370. Raemaekers J, Burgers M, Henry-Amar M, et al. Patients with stage III/IV Hodgkin's disease in partial remission after MOPP/ABV chemotherapy have excellent prognosis after additional involved-field radiotherapy: interim results from the ongoing EORTC-LCG and GPMC phase III trial. The EORTC Lymphoma Cooperative Group and Groupe Pierre-et-Marie-Curie. *Ann Oncol* 1997;8(Suppl 1):111.
371. Viviani S, Bonadonna G, Santoro A, et al. Alternating versus hybrid

MOPP and ABVD combinations in advanced Hodgkin's disease: ten-year results. *J Clin Oncol* 1996;14:1421.
372. Longo DL, Duffey PL, DeVita VT, et al. Treatment of advanced-stage Hodgkin's disease: alternating noncrossresistant MOPP/CABS is not superior to MOPP. *J Clin Oncol* 1991;9:1409.
373. Fabian CJ, Mansfield CM, Dahlberg S, et al. Low-dose involved field radiation after chemotherapy in advanced Hodgkin disease. A Southwest Oncology Group randomized study. *Ann Intern Med* 1994;120:903.
374. Horning SJ, Rosenberg SA, Hoppe RT. Brief chemotherapy (Stanford V) and adjuvant radiotherapy for bulky or advanced Hodgkin's disease: an update. *Ann Oncol* 1996;7(Suppl 4):105.

Hodgkin's Disease, edited by P. M. Mauch,
J. O. Armitage, V. Diehl, R. T. Hoppe, and L. M. Weiss.
Lippincott Williams & Wilkins, Philadephia ©1999.

CHAPTER 20

Unusual Syndromes in Hodgkin's Disease

Philip J. Bierman, Franco Cavalli, and James O. Armitage

Painless lymphadenopathy is the most common physical finding associated with Hodgkin's disease. However, a number of unusual manifestations of disease, unrelated to direct histologic involvement, may also be present at diagnosis or relapse. In some cases, these symptoms may be more distressing and life-threatening than Hodgkin's disease itself. Such manifestations may be present for long periods of time and lead to extensive evaluations before the underlying diagnosis of Hodgkin's disease is made. This chapter discusses some of the unusual syndromes associated with Hodgkin's disease.

SYSTEMIC SYMPTOMS

The presence of constitutional symptoms such as fever, weight loss, night sweats, pruritus, malaise, and weakness have been noted since the earliest descriptions of Hodgkin's disease. Early investigators recognized that these symptoms had prognostic significance and felt that their presence should be recorded in a systematic manner. The need for a standardized clinical staging system for Hodgkin's disease led to the development of the Rye staging system, which subclassified each stage as A or B to indicate the absence or presence of fever, night sweats, and pruritus (1). Later reports demonstrated the adverse prognostic significance of fever, night sweats, and weight loss, but they failed to document any adverse prognosis associated with pruritus (2). These findings led to the development of the commonly used Ann Arbor staging system, in which pruritus was no longer considered to be a B symptom (3). In this staging system, systemic symptoms consisted of (a) unexplained weight loss of more than 10% of body weight in the previous 6 months, (b) unexplained fever with temperatures above 38°, and (c) night sweats.

Fever was noted at the time of of diagnosis of Hodgkin's disease in 27% of patients at Stanford University (4), and it has been noted with higher frequency in other reports (5). Fever may be present for long periods of time and lead to prolonged evaluations and multiple courses of empiric antibiotic treatment before Hodgkin's disease is diagnosed. This diagnosis should be considered in any patient with fever of unknown origin. Fevers may be continuous or intermittent. They may be low-grade or may exceed 40°. Tachycardia frequently accompanies fever. Patients may be asymptomatic, or fevers may be associated with a sensation of discomfort or extreme fatigue. The classic Pel-Ebstein fever (Fig. 1) consists of cyclic episodes of high fevers lasting for 1 or 2 weeks, followed by afebrile periods of similar duration (6,7). This presentation is now rarely seen, but it may be the initial manifestation of relapse (8). Fevers invariably remit with the institution of treatment for Hodgkin's disease, and failure of fever to remit in the presence of responding disease should prompt a search for other causes of fever. Fevers also remit with administration of nonsteroidal antiinflammatory agents (9). Night sweats may take the form of mild dampness around the neck, but they are generally considered to be significant only if drenching in nature (4). Patients frequently report the need to change bedclothes or linens because of sweating. Night sweats may occur independently of other systemic symptoms but are usually accompanied by fevers (10). The etiology of night sweats is presumably related to defervescence. A slight rise in body temperature has been reported in the 30 minutes before sweating in patients with Hodgkin's disease (11).

The etiology of fever in Hodgkin's disease is uncertain and has been related to host immune response, lymph node necrosis, and damaged stromal cells (12). A variety

P. J. Bierman and J. O. Armitage: Department of Internal Medicine, Section of Oncology and Hematology, University of Nebraska, Omaha, Nebraska.

F. Cavalli: Division of Oncology, Ospedale San Giovanni, Bellinzona, Switzerland.

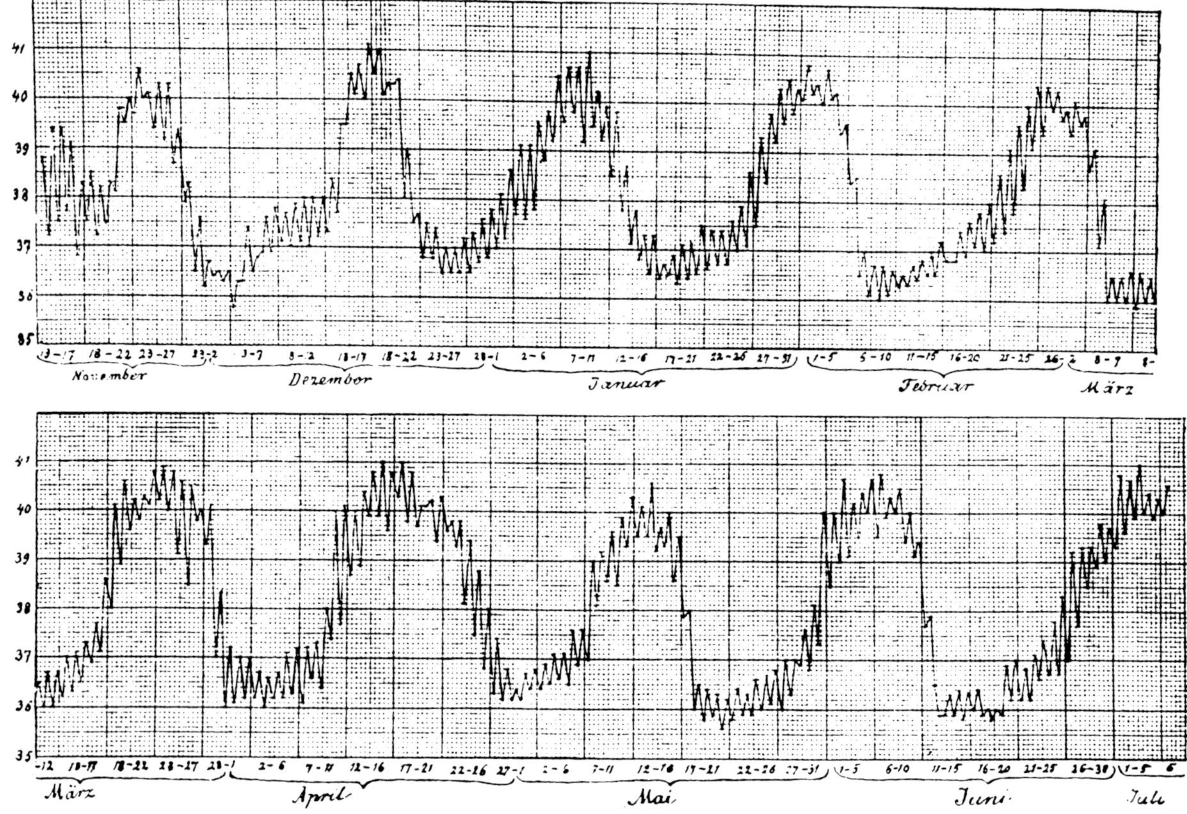

FIG. 1. Pel-Ebstein fever. (From ref. 6.)

of cytokines have been isolated from cell lines established from lymph nodes of patients with Hodgkin's disease (13). Patterns of cytokine expression are highly variable, but those most frequently produced include interleukin-6 (IL-6), tumor necrosis factor-α (TNF-α), and TNF-β (13). Other investigators have failed to find high levels of TNF protein expression in lymph nodes from patients with Hodgkin's disease, although nodes showed high levels of lymphotoxin expression (14). Variations in lymphokine expression, even among morphologically similar lymph nodes, have been noted by other investigators, although IL-1β expression correlated with systemic symptoms (15). Although elevated levels of serum IL-1α have been noted in Hodgkin's disease, cytokine levels did not correlate with B symptoms (16). Elevated serum levels of IL-6 have been associated with adverse prognostic factors and clinical outcomes, although the relation to systemic symptoms has been variable (17,18).

The presence of B symptoms is associated with adverse outcome (19) and continues to be included in newer staging systems (20). Patients who have all three B symptoms have poorer survival when compared with patients who have one or two symptoms (21). Night sweats may be less important than other systemic symptoms (2,10,21).

PRURITUS

Pruritus may be a symptom of renal disease, cholestatic liver disease, diabetes, and thyroid disorders. It is also seen in patients with polycythemia vera and is frequently a manifestation of AIDS. Systemic disease is ultimately identified in 30% of patients with unexplained itching, and 1% to 11% will have malignancies (22). Mild itching may be seen in 15% to 25% of patients with Hodgkin's disease, although severe itching is less common (4,23). Itching has been reported to occur in as many as 85% of patients at some time in the course of disease (5). Pruritus is generally more common in patients with advanced-stage disease and frequently accompanies other systemic symptoms (4,23). Itching may be more common in women (4). Itching associated with Hodgkin's disease is usually generalized and may be severe enough that excoriations are produced from scratching. Itching may be the first manifestation of Hodgkin's disease, and patients may visit several physicians before lymphoma is diagnosed. It is not unusual for patients with unexplained itching to be referred to a psychiatrist before a diagnosis of Hodgkin's disease is made (24). Patients with Hodgkin's disease may have itching related to cholestasis or to medications. In addition, various dermatologic manifestations of Hodgkin's disease may cause pruritus (*vide infra*). Finally, other causes of itching, such as scabies infection, which may mimic symptoms of active disease, should be considered in the differential diagnosis of pruritus in patients with Hodgkin's disease (25).

Although some early reports suggested that itching is not associated with poorer survival in patients with Hodgkin's disease (2,4), others have suggested that patients with significant pruritus do have inferior overall survival and that the importance of pruritus is similar to that of other B symptoms (23,24). Nonspecific therapy for itching is generally ineffective, although pruritus resolves when Hodgkin's disease is treated (23,24). Return of itching in treated patients may be the initial symptom of relapse (24).

The etiology of itching is poorly understood, although reports of resolution of itching accompanying spinal cord compression suggest that there may be a peripheral origin, with transmission of itching sensations through spinothalamic tracts (26).

CUTANEOUS MANIFESTATIONS

Cutaneous manifestations of Hodgkin's disease may appear in several forms (Table 1). Primary cutaneous Hodgkin's disease is felt to be a rare disorder (27). These patients may have an indolent course, and conservative treatment has been recommended. Lesions in these patients must be distinguished from those of other disorders, such as lymphomatoid papulosis and cutaneous T-cell lymphoma (27,28), which may contain cells that are morphologically similar to Reed-Sternberg cells. Furthermore, lymphomatoid papulosis may evolve into Hodgkin's disease. Cutaneous involvement of Hodgkin's disease associated with nodal sites of disease occurs in 0.5% to 7.5% of cases (29,30). Skin involvement in these patients is felt to be caused by obstruction of regional lymphatics, direct extension from underlying nodes, or hematogenous dissemination (29). Lesions usually consist of erythematous nodules or papules, which may ulcerate. These lesions may be a direct extension of nodal areas of involvement or may appear at distant sites. Lesions are most common on the trunk but may appear anywhere on the body. Dermal involvement of Hodgkin's disease is often accompanied by extensive involvement at other sites and has been associated with a poor prognosis (29).

TABLE 1. *Cutaneous manifestations of Hodgkin's disease*

Specific skin lesions
Primary cutaneous Hodgkin's disease
Lymphomatoid papulosis
Nonspecific skin lesions
Paraneoplastic lesions
Infections (e.g., varicella-zoster)

From ref. 31.

A large number of nonspecific erythematous, urticarial, vesicular, and bullous cutaneous manifestations of Hodgkin's disease have been described (31), mostly in case reports and small series. In some cases, these lesions are felt to represent a true paraneoplastic phenomenon, as they may be present at the time of diagnosis and remit with therapy. Reappearance of the lesions after treatment has heralded relapse. In other cases, the simultaneous appearance of skin lesions in association with Hodgkin's disease may be coincidental. It is postulated that cytokines secreted by tumor cells or accessory cells are responsible for the development of cutaneous paraneoplastic syndromes (31).

Erythema nodosum consists of inflammatory nodules that appear most commonly on the anterior surface of the legs. These lesions are usually associated with infections, drugs, or inflammatory bowel disease, but they have also been described in association with Hodgkin's disease (32). The lesions may be seen several months before relapse and respond to chemotherapy. Icthyosiform atrophy of the skin has also been associated with Hodgkin's disease and appears to respond to treatment for Hodgkin's disease (33). Acrokeratosis paraneoplastica is a paraneoplastic dermatosis most commonly associated with carcinomas of the lung or upper gastrointestinal system. This disorder has also been described in Hodgkin's disease and is reported to respond to chemotherapy (34). Granulomatous slack skin is a disorder associated with Hodgkin's disease as well as non-Hodgkin's lymphoma (35). Erythematous lesions gradually evolve into areas of pendulous skin. Although Hodgkin's disease responds to therapy, skin lesions do not usually regress. The multiple nevoid basal cell carcinoma is usually associated with solid tumors, although this syndrome has also been reported in association with Hodgkin's disease (36). Other skin lesions reported to occur in association with Hodgkin's disease and that regress with therapy include erythema annulare centrifugum (37), granulomatous dermohypodermitis (38), prurigo nodularis (39), and follicular mucinosis (40). The necrobiotic xanthogranuloma syndrome (41) and psoriasiform lesions (31) have also been described in association with Hodgkin's disease.

In addition to cutaneous lesions, nail changes have also been described in patients with Hodgkin's disease. One such abnormality consists of transverse white lines, which may be associated with poor prognosis (42). Hypertrophic osteoarthropathy has been reported to occur in patients with pulmonary and mediastinal Hodgkin's disease (43,44).

NEUROLOGIC MANIFESTATIONS

Neurologic manifestations of Hodgkin's disease are unusual and may be caused by parenchymal disease, meningeal disease, spinal cord compression, therapy-induced leukoencephalopathy, or central nervous system infection. In addition, neuropathies may be seen with administration of vinca alkaloids and following radiation therapy. However, a number of paraneoplastic manifestations that are relatively specific for Hodgkin's disease have been described (Table 2) (45). These syndromes are usually associated with autoimmunity, and it is postulated that tumor cells express antigens that are similar to molecules on neurons (46). It is thought that an autoimmune response arises against the tumor antigens and that this response spills over to attack normal neuronal tissue expressing similar antigens.

Paraneoplastic cerebellar degeneration is a condition associated with Hodgkin's disease and also with solid tumors, such as breast, lung and ovarian carcinomas (47, 48). The abrupt or subacute onset of gait ataxia is generally the initial complaint. Other symptoms include dysarthria, nystagmus, and diplopia. The onset of symptoms may precede the diagnosis of Hodgkin's disease by months or years (Fig. 2). Male patients are predominantly affected. In some cases, the onset of symptoms may herald a recurrence of lymphoma. Treatment is generally ineffective, although disease may stabilize, and improvements with plasma exchange or treatment for Hodgkin's disease have been reported (46,48,49).

The brains of patients with paraneoplastic cerebellar degeneration exhibit a diffuse loss of Purkinje cells throughout the cerebellar cortex (48). Serum antibodies directed against human and rodent Purkinje cells may be identified in patients with Hodgkin's disease who have cerebellar degeneration, although fewer than 50% have detectable antibodies (48,49). These antibodies are distinct from the anti-Yo and anti-Hu antibodies described in patients with breast, ovarian, and small-cell lung carcinomas. Antibody-negative patients may be slightly more likely to show neurologic improvement than patients with detectable anti-Purkinje cell antibodies in serum (46,48).

Limbic encephalitis is a syndrome of memory loss and amnesia. Anti-Hu antibodies have been described in patients who exhibit this syndrome in association with small-cell lung carcinoma (46). Limbic encephalitis has been described in association with Hodgkin's disease and may be reversible following chemotherapy (50).

Subacute myelopathy has rarely been associated with Hodgkin's disease (51). Most cases have been identified at autopsy and have been associated with spinal cord necrosis.

TABLE 2. *Paraneoplastic neurologic manifestations of Hodgkin's disease*

Subacute cerebellar degeneration
Limbic encephalitis
Subacute necrotic myelopathy
Subacute motor neuropathy

From ref. 45.

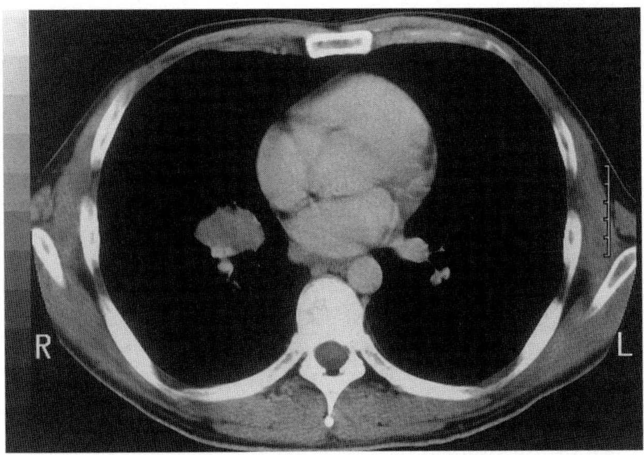

FIG. 2. Computed tomogram from a 31-year-old man with subacute cerebellar degeneration. Progressive diplopia, dysarthria, and ataxia developed in this patient in October 1994. In March 1995, his serum was found to contain anti-Purkinje cell antibodies and a right hilar mass was identified. Biopsy revealed nodular sclerosis Hodgkin's disease, and the patient achieved remission after combination chemotherapy. The patient remains in remission, although there has been no improvement in his neurologic status.

Subacute motor neuropathy associated with Hodgkin's disease is characterized by progressive, painless lower motor neuron weakness (52). The course of the disease is independent of Hodgkin's disease, and most patients stabilize or improve spontaneously. Motor neuron disease indistinguishable from amyotrophic lateral sclerosis has also been described in Hodgkin's disease (45,53). Patients have normal findings on nerve conduction studies and no sensory loss. Postmortem examination demonstrates loss of motor neurons in the spinal cord, brainstem, and motor cortex. Neurologic improvement after treatment of Hodgkin's disease is unusual.

Hodgkin's disease may also be associated with neuropathies involving peripheral nerves (54,55) and cranial nerves (54). These patients may respond to corticosteroids or Hodgkin's disease treatment. Other neurologic disorders that have been reported to occur in association with Hodgkin's disease include Guillain-Barré syndrome (56,57) and central pontine myelinolysis (58). Stiff-man syndrome has also been described in patients with Hodgkin's disease (46,59,60). This syndrome may be associated with autoantibodies and may remit after treatment of Hodgkin's disease (46,60). Opsoclonus (46), chorea (61), and autonomic dysfunction leading to orthostatic hypotension (62) have also been reported as paraneoplastic complications of Hodgkin's disease.

RENAL MANIFESTATIONS

Autopsy series have demonstrated that Hodgkin's disease may directly involve the kidney in as many as 13% of cases (63). Renal involvement may be unilateral or bilateral and may be present as diffuse involvement, discrete nodules, or microscopic disease. Renal involvement with Hodgkin's disease may go unrecognized, although parenchymal disease and ureteral obstruction may result in loss of function. Patients with Hodgkin's disease may also have renal dysfunction related to renal vein thrombosis, hypercalcemia, and hyperuricemia.

In addition to these direct and indirect effects on the kidney, Hodgkin's disease may be associated with glomerulonephritis. Although membranous nephropathy is generally associated with carcinomas, patients with Hodgkin's disease most commonly have minimal-change disease (64). However, membranous glomerulonephritis, focal glomerulosclerosis, membranoproliferative glomerulonephritis, proliferative glomerulonephritis, and crescentic glomerulonephritis have all been described in patients with Hodgkin's disease (65–67). Glomerulonephritis may also be associated with antiglomerular basement membrane antibody (67), or immune complex deposition with immunoglobulin and C3 (68).

Nephrotic syndrome generally occurs early in the course of disease and may predate the diagnosis of Hodgkin's disease (65,68). Patients with Hodgkin's disease and nephrotic syndrome frequently have mixed-cellularity histology (64). Nephrotic syndrome uniformly remits with successful treatment of Hodgkin's disease, even when radiation is used as the only means of therapy (68). Proteinuria will often return in association with relapse of Hodgkin's disease; however, nephrotic syndrome associated with minimal-change disease or other glomerulopathies may occur following successful treatment of Hodgkin's disease without relapse (69,70). In addition, minimal-change nephropathy may remit spontaneously in the face of Hodgkin's disease relapse (71).

The etiology of minimal-change disease in the setting of Hodgkin's disease is unknown. It is postulated that humoral factors produced by neoplastic cells may increase vascular permeability. Other investigators have suggested that disordered T-cell function may play a role in pathogenesis. The identity of the antigen associated with immune complex glomerulopathy is also unknown, although there is some evidence that virus-related antigens may play a role (68).

In addition to glomerulonephritis, amyloidosis has been associated with nephrotic syndrome in patients with Hodgkin's disease (65–68). Although common in the past, this association appears to be decreasing in frequency.

HEMATOLOGIC MANIFESTATIONS

A variety of hematologic abnormalities are associated with Hodgkin's disease. Myelosuppression in Hodgkin's disease may be caused by hypersplenism or bone marrow infiltration; however, some abnormalities have a clearly defined immunologic basis.

A positive Coombs' test result may be found at the time of diagnosis of Hodgkin's disease or at the time of relapse (72). A positive Coombs' test result may or may not be associated with overt hemolysis. Patients with a positive Coombs' test frequently have advanced-stage disease and systemic symptoms, although prognosis may or may not be poor. Other patients may have a hemolytic anemia that has been present for months before diagnosis, and these patients may have limited-stage disease (73,74). Cyclic hemolysis with exacerbations coinciding with Pel-Ebstein fever has been described (75).

Chemotherapy results in the fall of antibody titers and resolution of hemolysis, although other modalities, such as splenectomy, may also be successful. Recurrence of hemolysis may accompany relapse.

The antibody in patients with autoimmune hemolytic anemia and Hodgkin's disease is usually reactive against immunoglobulin G and C3. In one study, antibodies with anti-I^t specificity were identified (72).

Immune thrombocytopenia may accompany Hodgkin's disease in 1% to 2% of cases (76), and it may occur in association with autoimmune hemolytic anemia. Thrombocytopenia may develop before, concurrently with, or after the diagnosis of Hodgkin's disease (76,77). Immune thrombocytopenia may occur in patients with limited- or advanced-stage disease and with all histologic subtypes. Thrombocytopenia frequently occurs in patients in remission after Hodgkin's disease treatment, and the development of thrombocytopenia is not usually associated with relapse (76,77). The simultaneous appearance of immune thrombocytopenia and Hodgkin's disease may represent a chance occurrence.

The treatment of immune thrombocytopenia in patients with Hodgkin's disease should be approached in the same manner as in patients without malignancy. The response to therapy is similar to that of other patients, although corticosteroids or splenectomy alone is less likely to be beneficial in the presence of active lymphoma (77,78). Thrombotic thrombocytopenic purpura has also been described in Hodgkin's disease, and microangiopathic hemolytic anemia must be considered in any patient with thrombocytopenia (79).

Autoimmune neutropenia has also been described in patients with Hodgkin's disease (80–82). Neutropenia may occur before diagnosis and in patients who are apparently cured of lymphoma. Bone marrow aplasia in patients with Hodgkin's disease has been reported and may respond to therapy (83).

Eosinophilia is frequently associated with Hodgkin's disease. This complication was noted in 15% of patients who were entered in clinical trials conducted by the British National Lymphoma Investigation (84). Eosinophilia in the absence of general leukocytosis was associated with improved survival. The presence of eosinophilia does not appear to be related to stage or histology (85). *In situ* hybridization studies have demonstrated IL-5 production by Reed-Sternberg cells, which may explain the etiology of eosinophilia accompanying Hodgkin's disease (86).

Deficiencies of coagulation factors VII and XII in a patient with Hodgkin's disease have been reported (87). Reduction of factor levels was associated with disease progression, and levels returned to normal following successful treatment with both radiation and chemotherapy.

ENDOCRINE AND METABOLIC MANIFESTATIONS

The most common endocrine abnormality associated with Hodgkin's disease is hypercalcemia (88,89). The reported incidence of hypercalcemia in patients with Hodgkin's disease has ranged between 1% and 5% (89). Hypercalcemia is frequently associated with advanced stage and poor prognostic features, although hypercalcemia may accompany limited-stage disease. Bone involvement is unusual in patients with hypercalcemia. Little information on the prognostic significance of hypercalcemia is available, although long-term survival has been described and serum calcium levels return to normal with treatment.

The etiology of hypercalcemia in Hodgkin's disease appears to be related to altered levels of 1,25-$(OH)_2$-D_3 (calcitriol) levels in almost all cases (88,89). Elevated calcitriol levels and hypercalcemia may be associated with relapses, and levels will return to normal following chemotherapy (90). Infiltrating nonmalignant macrophages are felt to be the source of excess calcitriol. In some cases, hypercalcemia may be related to excess production of parathyroid hormone related-peptide (91), and reports of normalization of calcium levels with indomethacin suggest that prostaglandin synthesis may play a role in some cases of hypercalcemia (92).

Two cases of hypoglycemia caused by insulin receptor antibodies in patients with Hodgkin's disease have been described (93,94). In one case, immune hemolytic anemia had previously been described, and relapse of Hodgkin's disease was diagnosed after the onset of hypoglycemia (94).

The development of lactic acidosis at the time of Hodgkin's disease relapse has been described (95). Chemotherapy resolved the metabolic abnormality. Other metabolic abnormalities associated with Hodgkin's disease include hypouricemia (96) and syndrome of inappropriate secretion of antidiuretic hormone (97).

ALCOHOL-INDUCED PAIN

One of the most unusual syndromes associated with Hodgkin's disease is alcohol-induced pain. This symptom has been reported to occur in fewer than 5% of cases (4), and it may be less common in recent years (98). The pain may begin within minutes of ingestion and usually occurs in areas of nodal enlargement. Pain may occur in the chest with radiation to the arms, back, and legs (99). The pain may abate in minutes or rarely after several hours (99–100). Patients will frequently discontinue alcohol because of the discomfort. Symptoms may be elicited after ingestion of even small amounts of alcohol (99,101). The onset of alcohol-induced pain may precede the diagnosis of Hodgkin's disease by a long period of time (102). The pain diminishes with treatment of Hodgkin's disease and may recur before other signs or symptoms of relapse. In addition to pain, other symptoms, such as itching, flushing, nausea and vomiting, coughing, and dizziness, may be associated with alcohol ingestion (99). Although generally considered to be a syndrome that is relatively specific for Hodgkin's disease, alcohol-induced pain has been described in a wide variety of malignant conditions, as well as in nonmalignant conditions that may mimic Hodgkin's disease (101).

The mechanism of alcohol-induced pain is unknown, but edema of lesions, vasodilation, and release of histamine have been proposed as causes (101). It is interesting that pain may be elicited by intravenous as well as oral alcohol (99,100). Pain may also be blocked by administration of antihistamines (101).

MISCELLANEOUS ABNORMALITIES

A variety of miscellaneous abnormalities, in addition to those previously described, have been seen in association with Hodgkin's disease. Jaundice in patients with Hodgkin's disease may result from hepatic involvement, extrahepatic obstruction, infections, drugs, or hemolysis. Unexplained cholestasis has been described in several patients with Hodgkin's disease (103). Liver biopsies revealed cholestasis, and no evidence of extrahepatic obstruction was identified. Liver function normalized following mantle radiation. In other cases, cholestasis persisted following radiation therapy (104). The syndrome of adult bile ductopenia has also been described as a paraneoplastic complication of Hodgkin's disease (105). Chemotherapy resulted in morphologic and clinical improvement.

Patients with Hodgkin's disease frequently have noncaseating granulomas in uninvolved tissues as well as in those containing lymphoma (106). This finding may be associated with improved survival. Granulomatous angiitis of the brain (107) has been described in association with Hodgkin's disease, as has granulomatous angiitis of the spinal cord (108). A case of granulomatous uveitis in a patient with noncaseating splenic granulomas has also been reported (109). Uveitis persisted after successful lymphoma treatment.

Both polymyositis and scleroderma have been associated with Hodgkin's disease (110). Response of these conditions to therapy was poor. Hodgkin's disease has been associated with aortitis (111) and hypertension (112).

Blood pressure normalized when chemotherapy was initiated and then rose when Hodgkin's disease recurred.

REFERENCES

1. Rosenberg SA. Report of the committee on the staging of Hodgkin's disease. *Cancer Res* 1966;26:1310.
2. Tubiana M, Attié E, Flamant R, Gérard-Marchant R, Hayat M. Prognostic factors in 454 cases of Hodgkin's disease. *Cancer Res* 1971;31: 1801.
3. Carbone PP, Kaplan HS, Musshoff K, Smithers DW, Tubiana M. Report of the committee on Hodgkin's disease staging classification. *Cancer Res* 1971;31:1860.
4. Kaplan HS. *Hodgkin's disease*. Cambridge, MA: Harvard University Press, 1972.
5. Ultmann JE, Cunningham JK, Gellhorn A. The clinical picture of Hodgkin's disease. *Cancer Res* 1966;26:1047.
6. Ebstein W. Das chronische Rückfallsfieber, eine neue Infectionskrankheit. *Berlin Klin Wochenschr* 1887;24:565.
7. Pel PK. Pseudoleukaemie oder chronisches Rückfallsfieber? *Berlin Klin Wochenschr* 1887;24:644.
8. Racchi O, Rapezzi D, Ferraris AM, Gaetani GF. Unusual bone marrow relapse of Hodgkin's disease with typical Pel-Ebstein fever. *Ann Hematol* 1996;73:39.
9. Chang JC, Gross HM. Neoplastic fever responds to the treatment of an adequate dose of naproxen. *J Clin Oncol* 1985;3:552.
10. Gobbi PG, Cavalli C, Gendarini A, et al. Reevaluation of prognostic significance of symptoms in Hodgkin's disease. *Cancer* 1985;56:2874.
11. Gobbi PG, Pieresca C, Ricciardi L, et al. Night sweats in Hodgkin's disease: a manifestation of preceding minor febrile pulses. *Cancer* 1990;65:2074.
12. Ree HJ. Stromal macrophage-histiocytes in Hodgkin's disease. Their relation to fever. *Cancer* 1987;60:1479.
13. Klein S, Jücker M, Diehl V, Tesch H. Production of multiple cytokines by Hodgkin's disease derived cell lines. *Hematol Oncol* 1992;10:319.
14. Sappino A-P, Seelentag W, Pelte M-F, Alberto P, Vassalli P. Tumor necrosis factor/cachectin and lymphotoxin gene expression in lymph nodes from lymphoma patients. *Blood* 1990;75:958.
15. Perfetti V, Dragani TA, Paulli M, et al. Gene expression of pyrogenic cytokines in Hodgkin's disease lymph nodes. *Haematologica* 1992;77: 221.
16. Blay J-Y, Farcet J-P, Lavaud A, Radoux D, Chouaib S. Serum concentrations of cytokines in patients with Hodgkin's disease. *Eur J Cancer* 1994;30A:321.
17. Kurzrock R, Redman J, Cabanillas F, Jones D, Rothberg J, Talpaz M. Serum interleukin 6 levels are elevated in lymphoma patients and correlate with survival in advanced Hodgkin's disease and with B symptoms. *Cancer Res* 1993;53:2118.
18. Seymour JF, Talpaz M, Hagemeister FB, Cabanillas F, Kurzrock R. Clinical correlates of elevated serum levels of interleukin-6 patients with untreated Hodgkin's disease. *Am J Med* 1997;102:21.
19. Longo DL, Young RC, Wesley M, et al. Twenty years of MOPP therapy for Hodgkin's disease. *J Clin Oncol* 1986;4:1295.
20. Lister TA, Crowther D, Sutcliffe SB, et al. Report of a committee convened to discuss the evaluation and staging of patients with Hodgkin's disease: Cotswolds meeting. *J Clin Oncol* 1989;7:1630.
21. Crnkovich MJ, Hoppe RT, Rosenberg SA. Stage IIB Hodgkin's disease: the Stanford experience. *J Clin Oncol* 1986;4:472.
22. Kurzrock R, Cohen PR. Mucocutaneous paraneoplastic manifestations of hematologic malignancies. Am J Med 1995;99:207.
23. Gobbi PG, Attardo-Parrinello G, Lattanzio G, Rizzo SC, Ascari E. Severe pruritus should be a B-symptom in Hodgkin's disease. *Cancer* 1983;51:1934.
24. Feiner AS, Mahmood T, Wallner SF. Prognostic importance of pruritus in Hodgkin's disease. *JAMA* 1978;240:2738.
25. Seymour JF. Splenomegaly, eosinophilia, and pruritus: Hodgkin's disease, or . . .? *Blood* 1997;90:1719.
26. Olsson H, Brandt L. Relief of pruritus as an early sign of spinal cord compression in Hodgkin's disease. *Acta Med Scand* 1979;206:319.
27. Kadin ME. Lymphomatoid papulosis, Ki-1+ lymphoma, and primary cutaneous Hodgkin's disease. *Semin Dermatol* 1991;10:164.
28. Davis TH, Morton CC, Miller-Cassman R, et al. Hodgkin's disease, lymphomatoid papulosis, and cutaneous T-cell lymphoma derived from a common T-cell clone. *N Engl J Med* 1992;326:1115.
29. White RM, Patterson JW. Cutaneous involvement in Hodgkin's disease. *Cancer* 1985;55:1136.
30. Tassies D, Sierra J, Montserrat E, Marti R, Estrach T, Rozman C. Specific cutaneous involvement in Hodgkin's disease. *Hematol Oncol* 1992;10:75.
31. Milionis HJ, Elisaf MS. Psoriasiform lesions as paraneoplastic manifestation in Hodgkin's disease. *Ann Oncol* 1998;9:449.
32. Simon S, Azevedo SJ, Byrnes JJ. Erythema nodosum heralding recurrent Hodgkin's disease. *Cancer* 1985;56:1470.
33. Ronchese F, Gates DC. Ichthyosiform atrophy of the skin in Hodgkin's disease. *N Engl J Med* 1956;255:287.
34. Lucker GPH, Steijlen PM. Acrokeratosis paraneoplastica (Bazex syndrome) occurring with acquired ichthyosis in Hodgkin's disease. *Br J Dermatol* 1995;133:322.
35. Noto G, Pravatà G, Miceli S, Aricò M. Granulomatous slack skin: report of a case associated with Hodgkin's disease and a review of the literature. *Br J Dermatol* 1994;131:275.
36. Potaznik D, Steinherz P. Multiple nevoid basal cell carcinoma syndrome and Hodgkin's disease. *Cancer* 1984;53:2713.
37. Leimert JT, Corder MP, Skibba CA, Gingrich RD. Erythema annulare centrifugum and Hodgkin's disease. *Arch Intern Med* 1979;139: 486.
38. Benisovich V, Papadopoulos E, Amorosi EL, Zucker-Franklin D, Silber R. The association of progressive, atrophying, chronic, granulomatous dermohypodermitis with Hodgkin's disease. *Cancer* 1988;62: 2425.
39. Shelnitz, LS, Paller AS. Hodgkin's disease manifesting as prurigo nodularis. *Pediatr Dermatol* 1990;7:136.
40. Ramon DR, Jorda E, Molina I, et al. Follicular mucinosis and Hodgkin's disease. *Int J Dermatol* 1992;31:791.
41. Reeder CB, Connolly SM, Windelmann RK. The evolution of Hodgkin's disease and necrobiotic xanthogranuloma syndrome. *Mayo Clin Proc* 1991;66:1222.
42. Shahani RT, Blackburn EK. Nail anomalies in Hodgkin's disease. *Br J Dermatol* 1973;89:457.
43. Adler JJ, Sharma OP. Hypertrophic osteoarthropathy with intrathoracic Hodgkin's disease. *Am Rev Respir Dis* 1970;102:83.
44. Peck B. Hypertrophic osteoarthropathy with Hodgkin's disease in the mediastinum. *JAMA* 1977;238:1400.
45. Abate G, Corazzelli G, Ciarmiello A, Monfardini S. Neurologic complications of Hodgkin's disease: a case history. *Ann Oncol* 1997;8:593.
46. Dropcho EJ. Neurologic paraneoplastic syndromes. *J Neurol Sci* 1998;153:264.
47. Hammack J, Kotanides H, Rosenblum MK, Posner JB. Paraneoplastic cerebellar degeneration. II. Clinical and immunologic findings in 21 patients with Hodgkin's disease. *Neurology* 1992;42:1938.
48. Dropcho EJ. Autoimmune central nervous system paraneoplastic disorders: mechanisms, diagnosis, and therapeutic options. *Ann Neurol* 1995;37(Suppl 1):S102.
49. Cehreli C, Payzin B, Undar B, Yilmaz U, Alakavuklar MN. Paraneoplastic cerebellar degeneration in association with Hodgkin's disease: a report of two cases. *Acta Haematol* 1995;94:210.
50. Carr I. The Ophelia syndrome: memory loss in Hodgkin's disease. *Lancet* 1982;1:844.
51. Dansey RD, Hammond-Tooke GD, Lai K, Bezwoda WR. Subacute myelopathy: an unusual paraneoplastic complication of Hodgkin's disease. *Med Pediatr Oncol* 1988;16:284.
52. Schold SC, Cho E-S, Somasundaram M, Posner JB. Subacute motor neuropathy: a remote effect of lymphoma. *Ann Neurol* 1979;5:271.
53. Gordon PH, Rowland LP, Younger DS, et al. Lymphoproliferative disorders and motor neuron disease: an update. *Neurology* 1997;48:1671.
54. Vickers SM, Niederhuber JE. Hodgkin's disease associated with neurologic paraneoplastic syndrome. *South Med J* 1997;90:839.
55. Lachance DH, O'Neill BP, Harper CM, Cascino TL. Paraneoplastic brachial plexopathy in a patient with Hodgkin's disease. *Mayo Clin Proc* 1991;66:97.
56. Hughes RAC, Britton T, Richards M. Effects of lymphoma on the peripheral nervous system. *J R Soc Med* 1994;87:326.
57. Scully RE, Mark EJ, McNeely WF, McNeely BU. Case records of the Massachusetts Hospital. Case 39-1990. Presentation of case. *N Engl J Med* 1990;323:895.
58. Chintagumpala MM, Mahoney DH, McClain K, et al. Hodgkin's dis-

ease associated with central pontine myelinolysis. *Med Pediatr Oncol* 1993;21:311.

59. Grimaldi LME, Martino G, Braghi S, et al. Heterogeneity of autoantibodies in stiff-man syndrome. *Ann Neurol* 1993;34:57.
60. Ferrari P, Federico M, Grimaldi LM, Silingardi V. Stiff-man syndrome in a patient with Hodgkin's disease. An unusual paraneoplastic syndrome. *Haematologica* 1990;75:570.
61. Batchelor TT, Platten M, Palmer-Toy DE, et al. Chorea as a paraneoplastic complication of Hodgkin's disease. *J Neurooncol* 1998;36:185.
62. Levy Y, Barron SA, Shahin S, Haim N, Brook JG. Sympathetic dysautonomia as a remote effect of Hodgkin's lymphoma. Am J Med 1993; 95:340.
63. Richmond J, Sherman RS, Diamond HD, Craver LF. Renal lesions associated with malignant lymphomas. Am J Med 1962;32:184.
64. Fer MF, McKinney TD, Richardson RL, Hande KR, Oldham RK, Greco FA. Cancer and the kidney: renal complications of neoplasms. Am J Med 1981;71:704.
65. Dabbs DJ, Striker LMM, Mignon F, Striker G. Glomerular lesions in lymphomas and leukemias. Am J Med 1986;80:63.
66. Yum MN, Edwards JL, Kleit S. Glomerular lesions in Hodgkin's disease. *Arch Pathol* 1975;99:645.
67. Ma KW, Golbus SM, Kaufman R, Staley N, Londer H, Brown DC. Glomerulonephritis with Hodgkin's disease and herpes zoster. *Arch Pathol Lab Med* 1978;102:527.
68. Eagen JW, Lewis EJ. Glomerulopathies of neoplasia. *Kidney Int* 1977; 11:297.
69. Shapiro CM, Vander Laan BF, Jao W, Sloan DE. Nephrotic syndrome in two patients with cured Hodgkin's disease. *Cancer* 1985;55:1799.
70. Delmez JA, Safdar SH, Kissane JM. The successful treatment of recurrent nephrotic syndrome with the MOPP regimen in a patient with a remote history of Hodgkin's disease. *Am J Kidney Dis* 1994;23:743.
71. Korzets Z, Golan E, Manor Y, Schneider M, Bernheim J. Spontaneously remitting minimal change nephropathy preceding a relapse of Hodgkin's disease by 19 months. *Clin Nephrol* 1992;38:125.
72. Levine AM, Thornton P, Forman SJ, et al. Positive Coombs test in Hodgkin's disease: significance and implications. *Blood* 1980;55:607.
73. Björkholm M, Holm G, Merk K. Cyclic autoimmune hemolytic anemia as a presenting manifestation of splenic Hodgkin's disease. *Cancer* 1982;49:1702.
74. Majumdar G. Unremitting severe autoimmune haemolytic anaemia as a presenting feature of Hodgkin's disease with minimum tumour load. *Leuk Lymphoma* 1995;20:169.
75. Ranlö v P, Videbaek A. Cyclic haemolytic anaemia synchronous with Pel-Ebstein fever in a case of Hodgkin's disease. *Acta Med Scand* 1963;174:583.
76. Xiros N, Binder T, Anger B, Böhike J, Heimpel H. Idiopathic thrombocytopenic purpura and autoimmune hemolytic anemia in Hodgkin's disease. *Eur J Haematol* 1988;40:437.
77. Kirshner JJ, Zamkoff KW, Gottlieb AJ. Idiopathic thrombocytopenic purpura and Hodgkin's disease: report of two cases and a review of the literature. *Am J Med Sci* 1980;280:21.
78. Sonnenblick M, Kramer MR, Hershko C. Corticosteroid responsive immune thrombocytopenia in Hodgkin's disease. *Oncology* 1986;43: 349.
79. Linklater D, Voth A. Thrombocytopenic purpura. Importance of early diagnosis. *Can Fam Physician* 1996;42:1985.
80. Heyman MR, Walsh TJ. Autoimmune neutropenia and Hodgkin's disease. *Cancer* 1987;59:1903.
81. Fernández O, Morales E, Toledo J. Autoimmune processes terminating 24 years later in Hodgkin's disease. *Br J Haematol* 1992;81:308.
82. Hunter JD, Logue GL, Joyner JT. Autoimmune neutropenia in Hodgkin's disease. *Arch Intern Med* 1982;142:386.
83. Johnston PG, Ruscetti FW, Connaghan DG, Sullivan FJ, Longo DL. Transient reversal of bone marrow aplasia associated with lymphocyte depleted Hodgkin's disease after combination chemotherapy. *Am J Hematol* 1991;38:54.
84. Vaughan Hudson B, Linch DC, MacIntyre EA, et al. Selective peripheral blood eosinophilia associated with survival advantage in Hodgkin's disease (BNLI report no 31). *J Clin Pathol* 1987;40:247.
85. Desenne JJ, Acquatella G, Stern R, Muller A, Sanchez M, Somoza R. Blood eosinophilia in Hodgkin's disease. A follow-up of 25 cases in Venezuela. *Cancer* 1992;69:1248.
86. Samoszuk M, Nansen L. Detection of interleukin-5 messenger RNA in Reed-Sternberg cells of Hodgkin's disease with eosinophilia. *Blood* 1990;75:13.
87. Slease RB, Schumacher HR. Deficiency of coagulation factors VII and XII in a patient with Hodgkin's disease. *Arch Intern Med* 1977; 137:1633.
88. Rieke JW, Donaldson SS, Horning SJ. Hypercalcemia and vitamin D metabolism in Hodgkin's disease. *Cancer* 1989;63:1700.
89. Seymour JF, Gagel RF. Calcitriol: the major humoral mediator of hypercalcemia in Hodgkin's disease and non-Hodgkin's lymphomas. *Blood* 1993;82:1383.
90. Mercier RJ, Thompson JM, Harman GS, Messerschmidt GL. Recurrent hypercalcemia and elevated 1,25-dihydroxyvitamin D levels in Hodgkin's disease. Am J Med 1988;84:165.
91. Kremer R, Shustik C, Tabak T, Papavasiliou V, Goltzman D. Parathyroid-hormone-related peptide in hematologic malignancies. Am J Med 1996;100:406.
92. Laforga JB, Vierna J, Aranda FI. Hypercalcaemia in Hodgkin's disease related to prostaglandin synthesis. *J Clin Pathol* 1994;47:567.
93. Braund WJ, Williamson DH, Clark A, et al. Autoimmunity to insulin receptor and hypoglycaemia in a patient with Hodgkin's disease. *Lancet* 1987;1:237.
94. Walters EG, Denton RM, Tavare JM, Walters G. Hypoglycaemia due to an insulin-receptor antibody in Hodgkin's disease. *Lancet* 1987;1: 241.
95. Nadiminti Y, Wang JC, Chou S-Y, Pineles E, Tobin MS. Lactic acidosis associated with Hodgkin's disease. *N Engl J Med* 1980;303:15–17.
96. Bennett JS, Bond J, Singer I, Gottlieb AJ. Hypouricemia in Hodgkin's disease. *Ann Intern Med* 1972;76:751.
97. Eliakim R, Vertman E, Shinhar E. Case report: syndrome of inappropriate secretion of antidiuretic hormone in Hodgkin's disease. *Am J Med Sci* 1986;291:126.
98. Bichel J. Is the alcohol-intolerance syndrome in Hodgkin's disease disappearing? *Lancet* 1972;1:1069.
99. Bichel J. The alcohol-intolerance syndrome in Hodgkin's disease. *Acta Med Scand* 1959;164:105.
100. James AH. Hodgkin's disease with and without alcohol-induced pain. *Q J Med* 1960;113:47.
101. Custodi P, Cerutti A, Bagnato R, Cassani P. Alcohol-induced pain in tuberculous adenitis. *Haematologica* 1993;78:416.
102. Pinson P, Joos G, Praet M, Pauwels R. Primary pulmonary Hodgkin's disease. *Respiration* 1992;59:314.
103. Perera DR, Greene ML, Fenster LF. Cholestasis associated with extrabilliary Hodgkin's disease. *Gastroenterology* 1974;67:680.
104. Jansen PL, Van der Lelie H. Intrahepatic cholestasis and biliary cirrhosis associated with extrahepatic Hodgkin's disease. *Neth J Med* 1994;44:99.
105. Crosbie OM, Crown JP, Nolan NP, Murray R, Hegarty JE. Resolution of paraneoplastic bile duct paucity following successful treatment of Hodgkin's disease. *Hepatology* 1997;26:5.
106. Sacks EL, Donaldson SS, Gordon J, Dorfman RF. Epithelioid granulomas associated with Hodgkin's disease. *Cancer* 1978;41:562.
107. Younger DS, Hays AP, Brust JC, Rowland LP. Granulomatous angiitis of the brain. *Arch Neurol* 1988;45:514.
108. Inwards DJ, Piepgras DG, Lie JT, O'Neill BP, Scheithauer BW, Habermann TM. Granulomatous angiitis of the spinal cord associated with Hodgkin's disease. *Cancer* 1991;68:1318.
109. Mosteller MW, Margo CE, Hesse RJ. Hodgkin's disease and granulomatous uveitis. *Ann Ophthalmol* 1985;17:787.
110. Kedar A, Khan AB, Mattern QA, et al. Autoimmune disorders complicating adolescent Hodgkin's disease. *Cancer* 1979;44:112.
111. Fraumeni JF Jr, Herweg JC, Kissane JM. Panaortitis complicating Hodgkin's disease. *Ann Intern Med* 1967;67:1242.
112. Singh AP, Charan VD, Desai N, Choudhry VP. Hypertension as a paraneoplastic phenomenon in childhood Hodgkin's disease. *Leuk Lymphoma* 1993;11:315.

SECTION V

Treatment Principles and Techniques

Hodgkin's Disease, edited by P. M. Mauch, J. O. Armitage, V. Diehl, R. T. Hoppe, and L. M. Weiss. Lippincott Williams & Wilkins, Philadephia ©1999.

CHAPTER 21

Principles of Radiation Therapy in Hodgkin's Disease

Nancy P. Mendenhall, Richard T. Hoppe, Leonard R. Prosnitz, and Peter M. Mauch

Today, more than 75% of patients diagnosed with Hodgkin's disease will be cured with radiation therapy and/or chemotherapy given either initially or as salvage therapy. Many complex factors go into determining initial treatment decisions, including the efficacy of both chemotherapy and radiation therapy, the possibility of cure after relapse, the young age of most Hodgkin's disease patients, and the possible late effects of therapy. Medical oncologists and radiation oncologists face a myriad of staging and treatment choices. These choices are increasingly influenced by the goal of minimizing late effects of treatment. Because the risk of late effects increases with the intensity of initial treatment, tailored therapy has become an important concept to offer the best chance of cure with the least risk of toxicity. In many cases this can be accomplished with an approach of modified chemotherapy and radiation therapy. Radiation therapy in combined-modality regimens not only enhances disease control but also may allow for chemotherapy dose reduction. There is a role for radiation therapy alone or in conjunction with chemotherapy in almost all patients with Hodgkin's disease. Chemotherapy in combined-modality regimens reduces recurrence rates and allows for reduction of radiation dose and field size. For effective combined-modality therapy, both radiation therapy and chemotherapy must be delivered with precision and according to standard guidelines. It is critical that the efficacy of radiotherapy be maximized through a thorough understanding of the principles underlying appropriate field selection and design, dose prescription, and normal-tissue tolerance and protection as well as meticulous delivery of the planned treatment.

N. P. Mendenhall: Department of Radiation Oncology, University of Florida College of Medicine and Shands HealthCare at the University of Florida, Gainesville, Florida.

R. T. Hoppe: Department of Radiation Oncology, Stanford University, Stanford, California.

L. R. Prosnitz: Department of Radiation Oncology, Duke University Medical Center, Durham, North Carolina.

P. M. Mauch: Department of Radiation Oncology, Brigham and Women's Hospital and Dana-Farber Cancer Institute, Harvard Medical School, Boston, Massachusetts.

HISTORY

In his historic paper entitled "On Some Morbid Appearances of the Exorbant Glands and Spleen" presented to the Medical Chirurgical Society in London on January 10, 1832, Thomas Hodgkin described the clinical history and postmortem findings of the massive enlargement of lymph nodes and spleens of six patients studied at Guy's Hospital in London and of a seventh patient who had been seen by Carswell in 1828 (1) (see Chapter 1 for a biography of Thomas Hodgkin). For the next 70 years, most advances in Hodgkin's disease were descriptive. Wilks, Pel, Ebstein, and others contributed clinical information (2–4) (see Chapter 15 for more detail), and Greenfield, Sternberg, and Reed provided definition to the microscopic appearance of Hodgkin's disease (5–7) (see Chapter 7 for more detail).

The discovery of x-rays by Roentgen, radioactivity by Becquerel, and radium by the Curies in the late 19th century led to the early treatment of Hodgkin's disease with crude x-rays in 1901. Before 1900, arsenic, iodine, surgery, serum, and other biological preparations provided ineffective treatment. Thus, the first reports of dramatic shrinkage of enlarged lymph nodes with x-ray treatments produced both great excitement and premature predictions for the curability of Hodgkin's disease (8,9).

The German physicist Plucker was one of the first scientists to report on the production of x-rays (10). In 1854, he passed a high-voltage current through a vacuum tube, which produced an apple-green fluorescence on the inner wall of the tube. Other scientists observed that x-rays could pass through many different materials, including cloth, paper, wood, gold foil, and thin aluminum sheets. These rays also produced fluorescence of certain chemicals and changes on photographic plates. Roentgen, in 1895, building on these discoveries, dramatically demonstrated the ability of x-rays to pass through tissue by placing his hand between an x-ray tube and barium-platinum-cyanide crystals and reporting on the shadow outlining the bones of his hand in the glow of the crystals. He then "photographed" the bones in his hand by substituting a photographic plate for the crystals (11).

Within 2 years of Roentgen's discoveries, x-rays were used to treat patients. Radiation became popular for treating boils, fungal infections, lymph nodes swollen with tuberculosis, lupus of the skin, arthritis, and tumors. Some of radiation's powerful effects quickly became apparent; patients who endured long exposures and the operators who handled the x-ray equipment developed hair loss and superficial burns that affected the hands, eyelids, and skin.

Dr. William Pusey, a professor of dermatology at the University of Illinois Medical School in Chicago, first reported using x-rays to treat two patients with Hodgkin's disease. A 4-year-old boy with swelling in the neck was referred to Pusey on September 11, 1901. The boy's nodes, originally "as large as a fist," were "reduced to the size of an almond" 2 months after x-ray exposure. After a 50-year-old man with enlarged nodes under the right arm and at the elbow did not respond to arsenic injections, the nodes became so large that he could not bend his arm or put it at his side. With x-ray treatment, the nodes became smaller and softer, and Pusey noted that the patient could now "play billiards again" (8).

A year later, Nicholas Senn, a surgeon at Rush Medical College in Chicago, also reported on two patients with Hodgkin's disease. Photographs showed the shrinkage of massively swollen lymph nodes after treatment with radiation. One patient, a 43-year-old man with enlarged nodes in the neck, under the arms, and in the groin, received x-ray therapy after unsuccessful treatment with arsenic and iron. After 16 treatments, the radiation was stopped because of severe skin blistering, but by then the nodes had "nearly disappeared" (9).

Senn's other patient, a 53-year-old merchant with nodes enlarged for more than 10 years, had been treated unsuccessfully with arsenic, iodides, and liver oil. When referred for radiation, he had enlarged nodes in the neck, under the arms, and in the groin. He had also lost 45 lb and had become anemic from the Hodgkin's disease. Multiple x-ray treatments were separately applied to the neck, under the arms, elbows, chest, abdomen, and groin. After 15 days, the radiation was stopped because of severe skin redness, but the nodes continued to shrink, and the patient began to eat better and gain weight.

These responses encouraged Senn, who wrote that, "The eminent success attained in these two cases by the use of the x-ray can leave no further doubt of the curative effect of the Roentgen ray in the treatment of pseudoleukemia (Hodgkin's disease)." But his claims were premature, and more than 60 years would pass before it was generally accepted that Hodgkin's disease was a curable illness.

During the first two decades of the 20th century, crude x-ray equipment was used to treat Hodgkin's disease patients by administering either small doses of radiation to large fields at weekly intervals or a few large doses to small fields limited to the tumor. Neither controlled the Hodgkin's disease, and both caused complications, including local skin burns and ulceration. Enlarged nodes usually shrank with both techniques, but recurrence or extension to previously uninvolved nodes invariably followed. After several "successful" courses of radiotherapy, the Hodgkin's disease became more resistant to treatment, or patients developed systemic disease.

These multiple recurrences were not attributed to crude x-ray equipment or to suboptimal administration of radiation therapy but were viewed as inherent to the Hodgkin's disease itself. Most physicians, therefore, stopped using aggressive treatment to cure Hodgkin's disease by 1920. For the next four decades, treatment in most centers was mainly palliative—to shrink large nodes that were painful or that interfered with movement, eating, or breathing. Because Hodgkin's disease was invariably fatal, as little as possible was done to harm the patient or to treat the disease. Limited disease was treated either not at all or with only small doses of radiation.

Two technical advances in the 1920s, an improved cathode tube and deep therapy transformers capable of delivering higher-voltage x-rays, produced more deeply penetrating x-ray beams. These advances helped deliver larger doses to mediastinal and abdominal nodes than previously possible. However, even with the more powerful x-rays, adequate treatment of tumors deep in the abdomen or chest frequently was associated with complications to the skin, muscles, heart, or bowel. Machines powerful enough to treat deep tumors without delivering excessive dose to more superficial normal tissues would not be available until the late 1950s, when high-activity cobalt sources were produced.

The development of modern radiation therapy techniques for the treatment of Hodgkin's disease began with the work of Gilbert, a Swiss radiotherapist, in 1925 (12). Gilbert was one of the first physicians to point out specific clinical patterns in the spread of Hodgkin's disease, and he attempted to adapt his radiotherapy techniques to this knowledge. He advocated x-ray treatment of apparently uninvolved adjacent lymph node chains that might contain suspected microscopic disease as well as to the known sites of lymph node involvement. Initial treatment was concentrated on the regions known to be involved by

Hodgkin's disease, after which additional fields were used to encompass apparently healthy regions until low blood counts precluded further radiation. Gilbert and Babaiantz, in 1931, reported on 15 patients treated with fractionated and adjacent-site irradiation. Seven of the 15 were still alive, with an average survival time of 4.3 years for all patients (13), a survival rate that was unprecedented for that time. By the time of Gilbert's report in 1939 to the International Congress of Radiology (14), others had begun to adopt some of his ideas to the treatment of patients.

Craft, in 1940, published additional evidence that the survival of patients with Hodgkin's disease was significantly prolonged by treatment with x-rays. He reviewed 179 cases of Hodgkin's disease treated with Roentgen therapy at the University of Minnesota from 1926 to 1939 and compared their survival with that of 52 untreated cases discovered from autopsy files in the Department of Pathology from 1910 to 1939 (15). Forty-four percent of treated patients survived 3 years or longer compared to only 15% of the untreated patients. The 5-year survival rates of the two groups were 23% and 6%, respectively. Although the two groups were not entirely comparable, Craft concluded, "The difference between the three- and five-year survival rates, for the treated and the untreated groups, is very significant and attests to the therapeutic value of roentgen ray therapy. . . . The patients not only live longer, but their general well-being is tremendously improved in the large majority of cases." Craft's paper was not widely known or quoted, however. Even if it had been more widely circulated, the very low 10-year survival rate (10%) with the use of x-rays would have discouraged a more aggressive and potentially curative approach for Hodgkin's disease.

Vera Peters, in 1950, was the first physician to present definitive evidence that radiation therapy is a curative modality for early-stage Hodgkin's disease (16). She did this by identifying a group of patients with limited-stage Hodgkin's disease who were cured with high-dose, fractionated radiation therapy. She reviewed the records of 113 patients treated at The Ontario Institute of Radiotherapy from 1924 to 1942 and reported 5-year and 10-year survival rates of 88% and 79%, respectively, for patients with stage I Hodgkin's disease, rates that were notably high for a disease in which virtually no one survived 10 years. Thus, this was the first definitive report to demonstrate that patients with limited Hodgkin's disease could be cured with an aggressive treatment approach. In contrast, the 5-year and 10-year survival rates were 79% and 21%, respectively, for patients with stage II disease, and 9% and 0% for patients with stage III Hodgkin's disease.

Nonetheless, the results achieved in stage I Hodgkin's disease led to the eventual development of techniques to cure patients with more advanced disease. Patients received 1,800 to 5,000 Roentgen to areas of involvement, with the higher dose levels given to patients with early-stage disease. These doses were quite a bit higher than those recommended by others during this era. In addition, many patients received "prophylactic" irradiation with doses of 400 to 800 Roentgen to lymph node–bearing areas apparently uninvolved with disease. Peters and Middlemiss, in 1958, with longer follow-up of the cases they reported in 1950, observed no significant decrement in survival after the tenth year, thus providing additional support for the cure of early-stage Hodgkin's disease with radiation therapy (17).

Despite these studies, the concept that early-stage Hodgkin's disease might be curable with higher-dose and larger-field radiation therapy was slow to be accepted, and before the 1960s, most patients with limited Hodgkin's disease were not treated at all, or only with small doses of radiation. When in 1963 Easson and Russell published their paper, "The Cure of Hodgkin's Disease" (18), physicians were closer to accepting the effectiveness of radical treatment for this once fatal illness than they had been in 1950, the year Peters published her paper. Easson and Russell demonstrated a flat survival curve at 5, 10, and 15 years (50%, 42%, and 40%, respectively) for patients with localized Hodgkin's disease.

At Stanford, Henry S. Kaplan had become aware of the early work of Rene Gilbert (14) and Vera Peters (17) and was able to extend their concepts further, taking advantage of a new technology for cancer treatment—the linear accelerator. Henry Kaplan was a radiologist who began an illustrious career as a National Cancer Institute Fellow at the University of Minnesota, then became an Assistant Professor at Yale, and was 1 year into an appointment at the National Cancer Institute in Bethesda when he was recruited, at age 29, to become Professor and Chairman of the Department of Radiology at Stanford. Throughout his career, Kaplan emphasized the linkage between basic research and clinical medicine. He developed an early interest in the lymphomas and demonstrated that the lymphomagenic effect of whole-body irradiation in mice was related to the radiation leukemia virus (19). Kaplan was convinced that more effective radiation therapy for deep-seated cancers was essential to the advance of cancer treatment and became aware of the pioneering work in linear accelerator technology being conducted at the Stanford Microwave Laboratory by Edward Ginzton, William Hansen, and others. Kaplan and Ginzton had discussions that led them both to realize that the features of the linear accelerator would make it ideally suitable for cancer therapy (20). They initiated a collaboration in 1950 and, by 1952, had secured the requisite funding from the United States Public Health Service, the Office of Naval Research, and the American Cancer Society to develop a linear accelerator suitable for clinical radiation therapy (21). The project was successful, the unit was completed in 1956, and the first patient (with retinoblastoma) was treated shortly thereafter.

The development of the linear accelerator facilitated the evolution of high-dose, extended-field irradiation concepts in the management of Hodgkin's disease. As early as 1951, Kaplan had tried, with partial success, to treat patients with higher doses and extended fields using 200 kVp x-rays and experienced the usual skin reactions that limited patient tolerance and tumor dose. In 1956, immediately after the Stanford linear accelerator was commissioned, he began to treat patients with Hodgkin's disease utilizing these concepts of high-dose extended-field treatment and, in 1962, published his first observations on the radical radiotherapy of regionally localized Hodgkin's disease (22). In this paper, he compared his results (using 30 to 40 Gy, to extended fields) with the results of patients who were being treated palliatively (4 to 12 Gy, involved field) by other physicians at Stanford during the same period of time. He demonstrated dramatic improvement with the more aggressive approach. At 2 years, the freedom from recurrence or extension was 85% in the radically treated group but only 20% in the palliatively treated group ($p < 0.01$). Thirteen of the 16 patients treated radically were alive at the time of analysis, compared to only one of nine patients treated palliatively.

In 1961, Kaplan recruited Saul A. Rosenberg, an internist who had developed an interest in lymphoma while a fellow at the Memorial Hospital in New York, to join him at Stanford. Rosenberg was given a joint appointment in the Departments of Radiology and Medicine, and this marked the beginning of a fruitful collaboration. Rosenberg reviewed the work of Kaplan but insisted that his results be confirmed scientifically in a prospective randomized clinical trial. Kaplan agreed and, after obtaining funding from the National Cancer Institute to support this effort, initiated the first Stanford randomized clinical trials for Hodgkin's disease and the non-Hodgkin's lymphomas in 1962. At first, patients with both diseases were treated on the same protocols. The L1 Study, for patients with stage I to II disease, randomized treatment between involved-field (40 Gy) (the standard treatment arm) and extended-field (40 Gy) (the experimental arm) irradiation. The L2 Study, for patients with stage III disease, randomized between involved-field (15 Gy) (the standard palliative treatment at that time) and total lymphoid (40 Gy) irradiation. This was the first successful experimental treatment for patients with stage III Hodgkin's disease. Some of those patients remain alive, even today.

As outlined above, the development of the linear accelerator, which allowed higher doses and larger radiation fields to be used, the initiation of randomized clinical trials, the proposal of new classification systems for histologic subtyping (23) and staging (24), the pioneering of methods for more precise radiographic and surgical staging (bipedal lymphangiography and staging laparotomy) (25,26), and the development of an effective multiagent chemotherapy regimen (27) all contributed to the development of curative treatment for early Hodgkin's disease. Because of these advances, the philosophy and practice of managing early-stage Hodgkin's disease changed dramatically from no treatment in the early 1960s to extensive staging and radiation therapy with wide fields and high doses by the late 1960s (see Chapters 2, 3, and 4).

EQUIPMENT

Linear accelerators are the treatment machine of choice for radiotherapy of Hodgkin's disease with 6 MV, the desired energy in most instances, particularly for treatment above the diaphragm. A 6-MV beam is sufficiently penetrating to produce reasonable dose homogeneity throughout a large irregular treatment field with most accelerator beams characterized by reasonably flat beam profiles. The maximum dose point of a 6-MV beam is close enough to the skin surface to avoid underdosing superficially located lymph nodes, such as in the neck. The dose inhomogeneity measured in a mantle field treated with a 6-MV beam is, however, nonetheless still in the range of 10% to 20%, primarily as a result of the quite different separations in the superior and inferior portions of the field (28). This can be reduced by using extended source-to-skin distances (about 130 cm).

Four-megavolt linear accelerators and cobalt machines are less desirable than higher-energy supervoltage equipment. Many 4-MV accelerators have unusual beam profiles, particularly with large irregularly shaped fields in which the beam may be flat at a depth of 10 cm but, near the surface, the dose may be much greater at the edge of the field than it is at the center. When this effect is combined with the lesser separation in areas such as the neck and axillae, dose inhomogeneities of 20% to 30% may result (29). It is especially important, therefore, to calculate and measure doses at different points throughout the field if a 4-MV accelerator is being used and for the clinician to make the appropriate adjustments, either by shrinking the field or employing some type of filtration.

Cobalt-60 units, although seldom used in the United States today, are still common in many other areas of the world. Cobalt-60 machines have a different type of problem than 4-MV accelerators. The dose tends to fall off toward the edge of the field, so that larger nominal field sizes may be necessary. The risk is that of underdosing toward the field edges, not overdosing, as is generally the case with the 4-MV accelerator (30). Again, dose calculations and measurements throughout the field are mandatory. Additionally the penumbra on a cobalt unit makes evaluation of port films and calculation of gaps to avoid overlap more complex and difficult.

Beam energies greater than 6 MV may be desirable for larger patients for treatment of abdominal fields or limited chest fields when irradiation of superficial adenopathy in the neck or inguinal regions, for example, is not contemplated. High-energy beams will obviously result in better penetrability and greater dose homogeneity.

RADIATION THERAPY TECHNIQUES

Dose and Dose Delivery

The relationship between radiation dose and probability of tumor control has been the subject of an interesting and lengthy debate. Because of the long-term survival of most patients, and the association of tumor dose and field size to normal tissue complications, this debate is quite relevant.

The concept of 40 Gy as the tumoricidal dose for Hodgkin's disease has been well entrenched in radiation oncologic thinking for three decades, since the publication of Kaplan's landmark article (Fig. 1) (31). This paper reviewed a variety of dose–response data in the literature, most of which had been obtained with orthovoltage treatment, with some series including both Hodgkin's and non-Hodgkin's lymphomas and with some concern regarding the possibility of geographic misses as well as dose inhomogeneity. There was no consideration of whether different tumor burdens might require different doses; that is, was the dose necessary for control of subclinical disease the same as for clinically apparent disease. Prior studies of Peters (32) and Easson (18) in which doses of 3,000 R exerted a high degree of local control for clinically evident disease and much lower doses (1,000–1,500 R) effectively controlled subclinical disease receded into the background as radiation oncologists, now with the ability to readily deliver larger doses because of the advent of supervoltage equipment, enthusiastically embraced the Kaplan concepts.

A number of subsequent dose–response analyses, however, beginning with Fletcher and Shukovsky (33) and including the Patterns of Care Studies (34) as well as individual reports from Florida (35,36), Wisconsin (37),

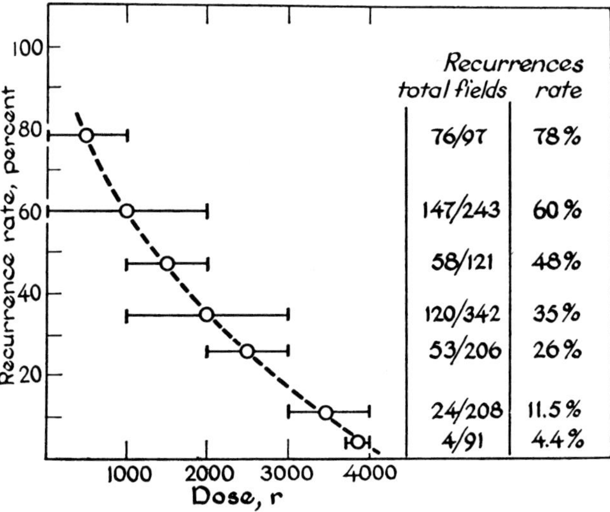

FIG 1. Evidence for a tumoricidal dose level in the radiotherapy of Hodgkin's disease. (Reproduced with permission from ref. 31.)

and Chicago (38), have questioned the Kaplan precepts. These reports suggest that the dose–response curve for Hodgkin's disease is sigmoid in nature and relatively flat with doses exceeding 30 Gy (Fig. 2). Also, Raubitschek and Glatstein (39) and Prosnitz (40) have proposed that there may be other factors affecting disease control that need to be taken into account in an analysis of dose; these include technical factors for accurate setup and field design, clinical and biological factors including tumor size and number of sites of involvement, and treatment factors such as combined-modality therapy and response to chemotherapy.

Although a few retrospective studies have attempted to address what radiation dose is needed for the prophylactic treatment of clinically uninvolved sites, the prospectively designed multicenter trial by the German Hodgkin's Study Group (GHSG), which evaluated the tumoricidal doses for subclinical involvement by Hodgkin's disease, provides definitive data (41). Only patients without risk factors were included in the trial (risk factors included any one of the following: large mediastinal adenopathy, massive splenic involvement, extranodal disease, an ESR of ≥30 with B symptoms, an ESR of ≥50 and no B symptoms, or three or more regions of involvement); 376 laparotomy-staged IA to IIB Hodgkin's disease patients were enrolled. Patients were randomized to receive 40 Gy extended-field radiation therapy or 30 Gy extended-field radiation therapy followed by an additional 10 Gy to involved lymph node regions (41). The 5-year freedom from treatment failure results favored the 30 Gy extended field plus 10 Gy arm over the 40 Gy extended field arm (81% vs. 70%, respectively, $p = 0.0263$). The 5-year survival results also favored the 30 Gy extended field arm (98% vs. 93%, respectively, $p = 0.0673$) (Fig. 3).

From these data, the following conclusions seem reasonable. (a) For clinical disease, the dose–response curve is sigmoid in nature, rising steeply above 20 Gy and flattening from about 30 Gy. With doses of 36 Gy, infield local control exceeds 95%. Equivalent local control rates are apparently achieved with doses of 30 to 35 Gy, although the number of patients treated in this dose range is not large. From 20 to 30 Gy, local control is achieved in 50% to 90% of instances. (b) For subclinical disease, local control is in excess of 90% for a broad range of doses exceeding 20 Gy. For doses exceeding 30 Gy, subclinical disease is controlled in more than 95% of instances. (c) For larger masses of disease, such as those exceeding 6 cm, the data are less clear, primarily because of the tendency for clinicians to use larger doses for larger masses. Many research programs use higher doses (36 Gy to 44 Gy) or combined chemotherapy and radiation therapy for patients with disease greater than 6 cm.

Equal doses should be administered from anterior and posterior fields; treatment of both fields daily minimizes the biological dose to normal tissues. Doses of

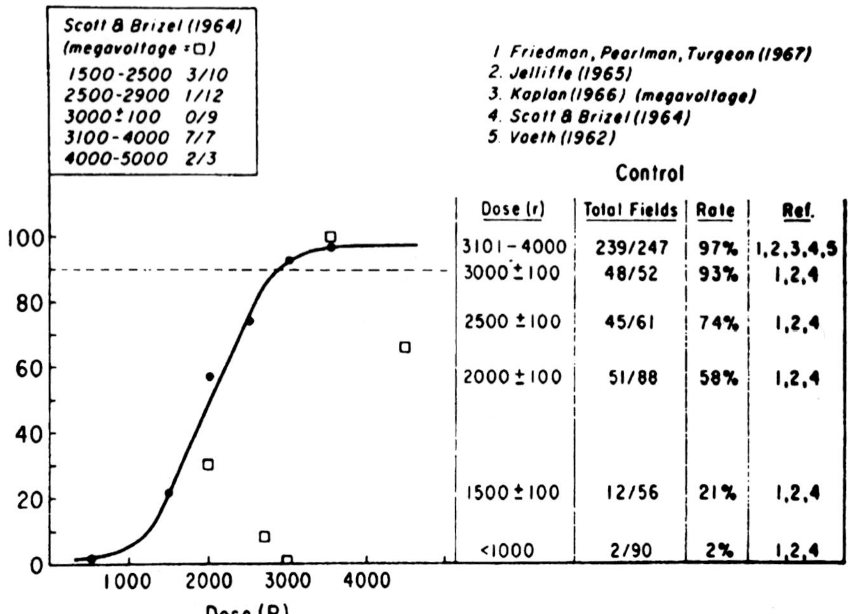

FIG. 2. Evidence for a tumoricidal dose level in the radiotherapy of Hodgkin's disease. (Reproduced with permission from ref. 33.)

1.8 to 2.0 Gy per day are recommended unless the treatment field includes the entire heart or entire lung, in which case the dose should be limited to 1.5 Gy or less per day.

Selecting the appropriate dose for radiotherapy of Hodgkin's disease is an important issue because long-term complications of treatment are clearly dose related. In particular, fatal cardiac complications were not seen in the large Stanford series with doses less than 30 Gy (42). One would similarly anticipate a lesser rate of nonfatal cardiac complications as the dose declines. The frequency of abdominal complications is diminished markedly as well with doses less than 30 Gy (43).

These dosimetric concepts have broad implications when radiation therapy is used in conjunction with combination chemotherapy. If doses of 25 to 30 Gy are adequate for subclinical disease, and 36 Gy is adequate for clinically apparent disease when radiotherapy alone is used, then in the presence of effective chemotherapy, radiation doses may theoretically be reduced even further. Determination of the optimal dose of radiation therapy in combination with chemotherapy may depend on the type and number of cycles of chemotherapy, and perhaps on the clinical response to chemotherapy. The German Hodgkin's Study Group (GHSG) found no differences among 20 Gy, 30 Gy, and 40 Gy given to involved nodal sites or for extended fields following remission from chemotherapy; initial bulky sites (> 7.5 cm) all received 40 Gy (44). Radiation doses in the range of 15 to 25 Gy given to pediatric patients, to patients with stage III to IV disease, and to patients with recurrent Hodgkin's disease have been very effective in terms of preventing in-field local relapse in patients who respond well to initial chemotherapy (45–47). The question of radiation dose when combined with chemotherapy is the subject of a number of ongoing trials by the European Organization for the Research and Treatment of Cancer (EORTC) and the GHSG (see Chapters 25 and 26). The principle that effective chemotherapy can replace a certain amount of radiation is also well documented in studies of a number of solid tumors such as esophageal, anal, and rectal carcinomas.

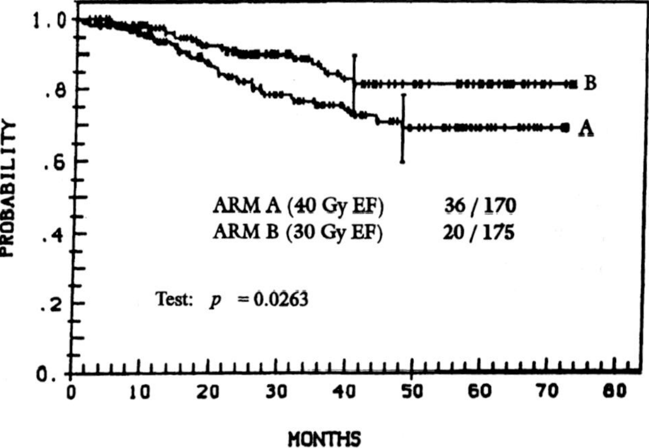

FIG. 3. Results from the German Hodgkin's Group Trial. The 5-year freedom from treatment failure results favored the 30-Gy extended field plus 10-Gy arm over the 40-Gy extended field arm (81% vs. 70%, respectively, $p = 0.0263$). The 5-year survival results also favored the 30-Gy extended field arm (98% vs. 93%, respectively, $p = 0.0673$), although the differences were not statistically significant. (Reprinted with permission from ref. 41.)

Positioning and Immobilization

One of the important lessons learned from three-dimensional treatment planning is that radiotherapy accuracy during a course of fractionated radiation is only as good as the immobilization of the patient. This is particularly important in patients with Hodgkin's disease in whom complex, large, irregularly shaped fields are most often used. With Cerrobend blocks attached to a standard machine block-holding tray, very small changes in patient position may result in considerable field variations. Accurate positioning requires reproducible neck and arm positioning and reproducible alignment and rotation of the torso and pelvis. Accurate knee and foot positioning may also be required under certain circumstances.

There are a number of acceptable methods to deliver radiation therapy accurately for Hodgkin's disease. These methods include different approaches to immobilization and block placement and to determination of field size and dose. Throughout this chapter we provide a spectrum of acceptable practice whenever possible. In terms of immobilization, the techniques used will in part depend on the experience and reliability of the therapists and the fields being treated. The techniques that utilize more rigid immobilization have the advantage of a more reproducible setup.

The following techniques can be used for immobilization of the head position. (a) For a patient treated in both the supine and prone positions, the head can rest in the supine position on a soft sponge with tape used to fix the chin position. In this way the light field can be visualized both anteriorly on the chin and laterally over the ears. In the prone position the chin can rest on the sponge, and again the light fields can be visualized. The advantage of this technique is that the head position can be changed between the supine and the prone positions to correspond to the divergence of the field; the disadvantage is in the day-to-day variation in setup. (b) When patients are treated in the supine position only, the head position can be reproduced with a head rest (Timo) and may be enhanced by the use of a bite block. Head rests are available in different sizes and shapes (Fig. 4A). Once the head rest is selected, the bite block position is set to secure reproducible head positioning. The mouthpiece for the bite block is customized to accommodate the shape of the individual patient's mouth. The settings on the bite block are recorded for daily replication on the treatment table (Fig. 4B). (c) An alternative method of immobilization is a customized upper body Styrofoam mold or an alpha cradle in conjunction with a chin band (28,47). The patient is simulated and treated in the cradle. A minor disadvantage of this system (aside from the time and expense required to make the cradles) is that some bolusing of the back results when the posterior field is treated through the cradle as well as the treatment couch, with some increase in the skin reaction posteriorly (47). Arm position varies according to the age of the patient and institutional preference. The akimbo arm position, selected for most children and some adults, can be reproduced by simply having the patient place his/her thumbs in the waistband or belt or on the table at that level. The arms-up position can be secured with an Alpha Cradle or customized upper body mold with hand grips for reproducible position (28), although in a cooperative patient the arm position may be secured with a less rigorous setup.

Wall-mounted lasers in the simulation and treatment rooms can aid in reproducing torso and pelvic alignment

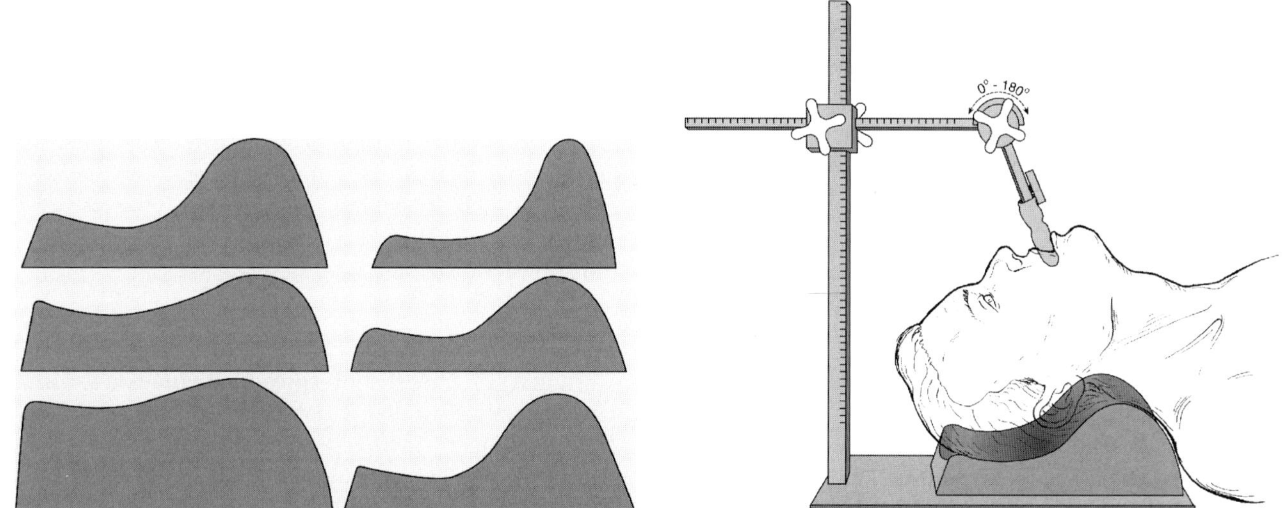

FIG. 4. Positioning and immobilization for mantle irradiation. **A:** Different headrests for patients being simulated for the mantle field. **B:** A bite-block apparatus used to facilitate reproduction of the head position. (Both parts drawn by Louis Clark.)

and rotation. Different techniques can be employed. Leveling tattoos can be used; one pair of lateral tattoos on each side of the central axis is used to aid in lining up with the side lasers. Another method involves the use of lasers without corresponding tattoos. One laser is used to place a straight line extending from the mid chin through the thyroid notch, suprasternal notch, xiphoid, umbilicus, and midsymphysis to secure cephalocaudad alignment. The table height is adjusted to place a second set of lateral lines (from midaxillae through the waist to the hips) that serve as leveling lines to prevent torso or pelvic rotation (the three-point setup).

Techniques to assure reproducibility of the knee and foot position are especially important for patients with subdiaphragmatic Hodgkin's disease. The ankles can be immobilized with tape or a bandage with a reproducible ankle separator that maintains ankle separation and thereby precludes knee or hip rotation. Many patients prefer a small amount of knee flexion for comfort. If this is required, it is best provided with a standard wedge under the knees that can be used each day along with an ankle separation device.

With extended distance travel couches and contemporary linear accelerators with large field sizes, patients can usually be treated to both anteroposterior and posteroanterior fields using an extended source-to-skin distance (SSD) technique while in the same supine position. Without the availability of the extended couch, the posterior fields may be treated with the patient prone. Because reproducibility in this position is more difficult, a customized body mold is helpful to secure reproducible shoulder, neck, and arm position. As in treatment in the supine position, wall-mounted lasers can be used to check leveling lines and a cephalocaudad line that will preclude vertical or horizontal rotation.

If the patient is to be treated with sequential radiation fields (e.g., a mantle followed later by upper abdominal fields), positioning for the two fields must be as consistent as possible to avoid inadvertent overlap with the previously treated field, created by shifts in patient position. The previous field position must be clearly documented. Inconspicuous tattoos placed at the field borders, use of the same patient position, radiographic documentation of the lower end of the mantle field with the use of spine films, and knowledge of previous field size and source-to-skin distance will allow calculation of an appropriate skin gap so that sequential fields may be treated safely.

Custom Blocks

Custom shielding blocks are essential to the delivery of high-quality radiation therapy. Divergent blocks are generally cast from a low-melting-point alloy such as Lipowitz metal (Cerrobend) and mounted on the collimator of the linear accelerator. These blocks are of a thickness calculated to reduce the transmitted beam by 5 half-values, that is, to approximately 3% of the prescribed dose.

Partial transmission blocks may also be employed. These are designed to appropriate thickness to permit partial transmission of a specific radiation dose. The use of partial transmission blocks permits the administration of a lower dose of radiation than the prescribed dose to selected portions of the radiation field. For example, when the mediastinum is being treated to a dose of 40 Gy, and there is an indication to deliver low-dose irradiation to the lung(s), a 37.5% transmission block may be used to deliver a dose of 15 Gy. Similar blocks can be used for low-dose treatment to the liver in conjunction with full-dose treatment to the paraaortic field (48).

Full-thickness Cerrobend blocks do not provide total protection for the blocked normal tissues such as the lung, heart, testicles, and ovaries. In addition to the 3% transmitted from the primary beam directly through the block, there is some dose delivered to the shielded areas from radiation scattered internally from other tissues within the direct path of the radiation beam. The amount of scatter depends on the amount of surrounding tissue within the primary beam (width of the area contributing scatter), the width of the block, the radiation energy (less scatter with higher-energy beams), and the distance from the edge of the protective block. For example, at the edge of the treatment field, the actual dose is about 50% of the prescribed dose; there is rapid dose falloff as the distance increases from the beam edge. Beneath the lung block in a typical mantle field, the actual dose to the lung may range from 5% to 20% of the prescribed dose.

Functional Field Definitions

Involved Field

The lymphatic system is arbitrarily divided into lymph node regions for the purpose of field design (Fig. 5). An *involved field* includes not only the individual clinically involved or enlarged nodes but also the other lymph nodes within the same lymph node region. For example, with a 2-cm node in the midright neck, an involved field technically would include the entire ipsilateral cervical/supraclavicular region, including all nodes from the base of the skull to the clavicle. The involved field is the minimum radiation field size used for Hodgkin's disease.

Extended Field

Studies of patterns of spread in Hodgkin's disease clearly established that lymph node sites adjacent to sites that are clinically involved are at high risk for subsequent involvement if left untreated (49). Based on these observations, the strict definition of an *extended field* is that it includes the involved field as well as all adjacent lymph node regions. Unfortunately, the term has occasionally been applied by some investigators to mean treatment of

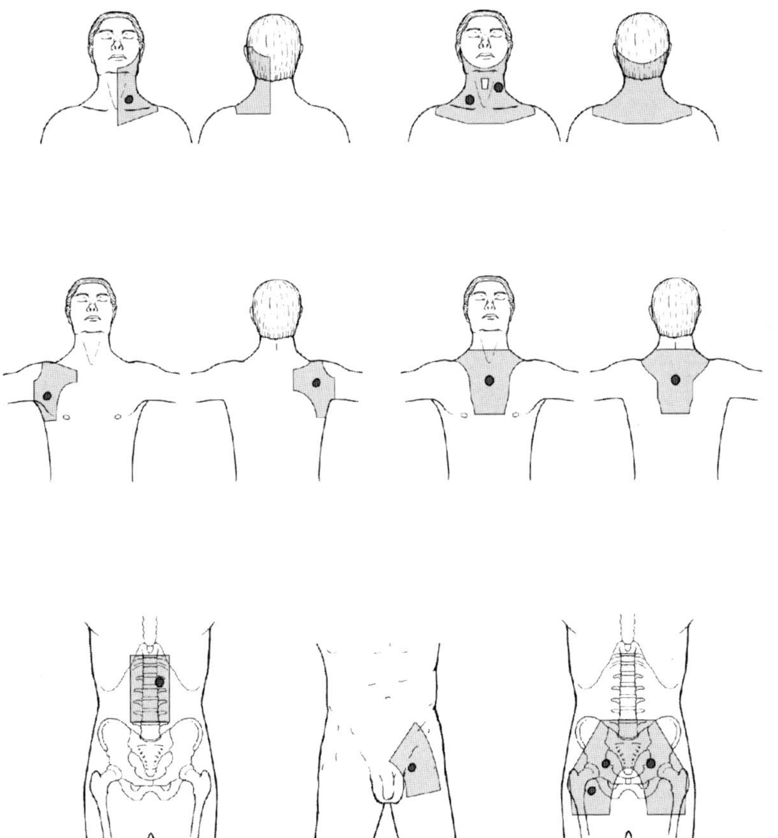

FIG. 5. Lymph node regions for involved field placement for patients with Hodgkin's disease. (Drawn by Louis Clark.)

a mantle field in a patient with disease in any supradiaphragmatic location, and by others to mean treatment both above and below the diaphragm. This has led to some confusion in the literature.

Another confusing issue relates to the contiguity of spread between supradiaphragmatic sites (mediastinum and supraclavicular areas) and the upper abdomen (retroperitoneal nodes and spleen). The interpretation of the early staging laparotomy studies at Stanford (50) was that there is contiguity between the low neck/supraclavicular region and the upper abdominal nodes/spleen, even in the absence of mediastinal disease (mediastinal skip), likely through spread of disease via the thoracic duct. Technically, therefore, an extended field would include the upper abdominal nodes and spleen whenever disease is present in the supraclavicular region.

Mantle/Paraaortic; Subtotal Lymphoid Irradiation; Subtotal Nodal Irradiation; Extended Mantle; Total Lymphoid Irradiation; and Total Nodal Irradiation

Most patients who are treated definitively with radiation therapy for early stage Hodgkin's disease require treatment both above and below the diaphragm. A variety of terms have been used to designate these fields. Any of these composite fields will include the spleen or splenic pedicle.

Mantle/paraaortic includes sequential treatment to the mantle and paraaortic fields, with the lower border of the field at the aortic bifurcation. The terms *subtotal lymphoid* and *subtotal nodal irradiation* (STLI and STNI) are synonymous and in most contexts represent the same fields as mantle and paraaortic/splenic radiation. However, on occasion these terms refer to the sequential treatment to the mantle and "spade" field, which differs from the paraaortic field by inclusion of the common iliac nodes.

Another technique of mantle and upper abdominal irradiation, particularly for patients with disease below the carina, is to treat both volumes in one field, an *extended mantle* (51). This technique requires an extended source-to-skin distance and may require a nonisocentric technique with the patient supine for the anterior and prone for the posterior field (Fig. 6). The large field size and extended distance increase the difficulty of daily setup. The two major advantages of this approach are the elimination of dose inhomogeneity associated with field matching and a significant shortening of the overall treatment time. The disadvantages are the increased probability of bone marrow suppression with the significantly larger treatment volume, the simultaneous acute morbidities associated with the mantle field (dysphagia and dermatitis) and the upper abdominal field (nausea), and the increased difficulty of accurate daily

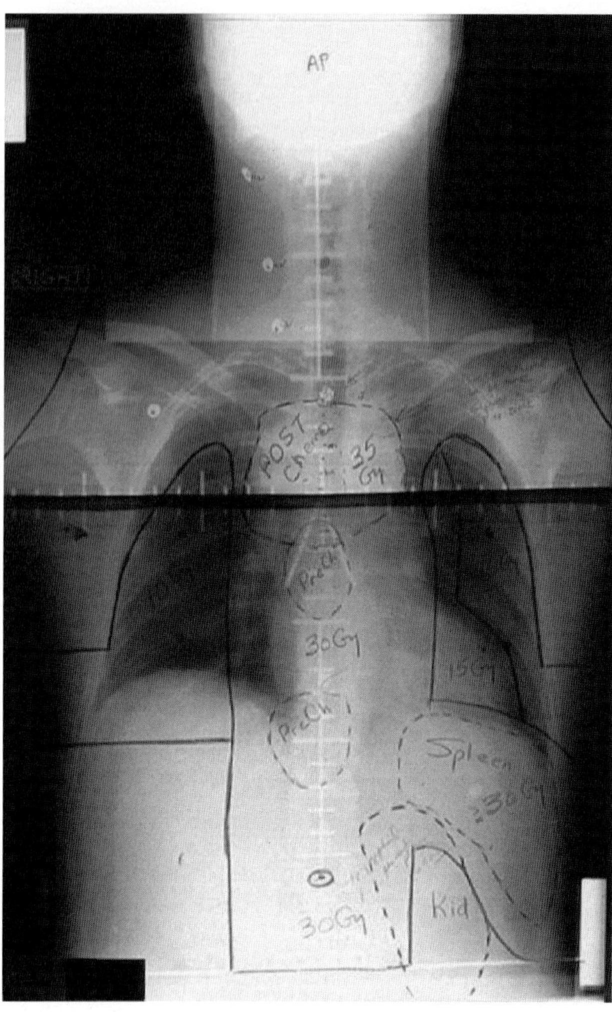

FIG. 6. Extended mantle field of a patient with mediastinal, subcarinal, and anterior cardiac nodal involvement. Note that the splenic and left kidney volumes have been outlined on the simulation film.

setup with a larger field size. These disadvantages are magnified if the spleen is included in the treatment volume or if the patient has received prior chemotherapy.

Total lymphoid and *total nodal irradiation* (TLI and TNI) are synonymous and imply treatment of all the major lymph node regions above and below the diaphragm. It is important to note that certain lymph node groups, including brachial, epitrochlear, popliteal, sacral, and mesenteric nodes, are rarely involved in Hodgkin's disease and are not included in these fields; involvement of these groups obviously requires modification of standard fields. In the postsplenectomy setting, total lymphoid fields include sequential treatment to the mantle and inverted Y. If a splenectomy has not been performed, the inverted Y spleen field usually must be divided into two components (paraaortic–spleen and pelvic fields) and treated sequentially to avoid excessive hematologic or gastrointestinal toxicity.

Mantle Field

The *mantle* is the most frequently treated field in Hodgkin's disease; it also is one of the most difficult to treat technically. The mantle includes all of the supradiaphragmatic lymph nodes commonly involved: the cervical, supraclavicular, axillary, infraclavicular, superior mediastinal, hilar, and subcarinal nodes. Many of these nodal areas overlie normal lung parenchyma and heart, providing a challenge to the clinician to design a field that adequately covers all clinically evident and subclinical disease while sparing sufficient normal tissue to avoid acute and late treatment sequelae. The irregular field shape, the different tissue densities, the depths of target nodes within the field, and the varying patient thickness throughout the thorax and neck complicate the dosimetry of the mantle field. Finally, the large field size, the extended distance from the source to the patient, and the irregular field shape make precise daily radiation delivery a challenge.

The mantle may be treated with the patient supine for treatment of both anterior and posterior fields using a fixed source–axis distance (SAD) or source–skin distance (SSD) technique. If the accelerator beam utilized is one with sufficient field size, the isocentric technique has the advantage of greater positioning accuracy, speed of setup, and simplicity. The disadvantages of the supine-only technique are smaller maximum field sizes, difficulty in verifying the appropriate skin gap for matched adjacent posterior fields, and the difficulty in providing ideal skin sparing in the posterior field. Optimally, if the patient is treated in the supine position, it should be on a 6-MV linear accelerator at extended distance (130 cm) by using a machine with an extended travel distance couch. The extended distance will minimize the dose inhomogeneity within the field. This can also be accomplished by using a higher energy, but with energies greater than 6 MV there is the risk of underdosing superficial nodes. Alternatively, the patient may be treated at a prescribed source-to-skin distance, supine for the anterior field and prone for the posterior field.

The arms may be placed akimbo or above the head (Fig. 7). The akimbo position is more comfortable and allows shielding of the humeral heads. Therefore, it is the preferred position for prepubertal children, as it allows protection of the epiphyseal plate of the humerus. There can be increased skin reaction in the folds of the axillary region with the arms-akimbo position. Figure 8 shows the simulation film of a patient with the arms akimbo. Note the strip of lung inside the ribs that is treated to include the axillary nodes with this technique.

Placement of the arms above the head pulls the axillary lymph nodes laterally and superiorly (Fig. 9), allowing increased shielding of the lung parenchyma, and is the preferred treatment for adults at some institutions. Figure 10 shows the simulation film of a patient with the arms

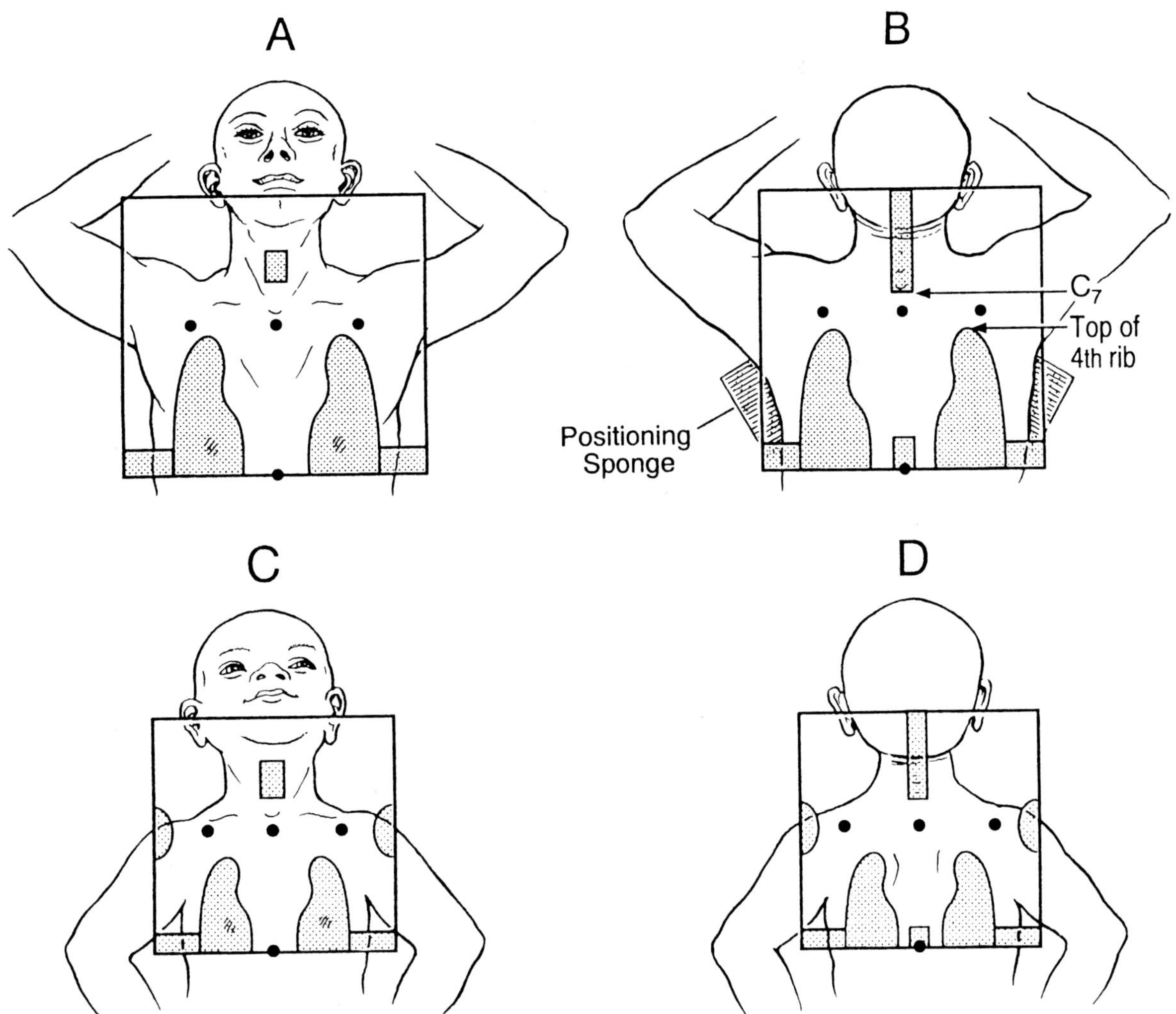

FIG. 7. Placement on the anterior **(A,C)** and posterior **(B,D)** mantle fields of the lung, wing, larynx, and cervical spine blocks in the arms-up position **(A,B)** and placement of the humeral head blocks in the arms-akimbo position **(C,D)** (tattoos indicated by ●). Note the positioning sponges placed under the shoulders on the posterior projection **(B)** to prevent medial rotation of the shoulders and axillary lymph nodes. (Reproduced with permission from ref. 84.)

above the head. With the arms above the head, the humeral heads should not be blocked, especially if there is evidence of axillary involvement. Note that the lung blocks laterally run along the inside of the ribs.

The upper border of the standard mantle field passes through the midmandible, midtragus, and mastoid. In general, the head is in the neutral position; too much extension will result in excessive treatment of the cerebellum; too much flexion will result in excessive treatment of the oral cavity. A superior central block may be customized for the posterior field to shield the occiput and oral cavity; however, care must be taken to avoid inadvertent shielding of medial neck nodes because the beam must pass through the posterior fossa before it reaches its target (the neck, submandibular, and submental nodes). Some institutions also recommend placing a cervical spine block after 30 Gy on the posterior field only. If neck disease is minimal, a small laryngeal block can be placed from the notch of the thyroid cartilage to the bottom of the cricoid cartilage. Most centers recommend placement of the larynx block after 18 to 20 Gy. If there is bulky disease or disease in the midneck, the larynx block should be omitted.

In the patient without clinically evident axillary disease, the lateral border just falls off the axillary skin, and shielding of the humerus may be added if the arms are akimbo. Without axillary involvement, the inferior border of the axillary portion of the field is usually placed at or a centimeter above the posterior inferior border of the scapula; soft tissue blocks are used below this region (see Fig. 7). With axillary involvement, the soft tissue blocks should be omitted, as isolated nodal recurrences have

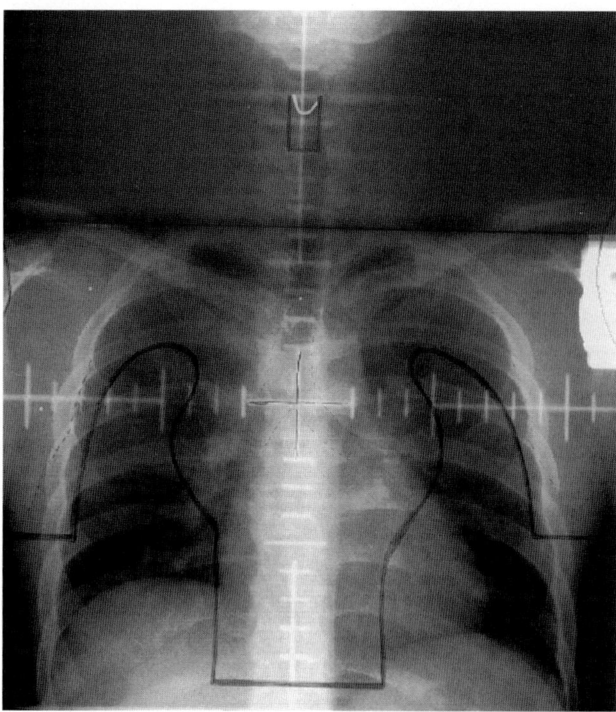

FIG. 8. A simulation film of a patient with the arms akimbo. Note the strip of lung inside the ribs that is treated to include the axillary nodes with this technique.

been noted outside the radiation portal posterior to the midaxillary line, below the scapula. The top of the lung block should be 1.5 to 2 cm below the clavicles to include the infraclavicular nodes. In patients with axillary disease, clinically evident axillary involvement often underestimates the extent of the adenopathy, and there is a risk that the standard lung blocks will block subpectoral or axillary nodes. The CT scan will help locate the adenopathy; ideally, these patients should undergo CT simulation to make sure that the axillary and subpectoral nodes are in the field. In patients with axillary involvement, special care should be taken to rule out brachial or epitrochlear involvement. The mantle lung blocks should include a generous margin on the hila and a 1.5- to 2-cm margin on the lateral borders of the tumor. Because the central axis usually rests at about T2 to T3, and the cord dose below that level will receive less than 100% of the central axis dose, it is rarely necessary to use a posterior thoracic spine block. The use of this block also risks blocking Hodgkin's disease in the mediastinal nodes.

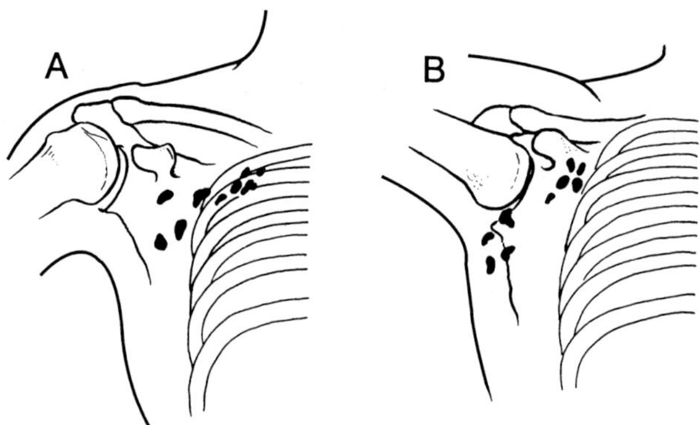

FIG. 9. The position of the axillary nodes varies with arm position. **A:** With arms akimbo. **B:** With arms up over the head. The arms-up position allows for more lung tissue to be shielded. (Reproduced with permission from ref. 84.)

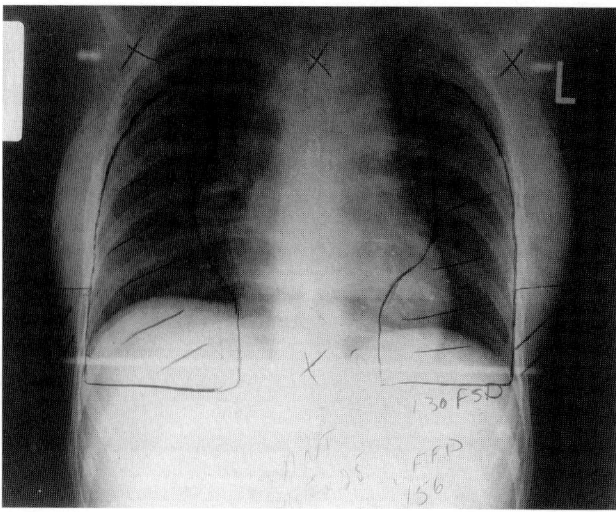

FIG. 10. A simulation film of a patient with arms above the head. Note that the lung blocks laterally run along the insides of the ribs.

The inferior margin of the mantle is determined by the inferior extent of disease and whether the patient also is receiving chemotherapy. In the patient with a clinically negative mediastinum receiving radiation therapy alone (mantle alone), the inferior border usually lies at approximately the bottom of T8 to T9, depending on individual patient anatomy (52). Under these circumstances, the field needs to cover only the hilar and subcarinal nodes, and the lower two-thirds of the heart is excluded from the field (see Fig. 11). This lower border also will suffice for a patient with upper mediastinal involvement receiving combined radiation therapy and chemotherapy.

In a patient with upper mediastinal nodes receiving mantle irradiation alone, the field should extend to the diaphragm (T10 to T11) to cover the central cardiac nodes (see Fig. 8) (52). Bulky mediastinal disease, subcarinal disease, and involvement of the hilar nodes indicate a moderate probability of subclinical disease in the adjacent pericardial and diaphragmatic nodes as well as the lung parenchyma and are considered indications for elective treatment of the cardiac silhouette, which includes the pericardial and diaphragmatic nodes in a patient not receiving chemotherapy. Large mediastinal and hilar adenopathy may also be considered indications for elective hemilung or whole-lung irradiation, espe-

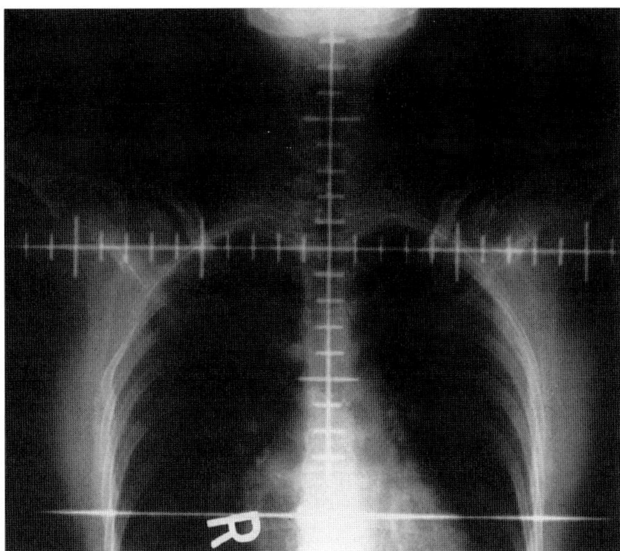

FIG. 11. Lower border of the mantle field in a 20-year-old patient with PS IA nodular sclerosis Hodgkin's disease with right cervical nodal involvement being treated with mantle irradiation alone. There was no mediastinal involvement on computed tomographic and gallium scanning. The mantle field includes the hilar and subcarinal nodes and is being treated with the arms above the head. The lung blocks are not shown. Note the large amount of the heart that is excluded from the field.

cially if the patient is being treated with radiation alone (although combined chemotherapy and radiation therapy is the treatment of choice in this setting).

With radiation therapy alone, if a patient is to receive mantle and paraaortic–splenic pedicle/splenic irradiation, the lower border of the mantle field must be high enough so that the spleen/splenic pedicle can be included in the abdominal field. This will not be feasible if the mantle field extends to the diaphragm. If there are low mediastinal nodes, the match will bridge an area of disease; this risks underdosing the tumor. Under these circumstances, an alternative technique may be used such as treatment with chemotherapy and a low mantle field without treatment of the abdomen or treatment with an extended mantle field that covers the upper abdomen.

The recommended prophylactic dose to the lung(s) and heart differs from the recommended dose for nodal disease in the remainder of the mantle field (Table 1). There are two techniques for delivering a differential dose to these areas: partial-transmission lung blocks and selective field blocking. Partial-transmission blocks may be used over the heart and lungs to reduce the dose per fraction and total dose to the desired level while permitting treatment of the standard mantle volume to the full dose and with standard-sized fractions. The use of this technique at Stanford has been associated with a decreased incidence of acute radiation pneumonitis (53). The disadvantage of this technique is the difficulty of accurate block fabrication.

The second technique, selective field blocking, is accomplished with multiple sets of blocks. If the blocks are inserted after the volume of interest has reached the prescribed total dose, then the region is treated with fractions of the same size as the remainder of the treatment volume. If the additional blocks are inserted for a portion of each daily treatment, then smaller fractions may be employed, analogous to the partial-transmission-block technique. However, the daily insertion of these additional blocks will significantly prolong the daily treatment time.

Patients who have large mediastinal masses and are being treated with radiation therapy alone may benefit from treatment using a shrinking-field technique. The initial field in these patients may include a large volume of the heart and lungs. Initial fractionation should be slow, 1.0 to 1.5 Gy per fraction to a total dose of 10 to 15 Gy. Time is then permitted for radiation-induced tumor regression, which allows an increase in the size of the subsequent lung and cardiac blocks.

Identification of the precise anatomic location of initial disease is crucial for determining the size and shape of the mantle blocks. Routine treatment-machine–generated verification films should be used to assure proper alignment. A mantle simulation film and the corresponding portal film are shown in Figure 12. Pretreatment computed tomographic and gallium studies will aid in this identification. After chemotherapy the lung blocks can be shaped to cover the residual mediastinal widening; it is not necessary to cover the prechemotherapy width of the mediastinal disease. However, areas of pleural, chest wall (Fig. 13), hilar (Fig. 14), axillary (Fig. 15), and cardiac nodal involvement should be treated with at least low-dose radiation even when there is a complete response to chemotherapy.

Some of the most difficult patients to treat are those with central or lateral cardiac nodes. These patients should be treated with combined chemotherapy and radiation therapy. In such cases, irradiation of large volumes of heart and lung to moderate or high doses should be avoided. However, even if the low mediastinal (cardiac) nodes completely resolve with chemotherapy, they should be treated with radiation therapy by delivering a low dose (15 Gy) to the whole heart followed by a cone down to the specific areas of cardiac nodal involvement if feasible. Review of the pretreatment computed tomographic studies is crucial for placement of the lower border of the field in this setting. In some cases, the lower border of the mantle field will need to be set as low as the bottom of T-12 because of the very low position of the nodes at the bottom of the diaphragm.

Two cases are shown for illustration. Figures 16A and 16B show the chest x-ray and magnetic resonance image of a patient with Hodgkin's disease along the left heart border. This patient received two cycles of chemotherapy (Fig. 16C) followed by a shrinking-field technique that

TABLE 1. *Recommended radiation dose (Gy)*[a]

	Prophylactic treatment				Involved sites				
					Maximum tumor dimension				
Treatment regimen	Nodal[b]	Lung	Heart	Liver	<6 cm	≥6 cm	Lung	Heart	Liver
Radiation alone (adults)	30–40	15–165	15	15–22	30–44	35–44	NA	NA	NA
Combined modality (adults)									
2–3 cycles of chemotherapy	25–30	10	15	15	30–36	35–40	15	25	25
≥6 cycles of chemotherapy									
PR	20–30	15–165	15	15–22	30–44	35–44	15	25	25
CR	NA	NA	NA	NA	20–30	30–36	15	20	20
Children[c]	NA	NA	NA	NA	15–25	15–25	10–15	10–15	10–15

[a]Recommended maximum dose per fraction: nodal areas, 1.5–1.8 Gy; cardiac silhouette, ≤1.5 Gy; lung 0.75–1.5 Gy; liver, 1.0–1.5 Gy.

[b]20–30 Gy in low-risk areas such as preauricular nodes and pelvis.

[c]Pediatric patients usually receive radiation therapy only to involved sites in conjunction with four to six cycles of chemotherapy.

NA, not applicable; PR, partial response; CR, complete response.

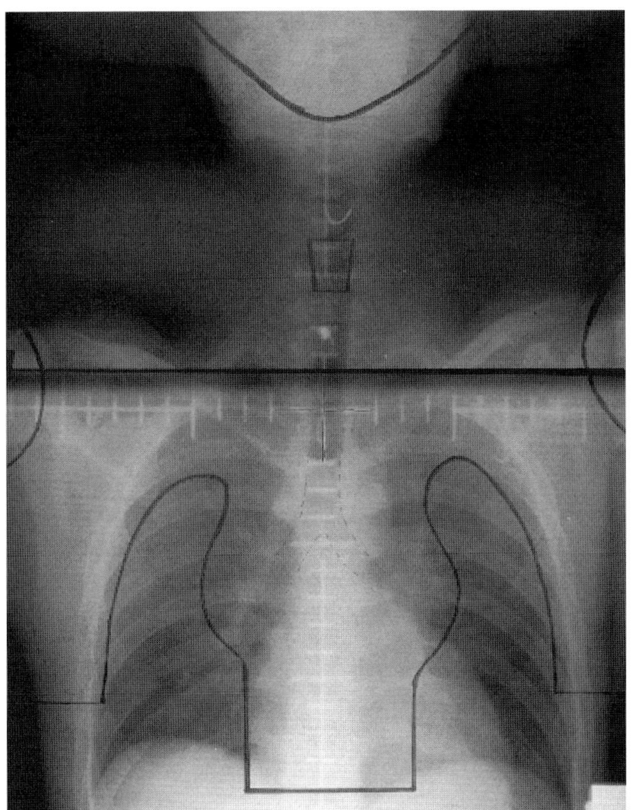

A

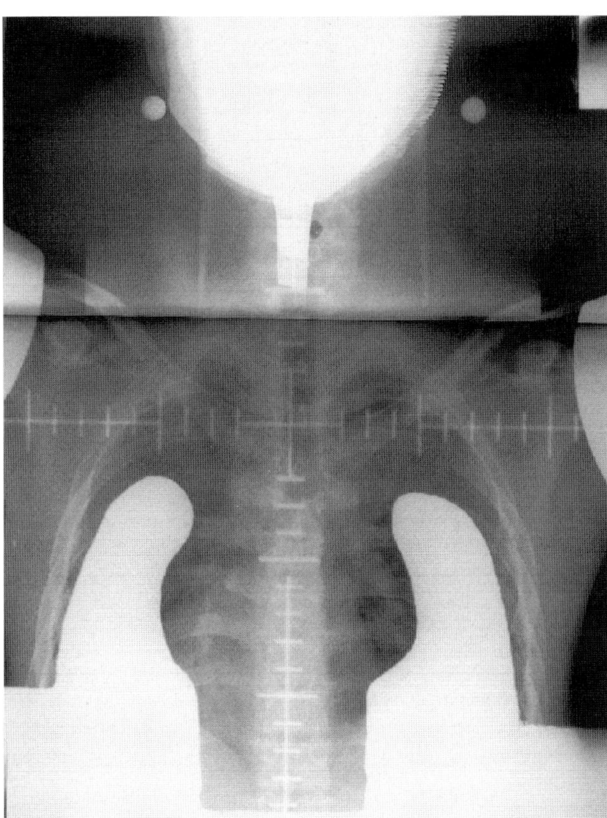

B

FIG. 12. An anterior–posterior mantle simulation film **(A)** and the corresponding portal film **(B)** of a patient with Hodgkin's disease treated in the arms-akimbo position.

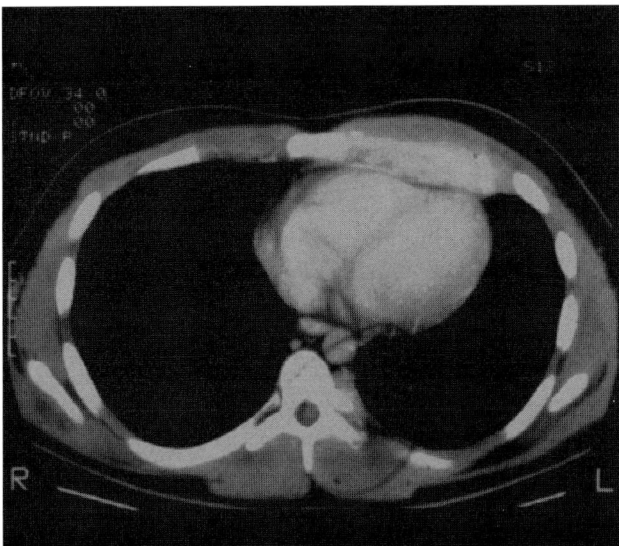

FIG. 13. Computed tomographic scan of chest wall involvement anterior and adjacent to the heart in a patient with Hodgkin's disease.

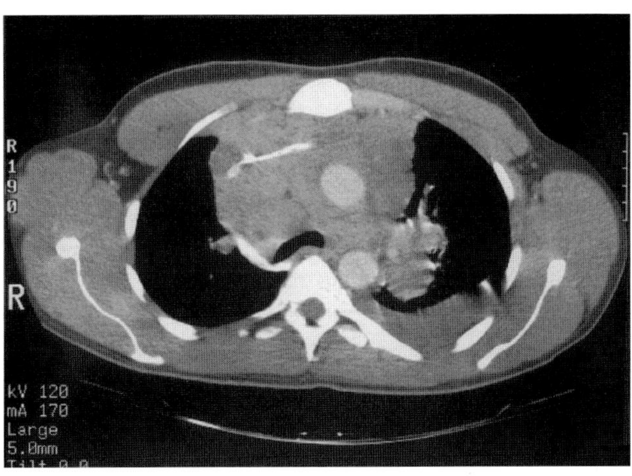

FIG. 14. Computed tomographic scan of large mediastinal, pleural, and left hilar involvement and a left pleural effusion in a 33-year-old man with Hodgkin's disease who presented with shortness of breath and tachycardia.

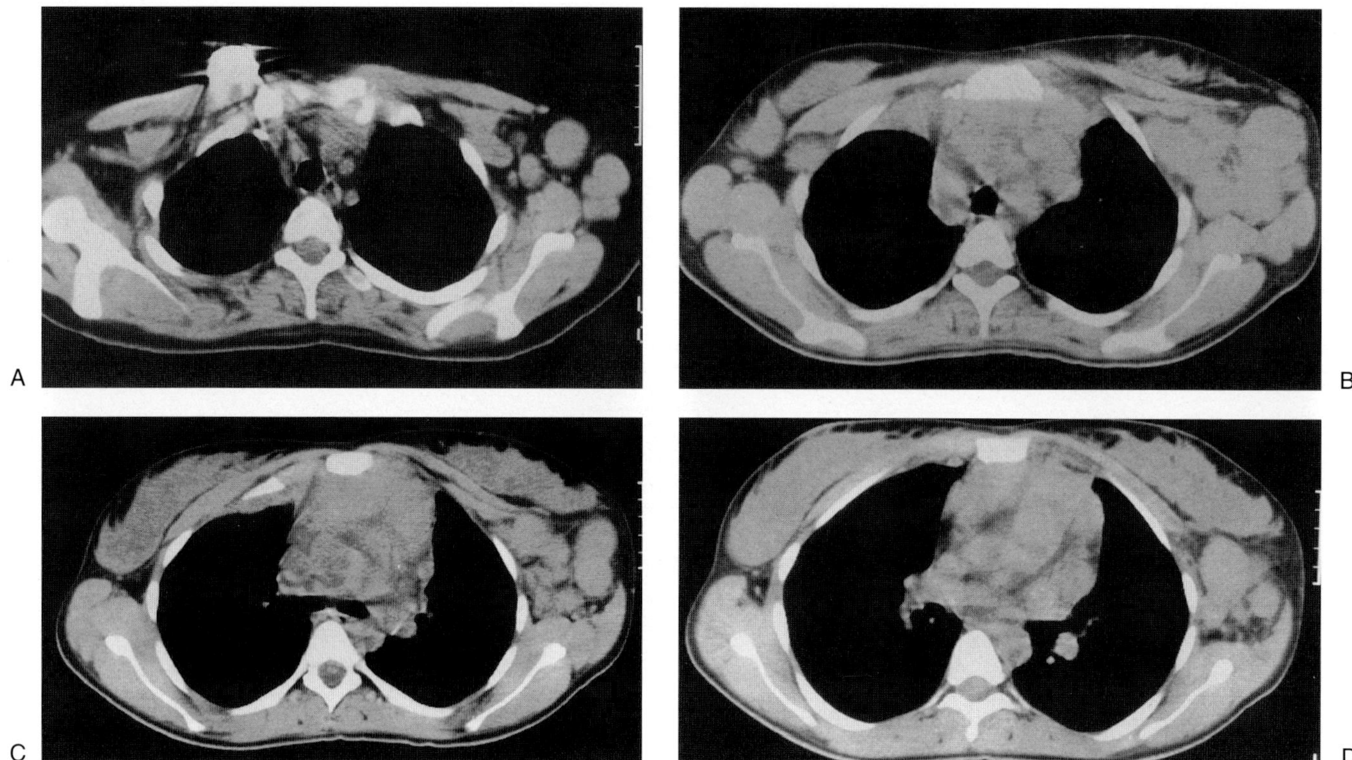

FIG. 15. Computed tomographic scans of bulky axillary involvement in a patient with Hodgkin's disease with cuts through the upper mediastinum **(A),** the mediastinum at T-4 **(B),** the mediastinum just below the carina **(C),** and the mediastinum at the hila **(D).** Left bulky axillary adenopathy is seen on all four cuts.

included 10 Gy to the entire cardiac silhouette and left lung (Fig. 16D), followed by an additional 10 Gy with a low heart block (Fig. 16E), followed by placement of a left ventricular block (Fig. 16F). The second case is a patient with CS IIA Hodgkin's disease with both medial and lateral cardiac nodes (Fig. 17A) treated with six cycles of ABVD. Following completion of chemotherapy, repeat computed tomographic scans showed a good response, but minimal evidence of cardiac adenopathy remained. The patient was treated with whole cardiac irradiation (15 Gy, ten fractions, 2 weeks) followed by a cone down (25 Gy) to a mantle field with left ventricular blocking (Fig. 17B), followed by a cone down to the mediastinum (site of bulky disease) to 36 Gy total dose (Fig. 17C).

The sloping surfaces, variation in patient thickness, tissue inhomogeneity, significant variation in distance from the source to the skin and distance from the central axis, irregular field shape, internal scatter, large blocks within the mantle volume, and transmission through the blocks may result in substantial dose inhomogeneity. Dose calculations off the central axis should be obtained, and adjustments made to improve the dose inhomogeneity that occurs from differences in patient separation within the large mantle field. For example, nodes in the axilla and neck receive a higher dose than the upper mediastinum because of decreased patient thickness. The subcarinal region receives a lower effective dose because of increased patient thickness and the loss of scatter from within the tissue protected by the lung blocks.

Dose calculations should be performed to identify the dose delivered to multiple points within the mantle field, especially the mid neck, axilla and low mediastinum. The calculations should include the effects of both primary and scattered radiation to each point of calculation (54). Unless such a variation in dose distribution is desired, the total dose to selected areas can be adjusted by the use of individually designed compensators or selective area blocking (54). One approach is to compensate treatment fields when the dose variation is greater than 7.5% to 10%. Alternatively, the prescription dose may be normalized to the mediastinum and the other site points (neck, supraclavicular region, axilla) are blocked after the prescribed dose is delivered. The subcarinal and pericardial doses should also be monitored and blocked when appropriate.

There are several situations in which treatment of the mantle in an upright position may be desirable. The first and most common is in patients with large, previously untreated mediastinal masses or large residual masses after chemotherapy, in whom it is difficult to shield sufficient lung and heart tissue (55). With the patient upright, the diaphragm frequently rests in a lower position, which stretches out the mediastinal contents,

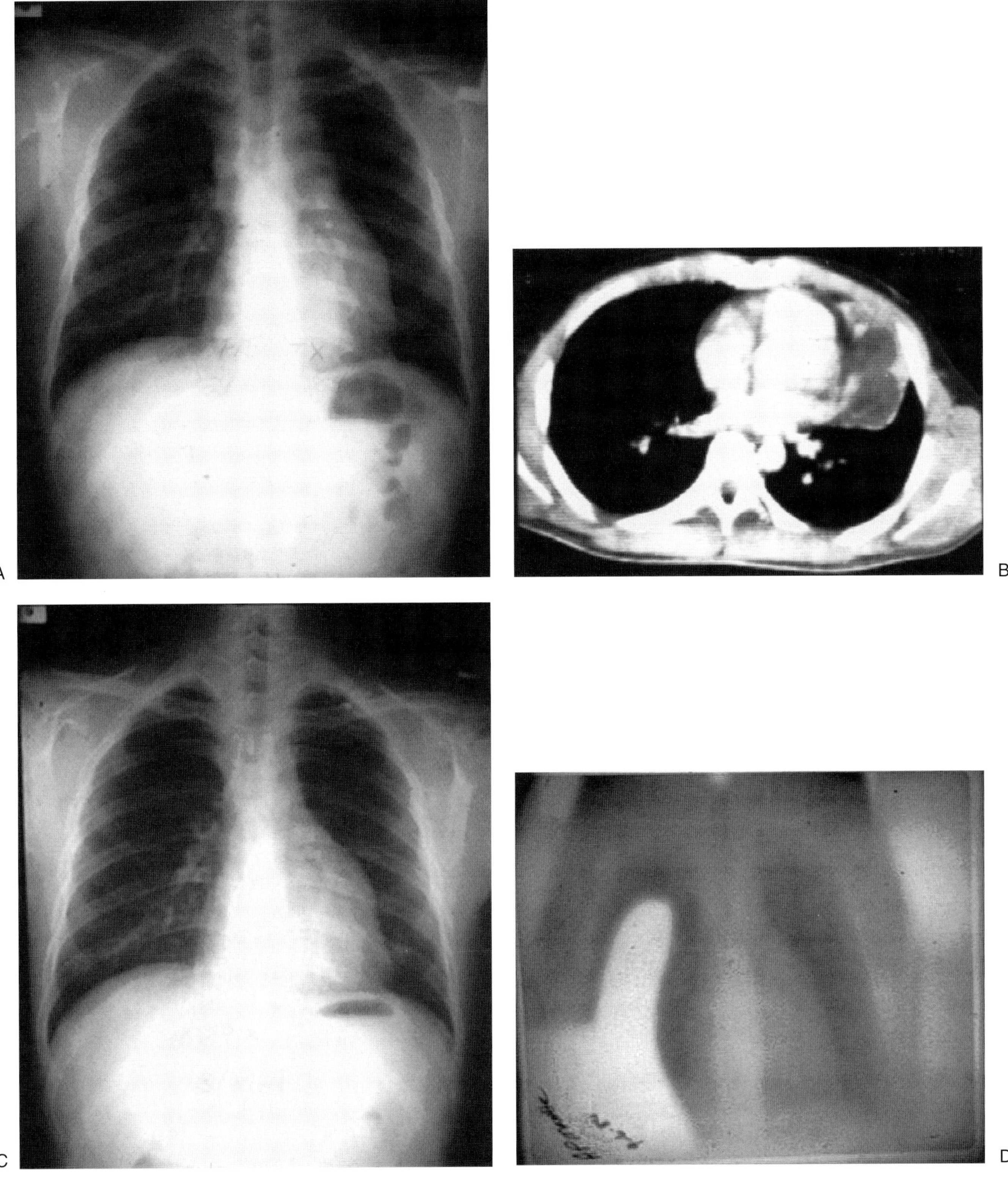

FIG. 16. Chest radiograph **(A)** and magnetic resonance image **(B)** of a patient with Hodgkin's disease along the left heart border. This patient received two cycles of chemotherapy and had a partial response **(C),** followed by a shrinking-field technique that included 10 Gy to the entire cardiac silhouette and left lung (port film, **D**), followed by an additional 10 Gy with a low heart block (port film, **E**), followed by placement of a left ventricular block (port film, **F**). *Continued on next page.*

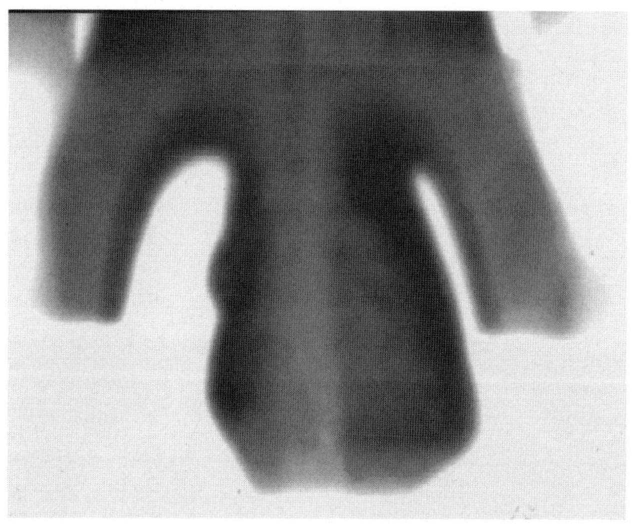
E

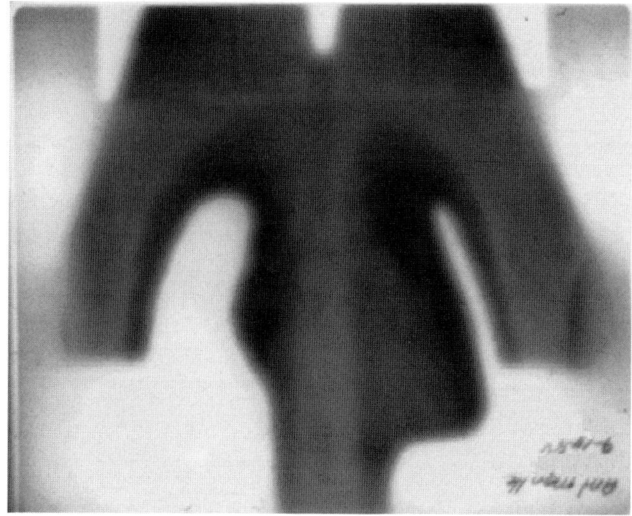
F

FIG. 16. *Continued.*

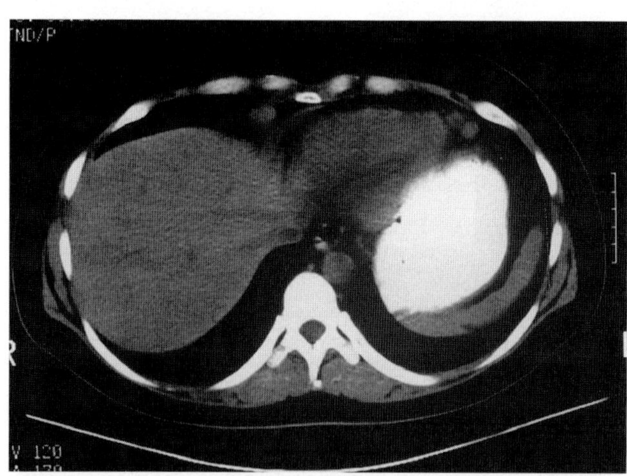
A

FIG. 17. A patient with CS IIA Hodgkin's disease with large mediastinal disease and both medial and lateral cardiac nodes on computed tomography (**A**) treated with 6 cycles of ABVD. Following completion of chemotherapy, repeat computed tomographic scans showed a good response, but minimal evidence of cardiac adenopathy remained. The patient was treated with whole cardiac irradiation (15 Gy, 10 fractions, 2 weeks) followed by a cone down to a mantle with left ventricular blocking to 25 Gy (see simulation film, **B**), followed by a cone down to the mediastinum (site of bulky disease) to 36 Gy (see simulation film, **C**).

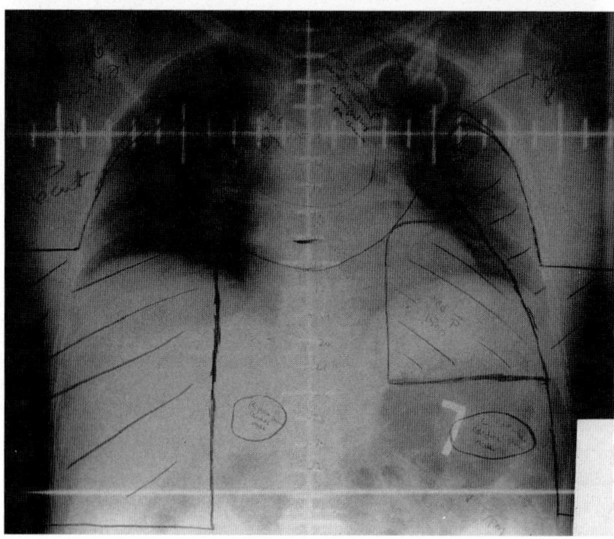
B

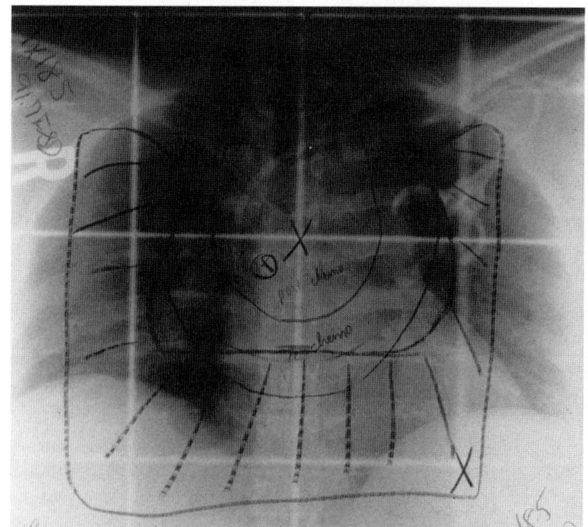
C

decreasing the width of the mediastinum. This permits increased pulmonary excursion and increases the amount of lung and heart that can be shielded (see Fig. 18). In addition, the patient may take a deep breath and hold it or breathe in a shallow manner during treatment. The chair may also be used for very large patients in whom pulmonary excursion is compromised or whose weight exceeds the treatment table limits. Other uncommon scenarios include the treatment of a patient whose medical condition precludes treatment in the supine position and a pregnant patient who requires maximal uterine shielding.

The major disadvantages of treatment in the upright position are increased difficulty in setup, reduced immobilization, reduced daily reproducibility, and difficulty in accurately matching the upright mantle treatment volume with upper abdominal radiation fields treated with the patient supine or prone. When the upright position is selected, immobilization and reproducibility can be significantly improved with the use of a special chair or standing rest. There are different versions (55); some are commercially available (56). Important features of the chair are shown in Figures 19 and 20. The setup time is substantially more than required for the supine position. The level of the seat must be adjustable and the height reproducible from day to day. The arm position must be maintained; one method is through adjustable axillary rests, forearm rests, and hand holders. The chest must be perpendicular to the beam; shoulder depressors keep the back flat against the backboard in the anterior position. In the posterior position, the chest may be pressed against the backboard. Adjustable chin rests or chin straps will achieve a reproducible degree of neck extension.

Minimantle Field

A *minimantle* excludes the mediastinum entirely and is designed to treat the bilateral cervical, supraclavicular, infraclavicular, and axillary nodes only. In young women without overt axillary involvement, some radiation oncol-

A

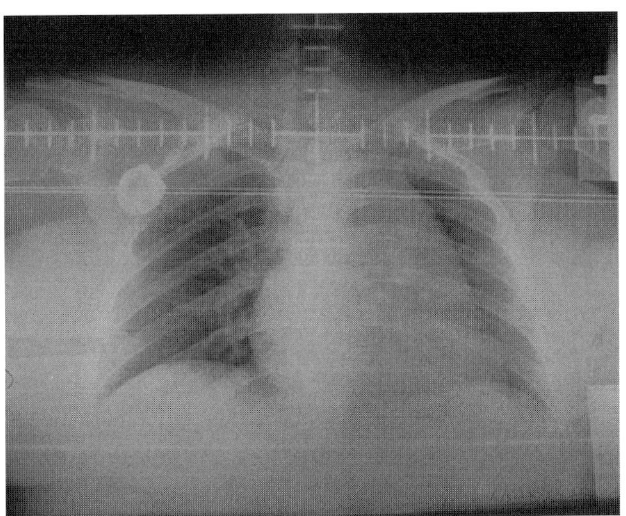

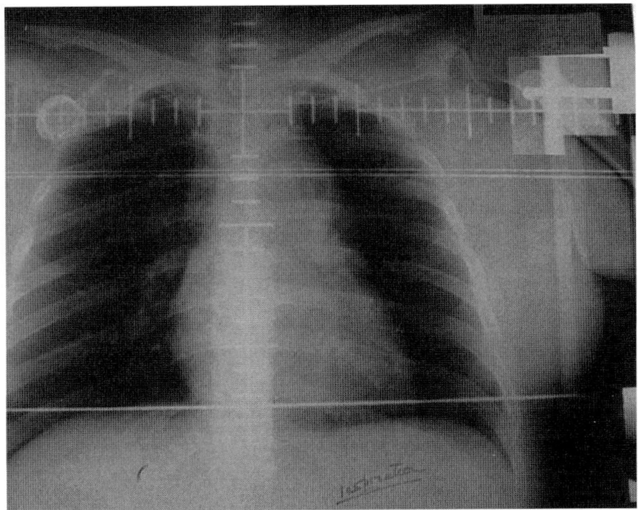

B

C

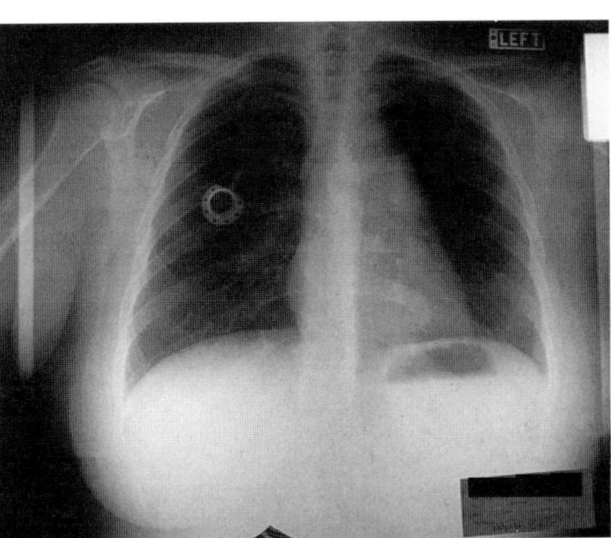

FIG. 18. Chest radiographs of a patient with mediastinal adenopathy showing the shift of the mass from the supine position **(A)** to the supine position at full inspiration **(B)** to the upright position **(C).** Note the increasing ability to block normal left lung with the change in inspiration and position.

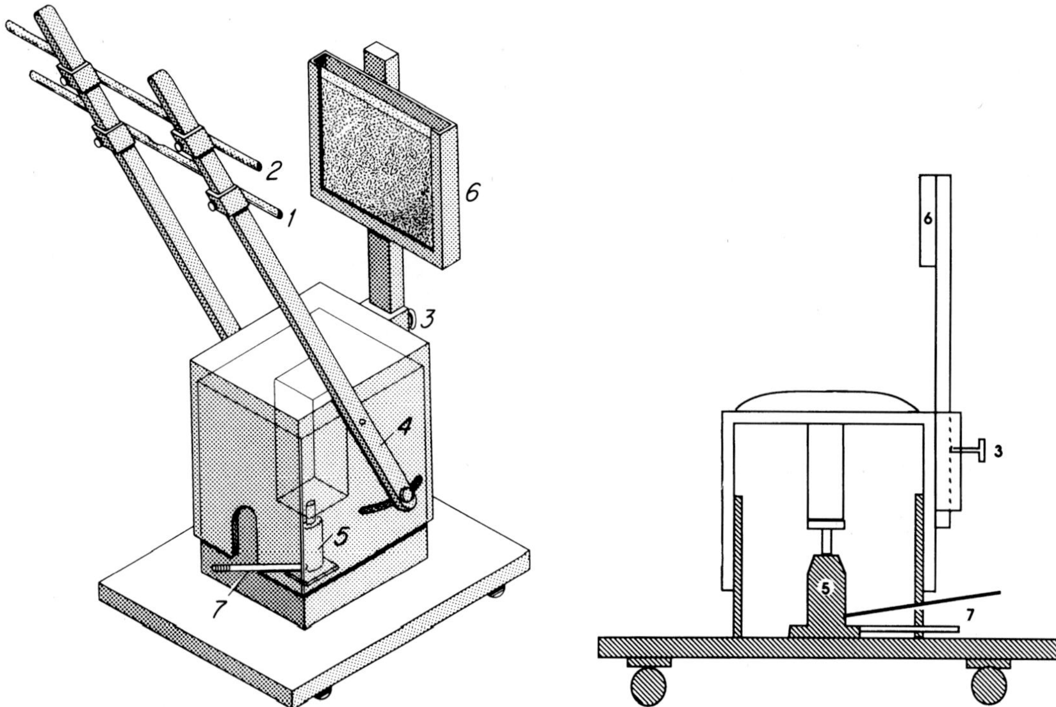

FIG. 19. Schematic representation of the chair used for upright mantle treatment: (1) chin rest;(2) bar for hand and arm support;(3) adjustment for back support;(4) angular adjustment of chin and arm support;(5) hydraulic lift;(6) back support and film holder;(7) hydraulic lift arm and release. (Reproduced with permission from ref. 55.)

ogists elect to exclude the axillae in an attempt to reduce the long-term risk of breast cancer. Such modifications of the mantle field may be employed more safely in the setting of combined-modality therapy because clinically uninvolved areas such as the axilla may be at high risk for harboring occult disease, especially in the presence of ipsilateral supraclavicular disease (57).

Involved Fields Above the Diaphragm

Involved fields can be used after combination chemotherapy to treat the initially involved lymph node region or after the mantle field to cone down to the regions of initial involvement. By definition, these fields treat the region of initial nodal involvement. The technique of treating the enlarged node without treating the region should be avoided.

Preauricular Field

The *preauricular field* includes the superficial lymph nodes just anterior to the tragus and therefore above or on the edge of standard anterior and posterior neck or mantle fields. This field may be added when a patient is being treated with radiation therapy alone and there is a moderate risk of subclinical involvement in the preauricular nodes because of disease in the upper neck (above the thyroid notch). One technique is to treat the patient with a lateral *en face* electron field that is usually approximately 4 cm in width and 4 to 6 cm in height, trapezoidal in shape, with the inferior border sloping to match the upper border of the mantle field. The upper border is approximately 2 cm above the tragus, usually just below the superior border of the helix; the posterior border is 1 cm behind the tragus; the anterior border is approximately 3 cm anterior to the tragus. If the area is being treated prophylactically, the dose is low, usually 20 to 30 Gy in 10 to 20 fractions, with low-energy electrons (6 to 9 MeV). If the region is clinically involved, the dose should be 30 to 36 Gy.

An alternative technique is to extend the superior border of the mantle field to encompass the preauricular region using a custom midline shielding block to protect the oral mucosa and block out the contralateral preauricular area completely (Fig. 21). An advantage of this technique is that it avoids dose inhomogeneity in the area of match between the anterior and posterior photon fields and the lateral electron field; however, it does require the capacity to treat an even larger field and is associated with potentially greater oral toxicity and occipital hair loss.

Waldeyer's Ring

There is little risk for subclinical disease in the extranodal lymphoid tissue of the nasopharynx, tonsil, and base

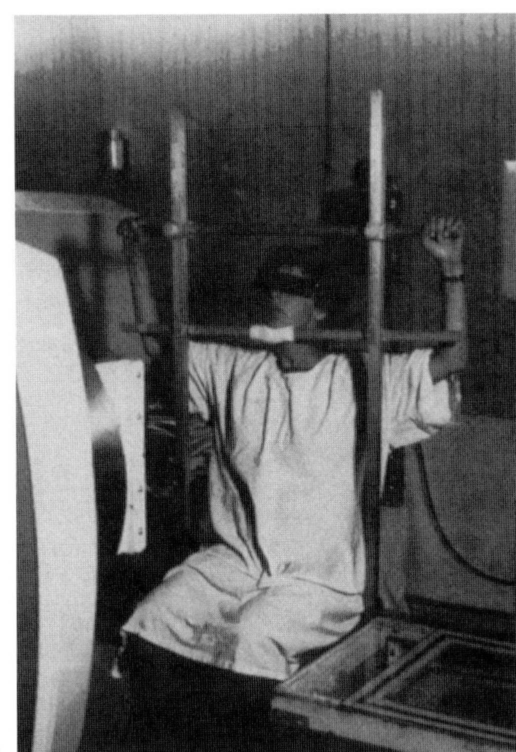

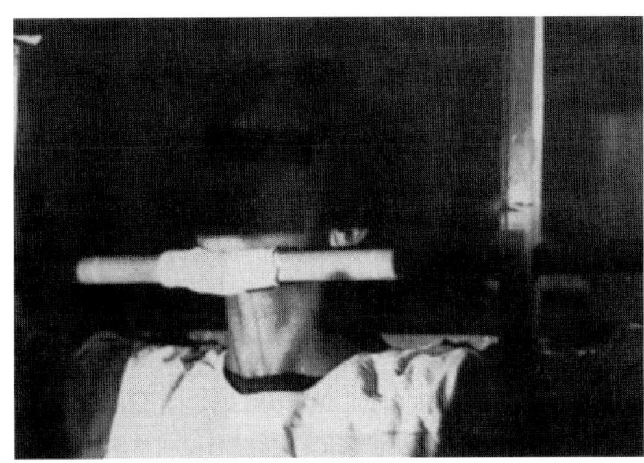

FIG. 20. Photographs of a patient in the treatment chair **(A)** and showing the upper border of the field **(B)**. (Reproduced with permission from ref. 55.)

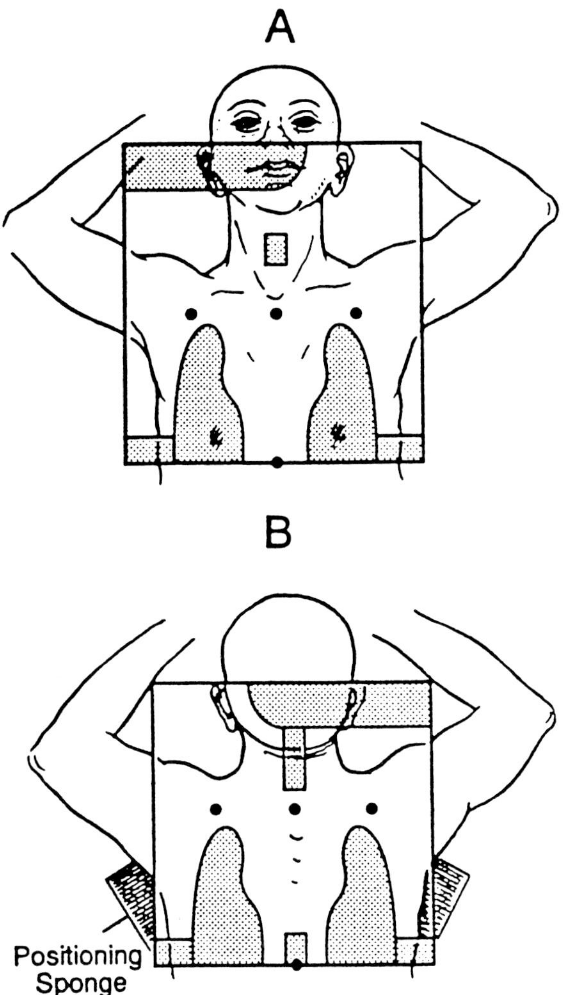

FIG. 21. Placement on the anterior **(A)** and posterior **(B)** "high" mantle of the superior border and mouth block when treating a patient with high neck disease. (Tattoos indicated by ●) (Reproduced with permission from ref. 84.)

of tongue, but occasionally there is biopsy proof of involvement in one of these sites. The most common indication for a *Waldeyer's field* in Hodgkin's disease is actually bulky disease in the upper neck, often in conjunction with preauricular, postauricular, submental, parotid, or retropharyngeal nodal involvement (Fig. 22A,B) that cannot be adequately encompassed with the standard mantle field. The typical Waldeyer field (Fig. 22C) includes extranodal lymphoid tissue in the nasopharynx, base of tongue, and tonsils as well as retropharyngeal, preauricular, postauricular, occipital, parotid, submandibular, and submental nodes. It is matched to the upper border of the neck or mantle fields at approximately the level of the thyroid notch. The easiest method of matching fields is to set the central axis of each field at the field junction to eliminate divergence. Extra protection may be provided by the inclusion of a short (2 cm) block over the superior portion of the spinal cord on the anterior and posterior neck or mantle fields. The most common energy chosen is 6 MV photons.

Cervical/Supraclavicular Fields

The *neck fields* include all nodal tissue from the base of the skull to the clavicles. The patient is positioned supine and treated with opposed anterior and posterior fields with the neck in the same position as for the upper border of the mantle; that is, the upper border of the field passes through midmandible, midtragus, and mastoid when the head is extended. The inferior border is 1 to 2 cm below the clavicles. The lateral border is set at the medial aspect of the acromion to encompass the supraclavicular and low neck

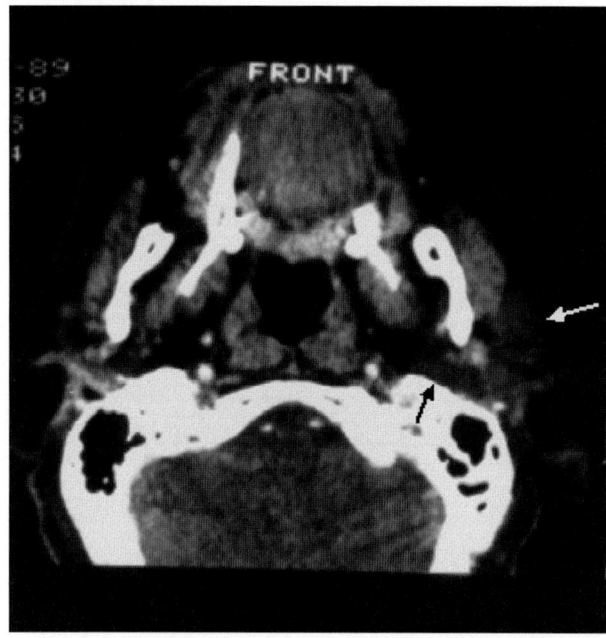

A

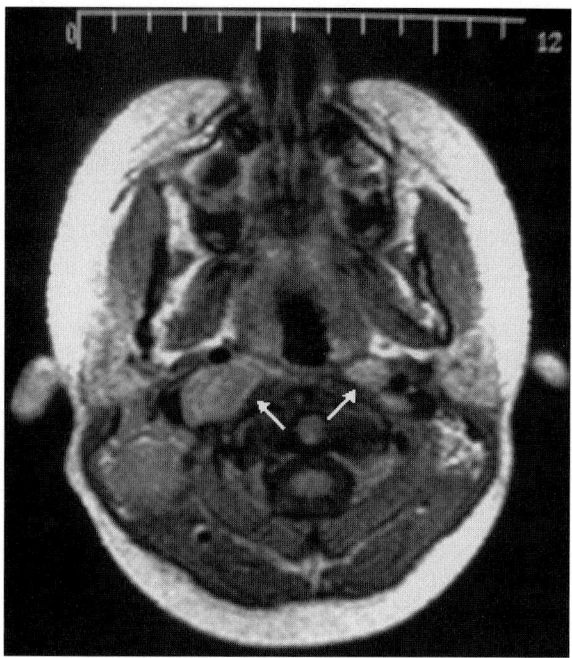

B

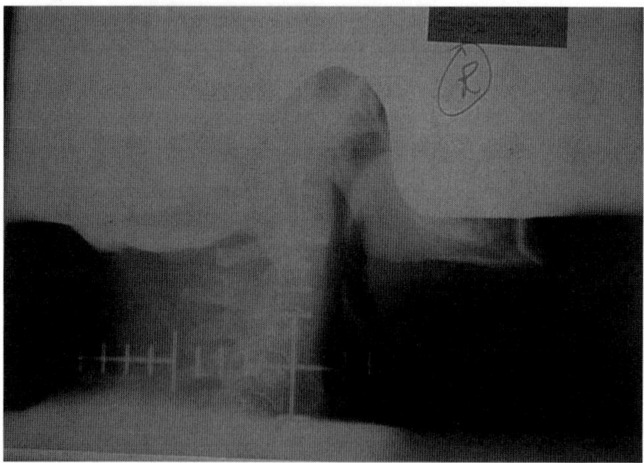

C

FIG. 22. The most common indication for a Waldeyer field in Hodgkin's disease is bulky disease in the upper neck, often in conjunction with preauricular **(A),** postauricular, submental, parotid, or retropharyngeal **(B)** nodal involvement that cannot be adequately encompassed with the standard mantle field. The typical Waldeyer field **(C)** includes extranodal lymphoid tissue in the nasopharynx, base of tongue, and tonsils as well as retropharyngeal, preauricular, postauricular, occipital, parotid, submandibular, and submental nodes. It is matched to the upper border of the neck or mantle fields at approximately the level of the thyroid notch.

nodes, and the beam tangentially irradiates the lateral neck skin and lower ear superiorly. The medial border for a single neck field is set at either the ipsilateral (cervical nodal involvement alone) or contralateral (with supraclavicular nodal involvement) vertebral pedicles, that is, either including or excluding the entire width of the spinal cord. When the contralateral vertebral pedicles are used, the pharynx and larynx can be blocked to approximately C5. Treatment should be given with 4- to 6-MV photons. If a higher energy is utilized, bolus may have to be applied because some of the nodes are located no more than 0.5 cm below the skin surface. Even with 6-MV photons, response of the supraclavicular nodes to radiation should be assessed midway into treatment. If the response is less than ideal, daily bolus over this region should be applied for the second half of the mantle treatment.

The fields should be equally weighted, given the normal location of lymph nodes within this field. If there is upper neck involvement (above the thyroid notch), a preauricular field may be added (see above). If there is confluent neck disease extending into the submandibular, preauricular, or postauricular regions, opposed lateral head and neck or Waldeyer's fields (see Waldeyer's Ring Fields) may be treated. This is because of the difficulty in obtaining an adequate margin on base-of-skull nodes, the risk of subclinical disease in the preauricular, postauricular, parotid, submental, and retropharyngeal nodes, as well as occasional extranodal involvement of the lymphatic tissues of Waldeyer's ring. The risk of Waldeyer's involvement is greater with bilateral preauricular or base of skull involvement.

Mediastinum

The *mediastinal field* includes anterior superior mediastinal, pretracheal, paratracheal, paraesophageal, hilar, internal mammary, and subcarinal nodes. The caudad/cephalad extent should cover from the top of T1 to the bottom of T8 (varies with patient anatomy) to cover the hilar and subcarinal nodes (Fig. 23). If the central cardiac and diaphragmatic nodes are involved, the field should extend to the level of the diaphragm (Fig. 24). The superior border should encompass the T1 vertebral body at the minimum. If there is extension into the deep supraclavicular fossa, the field should extend to the top of C7. Laterally, the fields should encompass any clinically evident tumor with a 1–2 cm margin as well as a 1–2 cm margin on the suerior mediastinal shadow, and the hila.

It is difficult on simulation films to visualize the sternum, which could serve as a landmark for setting an adequate lateral margin on the internal mammary nodes. Therefore, the spine is used as a surrogate landmark for the most lateral anterior and the most lateral posterior nodes in the mediastinal field. Any clinically evident disease on computed tomographic scanning in the internal mammary, pericardial, or diaphragmatic nodes must be mapped carefully and included with a 1–2 cm margin (see discussion on three dimensional treatment planning later in this chapter).

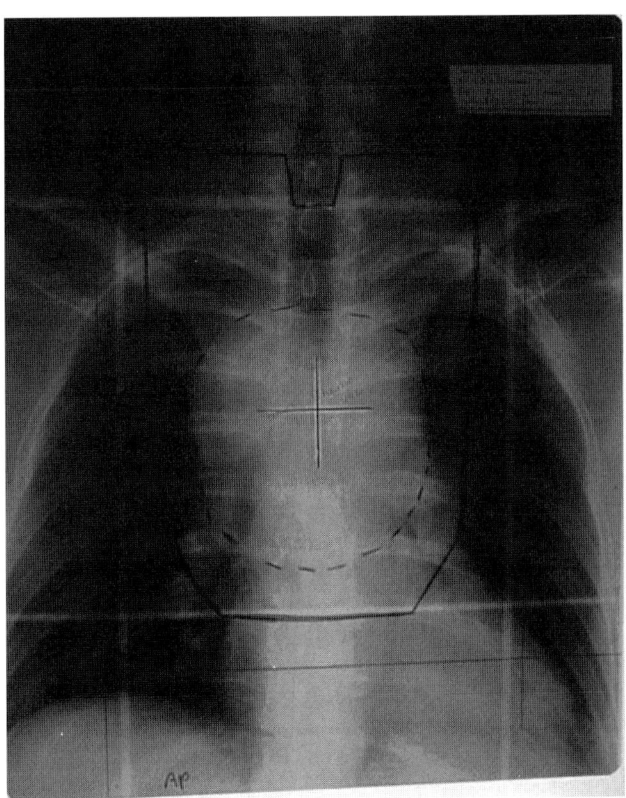

FIG. 23. Mediastinal field. The mediastinal field includes anterior superior mediastinal, pretracheal, paratracheal, paraesophageal, hilar, internal mammary, and subcarinal nodes. The caudad–cephalad extent should cover from the top of T-1 to T-8 or T-9 to cover the hilar and subcarinal nodes.

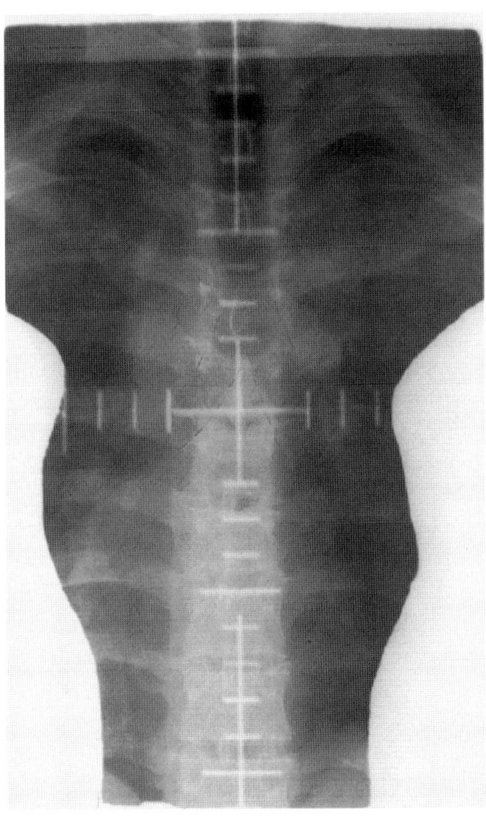

FIG. 24. Mediastinal field. If the central cardiac and diaphragmatic nodes are involved, the field should extend to the level of the diaphragm. Laterally, the fields should encompass any clinically evident tumor with a 1- to 2-cm margin as well as a 1- to 2-cm margin on the superior mediastinal shadow, the hila, and the vertebral bodies of the inferior thoracic spine.

Epitrochlear Nodes

Epitrochlear involvement in Hodgkin's disease is rare. With the arms rotated outward, the nodes lie in the medial half of the arm. The easiest way to treat the epitrochlear nodes is to use an involved field separate from the mantle field. Usually the lateral half of the arm can be blocked.

Paraaortic/Spleen Fields

The standard paraaortic treatment volume is treated through equally weighted, opposed anterior and posterior portals with the patient supine only or supine and prone (using the same setup as in the treatment of the mantle). The superior border matches the mantle field, with an appropriate gap to allow for divergence (see section on abutting fields later in this chapter). The inferior border is set at the bottom of L4 (bifurcation of the aorta). The paraaortic nodes normally lie within the most lateral extent of the transverse processes of the vertebral bodies. This normal position may be confirmed by computed tomographic scanning or lymphography. If the lateral borders of the field are set at the edges of the transverse processes (about 1.5 to 2 cm lateral to the border of the vertebral bodies), this will result in a field width of 8 to 9 cm. It is imperative that the location of each kidney be known and mapped and that no more than one-third of the total renal volume is included in the paraaortic field. Paraaortic irradiation is contraindicated in patients with horseshoe kidneys, as it is impossible to protect an adequate volume of kidney to assure subsequent normal kidney function. The spleen should be included in the paraaortic field as shown in Fig. 25A. The spleen is usually not visible on fluoroscopy or routine simulation films; in addition, splenic motion is associated with diaphragmatic motion. Computed tomographic scanning or magnetic resonance imaging should be utilized for treatment planning. Ideally, computed tomographic scanning is performed with the patient in the treatment position for improved accuracy. In most patients, a portion of the spleen abuts the diaphragm; inclusion of the diaphragm with a 0.5- to 1.0-cm border of lung will ensure adequate splenic coverage that can be verified with routine port films. The spleen also typically abuts the lateral abdominal wall; inclusion of rib cage or the lateral abdominal wall will ensure adequate lateral coverage. The medial and inferior borders of the spleen are determined by computed tomographic scanning or magnetic resonance imaging. On occasion, the inferior border of the spleen is clearly visible on the simulation film.

It is critical that the location of the kidneys be documented as a portion of the spleen and the left kidney are frequently superimposed. If more than one-third of the left kidney is included in the treatment field, an attempt should be made to minimize the amount of the right kidney in the paraaortic field. In cases in which more than half of the total renal volume would be included in the splenic and paraaortic fields, consideration should be given to the use of combined-modality therapy (permitting smaller radiation fields or lower radiation doses) or splenectomy.

Paraaortic/Splenic Pedicle Field

In the patient who has undergone a splenectomy, the paraaortic field is often extended laterally to include the splenic hilar region. Under ideal circumstances, the splenic hilum has been marked by the surgeon with radiopaque clips. In the absence of a splenic pedicle clip, the paraaortic field may be extended to the left at the level of the T12-L1 vertebral bodies to encompass the usual medial course of the splenic vasculature, along which the splenic hilar lymph nodes would be located. Alternatively, it may be possible to see residual splenic hilar nodes on computed tomographic scanning.

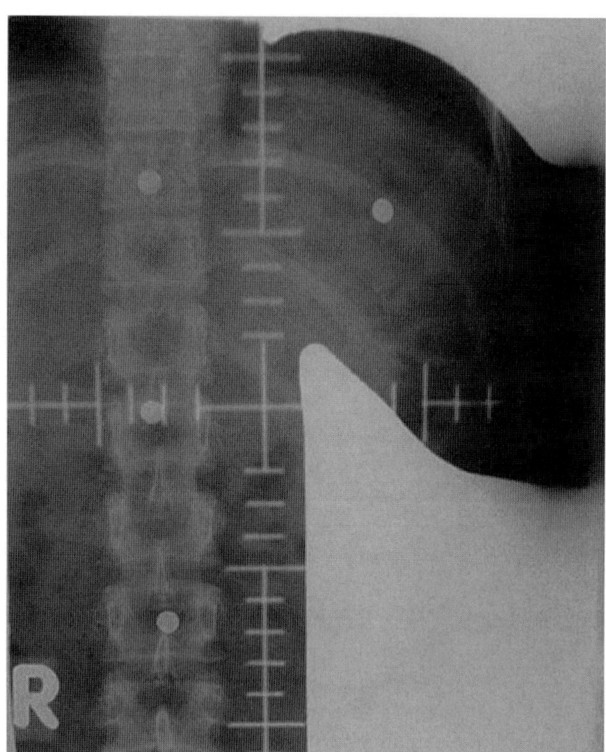

A

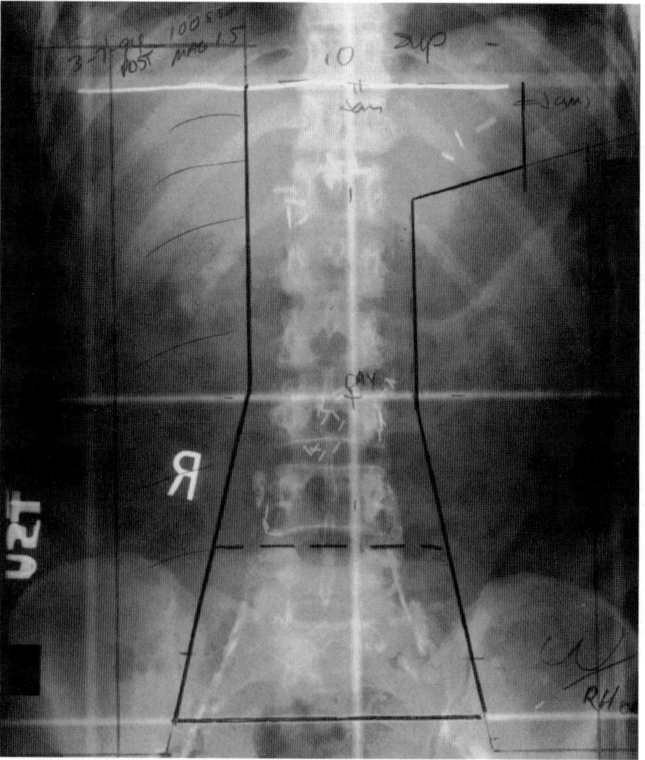

B

FIG. 25. A: Simulation film of a paraaortic and splenic field. **B:** Simulation film of a spade and splenic-pedicle field. (Reprinted from Leibel S, Phillips T. Hodgkin's disease. In *Clinical radiation oncology,* 1087.)

Spade Field

At some institutions, the paraaortic field is extended inferiorly, beyond the aortic bifurcation, to include the common iliac nodes. This extension is planned most readily in the presence of lymphographic contrast. In the absence of a lymphogram, the lateral borders of this extension should follow an oblique line from the lateral tip of each of the transverse processes of L-5 to a point 1-2 cm lateral to the widest point of the pelvis (Fig. 25B).

Pelvic Fields

The pelvic nodes are treated through opposed anterior and posterior fields with the patient supine (with an SAD or SSD technique) or supine and prone (SSD only). The superior border of the pelvic field matches the inferior border of the paraaortic field with an appropriate gap (see abutting fields) or, in the absence of other fields, extends to the top of L-5. The borders of the field are generally set to include the pelvic and inguinal nodes and inferiorly to extend to the bottom of the ischial tuberosities. For patients presenting with subdiaphragmatic Hodgkin's disease, the femoral nodes should be treated as well with the field extended inferiorly to include the palpable femoral triangle with a 1.5- to 2-cm margin, or approximately 5 cm below the inferior portion of the lesser trochanter (Fig. 26). A lymphogram is very helpful for ensuring inclusion of all external and common iliac nodes and maximizing central shielding (58). If a lymphogram is not available, the lateral border may be set laterally to the outer edge of the acetabulum with blocking of the iliac crests. A 4-cm central block extending superiorly to the level of the bottom of the sacroiliac joints should be added to shield the symphysis pubis, central bladder, and rectum.

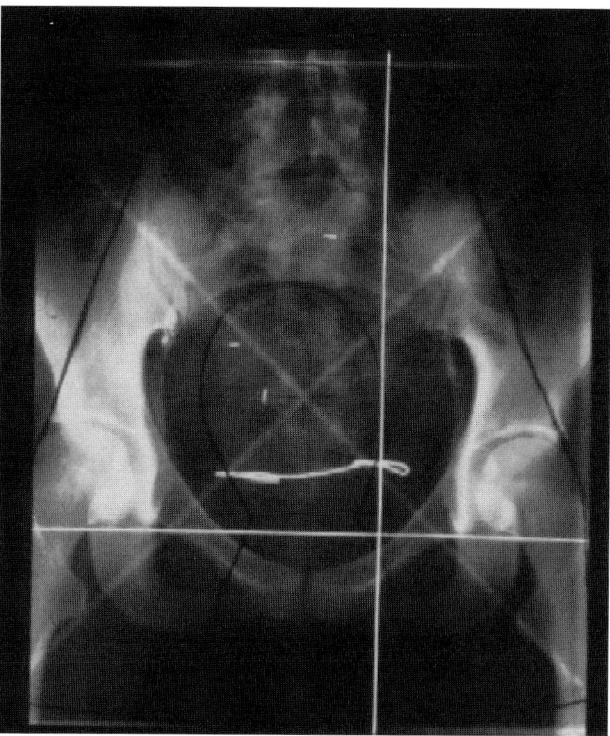

FIG. 26. Pelvic fields. Pelvic simulation film showing lymphangiogram dye and clips marking centrally transposed ovaries. The central pelvic and iliac wing blocks are not shown.

In the standard pelvic field, the testicles are not in the primary beam. However, scattered irradiation from the pelvic and inguinal fields is sufficient to produce permanent azoospermia in 20% to 50% of patients (59,60). The scattered dose received by the testicles depends on the total dose given to any field close enough to contribute scattered radiation, the distance from the edge of the contributing fields, and the design and positioning of special testicular shielding devices and is usually 2% to 3% of the total dose (61–63). When the femoral nodes are treated, the testes are often in the primary beam and receive just over 3% through the central pelvic block, as well as increased scatter from the open fields that lie on either side, so that the total dose to the testes is approximately 8%; this results in a much higher risk of sterility. The dose can be reduced with additional blocking of the primary beam. The dose decreases almost exponentially with distance from the edge of the field. Close to the edge of the field, the scattered dose is high at the surface, drops to a minimum at d_{max}, and increases with depth, but varies less with depth as the distance from the field edge increases. In addition to scattered dose, there is also a contribution from machine leakage resulting in scattered electrons at the skin surface.

To preserve fertility in the male patient treated with pelvic irradiation, the testicles must be shielded from as much internally scattered radiation as possible by using a special clamshell-like testicular shield (Fig. 27) (62–65). It is important that the testicles are positioned behind the front wall of the shield, and the lip of the shield lid must overlap the front wall of the shell. Clamshell shields will provide a 3- to 10-fold reduction in dose to the testes (63). Depending primarily on the distance from the field edge, the total dose to the testes often is no more than 2% to 3% of the prescribed pelvic dose. In patients with seminoma, Kubo and Shipley (65) employed a 10 cm lead scrotal block above the scrotum immediately outside the field that further reduced the testicular dose to 0.1% of the prescribed midplane pelvic dose by attenuating the scattered electrons from machine leakage. Whether this technique could be applied to the centrally shielded area of the pelvic field in Hodgkin's disease is unknown. The clamshell testicular shield should be coated with a 2-mm layer of rubber to attenuate the low-dose scattered electrons.

Normally, the ovaries lie just medial to the external iliac nodes and within a standard pelvic radiation field.

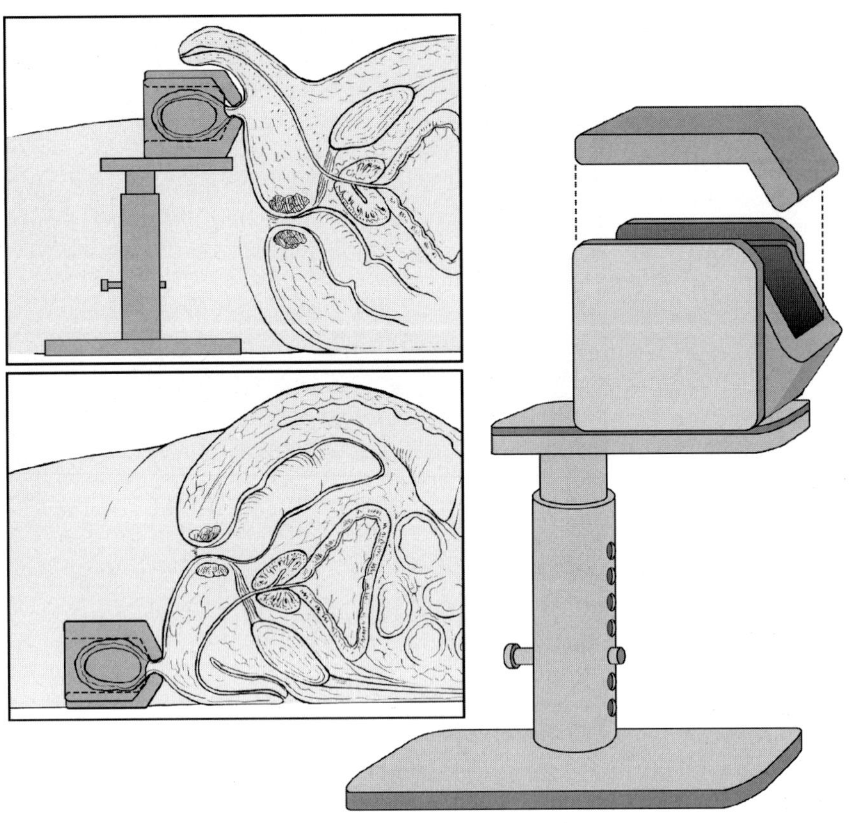

FIG. 27. Testicular shielding. Diagram of a scrotal shield. (Designed by Thomas P. Mitchell, M.S.; drawing by Louis Clark.)

The tolerance of the ovaries to radiation is well below the doses employed for Hodgkin's disease. If preservation of ovarian function, including fertility, is desired, the ovaries must be transposed to a location outside the primary radiation beam or to a location over which sufficient secondary shielding can be provided to prevent ovarian ablation. Surgical transposition or oophoropexy may be accomplished at laparotomy (66) or through a laparoscopic procedure (see Chapter 17) (67,68). Careful coordination between surgeon and radiation oncologist is required, with simulation and block outlining preceding surgery so that the surgeon understands exactly where the ovaries must be placed, marks them with radiopaque clips, and takes radiographs at the time of surgery on the operating room table to insure that the placement is correct. The most common method of ovarian protection is to transpose the ovaries to as low and medial a position in the pelvis as possible by fixing them to the posterior or anterior surface of the uterus (50,66,67,69,70). Even with excellent placement by the surgeon, the ovarian dose is still 10% to 20% of the prescribed dose because of scattered radiation under the block as well as transmission of the primary beam through the block (66,71–73). A number of technical factors affect the dose of scattered radiation delivered to the ovaries, including field size, distance from the edge of the unshielded beam, and the number of half-value layers blocking the primary beam. Too small a central block or suboptimal location beneath the block may result in inadequate reduction of the scatter component of radiation dose to protect ovarian function.

The possibility of oophoropexy failure has been noted by some investigators (69), mandating the use of radiopaque clips on the proximal and distal ends of the ovaries for precise localization at simulation. It has also been noted that ovaries can dislodge from the clips and return to anatomic position (58,69); ultrasound or other methods to verify ovarian position relative to the clips at the time of simulation will assure a greater likelihood that the ovaries will be adequately shielded to protect function. The central shield should provide a minimum margin of 1.5 cm for the pelvic lymph nodes; ideally, the central shield should also provide at least a 1.5- to 2-cm margin of shielding over the ovaries. If possible, lymphangiography should be performed before simulation, as an average of approximately 3 cm can be added to the central shield when the position of the lymph nodes is known precisely (58).

An alternative method to medial oophoropexy is to move the ovaries laterally and superiorly, out of the pelvic field; this reduces the scatter and eliminates the primary beam component (74–77). In one study (74), a comparison of actual doses registered on thermolucent dosimeters located in a phantom in medial and lateral oophoropexy positions shows that the dose to the ovaries can potentially be reduced to approximately 15% of the dose specified at midplane of the central axis of the pelvic field with the medialization technique and approximately 9% with the lateralization technique. Excellent results have been reported from the lateralization technique, although the follow-up period is short and there is less information available on the rate of subsequent pregnancy than with the medialization oophoropexy (74,75,77). Subsequent pregnancy with the lateral technique may also be problematic because of the distance of the ovaries from the fallopian tubes.

Ovarian function (hormonal function and menses) can be preserved in approximately 50% of women of childbearing age who receive pelvic irradiation for Hodgkin's disease (58,66,69,70,73) (Table 2). There has been less success in the preservation of fertility. Only 13 subsequent pregnancies were noted out of 94 patients reported in Table 2. Meticulous care in localization of the ovaries, design of the primary beam block, and daily execution of the treatment plan is required to minimize the dose to the ovaries. In some patients with limited Hodgkin's disease presenting below the diaphragm (unilateral pelvic nodal involvement or inguinal–femoral involvement without pelvic adenopathy), chemotherapy and involved field irradiation should be considered as an alternative to larger field irradiation, as fertility is more likely to be preserved with nonalkylating regimens and minimal radiation than with the larger field irradiation.

Inverted Y

The *inverted-Y* field is a combination of paraaortic, pelvic, and inguinal–femoral fields, with or without the spleen, and is most often used for patients with infradiaphragmatic Hodgkin's disease (see Chapter 41). The upper border may be set at the diaphragm in patients in whom only infradiaphragmatic fields will be treated; in patients who have had or will have treatment of supradiaphragmatic fields, the superior border must match the lower border of the supradiaphragmatic fields.

Selection of Treatment Fields

Radiation Alone

The greater the role of radiation in the treatment regimen, the greater the need for accurate staging procedures to define the extent of disease. If radiation therapy alone is to be used, the clinician must have a clear understanding of all sites of involvement as well as sites at risk for subclinical disease. Some areas at high risk for subclinical disease may need to be surgically evaluated in order to best tailor radiation fields to the extent of disease. The upper abdomen is a problematic area because, even with modern imaging, the false-negative and false-positive rates for noninvasive imaging studies range from 20% to 50% (78–82). For example, in a patient with three sites of supradiaphragmatic involvement, staging laparotomy data demonstrate that the probability of abdominal involvement is approximately 25% to 30%, even with negative imaging studies below the diaphragm. Without the information derived from staging laparotomy, elective treatment of the spleen and paraaortic nodes is indicated. If a staging laparotomy is performed and is negative, however, the radiation oncologist may in selected patients simply treat a mantle (52). Most patients who have disease above and below the diaphragm, whether based on imaging studies or the results of staging laparotomy, are treated with chemotherapy or combined-modality therapy.

Combined-Modality Therapy

Field selection in combined-modality regimens is dependent on the relative roles of radiation and chemotherapy and the specific defined treatment programs. Some protocols may call for radiation therapy only to sites that have responded incompletely (variably defined) to chemotherapy. In this setting, the irradiated fields would be involved fields based on postchemotherapy evaluation. Other programs call for irradiation of initially bulky (variably defined) sites only, irrespective of response. Still other programs call for irradiation of all initially involved regions. In programs with limited chemotherapy, extended field irradiation may be indicated (see Chapters 25 and 26).

Matching of Fields

The extent of the target volume in patients with Hodgkin's disease often necessitates the use of multiple abutting radiation fields (e.g., mantle, paraaortic–splenic/splenic hilar, and pelvis). The volume of normal tissue included, particularly the bone marrow, often mandates that these fields be treated sequentially to allow time for bone marrow recovery. Other abutting fields may be treated concurrently (e.g., simultaneous treatment of the Waldeyer's and mantle fields). Because of radiation beam divergence, significant areas of dose inhomogeneity can occur at the junction of these fields. There are three basic techniques that may be used to avoid or limit dose inhomogeneity at the field junction: half-beam, skin gap, and matching divergence.

Half-Beam Technique

The "half-beam" technique eliminates the problem of divergence by placing the central axes of the fields, where there is no divergence, at the edges of the abutting fields. This can be accomplished by using a block that eliminates half of the beam and leaves the central axis of the beam on the field edge (Fig. 28). Alternatively, on machines with asymmetric collimator jaws, one can simply close the col-

TABLE 2. *Ovarian function in women of childbearing age[a] after midline ovarian transposition and pelvic irradiation for Hodgkin's disease*

Institution, accrual dates	Chemotherapy	Radiation dose to pelvis (Gy)	Total no. of patients	Menstrual function			Subsequent pregnancies	Transient ablation
				Normal menses	Abnormal menses	Permanent amenorrhea		
Thomas (70) 1965–1974	No	35	12	1	2	9	1	3
Hunter (69) 1969–1977	No	No data	11	1	1	9	0	No data
Horning (73) 1968–1979	No	>40	19	9	9	1	7	No data
Horning (73) 1968–1979	Yes	30–40	50	10	14	26	5	No data
Mendenhall (58) 1964–1986	No	30–35	2	2	0	0	0	0

[a]Age was ≤35 years in all series except in Horning et al., where age was ≤40 years

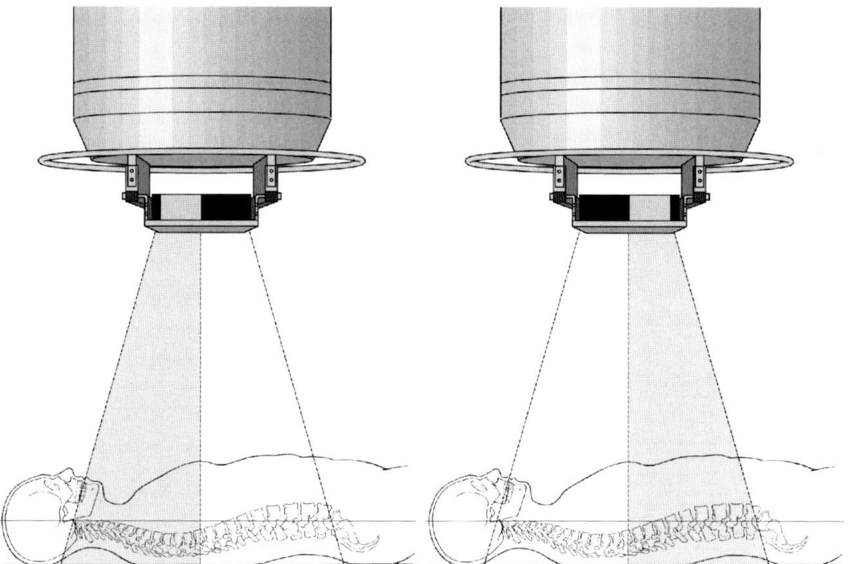

FIG. 28. Abutting field techniques. Half-beam technique. (Drawing by Louis Clark.)

limator jaw as far as the central axis of the beam on the border of the field that is to be matched. With the half-beam technique, the critical aspect of accuracy is patient immobilization for the duration of time required to complete treatment to the two fields during a single treatment setup. Day-to-day variation in setup does not matter as long as the two fields are matched perfectly each day. Half-beam blocking is ideal for matching the junction of the Waldeyer's and mantle fields, although too large a mantle field may preclude its use. In addition, if one field must be matched to two others (such as matching a mantle to both a Waldeyer's and a paraaortic field), the half-beam technique can be used for only one of the matches.

Skin-Gap Technique

The second method of dealing with abutting fields involves allowing a gap between the abutting fields on the skin that is calculated to result in matching of the fields at a desired depth, such as the midplane, the depth of tumor, or a critical structure such as the spinal cord (62,83). Ideally, all treated areas will be covered by two beams, one anterior and one posterior. The skin-gap method inherently has low-dose areas that are treated by only one of the four opposing beams (two anterior and two posterior) and high-dose areas that are treated by more than two opposing beams (Fig. 29). This method is often used for fields too large for the half-beam approach, and it may be utilized for patients treated either supine only or supine and prone; its best use is in situations where the target tissue is relatively deep with no superficial tissue at risk for tumor. Even in this setting, every effort should be made not to gap across areas of known disease, as this technique delivers 15% to 20%

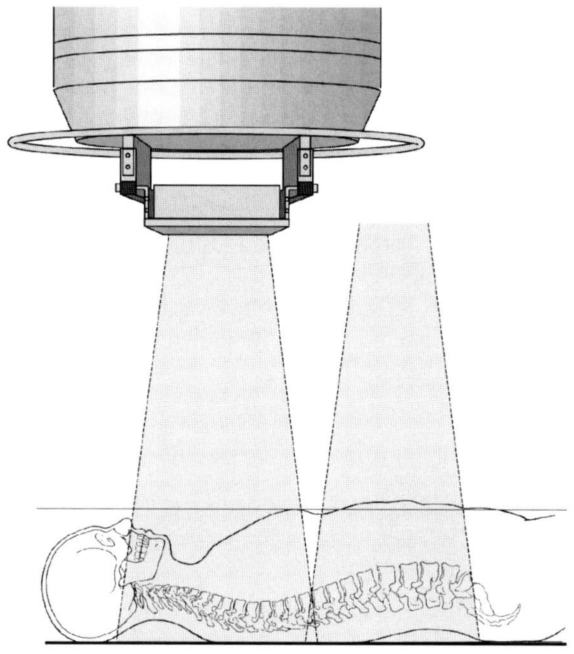

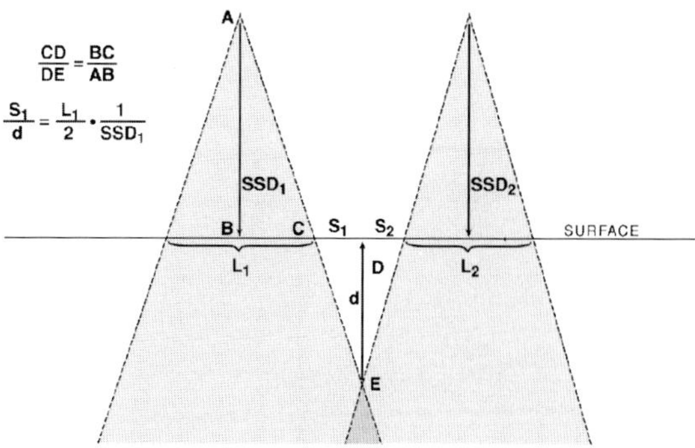

FIG. 29. Abutting field techniques. Skin-gap technique. (Drawing by Louis Clark.)

less dose than prescribed to the anterior pericardial nodes. One advantage of this technique is the ease of verifying the accuracy of daily setup. With the skin-gap method, the critical aspect of daily treatment accuracy is simply maintaining the specified skin gap between abutting fields; this is easily accomplished by placing small tattoos on the inferior border of the upper field and superior border of the lower field. This allows measuring of the skin gap before treatment if questions arise. The skin-gap method is commonly used in the matching of mantle and upper abdominal fields; in that situation it is common practice to include a small (2 cm wide × 1.5 cm long on skin) spinal cord block (either full thickness or 50% transmission). Others have proposed use of a wedge with the thickest portion at the edge of the field to allow extra blocking of the spinal cord near the match line (62). When the skin-gap technique is used, the clinician and physicist must determine the depth of the field match based on an understanding of the target volume (involved areas and those at risk for subclinical disease) as well as an understanding of the dose distribution in normal tissues. When the films are visually checked with the vertebral bodies used as anatomic landmarks, it is important to compare the inferior border of the anterior mantle field and the superior border of the posterior subdiaphragmatic field and similarly compare the inferior border of the posterior mantle field and the superior border of the anterior subdiaphragmatic field. If an overlap is seen on film, despite the calculated gap, an additional full-thickness block must be used.

The skin-gap technique has been published in detail (83–85). The key components include the following:

- Placement of tattoos to mark the lower border of the mantle field and upper border of the paraaortic field on skin.
- Determination of the same match point for both the anterior–posterior and posterior–anterior fields. This is especially crucial for patients treated in both the supine and prone positions. The match point is generally determined for a point in the middle of the patient and documented by projecting the point onto the spine using the nondivergent part of the beam.
- Documenting where the divergent edges of the four beams intersect the spine. This will add extra assurance that there is no overlap of the spinal cord.

Matching-Divergence Technique

A third, less commonly employed method for dealing with abutting fields is the "matching-divergence" technique, in which the inferior divergence from the superior posterior field is perfectly matched by the superior divergence from the inferior anterior field, and the inferior divergence from the superior anterior field is perfectly matched by the superior divergence of the inferior posterior field (Fig. 30). This can be accomplished only if patients are treated in the supine position only. Unlike the skin-gap method, if precisely executed, this method can achieve a perfect field match with no areas of underdosage or overdosage. Unlike the half-beam technique, it can be used for very large fields.

When the mantle and paraaortic fields are matched using the matching-divergence technique, the angle of divergence of the superior divergent edge of the paraaortic field and the inferior divergent angle of the mantle

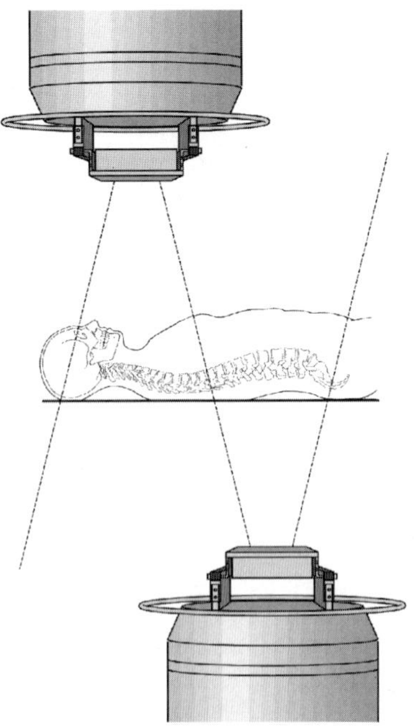

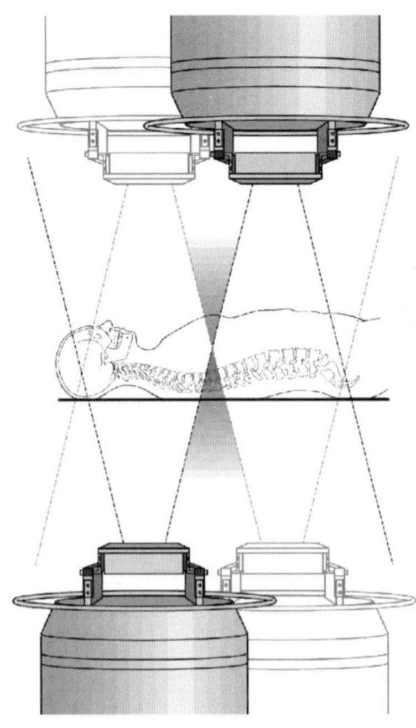

FIG. 30. Abutting field techniques. Matching divergence technique. (Drawing by Louis Clark.)

field must be coincident. To establish this congruency, the distance from the central axis to the field edge, at the edges of the fields to be matched, must be equivalent. This may be accomplished by using the independent jaws. The gap is calculated to the midplane and verified by using film. The vertebral bodies should be used as discussed above to verify the field position and lack of a field overlap. Often, a small block (1 to 2 cm in length and 1 to 1.5 cm in width) is inserted at the superior portion of the subdiaphragmatic field in order to limit the dose to the spinal cord and provide an extra measure of safety in that area of field abutment. The inferior border of the mantle field and superior border of the paraaortic field may be marked permanently with skin tattoos (or a single reference tattoo may be used).

Acceptable accuracy can be maintained easily with the half-beam technique through brief patient immobilization and with the skin-gap method by simple daily verification of the skin gap. Although it offers some theoretical advantages over the half-beam technique and the skin-gap technique, the matching-divergence technique is very labor-intensive.

Three-Dimensional Treatment Planning

The documentation of more extensive disease on computed tomography than is apparent from physical examination and plain chest radiography (86,87), the characterization of a high proportion of radiation treatment failures as marginal misses (34,88), and documented difficulties with reproducibility of planned treatment (89–91) all suggest that image-driven treatment planning and more precise treatment delivery would improve outcomes in patients with Hodgkin's disease receiving radiation therapy alone.

Three-dimensional treatment planning in Hodgkin's disease has been studied extensively at several institutions (87,92). With a beam's eye view to determine adequate coverage of involved areas, 16 patients with Hodgkin's disease were studied at the University of Michigan. Naida and co-workers (87) noted an overall error rate of 18% in the design of lung blocks based on simulation radiographs alone, which was reduced to 13% with the aid of computed tomographic images ($p = .038$) and theoretically reduced to 0 with the aid of beam's-eye-view verification of coverage. The areas at greatest risk for localization error were the axilla and the inferior mediastinum ($p = .0001$). In fact, the localization error rates in the axilla with and without computed tomography were 27% and 41.7%, respectively (Fig. 31). Localization errors were increasingly likely with increasing tumor size, particularly when computed tomographic scans were not available.

In a multiinstitutional study from the University of Pennsylvania and Fox Chase Cancer Center, Memorial Sloan-Kettering Cancer Center, Mallinckrodt Institute of Radiology, and Massachusetts General Hospital, three different treatment-planning methods for two patients with Hodgkin's disease were assessed for probability of tumor control and normal tissue complications (92). One patient had stage IA disease involving only small axillary nodes, and the other had extensive supradiaphragmatic disease with a mediastinal mass, just less than one-third the thoracic diameter, with sternal invasion and extensive paratracheal, axillary, and cervical lymphadenopathy. The pretreatment computed tomographic scans of each patient were entered into a three-dimensional planning system. Three kinds of treatment plans were generated from each of the four institutions by experienced clinicians. The first was a traditional plan employing standard

A 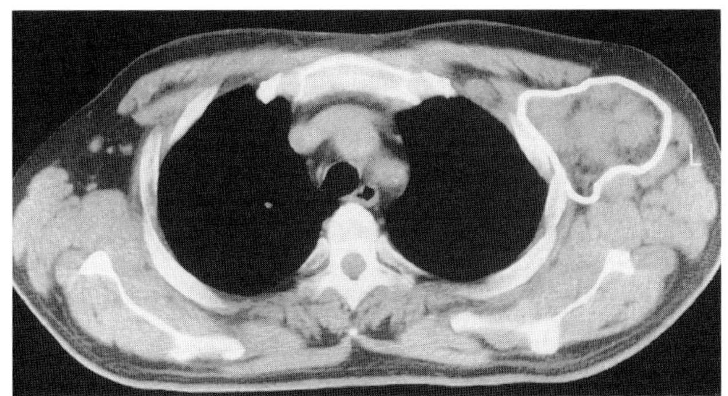

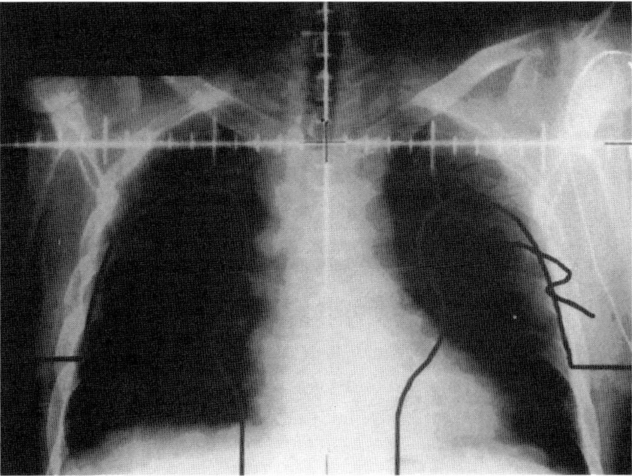 B

FIG. 31. Three-dimensional treatment techniques showing axillary lymphadenopathy on computed tomography **(A)** and the lower edge of the lymphadenopathy being blocked by the left lung block on the mantle simulation film **(B).** (From ref. 87.)

anterior and posterior fields based on a standard simulation film that was transferred into the three-dimensional planning system; the second employed standard anterior and posterior fields but was designed on the three-dimensional system based on the outlined target volumes; and the third was based on the outlined target volumes but not constrained in terms of field arrangement. The 24 treatment plans were then evaluated for tumor coverage and the probability of producing normal tissue complications. The conclusion of this complex analysis was that the use of three-dimensional techniques resulted in improved tumor coverage but increased doses to normal tissues such as the lung. The use of beam arrangements other than the standard anterior and posterior fields significantly increased the complexity of daily setup and verification. It was noted that the use of compensators reduced the dose variation within the treatment field. It was also noted that minimal patient misalignment had a profound effect on the dose actually received by target areas. Great variation was found among the clinicians in assessing the acceptability of the plans from different institutions for a given patient and of plans for a given patient using the three different methods, largely related to variance in opinion regarding normal-tissue tolerance.

Three-dimensional technology increases the accuracy of radiation therapy for Hodgkin's disease, but potentially at the expense of exposing a greater volume of normal tissue to radiation. Our current understanding of the minimum dose necessary for disease control in various clinical settings is based on past experience that has clearly been confounded by inaccuracies in field design and delivery. Likewise, our understanding of the relationship between volume and dose in determining normal-tissue tolerance is severely limited. The delicate balance that exists between the probabilities of normal-tissue tolerance and disease control must be better understood. Three-dimensional treatment planning and the ability to study normal-tissue tolerance through dose–volume histograms will undoubtedly improve outcomes with radiotherapy in Hodgkin's disease in the years to come.

Treatment Verification and Documentation

A number of studies have documented difficulty with accurate daily delivery of treatment (89,90,93–96), particularly with the mantle field, the one most commonly used in Hodgkin's disease. The large field size, irregular shape, extended distance between the source and target, and target motion related to respiratory and cardiac cycles (97) compound the difficulty of accurate setup. With the frequent use of imaging films, which document the volume of tissue actually exposed to radiation during a treatment, it is clear that both systematic errors and random errors may occur. Systematic errors result from a flawed simulation, perhaps because the patient was tense and later relaxed on the actual treatment table or because the initial simulation position was uncomfortable and not sustainable (89,93,95). Typically, systematic errors can be identified with an imaging film on the first day of treatment. Random errors are related to malposition of the patient or shielding blocks in daily treatment setups. Because of the large field size and the long distance from the source of the beam and the skin, significant errors can result from minimal rotation of the torso about the patient's cephalad–caudad axis or patient rotation with respect to the central axis of the beam, cephalad–caudad shifts caused by the respiratory cycles, and lateral shifts related to the width of skin marks or torso rotation. Random errors most commonly result in marginal miss in the axilla or inferior mediastinum. The points farthest away from the central axis are most affected by minimal rotation (90,94). The use of better positioning tools such as immobilization devices and lasers has aided in securing more accurate setups, and the use of frequent imaging films has focused attention on accuracy and identified systematic problems (89,91,94,98).

In Hodgkin's disease, local recurrence has been related to geographic miss in the Patterns of Care studies; geographic miss may occur because of errors in field design or errors in treatment delivery. Several studies of verification films have demonstrated a significant rate of localization errors (89,90,93,96,98) during the course of treatment. Two institutions reported on commencement of a policy of more frequent verification films; repeat studies showed an improvement in the error rate through better field design and increased use of verification films (91,99). In another institution, a policy of a detailed setup protocol and daily verification films led to a marked reduction in the number of deviations and unacceptable setups (94). Because of the emphasis on using the lowest effective doses to reduce the risk of late effects and the difficulty in setups, daily imaging films for patients being treated for Hodgkin's disease are recommended by some investigators. However, few institutions are willing to use daily imaging films because of the associated labor and costs.

Electronic portal imaging is under investigation for a number of tumor sites (100) and holds promise for reducing errors on the first day of treatment as well as increasing treatment efficiency. In Hodgkin's disease, where daily verification films are deemed necessary by some, electronic portal imaging is particularly appealing as a way of increasing accuracy throughout the course of treatment. It is possible that electronic on-line portal imaging will provide the best means of eliminating both systematic and random errors in the future (100).

SPECIAL TREATMENT CONSIDERATIONS

Pediatric Patients

In children, radiation therapy is used most commonly as a component of combined modality therapy programs (see Chapter 29). Potential risks to normal tissues are magnified in children compared to adults. Any asymmetry in field design or dose should be considered carefully in prepubertal children because of the potential for subsequent asymmetric growth. Radiation doses must be selected carefully, as there appears to be a very close correlation between soft-tissue growth impairment and dose, with a very steep dose response in the range of 20 to 40 Gy (81). It is also possible that the risk for radiation-related second cancers in children may be related to dose (101).

Pregnancy

Most women with Hodgkin's disease are of childbearing age. It is important to assess the possibility of pregnancy in any female patient who is initiating a diagnostic evaluation or treatment for Hodgkin's disease. In one series, coexisting pregnancy at diagnosis of Hodgkin's disease occurred in 3.2% of women (102). Concerns about carcinogenesis and induction of congenital abnormalities in the fetus complicate the management of the pregnant patient (see Chapter 38). When mantle treatment is required in the pregnant patient, treatment in the sitting or standing position may be advantageous. The force of gravity pulls the fetus lower and farther away from the mantle field. Additionally, the upright position offers the opportunity to significantly reduce radiation dose to the fetus by enhanced external shielding (Fig. 32A). The patient may be treated at an extended distance with the gantry rotated upward so that the inferior border of the beam does not diverge into the abdomen. A table may be placed between the patient and the machine, but below the field and in front of the uterus, to add additional blocking that would exceed the weight and safety limits for a normal blocking tray or table. With this method, the dose to the fetus during mantle field irradiation can be reduced to approximately 0.1% of the prescribed dose. Alternatively, the table may be placed over the patient in the supine position (Fig. 32B).

QUALITY CONTROL/ASSURANCE

The quality of radiation treatment depends on the successful completion of each of the following steps.

1. Identification of sites of involvement and sites at significant risk for microscopic disease. This requires an ability to perform an accurate and complete physical examination, to interpret the diagnostic images used in staging, and to understand the patterns of spread of Hodgkin's disease.
2. Selection and design of treatment fields that will adequately cover all areas requiring treatment and adequately spare normal tissues.
3. Prescription of the optimal dose for disease control and normal-tissue preservation.
4. Meticulous delivery of the treatment plan.

Failure to execute any of these steps properly will affect the quality and success of the overall treatment. Despite the excellent overall success rate with radiation therapy for Hodgkin's disease, a need for quality assurance programs to assure the success of each of these steps has been docu-

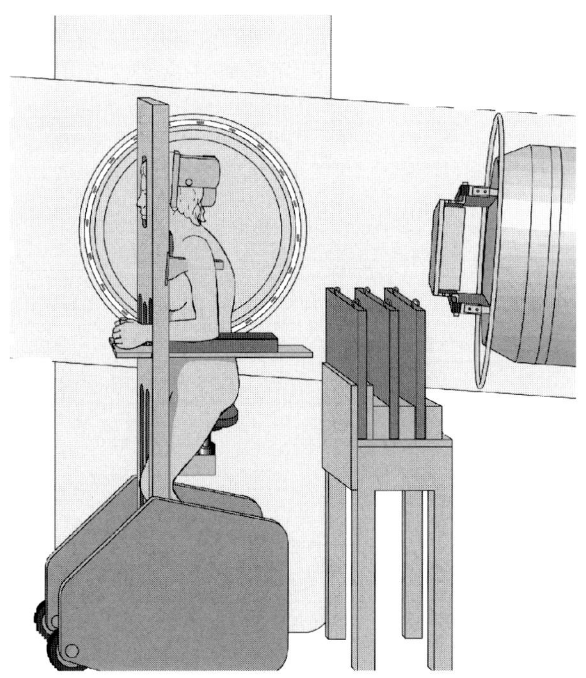
A

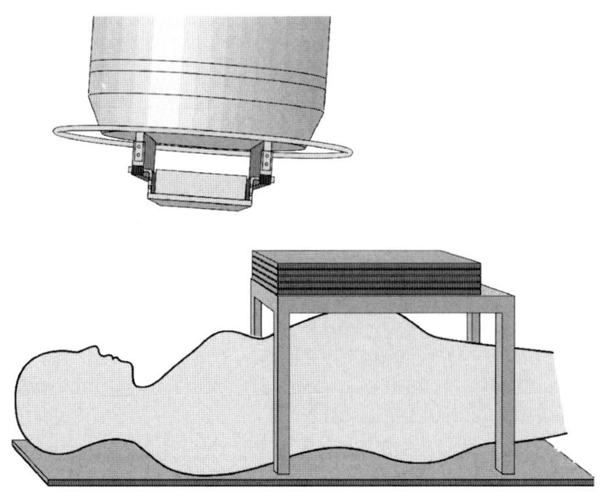
B

FIG. 32. Treatment of a pregnant patient in a standing position **(A)** or supine **(B)**. (Both parts drawn by Louis Clark.)

mented in the literature. Some cooperative groups, including the Pediatric Oncology Group (POG), now require pretreatment review of all imaging films in conjunction with all simulation or planning films to attempt to ensure that this critical step has been carried out successfully.

American College of Radiology Patterns of Care Study

In 1973, the American College of Radiology initiated the Patterns of Care Study for radiation oncology encompassing treatment of Hodgkin's disease and other malignancies. The first Patterns of Care Study (34,88) was a landmark report documenting excellent overall results in patients with Hodgkin's disease who were treated with radiotherapy. It also documented the difficulties of treatment-field design and delivery and their impact on treatment failure and death from Hodgkin's disease. The study aimed to provide a benchmark for the national practice in Hodgkin's disease. Records were reviewed on up to ten patients treated in 1973 in each of 163 facilities, randomly selected from a list of 1,021 facilities in the United States. Information was recorded regarding evaluation and treatment. Because of the substantial variation between the actual patterns of practice and the best current management according to the Patterns of Care concept, the benchmark data were then correlated with outcome data to determine whether the variations in patient evaluation and treatment had an impact on cure and complication-free survival in these patients. Two surveys were performed. The "regular" survey included data from 101 institutions of the original 163 randomly selected facilities and was considered to reflect the national practice. The "extended" survey included data on up to 50 cases from each of five of the largest institutions in the country and was considered to reflect academic practice.

From these surveys it was determined that lower recurrence rates were significantly associated with earlier disease stage, favorable histology, younger patient age, the use of chemotherapy, more comprehensive pretreatment evaluation, more comprehensive radiation fields, as well as factors reflecting the experience of the radiation oncologist, including larger new-patient loads, full-time practice, the use of treatment simulation, and the use of equipment with greater source-to-skin distance. In addition, higher complication rates were associated with patients of older age, the presence of coexisting disease, and radiation doses to subdiaphragmatic fields greater than 35 Gy.

Patients with early-stage disease had significantly better survival rates in the extended survey data than in the regular survey. The relative rate of recurrence from the five institutions in the extended survey was 0.75 as compared to 1.17 for the regular survey ($p \leq .01$), suggesting that treatment with radiation therapy alone yielded better results when given in institutions treating large numbers of Hodgkin's disease patients compared to centers seeing fewer patients (Table 3) (34). Portal films examined in the Patterns of Care study demonstrated that when there were inadequate margins between the protective lung and cardiac blocks and the tumor, both the overall recurrence rate (54% vs. 14%, $p \leq .0001$) and the infield or marginal recurrence rate increased dramatically (33% vs. 7%, $p \leq .001$). This suggested the possibility of better quality control at larger centers (Table 4) (88).

In 1994, Hoppe et al. (103) compared the 1973 Patterns of Care data with that of a second Patterns of Care survey, which included patients treated in 1983. Significant improvements were noted. Only 24% of patients were simulated on a dedicated simulator in 1973 compared with 82% in 1983 ($p < .001$). The use of routine port films increased from 91% to 99% ($p < .02$). The use of individually shaped blocks increased from 54% to 94% ($p < .001$). The extent of treatment increased; 11% of patients were treated only to involved fields in 1973, compared with just 3% in 1983 ($p = .024$). Fifty-five per-

TABLE 3. *The Patterns of Care Study in Hodgkin's disease: Variability in outcome associated with treatment facility*

	No. patients with recurrence/no. treated (by stage)				
Survey facility	IA	IIA	IIIA	I–IIIB	O/E rate of recurrence[a]
Regular survey[b]	19/102	34/133	28/61	23/38	1.17
Extended survey[c]	5/52	17/104	15/38	8/17	0.75
A	1/10	6/26	7/9	3/4	1.49
B	2/11	4/24	0/6	2/2	0.71
C	0/2	3/19	1/6	0/5	0.33
D	0/14	0/16	4/10	0/2	0.31
E	2/15	4/19	3/7	3/4	0.98

[a]Stage-adjusted recurrence rates are calculated, and the ratio of observed/expected is presented. Deviations above 1.0 indicate an increased recurrence rate over that expected; a ratio less than 1.0 indicates fewer recurrences than expected. The relative rates of recurrence for the regular and extended surveys are significantly different ($p \leq .01$).

[b]Regular survey is a sample of ten patients randomly chosen for review from each of 163 facilities randomly selected from 1,021 facilities in the United States.

[c]The extended survey is a random sample of 50 patients from each of five of the largest institutions.

Modified from ref. 3

TABLE 4. *The Patterns of Care outcome study in Hodgkin's disease: Relationship between treatment failure and adequacy of radiation treatment fields in patients treated with radiation therapy alone*

Radiation field margins	Any relapse		In-field or marginal recurrence	
	Yes	No	Yes	No
Adequate	14 (14%)	84 (86%)	7 (7%)	91 (93%)
Inadequate	31 (54%)	26 (46%)	19 (33%)	38 (67%)
Totals	45	110	26	129

Modified from ref. 88

cent of patients in 1973 received subtotal lymphoid irradiation (mantle and paraaortic or similar fields) compared with 73% in 1983 (p = .005). Port films were judged "adequate" in 63% of patients in 1973 compared with 92% of patients in 1983 (p < .01). The 5-year survival rate was 84% for patients treated in 1973 and 93% for patients treated in 1983 (p = .06). The 5-year freedom-from-relapse rate was 73% for patients treated in 1973 and 85% for patients treated in 1983 (p = .03). Further improvements in compliance with staging and treatment recommendations were demonstrated in the Patterns of Care Study survey completed in 1989 (104).

In 1993, Patterns of Care Study newsletters were published to report consensus statements on current guidelines for the management of Hodgkin's disease. These consensus statements were developed by a committee composed of recognized experts in the field, representing a broad range of radiation oncology practices across the United States. The guidelines included a decision tree for clinical evaluation and treatment schemes for each stage of disease as well as guidelines for treatment planning. In 1995, Hughes and colleagues (54) reported results of a survey carried out to assess compliance with treatment planning consensus guidelines. In many respects the consensus guidelines were common practice, but some discrepancies were noted that were thought to potentially influence outcome. The guidelines recommended dose calculation at multiple points in large, irregular fields such as the mantle, but 15% of patients in the 1988–1989 survey had dose calculations completed for only a single point. Thirty percent of patients did not have a gap calculation for the abutment of chest and abdominal fields. Very few patients received any kind of in vivo dosimetry check. No compensation was used in 70% of fields. Irregular-field dosimetry calculations did not take into account tissue inhomogeneities. Based on this survey, it was thought there were still opportunities for practice changes that would improve dose uniformity and treatment accuracy.

British National Lymphoma Investigation Patterns of Care Survey

Another survey, conducted by the British National Lymphoma Investigation and including institutions from the British National Lymphoma Investigation group, the United States, and Europe (105), queried radiation oncologists about their current practice in treating Hodgkin's disease. This survey demonstrated significant variations among practitioners regarding radiation technique, prescribed dose for involved and uninvolved areas, degree of spinal cord shielding, placement of the prescription point, appropriate modifications if radiation was given after chemotherapy, the true incidence of normal-tissue complications after radiation therapy, the total dose and dose per fraction considered necessary to produce an acceptable incidence of complications, and the recording of dose and dose per fraction delivered to critical normal tissues. Although there appeared to be a consensus among British and European practitioners for treatment with 40 Gy to clinically involved areas and 35 Gy to uninvolved areas, significant variation was found among practitioners from the United States, with 19% prescribing less than 35 Gy for uninvolved areas and less than 40 Gy for involved areas, and 25% to 31% prescribing more than 35 Gy for uninvolved areas and more than 40 Gy for involved areas.

The current emphasis in Hodgkin's disease is clearly on devising treatment regimens that not only produce excellent cure rates but also produce less normal-tissue damage. The British National Lymphoma Investigation study suggested that the late effects being observed today are the result of treatment techniques that are no longer in use. Many variations in current practice arose from observed complications of past treatment; these complications may not only be unnecessary but perhaps may obscure our understanding of true normal-tissue tolerance. The investigators concluded that well-designed quality-assurance programs were necessary to clarify areas of difference between practices that might affect normal tissues in particular. The availability of three-dimensional treatment planning and the ability to calculate dose volume histograms to describe normal tissue exposure provide excellent means for describing dose volume relationships, but will also provide significant opportunity for variability until clear guidelines for usage are established. Because it is clear that dose variations in the past may have led to excessive normal-tissue injury as well as problems with disease control, future quality assurance programs must address the subject of dose prescription.

Cooperative Group Trials

Within cooperative research groups, quality control in radiotherapy for Hodgkin's disease became a major focus of attention in the 1990s. Quality assurance programs identified noncompliance as a factor potentially affecting outcome in three trials: two dealing with adjuvant irradiation following chemotherapy in advanced disease and one dealing with radiation alone in early stage disease. These three trials are discussed here to underscore the importance of precise protocol compliance.

In a study by the Southwest Oncology Group (SWOG), adult patients with stage II to IV Hodgkin's disease who achieved a complete response to six cycles of MOP-BAP (mechlorethamine, vincristine, prednisone, bleomycin, doxorubicin, and procarbazine) chemotherapy were randomized to no further therapy or consolidative irradiation to all involved sites to a dose of 20 Gy (106). Of the 530 eligible patients entered on trial, 168 experienced a partial response and routinely went on to receive consolidative irradiation, whereas 322 patients had a complete response and were eligible for randomization. Of the 322 with a complete response, 44 refused randomization, leaving 135 patients randomized to receive radiation and 143 to receive no further therapy. The 5-year remission-duration estimate was 79% for patients randomized to receive radiation compared to 68% for those randomized to receive no further therapy (p = .09). The 5-year survival estimate for patients randomized to receive radiation was 86% compared to 79% for those randomized to no further treatment (p = .14). Although no significant difference was found in remission duration or overall survival between the treatment arms, several subsets of patients were identified that appeared to benefit from consolidative irradiation. The 5-year estimates of remission duration for patients with nodular sclerosis histology who were or were not randomized to receive radiation were 77% and 56%, respectively (p = .01). The benefit in patients with nodular sclerosis histology who received consolidative irradiation accrued both to patients with bulky disease (76% versus 46%) and those without bulky disease (88% versus 68%).

Because the overall analysis of the SWOG trial was based on "intent to treat" rather than actual treatment, 29 patients who were randomized to receive radiotherapy but did not were analyzed as though they had received radiation therapy per protocol. Additionally, the port films, dose calculations, and treatment records of all patients randomized to receive radiation were reviewed by the Quality Assurance Center, the Radiologic Physics Center, and the Medical and Radiation Oncology Protocol Coordinators, and treatment was evaluated as to whether it was in compliance with the protocol or included major or minor protocol violations. Dose infractions and failure to complete radiation therapy were considered minor radiation violations; failure to give any radiation at all to a previously involved site or concomitant administration of radiation and chemotherapy were considered major radiation therapy protocol violations. There is concern that poor radiation compliance may have had a significant impact on recurrence rates, the overall results of the trial, and conclusions about the potential role of radiotherapy in advanced Hodgkin's disease. As shown in Table 5, of the 135 patients who were randomized to receive radiation therapy on this trial, only 104 patients (77%) actually received radiation. Of the 104 who actually received any radiation, 18 patients (17%) were judged to have major protocol violations. Of patients who received radiation with a major protocol violation, 44% had a recurrence, compared with only 10% of patients who received radiation per protocol.

In the Pediatric Oncology Group (POG) between 1987 and 1992, 179 eligible pediatric patients with advanced

TABLE 5. *Cooperative group experience with quality assurance in RT for Hodgkin's disease: Association between outcome and prospective judgment of adequacy of RT field*

Cooperative group	Stage of disease	No. of patients randomized or allocated to RT arms	No. (%) of eligible patients who actually received RT on protocol	No. of patients receiving RT by protocol who were prospectively judged to have major RT protocol violations[a]/ No. receiving RT (%)	No. of patients with recurrence/ No. treated with RT protocol violations (%)	No. of patients with recurrence/ No. treated without RT protocol violations (%)
SWOG (106)	CS/PS III–IV	135	104 (77)	18/104 (17)	8/18 (44)	9/86 (10)
GHSG (41)	PS IA–IIB	393	393 (100)	118/393 (30)	22/118 (19)	26/229 (11)
POG (108)[b]	II–IVB, $IIIA_2$–IVA	90	70 (78)	25/70 (36)	4/25 (16)	3/45 (7)

[a]Major RT protocol violations: SWOG, failure to give RT to an involved site: GHSG, failure to use appropriate technique, adequate treatment volume, appropriate dose or dose fractionation schedule; POG, failure to use appropriate dose, dose per fraction, or treatment schedule, and failure to treat adequate treatment volume and all involved sites. RT, radiation therapy; SWOG, Southwest Oncology Group; GHSG, German Hodgkin's Study Group; POG, Pediatric Oncology Group.

[b]Written communication, POG Statistics Office, Gainesville, FL, June 1998.

Hodgkin's disease (stages IIB, $IIIA_2$, IIIB, and IV) were randomized to receive eight cycles of MOPP-ABVD (mechlorethamine, vincristine, procarbazine, prednisone, doxorubicin, bleomycin, vinblastine, and dacarbazine) chemotherapy followed by no further therapy or consolidative irradiation (21 Gy) to all involved sites (107,108). The randomization was done before initiating chemotherapy, and analysis was by "intent to treat." The estimated 5-year event-free survival rate was 80% for patients randomized to receive radiation and 79% for those randomized to no further therapy. The estimated 5-year overall survival rate was 87% for patients randomized to radiation therapy and 96% for those randomized to no further therapy. The apparent conclusion is that radiation therapy has no benefit in pediatric patients receiving eight cycles of MOPP-ABVD; however, the possibility has been raised that a potential benefit from radiation therapy could have been overlooked because of poor radiation therapy compliance. As shown in Table 5, only 70 of the 90 patients originally randomized to receive radiation actually received it on protocol. Ten patients randomized to receive radiation had disease progression or intercurrent disease during chemotherapy that took them off protocol before delivery of radiation; another 10 patients refused radiation therapy, had it off protocol, or developed AML before delivery of radiation under the protocol. Of the 70 patients who actually received radiotherapy on the POG protocol, 36% were judged to have major protocol violations by the same Quality Assurance Center used by SWOG. Of the 25 patients judged to have radiation protocol violations, the disease recurred in four (16%), compared with three of 45 patients (7%) judged to have received radiation in compliance with the protocol. In this trial, the results of chemotherapy alone were excellent, so there was little potential for the addition of radiation to improve survival. The POG Hodgkin's Disease Committee, however, believed that despite the excellent rate of disease control, there was room for improvement in regard to toxicity, and the near absence of recurrence with properly executed radiotherapy offered the possibility for chemotherapy dose reduction in future protocols. The Committee elected to retain low-dose irradiation in subsequent trials, requiring, however, central pretreatment review of all radiation fields and plans before treatment delivery to eliminate the problem of protocol compliance.

The third trial of interest is a randomized trial (HD4) of different radiation doses in patients with early-stage Hodgkin's disease treated with radiation alone conducted by the German Hodgkin Study Group between 1988 and 1993 (41). In this trial, a panel of four experienced chairpersons of different radiation therapy departments reviewed the radiation therapy treatment plan, simulation and verification films, technique, and dosimetry of 393 patients and classified each case as compliant with the protocol or in violation. As shown in Table 5, about 30% of cases were classified as having a major protocol violation; two thirds of violations were related to inadequate treatment volume, with most of the remainder of violations related to excessively protracted treatment time, technical inadequacies, and excessive radiation dose. Twenty-two patients (19%) with protocol violations subsequently had recurrence of Hodgkin's disease, compared with 26 patients (11%) whose treatment was consistent with the protocol. In this trial, prospective quality control was identified to be of prognostic value in that the probability of freedom from treatment failure at 5 years was 82% in patients treated without a protocol violation compared with 70% in patients with a protocol violation ($p <$ .04).

It is apparent from both the Patterns of Care Studies in the United States (34,88,103) and the cooperative group trials in both the United States and Germany that experienced radiation oncologists can identify treatment plans that are likely to be associated with treatment failure. Even early-stage Hodgkin's disease can be difficult for less experienced radiation oncologists to treat, resulting in significant variability in outcomes among institutions. Furthermore, those outcomes are predictable by experienced radiation oncologists on review of treatment fields. The encouraging finding from the Patterns of Care Study (103,104) is that in the 15 years following the first Patterns of Care Study, significant improvements occurred in many treatment parameters as well as in actual outcome for the national radiation oncology practice in treating Hodgkin's disease. It is probable that poor quality assurance for radiotherapy fields and techniques in the past have confounded the results of trials that were designed to determine the potential benefits of radiation alone or in combined modality regimens. It is hoped that with centralized pretreatment review, as instituted by POG, the true potential of radiation therapy, even in advanced disease, may be defined.

Palliative Therapy

With the curative potential of radiation therapy in Hodgkin's disease, it is easy to overlook its efficacy as a palliative therapy. Many patients with advanced Hodgkin's disease are treated initially with chemotherapy alone. High-dose-therapy salvage programs employed for patients who relapse may incorporate limited irradiation to sites of relapse. If disease recurs later in these patients, it may often be in sites not previously irradiated. Although systemic salvage regimens are often used in this setting, longer-term disease control may be provided by addition of palliative local irradiation. Some patients treated initially with extensive radiation may also relapse. Combination chemotherapy is often successful in salvaging many of these patients,while others may develop subsequent recurrences. Given the modest initial radiation doses that are often used in Hodgkin's disease, even these patients may be candidates for palliative irradiation to initial sites of disease. The original dose-control data for Hodgkin's disease published by Kaplan (31) indicated that long term local control could be achieved approximately 50% of the time with doses as low as 15 Gy. With many management programs employing initial radiation doses as low as 30 Gy, treatment to an additional 15 Gy as a palliative maneuver would rarely place any normal organs or tissues at risk for radiation injury. With careful three-dimensional planning, even higher doses may be utilized safely.

REFERENCES

1. Hodgkin T. On some morbid experiences of the absorbent glands and spleen. *Med-Chir Trans* 1832;17:68–97.
2. Wilks S. Cases of enlargement of the lymphatic glands and spleen (or Hodgkin's disease), with remarks. *Guy Hosp Rep* 1865;11:56–67.
3. Pel P. Zur Symptomatologie der sogenannten Pseudoleukamie. *Berl Klin Wochenschr* 1887;24:644–646.
4. Ebstein Wv. Das chronische Ruckfallsfieber eine neu Infectionskrankheit. *Berl Klin Wochenschr* 1887;24:565–568.
5. Greenfield W. Specimens illustrative of the pathology of lymphadenoma and leucocythemia. *Trans Pathol Soc Lond* 1878;29:272–304.
6. Sternberg C. Uber eine eigenartige unter dem Bilde der Pseudoleukamie verlaufende Tuberculose des lymphatischen Apparates. *Z Heilkd* 1898;19:21–90.
7. Reed D. On the pathological changes in Hodgkin's disease, with special reference to its relation to tuberculosis. *Johns Hopkins Hosp Rep* 1902;10:133–196.
8. Pusey W. Cases of sarcoma and of Hodgkin's disease treated by exposures to x-rays: a preliminary report. *JAMA* 1902;38:166–169.
9. Senn N. Therapeutical value of roentgen ray in treatment of pseudoleukemia. *NY Med J* 1903;77:665–668.
10. Plucker J. Quoted in Grubbe EH. Priority in the therapeutic use of x-rays. *Radiology* 1933;21:156–162.
11. Rontgen WG. Ueber eine neue Art von Strahlen Sitzungsberichte der physikalisch-medicinischen Gesellschaft zu Wurzburg. *Sitzung* 1895; 30:132–141.
12. Gilbert R. La roentgentherapie de la granulomatose maligne. *J Radiol Electrol* 1925;9:509–514.
13. Gilbert R, Babaiantz L. Notre methode de roentgentherapie de la lymphogranulomatose (Hodgkin); resultats eloignes. *Acta Radiol* 1931; 12:523–529.
14. Gilbert R. Radiotherapy in Hodgkin's disease (malignant granulomatosis); anatomic and clinical foundations; governing principles, results. *Am J Roentgenol* 1939;41:198–241.
15. Craft C. Results with roentgen ray therapy in Hodgkin's disease. *Bull Staff Meet Univ Miami Hosp* 1940;11:391–409.
16. Peters M. A study in survivals in Hodgkin's disease treated radiologically. *Am J Roentgenol* 1950;63:299–311.
17. Peters M, Middlemiss K. A study of Hodgkin's disease treated by irradiation. *Am J Roentgenol* 1958;79:114–121.
18. Easson E, Russell M. The cure of Hodgkin's disease. *Br Med J* 1963; 1:1704–1707.
19. Jones H, Illes J, Northway W. A history of the Department of Radiation Therapy at Stanford. *Am J Roentgenol* 1995;164:753–760.
20. Fuks Z, Feldman M. Henry S. Kaplan 1918–1984: A physician, a scientist, a friend. *Cancer Surv* 1985;4:295–311.
21. Ginzton E, Mallory K, Kaplan H. The Stanford medicallinear accelerator I: design and development. *Stanford Med Bull* 1957;15:123–140.
22. Kaplan H. The radical radiotherapy of Hodgkin's disease. *Radiology* 1962;78:553–561.
23. Lukes R, Butler J, Hicks E. Natural history of Hodgkin's disease as related to pathlogical picture. *Cancer* 1966;19:317–344.
24. Carbone P, Kaplan H, Musshoff K, Smithers D, Tubiana M. Report of the Committee on Hodgkin's Disease Staging Classification. *Cancer Res* 1971;31:1860–1861.
25. Glatstein E, Guernsey J, Rosenberg S, Kaplan H. The value of laparotomy and splenectomy in the staging of Hodgkin's disease. *Cancer* 1969;24:709–718.
26. Piro A, Hellman S, Moloney W. The influence of laparotomy on management decisions in Hodgkin's disease. *Arch Intern Med* 1972;130: 844–848.
27. DeVita V, Serpick A, Carbone P. Combination chemotherapy in the treatment of advanced Hodgkin's disease. *Ann Intern Med* 1970;73: 881–895.
28. Bentel G. Positioning and immobilization of patients undergoing radiation therapy for Hodgkin's disease. *Med Dosim* 1991;16:111–117.
29. Gray L, Prosnitz L. Mantle field dosimetry comparing 4 MV with cobalt. *Radiology* 1975;116:429–432.
30. Gray L, Prosnitz L. Dosimetry of Hodgkin's disease therapy using a 4 MV linear accelerator. *Radiology* 1975;116:423–428.
31. Kaplan H. Evidence for a tumoricidal dose level in the radiotherapy of Hodgkin's disease. *Cancer Res* 1966;26:1221–1224.
32. Peters M. Prophylactic treatment of adjacent areas in Hodgkin's disease. *Cancer Res* 1966;26:1232–1243.
33. Fletcher GH, Shukovsky LJ. The interplay of radiocurability and tolerance in the irradiation of human cancers. *J Radiol Electrol Med Nucl* 1975;56:383–400.
34. Hanks G, Kinzie J, White R, Herring D, Kramer S. Patterns of care outcome studies: Results of the national practice in Hodgkin's disease. *Cancer* 1983;51:569–573.
35. Thar T, Million R, Hausner R, McKetty M. Hodgkin's disease, stages I and II. *Cancer* 1979;43:1101–1105.
36. Mendenhall N, Rodrigue L, Moore G, Marcus R Jr, Million R. The optimal dose of radiation in Hodgkin's disease: An analysis of clinical and treatment factors affecting in-field disease control. *Int J Radiat Oncol Biol Phys* (in press).
37. Schewe K, Reavis J, Kun L, Cox J. Total dose, fraction size, and tumor volume in the local control of Hodgkin's disease. *Int J Radiat Oncol Biol Phys* 1988;15:25–28.
38. Vijayakumar S, Myrianthopoulos L. An updated dose–response analysis in Hodgkin's disease. *Radiother Oncol* 1992;24:1–13.
39. Raubitschek A, Glatstein E. The never-ending controversies in Hodgkin's disease. *Int J Radiat Oncol Biol Phys* 1989;17:1115–1117.
40. Prosnitz LR. Radiation complications for Hodgkin's disease and seminoma: assessing the risk:benefit ratio. *Int J Radiat Oncol Biol Phys* 1988;15:239–241.
41. Duhmke E, Diehl V, Loeffler M, et al. Randomized trial with early-stage Hodgkin's disease testing 30 Gy vs. 40 Gy extended field radiotherapy alone. *Int J Radiat Oncol Biol Phys* 1996;36:305–310.
42. Hancock S, Hoppe R. Long-term complications of treatment and causes of mortality after Hodgkin's disease. *Semin Radiat Oncol* 1996;6:225–242.
43. Coia L, Hanks G. Complications from large field intermediate dose infradiaphragmatic radiation: An analysis of the patterns of care outcome studies for Hodgkin's disease and seminoma. *Int J Radiat Oncol Biol Phys* 1988;15:29–35.
44. Loeffler M, Diehl V, Pfreundschuh M, et al. Dose–response relationship of complimentary radiotherapy following four cycles of combination chemotherapy in intermediate stage Hodgkin's disease. *J Clin Oncol* 1997;15:2275–2287.
45. Hudson MM, Greenwald C, Thompson E, et al. Efficacy and toxicity of multiagent chemotherapy and low-dose involved-field radiotherapy in children and adolescents with Hodgkin's disease. *J Clin Oncol* 1993;11:100–108.
46. Hunger SP, Link MP, Donaldson SS. ABVD/MOPP and low-dose involved-field radiotherapy in pediatric Hodgkin's disease: the Stanford experience. *J Clin Oncol* 1994;12:2160–2166.
47. Bentel GC, Marks LB, Krishnamurthy R, Prosnitz LR. Comparison of two repositioning devices used during radiation therapy for Hodgkin's disease. *Int J Radiat Oncol Biol Phys* 1997;38:791–795.
48. Schultz HP, Glatstein E, Kaplan HS. Management of presumptive or proven Hodgkin's disease of the liver: a new radiotherapy technique. *Int J Radiat Oncol Biol Phys* 1975;1:1–8.
49. Rosenberg S, Kaplan H. The evolution and summary results of the Stanford randomized clinical trials of the management of Hodgkin's disease: 1962–1984. *Int J Radiat Oncol Biol Phys* 1985;11:5–22.
50. Kaplan H. *Hodgkin's disease,* vol 2. Cambridge, MA: Harvard University Press, 1980.

51. Farah J, Ultmann J, Griem M, Golomb H, Kalokhe U. Extended mantle radiation therapy for pathologic stage I and II Hodgkin's disease. *J Clin Oncol* 1988;6:1047–1052.
52. Mauch P, Canellos G, Shulman L, et al. Mantle irradiation alone for selected patients with laparotomy-staged IA to IIA Hodgkin's disease: Preliminary results of a prospective trial. *J Clin Oncol* 1995;13: 947–952.
53. Carmel R, Kaplan H. Mantle irradiation in Hodgkin's disease: An analysis of technique, tumor eradication, and complications. *Cancer* 1976;37:2813–2825.
54. Hughes DB, Smith AR, Hoppe R, et al. Treatment planning for Hodgkin's disease: a patterns of care study. *Int J Radiat Oncol Biol Phys* 1995;33:519–524.
55. Marcus K, Svensson G, Rhodes L, Mauch P. Mantle irradiation in the upright position: A technique to reduce the volume of lung irradiated in patients with bulky mediastinal Hodgkin's disease. *Int J Radiat Oncol Biol Phys* 1992;23:443–447.
56. Klein EE, Wasserman T, Ermer B. Clinical introduction of a commercial treatment chair to facilitate thorax irradiation. *Med Dosim* 1995; 20:171–176.
57a. Hoppe RT. Hodgkin's disease. In: Leibel SA, Phillips TL (eds). *Textbook of radiation oncology.* Philadelphia: WB Saunders, 1998:1079–1094.
57. Mauch P, Kalish L, Kadin M, Coleman C, Osteen R, Hellman S. Patterns of presentation of Hodgkin's disease. *Cancer* 1993;71:2062–2071.
58. Mendenhall NP, Holland KW, Sombeck MD. The role of lymphangiography in designing fields for elective pelvic node irradiation in Hodgkin's disease. *Int J Radiat Oncol Biol Phys* 1994;30:993–995.
59. Centola GM, Keller JW, Henzler M, Rubin P. Effect of low-dose testicular irradiation on sperm count and fertility in patients with testicular seminoma. *J Androl* 1994;15:608–613.
60. Lushbaugh C, Casarett G. The effects of gonadal irradiation in clinical radiation therapy: A review. *Cancer* 1976;37:1111–1125.
61. Speiser B, Rubin P, Casarett G. Aspermia following lower truncal irradiation in Hodgkin's disease. *Cancer* 1973;32:692–698.
62. Fraass BA, van de Geijn J. Peripheral dose from megavolt beams. *Med Phys* 1983;10:809–818.
63. Fraass B, Kinsella T, Harrington F, Glatstein E. Peripheral dose to the testes: the design and clinical use of practical and effective gonadal shield. *Int J Radiat Biol Phys* 1985;11:609–615.
64. Million R. The lymphomatous diseases: Hodgkin's disease. In: Fletcher G, ed. *Textbook of radiotherapy.* Philadelphia: Lea & Febiger, 1980:584–621.
65. Kubo H, Shipley WU. Reduction of the scatter dose to the testicle outside the radiation treatment fields. *Int J Radiat Oncol Biol Phys* 1982; 8:1741–1745.
66. Ray G, Trueblood H, Enright L, Kaplan H, Nelsen T. Oophoropexy: A means of preserving ovarian function following pelvic megavoltage radiotherapy for Hodgkin's disease. *Radiology* 1970;96:175–180.
67. Williams RS, Mendenhall N. Laparoscopic oophoropexy for preservation of ovarian function before pelvic node irradiation. *Obstet Gynecol* 1992;80:541–543.
68. Clough KB, Goffinet F, Labib A, et al. Laparoscopic unilateral ovarian transposition prior to irradiation: prospective study of 20 cases. *Cancer* 1996;77:2638–2645.
69. Hunter M, Glees J, Gazet J. Oophoropexy and ovarian function in the treatment of Hodgkin's disease. *Clin Radiol* 1980;31:21–26.
70. Thomas PR, Winstanly D, Peckham MJ, Austin DE, Murray MA, Jacobs HS. Reproductive and endocrine function in patients with Hodgkin's disease: effects of oophoropexy and irradiation. *Br J Cancer* 1976;33:226–231.
71. Sharma S, Williamson J, Khan F, Lee C. Measurement and calculation of ovary and fetus dose in extended field radiotherapy for 10 MV x-rays. *Int J Radiat Oncol Biol Phys* 1981;7:843–846.
72. LeFloch O, Donaldson S, Kaplan H. Pregnancy following oophoropexy and total nodal irradiation in women with Hodgkin's disease. *Cancer* 1976;38:2263–2268.
73. Horning S. Female reproductive potential after treatment for Hodgkin's disease. *N Engl J Med* 1981;304:1377–1382.
74. Gaetini A, DeSimone M, Urgesi A, et al. Lateral high abdominal ovariopexy: an original surgical technique for protection of the ovaries during curative radiotherapy for Hodgkin's disease. *J Surg Oncol* 1988;39:22.
75. Nahhas WA, Nisce LZ, D'Angio GJ, Lewis JL Jr. Lateral ovarian transposition. Ovarian relocation in patients with Hodgkin's disease. *Obstet Gynecol* 1971;38:785–788.
76. Michel G, Lasser P, Castaigne D, Apelbaum H, Genin J, Lacour J. [Ovarian transposition. Technic, indications, results.] *Chirurgie* 1983; 109:55–60.
77. Hadar H, Loven D, Pearl P, Bairey O, Yagoda A, Levani H. An evaluation of lateral and medial transposition of the ovaries out of radiation fields. *Cancer* 1994;74:774–779.
78. Mendenhall NP, Cantor AB, Williams JL, et al. With modern imaging techniques, is staging laparotomy necessary in pediatric Hodgkin's disease? A Pediatric Oncology Group study. *J Clin Oncol* 1993;11: 2218–2225.
79. Mauch P, Larson D, Osteen R, et al. Prognostic factors for positive surgical staging in patients with Hodgkin's disease. *J Clin Oncol* 1990;8:257–265.
80. Schneeberger AL, Girvan DP. Staging laparotomy for Hodgkin's disease in children. *J Pediatr Surg* 1988;23:714–717.
81. Donaldson S, Link M. Combined modality treatment with low dose radiation and MOPP chemotherapy for children with Hodgkin's disease. *J Clin Oncol* 1987;5:742–749.
82. Leibenhaut M, Hoppe R, Efron B, Halpern J, Nelsen T, Rosenberg S. Prognostic indicators of laparotomy findings in clinical stage I–II supradiaphragmatic Hodgkin's disease. *J Clin Oncol* 1989;7:81–91.
83. Lutz W, Larsen R. Technique to match mantle and para-aortic fields. *Int J Radiat Oncol Biol Phys* 1983;9:1753–1756.
84. Marcus K, Buck B, Mauch P. Principles of radiation therapy in Hodgkin's disease and non-Hodgkin's lymphoma. In: Canellos GP, Lister T, Sklar J, ed. *The lymphomas.* Philadelphia: WB Saunders, 1998: 215–234.
85. Mauch P, Kalish L, Marcus K, et al. Second malignancies after treatment for laparotomy staged IA–IIIB Hodgkin's disease: long-term analysis of risk factors and outcome. *Blood* 1996;87:3625–3632.
86. Rostock R, Giangreco A, Wharam M, Lenhard R, Siegelman SS, Order SE. CT scan modification in the treatment of mediastinal Hodgkin's disease. *Cancer* 1982;49:2267–2275.
87. Naida JD, Eisbruch A, Schoeppel SL, Sandler HM, Turrisi AT, Lichter AS. Analysis of localization errors in the definition of the mantle field using a beam's eye view treatment-planning system. *Int J Radiat Oncol Biol Phys* 1996;35:377–382.
88. Kinzie J, Hanks G, Maclean C, Kramer S. Patterns of care study: Hodgkin's disease relapse rates and adequacy of portals. *Cancer* 1983;52:2223–2226.
89. McCord DL, Million RR, Northrop MF, Kavanaugh HV. Daily reproducibility of lung blocks in the mantle technique. *Radiology* 1973; 109:735–736.
90. Marks J, Haus A, Sutton H, Griem M. Localization error in the radiotherapy of Hodgkin's disease and malignant lymphoma with extended mantle fields. *Cancer* 1974;34:83–90.
91. Marks JE, Haus AG, Sutton HG, Griem ML. The value of frequent treatment verification films in reducing localization error in the irradiation of complex fields. *Cancer* 1976;37:2755–2761.
92. Brown A, Urie M, Barest G, et al. Three-dimensional photon treatment planning for Hodgkin's disease. *Int J Radiat Oncol Biol Phys* 1991;21:205–215.
93. Griffiths S, Pearcey R. The daily reproducibility of large complex-shaped radiotherapy fields to the thorax and neck. *Clin Radiol* 1986; 37:39.
94. Taylor BW Jr, Mendenhall NP, Million RR. Reproducibility of mantle irradiation with daily imaging films. *Int J Radiat Oncol Biol Phys* 1990;19:149–151.
95. Hulshof M, Vanuytsel L, Van Den Bogaert W, Van Der Schueren E. Localization errors in mantle-field irradiation for Hodgkin's disease. *Int J Radiat Biol Phys* 1989;17:679–683.
96. Rabinowitz I, Broomberg J, Goitein M, McCarthy K, Leong J. Accuracy of radiation field alignment in clinical practice. *Int J Radiat Oncol Biol Phys* 1985;11:1857–67.
97. Willet C, Linggood R, Stracher M, et al. The effect of the respiratory cycle on mediastinal and lung dimensions in Hodgkin's disease. Implications for radiotherapy gated to respiration. *Cancer* 1987;60: 1232–1237.
98. Byhardt RW, Cox JD, Hornburg A, Liermann G. Weekly localization films and detection of field placement errors. *Int J Radiat Oncol Biol Phys* 1978;4:881–897.

99. Taylor M, Kaplan H, Nelsen T. Staging laparotomy with splenectomy for Hodgkin's disease: The Stanford experience. *World J Surg* 1985;9: 449–460.
100. Cionini L, Bucciolini M. Role of portal imaging in clinical radiotherapy: Florence experience. *Radiother Oncol* 1993;29:230–236.
101. Tinger A, Wasserman TH, Klein EE, et al. The incidence of breast cancer following mantle field radiation therapy as a function of dose and technique. *Int J Radiat Oncol Biol Phys* 1997;37:865–870.
102. Woo SY, Fuller LM, Cundiff JH, et al. Radiotherapy during pregnancy for clinical stages IA–IIA Hodgkin's disease. *Int J Radiat Oncol Biol Phys* 1992;23:407–412.
103. Hoppe R, Hanlon A, Hanks G, Owen J. Progress in the treatment of Hodgkin's disease in the United States, 1973 versus 1983: The Patterns of Care Study. *Cancer* 1994;74:3198–3203.
104. Smitt M, Buzydlowski J, Hoppe R. Over 20 years of progress in radiation oncology: Hodgkin's disease. *Semin Oncol* 1997;7:127–134.
105. Sebag-Montefiore DJ, Maher EJ, Young J, Vaughan Hudson G, Hanks G. Variation in mantle technique: implications for establishing priorities for quality assurance in clinical trials. *Radiother Oncol* 1992;23: 144–149.
106. Fabian C, Mansfield C, Dahlberg S, et al. Low-dose involved field radiation after chemotherapy in advanced Hodgkin's disease. *Ann Intern Med* 1994;120:903–912.
107. Weiner MA, Leventhal BG, Marcus R, et al. Intensive chemotherapy and low-dose radiotherapy for the treatment of advanced-stage Hodgkin's disease in pediatric patients: a Pediatric Oncology Group study. *J Clin Oncol* 1991;9:1591–1598.
108. Weiner MA, Leventhal B, Brecher ML, et al. Randomized study of intensive MOPP-ABVD with or without low-dose total-nodal radiation therapy in the treatment of stages IIB, IIIA2, IIIB, and IV Hodgkin's disease in pediatric patients: a Pediatric Oncology Group study [see comments]. *J Clin Oncol* 1997;15:2769–2779.

Hodgkin's Disease, edited by P. M. Mauch, J. O. Armitage, V. Diehl, R. T. Hoppe, and L. M. Weiss. Lippincott Williams & Wilkins, Philadephia ©1999.

CHAPTER 22

Principles of Chemotherapy in Hodgkin's Disease

Rachel E. Hough and Barry W. Hancock

THE HISTORY OF CHEMOTHERAPY IN HODGKIN'S DISEASE

The advances made in the use of chemotherapy in Hodgkin's disease over the past half-century have been considerable, providing both the potential for cure in patients with advanced Hodgkin's disease and also a springboard for the development of modern chemotherapy in other malignancies.

By the early 1900s, it was recognized that arsenicals had some activity against Hodgkin's disease. However, the first real breakthrough came by way of an accident in World War II. Seamen exposed to mustard gas following the explosion of a military ship were found to have marrow and lymphoid hypoplasia. In the latter years of the war, nitrogen mustard was given to patients with Hodgkin's disease, and it resulted in a dramatic, albeit short-lived, clinical regression of disease (1). Development of mustard derivatives and other agents including antifolate antimetabolites, corticosteroids, vinca alkaloids, nitrosoureas, and procarbazine followed quickly. In 1964, the outlook for patients with Hodgkin's disease was dramatically improved with the development of the MOPP regimen (mechlorethamine, oncovin, procarbazine, and prednisone) (2), which achieved a complete remission in 84% of patients. Furthermore, unlike any treatment before it, these remissions were durable, with a 66% relapse-free survival at 20 years (3).

Since then, researchers have looked for ways of improving survival while minimizing both the short- and long-term side effects of treatment. Various MOPP-like and other combination regimens have been developed and given alone or as alternating or hybrid regimens. With the clear efficacy of radiotherapy in localized disease, a combined-modality approach has also been investigated in advanced Hodgkin's disease, using combination chemotherapy with radiotherapy to sites of bulky disease or slowly responding lymph nodes.

Today, the great success of these early researchers means that around 70% of patients with Hodgkin's disease will be cured. Regimens designed in the light of MOPP have provided some reduction in side effects but no significant gain in overall survival. Improving outcome and minimizing toxicity remain the challenges of today.

BASIC PRINCIPLES OF CHEMOTHERAPY AS APPLIED TO HODGKIN'S DISEASE

The ultimate aim of a cytotoxic drug is tumor cell death. This is achieved by a variety of mechanisms, which include causing structural change in the DNA, interference with enzymes central to DNA synthesis, and damage to the mitotic spindle.

The DNA structure can be altered by alkylation or intercalation of base pairs or by strand breakage. Nitrogen mustard and other alkylating agents form covalent bonds between the alkyl groups of the drug and the base pairs of the two DNA strands resulting in interstrand cross-links (4). These prevent the normal separation of DNA during mitosis. Intercalating agents such as the anthracyclines cause distortion of the DNA molecule by intercalation between adjacent nucleotide base pairs and prevent the action of DNA and RNA polymerases. Anthracyclines also cause double DNA strand breakage via inhibition of topoisomerase II (5,6).

Antimetabolite drugs inhibit DNA synthesis by binding to key enzymes in the purine or pyrimidine synthetic

R. E. Hough: Division of Oncology and Cellular Pathology, University of Sheffield and Department of Clinical Oncology, Weston Park Hospital, Sheffield, England.

B. W. Hancock: Division of Oncology and Cellular Pathology, University of Sheffield and Department of Medical Oncology, Weston Park Hospital, Sheffield, England.

pathways. A number of enzymes may be targeted, including thymidylate synthetase (fluorouracil), DNA polymerase (cytosine arabinoside), and dihydrofolate reductase (methotrexate) (7).

The vinca alkaloids (8) and taxanes (9) cause disruption of the mitotic spindle. The spindle is vital in the sorting and movement of chromosomes during mitosis, and these drugs result in metaphase arrest of dividing tumor cells.

Cytotoxic drugs are rarely, if ever, entirely selective for tumor cells and will inevitably affect normal cells passing through their cycle, particularly those in the bone marrow and gastrointestinal tract. Although normal cells are effective in repairing drug-induced DNA damage, they never develop drug resistance (10), and the maximum dose of any agent will be limited by its toxicity to normal tissues.

As our understanding of the biology of Hodgkin's disease increases, new drugs and strategies are developed. Initial efficacy is assessed using human tumor cell lines, and pharmacokinetic and toxicology data are obtained from animal studies. If a drug appears promising on the basis of these tests, it must be thoroughly investigated in at least three phases of human clinical trials before it can become widely available. In Hodgkin's disease, as with other cancers, Phase I and II studies are performed in patients with refractory, advanced disease for whom there is no effective alternative therapy.

Phase I trials are primarily concerned with drug safety. Initially a low dose of drug (as predicted from animal data) is used, and the dose is then escalated. Pharmacokinetic, pharmacodynamic, and toxicity data are analyzed to determine the optimum dose for further evaluation.

A Phase II trial is employed to determine whether the drug is effective against a particular malignancy. The optimum dose (determined in Phase I trial) is given to at least 14 patients with measurable disease. The principal endpoint is tumor shrinkage.

Any drug that has been shown to be both safe and effective must finally be compared to the standard treatment for that disease in a large number of patients by means of a prospective, randomized, controlled trial (Phase III). This chapter focuses on data accrued from such studies.

The incorporation of a new drug or drug regimen into standard practice must be based on data from all available clinical trials. This can be a difficult process, as trials often differ in patient selection, indices of response and survival, drug delivery, and lengths of follow-up; thus, only broad comparisons can be made. Patients should be carefully staged before and after treatment and response recorded in accordance with standard criteria, as follows:

A *complete response* is achieved when there is disappearance of all known disease on two identical evaluations not less than 4 weeks apart. A *partial response* is defined as a 50% or greater decrease in the sum of products of the largest perpendicular diameters of measurable lesions.

Stable disease describes less than a 50% decrease or 25% increase in measurable disease.

Progressive disease is defined as a 25% or greater increase in one or more of the measurable lesions or the appearance of a new lesion.

No cure can be achieved without the patient having first achieved a complete response, and this is an important goal for all cytotoxic drugs. However, the durability of this remission is central to long-term outcome, and progression-free survival following completion of chemotherapy is now considered to be an important measure of the quality of a response. In Hodgkin's disease, the cause-specific survival plateaus at between 5 and 10 years; such patients can be considered "cured." However, overall survival is, of course, influenced by other factors (second malignancy, increased heart and lung disease), and survival curves still show a downward trend even 20 to 25 years after treatment.

SINGLE AGENTS

Using the murine leukemia L1210, Skipper and colleagues provided a kinetic model for tumor growth and response to treatment (11,12). All the cells in this tumor were proliferating, and tumor growth was found to be logarithmic with a constant doubling time. It was seen that cell kill by drug administration was also logarithmic, following first-order kinetics; the proportion of tumor cells killed by a given dose of drug was constant irrespective of the number of tumor cells present initially. All tumor cells needed to be killed before cure could be achieved, as any remaining cells would inevitably proliferate. From these

TABLE 1. *Efficacy and toxicity of single agents in lymphoma*

Drug	Any response	Complete remission	Toxicity
Chlorambucil	60%	16%	Myelosuppression, teratogenesis
Cyclophosphamide	54%	12%	Myelosuppression, hemorrhagic cystitis, nausea, sterility, pulmonary fibrosis, alopecia
Nitrogen mustard	63%	13%	Nausea, vomiting, myelosuppression, thrombophlebitis, alopecia
Prednisolone	61%	0%	Cushing's syndrome, peptic ulceration, psychiatric disturbance, diabetes
Procarbazine	69%	38%	Nausea, myelotoxicity, neuropsychiatric disturbance, teratogenesis
Vinblastine	68%	30%	Myelotoxicity, neurotoxicity (infrequent)
Vincristine	64%	36%	Neurotoxicity

experiments, it was predicted that tumor eradication would be dependent on initial tumor burden, drug dose, and doubling time of residual tumor cells.

Following the discovery of the effects of nitrogen mustard in 1946 (1), a number of different drugs were developed and shown to be effective in Hodgkin's disease. Table 1 summarizes the response rates and toxicities associated with these agents when given to previously untreated patients (13,14). The majority of patients had regression of disease, with some achieving a complete remission. However, relapse was inevitable (14), and there have been no reports of cure of advanced Hodgkin's disease following administration of a single agent alone.

At least 10^9 to 10^{12} tumor cells must be present before disease becomes clinically detectable. It was clear that the drugs available by the early 1960s could reduce the tumor burden below this threshold. However, if they were used within the confines of acceptable toxicity, the tumor was not totally eradicated and quickly relapsed. To date, with the exceptions of choriocarcinoma (15) and Burkitt's lymphoma, human malignancies have proved to be incurable by single-agent chemotherapy (16).

COMBINATION CHEMOTHERAPY

Based on Skipper's model, it was postulated that the simultaneous use of more than one drug with different biological actions might have an additive killing effect. The combination of drugs could be tolerated if drugs with different toxicity profiles were used. DeVita has subsequently outlined principles that facilitate the selection of new effective combination regimens (16,17) (Table 2).

The first indication that such an approach was superior came in 1965. Lacher and Durant treated 16 patients with advanced Hodgkin's disease with a combination of chlorambucil and vinblastine (18). Thirteen had remissions (81%), which were complete in ten (63%). Median relapse-free survival was 7.5 months, a modest improvement from those previously treated with single agents, although the trial included no formal control group.

However, the true potential of combination chemotherapy in advanced Hodgkin's disease was first realized in 1967, when the effects of the quadruple regimen MOPP were first reported by DeVita and co-workers at the National Cancer Institute (NCI) (19). Of the 188 patients with histologically proven Hodgkin's disease receiving treatment, 157 (84%) achieved a complete remission. Subsequent follow-up has shown that this regimen gives a relapse-free survival of 66% and overall survival of 48% after more than 20 years (2,3). Patients received at least 6 cycles of MOPP or treatment to complete response followed by a further two cycles. Higher complete remission rates and longer survival were associated with the absence of B symptoms and with a higher dose of vincristine. Disease relapse tended to occur within 4 years of achieving a complete response and was uncommon after this time. Associated side effects were significant. Nausea, vomiting, phlebitis, myelosuppression, and reversible vincristine-related neuropathies were common acute toxicities. Long-term side effects included infertility and secondary malignancy. All men became azoospermic, and 41% of women over the age of 26 years became amenorrheic (3). Acute leukemia developed in 13 patients from the NCI series, but in all but one patient, radiotherapy had also been given. The efficacy of MOPP has been confirmed in a number of other studies (20–22), and this regimen quickly became the "gold standard" treatment in advanced Hodgkin's disease.

Since the development of the MOPP regimen, clinical research has striven to improve outcome while minimizing short- and long-term toxicity. A number of researchers attempted to improve MOPP by adding, removing, or substituting elements of the regimen (23) (Table 3). Mechlorethamine (nitrogen mustard) was replaced by less toxic agents including chlorambucil (24–26), cyclophosphamide (27), lomustine (28), and carmustine (29–32). Reduction in neurotoxicity was achieved by the substitution of vinblastine for vincristine, although none of the neurologic complications seen in the patients given MOPP caused permanent disability (3).

Substitution of vinblastine for vincristine in the MVPP regimen reduced neurotoxicity at the expense of myelotoxicity (33). Efficacy was comparable to that with MOPP. McElwain and colleagues found that substituting chlorambucil for nitrogen mustard in the MVPP regimen (ChlVPP) provided a better-tolerated, equally efficacious combination (24). Substitution of chlorambucil (Leukeran) for nitrogen mustard in the MOPP regimen in a randomized British National Lymphoma Investigation (BNLI) study confirmed that toxicity could be reduced without compromising efficacy (34–36). The Eastern Cooperative Oncology Group (ECOG) reported the only prospective randomized study in which there was any improved therapeutic benefit when compared to MOPP (20,37). They demonstrated an increase in disease-free survival following complete response with BCVPP (BCNU, cyclophosphamide, vinblastine, procarbazine, prednisone), although overall survival was no better. However, BCVPP was associated with a higher incidence of secondary acute leukemia. In a Southwest Oncology Group (SWOG) study, addition of

TABLE 2. *Important principles in the selection of combination chemotherapy regimens*

Only drugs known to cause tumor regression (partial or complete) when used alone should be included
When several equally effective drugs of the same class are available, the drug selection should be based on minimizing overlapping toxicities with the other elements of the regimen
Drugs should be used in their optimal doses and schedules
Drug combinations should be given at consistent intervals; these intervals should be as short as possible for renewal of normal tissue, usually the bone marrow

TABLE 3. *Efficacy and toxicity of MOPP variants in advanced Hodgkin's disease*

Regimen	Modification	Regimens compared	Complete remission	Freedom from relapse	Overall survival	Efficacy compared to MOPP	Toxicity compared to MOPP	Center (reference)
MVPP	Substitution of vinblastine for vincristine	MVPP	76%		65% (5 yr)	Equivalent	Less neurotoxicity	St Bartholomew's, London (33)
ChlVPP	Substitution of chlorambucil for nitrogen mustard and vinblastine for vincristine	ChlVPP	85%	71% (10 yr)	65% (10 yr)	Equivalent	Less nausea, vomiting, alopecia, and neurotoxicity	Royal Marsden, London (24–26)
LOPP	Substitution of chlorambucil for nitrogen mustard	LOPP MOPP	57% 63%	55% (10 yr) 60%	54% 52%	Equivalent	Less nausea, vomiting, and myelosuppression	BNLI (34–36)
BOPP	Substitution of BCNU for nitrogen mustard	BOPP MOPP	67% 63%	Approx 55% (5 yr) Approx 55%	Approx 50% Approx 50%	Equivalent	Equivalent	CALBG (29)
MOP	Deletion of prednisolone	MOP MOPP	36% 69%		30% (5 yr)* 60%	Reduced complete response rate and overall survival	Equivalent	BNLI (42)
BCVPP	Substitution of vinblastine for vincristine and BCNU and cyclophosphamide for nitrogen mustard	BCVPP MOPP	77% 73%	65% (5 yr)* 50%	65% 61%	Increased relapse-free survival Overall survival unchanged	Less nausea, vomiting, and neurotoxicity More myelotoxicity and leukemia	ECOG (20,37)
Bleo-MOPP	Addition of bleomycin	Bleo-MOPP MOPP	84% 70%	64% (3 yr) 53%	78% 58%	Equivalent		SWOG (38,39)

*Statistically significant.

TABLE 4. *Efficacy and toxicity of other combination chemotherapy regimens used in advanced Hodgkin's disease*

Regimen	Trial design and patients included	Complete remission	Freedom from relapse	Overall survival	Toxicity	Center (reference)
ABDIC	Phase II. Patients refractory to MOPP	35%	47 months in complete responders (median)	24 months (median)	Myelosuppression, vomiting, alopecia	MD Anderson (49)
B-Cave	Phase II. Patients refractory to MOPP	44%	24 months (median)		Thrombocytopenia	Stanford (50)
BCNU-VPP	Randomized trial comparing BCNU-VPP to BCNU alone as primary chemotherapy	83%	67% at 51+ months	92% at 51+ months	Myelosuppression, vomiting, peripheral neuropathy, encephalopathy	Northwest Oncology Group (51)
CABS	Phase II. Previously untreated patients	80%	8.6 years in complete responders (median)			Albert Einstein Center (52)
CCNU-VP	Randomized controlled trial comparing CCNU-VP to MOPP	72%		60% at 89+ months	Less nausea and emesis compared to MOPP	Western Cancer Study Group (53)
CEP	Phase II. Patients refractory to MOPP and ABVD	40%	15 months (median)	17 months (median)	Nausea, alopecia, myelosuppression	NCI (54)
CVPP	Randomized controlled trial comparing CVPP to MOPP, MVPP, or COPP	69%	71% of complete responders at 56 months	36% at 60 months	Myelosuppression; less gastrointestinal and neurotoxicity compared to MOPP	CALBG (55)
CVPP	Phase II. Previously untreated patients	74%	27 months (median)		Nausea, alopecia, myelosuppresion	Minnesota (56)
EVA	Phase II. Previously untreated patients	54%	44% at 2 years	86% at 2 years	Myelosuppression, leukemogenic	Duke University (57)
MIME	Phase II. Patients refractory to MOPP and ABVD	23%	25 months (median)	50 weeks (median)	Infections, hemorrhagic cystitis, neutropenia	MD Anderson (58)
MOP-BAP	Randomized controlled trial comparing MOP-BAP to MOPP-Bleomycin	77%		Superior to MOPP-Bleo in low risk patients		SWOG (39)
NOVP	Phase II. Early-stage disease with poor prognostic factors. Given with RT[a]	40% 44% (CRu)	93% at 1 year	100% at 1 year	Nausea, alopecia, myelosuppression, myalgia	MD Anderson (59)
PACEBOM	Phase II. Previously untreated patients	40% 16% (CRu)	64% at 3 years	92% at 3 years	Myelosuppression, skin reactions, mucositis, alopecia	CRC (60)
PAVE	Randomized controlled trial comparing PAVe+RT to MOPP+RT or ABVD+RT	93%	78% at 15 years	75% at 15 years	Myelosuppression, secondary malignancies	Stanford (61)
VAPEC B	Phase II. Patients refractory to Adriamycin-containing regimens, principally MVPP	30%			Myelosuppression	Christie (62)

[a]RT, radiotherapy.

bleomycin to MOPP was associated with no additional benefit (38,39). Although the role of prednisone had been debated, the prospective BNLI trial in which prednisolone was omitted from the MOPP regimen demonstrated significant reduction in the attainment of complete response and overall survival (40–42).

MOPP-like combination regimens significantly reduced some of the acute toxicities associated with MOPP but have failed to improve overall or disease-free survival.

A different approach was taken by Bonadonna and the Milan Cancer Institute Group. The ABVD regimen was developed as a non–cross-resistant alternative, initially for MOPP failures (43). It comprised Adriamycin, bleomycin, vinblastine, and dacarbazine, agents that had all been shown to have single-agent activity in Hodgkin's disease relapsing after MOPP. The regimen was shown to have good activity in patients with MOPP-resistant disease, causing less myelotoxicity, sterility, or acute leukemia. Side effects associated with ABVD included acute severe nausea and vomiting and long-term cardiac and pulmonary damage (44,45). In 1992, the Cancer and Leukemia Group B (CALGB) investigated the efficacy of this regimen in previously untreated patients with advanced Hodgkin's disease in a prospective randomized clinical trial (46,47). Complete remission rates were 82% in the ABVD arm compared with 66% for MOPP. Failure-free survival was also superior for ABVD (61% for ABVD and 50% for MOPP). However, no improvement in overall survival has been demonstrated. The lower response rate to MOPP probably resulted from drug delivery at a lower dose intensity than that originally described by the NCI, and this has led to some criticism of the trial (48).

Other alternative combination regimens have been shown to have activity as salvage regimens in relapsed or refractory Hodgkin's disease following MOPP and are summarized in Table 4. These include ABDIC (Adriamycin, bleomycin, DTIC, prednisolone, CCNU) (49), CABS (CCNU, Adriamycin, bleomycin, streptozocin) (53), CEP (CCNU, etoposide, prednimustine) (55), and MIME (methyl-GAG, ifosfamide, methotrexate, etoposide) (58). Their role in previously untreated patients has not yet been established in prospective randomized studies.

The use of maintenance chemotherapy to prevent regrowth of any residual tumor cells after complete remission has been achieved has not been shown to be beneficial in Hodgkin's disease. A number of studies have consistently failed to demonstrate any improvement in either disease-free or overall survival (37,63–65), and so maintenance chemotherapy is not routinely given in Hodgkin's disease.

ALTERNATING CHEMOTHERAPY

None of the combination regimens developed for the treatment of advanced Hodgkin's disease has shown clear superiority in efficacy when delivered close to the original intended dose and schedule. Goldie and Coldman hypothesized that this observation was a consequence of the development of chemotherapy resistance (66). They proposed that spontaneous mutations arise in tumor cells at a specific mutation rate related to the inherent genetic instability of a particular malignancy. The number of resistant cells in any tumor is therefore related to the total number of mitotic divisions that have occurred. Because at least 10^9 cells must be present before a tumor is clinically detectable, it is likely that cells resistant to at least one agent are present at the time of diagnosis. Further spontaneous mutations arising during treatment may result in additional resistance to other drugs. Goldie and Coldman predicted that the early introduction of as many effective agents as possible, before resistant clones emerged, would be more likely to eradicate the tumor (67). Taking into account acceptable toxicity, they advocated the use of alternating non–cross-resistant chemotherapy regimens.

The efficacy of ABVD in disease relapsing after treatment with MOPP is suggestive of non–cross-resistance between the two regimens. Bonadonna and colleagues in Milan randomized 88 patients with previously untreated stage IV Hodgkin's disease to monthly cycles of MOPP or MOPP alternating with ABVD (45,68–70). Relapse-free survival was better for the alternating regimen (Table 5), but the complete response rate was not significantly improved, and long-term follow-up has shown no overall survival advantage. A number of criticisms have been made of this study (48,71). MOPP was not administered in the standard manner described by the NCI group. A total of 12 cycles were given, rather than six, and the dose intensity was significantly reduced in more than half the patients. The outcome of patients on MOPP alone was worse than that described by other studies. In addition, half of the MOPP patients ultimately received ABVD.

The CALBG randomized a further 361 patients with stage III and IV Hodgkin's disease to six to eight cycles of MOPP or ABVD alone or 12 cycles of MOPP alternating with ABVD (46,47). Complete response rates and freedom from progression were equivalent for ABVD alone and the alternating regimen, both of which were superior to MOPP. No difference in overall survival was observed. Again, the dose intensity of MOPP was compromised.

A number of other studies, using a variety of alternating regimens, have failed to demonstrate a dramatic improvement in outcome when compared with properly administered four-drug combinations (Table 3). In fact, only the BNLI LOPP/EVAP versus LOPP study has shown a persisting advantage in overall survival for the alternating regimen (36).

However, these studies do not necessarily refute the Goldie–Coldman hypothesis, as the regimens used have not all been shown to be truly non–cross-resistant and have not always been administered at their optimal dose intensities.

TABLE 5. *Efficacy and toxicity of alternating chemotherapy in advanced Hodgkin's disease*

Regimen (no. of cycles)	Complete remission	Freedom from relapse	Overall survival	Efficacy	Toxicity	Center (reference)
MOPP (12) MOPP (6)/ABVD (6)	74% 89%	46% (10 yr)* 68%	58% 69%	No overall survival advantage MOPP given at reduced dose intensity	Greater alopecia and gastrointestinal disturbance with MOPP/ABVD; greater myelotoxicity with MOPP alone	Milan (45,68,69,70)
MOPP(6) ABVD (6) MOPP (6)/ABVD (6)	67%* 82% 83%	50% (5 yr)* 61% 65%	66% 73% 75%	MOPP had inferior CR and FFR to ABVD alone and alternating regimen; MOPP given at reduced dose intensity	Increased myelotoxicity in MOPP containing regimens; pulmonary and cardiac toxicity with ABVD; increased gastrointestinal toxicity with MOPP/ABVD	CALBG (46,47)
MOPP (6) MOPP (3)/CABS (3)	91% 92%	65% (12 yr) 72%	68% 54%	Equivalent	Greater gastrointestinal toxicity; increased risk of secondary leukemia	NCI (72)
MOPP (8) MOPP (2)/ABVD (2)	57% 59%	61% (6 yr) 69%	57% 65%	Alternating therapy had improved progression-free survival	Less secondary malignancy with MOPP/ABVD	EORTC (73)
MOPP (3)/ABV (3)/CAD (3) + RT MOPP (5)/ABVD (4)+RT	76% 83%	Approx 90% (3 yr) Approx 90%	80% 90%	Equivalent	Increased myelosuppression but less nausea and vomiting in MOPP/ABV/CAD+RT arm	MSKCC (74)
BVCPP-Bleo (6) BVCPP-Bleo (3)/ABVD (3)	Approx 73% Approx 73%	68% (5 yr) 77%	62% 64%	Equivalent Not truly cross-resistant regimens	Equivalent	SECSG (75,76)
CVPP (12) BAVS (12) CVPP (6)/BAVS (6)	72% 70% 82%	50% (5 yr) 59% 57%	55% 61% 68%	Equivalent	Increased myelosuppression with CVPP	CALBG (77,78)
LOPP (8) LOPP (4)/EVAP (4)	57% 64%	52% (5 yr)* 66%	66%* 75%	Alternating regimen superior	Increased alopecia and myelosuppression with LOPP/EVAP	BNLI (36,79)
ChlVPP (6) ChlVPP (3)/ABOD (3)	80% 80%	68% (5 yr) 69%	81% 80%	Equivalent	Increased life-threatening myelosuppression in elderly with ChlVPP	Norwegian Lymphoma Group (80)
PABLOE (6) ChlVPP (3)/PABLOE (3)	60% 75%		89% (2 yr) 93%	FFP at 2 years inferior for PABLOE (52%) compared with alternating regimen (72%)		BNLI/CLG (81,82)

CR, complete response; FFR, freedom from relapse; FFP, freedom from progression; *statistically significant.

TABLE 6. *Efficacy and toxicity of hybrid chemotherapy regimens in advanced Hodgkin's disease*

Regimen (no. of cycles)	Complete remission	Freedom from relapse	Overall survival	Efficacy	Toxicity	Center (reference)
MOPP (3)/ABVD (3) MA MA (6)	91% 89%	76% (10 yr) 78%	74% 75%	Equivalent	Equivalent	Milan (68,83,84)
MOPP (4)/ABVD (4) MOPP ABV (8)	83% 81%	67% (5 yr) 71%	83% 81%	Equivalent	Increased myelotoxicity with the hybrid	NCI, Canada (85,86)
MVPP (6) ChlVPP EVA (6)	55% 68%		71% (5 yr) 80%	Freedom from progression significantly better with hybrid	Equivalent	Christie/Barts (87)
MOPP (6)/ABVD (3)[a] MOPP ABV	73%* 82%	65% (8 yr)* 77%	82%* (3 yr) 89%	Hybrid superior	Increased risk of pulmonary toxicity and severe myelotoxicity but reduced incidence of secondary leukemia or myelodysplasia with hybrid	Intergroup, USA (88)
LOPP (3)/EVAP (3) LOPP EVA (6)	65%* 40%	85% (2 yr) 79%	88% 78%	Trial terminated early because of significantly inferior complete response for hybrid	Increased myelotoxicity with alternating regimen	BNLI (36,89)
ABVD (8) MOPP ABV (8)	73% 71%	67% (3 yr) 65%	85% 87%	Equivalent	Trial stopped early in view of excess deaths because of sepsis, pulmonary toxicity, and secondary malignancies in hybrid arm	Intergroup USA (90)

[a]Sequential therapy; *statistically significant.

HYBRID CHEMOTHERAPY

A further application of the Goldie-Coldman hypothesis was the development of hybrid chemotherapy, in which seven or eight drugs from effective non–cross-resistant regimens were consolidated into monthly cycles.

In 1982, the Milan group developed the MA/MA regimen, which consisted of half-cycles of MOPP on day 1 and half-cycles of ABVD on day 15 of a 28-day cycle. Four hundred and fifteen patients were randomized to receive either six cycles of MA/MA or six cycles of MOPP alternating with ABVD (68). After 9 years of follow-up, no significant difference between the two regimens could be demonstrated (Table 5) (83,84).

The MOPP/ABV regimen of Connors and Klimo comprised MOPP on day 1 and ABV on day 8 of a 28-day cycle. Dacarbazine was omitted, and the dose of doxorubicin was increased from 25 to 35 mg/m^2. Three hundred and one patients were randomized to receive eight cycles of MOPP/ABV or eight cycles of MOPP alternating with ABVD. Although the hybrid regimen initially appeared superior (85), long-term follow-up has shown that both regimens are equally effective (Table 5) (86).

Table 6 summarizes the efficacy and toxicity associated with other hybrid regimens that have been investigated. In general, these regimens appear to have equivalent efficacy to four-drug or alternating therapies but may be associated with increased toxicity.

DOSE INTENSITY

Skipper's laws were based on the L13210 mouse leukemia, in which 100% of the tumor cells were actively dividing and in cell cycle (11,12). In most human tumors there is a nonproliferating cell population as well as the proliferating population (91). As a result, most tumors follow a sigmoid-shaped Gompertzian growth curve rather than the logarithmic growth seen by Skipper (10). In this model, tumor growth is initially slow as the total number of cells is small. Growth rate reaches a maximum during the middle part of the curve and then slows to a plateau as the tumor reaches its maximum size. The concept of kinetic resistance in tumor response to chemotherapy was developed by Norton and Simon (92). They proposed that tumor cell kill also follows Gompertzian regression and is related to the dose of drug administered and the tumor growth rate at the start of treatment. Failure of a chemotherapy regimen to cure could reflect inadequate drug delivery, insufficient duration of treatment, or rapid doubling time of remaining tumor cells.

The dose intensity of a treatment was defined by Hryniuk and colleagues as the amount of drug delivered per unit of time, in milligrams per square meter per week (93). Dose intensity is therefore dependent on the dose of drug and the interval between successive cycles of treatment. The importance of dose intensity in determining outcome has been demonstrated in both animal studies and prospective clinical trials.

Based on data from experiments performed by Skipper and colleagues with the Ridgeway osteogenic sarcoma in mice (94), DeVita has emphasized that a reduction in dose intensity of the two-drug regimen cyclophosphamide and L-PAM by 27% reduces the cure rate by 80%, although the complete remission rate is unaffected (95). The results of these murine experiments become available in 90 days. The effects of delivering suboptimal therapy to humans in clinical trials may take up to 10 years to be realized.

The effects of altered dose intensity on outcome in the Skipper model are indeed, paralleled in prospective clinical trials. DeVita et al. have calculated the actual dose intensities of MOPP delivered in published prospective clinical trials (95). In keeping with the animal data, reduction in dose intensity had no consistent effect on complete response rate but significantly reduced ongoing disease-free survival. In the NCI study, the rate of delivery of vincristine was found to be the most important variable in predicting outcome (3). The Stanford group found that the dose and dose rate of nitrogen mustard, vincristine, and procarbazine were important in the attainment of a complete remission, and reduction in the dose of nitrogen mustard was associated with a significantly poorer outcome (96). DeVita points out that the loss of life to disease resulting from suboptimal therapy could far exceed the morbidity and mortality associated with a properly administered regimen (95).

Dose intensity of chemotherapy regimens can be increased by shortening the interval between cycles and escalating the dose of individual agents. Intensified (escalated) chemotherapy regimens and high-dose chemotherapy supported by hematopoietic stem-cell transplants are practical applications of this theory and are currently under evaluation.

INTENSIFIED (ESCALATED) CHEMOTHERAPY

One of the major dose-limiting toxicities of chemotherapy is myelosuppression. The recent advent of hematologic growth factors (97) to support treatment may allow regimens with higher dose intensity to be tolerated. According to the models of kinetic and genetic resistance previously discussed, this approach should, theoretically, increase the likelihood of total tumor eradication or cure. Indeed, Goldie and Coldman hypothesized that the most effective treatment strategies would be those that allowed the minimum amount of regrowth of residual cells between cycles of treatment (67).

Intensified regimens may have the additional advantage of reduced long-term morbidity. Most late side effects of chemotherapy agents are a function of the total dose delivered (98–100). Increasing the dose intensity of specific drugs can reduce the overall cumulative dose.

TABLE 7. *The Stanford V chemotherapy regimen*[a]

Doxorubicin 25 mg/m^2 day 1 + 15
Vinblastine 6 mg/m^2 day 1 + 15
Mechlorethamine 6 mg/m^2 day 1
Vincristine 1.4 mg/m^2 (max. dose 2 mg) day 8 + 22
Bleomycin 5 U/m^2 day 8 + 22
Etoposide 60 mg/m^2 day 15 + 16
Prednisolone 40 mg/m^2 (reducing from week 10) alternate days

[a]Vinblastine dose decreased to 4 mg/m^2 and vincristine dose to 1 mg/m^2 during cycle 3 in those 50 years or older. Treatment repeated every 28 days for a total of three cycles.

Starting in May 1989, the Stanford group treated 65 previously untreated patients with an intensified approach (101). The Stanford V regimen included weekly chemotherapy for 12 weeks, alternating myelosuppressive and nonmyelosuppressive drugs (Table 7). All patients received prophylactic, daily oral trimethoprim and, from May 1991, all patients with significant hematologic toxicity received granulocyte colony-stimulating factor (G-CSF). In the first 25 patients, consolidative radiotherapy was given to sites of initial bulky disease or persistent radiologic abnormalities following chemotherapy. In the others, radiotherapy was limited to sites of bulky disease alone. Radiotherapy was given at an attenuated dose to prevent unacceptable toxicity. Bartlett et al reported preliminary results in 1995 after a median of 2 years follow-up. The 3-year failure-free survival was 100% for stage II patients with bulky mediastinal disease and 82% with stage III and IV disease. Overall survival was 96%, and failure-free survival was 87% at 3 years. At present, fertility appears to be preserved, and no symptomatic pulmonary or cardiac toxicities have been observed.

Seventy-three patients with stage IIB to IV Hodgkin's disease have been treated with the Milan group's VEBEP regimen (Table 8) (102). Eight cycles were given every 21 days, followed by involved-field radiotherapy. All patients received prophylactic antibacterial and antifungal therapy. Complete response was achieved in 94%. After 3 years of follow-up, freedom from progression was 82%, with an overall survival of 84%.

The German Hodgkin's Lymphoma Study Group have developed an alternative intensified regimen (103). Thirty untreated patients with stage IIB to IV Hodgkin's disease were treated with eight cycles of a seven-drug BEACOPP regimen every 21 days (Table 9). Consolidative radiotherapy was restricted to sites of bulky disease pretreatment and residual tumor following chemotherapy.

TABLE 8. *The VEBEP regimen*

VP16 120 mg/m^2 days 1 + 2
Epidoxorubicin 40 mg/m^2 days 1 + 2
Bleomycin 10 mg/m^2 day 1
Cyclophosphamide 500 mg/m^2 days 1 + 2
Prednisolone 50 mg days 1–7

TABLE 9. *The BEACOPP regimens*

BEACOPP 1 from August 1991 to May 1992
Cyclophosphamide 650 mg/m^2 day 1
Doxorubicin 40 mg/m^2 day 1
Etoposide 50 mg/m^2 days 3–12
Procarbazine 100 mg/m^2 days 1–7
Prednisolone 40 mg/m^2 days 1–14
Vincristine 1.4 mg/m^2 (max. dose 2 mg) day 8
Bleomycin 10 mg/m^2 day 8
BEACOPP 2 from May 1992 to January 1993 as growth factor support became available
Cyclophosphamide 650 mg/m^2 day 1
Doxorubicin 25 mg/m^2 day 1
Etoposide 100 mg/m^2 days 1–3
Procarbazine 100 mg/m^2 days 1–7
Prednisolone 40 mg/m^2 days 1–14
Vincristine 1.4 mg/m^2 (max. dose 2 mg) day 8
Bleomycin 10 mg/m^2 day 8

Diehl et al. have recently reported the preliminary findings (103). Complete response was achieved in 93%, and freedom from treatment failure was 89% at a median follow-up of 40 months. Moderate toxicity was observed, particularly hematologic, but there were no treatment-related deaths.

BEACOPP has been shown to be at least equally as effective as COPP/ABVD in an ongoing multicenter randomized trial (104). Patients have been randomized to receive four double cycles of COPP/ABVD or BEACOPP at standard dose or escalated dose. An interim analysis of the first 321 patients showed a nonsignificantly poorer complete response rate in the alternating arm compared with the BEACOPP arm (76% vs. 89%). Progression rates and overall survival were significantly worse in the alternating arm, which has been closed early (104).

The risk of long-term complications in dose-intense regimens remains uncertain. An interim analysis of the BEACOPP regimens at 7 years from the start of trials gives an incidence of 0.7% for secondary neoplasia (V. Diehl, *unpublished data,* 1998). However, secondary leukemias usually do not usually develop until 5 to 10 years after chemotherapy, and these patients continue to be monitored closely.

These early results with intensified regimens are very promising but will need to be fully substantiated in prospective randomized trials before they can be considered as acceptable alternatives to standard therapies.

HIGH-DOSE CHEMOTHERAPY

Throughout the development of chemotherapy strategies in advanced Hodgkin's disease, bone marrow suppression has been the major dose-limiting toxicity. How-

TABLE 10. *Efficacy and toxicity of high-dose chemotherapy in resistant and refractory Hodgkin's disease*

Preparatory regimens[a]	Source of progenitors	CR (PR)	Progression/ disease/event-free survival	Overall survival	Treatment-related deaths	Investigator (reference)
CBV	ABMT	50%			7%	Jagannath (108)
CBV	ABMT	57% (18%)	25%	45% (4 yr)	9%	Bierman (109)
CBV	ABMT	48% (32%)	40–50%		4%	Carella (110)
Augmented CBV	ABMT	80% (4%)	47%	53% (3.5 yr)	21%	Reece (111)
CBV or BEAM	ABMT and/or PBSCT	72% (14%)	44%	61% (12 mo)	21%	Schmitz (112)
BEAM	ABMT	28% (46%)	50%	50%	55%	Chopra (113)
Cyclophosphamide, methotrexate, etoposide, TBI, melphalan	PBSCT and ABMT		48%	54% (6 yr)	0%	Gianni (114)
MINE +/- BEAM/CBV	ABMT or PBSCT	34% (39%)	46%	59% (2 yr)	3%	Ferme (51)
Etoposide, melphalan	ABMT	75% (3%)	39%		10%	Crump (115)
TLI, etoposide, cyclophosphamide	ABMT	74% (21%)	50%		17%	Yahalom (116)

[a]CBV, cyclophosphamide; BCNU, (carmustine); VP 16, (etoposide); TLI, total lymphoid irradiation.

ever, dose intensity can be maximized by administering myeloablative doses of effective agents, if rescued by the infusion of hematopoietic stem cells. These progenitor cells can now be harvested from the peripheral blood, obviating the need for the general anesthetic necessary for bone marrow collection (105). Peripheral blood stem cells engraft earlier, reducing the morbidity and mortality associated with prolonged neutropenia and thrombocytopenia. With the simultaneous advances made in supportive care, high-dose chemotherapy is now a safer, less expensive procedure which is becoming more widely available (106,107).

High-dose chemotherapy has been consistently shown to be effective in the treatment of relapsed or primary refractory Hodgkin's disease in a number of studies (Table 10). Complete remission can be achieved in 28% to 80% of patients whose prognosis would otherwise be poor (117). Only one prospective randomized controlled trial comparing high-dose chemotherapy to conventional salvage chemotherapy in relapsed disease has been reported to date. The BNLI randomized 20 patients to receive subablative chemotherapy with mini-BEAM (BCNU, etoposide, Ara-C, melphalan) and a further 20 patients to BEAM (BCNU, etoposide, Ara-C, melphalan at ablative doses) with autologous bone marrow transplantation (118). A significant superiority for BEAM with autologous bone marrow transplantation was demonstrated for 3-year event-free and progression-free survivals. A trend for improved overall survival in the same arm was not statistically significant. The study was closed early because of poor recruitment.

The risk of serious or lethal toxicity from high-dose chemotherapy is particularly pertinent in relapsed or refractory Hodgkin's disease. These patients have generally been heavily pretreated, often with both chemotherapy and radiotherapy. In the past, treatment-related deaths have been reported in up to 21% of patients (111,112). However, with recent advances, the mortality associated with high-dose chemotherapy is now less than 5% in the majority of centers.

The ultimate role of high-dose chemotherapy in advanced Hodgkin's disease is yet to be defined. Ongoing and future studies will need to clarify the optimum preparative regimens, source and treatment of progenitor cells and whether high-risk patients should receive earlier high-dose chemotherapy.

COMBINED-MODALITY THERAPY

Approximately one third of patients achieving a complete response with conventional combination chemotherapy will subsequently relapse, most often at sites of previous bulk disease (119). Radiotherapy is curative in early stage Hodgkin's disease and appears to be non-cross-resistant with the chemotherapy regimens currently used in widespread disease. It would be reasonable to anticipate that combining chemotherapy with radiotherapy to involved nodes would improve the potential for cure in advanced Hodgkin's disease.

A number of retrospective studies support this hypothesis (Table 11), demonstrating improved disease-free and overall survival with this approach. However, prospective

TABLE 11. *Efficacy and toxicity of combined modality therapy in advanced Hodgkin's disease*

Regimens (no. cycles)	Complete response	Freedom from relapse	Overall survival	Efficacy	Toxicity	Center (reference)
TNI	60–96%	60% (3 yr)*		FFR superior for TNI + BOPP; no significant differences in overall survival		CALGB (77)
TNI + BOPP (6)	79–84%	80%				
BOPP(6) + TNI	88–94%	55%				
BOPP (6)	74–77%					
TNI	86%	55% (15 yr)*	60%	FFR superior for TNI + LOPP		BNLI (120,121)
TNI + LOPP	86%	75%	60%			
MOPP-Bleo (10)	89%	84% (5 yr)	87%	Equivalent	Increased risk of infection, pulmonary toxicity and possibly secondary leukemia with combined modality; increased neurotoxicity with MOPP alone	SWOG (122)
MOPP-Bleo (3) + TNI	96%	70%	89%			
CVPP (6 or 12)	68% or 59%	60% or 55% (3 yr)		Possible survival advantage to sandwich therapy arm		CALBG (77)
CVPP (6) + low dose RT	57%	55%				
CVPP (3)/RT/CVPP (3)	65%	65%				
MVPP (6)	88%	80% (5 yr)	85%	Equivalent	Equivalent	Christie (123)
MVPP (6) + RT	100%	80%	85%			
MOPP-Bleo (6) + ABVD (3)	74%	68% (5 yr)	92%*	Survival advantage to chemotherapy alone	Increased hematological toxicity with combined modality; increased emesis with ABVD	ECOG (37,123)
MOPP-Bleo (6) + RT	74%	66%	83%			
CVPP (6)	73%	23% (7 yr)*	58%	FFR superior for CVPP + RT	Equivalent	GATLA (124)
CVPP (6) + RT	86%	51%	71%			
MOP-BAP (6)	CR with MOPP-BAP prerequisite for entry	66% (5 yr)	79%	Equivalent	Increased risk of secondary malignancy with combined modality approach	SWOG (125)
MOP-BAP (6) + RT		74%	86%			
COPP/ABVD (6) + COPP/ABVD (2)	CR with COPP/ABVD (6) prerequisite for entry	81% (21 mo)		Equivalent		GHSG (126)
COPP/ABVD (6) + RT		87%				

TNI, total nodal irradiation; RT, radiotherapy; CR, complete response; FFR, freedom from relapse;
*statistically significant.

studies have been unable to substantiate these observations convincingly (Table 11). Current philosophies range from the routine administration of radiotherapy to all initially involved sites once chemotherapy is complete to the restriction of radiotherapy to bulky mediastinal involvement or poorly responding nodes.

Loeffler et al. have recently reported a meta-analysis on the outcome of 1,740 patients treated in 14 randomized trials comparing chemotherapy with combined-modality treatment (127). Additional radiotherapy showed a significant improvement in tumor control rate but no difference in overall survival. In contrast, when compared with extended chemotherapy, combined-modality treatment had a significantly inferior long-term survival (127).

The combined use of radiotherapy and chemotherapy is also associated with an increased risk of both short- and long-term side effects including mucositis, neuropathies, secondary leukemia, other cancers (128), and cardiac and pulmonary toxicity. Attempts to minimize toxicity by reducing the dose of radiation delivered have been ineffective (48). The role of the combined-modality approach in the treatment of advanced Hodgkin's disease remains a controversial issue.

The use of neoadjuvant chemotherapy before radiotherapy in localized disease, in an attempt to reduce the toxicity of combined modality programs and eliminate any need for staging by laparotomy, is also subject to debate (129,130) and ongoing investigation (131). For example, in patients with early-stage Hodgkin's disease with large mediastinal adenopathy, the M. D. Anderson group successfully used a short course of a novel chemotherapy regimen, NOVP (novantrone, Oncovin, vinblastine, procarbazine), followed by radical radiotherapy to areas of bulk nodal involvement (132).

This "minimal invasive treatment" philosophy has been applied to other groups of "good prognosis" localized Hodgkin's disease. As yet, there is no randomized controlled trial evidence of survival benefit. Such data will be difficult to obtain, given the long and favourable natural history in this group. Perhaps the best model for this approach is in Hodgkin's disease of childhood, where it has revolutionized clinical management

See Table 12 for a listing of chemotherapy agent synonyms.

TABLE 12. *Chemotherapy agent synonyms*

Bleomycin, blenoxane
Carmustine, BCNU
Cyclophosphamide, cytoxan
Cytarabine, cytosine arabinoside, ara-C
Dacarbazine, DTIC
Doxorubicin, adriamycin
Etoposide, VP16
Lomustine, CCNU
Mechlorethamine, nitrogen mustard, mustine
Methotrexate, mexate
Procarbazine, matulane, natulan
Streptozocin, zanosar
Vinblastine, velban, velbe
Vincristine, oncovin

PATIENT SELECTION

Several groups have attempted to identify prognostic groupings for advanced Hodgkin's disease, with limited success. Such studies have not yet managed to define a wide separation of risk categories using conventional prognostic indices. Even with the large International Prognostic Index Study presented by Hasenclever at the 4th International Symposium on Hodgkin's Lymphoma, only a relatively small number of patients can be identified as having a very poor prognosis (fewer than 10% of patients were expected to have a progression-free survival of less than 5 years). If it were possible to identify patient groups with significant difference in survival, it would be feasible to devise different strategies for initial treatments. For example, in those with a favorable prognosis, therapy could be kept to a minimum with the least possible number of courses of relatively nontoxic chemotherapy or short-course chemotherapy (plus minimum-field radiotherapy) as an extension of the principles already being applied to localized Hodgkin's disease. For those with poor prognosis, very intensive chemotherapy regimens (high-dose or accelerated) might be employed up front. As we have seen, however, as yet the numbers of patients that can be identified in these very good and very poor prognostic groups are relatively small, and therapies could only be validated by international collaboration in clinical trials.

CHEMOTHERAPY ADMINISTRATION

Patients with Hodgkin's disease should be treated by multidisciplinary teams. Certain skills and resources are mandatory to their optimal care. The senior clinicians directing care should have a clear understanding of treatment protocols, the importance of maintaining dose intensity, the acute and chronic side effects of treatment, and what action should be taken if the disease does not respond or complications of therapy arise. Expert nursing support is essential, as patients with Hodgkin's disease are often sick and have very specific needs. Specialist knowledge and experience of intravenous drug administration (including indwelling catheters), complications of chemotherapy, and the associated emotional difficulties are central to good patient care. Dedicated pharmacy facilities are also important for the preparation and checking of drug doses and schedules. Radiotherapy presence is important from the start, and other oncologists should be aware of the crucial importance of radiotherapy as part of the planned management of patients.

MANAGEMENT OF PATIENTS RECEIVING CHEMOTHERAPY FOR HODGKIN'S DISEASE

The dose intensity of chemotherapy in Hodgkin's disease has clearly been shown to influence outcome. Inappropriate dose reductions or delays potentially reduce disease-free and overall survival. Deviations from drug protocols are usually in response to side effects but may occasionally anticipate expected side effects. In a less well supported and experienced setting, the risk of delivering a suboptimal regimen may be greater.

Therefore, every effort should be made to deliver chemotherapy regimens at the intended dose and schedule. A thorough clinical assessment should be performed before any treatment. Simple noninvasive tests should be used to monitor for toxicity; for example, full blood count for marrow suppression, pulmonary function tests in regimens incorporating bleomycin and those receiving mantle radiotherapy, and echocardiography for those receiving anthracyclines (particularly if there is a history of cardiac disease). A male patient to be treated with an alkylating agent should be offered sperm storage, and in female patients the possibility of cryopreservation of ovarian tissue or embryo should be discussed.

When toxicity occurs, the following should be considered:

- Hematopoietic growth factors to prevent neutropenia.
- Prophylactic antibiotics during periods of neutropenia, particularly following a previous episode of neutropenic sepsis, or in those of high risk of infection (i.e., those who are elderly and/or have poor performance status).
- Substitution of vinblastine for vincristine in neuropathy.
- Dose reduction or delay in therapy may be inevitable but should be as minimal as possible; it may be necessary to consider adopting an alternative regimen that does not include the likely offending drug.

CLINICAL SETTING

There is no cause for complacency in the management of Hodgkin's disease; over one-fourth of patients still die of their disease. Where possible patients should be offered treatment in the context of a well-designed clinical trial (133). Even where this is not feasible they should be managed by a skilled multidisciplinary team; optimal resources include facilities for high-dose chemotherapy, state-of-the-art radiotherapy, specialized nursing and other supporting resources. Such criteria are more likely to be met in comprehensive cancer treatment centers, and these centers are more likely to offer their patients involvement in clinical trials. It does seem (though it is still much debated) that patients treated at such centers are likely to have a better outcome than those treated elsewhere (134). For example, Davis et al. found that survival in 3,607 patients entered into the Surveillance, Epidemiology and End Results program of the National Cancer Institute was about 1.5 times better than in the 2,278 patients treated in community general hospitals (135).

FUTURE PROSPECTS FOR CHEMOTHERAPY IN HODGKIN'S DISEASE

It is 30 years since cyclic combination chemotherapy (MOPP or MVPP) was established as effective treatment for Hodgkin's disease. Long-term survival was observed in approximately one-half of patients treated with these regimens. The substitution of chlorambucil for mustine gave each equally favorable results with less toxicity. However, such regimens and others containing alkylating agents (such as the nitrosoureas) have given concern regarding long-term toxicities. ABVD appeared at least as efficacious with less gonadal toxicity and second cancers. Alternating or hybrid regimens may give marginal benefits in terms of overall survival, but the jury is still out on this. The role of combined modality therapy remains controversial, particularly where there is complete remission after chemotherapy.

In general, the regimens that have been most widely adopted are those shown in prospective, randomized clinical trials to be equally efficacious or better than MOPP, with less short- and long-term toxicity and that can be successfully administered in a number of centers (not only at heavily resourced academic units).

It is unlikely that the introduction of new chemotherapeutic agents will improve the outlook in Hodgkin's disease; more likely, raising the doses or intensifying the schedules of established agents will lead to further modest improvement in overall survival. Hence, escalated, intensified regimens (often growth factor supported) are being evaluated in randomized studies; appropriately and skillfully administered radiotherapy seems crucial to the preliminary excellent results described in pilot studies.

High-dose chemotherapy with stem-cell rescue is finding its niche, particularly for chemorefractory or relapsed patients; however, the role for high-dose chemotherapy up front or in first remission remains to be established. It would be nice to be able to identify and select patients for different approaches on the basis of prognostic factors; unfortunately, this is still not possible except for a small proportion of very high-risk patients.

For localized Hodgkin's disease, radiotherapy can be curative. The use of minimally invasive approaches, usually in the form of a short course of relatively nontoxic chemotherapy before involved field radiotherapy, is likely to reduce relapse and long-term toxicity but unlikely to have a major effect on survival (given the already recognized excellent prognosis in this group).

The majority of patients with Hodgkin's disease can now be cured; however, a significant percentage still die. For this reason, patients should be given the opportunity to be involved in clinical trials whenever possible. They should be treated by multidisciplinary teams working in well-resourced centers.

REFERENCES

1. Goodman LS, Wintrobe MM, Dameshek W, et al. Nitrogen mustard therapy. *JAMA* 1946;132:126–132.
2. De Vita VT, Serpick AA, Carbone PP. Combination chemotherapy in the treatment of advanced Hodgkin's disease. *Ann Intern Med* 1970; 73:881–895.
3. Longo DL, Young RC, Wesley M, et al. 20 years of MOPP therapy for Hodgkin's disease. *J Clin Oncol* 1986;4:1295–1306.
4. Bubley GJ, Ogata GK, Dupuis NP, et al. Detection of sequence specific antitumor alkylating agent DNA damage from cells treated in culture and from a patient. *Cancer Res* 1994;54:6325–6329.
5. D'Incalci M. DNA topoisomerase inhibitors. *Curr Opin Oncol* 1993; 5:1023–1028.
6. Smith PJ, Soues S. Multilevel therapeutic targeting by topoisomerase inhibitors. *Br J Cancer* 1994;23(Suppl):47–51.
7. Bleyer WA. The clinical pharmacology of methotrexate: new applications of an old drug. *Cancer* 1978;41:36–51.
8. Jordan MA, Thrower D, Wilson L. Mechanisms of inhibition of cell proliferation by vinca alkaloids. *Cancer Res* 1991;51:2212–2222.
9. Schiff PB, Fant J, Horwitz SB. Promotion of microtubule assembly *in vitro* by taxol. *Nature* 1979;277:665–667.
10. Yarbro JW. The scientific basis of cancer chemotherapy. In Perry MC, ed. *The chemotherapy source book.* Baltimore: Williams & Wilkins, 1992:2–15.
11. Skipper HE, Schabel FM, Wilcox WS. Experimental evaluation of potential anti-cancer agents. XII. On the criteria and kinetics associated with "curability" of experimental leukemia. *Cancer Chemother Rep* 1964;35:1–111.
12. Skipper HE. Historic milestones in cancer biology: a few that are important to cancer treatment (revisited). *Semin Oncol* 1979;6: 506–514.
13. Carter SK, Livingstone RB. Single-agent therapy for Hodgkin's disease. *Arch Intern Med* 1973;131:377–387.
14. Coltman CA. Chemotherapy of advanced Hodgkin's disease. *Semin Oncol* 1980;7:155–173.
15. Sheridan E, Hancock BW, Smith SC. Gestational trophoblastic disease: Experience of the Sheffield (United Kingdom) supraregional screening and treatment service (Review). *Int J Oncol* 1993;3: 149–155.
16. DeVita VT Jr, DeVita VT. Principles of cancer management: Chemotherapy. In DeVita VT, Hellman S, Rosenberg SA, eds. *Cancer, principles and practice of oncology,* 5th ed. Philadelphia: Lippincott-Raven, 1997:333–348.
17. De Vita VT, Schein PS. The use of drugs in combination for the treatment of patients with cancer: Rationale and results. *N Engl J Med* 1973;288:998–1006.
18. Lacher MU, Durant JR. Combined vinblastine and chlorambucil therapy of Hodgkin's disease. *Ann Intern Med* 1965;62:468–476.
19. DeVita VT, Serpick A. Combination chemotherapy in the treatment of advanced Hodgkin's disease (abstract). *Proc Am Assoc Cancer Res* 1967;8:13.
20. Bakemeier RF, Anderson JR, Costello W, et al. BCVPP chemotherapy for advanced Hodgkin's disease: Evidence for greater duration of complete remission, greater survival, and less toxicity than with a MOPP regimen. *Ann Intern Med* 1984;101:447–456.
21. Bonadonna G, Valagussa P, Santoro A. Alternating non-cross-resistant combination chemotherapy or MOPP in stage IV Hodgkin's disease. A report of 8 year results. *Ann Intern Med* 1986;104:739–746.
22. Rosenberg SA, Kaplan HS, Hoppe RT, et al. The Stanford randomized trials of the treatment of Hodgkin's disease 1967–1980. In: Rosenberg SA, Kaplan HS, eds. *Malignant lymphomas.* New York: Academic Press, 1982:513–522.
23. Longo DL, Young RC, DeVita VT Jr. Chemotherapy for Hodgkin's disease: the remaining challenges. *Cancer Treat Rep* 1982;66: 925–936.
24. McElwain TJ, Toy J, Peckham MJ, Austin DE. A combination of chlorambucil, vinblastine, procarbazine and prednisolone for treatment of Hodgkin's disease. *Br J Cancer* 1977;36:276–280.
25. Selby P, Patel P, Milan S, et al. ChlVPP combination chemotherapy for Hodgkin's disease; long-term results. *Br J Cancer* 1990;62:279–285.
26. The International ChlVPP Treatment Group. ChlVPP therapy for Hodgkin's disease: Experience of 960 patients. *Ann Oncol* 1995;6: 167–172.
27. Bloomfield CS, Weiss RB, Fortuny I, et al. Combined chemotherapy with cyclophosphamide, vinblastine, procarbazine and prednisone (CVPP) for patients with advanced Hodgkin's disease: An alternative program to MOPP. *Cancer* 1976;38:42–48.
28. Cooper MR, Pajak TF, Nissen NI, et al. A new effective four-drug combination of CCNU (1-[2-chloroethyl]-3-cyclohexyl-1-nitrosourea) (NSC-79038), vinblastine, prednisone and procarbazine for the treatment of advanced Hodgkin's disease. *Cancer* 1980;46: 654–662.
29. Nissen NI, Pajak TF, Glidewell O, et al. A comparative study of a BCNU containing 4-drug programme versus 3-drug combinations in advanced Hodgkin's disease. A comparative study by the Cancer and Leukaemia Group B. *Cancer* 1979;43:31–40.
30. Bennett JM, Bakemeier RF, Carbone PP, et al. Clinical trials with BCNU (NSC-409962) in malignant lymphomas by the Eastern Cooperative Oncology Group. *Cancer Treat Rep* 1976;60:739–745.
31. Durant JR, Gams RA, Velez-Garcia E, et al. BCNU, velban, cyclophosphamide, procarbazine and prednisone (BVCPP) in advanced Hodgkin's disease. *Cancer* 1978;42:2101–2110.
32. Harrison DT, Neiman PE. Primary treatment of disseminated Hodgkin's disease with BCNU alone and in combination with vincristine, procarbazine and prednisone. *Cancer Treat Rep* 1977;61: 789–795.
33. Sutcliffe SB, Wrigley RF, Peto J, et al. MVPP chemotherapy regimen for advanced Hodgkin's disease. *Br Med J* 1978;1:679–683.
34. Hancock BW. Randomised study of MOPP (mustine, oncovin, procarbazine, prednisone) against LOPP (leukeran substituted for mustine) in advanced Hodgkin's disease. British National Lymphoma Investigation. *Radiother Oncol* 1986;7:215–221.
35. Hancock BW, Vaughan Hudson G, Vaughan Hudson B, et al. British National Lymphoma Investigation randomised study of MOPP (mustine, oncovin, procarbazine, predisolone) against LOPP (leukeran substituted for mustine) in advanced Hodgkin's disease—long term results. *Br J Cancer* 1991;63:579–582.
36. Hancock BW, Vaughan Hudson G, Vaughan Hudson B, et al. British National Lymphoma Investigation (BNLI) randomised trial in advanced Hodgkin's disease: update of the MOPP v LOPP (1979–1983), LOPP v LOPP/EVAP (1983–1989), and LOPP/EVAP v LOPP/EVA (1990–1991) studies. *Proc XVI Int Cancer Cong New Delhi* 1994;2611–2615.
37. Glick JH, Barnes JM, Bakemeier RF, et al. Treatment of advanced Hodgkin's disease: 10 years experience in the Eastern Cooperative Oncology Group. *Cancer Treat Rep* 1982;66:855–870.
38. Coltman CA, Jones SE, Grozea P, et al. Bleomycin in combination with MOPP for the management of Hodgkin's disease: Southwest Oncology Group experience. In Carter SK, Crooke ST, Umezawa H, eds. *Bleomycin: Current status and new developments.* New York: Academic Press, 1978:227–242.
39. Jones SE, Coltman CA, Grozea PN, et al. Conclusions from clinical trials of the Southwest Oncology Group. *Cancer Treat Rep* 1982;66: 847–853.
40. Goldman JM. Combination chemotherapy for stage IV Hodgkin's disease. *Clin Radiol* 1981;32:531–536.
41. Hancock BW. Advanced Hodgkin's disease—British National Lymphoma Investigation results. Oncology section of Royal Society of Medicine. British Institute of Radiology and Royal College of Radiologists. *J R Soc Med* 1986;80:122–123.
42. British National Lymphoma Investigation. Value of prednisolone in combination chemotherapy of stage IV Hodgkin's disease. *Br Med J* 1975;3:413–414.
43. Santoro A, Bonfante V, Bonadonna G. Salvage chemotherapy with ABVD in MOPP-resistant Hodgkin's disease. *Ann Intern Med* 1982; 96:139–143.
44. Bonnadonna G, Zucali R, Monfardini S, et al. Combination chemotherapy of Hodgkin's disease with adriamycin, bleomycin, vinblastine, and imidazole carboxamide versus MOPP. *Cancer* 1975; 36:252–259.
45. Bonadonna G. Modern treatment of malignant lymphomas: A multidisciplinary approach? *Ann Oncol* 1994;5(Suppl 2):S5–S16.

46. Canellos GP, Propert K, Cooper R, et al. Cancer and leukemia group B. MOPP vs ABVD vs MOPP alternating with ABVD in advanced Hodgkin's disease: A prospective randomized CALGB trial (abstract 888). *Proc Am Soc Clin Oncol* 1988;7:230.
47. Canellos GP, Anderson JR, Propert KJ, et al. Chemotherapy of advanced Hodgkin's disease with MOPP, ABVD, or MOPP alternating with ABVD. *N Engl J Med* 1992;327:1478–1484.
48. Urba WJ, Longo DL. Hodgkin's disease in adults: part I. *Invest Radiol* 1993;28:737–752.
49. Tannir N, Hagemeister F. et al. (1983) Long-term follow-up with ABDIC salvage chemotherapy of MOPP-resistant Hodgkin's disease. *J Clin Oncol* 1983;1:432–438.
50. Harker GW, Kushlan P, Rosenberg SA. Combination chemotherapy for advanced Hodgkin's disease after failure of MOPP: ABVD and B-CAVe. *Ann Intern Med* 1984;101:440–446.
51. Harrison DT, Neiman PE. Primary treatment of disseminated Hodgkin's disease with BCNU alone and in combination with vincristine, procarbazine and prednisolone. *Cancer Treat Rep* 1977;61:789–795.
52. Wiernik PH, Schiffer CA. Long-term follow-up of advanced Hodgkin's disease patients treated with a combination of streptozotocin, lomustine (CCNU) and bleomycin (SCAB). *J Cancer Res Clin Oncol* 1988;114:105–107.
53. Liebman HA, Hum GJ, Sheehan WW, et al. Randomized study for the treatment of adult advanced Hodgkin's disease: Mechlorethamine, vincristine, procarbazine and prednisolone (MOPP) versus lomustine, vinblastine and prednisolone. *Cancer Treat Rep* 1983;67:413–419.
54. Santoro A, Viviani S, Valagussa P, et al. CCNU, etoposide and prednimustine (CEP) in refractory Hodgkin's disease. *Semin Oncol* 1986; 13:23–26.
55. Cooper MR, Pajak TF, Nissen NI, et al. A new effective four-drug combination of CCNU, vinblastine, prednisolone and procarbazine for the treatment of advanced Hodgkin's disease. *Cancer* 1980;46: 654–662.
56. Bloomfield CD, Weiss RB, Fortuny I, et al. Combined chemotherapy with cyclophosphamide, vinblastine, procarbazine and prednisolone (CVPP) for patients with advanced Hodgkin's disease. *Cancer* 1976; 38:42–48.
57. Brizel DM, Gockerman JP, Crawford J, et al. A pilot study of etoposide, vinblastine, and doxorubicin plus involved field irradiation in advanced, previously untreated Hodgkin's disease. *Cancer* 1994;74: 159–163.
58. Hagemeister FB, Tannir N, McLaughlin P, et al. MIME chemotherapy (methyl-GAG, ifosfamide, methotrexate, etoposide) as treatment for recurrent Hodgkin's disease. *J Clin Oncol* 1987;5:556–561.
59. Hagemeister FB, Cabanillas F, Velasquez WS, et al. NOVP: A novel chemotherapeutic regimen with minimal toxicity for treatment of Hodgkin's disease. *Semin Oncol* 1990;17:34–40.
60. Simmonds PD, Mead GM, Sweetenham JW, et al. PACEBOM chemotherapy: A twelve week alternating regimen for advanced Hodgkin's disease. *Ann Oncol* 1997;8:259–266.
61. Horning SJ, Ang PT, Hoppe RT, et al. The Stanford experience with combined procarbazine, alkeran and vinblastine (PAVe) and radiotherapy for locally extensive and advanced stage Hodgkin's disease. *Ann Oncol* 1992;3:747–754.
62. Radford JA, Crowther D. Treatment of relapsed Hodgkin's disease using a weekly chemotherapy of short duration: Results of a pilot study in 20 patients. *Ann Oncol* 1991;2:505–509.
63. Coltman CA, Frei E III, Delaney FC. Effectiveness of actinomycin (A), methotrexate (MTX) and vinblastine (V) in prolonging the duration of combination chemotherapy (MOPP) induced remission in advanced Hodgkin's disease (HD). *Proc Am Soc Clin Oncol* 1973;9:78.
64. Medical Research Council's Working Party on Lymphomas. Randomised trial of two-drug and four-drug maintenance chemotherapy in advanced or recurrent Hodgkin's disease. *Br Med J* 1979;1: 1105–1108.
65. Young RC, Canellos GP, Chabner BA, et al. Maintenance chemotherapy for advanced Hodgkin's disease in remission. *Lancet* 1973;1: 1339–1343.
66. Goldie JH, Coldman AJ. A mathematical model for relating the drug sensitivity of tumors to their spontaneous mutation rate. *Cancer Treat Rep* 1979;63:1727–1733.
67. Goldie JH, Coldman AJ, Gudauskas GA. Rationale for the use of alternating non-cross-resistant chemotherapy. *Cancer Treat Rep* 1982;66:439–449.
68. Bonadonna G, Santoro A, Valagussa P, et al. Current status of the Milan trials for Hodgkin's disease in adults. In Cavalli F, Bonadonna G, Rozencweig M, eds. *Malignant lymphomas and Hodgkin's disease: Experimental and therapeutic advances. Proceedings of the Second International Conference on Malignant Lymphomas, Lugano, Switzerland, June 13–16, 1984.* Boston: Martinus Nijhoff, 1985: 299–307.
69. Santoro A, Bonadonna G, Bonfante V, Valagussa P. Alternating drug combinations in the treatment of advanced Hodgkin's disease. *N Engl J Med* 1982;306:770–775.
70. Bonadonna G, Valagussa P, Santoro A. Alternating non-crossresistant combination chemotherapy or MOPP in stage IV Hodgkin's disease: A report of 8-year results. *Ann Intern Med* 1986;104:739–746.
71. Longo DL. The use of chemotherapy in the treatment of Hodgkin's disease. *Semin Oncol* 1990;6:716–735.
72. Longo DL, Duffey PL, DeVita VT, et al. Treatment of advanced-stage Hodgkin's disease: alternating non-crossresistant MOPP/CABS is not superior to MOPP. *J Clin Oncol* 1991;9:1409–1420.
73. Somers R, Carde P, Henry-Amar M, et al. A randomised study in stage IIIB and IV Hodgkin's disease comparing eight courses of MOPP versus an alternation of MOPP with ABVD: A European Organisation for Research and Treatment of Cancer Lymphoma Co-operative Group and Groupe Pierre et Marie Curie Controlled Clinical Trial. *J Clin Oncol* 1994;12:279–287.
74. Straus DJ, Myers J, Lee BJ, et al. Treatment of advanced Hodgkin's disease with chemotherapy and irradiation. Controlled trial of two versus three alternating, potentially non-cross-resistant drug combinations. *Am J Med* 1984;76:270–278.
75. Gams RA, Omura GA, Velez-Garcia E, et al. Alternating sequential combination chemotherapy in the management of advanced Hodgkin's disease. A Southeastern Cancer Study Group Trial. *Cancer* 1986;58:1963–1986.
76. Gams RA, Durant JR, Bartolucci AA. Chemotherapy for advanced Hodgkin's disease: Conclusions from the Southeastern Cancer Study Group. *Cancer Treat Rep* 1982;66:899–905.
77. Bloomfield CD, Pajak TF, Glicksman AS, et al. Chemotherapy and combined modality therapy for Hodgkin's disease: A progress report on Cancer And Leukaemia Group B studies. *Cancer Treat Rep* 1982;66:835–846.
78. Vinciguerra V, Propert KJ, Coleman M, et al. Alternating cycles of combination chemotherapy for patients with recurrent Hodgkin's disease following radiotherapy. A prospectively randomized study by the Cancer and Leukaemia Group B. *J Clin Oncol* 1986;4:838–846.
79. Hancock BW, Vaughan Hudson G, Vaughan Hudson B, et al. LOPP alternating with EVAP is superior to LOPP alone in the initial treatment of advanced Hodgkin's disease: Results of a British National Lymphoma Investigation Trial. *J Clin Oncol* 1992;10:1252–1258.
80. Holte H, Mella O, Telhaug R, et al. Randomised study in stage III–IV Hodgkin's disease: ChlVPP is as effective as alternating ChlVPP/ABOD chemotherapy. In *3rd International Symposium on Hodgkin's Lymphoma, September 18–23, Köln, Germany.* 1995:113.
81. Cullen MH, Stuart NSA, Woodroffe C, et al. ChlVPP/PABlOE and radiotherapy in advanced Hodgkin's disease. *J Clin Oncol* 1994; 12:779–787.
82. Hancock BW, Cullen MH, Vaughan Hudson G. Alternating ChlVPP/PABlOE is better than PABlOE alone as initial chemotherapy for advanced HD: First results of a BNLI/CLG study (abstract). *Br J Cancer* 1997;76(Suppl):32.
83. Viviani S, Bonadonna G, Devizzi L, et al. Ten year results of alternating vs hybrid administration of MOPP–ABVD in Hodgkin's disease (HD). In *3rd International Symposium on Hodgkin's Lymphoma. September 18–23, Köln, Germany.* 1995:74.
84. Viviani S, Bonadonna G, Santoro A, et al. Alternating versus hybrid MOPP and ABVD combinations in advanced Hodgkin's disease: ten-year results. *J Clin Oncol* 1996;14:1421–1430.
85. Klimo P, Connors JM. MOPP/ABV hybrid program: combination chemotherapy based on early introduction of seven effective drugs for advanced Hodgkin's disease. *J Clin Oncol* 1985;3:1174–1182.
86. Connors JM, Klimo P, Adams G, et al. Treatment of advanced Hodgkin's disease with chemotherapy—comparison of MOPP/ABV hybrid regimen with alternating courses of MOPP and ABVD: A report from the National Cancer Institute of Canada Clinical Trials Group. *J Clin Oncol* 1997;15:1638–1645.
87. Radford JA, Crowther D, Rohatiner AZS, et al. Results of a ran-

domised trial comparing MVPP chemotherapy with a hybrid regimen, ChlVPP/EVA, in the initial treatment of Hodgkin's disease. *J Clin Oncol* 1995;13:2379–2385.

88. Glick J, Tsiatis R, Schilsky T, et al. A randomised phase III trial of MOPP/ABV hybrid vs sequential MOPP/ABVD in advanced Hodgkin's disease: Results of the intergroup trial (abstract 59). In *Fifth International Conference on Malignant Lymphoma, Lugano, 1993.*
89. Hancock BW, Vaughan Hudson G, Vaughan Hudson B, et al. Hybrid LOPP/EVA is not better than LOPP alternating with EVAP: A prematurely terminated British National Lymphoma Investigation randomized trial. *Ann Oncol* 1994;5(Suppl 2):S117–S120.
90. Duggan D, Petroni G, Johnson J, et al. MOPP/ABV versus ABVD for advanced Hodgkin's disease—a preliminary report of CALGB 8952 (with SWOG, ECOG, NCIC) (abstract 43). *Proc Am Soc Clin Oncol* 1997;16:12a.
91. Tannock IF. The relationship between proliferation and the vascular system in a transplanted mouse mammary tumor. *Br J Cancer* 1968;22:258–273.
92. Norton L, Simon R. The Norton–Simon hypothesis revisited. *Cancer Treat Rep* 1986;70:163–169.
93. Hryniuk W, Bush H. The importance of dose intensity in chemotherapy of metastatic breast cancer. *J Clin Oncol* 1984;2:1281–1288.
94. Skipper HS. *Analyses of 42 arms of 4 multiarmed trials in which animals bearing 2–3g ROS tumors were treated with simultaneous cyclophosphamide and L-PAM with systemic variations of the relative dose intensity of each drug and the average relative dose intensity.* Booklet 5, AL. Southern Research Institute, 1986.
95. DeVita VT, Hubbard SM, Longo DL. The chemotherapy of lymphomas: Looking back, moving forward—The Richard and Hinda Rosenthal Foundation award lecture. *Cancer Res* 1987;47:5810–5824.
96. Carde P, MacKintosh R, Rosenberg SA. A dose and time response analysis of the treatment of Hodgkin's disease with MOPP therapy. *J Clin Oncol* 1983;1:146–153.
97. Clark SC, Kamen R. The human hematopoietic colony-stimulating factors. *Science* 1987;236:1229–1237.
98. Bristow MR, Billingham ME, Mason JW, et al. Clinical spectrum of anthracycline cardiotoxicity. *Cancer Treat Rep* 1978;62:873–879.
99. Schaeppi U, Phelan R, Stadnicki SW, et al. Pulmonary fibrosis following multiple treatment with bleomycin (NSC-125066) in dogs. *Cancer Chemother Rep* 1974;58:301–310.
100. Pedersen-Bjergaard J, Larsen SO, Struck J, et al. Risk of therapy-related leukaemia and pre-leukaemia after Hodgkin's disease: relation to age, cumulative dose of alkylating agents, and time for chemotherapy. *Lancet* 1987;2:83–88.
101. Bartlett NL, Rosenberg SA, Hoppe RT, et al. Brief chemotherapy, Stanford V, and adjuvant radiotherapy for bulky or advanced-stage Hodgkin's disease: a preliminary report. *J Clin Oncol* 1995;13:1080–1088.
102. Viviani S, Santoro A, Devizzi L, et al. VEBEP plus involved field RT: Efficacy and feasibility of an intensive regimen for advanced Hodgkin's disease (abstract 1239). *Proc Am Soc Clin Oncol* 1995;14:395.
103. Diehl V, Sieber M, Rüffler U, et al. BEACOPP: An intensified chemotherapy regimen in advanced Hodgkin's disease. *Ann Oncol* 1997;8:143–148.
104. Diehl V, Tesch H, Lathan B, et al. BEACOPP, a new intensified hybrid regimen, is at least equally effective compared with COPP/ABVD in patients with advanced stage Hodgkin's lymphoma (abstract 5). *Proc Am Soc Clin Oncol* 1997;16:2a.
105. Kessinger A, Armitage JO, Landmark JD, et al. Autologous peripheral hematopoietic stem cell transplantation restores hematopoietic function following marrow ablative therapy. *Blood* 1988;71:723–727.
106. Bennett CL, Armitage JL, Armitage GO, et al. Costs of care and outcomes for high-dose therapy and autologous transplantation for lymphoid malignancies: Results from the University of Nebraska 1987 through 1991. *J Clin Oncol* 1995;13:969–973.
107. Smith TJ, Hillner BE, Schmitz DC, et al. Economic analysis of a randomised clinical trial to compare filgrastim-mobilised peripheral blood progenitor cell transplantation in patients with Hodgkin's and non-Hodgkin's lymphoma. *J Clin Oncol* 1997;15:5–10.
108. Jagannath S, Dicke DA, Armitage JO, et al. High dose cyclophosphamide, carmustine and etoposide and autologous bone marrow transplantation for relapsed Hodgkin's disease. *Ann Intern Med* 1986;104:163–168.
109. Bierman PJ, Bagin RG, Jagannath S, et al. High dose chemotherapy followed by autologous hematopoietic rescue in Hodgkin's disease: Long-term follow-up in 128 patients. *Ann Oncol* 1993;4:767–773.
110. Carella AM, Congiu AM, Gaozza E, et al. High dose chemotherapy with autologous bone marrow transplantation in 50 advanced resistant Hodgkin's disease patients: An Italian study group report. *J Clin Oncol* 1988;6:1411–1416.
111. Reece DE, Barnett MJ, Connors JM, et al. Intensive chemotherapy with cyclophosphamide, carmustine and etopside followed by autologous bone marrow transplantation for relapsed Hodgkin's disease. *J Clin Oncol* 1991;9:1871–1879.
112. Schmitz N, Glass B, Haferlach T, et al. High dose chemotherapy and hematopoietic stem cell rescue in patients with relapsed Hodgkin's disease. *Ann Hematol* 1993;66:251–256.
113. Chopra R, McMillan AK, Linch DC, et al. The place of high-dose BEAM therapy and autologous bone marrow transplantation in poor-risk Hodgkin's disease. A single center eight year study of 155 patients. *Blood* 1993;81:1137–1145.
114. Gianni AM, Siena S, Bregni M, et al. High-dose sequential chemo-radiotherapy with peripheral blood progenitor cell support for relapsed or refractory Hodgkin's disease—a 6 year update. *Ann Oncol* 1993;4:889–891.
115. Crump M, Smith AM, Brandwein J, et al. High-dose etoposide and melphalan, and autologous bone marrow transplantation for patients with advanced Hodgkin's disease: Importance of disease status at transplant. *J Clin Oncol* 1993;11:704–711.
116. Yahalom J, Gulati SC, Toia M, et al. Accelerated hyperfractionated total lymphoid irradiation, high dose chemotherapy, and autologous bone marrow transplantation for refractory and relapsing patients with Hodgkin's disease. *J Clin Oncol* 1993;11:1062–1070.
117. Longo DL, Duffey PL, Young RC, et al. Conventional-dose salvage combination chemotherapy in patients relapsing with Hodgkin's disease after combination chemotherapy: the low probability of cure. *J Clin Oncol* 1992;10:210–218.
118. Linch DC, Winfield D, Goldstone AH, et al. Dose intensification in relapsed and resistant Hodgkin's disease: results of a BNLI randomised trial. *Lancet* 1993;341:1051–1054.
119. Young RC, Canellos GP, Bruce A, et al. Patterns of relapse in advanced Hodgkin's disease treated with combination chemotherapy. *Cancer* 1978;42:1001–1007.
120. Strickland P. Radiotherapy or chemotherapy as the initial treatment for stage IIIA Hodgkin's disease. *Clin Radiol* 1981;32:527–530.
121. Hancock BW, Vaughan Hudson G, Vaughan Hudson B, et al. British National Lymphoma Investigation studies of pathological stage IIIA Hodgkin's disease: Long term follow up. No role for total nodal irradiation? (abstract). *Br J Cancer* 1990;62(Suppl 11):9.
122. Grozea PN, Depersio EJ, Coltman CA Jr, et al. Chemotherapy alone versus combined modality therapy for Stage III Hodgkin's disease: A five-year follow-up of a Southwest Oncology Group study (SWOG-7518). In *Proceedings of the Second International Conference on Malignant Lymphomas, Lugano, Switzerland, June 13–16.* 1984: 345–351.
123. Glick J, Tsiatis A, Prosnitz L, et al. Improved survival with sequential Bleo-MOPP followed by ABVD for advanced Hodgkin's disease (abstract 926). *Proc Am Soc Clin Oncol* 1984;3:237.
124. Pavlovsky S, Santarelli MT, Sackmann MF, et al. Randomized trial of chemotherapy versus chemotherapy plus radiotherapy for stage III–IV A & B Hodgkin's disease. *Ann Oncol* 1992;3:533–537.
125. Fabian CJ, Mansfield CM, Dahlberg S, et al. Low dose involved field radiation after chemotherapy in advanced Hodgkin's disease. A Southwest Oncology Group Randomised study. *Ann Intern Med* 1994;120: 903–912.
126. Diehl V, Pfreundschuh M, Löffler M, et al. Chemotherapy vs involved-field (IF) radiotherapy for consolidation of remission achieved with three double cycles of cyclophosphamide, vincristin procarbazine, prednisolone (COPP) and doxorubicin, bleomycin, vinblastine, dacarbazine (ABVD) for stages IIIB/IV Hodgkin's disease: A randomized trial of the German Hodgkin's Study Group (abstract 1057). *Proc Am Soc Clin Oncol* 1990:9:273.
127. Loeffler M, Brosteanu O, Hasenclever D, et al. Meta-analysis of chemotherapy versus combined modality treatment trials in Hodgkin's disease. *J Clin Oncol* 1998;6:818–829.
128. Tucker M, Coleman CN, Cox RS, et al. Risk of second cancers after treatment for Hodgkin's disease. *N Engl J Med* 1988;318:76–81.
129. Horning SJ, Hoppe RT, Hancock SL, et al. Vinblastine, bleomycin and

methotrexate: An effective adjuvant in favorable Hodgkin's disease. *J Clin Oncol* 1988;6:1822–1831.
130. Radford JA, Cowan RA, Ryder WDJ, et al. Four weeks of neo-adjuvant chemotherapy significantly reduces the progression rate in patients treated with limited field radiotherapy for clinical stage I/IIA Hodgkin's disease. Results of a randomized pilot study (abstract 21). *Ann Oncol* 1996;7(Suppl 3):21.
131. United Kingdom Lymphoma Group (UKLG) trial. Minimal initial therapy (MIT) for "early" supradiaphragmatic Hodgkin's disease. In: Hancock B, ed. *Proceedings of the Northern UK Highlights Meeting, July 17, 1998.* Sheffield, UK: 3–4.
132. Preti A, Hagemeister FB, McLaughlin P, et al. Hodgkin's disease with a mediastinal mass greater than 10 cm: Results of four different treatment approaches. *Ann Oncol* 1994;5:S97–S100.
133. Hancock BW, Aitken M, Radstone C, et al. Why don't cancer patients get entered into clinical trials? Experience of the Sheffield Lymphoma Group's collaboration in British National Lymphoma Investigation studies. *Br Med J* 1997;314:36–37.
134. Selby P, Gillis C, Haward R. Benefits of specialised cancer care. *Lancet* 1996;348:313–318.
135. Davis S, Dahlberg S, Myers M, et al. Hodgkin's disease in the United States: comparison of patient characteristics and survival in the centralized cancer patient data system and the Surveillance, Epidemiology and End Results program. *J Natl Cancer Inst* 1987;78:471–478.

Hodgkin's Disease, edited by P.M. Mauch,
J.O. Armitage, V. Diehl, R.T. Hoppe, and L.M. Weiss.
Lippincott Williams & Wilkins, Philadephia ©1999.

CHAPTER 23

Principles of Combined-Modality Therapy in Hodgkin's Disease

Joseph M. Connors, Joachim Yahalom, and Evert M. Noordijk

Hodgkin's disease was initially described 170 years ago (1), and its diagnostic histologic appearance was detailed almost a century ago (2,3). Initial treatment consisted of palliative medication for symptoms and occasional noncurative surgery to remove accessible bulky involved lymph nodes. Shortly after the introduction of irradiation as a new therapy almost 100 years ago, it was recognized as a useful intervention to reduce enlarged lymph nodes and ameliorate locally symptomatic lesions (4). However, the curative potential of irradiation was not realized until a number of innovations and observations had become available: reliable dosimetry (5); adequate design of radiation fields using shaped blocks (6); appreciation of the need for fractionation to best balance efficacy and toxicity (7); and maintenance of follow-up records adequate to demonstrate a change in the natural history of the disease and improved survival probability for the patients (8). Over the past 50 years continued refinement of the technique of radiation treatment has made it a cornerstone of the curative treatment of Hodgkin's disease (9). Current state-of-the-art treatment rests firmly on its appropriate use.

The very first chemotherapeutic agents introduced into clinical practice, corticosteroids (10), alkylating agents (11), vinca alkyloids (12), and later procarbazine (13), were all effective against Hodgkin's disease but were employed for palliation of symptomatic or threatening disease. The curative potential of multiagent chemotherapy was realized only with the design of combinations such as MOPP (mechlorethamine, vincristine, procarbazine, and prednisone) (14,15). Since then many other combinations have been devised, tested, used in clinical practice, and shown to have curative potential even when the disease is bulky, widely disseminated, or recurrent despite previous irradiation. The numerous regimens devised can be divided into three main types: those similar to MOPP; those incorporating newer antibiotic antineoplastic agents such as ABVD (doxorubicin, bleomycin, vinblastine, and dacarbazine) (16); and combinations of the two into alternating (MOPP/ABVD) (17) or hybrid (MOPPABV) (18,19) regimens. Recently completed large clinical trials have established that the ABVD (20) and MOPPABV (20–25) regimens have the greatest effectiveness against Hodgkin's disease and that ABVD, lacking potent alkylating agents and therefore neither sterilizing (26) nor leukemogenic (27), is the best combination for current clinical practice. Thus, clinicians have two powerful but quite different tools available for effective, often curative, treatment of Hodgkin's disease: irradiation and multiagent chemotherapy. It is reasonable to hope that the careful use of both of these modalities together might achieve even more than either can separately. Such combined-modality therapy holds substantial potential to improve treatment results and, at the same time, reduce toxicity, but this potential can be realized only with careful integration of both techniques.

J.M. Connors: Division of Medical Oncology, University of British Columbia, British Columbia, Canada.

J. Yahalom: Department of Medicine, Cornell University Medical College and Department of Radiation Oncology, Memorial Sloan-Kettering Cancer Center, New York, New York.

E.M. Noordijk: Department of Clinical Oncology, Leiden University Medical Center, Leiden, The Netherlands.

RATIONALE FOR COMBINED-MODALITY TREATMENT OF HODGKIN'S DISEASE

Why combine chemotherapy and irradiation when treating Hodgkin's disease? Table 1 lists the potential benefits of such an approach. The most obvious is the

TABLE 1. *Potential benefits of combining chemotherapy and irradiation for the treatment of Hodgkin's disease*

Additive curative effect
Treatment addresses both disseminated and local disease
Simplification of staging, eliminating the need for extensive or invasive testing such as staging laparotomy
Reduction of overall time and extent of treatment with subsequent reduction in toxicity and overall cost
Reduction in time to initiation of treatment
Elimination of dependence on complex, potentially error-prone, prognostic models
Elimination of relapses, allowing avoidance of costly and toxic secondary treatment
Ability to reduce amount and toxicity of both radiation and chemotherapy

potential for an additive curative effect on known or even unknown sites of disease. Are these treatments genuinely additive in effect? Yes. Multiagent chemotherapy can cure disease that has not been eradicated by irradiation (28–30), even when the disease recurs in a previously irradiated site. This establishes unequivocally that disease that is resistant to radiation is only partially cross-resistant to chemotherapy. In addition, several authors have shown that irradiation can cure Hodgkin's disease after multiagent chemotherapy has failed to do so (31–36). Thus, non–cross-resistance is present for either sequence, indicating that the combination of both modalities should be at least partially additive in curative potential. This, in turn, should increase the frequency with which such presentations as bulky mediastinal disease can be cured despite frequent failure of single-modality treatment.

Another reason it is attractive to combine chemotherapy and irradiation is the way each complements the other in terms of disease coverage. When irradiation fails to cure Hodgkin's disease, relapse most usually occurs outside of the irradiated site (37), but when chemotherapy fails, relapse is most common in previous, especially nodal, sites of disease (38). Together the two modalities ought to be able to eradicate extensive disease by employing the wide reach of chemotherapy and regional disease by relying on the local effectiveness of irradiation.

Although the ability of combined-modality treatment to be more effective than either single modality, by itself, would justify investigation of such a treatment approach, there are other reasons to explore its use. One is the tendency for the disease to metastasize even in its early stages. Even the most meticulous staging evaluation, including staging laparotomy, fails to discover all the disease in at least 20% of patients (25,30,37,39,40). Chemotherapy has the potential to eradicate this micrometastatic disease while the irradiation deals with the localized tumor. Combining both modalities may also, somewhat paradoxically, reduce toxicity. This is accomplished by depending on their additive and complementary effects. For example, if chemotherapy is added to the management of early-stage disease or used to reduce the bulkiness of mediastinal disease, less extensive irradiation may be required (41,42), reducing toxicity related to field size, an important consideration with intrathoracic disease, where pulmonary and cardiac function are at risk. Likewise, the use of irradiation to complete treatment when bulky disease is present may allow foreshortening of the chemotherapy and avoidance of toxicity related to total accumulated drug dose.

Other benefits accrue when combined-modality treatment is used to treat early-stage disease. Because the chemotherapy reliably eliminates modest or microscopic amounts of metastatic disease, it is not necessary or desirable to employ exhaustive or highly invasive staging tests. If standard imaging techniques such as chest radiography and abdominopelvic computed tomography fail to visualize disease, then the maximum amount that might be present should be well within that which chemotherapy can reliably eliminate. Although chemotherapy should never be relied on to undo the consequences of careless or incomplete evaluation, it can complement an efficiently abbreviated, less invasive series of staging tests without compromising the overall effectiveness of the treatment program. Another advantage conferred by adding the chemotherapy relates to time spent in staging and initiating treatment. Promptly initiating the chemotherapy in the combined-modality treatment eliminates delay in starting treatment. As soon as the diagnosis is firm and a short list of staging tests are complete, treatment can begin rather than being delayed while the patient recovers from invasive tests such as staging laparotomy or awaits the planning and initiation of complex radiation treatment. Such a prompt start to treatment is of psychological and financial benefit and should, at least theoretically, improve the likelihood of cure by depriving the malignancy of any further chance to develop treatment resistance, an event that must at least in part be a function of time.

Combined-modality treatment also permits elimination of reliance on complex prognostic models. When unimodality treatment is used to treat Hodgkin's disease, a large number of prognostic factors potentially affect outcome (25,39,40,43–45). There is no universal agreement, however, on the specific factors of greatest importance. In addition, it is clear that the factors identified are related to the precise details of the treatment employed, with many factors losing their significance when more effective treatments are used. Thus, the clinician cannot be assured that any specific set of prognostic factors applies reliably to any individual patient. However, when combined-modality therapy, with its greater potential to control both local and distant disease, is employed, many of these factors lose their impact (46). This obviates the need to develop long lists and complex models of prognostic factors and, by simplifying the assignment of optimal treatment, helps clinicians avoid error in this choice. Because there is some evidence that overreliance on such models leads to inferior outcomes (47,48), simpler schemes for choosing treatment are more desirable. Finally, if it is a more effective primary treatment, combined-modality intervention may eliminate the occurrence of at least some relapses and all of the fear, cost, toxicity, and potential for treatment failure associated with them. Elimination of relapses, if achieved, is obviously beneficial. Relapse of disease provokes justifiable anxiety, precipitates another round of expensive, uncomfortable tests, and requires a return to toxic treatments often made more noxious psychologically by memories of previous treatment and physically by long-term effects of prior treatment on organ function, especially that of the lungs, heart, liver, or bone marrow. Although treatment of relapse in Hodgkin's disease can be successful after primary irradiation, chemotherapy, or even combined-modality treatment, it is often more difficult and less effective than what can be achieved by maximizing the effectiveness of the primary therapy. Although this effect of initial treatment on the tolerance for and efficacy of secondary treatment is most clear in the case of primary chemotherapy or combined-modality therapy, it is also true even when the initial treatment is with radiation alone because of its effects on bone marrow function and peripheral blood count recovery during subsequent chemotherapy.

For all of its benefits, there are some countervailing drawbacks to combining radiation and chemotherapy for Hodgkin's disease. These may include increased cost, inconvenience of treatment, or, as discussed below, enhanced toxicity. Combined-modality treatment is certainly not the best treatment for all patients but may produce the most desirable blend of high efficacy and reduced toxicity and cost for appropriately selected subgroups. The choice of candidates for combined-modality treatment must rest on a full appreciation of the specific techniques for integrating the two types of treatment, adoption of methods for maximizing effectiveness and minimizing toxicity, and an understanding of the implications of sequencing and the potential for additive toxicity. The next two sections discuss these issues and the identification of optimal stage-specific treatment plans.

SPECIAL ASPECTS OF COMBINED-MODALITY TREATMENT: DOSE, FIELD SIZE, SEQUENCING, AND TOXICITY

Radiation Dose and Field Size

In addition to the many factors that affect either chemotherapy or radiation therapy when used alone, there are several issues that arise specifically because of potential interaction and summing of effects when they are combined. In particular, clinicians must consider such aspects as dose of treatment, sequencing of each modality, special populations such as children, and the potential for enhanced toxicity. Only when these special aspects are fully considered can an optimal balance of increased effectiveness and manageable toxicity be found.

The likelihood of recurrence of Hodgkin's disease within an irradiated field falls to less than 5% when a dose of 35 Gy or higher is given, establishing a standard dose for unimodality treatment (5). There is, however, no consensus on whether this dose can be reduced when irradiation is combined with multiagent chemotherapy and still maintain a high likelihood of eradicating disease. Theoretical arguments have been advanced both in favor of and against acceptance of a reduced dose (5,49). On the one hand, it seems intuitively likely that adding two highly effective treatments together should so enhance overall potency that the dose of one of them, in this case the irradiation, could be reduced while preserving effectiveness. On the other, it is important to remember that the purpose of adding a second modality is to overcome resistance to the first, and in the case of adding irradiation to chemotherapy for Hodgkin's disease, it seems likely that full-dose irradiation may be needed to overcome primary resistance to chemotherapy. This question can only be resolved by being tested in clinical trials. When it is the only modality, the dose of radiation can be safely reduced to 30 Gy for the uninvolved areas being treated prophylactically, as was well demonstrated in a large German Hodgkin's Study Group trial (50). Unfortunately, there have been few trials specifically designed to determine the minimum necessary dose of irradiation to known disease when combined with multiagent chemotherapy for Hodgkin's disease. Of particular interest are two German trials recently summarized by Loeffler and colleagues (51) in which patients with stage IA, IB, IIA, IIB, or IIIA disease with extensive mediastinal or splenic involvement or E lesions were treated with COPP/ABVD followed by irradiation. In the first trial (HD1), responders to chemotherapy were then given extended-field irradiation with the dose to nonbulky sites assigned randomly to be either 20 Gy or 40 Gy. In the second study (HD5), a similar group of patients received 30 Gy to the nonbulky sites. Bulky sites received 40 Gy in both trials. Freedom from treatment failure was the same in all three groups, strongly implying that after optimal chemotherapy, irradiation dose, at least to nonbulky sites, can be reduced without sacrificing efficiency. However, bulky sites received 40 Gy, leaving open the question of whether that dose might also be reduced. Until more results become available, the most prudent course will be that guided by focusing on toxicity.

The risk of two important late complications of irradiation may be reduced by lowering the dose. Studies of late sequelae of treatment for Hodgkin's disease (52,53) suggest that the risk of second neoplasms, especially breast cancer in women, may be reduced by using a lower radiation dose. In particular, the risk of second neoplasms was found to be substantially higher after a dose greater than 40 Gy than after 15 to 25 Gy (53). The other late toxicity possibly associated with radiation dose is cardiovascular. The Stanford University group found that a higher dose of irradiation to the mediastinum was associated with increased mortality from cardiac disease (54). Thus, for adults, in whom a radiation dose of 30 Gy is usually acceptably tolerated even after chemotherapy but a dose above 40 Gy leads to increased toxicity (51), the dose should be reduced to 30 Gy to uninvolved or nonbulky sites, although a higher dose, preferably not to exceed 40 Gy, should be reserved for bulky sites if used at all. However, for children, who have not yet completed bone growth, the gain in reducing long-term toxicity appears to justify the theoretical risk of lowered efficacy, and doses of 20 to 25 Gy have become accepted practice (55–57).

An alternative way to reduce toxicity from irradiation when used in combined-modality treatment is to reduce not the dose but the extent of the fields encompassed. Here theory and clinical trial results match nicely. Several trials involving patients with limited-stage Hodgkin's disease have shown that as good or superior results can be achieved when chemotherapy is combined with involved-region radiation compared to irradiation alone to an extended field, even full mantle or inverted-Y or subtotal nodal irradiation (37,41,47,58,59). The ability to preserve efficacy while limiting toxicity by reducing the size of the treatment fields is one of the most attractive aspects of using combined-modality treatment. Because 90% of cases of Hodgkin's disease present above the diaphragm, field size directly affects long-term pulmonary and cardiac toxicity. Thus, while evidence that radiation dose can be reduced in combined-modality therapy without compromising efficacy is lacking, ample experience has been accumulated in clinical trials to provide assurance that when effective chemotherapy is part of the treatment program the radiation field size can be safely reduced to just include the known region of disease, avoiding the extra toxicity that results from wide field treatment. The precise extent to which the field size of the radiation treatment can be reduced when the chemotherapy duration is also reduced remains a subject of active clinical investigation (41,60).

Chemotherapy Dose and Duration

The same theoretical considerations that apply to irradiation are also relevant when one considers reduction of the dose of chemotherapy used in combined-modality treatment. Once again it seems theoretically possible that efficacy might be preserved while reduced doses are used in a combined program, thus resulting in less toxicity. On the other hand, compromising the chemotherapy that is supposed to eliminate Hodgkin's disease that is resistant to full-dose irradiation may sacrifice overall effectiveness. To add complexity, chemotherapy doses may be reduced by using lower individual doses or abbreviating the course of treatment. Influenced by a desire to preserve dose intensity, most investigators have chosen to keep individual doses at full standard levels, and reductions in the chemotherapy have been accomplished by using fewer cycles of treatment. After initial trials of combined-modality treatment for early-stage Hodgkin's disease showed that the addition of six monthly cycles of chemotherapy allowed reduction of radiation field size to just an involved field (37,58), other investigators went on to demonstrate that shortening the chemotherapy to four or even two monthly cycles also produces excellent results (41,60). The section on early-stage disease below examines these results in more detail.

The potential advantage of reducing the extent of chemotherapy in early-stage Hodgkin's disease seems clear because the focus is appropriately on reducing toxicity while maintaining high efficacy. However, the failure of even combined-modality treatment to cure more than 70% to 75% of patients with advanced disease mitigates against exploring reduction of chemotherapy in this setting, although a special approach to stage III disease in which two cycles of chemotherapy are followed by full-dose extended-field irradiation has been studied at M. D. Anderson Hospital with good results (61). Further such investigation will await development of more effective programs, after which it will be appropriate to shift focus to reducing toxicity. A novel type of regimen in which chemotherapy is abbreviated has been tested at Stanford University and found promising. The Stanford V regimen employs chemotherapy for only 3 months followed by extensive irradiation (62). However, although the chemotherapy course has been shortened, the dose intensity has been increased substantially such that this regimen is not actually an attempt to examine the reduction of chemotherapy but rather its redesign into a briefer, more intensive program.

Sequence

In theory, either the chemotherapy or the radiation could come first in the sequence of combined-modality treatment. In practice, it is almost always desirable for the chemotherapy to do so. The reasons for this include early effective treatment of metastatic disease, delay in induction of irreversible loss of bone marrow function, and the opportunity to use smaller potentially less toxic radiation treatment fields after chemotherapy has induced tumor regression.

In addition to its desired impact on the known sites of disease, a major reason for the inclusion of chemotherapy is to deal with metastatic or subclinical deposits whether known or unappreciated. Any such subclinical disease that lies outside the radiation treatment field is left untreated during irradiation and thus permitted to progress if that modality is employed first. Thus chemotherapy, which exerts its impact on both the known primary tumor and potential subclinical disease at the same time is the more desirable first modality. Another reason to put irradiation second is that it ablates bone marrow function within the treatment field, which often includes clavicles, sternum, parts of the ribs and spine, and may extend to proximal humeri or pelvis. Compromise of the bone marrow to this extent may reduce tolerance for chemotherapy and thus impair the effectiveness of the overall treatment regimen. While chemotherapy also affects marrow function, with nonalkylating agent regimens there is usually little difficulty delivering involved field irradiation after chemotherapy. Finally, the irradiation is frequently incorporated in the combined-modality plan because bulky disease is present at diagnosis. If irradiation is used first in such cases, the treatment field must be quite large, substantially overlapping radiation-sensitive organs such as the lung, heart, liver, or kidneys. Using radiation after chemotherapy has induced substantial tumor shrinkage may permit a smaller treatment field without sacrificing the need to maintain adequate margins. This field reduction in turn reduces toxicity to surrounding tissue. In practice, one of two approaches has been taken: either the chemotherapy is completed entirely before the irradiation or a sandwich technique is used with three or four cycles before the irradiation and the rest of the planned chemotherapy after it. This latter approach has been employed in several of the major trials undertaken by the European Organization for Research and Treatment of Cancer (EORTC) (25, 63). However, these investigators found that hematologic and pulmonary toxicity from the radiation interfered with delivery of full doses of the chemotherapy in the latter cycles and they have abandoned it for future trials. Thus, for three major reasons, earliest possible treatment of potential subclinical disease, delay of bone marrow injury and reduction of toxicity to surrounding organs, the standard sequence for combined-modality treatment of Hodgkin's disease should be chemotherapy followed by irradiation.

Toxicity

Hodgkin's disease cannot be cured without the use of treatments associated with significant short- and long-term toxicity (64,65). The appropriate use of combined-modality treatment may help to reduce this toxicity by permitting reductions in radiation treatment field size, by maintaining high levels of efficacy even when chemotherapy is abbreviated, or by preventing relapse, which then requires additional cumulatively toxic retreatment. However, the combination of two separate potently cytotoxic interventions may increase toxicity by adding together the impacts of each treatment (66–68). Table 2 lists types of toxicity that might be increased by combined-modality treatment. With the recognition of the superiority of chemotherapy regimens that include doxorubicin and bleomycin (20–22,25), the potential interaction of these two drugs with radiation to produce enhanced cardiac or pulmonary toxicity is of concern. Although some observers have felt that the likelihood of doxorubicin-associated cardiomyopathy is increased if the heart is irradiated, especially if the left ventricle is included in the field (69), strong evidence for this additive effect is lacking at doses usually used for Hodgkin's disease. Because doxorubicin causes myofibril damage and irradiation endothelial and small vessel injury, their effects may not be additive. Similar concerns arise concerning bleomycin, because it and radiation each independently cause pulmonary toxicity (70). Combining them raises concern about increased damage to the lungs. Likewise, both chemotherapy and radiation are toxic to the bone marrow and independently carcinogenic. At least in theory, combining them could lead to increased rates of myelodysplasia, leukemia, and secondary solid tumors. Whether these adverse late effects occur sufficiently often to offset the gains brought by the combined-modality approach can only be determined with careful long-term follow-up of patients successfully cured of Hodgkin's disease. Fortunately, what data are available provide reassurance. Long-term follow-up studies of adult patients treated with six cycles of ABVD and irradiation have not revealed rates of clinically significant cardiotoxicity above those seen with chemotherapy alone (25,71). This may indicate either a lack of any additive effect at all or avoidance of significant additive effects when the doxorubicin dose is kept to a maximum of 300 mg/m^2 and the radiation to less than 30 to 40 Gy and the radiation field includes as little of the myocardium as possible. Likewise, the rates of symptomatic pulmonary toxicity seen when bleomycin-containing regimens are combined with radiation do not seem to be greater than those seen after radiation alone (71,72). However, caution is still necessary. These data are based on cumulative doses of doxorubicin that did not usually exceed 300 mg/m^2, and bleomycin that did not exceed 120 $units/m^2$. Combining higher doses with radiation may be less safe. Also, these conclusions apply only to adults. The increased sensitivity of these same tissues in children to damage from doxorubicin (69) and possibly bleomycin (73) may well lead to enhanced toxicity after combined-modality treatment. Until better long-term data from children are available, combining these drugs with radiation in the pediatric setting should be done with great caution. Finally, not all reported data are as reassuring. The combination of VBM (vinblastine, bleomycin, and methotrexate) with irradiation caused unacceptable pulmonary toxicity in the hands of two groups testing this combination

TABLE 2. *Types of toxicity potentially increased by combined-modality treatment for Hodgkin's disease*

Type	Agents
Cardiac	Anthracyclines, radiation
Pulmonary	Bleomycin, radiation
Hematopoietic	Multiple drugs, radiation
Gonadal	Alkylating agents, procarbazine, radiation
Second neoplasms	Multiple drugs, radiation

(74,75), although this was not seen by investigators at the original center where it was designed (58).

Does combining radiation and chemotherapy increase rates of myelodysplasia or secondary neoplasms over that seen when chemotherapy is used alone? This question is unanswered because we do not have the long follow-up in large numbers of patients required to address it. Although it is clear that patients cured of Hodgkin's disease have an increased risk of later hematologic and solid neoplasms (76) and that secondary myelodysplasia and leukemia are most related to exposure to alkylating agents such as mechlorethamine, cyclophosphamide, procarbazine, and chlorambucil (76), what contribution to this secondary carcinogenesis comes from factors that caused the development of the Hodgkin's disease itself, which from chemotherapy, and which from radiation remains unclear. None of the long-term studies has clearly shown an increase in risk of secondary cancer specifically attributable to the use of combined-modality treatment as opposed to chemotherapy alone, although rates of second neoplasms are usually higher than those seen in patients treated with irradiation alone (66,68,77). In the end it is important to keep this problem in perspective. The greatest single threat to the life of a patient with Hodgkin's disease is that the disease not be cured. Thus, the highest possible level of treatment effectiveness must be maintained while efforts to reduce toxicity are made, even toxicity as serious as secondary cancer. Also, the marginal increase in incidence of secondary neoplasms that might be caused by the use of combined-modality treatment must be weighed against the potential to increase the rate of cure of the Hodgkin's disease itself. Even if secondary carcinogenesis is increased, an effect not apparent from currently available data, this undesirable effect may be more than offset by improved control of the Hodgkin's disease. Only long-term follow-up of patients treated with the currently recognized best protocols will settle these issues.

COMBINED-MODALITY TREATMENT IN CLINICAL PRACTICE

The rationale for the use of combined-modality treatment for Hodgkin's disease differs with the stage and presentation. When it is employed in early-stage disease, its purpose is to help minimize invasive staging procedures and reduce extent of treatment while maintaining very high cure rates. When it is used for patients with bulky disease at presentation, the goal is to augment the effectiveness of unimodality treatment by enhancing both local and overall disease control. Combining chemotherapy and irradiation to treat advanced disease has the straightforward goal of increasing overall treatment efficacy. Finally, irradiation can be added to high-dose chemotherapy and hematopoietic stem cell transplantation for persistent or recurrent disease after failure of primary chemotherapy. Results from clinical trials provide useful guidance to delineate the role of combined-modality treatment in each of these settings.

Early-Stage Disease

Approximately 35% of patients with Hodgkin's disease present free of the constitutional symptoms of fever, night sweats, or weight loss and with disease confined to one side of the diaphragm, that is, stage I or II, without any tumor mass greater than 10 cm or a mediastinal tumor diameter exceeding one-third of the greatest transthoracic diameter. These patients constitute a group with early Hodgkin's disease and have a very favorable prognosis (see Chapter 25). Traditionally these patients have been subjected to rigorous, often invasive, staging procedures. If they proved to have limited disease, they were treated with unimodal radiation therapy. Such an approach cures about 80% of patients (25,37,39) and permits approximately 60% to avoid chemotherapy (at least 20% require chemotherapy because of upstaging at laparotomy and 20% because of relapse after irradiation). Some institutions and cooperative groups have omitted staging laparotomy and substituted assignment of treatment based on prognostic factors, which are useful at predicting the findings expected at laparotomy (30), instead of actually using surgical staging. However, even when quite favorable groups are thus chosen, relapse rates reach or exceed 20% if radiation is used alone (78,79).

After it became apparent that even meticulously staged patients with early-stage Hodgkin's disease experience at least a 20% relapse rate despite wide-field irradiation and that multiagent chemotherapy can cure disseminated disease, clinical trials were launched to compare the use of combined-modality treatment versus radiation alone. These trials have consistently shown a substantial reduction in risk of relapse but only modest or no effect on overall survival, presumably because the effectiveness of salvage chemotherapy is greater in patients who have not received chemotherapy as part of their primary treatment (80–92). Specht and her co-workers, on behalf of the International Hodgkin's Disease Collaborative Group, have obtained updated individual patient results from 12 randomized controlled trials that enrolled 1,666 patients with early-stage Hodgkin's disease comparing chemotherapy plus radiation with radiation alone (93). They performed a detailed meta-analysis that confirmed that adding chemotherapy to irradiation for early-stage Hodgkin's disease reduces the risk of treatment failure by approximately 50% but has only very modest impact on survival, if any. In the pooled results, the 10-year risk of treatment failure after radiation alone of 33% was reduced to 16% by the addition of chemotherapy. However, because of excellent salvage treatments, the 10-year overall survival was 79% after combined-modality treatment and 76% after radiation alone, with only a trend for less likelihood of death from Hodgkin's disease (15% after irradiation,

12% after chemotherapy plus irradiation; p = .07). Despite their importance, several factors reduce the current applicability of these results. The trials enrolled a mixture of clinically and laparotomy staged patients; the chemotherapy was almost always MOPP or a close variant and was usually given for six cycles, which may have contributed to the approximately 10% increase in the odds of death from causes other than Hodgkin's disease seen in the combined-modality group; and some patients with B symptoms or bulky or stage III disease were included. These aspects make the observations from these trials mostly of historic interest but do not obscure the major potential for combined-modality treatment to reduce risk of relapse in early-stage Hodgkin's disease.

An alternative approach to these same patients employs clinical staging followed by brief chemotherapy and then irradiation. This latter approach has several advantages: invasive staging tests such as lymphangiography and staging laparotomy are unnecessary, splenectomy is avoided, treatment can be initiated promptly, and because systemic therapy is given to all patients, relapse because of undiscovered micrometastatic disease can be prevented. Table 3 summarizes the results that can be achieved using such combined-modality treatment for early-stage Hodgkin's disease. Older studies using MOPP-type chemotherapy have been omitted because the inferiority of such chemotherapy regimens in terms of lesser efficacy and greater toxicity is now well documented (20–22,25). Several important lessons can be drawn from these studies. First, adding chemotherapy to the primary treatment of early-stage Hodgkin's disease improves disease control despite the fact that at least 20% of patients actually harbor stage III disease, which was missed because laparotomy was omitted. Second, if highly effective chemotherapy such as ABVD is used, the course of chemotherapy can be quite short, certainly as few as 4 or even 2 months. Third, the addition of the chemotherapy allows reduction in the field size for the radiation, an outcome nicely delineated by the Milan trial showing in a randomized prospective comparison that after four months of ABVD, involved field is just as effective as extended-field mantle irradiation (41). Finally, these excellent outcomes can be achieved without staging laparotomy thus avoiding the toxicity, cost, treatment delay and late complications associated with that surgery. These results indicate that abbreviated chemotherapy and reduced volume irradiation can be combined into highly effective treatment for early stage Hodgkin's disease. Future investigations will be needed to define the optimal composition and minimum duration of chemotherapy necessary, the maximum extent of disease that can be controlled in this fashion, and, finally, whether some or all of these patients could be managed as well relying solely on a brief course of chemotherapy without any irradiation, a question now being tested in clinical trials.

Bulky Disease

Bulky Hodgkin's disease usually presents in the mediastinum and occasionally in the retroperitoneum or peripheral lymph nodes. Although definitions vary, disease at any site exceeding 10 cm in diameter or in the mediastinum exceeding one-third of the greatest transthoracic diameter is widely accepted as constituting bulky disease. Because the likelihood of controlling such disease is only about 50% with irradiation or chemotherapy alone (37,94–99), and given the often localized nature of this presentation, bulky Hodgkin's disease was the first type to be treated with combined-modality therapy. Conceptually it is useful to separate patients into those with localized bulky disease, usually stage II, and those with widely disseminated disease where a bulky site is just one among several, usually stage III or IV. Table 4 summarizes selected studies addressing the role of combined-modality treatment for patients with localized but bulky presentation. In addition, Hughes-Davies and colleagues have provided a useful overview of the recent and older studies that have focused on this specific issue (100). These studies have repeatedly shown that combined chemotherapy and irradiation is more effective at eradicating disease than single-modality treatment, usually increasing disease-free survival from approximately 50% to over 75% (37,42,46,101–103). However, the same studies have failed to show more than a trend toward better survival in the combined-modality group, presumably because of the effective use of chemo-

TABLE 3. *Combined-modality treatment for early-stage Hodgkin's disease*

Group	Age (yr)	Stage[a]	Chemotherapy	Radiation	n	5- to 6-yr DFS (%)	5- to 6-yr OS (%)	Reference
EORTC	<50	CS I,II Fav	EBVP × 6	IFRT	168	92	98	48
BCCA	<65	CS I, II	ABVD × 2	Mantle/STNI	97	100	96	60
Stanford	<65	CS I, II	VBM × 6	IFRT	35	87	96	58
Milan	<65	CS IA, IB, IIA	ABVD × 4	Mantle or IFRT	114	94	100	41

[a]Patients with bulky disease or B symptoms were excluded unless noted; DFS, disease-free survival; OS, overall survival; EORTC, European Organization for Research and Treatment of Cancer; Fav, favorable; CS, clinical stage; EBVP, epirubicin, bleomycin, vinblastine and prednisone; IFRT, involved field radiation therapy; BCCA, British Columbia Cancer Agency; ABVD, doxorubicin, bleomycin, vinblastine, and dacarbazine; STNI, subtotal nodal irradiation; VBM, vinblastine, bleomycin, and methotrexate.

TABLE 4. *Comparative trials addressing the utility of combined-modality treatment for localized Hodgkin's disease presenting with bulky tumor*[a]

Group	Mediastinal mass ratio	Treatment	*n*	6- to 10-yr FFR (%)	6- to 10-yr OS (%)	Reference
Stanford	>0.33	RT alone	14	45	82	37
		RT + CT	27	81	81	
Milan	>0.33	RT + MOPP	66	55	59	101
		RT + ABVD	78	73	66	
St. Luc, Brussels	>0.35	RT + MOPP	26	46	46	102
NCI-US	>0.33	RT + MOPP/ABVD	80	55	75	103
Paris-Ouest, France	>0.33	RT + ABVD + P	91	(71)	(81)	46
Stanford	>0.33	RT + CT	48	88	84	42

[a]FFR, freedom from relapse; OS, overall survival; RT, radiation therapy; CT, mixture of chemotherapy regimens including MOPP, ABVD, or PAVe (procarbazine, melphalan, vinblastine); percentages in parentheses are estimated from the original report.

therapy for relapse in the group initially managed with irradiation alone. The advantages of much better disease control with primary treatment, reduction in the financial and psychological costs of dealing with a relapse, and possibly better survival have persuaded most clinicians to incorporate both chemotherapy and radiation into the primary management of patients with bulky but otherwise localized Hodgkin's disease.

The role of a combined-modality approach in the treatment of patients with advanced disease, usually stage III or IV, and at least one bulky site, is less clearly defined. It is best considered within the overall topic of the usefulness of adding irradiation to the chemotherapeutic treatment of patients with advanced Hodgkin's disease, which is discussed in the next section. Similarly, the use of radiation for residual masses, whether bulky at presentation or not, persisting after completion of a full planned course of chemotherapy is best considered as part of the section on treatment of advanced disease. Regardless of conclusions applicable to advanced disease, however, combined-modality therapy in which the patient first receives an extended course of chemotherapy, usually four to six monthly cycles, followed by involved-field irradiation has been shown to be the best strategy to produce the highest disease- and relapse-free survival for patients with localized but bulky presentations and is currently the standard of practice.

Advanced Disease

There are several possible roles for radiation in the treatment of advanced Hodgkin's disease. One is that of a planned addition to the primary chemotherapy, either as an adjuvant at the end of systemic treatment or integrated into the basic program. Another role for irradiation is for treatment of apparent residual disease, essentially reserving its use for disease that does not enter complete remission after the chemotherapy. This is often characterized as using irradiation to convert partial responders or nonresponders to complete responders. Finally, radiotherapy can be used for relapsed disease either by itself for selected patients with recurrence in lymph nodal tissue only or included in a program of standard or high-dose chemotherapy, a setting in which hematopoietic stem cell transplantation is often also employed. Each of these roles poses its own opportunities and problems and requires separate analysis.

The most widely explored use of the addition of radiation treatment to chemotherapy for advanced Hodgkin's disease is as an adjuvant to the primary systemic treatment. Retrospective analyses provided support for the hypothesis that adding irradiation to a full course of chemotherapy compared to solely using chemotherapy improves outcome, but these data are useful only for generation of that hypothesis (97,104–107). Patient selection and the tendency for only positive observations to be published could easily explain the observed differences in outcome. Analysis of patterns of relapse also supports the use of radiation because the apparent sites of relapse after chemotherapy alone tend to be in sites of prior nodal, often bulky, disease (38,107,108). However, it must be remembered that these studies necessarily noted only the clinically detectable first sites of disease apparent at the time of relapse. It seems likely that relapse will be first noted at sites where the most disease was present originally. That does not mean, however, that these sites constitute all of the sites of recurrence, just those most apparent and clinically detectable at that time. Thus, failure analysis, like retrospective comparison of irradiated and unirradiated patients, can suggest, but does not prove, that adding irradiation improves outcome.

The definitive answer to whether adjuvant irradiation adds to disease control and patient survival for those with advanced Hodgkin's disease should have emerged from clinical trials. Unfortunately, the available randomized trials so far reported (108–117) have often been small and varied widely in patient eligibility; type and extent of chemotherapy; dose, timing, and field size of radiotherapy; nature of salvage treatment; and duration and quality of follow-up and outcome reporting. In general these trials provide support for the assertion that when irradiation is added to primary chemotherapy for advanced disease it improves disease control, reduces and delays relapse, and improves disease-free, relapse-free, and treatment failure-free survival. However, none convincingly demonstrated improved overall survival. Recently, in a landmark meta-analysis using updated primary data on all enrolled patients, Loeffler, on behalf of the International Database on Hodgkin's Disease Overview Study Group, conducted a detailed analysis of the pooled data from most of the relevant trials. This analysis has shed much light on a previously murky subject (67). Several observations from it are relevant to the use of adjuvant irradiation in advanced Hodgkin's disease.

Loeffler and his colleagues divided the trials with available data into two groups. The first, labeled "additional radiation therapy" studies, included those in which the control treatment was chemotherapy alone and the experimental treatment the same chemotherapy plus irradiation. The second group of studies, labeled "parallel radiation therapy/chemotherapy" studies, were those in which both groups of patients received the same chemotherapy and then patients were assigned to more chemotherapy (occasionally the same but more usually different chemotherapy) versus irradiation. For historical reasons most of the patients in the additional radiation therapy trials received MOPP-type chemotherapy regimens, whereas most on the parallel radiation therapy/chemotherapy studies were treated with regimens including doxorubicin such as ABVD or MOPP/ABV hybrids. The major observations from the meta-analysis are summarized in Table 5. When MOPP-type chemotherapy was used, additional irradiation improved disease control and disease-free survival but had no discernible impact on overall survival. When better, doxorubicin-containing, chemotherapy was used, not only did added irradiation fail to improve disease control or disease-free survival but survival was significantly decreased, with an 8% lower 10-year overall survival after chemotherapy plus irradiation. The reason for this reduced likelihood of survival was a consistently increased relative risk of dying from causes other than Hodgkin's disease after combined-modality treatment (1.64, 95% CI 0.94 to 2.85 for additional radiation therapy trials; 1.72, 95% CI 1.04 to 2.82 for parallel radiation therapy/chemotherapy trials; and 1.73, 95% CI 1.17 to 2.53, $p = 0.0051$, for all trials combined). The most reasonable conclusion from this exhaustive analysis is that when modern doxorubicin-containing chemotherapy is used, the routine addition of irradiation does not improve disease control and probably increases risk of death from other causes. Unfortunately, several intrinsic methodologic deficiencies inherent to this type of meta-analysis reduce the strength of the conclusions that can be drawn from it (118). These include the unquantifiable impact of failure to irradiate substantial numbers of patients assigned to the radiation arm in several of the trials; differences in numbers of patients with and definitions of bulky disease across the trials; lack of detailed information on specific causes of death in large numbers of the patients; likely variations in dosing and intensity of delivered chemotherapy over the decades from inception of these trials to this analysis; variable quality control of dosimetry and treatment field simulation; lack of regular use of precise CT-scan–guided shaping of treatment fields; and variable availability of all the other important improvements in Hodgkin's disease management that have occurred since these trials were conceived, including better diagnosis, more sophisticated staging, more accurate disease localization, improved dosimetry calculations, greater attention to maintenance of chemotherapy dose intensity, enhanced supportive care for acute and late toxicity, and others difficult to quantify. Thus, even this major meta-analysis can only be seen as strongly suggestive, not definitive. Presently it is reasonable to avoid routinely adding irradiation to chemotherapy in the treatment of advanced-stage Hodgkin's disease. Whether specifically targeting patients with locally bulky tumor, such as those with stage II bulky disease, improves outcome remains unclear pending additional trials and analyses.

Persistent or Recurrent Disease

When Hodgkin's disease persists after or recurs despite optimal initial chemotherapy or combined-modality treatment, only an occasional patient can be cured with standard irradiation (31–36) or chemotherapy (119–123). For this reason it has become common practice to treat such patients with high-dose chemotherapy and hematopoietic stem cell transplantation. This topic is examined in detail in the chapters devoted to secondary or salvage treatment approaches (Chapters 28 and 29), but it is appropriate to

TABLE 5. *Impact of addition of irradiation to primary chemotherapy for advanced Hodgkin's disease*

Strategy	*n*	Treatment	10-yr % DSF	*p*	10-yr % OS	*p*
Additional RT studies	>900	CT	50	0.001	63	0.6
		CT + RT	61		65	
Parallel RT/CT studies	>800	CT_1 + CT_2	59	0.43	68	0.045
		CT_1 + RT	61		60	

n, number of patients available for analysis; DFS, disease-free survival; OS, overall survival; RT, radiation therapy; CT, chemotherapy; CT1, first chemotherapy regimen; CT2, second chemotherapy regimen; percentages in parentheses are estimated from the original report. Data from ref. 67.

note the potential role of a combined-modality approach to such patients. In particular, patients with persistence or relapse of Hodgkin's disease in previously unirradiated nodal sites, especially if bulky, may do better if also given involved-field irradiation to these sites (124–127). Even in the setting of recent recovery from high-dose chemotherapy and hematopoietic stem-cell transplantation, irradiation to modest size involved fields is usually acceptably tolerated (126). Because of increased risk of interstitial pneumonitis or enhanced gastrointestinal toxicity if the irradiation is given before the high-dose chemotherapy, it is probably safer to reserve it until after hematologic recovery has occurred. Given the clear necessity to maximize disease control in these patients whose lymphoma could not be cured with standard-dose chemotherapy, it is appropriate to intensify treatment even in the face of considerable acute and chronic toxicity. The judicious addition of involved-field irradiation to the high-dose program appears to improve disease control within acceptable bounds of toxicity and is a valuable tool in the management of this treatment-resistant disease.

CONCLUSION

Over the past several decades, the goal of curing the majority of patients with Hodgkin's disease has been reached. However, much still needs to be accomplished. Not all patients are cured, and even the best available programs carry substantial acute and chronic toxicity. Two powerful tools, irradiation and multiagent chemotherapy, have emerged as the mainstays of modern treatment. Although irradiation was developed primarily to control localized tumors and chemotherapy to eradicate disseminated disease, in the treatment of Hodgkin's disease their best use is often complementary, emphasizing each modality's major strengths. A clear role for combined-modality treatment can be defined in the management of patients with early-stage disease and for those with bulky tumors. Likewise, irradiation can add to what can be accomplished by high-dose chemotherapy for primarily refractory or relapsed disease. The use of routine irradiation for advanced disease remains controversial, with the available data cautioning against its use but falling short of settling the issue clearly. Continued careful clinical investigation of how best to combine chemotherapy and irradiation for all stages of Hodgkin's disease should remain a priority of oncologists and hematologists. If this happens, the potential of combined-modality treatment to maximize the likelihood of cure while minimizing long-term toxicity will be even further enhanced.

REFERENCES

1. Hodgkin T. On some morbid appearances of the absorbent glands and spleen. *Med-Chir Trans* 1832;17:68–114.
2. Reed DM. On the pathologic changes in Hodgkin's disease, with especial reference to its relation to tuberculosis. *Johns Hopkins Hosp Rep* 1902;10:133–196.
3. Sternberg C. Uber eine eigenartige unter dem Bilde der Pseudoleukamie verlaufende Tuberculose des lymphatischen Apperates. *Z Heilkd* 1898;31:21–90.
4. Pusey WA. Cases of sarcoma and of Hodgkin's disease treated by exposure to X-rays: A preliminary report. *JAMA* 1902;38:166–169.
5. Kaplan HS. Evidence for a tumoricidal dose level in the radiotherapy of Hodgkin's disease. *Cancer Res* 1966;26:1221–1224.
6. Kaplan HS. The radical radiotherapy of regionally localized Hodgkin's disease. *Radiology* 1962;78:553–561.
7. Friedman M, Pearlman AW, Turgeon L. Hodgkin's disease: Tumor lethal dose and iso-effect recovery curve. *Am J Roentgenol* 1967;99: 843–850.
8. Peters MV. A study in survival of Hodgkin's disease treated radiologically. *Am J Roentgenol* 1950;63:299–311.
9. DeVita VT Jr., Hubbard SM. Hodgkin's disease. *N Engl J Med* 1993; 328(8):560–565.
10. Hall TC, Choi OS, Abadi A, et al. High dose corticoid therapy in Hodgkin's disease and other lymphomas. *Ann Intern Med* 1967;66: 1144–1150.
11. Jacobson LO, Spurr CL, Guzman Barron ES, Smith T, Lushbaugh C, Dick GF. Nitrogen mustard therapy; studies on the effect of methyl-(beta-chloroethyl) amine hydrochloride on neoplastic disorders and allied disorders of the hemopoietic system. *JAMA* 1946;132:263–271.
12. Carbone PP, Spurr C. Management of patients with malignant lymphoma: A comparative study with cyclophosphamide and vinca alkaloids. *Cancer Res* 1968;28:811–822.
13. Brunner KW, Young CW. A methylhydrazine derivative in Hodgkin's disease and other malignant neoplasms. *Ann Intern Med* 1965;62: 69–86.
14. DeVita VT, Serpick A, Carbone PP. Combination chemotherapy in the treatment of Hodgkin's disease. *Ann Intern Med* 1970;73:881–895.
15. Longo DL, Young RC, Wesley M, et al. Twenty years of MOPP therapy for Hodgkin's disease. *J Clin Oncol* 1986;4(9):1295–1306.
16. Bonadonna G, Zucali R, Monfardini S, DeLena M, Uslenghi C. Combination chemotherapy of Hodgkin's disease with Adriamycin, bleomycin, vinblastine and imidazole carboxamide. *Cancer* 1975;36: 252–259.
17. Santoro A, Bonadonna G, Bonfante V, Valagussa P. Alternating drug combinations in the treatment of advanced Hodgkin's disease. *N Engl J Med* 1982;306:770–775.
18. Klimo P, Connors JM. MOPP/ABV hybrid program: combination chemotherapy based on early introduction of seven effective drugs for advanced Hodgkin's disease. *J Clin Oncol* 1985;3(9):1174–1182.
19. Viviani S, Bonadonna G, Santoro A, et al. Alternating versus hybrid MOPP and ABVD combinations in advanced Hodgkin's disease: ten-year results. *J Clin Oncol* 1996;14(5):1421–1430.
20. Canellos GP, Anderson JR, Propert KJ, et al. Chemotherapy of advanced Hodgkin's disease with MOPP, ABVD, or MOPP alternating with ABVD. *N Engl J Med* 1992;327(21):1478–1484.
21. Duggan D, Petroni G, Johnson J, et al. MOPP/ABV versus ABVD for advanced Hodgkin's disease. *Proc Am Soc Clin Oncol* 1997;16:13a (abstract 43).
22. Glick JH, Young ML, Harrington D, et al. MOPP/ABV hybrid chemotherapy for advanced Hodgkin's disease significantly improves failure-free and overall survival: The 8-year results of the Intergroup trial. *J Clin Oncol* 1998;16:19–26.
23. Connors JM. Is cyclic chemotherapy better than standard four-drug chemotherapy for Hodgkin's disease? Yes. *Important Adv Oncol* 1993: 189–195.
24. Somers R, Carde P, Henry-Amar M, et al. A randomized study in stage IIIB and IV Hodgkin's disease comparing eight courses of MOPP versus an alternation of MOPP with ABVD: a European Organization for Research and Treatment of Cancer Lymphoma Cooperative Group and Groupe Pierre-et-Marie-Curie controlled clinical trial. *J Clin Oncol* 1994;12(2):279–287.
25. Carde P, Hagenbeek A, Hayat M, et al. Clinical staging versus laparotomy and combined modality with MOPP versus ABVD in early-stage Hodgkin's disease: the H6 twin randomized trials from the European Organization for Research and Treatment of Cancer Lymphoma Cooperative Group. *J Clin Oncol* 1993;11(11):2258–2272.
26. Viviani S, Santoro A, Ragni G, Bonfante V, Bestetti O, Bonadonna G. Gonadal toxicity after combination chemotherapy for Hodgkin's disease. Comparative results of MOPP vs ABVD. *Eur J Cancer Clin Oncol* 1985;21(5):601–605.

27. Bonadonna G, Valagussa P, Santoro A, Viviani S, Bonfante V, Banfi A. Hodgkin's disease: the Milan Cancer Institute experience with MOPP and ABVD. *Recent Results Cancer Res* 1989;117:169–174.
28. Weller SA, Glatstein E, Kaplan HS, Rosenberg SA. Initial relapses in previously treated Hodgkin's disease. I. Results of second treatment. *Cancer* 1976;37:2840–2846.
29. Healey EA, Tarbell NJ, Kalish LA, et al. Prognostic factors for patients with Hodgkin disease in first relapse. *Cancer* 1993;71(8):2613–2620.
30. Mauch P, Larson D, Osteen R, et al. Prognostic factors for positive surgical staging in patients with Hodgkin's disease. *J Clin Oncol* 1990;8(2):257–265.
31. Roach MD, Kapp DS, Rosenberg SA, Hoppe RT. Radiotherapy with curative intent: an option in selected patients relapsing after chemotherapy for advanced Hodgkin's disease. *J Clin Oncol* 1987;5(4):550–555.
32. Mauch P, Tarbell N, Skarin A, Rosenthal D, Weinstein H. Wide-field radiation therapy alone or with chemotherapy for Hodgkin's disease in relapse from combination chemotherapy. *J Clin Oncol* 1987;5(4): 544–549.
33. Uematsu M, Tarbell NJ, Silver B, et al. Wide-field radiation therapy with or without chemotherapy for patients with Hodgkin disease in relapse after initial combination chemotherapy. *Cancer* 1993;72(1): 207–212.
34. MacMillan CH, Bessell EM. The effectiveness of radiotherapy for localized relapse in patients with Hodgkin's disease (IIB–IVB) who obtained a complete response with chemotherapy alone as initial treatment. *Clin Oncol (R Coll Radiol)* 1994;6(3):147–150.
35. Diehl LF, Perry DJ, Terebelo H, et al. Radiation as salvage therapy for patients with Hodgkin's disease relapsing after MOPP (mechlorethamine, vincristine, prednisone, and procarbazine) chemotherapy. *Cancer Treat Rep* 1983;67(9):827–829.
36. Fox KA, Lippman SM, Cassady JR, Heusinkveld RS, Miller TP. Radiation therapy salvage of Hodgkin's disease following chemotherapy failure. *J Clin Oncol* 1987;5(1):38–45.
37. Hoppe RT, Coleman CN, Cox RS, Rosenberg SA, Kaplan HS. The management of stage I–II Hodgkin's disease with irradiation alone or combined modality therapy: the Stanford experience. *Blood* 1982;59 (3):455–465.
38. Young RC, Canellos GP, Chabner BA, Hubbard SM, DeVita VT, Jr. Patterns of relapse in advanced Hodgkin's disease treated with combination chemotherapy. *Cancer* 1978;42(2 Suppl):1001–1007.
39. Mauch P, Tarbell N, Weinstein H, et al. Stage IA and IIA supradiaphragmatic Hodgkin's disease: prognostic factors in surgically staged patients treated with mantle and paraaortic irradiation. *J Clin Oncol* 1988;6(10):1576–1583.
40. Leibenhaut MH, Hoppe RT, Efron B, Halpern J, Nelsen T, Rosenberg SA. Prognostic indicators of laparotomy findings in clinical stage I–II supradiaphragmatic Hodgkin's disease. *J Clin Oncol* 1989;7(1): 81–91.
41. Santoro A, Bonfante V, Viviani S, et al. Subtotal nodal (STNI) vs. involved field (IFRT) irradiation after 4 cycles of ABVD in early stage Hodgkin's disease (HD). *Proc Am Soc Clin Oncol* 1996;15:415 (abstract 1271).
42. Behar RA, Horning SJ, Hoppe RT. Hodgkin's disease with bulky mediastinal involvement: effective management with combined modality therapy. *Int J Radiat Oncol Biol Phys* 1993;25(5):771–776.
43. Gobbi PG, Comelli M, Grignani GE, Pieresca C, Bertoloni D, Ascari E. Estimate of expected survival at diagnosis in Hodgkin's disease: a means of weighting prognostic factors and a tool for treatment choice and clinical research. A report from the International Database on Hodgkin's Disease (IDHD). *Haematologica* 1994;79(3):241–255.
44. Vlachaki MT, Hagemeister FB, Fuller LM, et al. Long-term outcome of treatment for Ann Arbor Stage I Hodgkin's disease: prognostic factors for survival and freedom from progression. *Int J Radiat Oncol Biol Phys* 1997;38(3):593–599.
45. Tubiana M, Henry-Amar M, Carde P, et al. Toward comprehensive management tailored to prognostic factors of patients with clinical stages I and II in Hodgkin's disease. The EORTC Lymphoma Group controlled clinical trials: 1964–1987. *Blood* 1989;73(1):47–56.
46. Colonna P, Jais JP, Desablens B, et al. Mediastinal tumor size and response to chemotherapy are the only prognostic factors in supradiaphragmatic Hodgkin's disease treated by ABVD plus radiotherapy: ten-year results of the Paris–Ouest–France 81/12 trial, including 262 patients. *J Clin Oncol* 1996;14(6):1928–1935.
47. Noordijk EM, Carde P, Mandard AM, et al. Preliminary results of the EORTC–GPMC controlled clinical trial H7 in early-stage Hodgkin's disease. EORTC Lymphoma Cooperative Group. Groupe Pierre-et-Marie-Curie. *Ann Oncol* 1994;5(Suppl 2):107–112.
48. Hagenbeek A, Carde P, Noordijk EM, et al. Prognostic factor tailored treatment of early stage Hodgkin's disease. Results from a prospective randomized phase III clinical trial in 762 patients (H7 study). *Blood* 1997;90(Suppl 1):585a.
49. Prosnitz LR, Brizel DM, Light KL. Radiation techniques for the treatment of Hodgkin's disease with combined modality therapy or radiation alone. *Int J Radiat Oncol Biol Phys* 1997;39(4):885–895.
50. Duhmke E, Diehl V, Loeffler M, et al. Randomized trial with early-stage Hodgkin's disease testing 30 Gy vs. 40 Gy extended field radiotherapy alone. *Int J Radiat Oncol Biol Phys* 1996;36(2):305–310.
51. Loeffler M, Diehl V, Pfreundschuh M, et al. Dose–response relationship of complementary radiotherapy following four cycles of combination chemotherapy in intermediate-stage Hodgkin's disease. *J Clin Oncol* 1997;15(6):2275–2287.
52. Bhatia S, Robison LL, Oberlin O, et al. Breast cancer and other second neoplasms after childhood Hodgkin's disease. *N Engl J Med* 1996;334(12):745–751.
53. Salloum E, Doria R, Schubert W, et al. Second solid tumors in patients with Hodgkin's disease cured after radiation or chemotherapy plus adjuvant low-dose radiation. *J Clin Oncol* 1996;14(9):2435–2443.
54. Hancock SL, Tucker MA, Hoppe RT. Factors affecting late mortality from heart disease after treatment of Hodgkin's disease. *JAMA* 1993; 270(16):1949–1955.
55. Hunger SP, Link MP, Donaldson SS. ABVD/MOPP and low-dose involved-field radiotherapy in pediatric Hodgkin's disease: the Stanford experience. *J Clin Oncol* 1994;12(10):2160–2166.
56. Cleary SF, Link MP, Donaldson SS. Hodgkin's disease in the very young. *Int J Radiat Oncol Biol Phys* 1994;28(1):77–83.
57. Schellong G. The balance between cure and late effects in childhood Hodgkin's lymphoma: the experience of the German-Austrian Study-Group since 1978. German-Austrian Pediatric Hodgkin's Disease Study Group. *Ann Oncol* 1996;7(Suppl 4):67–72.
58. Horning SJ, Hoppe RT, Mason J, et al. Stanford-Kaiser Permanente G1 study for clinical stage I to IIA Hodgkin's disease: subtotal lymphoid irradiation versus vinblastine, methotrexate, and bleomycin chemotherapy and regional irradiation. *J Clin Oncol* 1997;15(5): 1736–1744.
59. Straus DJ, Yahalom J, Gaynor J, et al. Four cycles of chemotherapy and regional radiation therapy for clinical early-stage and intermediate-stage Hodgkin's disease. *Cancer* 1992;69(4):1052–1060.
60. Klasa RJ, Connors JM, Fairey R, et al. Treatment of early stage Hodgkin's disease: Improved outcome with brief chemotherapy and radiotherapy without staging laparotomy (abstract 67). *Ann Oncol* 1996;7(Suppl 3):21.
61. Hagemeister FB, Fuller LM, Velasquez WS, et al. Two cycles of MOPP and radiotherapy: effective treatment for stage IIIA and IIIB Hodgkin's disease. *Ann Oncol* 1991;2(1):25–31.
62. Horning SJ, Rosenberg SA, Hoppe RT. Brief chemotherapy (Stanford V) and adjuvant radiotherapy for bulky or advanced Hodgkin's disease: an update. *Ann Oncol* 1996;7(Suppl 4):105–108.
63. Carde P, Burgers JM, Henry-Amar M, et al. Clinical stages I and II Hodgkin's disease: a specifically tailored therapy according to prognostic factors. *J Clin Oncol* 1988;6(2):239–252.
64. Mauch PM, Kalish LA, Marcus KC, et al. Long term survival in Hodgkin's disease: Relative impact of mortality, second tumors, infection, and cardiovascular disease. *Cancer J Sci Am* 1995;1(1): 33–42.
65. Swerdlow AJ, Douglas AJ, Vaughan Hudson G, Vaughan Hudson B, Bennett MH, MacLennan KA. Risk of second primary cancers after Hodgkin's disease by type of treatment: analysis of 2846 patients in the British National Lymphoma Investigation. *Br Med J* 1992;304: 1137–1143.
66. Biti G, Cellai E, Magrini SM, Papi MG, Ponticelli P, Boddi V. Second solid tumors and leukemia after treatment for Hodgkin's disease: an analysis of 1121 patients from a single institution. *Int J Radiat Oncol Biol Phys* 1994;29(1):25–31.
67. Loeffler M, Brosteanu O, Hasenclever D, et al. Meta-analysis of chemotherapy versus combined modality treatment trials in Hodgkin's disease. International Database on Hodgkin's Disease Overview Study Group. *J Clin Oncol* 1998;16(3):818–829.
68. Mauch PM, Kalish LA, Marcus KC, et al. Second malignancies after

treatment for laparotomy staged IA-IIIB Hodgkin's disease: long-term analysis of risk factors and outcome. *Blood* 1996;87(9):3625–3632.
69. Dunn J. Doxorubicin-induced cardiomyopathy. *J Pediatr Oncol Nurs* 1994;11(4):152–160.
70. Horning SJ, Adhikari A, Rizk N, Hoppe RT, Olshen RA. Effect of treatment for Hodgkin's disease on pulmonary function: results of a prospective study. *J Clin Oncol* 1994;12(2):297–305.
71. Santoro A, Bonadonna G, Valagussa P, et al. Long-term results of combined chemotherapy-radiotherapy approach in Hodgkin's disease: superiority of ABVD plus radiotherapy versus MOPP plus radiotherapy. *J Clin Oncol* 1987;5(1):27–37.
72. Hirsch A, Vander Els N, Straus DJ, et al. Effect of ABVD chemotherapy with and without mantle or mediastinal irradiation on pulmonary function and symptoms in early-stage Hodgkin's disease. *J Clin Oncol* 1996;14(4):1297–1305.
73. Lazo JS, Sebti SM, Schellens JH. Bleomycin. *Cancer Chemother Biol Response Modif* 1996;16:39–47.
74. Gobbi PG, Pieresca C, Frassoldati A, et al. Vinblastine, bleomycin, and methotrexate chemotherapy plus extended-field radiotherapy in early, favorably presenting, clinically staged Hodgkin's patients: the Gruppo Italiano per lo Studio dei Linfomi experience. *J Clin Oncol* 1996;14(2):527–533.
75. Bates NP, Williams MV, Bessell EM, Vaughan Hudson G, Vaughan Hudson B. Efficacy and toxicity of vinblastine, bleomycin, and methotrexate with involved-field radiotherapy in clinical stage IA and IIA Hodgkin's disease: a British National Lymphoma Investigation pilot study. *J Clin Oncol* 1994;12(2):288–296.
76. Connors JM. Induction of secondary neoplasms by the treatment of malignant disease: lessons from Hodgkin's disease. *Prog Clin Biol Res* 1990;354B:219–226.
77. Tucker MA, Coleman CN, Cox RS, Varghese A, Rosenberg SA. Risk of second cancers after treatment for Hodgkin's disease. *N Engl J Med* 1988;318(2):76–81.
78. Gospodarowicz MK, Sutcliffe SB, Clark RM, et al. Analysis of supradiaphragmatic clinical stage I and II Hodgkin's disease treated with radiation alone. *Int J Radiat Oncol Biol Phys* 1992;22(5):859–865.
79. Noordijk EM, Mellink WAM, Carde P, et al. Very favorable Hodgkin's disease: does it really exist? (abstract). *Lymph Leuk* 1998;29(Suppl 1):49.
80. Coltman CA, Myers JW, Montague E, et al. The role of combined radiotherapy and chemotherapy in the primary management of Hodgkin's disease: Southwest Oncology Group Studies. In: Rosenberg SA, Kaplan HS, eds. *Malignant lymphomas: Etiology, immunology, pathology, treatment.* New York: Academic Press, 1982:523–535.
81. Haybittle JL, Hayhoe FG, Easterling MJ, et al. Review of British National Lymphoma Investigation studies of Hodgkin's disease and development of prognostic index. *Lancet* 1985;1:967–972.
82. Gomez GA, Panahon AM, Stutzman L, et al. Large mediastinal mass in Hodgkin's disease. Results of two treatment modalities. *Am J Clin Oncol* 1984;7(1):65–73.
83. Somers R, Tubiana M, Henry-Amar M. EORTC Lymphoma Cooperative Group studies in clinical stage I–II Hodgkin's disease 1963–1987. *Recent Results Cancer Res* 1989;117:175–181.
84. Anderson H, Crowther D, Deakin DP, Ryder WD, Radford JA. A randomised study of adjuvant MVPP chemotherapy after mantle radiotherapy in pathologically staged IA–IIB Hodgkin's disease: 10-year follow-up. *Ann Oncol* 1991;2(Suppl 2):49–54.
85. Hoppe RT, Horning SJ, Hancock SL, Rosenberg SA. Current Stanford clinical trials for Hodgkin's disease. *Recent Results Cancer Res* 1989; 117:182–190.
86. Gehan EA, Sullivan MP, Fuller LM, et al. The intergroup Hodgkin's disease in children. A study of stages I and II. *Cancer* 1990;65(6): 1429–1437.
87. Wiernik PH, Lichtenfeld JL. Combined modality therapy for localized Hodgkin's disease. A seven-year update of an early study. *Oncology* 1975;32(5–6):208–213.
88. Diehl V, Pfreundschuh M, Loffler M, et al. Therapiestudien der deutschen Hodgkin-Studiengruppe. Zwischenergebnisse der Studienprotokolle HD1, HD2 und HD3. *Onkologie* 1987;10(2):62–66.
89. Dutcher JP, Wiernik PH. Combined modality treatment of Hodgkin's disease confined to lymph nodes. In: Cavalli F, Bonadonna G, Rosencweig M, eds. *Malignant lymphomas and Hodgkin's disease; experimental and therapeutic advances.* Boston: Martinus Nijhoff, 1985:317–327.
90. Nissen NI, Nordentoft AM. Radiotherapy versus combined modality treatment of stage I and II Hodgkin's disease. *Cancer Treat Rep* 1982;66(4):799–803.
91. Longo DL, Glatstein E, Duffey PL, et al. Radiation therapy versus combination chemotherapy in the treatment of early-stage Hodgkin's disease: seven-year results of a prospective randomized trial. *J Clin Oncol* 1991;9(6):906–917.
92. Bloomfield CD, Pajak TF, Glicksman AS, et al. Chemotherapy and combined modality therapy for Hodgkin's disease: a progress report on Cancer and Leukemia Group B studies. *Cancer Treat Rep* 1982; 66(4):835–846.
93. Specht L, Gray RG, Clarke MJ, Peto R. Influence of more extensive radiotherapy and adjuvant chemotherapy on long-term outcome of early-stage Hodgkin's disease: a meta-analysis of 23 randomized trials involving 3,888 patients. International Hodgkin's Disease Collaborative Group. *J Clin Oncol* 1998;16(3):830–843.
94. Lee CK, Bloomfield CD, Goldman AI, Levitt SH. Prognostic significance of mediastinal involvement in Hodgkin's disease treated with curative radiotherapy. *Cancer* 1980;46(11):2403–2409.
95. Liew KH, Easton D, Horwich A, Barrett A, Peckham MJ. Bulky mediastinal Hodgkin's disease management and prognosis. *Hematol Oncol* 1984;2(1):45–59.
96. Schomberg PJ, Evans RG, O'Connell MJ, et al. Prognostic significance of mediastinal mass in adult Hodgkin's disease. *Cancer* 1984; 53(2):324–328.
97. Longo DL, Russo A, Duffey PL, et al. Treatment of advanced-stage massive mediastinal Hodgkin's disease: the case for combined modality treatment. *J Clin Oncol* 1991;9(2):227–235.
98. Mauch P, Gorshein D, Cunningham J, Hellman S. Influence of mediastinal adenopathy on site and frequency of relapse in patients with Hodgkin's disease. *Cancer Treat Rep* 1982;66(4):809–817.
99. Leslie NT, Mauch PM, Hellman S. Stage IA to IIB supradiaphragmatic Hodgkin's disease. Long-term survival and relapse frequency. *Cancer* 1985;55(9 Suppl):2072–2078.
100. Hughes-Davies L, Tarbell NJ, Coleman CN, et al. Stage IA–IIB Hodgkin's disease: management and outcome of extensive thoracic involvement. *Int J Radiat Oncol Biol Phys* 1997;39(2):361–369.
101. Bonadonna G, Valagussa P, Santoro A. Prognosis of bulky Hodgkin's disease treated with chemotherapy alone or combined with radiotherapy. *Cancer Surv* 1985;4(2):439–458.
102. Ferrant A, Hamoir V, Binon J, Michaux JL, Sokal G. Combined modality therapy for mediastinal Hodgkin's disease. Prognostic significance of constitutional symptoms and size of disease. *Cancer* 1985;55(2):317–322.
103. Longo DL, Glatstein E, Duffey PL, et al. Alternating MOPP and ABVD chemotherapy plus mantle-field radiation therapy in patients with massive mediastinal Hodgkin's disease. *J Clin Oncol* 1997;15: 3338–3346.
104. Prosnitz LR, Farber LR, Kapp DS, et al. Combined modality therapy for advanced Hodgkin's disease: 15-year follow-up data. *J Clin Oncol* 1988;6(4):603–612.
105. Brizel DM, Winer EP, Prosnitz LR, et al. Improved survival in advanced Hodgkin's disease with the use of combined modality therapy. *Int J Radiat Oncol Biol Phys* 1990;19(3):535–542.
106. Young CW, Straus DJ, Myers J, et al. Multidisciplinary treatment of advanced Hodgkin's disease by an alternating chemotherapeutic regimen of MOPP/ABDV and low-dose radiation therapy restricted to originally bulky disease. *Cancer Treat Rep* 1982; 66(4):907–914.
107. Yahalom J, Ryu J, Straus DJ, et al. Impact of adjuvant radiation on the patterns and rate of relapse in advanced-stage Hodgkin's disease treated with alternating chemotherapy combinations. *J Clin Oncol* 1991;9(12):2193–2201.
108. Fabian CJ, Mansfield CM, Dahlberg S, et al. Low-dose involved field radiation after chemotherapy in advanced Hodgkin disease. A Southwest Oncology Group randomized study. *Ann Intern Med* 1994; 120(11):903–912.
109. Crowther D, Wagstaff J, Deakin D, et al. A randomized study comparing chemotherapy alone with chemotherapy followed by radiotherapy in patients with pathologically staged IIIA Hodgkin's disease. *J Clin Oncol* 1984;2(8):892–897.
110. Pavlovsky S, Maschio M, Santarelli MT, et al. Randomized trial of chemotherapy versus chemotherapy plus radiotherapy for stage I–II Hodgkin's disease. *J Natl Cancer Inst* 1988;80(18):1466–1473.

111. Pavlovsky S, Santarelli MT, Muriel FS, et al. Randomized trial of chemotherapy versus chemotherapy plus radiotherapy for stage III–IV A & B Hodgkin's disease. *Ann Oncol* 1992;3(7):533–537.
112. Glick JH, Tsiatis A. MOPP/ABVD chemotherapy for advanced Hodgkin's disease. *Ann Intern Med* 1986;104(6):876–878.
113. Rosenberg SA, Kaplan HS. The evolution and summary results of the Stanford randomized clinical trials of the management of Hodgkin's disease: 1962–1984. *Int J Radiat Oncol Biol Phys* 1985;11(1):5–22.
114. Yelle L, Bergsagel D, Basco V, et al. Combined modality therapy of Hodgkin's disease: 10-year results of National Cancer Institute of Canada Clinical Trials Group multicenter clinical trial. *J Clin Oncol* 1991;9(11):1983–1993.
115. Glick JH, Barnes JM, Bakemeier RF, et al. Treatment of advanced Hodgkin's disease: 10-year experience in the Eastern Cooperative Oncology group. *Cancer Treat Rep* 1982;66(4):855–870.
116. Diehl V, Loeffler M, Pfreundschuh M, et al. Further chemotherapy versus low-dose involved-field radiotherapy as consolidation of complete remission after six cycles of alternating chemotherapy in patients with advance Hodgkin's disease. German Hodgkins' Study Group (GHSG). *Ann Oncol* 1995;6(9):901–910.
117. Jones SE, Coltman CA Jr, Grozea PN, DePersio EJ, Dixon DO. Conclusions from clinical trials of the Southwest Oncology Group. *Cancer Treat Rep* 1982;66(4):847–853.
118. Mauch P. What is the role for adjuvant radiation therapy in advanced Hodgkin's disease? *J Clin Oncol* 1998;16(3):815–817.
119. Buzaid AC, Lippman SM, Miller TP. Salvage therapy of advanced Hodgkin's disease. Critical appraisal of curative potential. *Am J Med* 1987;83(3):523–532.
120. Bonfante V, Santoro A, Viviani S, et al. Outcome of patients with Hodgkin's disease failing after primary MOPP-ABVD. *J Clin Oncol* 1997;15(2):528–534.
121. Bonadonna G, Santoro A, Gianni AM, et al. Primary and salvage chemotherapy in advanced Hodgkin's disease: the Milan Cancer Institute experience. *Ann Oncol* 1991;2(Suppl 1):9–16.
122. Longo DL, Duffey PL, Young RC, et al. Conventional-dose salvage combination chemotherapy in patients relapsing with Hodgkin's disease after combination chemotherapy: the low probability for cure. *J Clin Oncol* 1992;10(2):210–218.
123. Yuen AR, Rosenberg SA, Hoppe RT, Halpern JD, Horning SJ. Comparison between conventional salvage therapy and high-dose therapy with autografting for recurrent or refractory Hodgkin's disease. *Blood* 1997;89(3):814–822.
124. Mundt AJ, Sibley G, Williams S, Hallahan D, Nautiyal J, Weichselbaum RR. Patterns of failure following high-dose chemotherapy and autologous bone marrow transplantation with involved field radiotherapy for relapsed/refractory Hodgkin's disease. *Int J Radiat Oncol Biol Phys* 1995;33(2):261–270.
125. Poen JC, Hoppe RT, Horning SJ. High-dose therapy and autologous bone marrow transplantation for relapsed/refractory Hodgkin's disease: the impact of involved field radiotherapy on patterns of failure and survival. *Int J Radiat Oncol Biol Phys* 1996;36(1):3–12.
126. Yahalom J. Integrating radiotherapy into bone marrow transplantation programs for Hodgkin's disease. *Int J Radiat Oncol Biol Phys* 1995;33(2):525–528.
127. Yahalom J, Gulati SC, Toia M, et al. Accelerated hyperfractionated total-lymphoid irradiation, high-dose chemotherapy, and autologous bone marrow transplantation for refractory and relapsing patients with Hodgkin's disease. *J Clin Oncol* 1993;11(6):1062–1070.

Hodgkin's Disease, edited by P. M. Mauch,
J.O. Armitage, V. Diehl, R.T. Hoppe, and L.M. Weiss.
Lippincott Williams & Wilkins, Philadelphia ©1999.

CHAPTER 24

Novel Techniques in Hodgkin's Disease

Ute Winkler, Andreas Engert, and Volker Diehl

While most patients with early-stage Hodgkin's disease are cured by conventional chemo- and/or radiotherapy, there are still a considerable number of patients who do not respond to standard therapy or relapse after first-line treatment. Intensification of the chemotherapy schedule produces superior results, but is associated with increased toxicity. Today, most patients with relapsed Hodgkin's disease are treated by using autologous bone marrow transplantation or peripheral blood stem cell transplantation. However, high-dose chemotherapy is only feasible for patients younger than 60 years with no major organ dysfunction. Patients who relapse after second-line treatment cannot be cured by any treatment modality that is available at present. The main reason for tumor relapse is the development of resistant cell clones. These cells might be eradicated by new immunotherapeutic agents, such as monoclonal antibodies for specific targeting of the malignant cells or various cytokines for modulation of the cellular-based immune response to tumor cells.

For several malignancies new immunotherapeutic approaches have already been acknowledged as one modality of standard oncologic therapy in addition to surgery, chemotherapy, and radiation. The chimeric anti-CD20 antibody rituximab, for example, has been approved by the Food and Drug Administration (FDA) for therapy of relapsed low-grade non-Hodgkin's lymphoma (1). Interferon-α (IFN-α) is used for first-line treatment in hairy-cell leukemia. The combination of immunotherapeutic drugs with standard regimens seems to be promising as well. Due to the different mechanisms of action of both treatment modalities, cross-resistance of malignant cells is expected to be rare. Side effects of both strategies also differ, so that toxicity usually does not add up. Examples of the combination of immunotherapeutic agents with conventional treatment procedures are the perioperative application of the monoclonal antibody 17-1A in patients with colorectal carcinoma (2) or the use of granulocyte-colony stimulating factor (G-CSF) to allow further dose-time escalation in conventional chemotherapy for leukemia and lymphoma. Several other immunotherapeutic strategies, including interleukins, interferons, native monoclonal antibodies, immunotoxins, radioimmunoconjugates, bi-specific antibodies, and tumor vaccines, have proven to be successful *in vitro* and in animal models. Most of these agents are currently being investigated in clinical phase I/II studies for toxicity and efficacy in Hodgkin's disease or other malignancies.

EARLY APPROACHES TO IMMUNOTHERAPY OF HODGKIN'S DISEASE

Hodgkin's disease is clinically characterized by the presence of a cellular immune deficiency that is evident at any time during the course of the disease. It was Dorothy Reed (3) who noted as early as 1902 that "tuberculin was given in five cases (of Hodgkin's disease) but without reaction." Since then it has been demonstrated in patients with Hodgkin's disease that T- and B-cell function are highly impaired *in vitro* and *in vivo* (4). The ineffective immune response of the host toward Reed-Sternberg cells in the involved tissue has even been discussed as one mechanism in the pathogenesis of Hodgkin's disease. Therefore, therapeutic strategies modulating the cellular immune response have been investigated in lymphoma patients for more than 25 years.

Bacillus Calmette-Guérin (BCG) as well as the partial purification product of its immunizing component, BCG/MER (methanol extraction residue), has exhibited antitumor effects in both animals and humans (5). Although the exact mechanism of action has never been completely defined, BCG and BCG/MER are known to increase reticuloendothelial activity and stimulate both humoral and cellular immune response (6). Preliminary observations using immunotherapy with BCG/MER have suggested therapeutic effects when combined with

U. Winkler, A. Engert, and V. Diehl: Klinik I für Innere Medizin, der Universität zu Köln, Köln, Germany.

chemotherapy in patients with acute myelocytic leukemia and breast cancer (7,8).

Cooper et al. (9) randomized 196 patients with stage III and IV Hodgkin's disease to receive either treatment with the MER/BCG or no immunotherapy after six courses of induction therapy and 2 years of maintenance chemotherapy. During the first 2 years of immunotherapy, the MER/BCG group had a relapse frequency twice that of the controls. The overall crude relapse frequency and disease-free survival were similar in both treatment groups. The MER/BCG dose schedule was associated with a high frequency of unacceptable toxicity and thus a high degree of patient noncompliance.

Similar findings were observed in a Cancer and Leukemia Group B (CALGB) randomized study (10); 167 patients with previously treated advanced Hodgkin's disease received chemotherapy either alone or in combination with BCG/MER administered intradermally on the first day of each cycle. The chemoimmunotherapy did not improve complete response frequency and was associated with severe toxicity (slow healing, painful ulcers; fever). Because of the documented lack of therapeutic benefit and a higher morbidity, BCG/MER treatment was discontinued in the CALGB trial. In the early 1980s the consensus was to no longer recommend BCG/MER for combined treatment of Hodgkin's disease (9,10).

HODGKIN AND REED-STERNBERG CELLS AS TARGETS FOR SELECTIVE IMMUNOTHERAPY

Today, selective immunotherapy is feasible after monoclonal antibodies have become available in unlimited amounts (11). While systemically administered chemotherapeutics kill all rapidly dividing cells in the body, monoclonal antibodies can target tumor cells selectively. Normal cells that lack specific tumor antigens are not harmed. Lymphomas, especially Hodgkin's lymphomas, seem to be an ideal target for antibody-based therapeutic approaches for several reasons: (a) Hodgkin–Reed-Sternberg cells express many different cell surface antigens, such as CD15 (12), CD25 (13,14), CD30 (15), CD40 (16), and CD80 (B7-1) (17), which are present only on a minority of normal human cells. Due to low cross-reactivity with healthy human tissue, side effects are expected to be rare. (b) Since Hodgkin–Reed-Sternberg cells express many different surface markers, "cocktails," i.e., a combination of various antibody conjugates targeting different Hodgkin-specific antigens, might be useful for selective immunotherapy. If one malignant cell clone is resistant to one antibody due to lack of antigen, cells might still be targeted by the second or third antibody conjugate administered at the same time. (c) The number of malignant cells that need to be killed is small in Hodgkin's disease, since the majority of cells in the involved lymph nodes are innocent bystander cells. (d) Hodgkin's lymphomas are very well vascularized (18), so that intravenously administered antibody conjugates can easily reach their target cells. (e) Hodgkin's disease is known to respond very well to standard therapeutic regimens; thus bulky disease can be eliminated by chemo- and/or radiotherapy, while remaining cells are to be targeted by immunotherapeutics.

MINIMAL RESIDUAL DISEASE

In the treatment of Hodgkin'sdisease, clinical complete remission is often achieved after standard-dose therapy; a considerable number of patients, however, relapse. These clinical complete remission patients obviously still harbored lymphoma cells in insufficient numbers to be detected by standard diagnostic techniques, but sufficient to induce an early or late relapse after initial remission. Tumor cells that survive intensive therapy are defined as minimal residual disease (19). Since minimal residual disease is almost certainly the source of recurring Hodgkin's disease, detectable residual cells after therapy might be expected to be a prognostic factor. For non-Hodgkin's disease, a strong correlation between minimal residual disease and poor outcome has already been demonstrated in several clinical trials (20–22). The highest sensitivity in detecting residual tumor cells can be reached by using polymerase chain reaction (PCR). For Hodgkin's disease Küppers et al. (23,24) have established a method for isolating single cells from frozen tissue sections and analyzing those cells for immunoglobulin (Ig) gene rearrangements by PCR. Using tumor clone specific oligonucleotides as primers in PCR analyses, blood and bone marrow of the same patient can be examined for the presence of small numbers of Hodgkin and Reed-Sternberg cells (25). Furthermore, autologous stem cell preparations could be investigated for contamination by malignant cells before peripheral blood stem cell transplantation is carried out. If it were shown that eradication of occult tumor cells was necessary for cure, assessment of minimal residual disease by means of this newer, more sensitive method would become a novel component of routine posttherapy staging procedures. To date, no study has determined conclusively that eradication of minimal residual tumor cells is necessary for the cure of lymphoma. However, clinical observations reveal that patients with Hodgkin's disease who relapse but achieve a second remission usually relapse again. Since lymphomas are among the tumors most sensitive to our currently available treatment modalities, the ability to identify patients with residual disease who are likely to relapse would be important.

Recently, clonal dissemination of Reed-Sternberg cells and reappearance in relapsing disease was demonstrated for the first time *in vivo* (26). In one patient with mixed-cellularity Hodgkin's disease, Reed-Sternberg cells of the same clone were detected in the initial biopsy specimen from the patient's cervical lymph node as well as from the bone marrow and the peripheral blood obtained 4 years later when the disease had progressed to stage IV despite complete remission after aggressive treatment.

INTERLEUKIN-2

The 15- to 17-kd glycoprotein interleukin-2 (IL-2) is a pleiotropic cytokine secreted by T lymphocytes. It plays an essential role in clonal T-cell proliferation. The receptor for IL-2 (IL-2R) is composed of three different membrane components (the α, β, and γ chains) and is expressed on most T lymphocytes upon activation. The combination of the α chain (CD25, 55-kd glycoprotein), the β chain (75 kd), and the γ chain (50 to 64 kd) results in different forms of the IL-2 receptor with distinct binding affinities. IL-2R has been detected at high levels on cells of different hemopoietic malignancies and various autoimmune disorders (27). Therefore, IL-2 was one of the first immunotherapeutic agents used for anticancer therapy. It augments the cytotoxicity of natural killer (NK) cells, induces lymphokine-activated killer (LAK) cells, and activates T lymphocytes, B lymphocytes, and monocytes. Antitumor effects have been demonstrated *in vitro* and in various animal models. After recombinant DNA technology made IL-2 available in large amounts, Rosenberg et al. (28) initiated the first clinical trials in 1984. Since then, recombinant IL-2 (rIL-2) has been used alone and in combination with autologous LAK cells (adoptive immunotherapy) or other cytokines for the treatment of various malignancies. The highest response rates after systemic application of rIL-2 were observed in metastatic renal cell carcinoma (25%) and in malignant melanoma (20%) (29).

Several clinical trials have been initiated to study the efficacy of rIL-2 alone or in combination with LAK cells in patients with refractory Hodgkin's disease (Table 1). Paciucci et al. (30) treated three patients with advanced refractory Hodgkin's disease with rIL-2 and LAK cells. Leukapheresis was performed on the first day of each cycle, and the lymphocytes were subsequently cultured with IL-2 overnight. On day 2 a continuous infusion of escalating doses of IL-2 (1×10^6 U/m²/day up to 5×10^6 U/m²/day) was started just after reinfusion of LAK cells and continued for 6 days in an escalating dose regimen. One out of three Hodgkin's disease patients achieved a partial remission with a duration of 11 months. One patient had a minor response lasting 20 months. Side effects were moderate and transient and included renal as well as hepatic dysfunction, dyspnea, fatigue, fever, hypotension, edema, mucositis, anemia, and thrombocytopenia.

Margolin et al. (31) treated 12 patients with relapsed Hodgkin's disease to explore the activity of high-dose rIL-2 (600 IU/kg per dose) and autologous LAK cells. One schedule consisted of a bolus injection of rIL-2 on days 1 to 5 and 12 to 16. Leukapheresis was performed between days 7 and 10; LAK cells were reinfused on days 12, 13, and 15. Another schedule consisted of a bolus

TABLE 1. *Results of clinical trials with recombinant interleukin-2 (IL-2) in patients with Hodgkin's disease*

n	Dosing regimen of IL-2	Toxicity	Response (duration)	Reference
1	CIV 24 h 1×10^6 IU/m²/day up to 5×10^6 IU/m²/day on days 1–5 and 10–15 + LAK cells	Rash, anemia, hypoalbuminemia, nausea, diarrhea, stomatitis, renal, hypotension	1 PR	34
3	CIV 24 h 1×10^6 IU/m²/day up to 5×10^6 IU/m²/day over 4×6 days + LAK cells	Renal, hepatic, dyspnea, mild fatigue, fever, hypotension, mucositis, anemia	1 PR (11 months)	30
3	CIV 24 h 3×10^6 IU/m²/day on days 1–5 and 12–16 + LAK cells	Fever, rash, diarrhea	1 PR	32
4	CIV 24 h 18×10^6 IU/m²/day on days 1–5 and 12–16 + LAK cells	Renal, cardiovascular, fever, rash, thrombocytopenia	No response	33
12	600 IU/kg/day on days 1–5 and 12–16 + LAK cells vs. 600 IU/kg/day bolus days 1–3 + CIV 24 h 600 IU/kg/day on days 9–15 + LAK cells	Fever, rash, renal, hepatic, hematodynamic, cardiopulmonary	2 PR (6 + 12 weeks)	31
4	CIV 24 h 3×10^6 IU/m²/day on days 1–5 and 13–17.5	Anemia, thrombocytopenia, neutropenia, septicemia, fever, diarrhea	No response	177
7	CIV 24 h 20×10^6 IU/m² over 5, 4, 3 days	Vascular leak syndrome, cardiac, renal, thrombocytopenia, neutropenia	No response	178

CIV 24 h, continuous intravenous infusion over 24 hours; PR, partial remission; *n,* number of patients; LAK, lymphokine-activated killer cells.

injection of rIL-2 on days 1 to 3 and continuous infusion on days 9 to 15. Leukapheresis was performed on days 5 to 8, and LAK cells were reinfused on days 9, 10, and 12. The toxicities were flu-like symptoms, fever, rash, and cardiopulmonary, renal, and hepatic dysfunction. Two out of 12 patients achieved partial remission lasting 6 and 12 weeks.

Another three Hodgkin's disease patients were treated with 3×10^6 IU/m^2 rIL-2 per day administered as a continuous infusion over 5 days (32). Patients underwent leukapheresis on days 6 to 9, and LAK cells were reinfused on days 12 to 14. IL-2 was applied again on days 12 to 16. One partial remission was reported.

In a clinical phase I/II study directed by Tourani et al. (33), four patients with relapsed Hodgkin's disease were treated with a continuous rIL-2 infusion at 18×10^6 IU/m^2/day on days 1 to 5 and days 12 to 16. No response was observed in any of these patients.

A different treatment schedule with constant infusion of rIL-2 and adoptive immunotherapy was investigated in 48 patients with advanced cancer (34). They were treated with escalating doses of rIL-2 as continuous infusion for 5 days followed by 1 day of rest and 4 days of leukapheresis. The second and third 5-day cycles of rIL-2 in a higher dose were accompanied by reinfusion of activated cells. A 42-year-old woman with nodular sclerosis Hodgkin's disease who had received intermittent chemotherapy for 15 years was treated and achieved a partial remission lasting 1.5 months. Despite extensive prior treatment with immunosuppressive drugs, this patient had a rebound lymphocytosis involving 25,000 cells per cubic millimeter after the priming cycle rIL-2. As demonstrated by serial gallium scan, disease began to regress after the priming cycle of rIL-2 and almost totally resolved with the reinfusion of activated cells and additional rIL-2.

In these clinical pilot trials, rIL-2 was mainly administered to heavily pretreated patients with relapsed or refractory Hodgkin's disease. Considering that these patients are unfavorable candidates for (adoptive) immunotherapy, these preliminary results are quite promising. Therefore, rIL-2 is currently under clinical investigation for efficacy as a maintenance regimen alone or in combination with other cytokines after high-dose chemotherapy.

INTERFERONS

Interferons are naturally occurring glycoproteins and were initially discovered as inhibitors of viral replication. IFN-α is produced by leukocytes, IFN-β by fibroblasts, and IFN-γ by activated T and NK cells. Recently, IFN-α_2 has been reclassified as a distinct leukocyte IFN-ω on the basis of gene sequencing. The mechanisms of action are multifaceted and include immunoregulatory activity as well as antiproliferative effects (35) that might be due to modulation of certain oncogenes (36). While single-agent IFN-α can induce remissions in a large number of patients with low-grade lymphoma (37), experience with interferon treatment in Hodgkin's disease patients is limited. Case reports of a few patients who received interferon for treatment of viral infection observed minor responses of Hodgkin's disease. Therefore, some pilot studies were initiated to investigate the efficacy of interferon in the salvage or maintenance therapy of Hodgkin's disease (Table 2).

Preliminary results suggest limited activity of IFN-α in patients with relapsed or refractory Hodgkin's disease: one partial remission among four patients was reported in one trial (38), and four partial remissions among 13 in another (39). Horning et al. (40) observed only minor responses in two out of eight patients. Three of four patients with refractory Hodgkin's disease achieved partial remission after combination therapy of interferon and chlorambucil (41). In a small series from Argentina, one partial remission in five patients was reported after single-agent IFN-α (42).

In a multiinstitutional trial conducted by the CALGB (study 8652), 19 patients were treated with 10×10^6 IU/m^2 IFN-α_{2b} subcutaneously three times per week (43). All patients were heavily pretreated with a median of four previous chemotherapeutic programs. Three patients had undergone high-dose therapy and autologous bone mar-

TABLE 2. *Results of clinical trials with interferon-α (IFN-α) in patients with Hodgkin's lymphoma*

n	Dosing regimen of IFN-α	Toxicity	Response (duration)	Reference
4	5×10^6–10×10^6 IU/day . every 3 days i.m.	Fatigue, fever, nausea, severe neurotoxicity, mental changes, dizziness, myalgia	1 PR	38
8	1×10^6 IU–9×10^6 IU daily i.m. for 30 days	Fatigue, fever, myalgias, weight loss	No response	40
13	10×10^6 IU/m^2 s.c. 3×/week or 30–50 $\times 10^6$ IU over 5 days every 3 weeks i.v.	Fever, chills, headache, anorexia, myalgia	4 PR (1–6 months)	39
19	10×10^6 IU/m^2 s.c. 3×/week	Myelosuppression	1 PR (3 weeks)	43
6	5×10^6 IU/m^2/day s.c. 5 days/week	Increase in liver enzymes, fever, chills, headache	No response	42

PR, partial remission; s.c., subcutaneously; i.v., intravenously; i.m., intramuscularly; *n,* number of patients.

row transplantation. There was one partial remission, and four patients had reduction in measurable disease not meeting the criteria for partial response. Myelosuppression was the major toxicity.

Redman et al. (44) documented remissions in 37% of pretreated patients after intramuscular application of escalating doses of IFN-α_{2b}. Remissions were even documented in 17% of all patients who had undergone prior autologous bone marrow transplantation.

The toxicity of single-agent interferon has been well described (45). Many of the initial flu-like symptoms, such as fever and myalgias, are self-limited and reasonably well controlled with symptomatic therapy such as acetaminophen. Some of the more troublesome side effects associated with chronic interferon therapy are anorexia, fatigue, and depression. When interferon is used with chemotherapy, increased myelotoxicity, especially neutropenia, has been a consistent observation (46,47). An increased incidence of infection has also been reported (47).

While further clinical trials in heavily pretreated patients do not appear to be indicated, studies of interferon in conjunction with other biologic agents or chemotherapeutic agents are warranted. Patients with less advanced disease or with low tumor burden after prior standard therapy may be more amenable to the immunologic effects of interferon. Based on the evidence of some efficacy and on the potentially favorable immunomodulatory effects of interferon, one group has adopted a strategy of interferon maintenance after chemotherapy for high-risk Hodgkin's disease patients; in a preliminary report on this trial, follow-up was too short to draw conclusions (48).

High-dose chemotherapy in conjunction with autologous bone marrow or peripheral blood stem cell transplantation is increasingly being used for treatment of patients with relapsed or refractory Hodgkin's disease. Although some patients may achieve a continuous complete remission after peripheral blood stem cell transplantation, the relapse rate after high-dose chemotherapy still remains high. It is believed that this is due to the lack of immune response of immunocompetent cells to residual tumor cells. Currently, it has been demonstrated that an immune-mediated graft-versus-lymphoma effect may be induced in certain categories of lymphoma recipients of allogeneic marrow grafts (49). This suggests that one of the ways to reduce relapse rates after peripheral blood stem cell transplantation may be to intensify immune-mediated effector mechanisms against residual malignant cells. In a phase II trial, 24 Hodgkin's disease patients were treated with repeating cycles of IFN-α subcutaneously 3×10^6 IU/day × 5 days/week combined with rIL-2 s.c. 3 to 6×10^6 IU/m^2/d × 5 days/week for 4 weeks following autologous stem cell transplantation (50). The median time from autologous blood stem cell transplantation until the onset of immunotherapy was 4 months. Survival and disease-free survival were significantly higher in the group with the combined immunologic maintenance therapy compared to historical controls without cytokine treatment. Three out of 24 Hodgkin's disease patients (12.5%) relapsed after antologous stem cell transplantation combined with maintenance immunotherapy, while in the control group eight out of 25 patients (32%) who did not receive immunotherapy relapsed. Side effects were those expected from IFN-α and rIL-2 when given as single agents (51). They included fever, chills, fatigue, flu-like symptoms, anorexia, nausea, vomiting, and diarrhea, and were transient and reversible. Prospective randomized studies are planned to confirm the promising treatment results of this combined IFN-α/rIL-2 maintenance therapy after autologous bone marrow transplantation.

NATIVE MONOCLONAL ANTIBODIES

The vision of selective immunotherapy of cancer first proposed by Paul Ehrlich about a hundred years ago (52) has turned into reality, after monoclonal antibodies and their derivatives have become available in limitless amounts (11). Ideally, the antibody targets an antigen only present on the tumor cells with high specificity and has no cross-reactivity with normal human tissue. The mechanisms of action of native antibodies include complement activation, antibody-dependent cellular cytotoxicity (ADCC), phagocytosis of antibody-coated target cells, inhibition of cell cycle progression, and induction of apoptosis (53,54). Alternatively, antibodies can destroy tumor cells by blocking structures such as growth factor receptors involved in signal transduction or cell proliferation. The cytotoxic activity of an individual antibody is determined by many different components, such as affinity and specificity of the antibody, density and quantity of the antigen on the target cell, distance of the epitope to the cell surface membrane, heterogeneity of antigen expression on the tumor cell, presence of shed antigen in the serum, antigen modulation, natural function of the antigen, tumor size, internalization rate, and metabolism of the antigen structure.

After treatment of the first patients with monoclonal antibodies in 1979, several phase I/II trials have been initiated to evaluate efficacy of antibody therapy in various malignancies. Adverse effects were moderate and included chills, fever, dyspnea, nausea, diarrhea, and myalgia. Toxicity was usually related to the number of circulating tumor cells and the development of human antimouse antibodies (HAMAs). HAMAs are produced by the functioning human immune system after reexposure to the Fc part of murine antibodies. Chimeric antibodies, which consist of human constant IgG1 and kappa constant regions and murine variable regions, rarely induce HAMA formation (55).

In various multicenter trials different native antibodies have proven effective in patients with non-Hodgkin's lymphoma. Response rates up to 70% were reported after the ADCC-mediating and complement-dependent cytotoxicity-mediating anti-CD52 antibody Campath-1H had been used as first- or second-line treatment in patients with chronic lymphocytic leukemia (56,57). The chimeric anti-CD20 antibody IDEC-C2B8 (rituximab) was approved by the FDA after a pivotal trial had demonstrated partial remission in 50% of patients with relapsed follicular non-Hodgkin's lymphoma (1).

Engert et al. (58,59) evaluated more than 40 different monoclonal antibodies for their antitumor activity toward Hodgkin's-derived cell lines *in vitro.* In most cases cytotoxicity was considerably improved by coupling the native antibody to potent toxins, such as ricin A chain or saporin. Even new anti-CD30 antibodies with promising cytotoxic effects *in vitro* (60) demonstrated improved antitumor activity *in vivo* when coupled with toxic substances (61). So far it has not been possible to identify a monoclonal antibody against Hodgkin-specific antigens that exhibited enough potency *in vitro* or *in vivo* to be used as native molecule in the treatment of patients with Hodgkin's disease. Thus, only antibodies conjugated to plant or bacterial toxins, radioisotopes, enzymes, or a second antibody have been chosen for clinical trials in patients with Hodgkin's disease so far.

IMMUNOTOXINS

Immunotoxins generally consist of a binding moiety and a toxin moiety, which are either covalently linked via a chemical linker or generated by recombinant fusion technology. The binding domain is usually a monoclonal antibody, a Fab fragment of an antibody, a single-chain variable fragment (scFv), or a cytokine. The toxin moiety is of bacterial or plant origin. Ribosome-inactivating proteins (RIPs) from various plants possess specific adenosine nucleosidase activity toward rRNA, thus damaging ribosomes and arresting protein synthesis (62). Type-1 RIPs are single-chain proteins; type-2 RIPs contain two polypeptide chains, one of which (A chain) confers RNA *N*-glycosidase activity. The galactose-specific lectin-binding B chain mediates unspecific uptake of RIPs into human cells (63). For the construction of immunotoxins, the B chain must be replaced by a specific binding structure. Then, immunotoxins can bind selectively to their target cells, which are destroyed upon internalization of the construct (Fig. 1). Theoretically, one toxin molecule is sufficient in killing a single given cell (64).

The plant toxin used most frequently for the construction of chemically linked immunotoxins is the type-2 RIP ricin. It has to be extracted from the seeds of *Ricinus communis* (castor bean) and is the most toxic molecule isolated from eukaryotic organisms to date. First-generation ricin–A chain immunotoxins showed potent antitumor effects *in vitro,* but poor efficacy when administered *in vivo* (65). Subsequently, immunotoxins of the second generation were developed. These constructs were characterized by a higher grade of purity (66), reduced unspecific binding capacity (67), and improved stability *in vivo* (68). For these second-generation immunotoxins Fulton et al. (69) demonstrated significantly better antitumor effects in animal models compared to their predecessors.

About 40 different monoclonal antibodies have been evaluated for their potential clinical use as ricin–A chain immunotoxins against Hodgkin's disease (70). Many of them were directed toward the CD30 antigen, a 120-kd member of the tumor necrosis factor (TNF) receptor superfamily. It is present on the surface of the majority of Hodgkin–Reed-Sternberg cells and on large-cell anaplastic lymphoma cells (Ki-1 lymphoma). The first five monoclonal anti-CD30 antibodies (HRS-1, HRS-3, HRS-4, Ber-H2, and Ki-1) that were conjugated to deglycosylated ricin A chain (dgA) showed only minor cross-reactivity with vital human organs, apart from HRS-4, which bound to pancreas and kidney cells on frozen tissue sections (58). HRS-3.dgA and Ber-H2.dgA, the immunotoxins that showed highest cytotoxicity toward Hodgkin-derived cell lines *in vitro* were subsequently evaluated against heterotransplanted subcutaneous Hodgkin's disease in triple-beige nude mice (71). One intravenous injection of HRS-3.dgA rendered 69% of the animals tumor free, while Ber-H2.dgA was less effective with a response rate of 38% *in vivo.* Several new high-affinity monoclonal antibodies toward different epitopes of CD30 have been developed recently (60). Six of them (Ki-2 to Ki-7) were linked to dgA. The most potent immunotoxin, Ki-4.dgA, achieved a 50% reduction of protein syntheses relative to untreated central cultures (IC_{50}) at a concentration of 4 $\times 10^{-11}$ M and was 5- and 7.5-fold more effective *in vitro* than HRS-3.dgA or Ber-H2.dgA, respectively. Fifty percent continuous complete remissions were achieved by treatment of disseminated human Hodgkin's disease in mice with severe combined immunodeficiency (SCID) with Ki-4.dgA (61). This highly effective immunotoxin is currently being prepared for clinical trials.

Another interesting target for selective immunotherapy in Hodgkin's disease is the IL-2 receptor (CD25), which is expressed on the majority of Hodgkin–Reed-Sternberg cells (72). Several anti-CD25 monoclonal antibodies have been evaluated for their potential clinical use in Hodgkin's disease (59). From a panel of more than 30 antibodies, five exhibited promising cytotoxicity *in vitro* and were therefore coupled to dgA. The most potent immunotoxin, RFT5.dgA, inhibited the protein synthesis of Hodgkin-derived cell lines at a concentration of 7×10^{-12} M, which is nearly identical to that of native ricin under the same experimental conditions (59). In triple-beige nude mice with subcutaneous human Hodgkin's tumors, RFT5.dgA was superior compared to the CD30 immunotoxins, HRS-3.dgA or Ber-H2.dgA (59). In SCID mice with disseminated Hodgkin's disease, CRs were observed in 95% of animals after a single intraperitoneal injection of 8 μg RFT5.dgA (73). The

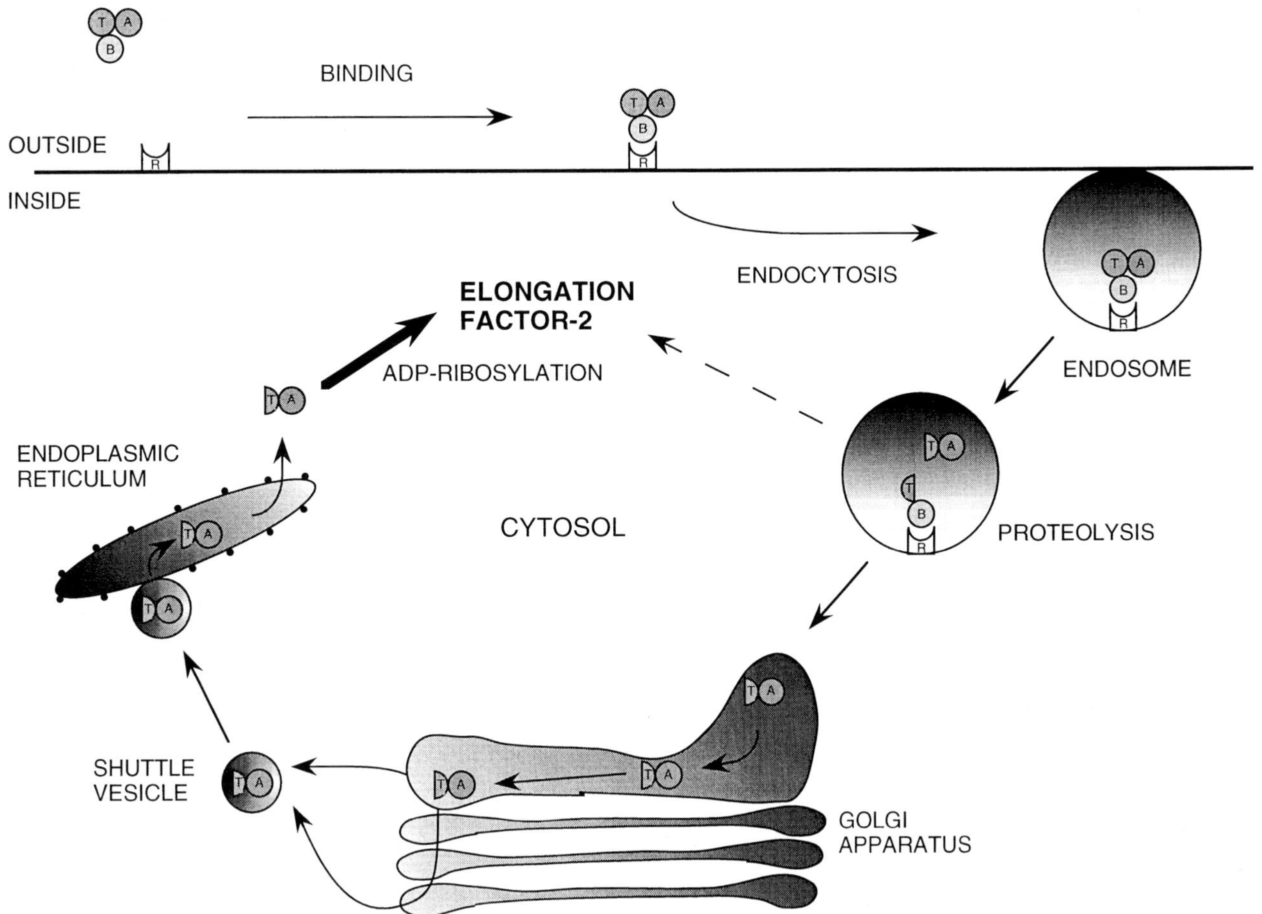

FIG. 1. Schematic model of the interaction of a recombinant fusion toxin with its target cell. After binding of the immunotoxin (IT) to a specific cell surface receptor, the toxin-receptor complex is internalized into an endosome. Low pH induces unfolding of the IT followed by specific proteolytic cleavage. The released 37-kd carboxy-terminal fragment finally reaches the cytosol and inhibits protein synthesis by adenosine diphosphate (ADP)-ribosylation of elongation factor 2. R, receptor on cell surface of specific target cell; B, binding moiety (cytokine or antibody fragment); T, translocation domain of *Pseudomonas* exotoxin A; C, catalytically active component of the exotoxin.

mean survival time of immunotoxin-treated mice was >150 days as compared to 36 days in phosphate buffered saline- or RFT5-treated controls. Some mice relapsed after initial response to immunotoxin treatment. Cells of these tumors were cultivated and evaluated for expression of cell surface antigen. The density of CD25 was significantly lower on these cells than on the parental Hodgkin-derived cell line L540Cy or on disseminated lymphomas in untreated mice (73). These findings suggest the existence of antigen-deficient cell clones surviving immunotherapy with only one antibody and causing late relapses. Thus cocktails consisting of two or more immunotoxins targeting different antigens on the surface of the Hodgkin–Reed-Sternberg cells are expected to be more effective, since cells lacking one antigen might still be killed by an immunotoxin directed toward a second epitope. *In vitro* immunotoxin cocktails consisting of RFT5.dgA (CD25), HRS3.dgA (CD30), and IRac.dgA (unclustered 70 kd) were more efficient in inhibiting protein synthesis of Hodgkin's-derived cell lines than either immunotoxin alone or a combination of only two of them, respectively (74).

In a phase I dose-escalation study, 15 patients with refractory Hodgkin's disease were treated with the anti-CD25 immunotoxin RFT5.dgA (75). All patients in this trial were heavily pretreated with a mean of five prior chemotherapeutic regimens, including autologous bone marrow transplantation in eight of 15 patients. The immunotoxin was administered intravenously over 4 hours on days 1, 3, 5, and 7 for total doses per cycle of 5, 10, 15, or 20 mg/m^2. Side effects were related to vascular leak syndrome. Two patients had a World Health Organization (WHO) grade 2 allergic reaction with generalized urticaria and mild bronchospasm. The maximal tolerated dose was 15 mg/m^2, since in higher doses grade 3 and 4 toxicities, specifically a concerning vascular leak syndrome, and myalgia, occurred. HAMAs were detected in six out of 15 cases, while seven of 15 patients developed human antiricin antibodies (HARAs). Clinical response included two PRs, one minor response, three stable diseases, and nine progressive diseases. A multicenter phase II clinical trial with the same anti-CD25 immunotoxin for the treatment of patients with advanced refractory Hodgkin's disease has just been finished; response rates are expected to be higher than in the phase I trial, since RFT5.dgA was only administered to patients with Hodgkin cells expressing the CD25 antigen in high density.

The only anti-CD30 immunotoxin that has been investigated in clinical trials for the treatment of Hodgkin's disease patients so far is Ber-H2-Sap6 (Table 3). Saporin-S6 (Sap6) is a type-1 RIP extracted from the seeds of *Saponaria officinalis* (Soapwort). For use in Hodgkin's disease Saporin-S6 was chemically conjugated to the anti-CD30 antibody Ber-H2. Pasqualucci et al. (76) reported continuous CRs in 79% of SCID mice with subcutaneous CD30-positive lymphoma xenografts after application of 3.3 μg Ber-H2-Sap6 per day for 3 days. Even in mice with established subcutaneous tumors, a single course of 10 μg immunotoxin induced a significant growth delay with 29% of all animals achieving CR. In a clinical phase I/II trial, 12 patients with advanced refractory Hodgkin's disease were treated with one or two infusions of 0.8 mg/kg Ber-H2-Sap6 over 4 hours (77,78). Four patients achieved a PR with a substantial decrease of tumor mass lasting 6 to 10 weeks. Fever, malaise, anorexia, fatigue, mild myalgias, weight gain, and a four- to fivefold increase in liver enzymes were the main toxicities. The maximal tolerated dose was reached at 0.8 mg/kg. Since responses were only short and partial, two new anti-CD30 immunotoxins were developed by covalently linking murine Ber-H2 to the type 1 RIPs momordin and pokeweed antiviral protein from seeds, respectively (79). Both immunotoxins inhibited protein synthesis of CD30-positive target cell lines with high efficiency and prevented tumor growth in about 40% of SCID mice with xenografted CD30-positive anaplastic large-cell lymphoma. The main toxicity in mice and rabbits was a dose-related increase of transaminases and creatine phosphokinase. Sequential administration of Ber-H2 coupled to momordin and Ber-H2-Sap6 was well tolerated and did not result in formation of antibodies cross-reacting with the two plant toxins, respectively. In humans sequential application of anti-CD30 antibodies linked to distinct type 1 RIPs should prevent formation of human antibodies against the toxins.

Highly potent immunotoxins were also generated by conjugation of Ber-H2 (anti-CD30) to native or recombinant dianthin 30, a RIP extracted from *Dianthus caryophyllus* (carnation). The effect of either immunotoxin on protein synthesis of the CD30-positive cell line K562 (from a patient with chronic myeloid leukemia) was not different from that of free dianthin (80).

Recombinant DNA technology has allowed the construction of third-generation immunotoxins by fusing coding regions of toxins such as diphtheria toxin (DT) or *Pseudomonas* exotoxin-A (81) to ligand genes. These fusion gene products are highly homogeneous compared to chemically linked conjugates, which usually contain molecules connected at unfavorable positions on the toxin or the antibody. The recombinant toxins are defined, compact molecules, easy to modify and much more economical to produce when compared to chemical immunoconjugates (82). Thus, some recombinant immunotoxins are now being evaluated for their antitumor activity in clinical trials (Table 3).

DAB486IL-2, an immunotoxin generated by fusing a cytokine to the truncated form of diphtheria toxin, was tested in a phase I/II clinical study for treatment of CD25-positive hematologic malignancies including chronic

TABLE 3. *Results of clinical trials with immunotoxins in patients with Hodgkin's disease*

Immunotoxin	Antigen	*n*	Dosing regimen	Toxicity	Immune response	Response	Reference
Ber-H2-Sap6	CD30	12	1 bolus (0.8 mg/kg)	Hepatic, VLS, myalgia, fever	12 HAMA	4 PR	77,78
RFT5-dgA	CD25	15	4-hour infusion, days 1, 3, 5, and 7 (15 mg/m^2)	ULS, myalgia, nausea, fatigue	6 HAMA, 7 HARA	2 PR	75
DAB389IL-2	CD25	21	Bolus infusion days 1–5 (0.1 μg/kg/day)	Hepatic, chills, fever, fatigue	15 anti-DT-A	No response	85
DAB486IL-2	CD25	3	10 bolus infusions (0.1 mg/kg/day)	Hepatic, renal, nausea, rash, fever, fatigue	2 anti-DT-A, 2 anti-DAB-A, 2 anti-IL-2-A	No response	83
DAB486IL-2	CD25	4	Bolus infusion days 1–5 (0.2 mg/kg/day)	Hepatic, renal, proteinuria, hypoalbuminemia, rash	2 anti-DT-A, 2 anti-DAB-A	1 CR	84

VLS, vascular leak syndrome; HAMA, human antimouse antibodies; HARA, human antiricin antibodies; anti-DT-A, anti–diphtheria toxin antibodies; anti-DAB-A, anti-DAB-antibodies; anti-IL-2-A, anti–interleukin-2 antibodies; CR, complete remission; PR, partial remission.

lymphocytic leukemia, Sézary syndrome, and Hodgkin's and non-Hodgkin's lymphoma (83). A complete remission lasting more than 2 years was reported in one patient with Hodgkin's disease after this immunotoxin had been administered as a 30- to 60-minute i.v. infusion at dose levels of 0.2 mg/kg daily for 5 days (84). Six other patients with refractory Hodgkin's disease did not respond to immunotoxin treatment. Side effects were hypersensitivity-like symptoms and reversible transaminase elevations. The major toxicity in a phase I/II trial with the recombinant DAB389IL-2 was fatigue. This fusion toxin was constructed by deletion of amino acids 389 to 485 of the diphtheria toxin, which renders it approximately tenfold more toxic than DAB486IL-2 (85). Thus far, 73 patients with IL-2 receptor-expressing lymphoma (non-Hodgkin's lymphoma, Hodgkin's disease, cutaneous T-cell lymphoma) have been treated with escalating doses of DAB389IL-2. None of the 21 patients with Hodgkin's disease responded to immunotoxin therapy. Formation of antiimmunotoxin antibodies by the patient's functioning immune system is a major problem in fusion toxin therapy as well. In the phase I clinical study with the diphtheria toxin–containing immunotoxin DAB486IL-2, a correlation between the concentrations of antiimmunotoxin antibody and the incidence of side effects was demonstrated in 50% of all patients presenting with preexisting antibodies after immunization in early childhood (83). Therefore, repeated application of the immunotoxin was impossible in some of the patients. Nevertheless, responses after immunotoxin therapy have been observed even in the face of antibodies. Diminishing the immunogenicity of immunotoxins might decrease HAMA formation in humans. Promising approaches include deleting certain immunodominant epitopes or humanizing the antibody moiety of the immunotoxin. Antibodies consisting of human constant regions have already been generated using DNA technology (86). Totally humanized antibodies can be isolated from the serum of transgenic mice (87) or can be produced by targeted selection utilizing phage display (88).

Based on the encouraging results with the chemically linked anti-CD25 immunotoxin RFT5.dgA in Hodgkin's disease patients, a new recombinant RFT5(scFv)-ETA′ was constructed (89) by fusing RFT5(scFv) to a deletion mutant of *Pseudomonas aeruginosa* exotoxin A (ETA′) (90). Binding of this construct to the CD25 antigen was demonstrated and resulted in cytotoxicity toward CD25-positive Hodgkin's-derived cell lines. The same modified ETA was fused with a single chain variable fragment from the murine anti-CD30 antibody Ki-4 (91). The functional high-affinity single chain was produced using the phage display technique and was selected for binding on the Hodgkin cell line L540Cy. The complete recombinant Ki-4(scFv)-ETA′ fusion toxin inhibited protein synthesis of L540Cy cells by 50% at concentrations of 3 ng/ml and will be further investigated *in vivo.* The coding regions for ETA′ have also been successfully fused to cDNA for the human IL-9 receptor (92), which is expressed on a variety of malignant cells, including Hodgkin's Reed-Sternberg cells. The cytotoxic effect against the Hodgkin cell line L1236 suggests a potential use of recombinant hIL-9-ETA′ in immunotherapy, both alone and in combination with other immunotoxins. Another single-chain fusion immunotoxin for potential clinical use in Hodgkin's disease is G28-5 sFv-PE40 (93), which targets the CD40 antigen expressed on B-cell malignancies, Hodgkin's disease, and multiple myeloma. This immunotoxin was effective in treating SCID mice bearing human Burkitt's lymphoma, with complete remissions obtained at doses of 0.13 to 0.26 mg/kg. CD40 is also expressed on a variety of normal human tissues. However, G28-5 sFv-PE40 was well tolerated in monkeys at doses that provided complete antitumor responses in mice. Thus, expression of CD40 on normal tissue may not limit the potential use of anti-CD40 immunotoxins in immunotherapy of Hodgkin's disease and other hematologic malignancies.

RADIOIMMUNOCONJUGATES

Radiolabeled antibodies have been extensively studied for diagnostic and therapeutic use in malignant tumors. These radioimmunoconjugates are constructed by linking a monoclonal antibody to radioisotopes without significantly altering the immunologic specificity of the protein.

The most important advantage of radioimmunoconjugates compared to all other antibody-based therapeutic strategies is that beta particles emitted by radionuclides can kill adjacent tumor cells through a crossfire effect, regardless of whether cells express the target antigen (94). Radioimmunotherapy differs from external-beam radiation therapy in several respects. First, with radioimmunotherapy radiation is continuously delivered at a low dose rate that initially increases as radiolabeled antibodies accumulate in a tumor and then decreases because of physical decay and biologic clearance (95). Second, radioimmunotherapy delivers radiation to the whole body including occult micrometastases. Finally, antibodies themselves may, in some cases, exert antitumor effects. Nevertheless, radioimmunotherapy is suggested to be 20% less effective than dose-equivalent external beam radiation therapy, since the low dose rates characteristic of radioimmunotherapy allow time for repair of sublethally damaged tumor cells. Tumor cell proliferation may also reduce the effectiveness of radioimmunotherapy, particularly if a radioisotope with a long physical half-life is used.

Antibodies can be directly labeled either using iodine (96) or technetium-99m (97). In these constructs, the radionuclide is directly attached to the protein by endogenous groups. Alternatively, radionuclides such as technetium-99m, yttrium-90, or indium-111 can be coupled indirectly via bifunctional chelating agents (98). Rhenium-186 has been determined to be a leading radionuclide for radioimmunotherapy because of its physical half-life of 90 hours and beta emission of 1.07 MeV. Thus, rhenium-186 delivers sufficient doses over a distance of 100 to 1,000 cell diameters without the need for hospitalization. The additional 137 keV (9%) gamma emission also allows simultaneous scintigraphic imaging. However, use has been limited due to the lack of a convenient and efficient method for conjugation of rhenium-186 to antibody. Recently, a new simple labeling technique has been developed by John et al. (99), so that ^{186}Re-labeled antibodies will be more frequently used for clinical application in the future.

Clinical trials investigating radioimmunotherapy began in the 1950s when Beierwaltes (100) administered ^{131}I-labeled rabbit antibodies to 14 patients with metastatic melanoma and achieved a pathologically documented complete remission in one patient. Since then many different epithelial tumors as well as hematologic malignancies have been treated with radiolabeled antibodies. The highest complete response rates (overall about 50%) have been achieved in patients with B-cell non-Hodgkin's lymphoma.

Currently, both nonmyeloablative and myeloablative strategies involving radiolabeled antibodies are being investigated for imaging and treatment of Hodgkin's disease (Table 4). Low-energetic radionuclides are coupled to monoclonal antibodies either for diagnostic use, e.g., immunoscintigraphy, or for low-dose radioimmunotherapy without severe myelosuppression. Thirty-eight Hodgkin's disease patients were treated with ^{131}I-labeled polyclonal ferritin-directed antibodies in a phase I trial (101). Ferritin is a tumor-associated protein that was first described in Hodgkin's disease (102). Patients received 30 mCi of the ^{131}I-labeled antibodies intravenously, followed by an additional 20 mCi 5 days later; 77% of those patients experienced symptomatic improvement and 40% objective tumor regression. Treatment was limited due to chronic bone marrow toxicity.

Herpst et al. (103) administered multiple 10- to 50-mCi infusions of ^{90}Y-antiferritin polyclonal antibodies to patients with recurrent Hodgkin's disease who had previously failed to respond to two or more multiagent chemotherapy regimens. Tumor doses ranged from 3 to 30 Gy. A CR was observed in 10 of 39 patients (26%), and a PR was observed in 10 of 39 patients (26%). The small quantity of antibodies (2 to 5 mg) used in this study suggests that the responses were due to radiation rather than complement-mediated cytotoxicity or ADCC. Some of the patients were supported with autologous bone marrow transplantation. Patients did not develop neutralizing antibodies against the polyclonal antibodies. The median survival time was 6 months.

HRS-1 (anti-CD30) has been labeled with radioiodine (^{123}I, ^{131}I) and administered to ten patients with Hodgkin's disease for immunoscintigraphy (104). Six out of eight patients had a true positive scan. Imaging was equivocal or failed in two other patients. In the last two patients immunoscintigraphic imaging was true negative due to the absence of residual Hodgkin's disease in one patient and to an erroneous histologic diagnosis of Hodgkin's disease in the other.

Immunoscintigraphy using the HRS-3 (anti-CD30) monoclonal antibody was performed in 18 patients with Hodgkin's disease at staging or restaging examinations (105). Either F(ab')^2 fragments (14 patients) or whole HRS-3 (4 patients) labeled with 77-260Mbq iodine-131 were used. Fourteen out of 17 evaluable patients showed a true positive result including two cases that were reviewed as anaplastic large-cell lymphoma. Nodal, splenic, bone marrow, and muscle involvement were imaged, and many of these sites were previously undetected. In two patients, imaging was true negative due to the absence of active Hodgkin's disease, and one false-negative result occurred (inguinal node). A false-positive image was observed in none of the patients. To rule out nonspecific iodine uptake, a ^{125}I-labeled anti-

TABLE 4. *Results of clinical trials with radioimmunoconjugates in patients with Hodgkin's disease*

Antibody	Clonality	Antigen	Radioisotope	*n*	Diagnostic tumor labeling	Response	Reference
HRS-1	Monoclonal	CD30	Iodine-131 Iodine-123	8	6/8 true positive 2/8 false negative		104
HRS-3	Monoclonal IgG Monoclonal Fab	CD30	Iodine-131	4 13	14/17 true positive 1/17 false negative		105
Antiferritin	Polyclonal	Ferritin	Iodine-131	38		No response	101
Antiferritin	Polyclonal	Ferritin	Yttrium-90	39		10 CR, 10 PR	103
Antiferritin	Polyclonal	Ferritin	Indium-111	45	40/45 true positive		107
Antiferritin	Polyclonal	Ferritin	Yttrium-90	17		7 CR (2–26+ months) 4 PR (2–6 months)	107
Ber-H2	Monoclonal	CD30	Technetium-99m	15	Only preliminary results		106

CR, complete remission; PR, partial remission; IgG, immunoglobulin G.

angiotensin-converting enzyme control antibody was injected simultaneously in ten patients. The evaluation of the study revealed a sensitivity of 87% and a good specificity. There were no major side effects; only one patient had to drop out because of iodine intolerance.

Recently, a clinical trial has been initiated for investigation of the safety of the ^{99m}Tc-labeled anti-CD30 antibody Ber-H2 for immunotherapeutic and immunoscintigraphic application in patients with refractory Hodgkin's disease and large-cell anaplastic lymphoma. Preliminary results (106) suggest good tolerance of the therapy with no major side effects and satisfactory efficacy for imaging Hodgkin's disease lesions (Fig. 2).

Because low-dose radioimmunotherapy has demonstrated promising results in many malignancies, dose escalation seems reasonable. Stem-cell support for hematopoietic recovery might be necessary in high-dose radioimmunotherapy. A phase I/II study with ^{90}Y-labeled polyclonal antiferritin antibodies for refractory Hodgkin's disease followed by autologous bone marrow transplantation was performed by Vriesendorp et al. (107). Forty out of 45 patients showed positive imaging with ^{111}In-labeled antiferritin and were subsequently treated with ^{90}Y-labeled antibodies. Nineteen out of 35 patients received doses ranging from 20 to 50 mCi in one to three cycles followed by autologous bone marrow transplantation. Seven out of 17 patients achieved complete remission (lasting 2–26+ months) and four patients partial remission (2–6 months). Twelve patients received a reduced dose (20 mCi) due to bone marrow involvement or unsuccessful marrow harvest. Two of them achieved complete remission, five partial remission. For all doses, response rates were better with small tumor burden (<30cm^3). Relapses occurred in new areas or in sites of previous bulky disease.

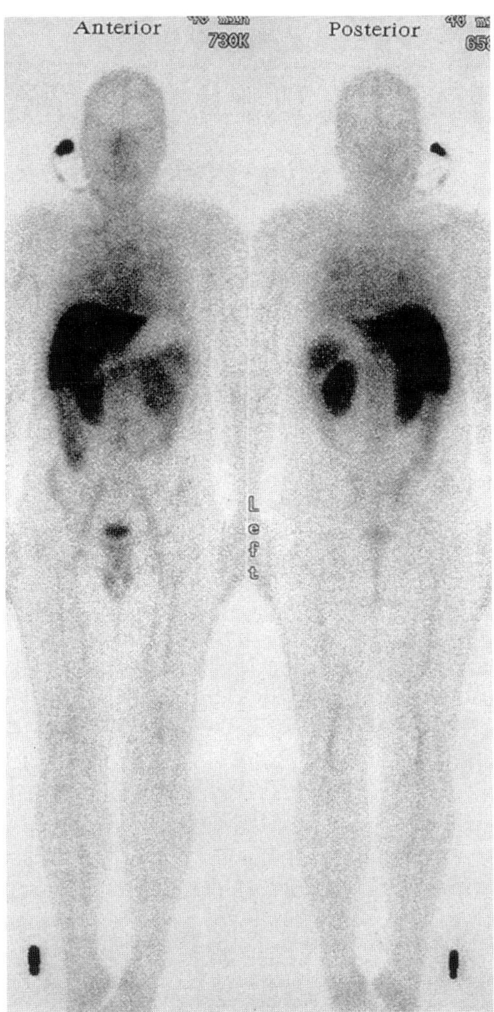

FIG. 2. Technetium-99m (Tc-99m) immunoscintigraphic image (anterior and posterior view) of a patient with active relapsed Hodgkin's disease. Positive scan (involved Hodgkin's disease at both pulmonary hili) recorded with a large field-of-view gamma camera 24 hours after intravenous bolus injection of 2 mg Tc-99m-Ber-H2 (anti-CD30) to a 36-year-old man with relapsed Hodgkin's disease.

Due to the encouraging response rates in lymphoma, high-dose and low-dose radioimmunotherapy appear to be promising approaches (108). More clinical studies are necessary to solve problems that are still posed by radioimmunotherapeutic approaches and to address the following issues: (a) Only small amounts of radiolabeled antibodies, ranging between 0.001% and 0.01% of the total injected dose, accumulate at the tumor site. DeNardo et al. (109) reported increased radioimmune conjugate uptake in the tumor after induction of IL-2–mediated vascular leak syndrome in mice. (b) Chelation techniques have to be improved for yttrium-90 and new promising radioisotopes, such as rhenium-186, so that radioimmunotherapy can be more widely used for cancer treatment. (c) New carrier molecules have to be investigated for their efficacy as radionuclide carriers *in vivo.* In addition to murine monoclonal and polyclonal antibodies, chimeric and humanized antibodies or Fab′ fragments might be used for conjugation. (d) Dose escalation seems to be promising in radioimmunotherapy as well and has to be studied in animals and humans with support of hematopoietic stem cells and growth factors. (e) Whenever feasible, radioimmunotherapy should not be used as a single-agent treatment regimen for patients with refractory disease, but should be applied in combination with other therapeutic strategies in early stages.

BI-SPECIFIC MONOCLONAL ANTIBODIES

Bi-specific monoclonal antibodies contain two different recognition sites, one for antigens on tumor cells and one for antigens on immunologic effector cells, such as macrophages, T lymphocytes, or NK cells. Thus, they have the potential to combine the advantages of antibody specificity with the cytotoxic capabilities of the immune-competent cells (110) (Fig. 3). Besides their ability to enrich effector cells at the tumor site, bi-specific mono-

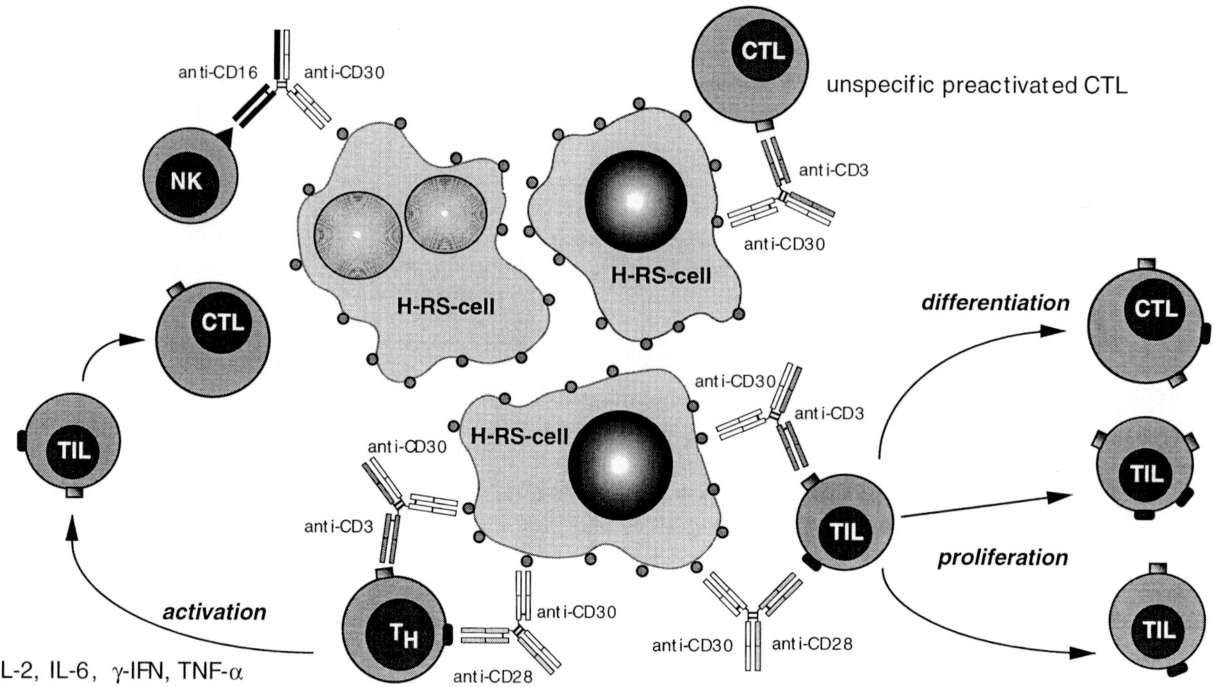

FIG. 3. Potential mechanisms of action of bi-specific antibodies in Hodgkin's disease. 1: Natural killer (NK)-cell mediated tumor lysis induced by a bi-specific antibody directed against the CD16 antigen on NK-cells and the CD30 antigen on Hodgkin–Reed-Sternberg cells. 2: Activation of cytotoxic T lymphocytes via bi-specific antibodies against the T-cell receptor/CD3 complex, and the CD30 antigen induces cytolysis. 3: Co-stimulation of resting T cells or tumor-infiltrating lymphocytes with a second bi-specific antibody directed against the CD28 and CD30 antigen. CTL, cytotoxic T lymphocyte; TIL, tumor infiltrating lymphocyte; TH, T helper cell; H-RS-cell, Hodgkin–Reed-Sternberg cell; IL, interleukin; IFN, interferon; TNF, tumor necrosis factor.

clonal antibodies can make an additional contribution to the immune recruitment by their potential to activate tumor-bound effector cells. This is possible if the arm of the bi-specific antibody that binds to the effector cell is directed toward and able to activate trigger molecules expressed on the surface of these cells. Bi-specific monoclonal antibodies can be obtained in two different ways: so-called heteroconjugates are generated first by the chemical cross-linking of two monoclonal antibodies with distinct specificities, and second by hybrid-hybridomas (tetradomas), which are established by somatic fusion of two hybridomas secreting the proper antibodies. Recently, new recombinant technology has been used for construction of bi-specific monoclonal antibodies.

Most bi-specific monoclonal antibodies involve the T-cell receptor (TCR)/CD3 complex, thus activating and recruiting cytotoxic T cells against the tumor (111,112). For T-cell proliferation, antigen-presenting cells as well as co-stimulatory signals are needed. Without co-stimulation, exposure of T cells to an antigen may cause unresponsiveness and clonal anergy or deletion. Co-stimulation can be provided by a variety of cytokines or membrane-bound molecules, most of which belong to the group of adhesion molecules, e.g., the B7 family, which represent the natural ligands for the CD28 and the CTLA-4 counterreceptors on T cells. Therefore, preactivation via cytokines or antigen-presenting cells is necessary before T lymphocytes stimulated by bi-specific monoclonal antibodies can fully exert their cytotoxic activity *in vivo* (113).

Since it is possible to stimulate resting T cells by the combined triggering of the TCR complex and CD28, a combination of CD3/CD30 (HRS-3/OKT3) and CD28/CD30 (HRS-3/15E8) bi-specific antibodies was used for targeting Hodgkin cell lines *in vitro* (114) (Fig. 3). Tumor cell lysis was clearly antigen dependent and not major-histocompatibility-complex (MHC) restricted, as only CD30-positive tumor cells or monkey kidney COS cells transfected with cDNA coding for the CD30 antigen served as targets for bi-specific antibody activated lymphocytes. These CD3/CD30 and CD28/CD30 bi-specific antibodies were also able to modify impaired T-cell function in Hodgkin's disease. Renner (115) demonstrated that peripheral blood T cells from patients with untreated Hodgkin's disease expressed decreased levels of the TCRζ chain. In T lymphocytes it seems to play the primary role in signal transduction. A ζ chain negative mutant cell line was incapable of responding to antigen and was poorly responsive to anti-CD3 antibodies (116,117). After stimulation by

CD3/CD30 and CD28/CD30 bi-specific antibodies, T cells from Hodgkin's disease patients upregulated ζ chain protein expression to normal values within 48 hours and achieved a cytolytic potential and levels of IL-2 secretion that were no different from T cells obtained from healthy controls. However, only activation of T cells by simultaneous CD3 and CD28 cross-linking was able to upregulate the defective expression of the TCR ζ chain.

SCID mice with subcutaneous Hodgkin's-derived tumors were treated with an intravenous injection of bi-specific antibodies CD3/CD30 and CD28/CD30. Tumor-bearing animals also received previously stimulated human peripheral lymphocytes 24 hours after administration of the antibody. All 20 animals that received both bi-specific monoclonal antibodies were cured of the xenografted tumors. All other animals that received the parental antibodies or either bi-specific antibody alone died of progressive tumor growth (118). To adapt this model to the clinical situation, SCID mice bearing disseminated CD30-positive tumors established by intravenous injection of the Hodgkin's-derived cell line L540Cy were also treated with the combination of CD3/CD30 and CD28/CD30 bi-specific antibodies and naive human T cells (119). All animals were cured with T lymphocytes obtained from patients, with advanced-stage untreated Hodgkin's disease being as effective as lymphocytes from healthy controls. Treatment was effective when delayed until 2 weeks after tumor cell inoculation. Results with isolated CD4+ and CD8+ human T cells suggest that both subsets are necessary for the bi-specific antibody-mediated cure of xenografted human Hodgkin tumors in SCID mice.

One of the most frequently used cell types in preclinical studies involving bi-specific antibody and effector cells are NK cells. In contrast to T lymphocytes, NK cells represent a subset of lymphocytes that do not need specific activation as they constitutively express cytolytic functions against a number of NK-susceptible tumor target cells. However, NK-cell activation, e.g., by addition of IL-2, is necessary for active tumor lysis. Binding of anti-CD16 antibodies to the receptor for the Fc part of IgG (Fcγ-RIII) expressed by human large granular lymphocytes can induce NK cell–mediated cytotoxicity (120), which is not restricted by MHC gene products.

For treatment of Hodgkin's disease with NK cell–activating bi-specific antibodies, a CD16/CD30 bi-specific antibody was chosen that is produced by a A9/HRS-3 hybridoma (121), with A9 being the anti-CD16 producing cell line and with HRS-3 producing antibodies toward the CD30 molecule. Crude supernatant as well as the purified HRS-3/A9 bi-specific antibody triggered specific lysis of the CD30-positive Hodgkin's derived cell line L540, but not of the CD30-negative cell line HPB-ALL after incubation with unstimulated peripheral blood lymphocytes as well as NK cell–enriched populations. Moreover, SCID mice bearing subcutaneous Hodgkin's cell tumors received 100 μg of bi-specific antibody HRS-3/A9 together with 10^7 unstimulated peripheral human blood lymphocytes. Complete remission of the tumors was achieved in all animals treated this way; 60% of the animals relapsed. Moreover, it seems possible to increase the cure rate of established human xenografted tumors using NK cell–activating bi-specific monoclonal antibodies in combination with IL-2 and IL-12 (122). The augmented tumor cell lysis was achieved with IL-12 at considerably lower concentrations than with IL-2 and was associated with a significantly increased bi-specific antibody-mediated intracellular Ca^{2+} mobilization. These findings are important because expensive bi-specific monoclonal antibodies can be spared by addition of cytokines. Dose reduction of CD16-specific bi-specific monoclonal antibodies *in vivo* is also useful, since these constructs have exerted dose-limiting toxicities in early clinical trials at very low doses (123). In contrast, the side effects of IL-12 were moderate after systemic application in primates and humans compared to IL-2–associated toxicity (124).

The humanized bi-specific antibody anti-CD3 x anti-1D10 F(ab′)2 was also utilized to redirect cytokine induced killer cells toward Hodgkin's disease cells (125). The 1D10 antigen is a variant of human leukocyte antigen (HLA)-DR expressed on the surface of a variety of lymphoid malignancies, but not on normal hematopoietic cells. The bi-specific anti-CD3 x 1D10 Bs F(ab′)2 was constructed from anti-CD3 and 1D10 using the leucine zipper technique. It consistently enhanced cytokine-induced NK cell–mediated killing of the Hodgkin's-derived cell line L541 as measured in a ^{51}Cr-release assay. The enhanced cytotoxicity was also observed using lymphoblastoid and Burkitt's lymphoma cell lines as targets. Thus, this strategy might represent a new therapeutic tool for 1D10-positive lymphoid malignancies.

The first clinical trial using bi-specific monoclonal antibodies for the treatment of Hodgkin's disease was initiated in 1995. Heavily pretreated patients with refractory Hodgkin's disease received a 1-hour i.v. infusion of the CD16/CD30 (A9/HRS-3) antibody four times every 3 or 4 days (126). Fifteen patients with refractory Hodgkin's disease were treated with an escalating dosing schedule. The maximum tolerated dose was not reached at 64 mg/m^2. Side effects were rare and consisted of short-lasting fever, pain in involved lymph nodes, and a maculopapulous rash. HAMAs were detected in a total of nine patients, and four patients developed an allergic reaction after attempted retreatment. A total of one complete remission and one partial remission (lasting 16 and 3 months, respectively), three minor responses (one to 11+ months), and one mixed response were achieved.

Major obstacles for a successful bi-specific antibody therapy in human malignancies are the development of HAMA in the majority of patients and the high incidence of allergic reactions even in HAMA-negative patients who are reexposed to bi-specific antibodies. These problems might be resolved by the construction of less immunogenic bi-specific single-chain antibodies (127) or so-called diabodies (128). Diabodies are formed by linking the variable domains of heavy and light chain immunoglobulin (V_H and V_L) of two different antibodies A and B to form two different crossover chains V_HA-V_LB and V_HB-V_LA. Because of their small size and the absence of the Fc fragment, biodistribution of these recombinant bi-specific peptides should be superior to that of bi-specific antibodies established by the tetradoma technique. In addition, recombinant DNA technology might reduce the difficulties in producing bi-specific antibodies in sufficient quantity and quality needed for administration in humans. Costs are also lower compared to production of bi-specific monoclonal antibodies by the tetradoma technology . The value of co-stimulation of effector cells with cytokines such as IL-2 or IL-12 also requires further investigation. Cytotoxicity of bi-specific monoclonal antibodies can also be enhanced by constructing bi-specific immunotoxins combining toxin-mediated and T cell–mediated killing (129).

PRODRUGS

Due to the limited number and size of cytotoxic molecules that can be bound to an immunoglobulin without interfering with the antigen-binding capacity of the antibody, sufficient concentrations of cytotoxic drugs in the tumor are achieved with great difficulty (130). It has been shown that one single ricin–A chain immunotoxin molecule can kill an effector cell if the toxin reaches its specific site of action (131). However, this is not possible if a given antibody binds to an antigen that is not internalized or is degraded in the lysosymes of the target cells. Moreover, prerequisite for the effectiveness of immunotoxins for

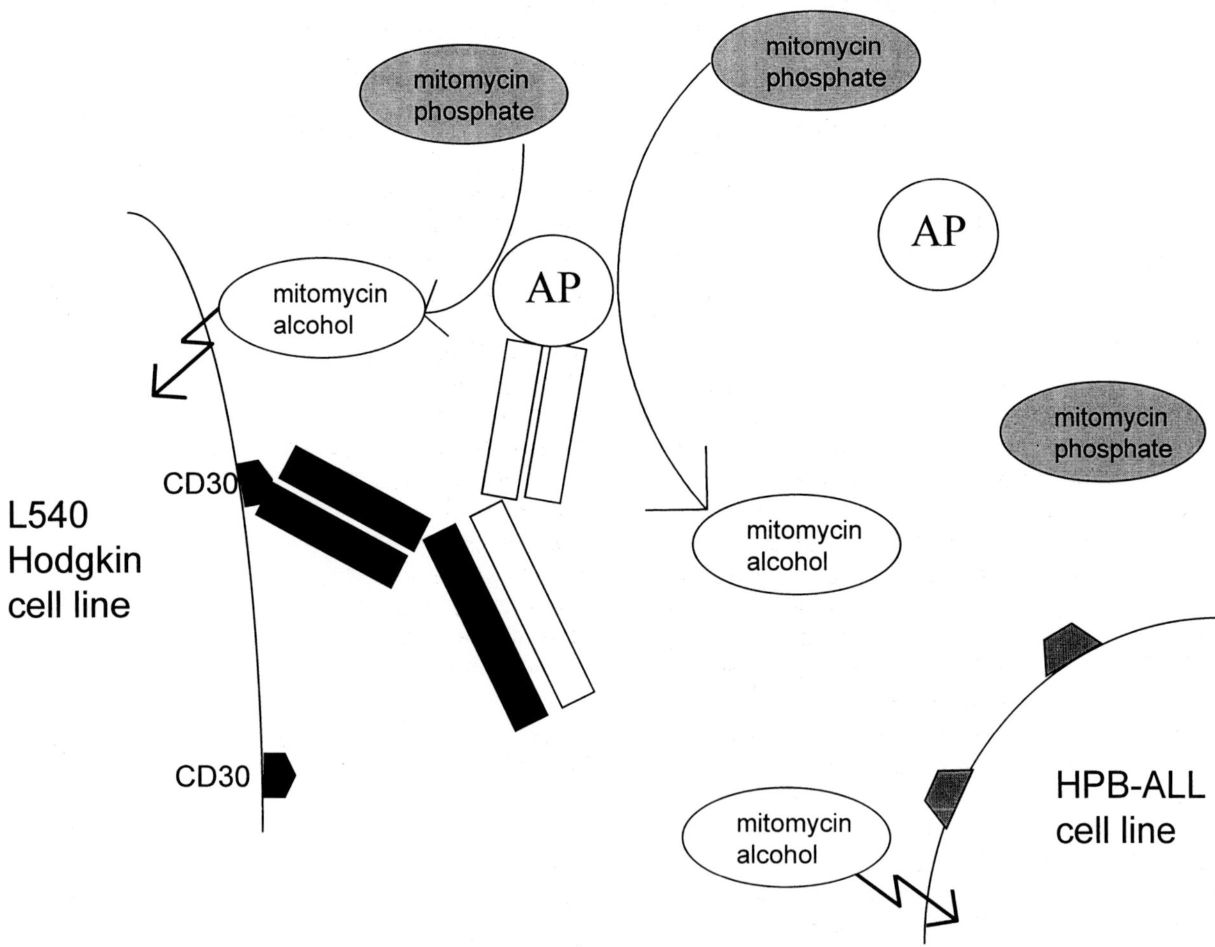

FIG. 4. Prodrug activation of mitomycin phosphate using the HRS-3/AP-1 bi-specific antibody. To overcome malignant cell escape due to antigen deficiency of some Hodgkin–Reed-Sternberg cells, Sahin et al. (135) constructed a bi-specific monoclonal antibody targeting the CD30 antigen (HRS-3) and alkaline phosphatase (AP-1). Mitomycin phosphate was converted to the 100-fold more cytotoxic mitomycin alcohol by the alkaline phosphatase bound to the bi-specific antibody. The cytostatic drug mitomycin alcohol killed not only the CD30-positive target cells but also antigen-deficient mutants nearby.

treating tumors is the expression of the immunotoxin-binding antigen on nearly all of the tumor cells, an event that is unlikely to occur as a result of the heterogeneity and instability of the malignant cell population within a given tumor. Finally, the modification of antibodies with toxins or cytotoxic drugs by chemical means carries the risk of changing the binding properties of the antibody moiety.

An approach to address these problems is the construction of antibodies carrying enzymes that are capable of converting relatively nontoxic prodrugs into active anticancer agents (132–134). It was postulated that the drugs thus formed at the surface of the antigen-positive tumor cells should be able to act also on antigen-negative cells nearby (132,133) (Fig. 4). Alkaline phosphatase (AP) is the most frequently used enzyme for converting relatively noncytotoxic prodrugs such as mitomycin phosphate or etoposide phosphate into the active cytostatic drugs mitomycin and etoposide.

For experimental use in Hodgkin's disease Sahin et al. (135) constructed the HRS-3/AP-1 bi-specific monoclonal antibody directed against the CD30 antigen and alkaline phosphatase (Fig. 4). Bi-specific monoclonal antibodies were used to preclude the need for forming antibody-enzyme conjugates chemically; in addition, such bi-specific antibodies might be superior due to their uniform composition and low molecular weight. After incubation of HRS-3/AP-1 and alkaline phosphatase with the Hodgkin's-derived cell line L540, mitomycin phosphate was converted into mitomycin alcohol, which was 100 times more toxic to L540 cells than mitomycin phosphate. The cytotoxic activity of mitomycin phosphate was unaffected when the cells were pretreated with either the bi-specific monoclonal antibody or the enzyme alone. HRS-3/AP-1 did not bind to the CD30-negative cell line HPB-ALL and was not able to activate mitomycin phosphate on these cells. In cocultivation experiments with HPB-ALL and L540 cells, the activation of mitomycin phosphate by the bi-specific monoclonal antibody HRS-3/AP-1 and alkaline phosphatase led to considerable cytotoxicity toward the antigen-negative bystander cells. Thus, this immunotherapeutic approach might be effective *in vivo,* with not all the tumor cells carrying the respective tumor antigen. It is expected that this approach will lead to less destruction of normal cells than after a conventional systemic therapy with the same drugs, since the major portion of the active drug will be released at the target site. The alkaline phosphatase-mediated activation of cytotoxic prodrug on tumor cells is not restricted to phosphates of etoposide or mitomycin, as other hydroxyl-containing cytotoxic drugs may be amenable to phosphorylation, thus opening the possibility of polychemoimmunotherapy.

VASCULAR TARGETING

Instead of targeting tumor cells directly, immunoconjugates can also be used for selectively occluding tumor vasculature. Since malignant cells are highly dependent on sufficient blood supply, local interruption of the tumor vasculature will result in death of the majority of dependent cells. Endothelial cells of tumor vessels are in direct contact with the bloodstream, whereas tumor cells are often poorly accessible to circulating immunoconjugates. Since tumor endothelial cells are not transformed, it is unlikely that they acquire mutations that render them resistant to therapy. It might even be possible to identify antigens that are universally expressed on the endothelial cells of all different types of tumors. Vascular targeting is of special interest in the treatment of solid tumors or bulky lymphoma, since penetration of tumor cell-specific immunoconjugates is often poor in these disease entities. This is partly due to the dense packing of tumor cells surrounded by large amounts of fibrous stroma. In addition, interstitial pressure in the tumor tissue is usually high, lymphatic tumor drainage is insufficient, and antibodies are usually absorbed early by perivascular tumor cell layers.

Initial data from *in vivo* experiments were highly promising: Mice were inoculated with neuroblastoma cells transfected with the IFN-γ gene, which induces expression of MHC class II antigens on the surface of endothelial cells in solid xenografted neuroblastoma tumors (136). Application of anti–MHC-II ricin–A chain immunotoxins to tumor-bearing mice induced thrombosis of tumor vessels and impressive reduction of tumor mass. Only some cell layers at the border of the tumor survived immunotoxin therapy. Combination of anti–MHC-II immunotoxin with immunotoxins targeting neuroblastoma-specific antigens induced complete remission in all treated mice.

Bi-specific antibodies have also been successfully used for vascular targeting *in vivo.* Since naturally occurring markers of tumor vasculature endothelium have not been identified in mice, the above-mentioned animal model with subcutaneous tumors of transfected neuroblastoma cells was used for *in vivo* experiments as well. Mice were treated with a bi-specific antibody targeting I-Ad, one epitope of the MHC-II antigen complex, as well as a noninhibitory epitope of the human tissue factor (137). The truncated form of tissue factor had a limited ability in initiating thrombosis when free in circulation, but became an effective and selective thrombogen when targeted to tumor endothelial cells. Intravenous administration of the bi-specific antibody to mice with large neuroblastoma tumors resulted in complete tumor regressions in 38% of the animals. These experiments illustrate the therapeutic potential of selective initiation of the blood coagulation cascade in tumor vasculature by targeting a thrombogen to tumor endothelial cell markers. For clinical application, it is crucial to identify target molecules that are present in sufficient density on the surface of tumor vessel endothelium but absent from normal vascular endothelium.

Recently, endoglin has been identified as a potential target for selective immunotherapy in Hodgkin's disease

(138). This homodimeric membrane glycoprotein is part of the transforming growth factor (TGF)-β receptor and is expressed on proliferating endothelial cells in humans and mice (139). The antibody MJ7/18, which binds selectively to murine endoglin, has been used for investigating expression of endoglin on vascular endothelia of SCID mice bearing human Hodgkin's disease. Immunohistochemical examinations revealed that tumor blood vessels gave distinct staining using this antibody. In addition, *in vivo* localization studies were performed with MJ7/18 as well as with the positive control pan-endothelial antibody MECA32. After intravenous injection of these antibodies into tumor-bearing mice, animals were sacrificed and cryosections of lymphomas and different organs were subjected to an indirect immunoperoxidase staining. Endoglin was significantly upregulated on tumor vessels. In normal organs, vessels were not stained or were only weakly stained with MJ7/18 (except for the kidney and the small intestine where the glomeruli and villous endothelial cells, respectively, were stained). The pan-endothelial MECA32-antigen was not restricted to the tumor site. These results suggest that endoglin can serve as a target for selective immunotherapy of human Hodgkin's disease using MJ7/18, for example, but careful determination of cross-reactivities with normal human tissue is necessary.

VACCINATION

Active specific immunotherapy is the main principle of tumor cell vaccination. Tumor cell antigens or their antiidiotype vaccine are administered to the patient for stimulation of a specific immune response. Problems with vaccination are the limited availability of purified material and the development of immune tolerance against autogenic tumor antigens (140,141). In Hodgkin's disease, the presence of soluble CD30 in the sera of Hodgkin's disease patients might be one example (142). However, active specific immunotherapy circumventing tumor tolerance is implied by the network theory proposed by Nils Jerne (143). This concept provides a theoretical basis for replacing tumor antigen with monoclonal antibodies that carry structures of the tumor antigen as an internal image. According to the network theory, any nominal antigen can induce a cascade of specific antibodies called Ab1, Ab2, Ab3, etc. The second generation of antibodies (Ab2) raised against the antigen-binding site of the antitumor antibody (Ab1) can mimic the confirmation of the original antigen like an internal image. These internal images can induce specific antitumor responses like the nominal antigen and can thus substitute for tumor antigen as vaccine material (Fig. 5).

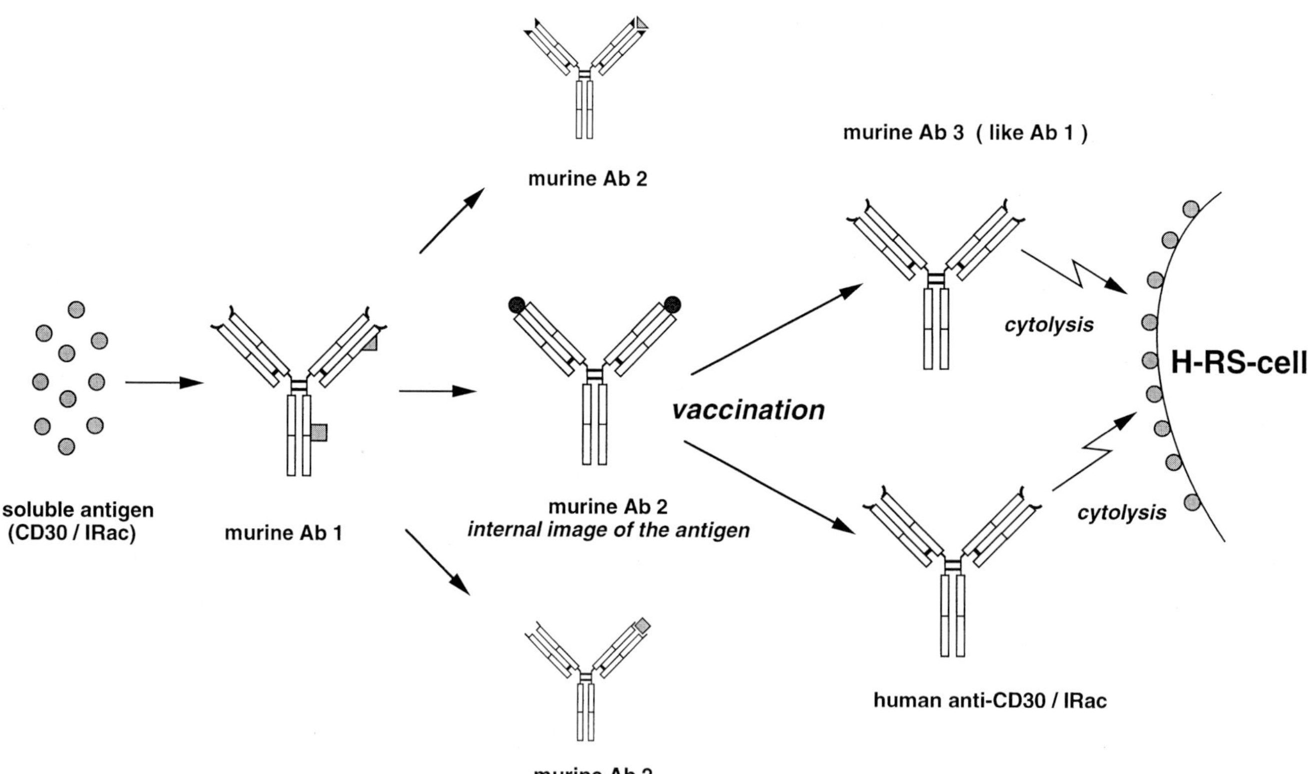

FIG. 5. Ab1-Ab2-Ab3 internal image antibody network as antiidiotype vaccine against Hodgkin's lymphoma. Tumor-associated antigen induces murine monoclonal antibodies (Ab1). Internal antibodies (Ab2) against the binding site of Ab1 mimic structures of the nominal antigen and can be used to generate monoclonal or polyclonal antibodies, Ab3, which can induce cytolysis by complement activation and antibody-dependent cell-mediated mechanisms. Ab, antibody; H-RS-cell, Hodgkin–Reed-Sternberg cell.

In several tumor models Ab2β has been reported to induce specific immunity to tumor-associated antigens. In clinical trials, promising results were obtained with polyclonal goat Ab2 as surrogate vaccines in patients with colorectal carcinoma (144) as well as with syngeneic murine monoclonal antiidiotypic antibody mimicking epitope structures of melanoma-associated antigens (145).

For the development of a vaccine for Hodgkin's disease, different monoclonal antibodies, such as HRS-3 and HRS-4 (both anti-CD30) and IRac (146), were evaluated as tumor-specific Ab1 for the induction of internal image antibodies mimicking structures of the tumor antigen. Several murine monoclonal Ab2 directed against HRS-3, HRS-4, and IRac were established as antiidiotypic Ab2β carrying the internal image of the CD30 or IRac antigen (147,148). These antibodies bound specifically to HRS-3, HRS-4, and IRac, respectively, and inhibited their binding to CD30 and IRac antigen preparations effectively at concentrations as low as 50 ng/ml. The Ab2β antibodies induced a polyclonal humoral response against the 120-kd band of the CD30 antigen or the IRac antigen in different animal models. The polyclonal Ab3 preparations induced ADCC-mediated specific cytotoxicity to the Hodgkin's-derived cell line L540 as measured in a Cr_{51} release assay.

The most promising internal image antibody, 9G10, against HRS-4 was used to generate monoclonal anti-anti-idiotypic antibodies (Ab3). Analyses of Ab3 hybridoma (4A4) showed specific binding to the CD30 antigen; 4A4 induced complement-dependent cytotoxicity to CD30-positive Hodgkin cells and prevented subcutaneous growth of solid human Hodgkin tumors in NK cell–depleted SCID mice (149).

The murine monoclonal antibody anti-IRac binds to a surface antigen structure (70 kd) on Hodgkin–Reed-Sternberg and interdigitating reticulum cells and was used to generate a cascade of antiidiotypic antibodies as well as cellular immunity to Hodgkin–Reed-Sternberg cells in syngeneic BALB/c-mice (150). The antiidiotypic antibody 4B4 demonstrated characteristics of an internal image Ab2β. Ab2β 4B4 bound specifically to anti-IRac and inhibited anti-IRac binding to antigen-bearing cells effectively; 4B4 induced an IRac-specific humoral polyclonal immune response in animal models. BALB/c-mice immunized with 4B4 showed statistically significant delayed-type hypersensitivity reaction to IRac-expressing Hodgkin cell lines. In addition, Ab2β 4B4 induced in syngeneic mice a monoclonal anti-antiidiotypic antibody (Ab3) that mimicked the specificities of Ab1 anti-IRac and thus confirmed the internal image nature of Ab2β 4B4. The antiidiotype-induced tumor cell specific immune response against the Hodgkin's disease–associated antigens CD30 and IRac as described in animal models even across species barriers might indicate a possible role for an active specific immunotherapy in Hodgkin's disease.

A newer vaccination approach uses dendritic cells, which are the most effective antigen-presenting cells. They express high levels of adhesion molecules such as ICAM-1 (intercellular adhesion molecule) and LFA-3 (lymphocyte function-associated antigen 3), as well as MHC class I and II proteins (151). Recently, Hsu et al. (152) treated four non-Hodgkin's disease patients with autologous dendritic cells. These cells were first pulsed with idiotypic protein, then matured *in vitro* in the presence of antigen, and administered to the patients subcutaneously up to four times. Treatment was well tolerated, and all patients generated lymphocytes with specific response to the Ig idiotype *in vitro*. One patient had a complete remission, one achieved a partial remission, and one with minimal residual disease only detected using PCR became PCR-negative after treatment with dendritic cells. Since treatment results in patients with non-Hodgkin's lymphoma are quite encouraging, this vaccination approach using dendritic cells might be successful in Hodgkin's disease as well.

GENE THERAPY

Attempts to alter immune reactivity in cancer patients have recently turned to genetic manipulation of immune-competent and malignant cells. Gene therapy can be defined as a therapeutic technique in which a functioning gene is inserted into the cells of a patient to correct an inborn genetic error or to provide a new function of a given cell. The development of novel techniques for inserting foreign genes in eukaryotic cells and an increased understanding of the regulation of gene expression have opened new possibilities for cancer therapy.

A very promising strategy in cellular immunotherapy is the combination of target specificity and MHC independence of monoclonal antibodies with the cellular activation potential of the TCR complex to generate chimeric receptors that are capable of both targeting and activating the autologous host T cells. This strategy is based on the similarity of the primary structure and the basic spatial conformation of the variable regions of Ig and TCR molecules (153). T cells are equipped with a chimeric receptor molecule, the extracellular moiety of which consists of a binding domain, e.g., a single chain fragment of the variable Ig domain (scFv), and the transmembrane and intracellular domain of which consist of a signaling unit, e.g., derived from the γ chain of the FcεRI receptor. After specific binding of the scFv to the antigen expressed on the target cell, the γ chain of the chimeric receptor transduces a cellular activation signal resulting in T-cell activation indicated by proliferation, increased IL-2 secretion, and specific cytotoxicity of the T cell to the target cell. Thus the chimeric receptor has combined the non–MHC-restricted specificity of the antibody molecule with the ability of the TCR complex to trigger T-cell activation. Moreover, the low affinity of the authentic TCR to antigen is changed to the high-affinity binding domain of the Ig.

Hodgkin–Reed-Sternberg cells exhibit high amounts of CD30 antigen on the cell surface, express normal amounts of MHC class I molecules, and are surrounded by a high number of cytotoxic T cells. However, Hodgkin's disease patients fail to establish an efficient cellular response to the CD30-positive lymphoma cells. Recently, peripheral T cells of patients with Hodgkin's disease were reported to have a reduced CD3ζ chain expression, which is thought to be pathogenetically involved in the impaired TCR-mediated cellular activation (115). An anti-CD30 scFv-γ (FcγRI) recombinant TCR was designed for TCR/CD3ζ independent T-cell activation by Hombach et al (154). Specific receptor cross-linking by interaction of transfected MD45 T cells with CD30-positive Hodgkin's cells resulted in cellular activation indicated by increase of IL-2 secretion and in specific target cell lysis *in vitro.* Currently, the recombinant anti-CD30-γ receptor is being assessed for bypassing the impaired CD3ζ signaling in T cells of Hodgkin's disease patients, providing a perspective for cellular immunotherapy of Hodgkin's disease. Before this immunotherapeutic approach can enter clinical trials in humans, several parameters have to be optimized: Reinfusion of an estimated 10^8 to 10^9 transduced T cells seems to be necessary for efficient elimination of residual tumor cells *in vivo.* Therefore, lymphocyte expansion prior to application has to be prolonged and/or a higher proportion of lymphocytes has to be effectively transduced. However, transgene expression in normal T cells is one of the most crucial steps in the chimeric receptor approach. Retroviral vectors were most successful in gene transfer into normal lymphocytes, but the efficiency of transduction is quite poor in T cells compared to other cells. However, expression constructs for chimeric receptors have been successfully transferred to primary T cells from peripheral blood (155–157). Although DNA is inserted nearly randomly into the host genome, no major abnormality, side effect, or pathology due to retroviral gene transfer has been reported from *in vitro* experiments, animal models, or more than 30 patients who have now received gene transfected autologous T cells in clinical phase I protocols (158).

One important, though not yet fully understood, mechanism in the pathogenesis of Hodgkin's disease, is the frequent association with Epstein-Barr virus (EBV) infection (159). In industrialized countries EBV-coding genes can be detected in Hodgkin–Reed-Sternberg cells of 50% to 60% of all lymphoma patients (159,160). While EBV-infected B cells can be controlled by T lymphocytes of immune-competent individuals, T-cell–mediated elimination of infected Hodgkin–Reed-Sternberg cells is impaired in Hodgkin's disease patients. Therefore, modulation of T-cell activity might be another interesting new approach to cell-mediated immunotherapy of Hodgkin's lymphoma. Heslop et al. (161) developed EBV-specific cytotoxic T lymphocytes (CTLs) for treatment of EBV-associated lymphoma after bone marrow transplantation. Donors' blood samples were used for generation of EBV-transformed B-cell lines [lymphoblastoid cell lines (LCLs)] and for production of CTLs. Incubation of activated CTLs with LCLs of the same probe induced formation of EBV-specific CTLs. After insertion of the neomycin-resistance gene into the specific CTLs, cells were administered to the bone marrow recipients. In this preliminary study three of ten patients developed elevated levels of EBV-DNA after allogeneic transplantation, indicating reactivation of an EBV-infection. DNA levels normalized after infusion of the EBV-specific CTLs. One patient with immunoblastic non-Hodgkin's lymphoma even achieved complete remission after this kind of treatment. *In vitro* EBV-specific CTLs consist of polyclonal populations of CD4+ and CD8+ T lymphocytes.

Since EBV-infected Hodgkin–Reed-Sternberg cells might also be suitable as targets for T-cell–mediated immune response (162), EBV-specific CTLs were isolated for an adoptive transfer in patients with EBV-positive Hodgkin's disease (163). Nine patients with active relapsed Hodgkin's disease and four who were in complete remission after first or subsequent therapy were treated with autologous EBV-specific CTLs. For detection of persistent CTLs, T cells were transfected with the gene for neomycin-resistance before reinfusion. It could be detected in circulating mononuclear cells for more than 3 months after the first application. A 100-fold reduction of EBV-DNA was achieved due to this adoptive treatment strategy. In two of nine patients, B symptoms ceased after therapy with specific CTLs.

Induction of a latent membrane protein (LMP)-2–specific immune response has also been evaluated for immunotherapy of Hodgkin's disease (164). LMP1, 2a, and 2b are expressed on the surface of EBV-infected Hodgkin–Reed-Sternberg cells. Autologous dendritic cells were transfected with the EBV gene LMP-2a using retroviral vectors. LMP2A expressing dendritic cells was then used for generation of LMP2A–specific monoclonal CTLs *ex vivo.* This method was feasible for isolation of specific T cells from EBV-seropositive as well as from EBV-seronegative patients (165).

PERSPECTIVES

Many new approaches involving immunotherapeutic agents have given promising results *in vitro* and in experimental Hodgkin's disease models. First clinical trials with IL-2, bi-specific antibodies, immunotoxins, and radioimmunoconjugates have been initiated. In these phase I/II studies only patients with advanced refractory disease have been treated. Although antigen expression is often altered after polychemotherapy and patients usually present with bulky disease at this stage of disease, some clinical efficacy was demonstrated in most of the trials. However, it is very unlikely that patients with larger tumor masses will be cured by single-agent immunotherapy. It might be more effective to eradicate bulky disease by conventional therapeutic methods first and then administer biologic drugs in order to kill residual Hodgkin–Reed-Sternberg cells. Future phase III trials will have to prove whether patients with Hodgkin's disease benefit from the combination of conventional and immunobiologic therapy at first diagnosis or in relapsed disease. The sequential or simultaneous use of immunoconjugates targeting different antigens on Hodgkin cells might also result in superior therapeutic efficacy. Malignant cells deficient of one antigen might survive treatment with the specific immunoconjugate. Concurrent administration of a second conjugate targeting a different antigen might avoid malignant cell escape.

Immunotherapy is expected to be highly efficient in eliminating minimal residual disease after successful first- or second-line treatment. It is known that residual Hodgkin cells not detected by standard diagnostic procedures might survive initial therapy and can cause early or late relapses. Diagnostic tools for detection of minimal residual disease in Hodgkin's disease have to be improved, so that patients at high risk for relapse can be identified and treated with biologic drugs for prophylaxis of recurring disease.

While many immunotherapeutic approaches have finally entered clinical trials, the search for more promising immunologic strategies continues. Most antibody-derived conjugates used today are of murine origin. However, humanized constructs are much better tolerated; formation of antibodies by the patient's immune system is rare. Therefore, neutralization of the therapeutic agent or anaphylactic reactions are expected to occur less frequently. In addition, the immune response is more efficient when the Fc part of the antibody conjugate is humanized. New technologies involved in designing high-affinity human monoclonal antibodies include the phage display technique (166) or transgenic humanized mice (87). The first fully human anti-CD30 antibody is Ki-4 scFv, which has been produced by guided selection using phage display (167). It competes with the murine Ig Ki-4 for binding CD30 on Hodgkin's-derived cell lines and will be used to create immunotherapeutics with minimal immunogenicity and maximal anti-tumor efficacy.

Highly cytotoxic immunotoxins are created by conjugation of conventional or single-chain antibodies to toxins of bacterial or plant origin. After intravenous administration of an immunotoxin to patients with malignant tumors, however, the human immune system often produces neutralizing antibodies against the antibody as well as the toxin part. In addition to using humanized single-chain antibodies for the production of less immunogenic fusion toxins, several human proteins have been investigated for conjugation to antibodies as well. Human ribonucleases (RNases), for example, could provide an alternative basis for the construction of better tolerated immunotoxins. Two members of the human RNase family, angiogenin and eosinophil-derived neurotoxin, were fused to a single-chain antibody against the human transferrin receptor (168). Both fusion toxins inhibited the protein synthesis of three human tumor cell lines derived from a melanoma, a renal carcinoma, and a breast carcinoma with high efficacy. These results suggest that human ribonucleases, which are expected to have a very low immunogenic potential in humans with no inherent toxicity, might be used as a potent toxic moiety for the generation of new fusion proteins.

Multiple monoclonal antibodies have been detected for targeting different antigens on the surface of Hodgkin–Reed-Sternberg cells. Recent advances in genetic engineering have allowed the genes encoding antibodies to be manipulated so that it is possible to produce antibodies to virtually any target molecule whether it be self or foreign, protein or nucleic acid, carbohydrate or protein. Intracellular antibodies, or intrabodies, are single-chain antibodies synthesized by the cell and targeted to a particular cellular compartment (169). They are able to interfere in a highly specific manner with cell growth and metabolism. Intrabodies may be used to divert proteins from their cellular compartment, for example, by sequestering transcription factors in the cytoplasm, or by retention in the endoplasmatic reticulum (ER) of proteins that are destined for the cell surface. An ER-targeted intrabody was used to down-regulate the α subunit of the IL-2R, which is overexpressed in some T- and B-cell leukemias (170). In Hodgkin's disease this strategy of modulating surface receptor expression would be especially interesting, because proliferation of Hodgkin–Reed-Sternberg cells seems to be highly dependent on cytokine-mediated regulatory mechanisms. As is the case for other gene-based therapies, the greatest challenge with this approach is the problem of efficient gene delivery to, and correct gene expression in, a sufficient number of target cells (171). Once these problems are solved, gene transfer into tumor cells will be a powerful tool in modern oncologic treatment. Further strategies that might be applicable in gene therapy of Hodgkin's disease include the transfection of malignant cells with genes coding for certain cytokines, adhesion molecules, or surface markers. Additional application of the corresponding ligands might inhibit tumor growth then, as was demonstrated *in vivo* for ovarian carcinoma cell lines transfected with the gene for the monocyte chemoattractant and activating factor (172). In virally directed enzyme/prodrug therapy, a gene for a prodrug-activating enzyme is inserted into tumor cells using retroviral vectors (173). 5′-Fluorocytosine, for example, was transformed into the highly toxic 5′-fluorouracil in mammalian tumor cells transfected with a gene coding for the enzyme cytosine deaminase (174). Though these genes are of bacterial origin, transfected human cells do not exhibit proliferation properties that differ from those of the original cells (175).

One of the most promising strategies in gene therapy at the moment is the insertion of genes into immune-competent cells. Since the majority of these cells circulates in the blood, they are easily accessible for *in vivo* or *ex vivo* gene transfer. Genetically modified CTLs are currently investigated for clinical use in patients with Hodgkin's disease (see above). Recently, a new class of antigen-specific killer cells has been generated that combines the features of antibody-mediated and cell-mediated immunity. Yang and Chen (176) transduced a bicistronic expression vector into a CD4-positive human T-lymphocyte cell line. The vector contained the genes coding for the Fd fragment of a human monoclonal antibody against the CD4-binding site of gp120 expressed on the surface of HIV-1 infected cells as well as for the domains II and III of *Pseudomonas* exotoxin A, including an internal sequence preventing the toxin molecule from being secreted into the cytosol where it would block protein synthesis at the ribosomes. These transfected cells were found to have selective and potent cytotoxicity to HIV-infected cells. This approach may also be used for selectively killing tumor cells that express specific target antigens.

All these new and interesting strategies in immunotherapy and gene transfer will be further investigated *in vitro* and in patients with Hodgkin's disease and other malignancies. These innovative methods not only are promising tools in cancer therapy, but also serve basic science in attaining further insight into the pathogenesis and physiologic regulation mechanisms of tumor cell growth and proliferation. Only a thorough understanding of immunologic and molecular-biologic processes concerning Hodgkin–Reed-Sternberg cells and their microenvironment will give rise to new treatment modalities that might complement conventional therapeutic regimens in Hodgkin's disease in the future. Chemo- and radiotherapy are most efficient in killing large amounts of tumor cells at once; these strategies are not specific and therefore are able to induce severe acute as well as long-term toxicities, including secondary cancer. To date, replacement of standard therapeutic principles in Hodgkin's disease with novel biologic strategies is impossible, but simultaneous application of powerful conventional regimens and adjuvant immunotherapeutics with more specificity might reduce side effects, lower relapse rates, and extend overall survival.

REFERENCES

1. McLaughlin P, Cabanillas F, Grillo-Lopez AJ, et al. IDEC-C2B8 anti-CD20 antibody: final report on a phase III pivotal trial in patients with relapsed low-grade or follicular lymphoma. *Blood* 1996;88(S1),349a(abst).
2. Riethmüller G, Schneider-Gädicke E, Schlimok G, et al. Randomised trial of monoclonal antibody for adjuvant therapy of resected Dukes C colorectal carcinoma. *Lancet* 1993;343:1177.
3. Reed D. On the pathological changes in Hodgkin's disease with especial reference to its relation to tuberculosis. *Johns Hopkins Hosp Rep* 1902;10:133.
4. Poppema S. Immunology of Hodgkin's disease. *Baillieres Clin Haematol* 1996;9:447.
5. Moertel CG, Ritts RE Jr, Schutts AJ, Hahn RG. Clinical studies of methanol extraction residue fraction of bacillus Calmette-Guerin as immuno-stimulant in patients with advanced cancer. *Cancer Res* 1975; 35:3075.
6. Jacobs D, Yashphe DT, Abraham C. Stimulation of T-cell activity by a methanol-extraction residue (MER) of BCG. *Recent Results Cancer Res* 1974;47:183.
7. Cuttner J, Holland JF, Bekesi JG. Chemoimmunotherapy of acute myelocytic leukemia. *Proc Am Assoc Cancer Res* 1975;16:264.
8. Perloff M, Holland J, Bekesi JG. Chemoimmunotherapy of breast cancer. *Proc Am Assoc Cancer Res* 1976;17,308.
9. Cooper MR, Pajak TF, Nissen NI, et al. Effect of the methanol extraction residue of bacillus Calmette-Guerin in advanced Hodgkin's disease. *Cancer* 1982;49:2226.
10. Vinciguerra V, Coleman M, Pajak TF, et al. MER immunotherapy and combination chemotherapy for advanced, recurrent Hodgkin's disease. *Cancer Clin Trials* 1981;4:99.
11. Köhler G, Milstein C. Continuous cultures of fused cells secreting antibody of pre-defined specificity. *Nature* 1975;256:495.
12. Hsu SM, Jaffe ES. Leu M1 and peanut agglutinin stain the neoplastic cells of Hodgkin's disease. *Am J Clin Pathol* 1984;82:29.
13. Agnarrson BA, Kadin ME. The immunophenotype of Reed-Sternberg cells. A study of 50 cases of Hodgkin's disease using fixed frozen tissue. *Cancer* 1989;63:2083.
14. Casey TT, Olson SJ, Cousar JB, Collins RD. Immunophenotypes of Reed-Sternberg cells: a study of 19 cases of Hodgkin's disease in plastic-embedded sections. *Blood* 1989;74:5042.
15. Stein H, Mason DY, Gerdes J, et al. The expression of the Hodgkin's-disease-associated antigen Ki-1 in reactive and neoplastic lymphoid tissue: evidence that Sternberg-Reed cells and histiocytic malignancies are derived from activated lymphoid cells. *Blood* 1985;66:848.
16. Kennedy IC, Hart DN, Colls BM, et al. Nodular sclerosing, mixed cellularity and lymphocyte-depleted variants of Hodgkin's disease are probable dendritic cell malignancies. *Clin Exp Immunol* 1989;76:324.
17. Delabie J, Ceuppens JL, Vandenberghe P, et al. The B7/BB1 antigen is expressed by Reed-Sternberg cells of Hodgkin's disease and contributes to the stimulating capacity of Hodgkin's disease-derived cell lines. *Blood* 1993;82:2845.
18. Kaplan HS. Hodgkin's disease: unfolding concepts concerning its nature, management and prognosis. *Cancer* 1980;45:2439.
19. Hagenbeek A, Martens ACM. Cryopreservation of autologous marrow grafts in acute leukemia: survival of *in vivo* clonogenic leukemic cells and normal hematopoietic stem cells. *Leukemia* 1989;3:535.
20. Gribben JG, Freedman AS, Neuberg D, et al. Immunological purging of marrow assessed by PCR before autologous bone marrow transplantation for B-cell lymphoma. *N Engl J Med* 1991;325:1525.
21. Sharp JG, Joshi SS, Armitage JO, et al. Significance of detection of occult non-Hodgkin's lymphoma in histologically uninvolved bone marrow by a culture technique. *Blood* 1992;79:1074.
22. Campana D, Pui CH. Detection of minimal residual disease in acute leukemia: methodological advances and clinical significance. *Blood* 1995;85:1416.
23. Küppers R, Zhao M, Hansmann ML, Rajewsky K. Tracing B cell development in human germinal centres by molecular analysis of single cells picked from histological sections. *EMBO J* 1993;12:4955.
24. Küppers R, Hansmann ML, Rajewsky K. Micromanipulation and PCR analysis of single cells from tissue sections. In: Weit DM, Blackwell C, Henneberg LA, eds. *Handbook of experimental immunology,* 5th ed. Cambridge, MA: Blackwell Scientific, 1996:206.
25. Küppers R, Hansmann ML, Diehl V, Rajewsky K. Molecular single-cell analysis of Hodgkin and Reed-Sternberg cells. *Mol Med Today* 1995;1:26.
26. Jox A, Zander T, Diehl V, Wolf J. Clonal relapse of Hodgkin's disease. *N Engl J Med* 1997;337:499.
27. Kreitman RJ, Pastan I. Recombinant single-chain immunotoxins against T and B cell leukemias. *Leuk Lymph* 1994;13:1.
28. Rosenberg SA, Lotze MT, Muul LM, et al. Observations on the systemic administration of autologous lymphokine-activated killer cells and recombinant interleukin-2 to patients with metastatic cancer. *N Engl J Med* 1985;313:1485.
29. Rosenberg SA, Lotze MT, Muul LM, et al. A progress report on the treatment of 157 patients with advanced cancer using lymphokine-

activated killer cells and interleukin-2 or high-dose interleukin-2 alone. *N Engl J Med* 1987;316:889.
30. Paciucci PA, Holland JF, Gildwell O, Odechimar R. Recombinant IL-2 by continuous infusion and adoptive transfer of recombinant interleukin-2 activated cells in patients with advanced cancer. *J Clin Oncol* 1989;7:869.
31. Margolin KA, Aronson FR, Sznol M, et al. Phase II trial of high-dose interleukin-2 and lymphokine-activated killer cells in Hodgkin's disease and non-Hodgkin's lymphoma. *J Immunother* 1991;10:214.
32. Bernstein ZP, Vaickus L, Friedman N, et al. Interleukin-2 lymphokine-activated killer cell therapy of non-Hodgkin's lymphoma and Hodgkin's disease. *J Immunother* 1991;10:141.
33. Tourani JM, Levy V, Briere J, et al. Interleukin-2 therapy for refractory and relapsing lymphoma. *Eur J Cancer* 1991;27:1676.
34. West WH, Tauer KW, Yannelli, JR, et al. Constant-infusion of recombinant interleukin-2 in adoptive immunotherapy of advanced cancer. *N Engl J Med* 1987;316:898.
35. Baron S, Tyring SK, Fleischmann R, et al. The interferons: mechanism of action and clinical applications. *JAMA* 1991;266:1375.
36. Einat M, Resnitzky D, Kimchi A. Close link between reduction of c-myc expression by interferon and G0/G1 arrest. *Nature* 1985;313:597.
37. McLaughlin P. The role of interferon in the therapy of malignant lymphoma. *Biomed Pharmacother* 1996;50:140.
38. Janssen JT, Ludwig H, Scheithauer W, et al. Phase I study of recombinant human interferon 2C in patients with chemotherapy refractory malignancies. *Oncology* 1985;42(S1):3.
39. Leavitt RD, Ratanatharathorn V, Ozer H, et al. Alfa-2b interferon in the treatment of Hodgkin's disease and non-Hodgkin's lymphoma. *Semin Oncol* 1987;14(S2):18.
40. Horning SJ, Merigan TE, Krown SE, et al. Human interferon alpha in malignant lymphoma and Hodgkin's disease. *Cancer* 1985;56:1305.
41. Clark RH, Dimitrov NV, Axelson JA, Charamella LJ. Leukocyte interferon as a possible biological response modifier in lymphoproliferative disorders resistant to standard therapy. *J Biol Response Mod* 1984;3:613.
42. Koziner B. Alpha interferon in patients with progressive and/or recurrent Hodgkin's disease. *Eur J Cancer* 1991;27(S4):S79.
43. Rybak ME, McCarroll K, Bernard S, et al. Interferon therapy of relapsed and refractory Hodgkin's disease: Cancer and Leukemia Group B Study 8652. *J Biol Response Mod* 1990;9:1.
44. Redman J, Hagemeister F, McLaughlin P, et al. Alpha-interferon treatment of Hodgkin's disease (HD). *Am Soc Clin Oncol* (ASCO) 1990; 256:993a(abst).
45. Queseda JR, Talpaz M, Rios A, et al. Clinical toxicity of interferons in cancer patients: a review. *J Clin Oncol* 1986;4:234.
46. Smalley RV, Andersen JW, Hawkins MJ, et al. Interferon α combined with cytotoxic chemotherapy for patients with non-Hodgkin's lymphoma. *N Engl J Med* 1992;327:1335.
47. Solal-Céligny P, LePage E, Brousse N, et al. Recombinant interferon α-2b combined with a regimen containing doxorubicin in patients with advanced follicular lymphoma. *N Engl J Med* 1993;329:1608.
48. Mazza P, Tura S, Bocchia M, et al. Alpha-2b recombinant interferon (Intron) in Hodgkin's lymphoma: therapeutic perspective. *Eur J Haematol* 1990;45(S10):17.
49. Jones RJ, Ambinder RF, Piantadosi S, Santos GW. Evidence of a graft versus lymphoma effect associated with allogeneic bone marrow transplantation. *Blood* 1991;77:649.
50. Nagler A, Ackerstein A, Or R, Naparstek E, Slavin S. Immunotherapy with recombinant human interleukin-2 and recombinant interferon-α in lymphoma patients postautologous marrow or stem cell transplantation. *Blood* 1997;89:3951.
51. Atzpodien J, Korfer A, Franks CR, Poliwoda H, Kirchner H. Home therapy with recombinant interleukin-2 and interferon-α2b in advanced human malignancies. *Lancet* 1990;335:1509.
52. Ehrlich P. The relations existing between chemical constitution, distribution, and pharmacological action. In: Himmelweite F, Marquardt M, Dale Sir Henry, eds. *The collected papers of Paul Ehrlich,* vol I. Oxford, London, New York: Pergamom Press, 1956:596.
53. Tedder TF, Engel P. CD20: a regulator of cell-cycle progression and B-lymphocytes. *Immunol Today* 1994;15:450.
54. Yao XR, Scott DW. Expression of protein tyrosine kinases in the Ig complex of anti-mu-sensitive and anti-mu-resistant B-cell lymphomas: role of the p55blk kinase in signaling growth arrest and apoptosis. *Immunol Rev* 1993;132:163.
55. Maloney D, Grillo-López A, White C, et al. IDEC-C2B8 (rituximab) anti-CD20 monoclonal antibody therapy in patients with relapsed low-grade non-Hodgkin's lymphoma. *Blood* 1997;90:2188.
56. Österborg A, Fassa A, Agnostopoulos A, et al. Humanized CD52 monoclonal antibody Campath-1H as first-line treatment in chronic lymphocytic leukemia. *Br J Haematol* 1996;93:151.
57. Österborg A, Dyer M, Bunjes M, et al. Phase II multicenter study of human CD52 antibody in previously treated chronic lymphocytic leukemia. *J Clin Oncol* 1997;15:1567.
58. Engert A, Burrows F, Jung W, et al. Evaluation of ricin-A chain-containing immunotoxins directed against the CD30 antigen as potential reagents for the treatment of Hodgkin's disease. *Cancer Res* 1990;50:84.
59. Engert A, Martin G, Amlot P, et al. Immunotoxins constructed with anti-CD25 monoclonal antibodies and deglycosylated ricin A-chain have potent anti-tumour effects against human Hodgkin cells in vitro and solid Hodgkin tumours in mice. *Int J Cancer* 1991;49,450.
60. Horn-Lohrens O, Tiemann M, Lange H, et al. Shedding of the soluble form of CD30 from the Hodgkin-analogous cell line L540 is strongly inhibited by a new CD30-specific antibody (Ki-4). *Int J Cancer* 1995; 60:539.
61. Schnell R, Linnartz C, Katouzi AA, et al. Development of new ricin-A chain immunotoxins with potent anti-tumor effects against human Hodgkin cells in vitro and disseminated Hodgkin tumors in SCID mice using high-affinity monoclonal antibodies directed against the CD30 antigen. *Int J Cancer* 1995;63:238.
62. Endo Y, Tsurugi K. RNA N-glycosidase activity of ricin-A chain. Mechanism of action of the toxic lectin ricin on eukaryotic ribosome. *J Biol Chem* 1987;262:8128.
63. Lewis MS, Youle RJ. Ricin subunit association. Thermodynamics and the role of the disulfide bond in toxicity. *J Biol Chem* 1986;261:11571.
64. Eiklid K, Olsnes S, Phil A. Entry of lethal doses of abrin, ricin and modeccin into the cytosol of HeLa cells. *Exp Cell Res* 1980;126:321.
65. Byers VS, Baldwin RW. Therapeutic strategies with monoclonal antibodies and immunoconjugates. *Immunology* 1988;65:329.
66. Knowles PP, Thorpe PE. Purification of immunotoxins containing ricin A-chain and abrin A-chain using Blue Sepharose CL-6B. *Ann Biochem* 1987;160:440.
67. Thorpe PE, Detre SI, Foxwell BMJ, et al. Modification of the carbohydrate in ricin with metaperiodate-cyanoborohydride mixtures. Effects on toxicity and *in vivo* distribution. *Eur J Biochem* 1985;147:197.
68. Thorpe PE, Wallace PM, Knowles PP, et al. New coupling agents for the synthesis of immunotoxins containing a hindered disulphide bond with improved stability *in vivo. Cancer Res* 1987;47:5924.
69. Fulton RJ, Uhr JW, Vitetta ES. *In vivo* therapy of BCL_1 tumor: effect of immunotoxin valency and deglycosylation of the ricin-A chain. *Cancer Res* 1988;48:2626.
70. Engert A, Gottstein C, Winkler U, et al. Experimental treatment of human Hodgkin's disease with ricin A-chain immunotoxins. *Leuk Lymph* 1994;13:441.
71. Engert A, Martin G, Pfreundschuh M, et al. Antitumor effects of ricin A-chain immunotoxins prepared from intact antibodies and Fab′ fragments on solid human Hodgkin's disease tumors in mice. *Cancer Res* 1990;50:2929.
72. Strauchen JA, Breakstone BA. IL-2 receptor expression in human lymphoid lesions. Immunohistochemical study of 166 cases. *Am J Pathol* 1987;126:506.
73. Winkler U, Gottstein C, Schön G, et al. Successful treatment of disseminated human Hodgkin's disease in SCID mice with deglycosylated ricin A-chain immunotoxins. *Blood* 1994;83:466.
74. Engert A, Gottstein C, Bohlen H, et al. Cocktails of ricin A-chain immunotoxins against different antigens on Hodgkin and Sternberg-Reed cells have superior effects against H-RS cells in vitro and solid Hodgkin's tumors in mice. *Int J Cancer* 1995;63:304.
75. Engert A, Diehl V, Schnell R, et al. A Phase-I study of an anti-CD25 ricin A-chain immunotoxin (RFT5-SMPT-dgA) in patients with refractory Hodgkin's lymphoma. *Blood* 1997;89:403.
76. Pasqualucci L, Wasik M, Teicher BA, et al. Antitumor activity of anti-CD30 immuntoxin (Ber-H2/saporin) *in vitro* and in severe combined immunodeficiency disease mice xenografted with human $CD30^+$ anaplastic large-cell lymphoma. *Blood* 1995;85:2139.
77. Falini B, Bolognesi A, Flenghi L, et al. Response of refractory Hodgkin's disease to monoclonal anti-CD30 immunotoxin. *Lancet* 1992;339:1195.
78. Falini B, Pasqualucci L, Flenghi L, et al. Anti-CD30 immunotoxins: experimental and clinical studies (Abstract). In: *Abstracts of the*

Fourth International Symposium on Immunotoxins, Myrtle Beach, SC, June 8–14, 1991:160.

79. Terenzi A, Bolognesi A, Pasqualucci L, et al. Anti-CD30 (Ber-H2) immunotoxins containing the type-1 ribosome-inactivating proteins momordin and PAP-S (pokeweed antiviral protein from seeds) display powerful antitumour activity against CD30+ tumour cells in vitro and in SCID mice. *Br J Haematol* 1996;92:872.
80. Bolognesi A, Stirpe F, Conte R, et al. Anti-CD30 immunotoxins with native or recombinant dianthin 30. *Cancer Immunol Immunother* 1995; 40:109.
81. FitzGerald D, Pastan I. Targeted toxin therapy for the treatment of cancer. *J Natl Cancer Inst* 1989;81:1455.
82. Kreitman RJ, Pastan I. Recombinant toxins. *Adv Pharmacol* 1994; 28:193.
83. LeMaistre CF, Meneghetti C, Rosenblum M, et al. Phase I trial of an interleukin-2 (IL-2) fusion toxins ($DAB_{486}IL$-2) in hematologic malignancies expressing the IL-2 receptor. *Blood* 1992;79:2547.
84. Tepler I, Schwartz G, Parker K, et al. Phase I trial of an interleukin-2 fusion toxin ($DAB_{486}IL$-2) in hematologic malignancies: complete response in a patient with Hodgkin's disease refractory to chemotherapy. *Cancer* 1994;73:1276.
85. Foss F, Nichols J, Parker K, Seragen Lymphoma Study Group. Phase I/II trial of DAB389IL-2 in patients with NHL, HD and CTCL (Abstract). In: *Abstracts of the Fourth International Symposium on Immunotoxins,* Myrtle Beach, SC, June 8–14, 1994:159.
86. Riechmann L, Clark M, Waldmann H, et al. Reshaping human antibodies for therapy. *Nature* 1988;332:323.
87. Lonberg N, Taylor LD, Harding FA, et al. Antigen-specific human antibodies from mice comprising four distinct genetic modifications. *Nature* 1994;368:856.
88. Barbas III CF, Amberg W, Simonesits A, et al. Selection of human antihapten antibodies from semisynthetic libraries. *Gene* 1993;137:57.
89. Barth S, Huhn M, Wels W, Diehl V, Engert A. Construction and in vitro evaluation of RFT5(scFc)-ETA′, a new recombinant single-chain immunotoxin with specific cytotoxicity toward $CD25^+$ Hodgkin-derived cell lines. *Int J Mol Med* 1998;1:249.
90. Wels W, Harwerth IM, Müller M, et al. Selective inhibition of tumor cell growth by a recombinant single-chain antibody-toxin specific for the erbB-2 receptor. *Cancer Res* 1992;52:6310.
91. Klimka A, Barth S, Matthey B, et al. The new recombinant immunotoxin Ki-4(scFv)-ETA′ shows specific cytotoxicity against CD30-positive Hodgkin lymphoma cells. *Onkologie* 1997;20(suppl I):405a(abst).
92. Klimka A, Barth S, Drillich S, et al. A deletion mutant of Pseudomonas exotoxin-A fused to recombinant human interleukin-9 (rhIL-9-ETA′) shows specific cytotoxicity against IL-9-receptor-expressing cell lines. *Cyto Mol Ther* 1996;2:139.
93. Francisco JA, Schreiber GJ, Comereski CR, et al. *In vivo* efficacy and toxicity of a single-chain immunotoxin targeted to CD40. *Blood* 1997; 89:4493.
94. Nourigat C, Badger CC, Bernstein ID. Treatment of lymphoma with radiolabeled antibody: elimination of tumor cells lacking target antigen. *J Natl Cancer Inst* 1990;82:47.
95. O'Donoghue JA. The impact of tumor cell proliferation in radioimmunotherapy. *Cancer* 1994;73:974.
96. Eary JF, Krohn KA, Kishore R, Nelp WB. Radiochemistry halogenated antibodies. In: Zalutsky M, ed. *Antibodies in radiodiagnosis and therapy.* Boca Raton, FL: CRC Press, 1989:84.
97. Rhodes BA, Zamora PA, Newell KD, et al. Tc-99m labeling of murine monoclonal antibody fragments. *J Nucl Med* 1986;27:685.
98. Zimmer AM, Spies SM. New approaches to radiolabeling monoclonal antibodies. In: Rosen ST, Kuzel TM, eds. *Immunoconjugate therapy of hematologic malignancies.* Amsterdam: Kluwer Academic, 1993:100.
99. John E, Thakur ML, DeFulvio J, McDevitt, Damjanov I. Rhenium-186-labeled monoclonal antibodies for radioimmunotherapy: preparation and evaluation. *J Nucl Med* 1993;34:260.
100. Beierwaltes WH. Radioiodine-labelled compounds previously or currently used for tumour localization, in Agency IAE. In: Beierwaltes WH, ed. *Proceedings of an advisory group meeting on tumour localization with radioactive agents.* Panel Proceedings Series. Vienna, Austria: International Atomic Energy Agency, 1974:47.
101. Lenhard RE, Order SE, Spunberg JJ, et al. A new systemic therapy for advanced Hodgkin's disease. *J Clin Oncol* 1985;3:1296.
102. Order SE, Porter M, Hellmann S. Evidence for a tumor associated antigen. *N Engl J Med* 1971;285:471.
103. Herpst JM, Klein JL, Leichner PK, et al. Survival of patients with resistant Hodgkin's disease after polyclonal yttrium-90 labeled antiferritin treatment. *J Clin Oncol* 1995;13:2394.
104. Carde P, Da Costa L, Manil L, et al. Immunoscintigraphy of Hodgkin's disease: in vivo use of radiolabelled monoclonal antibodies derived from Hodgkin cell lines. *Eur J Cancer* 1990;26:474.
105. Da Costa L, Carde P, Lumbroso JD, et al. Immunoscintigraphy in Hodgkin's disease and anaplastic large cell lymphoma: results in 18 patients using the iodine radiolabeled monoclonal antibody HRS-3. *Ann Oncol* 1992;3(S4):53.
106. Winkler U, Stein H, Scheidhauer K, et al. Radioimmunoconjugates for the therapy of Hodgkin's lymphoma: preliminary data of a clinical study using the anti-CD30 antibody 99mTc-BerH2 (Abstract). *Leuk Lymphoma,* 1998;29:115.
107. Vriesendorp HM, Herpst JM, Germack MA, et al. Phase I-II studies of yttrium-labeled anti-ferritin treatment for end-stage Hodgkin's disease, including Radiation Therapy Oncology Group 87-01. *J Clin Oncol* 1991;9:918.
108. Press OW, Eary J, Badger CC, et al. High-dose radioimmunotherapy of lymphomas. In: Rosen ST, Kuzel TM, eds. *Immunoconjugate therapy of hematologic malignancies.* Amsterdam: Kluwer Academic, 1993:13.
109. DeNardo GL, DeNardo SJ, Lamborn KR, et al. Enhancement of tumor uptake of monoclonal antibody in nude mice with PEG-IL-2. *Antibodies Immunoconj Radiopharm* 1991;4:859.
110. Milstein C, Cuello AC. Hybrid hybridomas and their use in immunohistochemistry. *Nature* 1983; 305:537.
111. Perez P, Hoffman RW, Shaw S. Specific targeting of cytotoxic T cells by anti-T3 conjugates. *Nature* 1985;316:354.
112. June CH, Ledbetter JA, Linsley P, Thompson CB. Role of the CD28 receptor in T-cell activation. *Immunol Today* 1990;11:211.
113. Segal DM, Garrido MA, Perez P, et al. Targeted cytotoxic cells as a novel form of cancer immunotherapy. *Mol Immunol* 1988;25:1099.
114. Pohl C, Denfeld R, Renner C, et al. CD30-antigen-specific targeting and activation of T cells via murine bispecific monoclonal antibodies against CD3 and CD28: potential use for the treatment of Hodgkin's lymphoma. *Int J Cancer* 1993;54:820.
115. Renner C, Ohnesorge S, Held G, et al. T cells from patients with Hodgkin's disease have a defective T-cell receptor ζ chain expression that is reversible by T-cell stimulation with CD3 and CD28. *Blood* 1996;88:236.
116. Romeo C, Amiot M, Seed B. Sequence requirements for induction of cytolysis by the T cell antigen/Fc receptor ζ chain. *Cell* 1992;69:889.
117. Sussman JJ, Bonifacino JS, Lippincott-Schwartz J, et al. Failure to synthesize the T cell CD3 ζ chain: structure and function of a partial T cell receptor complex. *Cell* 1988;52:85.
118. Renner C, Jung W, Sahin U, et al. Cure of xenografted human tumors by bispecific monoclonal antibodies and human T cells. *Science* 1994; 264:833.
119. Renner C, Bauer S, Sahin U, et al. Cure of disseminated xenografted human Hodgkin's tumors by bispecific monoclonal antibodies and human T cells: the role of human T-cell subsets in a preclinical model. *Blood* 1996;87:2930.
120. Fanger MW, Shen L, Grazaino RF, Guyre PM. Cytotoxicity mediated by human Fc receptors for IgG. *Immunol Today* 1989;10:92.
121. Hombach A, Jung W, Pohl C, et al. A CD16/CD30 bispecific monoclonal antibody induces lysis of Hodgkin's cells by unstimulated natural killer cells in vitro and in vivo. *Int J Cancer* 1993;55:830.
122. Sahin U, Kraft-Bauer S, Ohnesorge S, et al. Interleukin-12 increases bispecific-antibody-mediated natural killer cell cytotoxicity against human tumors. *Cancer Immunol Immunother* 1996;42:9.
123. Wallace PK, Howell AL, Fanger MW. Role of Fcg receptors in cancer and infectious disease. *J Leukoc Biol* 1994;55:816.
124. Trinchieri G. Interleukin-12 and its role in the generation of Th_1 cells. *Immunol Today* 1993; 14:335.
125. Kornacker M, Tso J, Weiner G, Negrin R. Anti-CD3 x anti-1D10 bispecific antibody enhances cytotoxicity of cytokine induced killer cells against Hodgkin's derived cells (Abstract). *Leuk Lymphoma* 1998;29: 116.
126. Hartmann F, Renner C, Jung W, et al. Treatment of refractory Hodgkin's disease with an anti-CD16/CD30 bispecific antibody. *Blood* 1997; 89:2042.
127. Mack M, Riethmüller G, Kufer P. A small bispecific antibody construct expressed as a functional single-chain molecule with high tumor cell cytotoxicity. *Proc Natl Acad Sci USA* 1995;92:7021.
128. Holliger P, Prospero T, Winter G: Diabodies: small bivalent and bispecific antibody fragments. *Proc Natl Acad Sci USA* 1993;90:6444.

129. Shen GL, Li JL, Ghetie MA, et al. Evaluation of four CD22 antibodies as ricin A-chain-containing immunotoxins for the in vivo therapy of human B-cell leukemias and lymphomas. *Int J Cancer* 1988;42:792.
130. Thorpe PE.Antibody carriers of cytotoxic agents in cancer therapy: a review. In: Pinchera A, Doria G, Dammacco F, Bargellesi A, eds. *Monoclonal antibodies 84:* biological and clinical applications. Milan, Italy: Editrice Kurtis S.R.I., 1985:475.
131. Vitetta ES, Fulton RJ, May RD, Till M, Uhr J. Redesigning nature's poisons to create anti-tumor agents. *Science* 1987;238:1098.
132. Senter PD, Saulnier MG, Schreiber GJ, et al. Anti-tumor effects of antibody alkaline phosphatase conjugates in combination with etoposide phosphate. *Proc Natl Acad Sci USA* 1988;85:4842.
133. Senter PD, Schreiber GJ, Hirschberg DL, Ashe SA, Hellström KE, Hellström I. Enhancement of the *in vitro* and *in vivo* antitumor activities of phosphorylated mitomycin and etoposide derivatives by monoclonal antibody-alkaline phosphatase conjugates. *Cancer Res* 1988;49:5789.
134. Bagshawe KD, Springer CJ, Searle F, et al. A cytotoxic agent can be generated selectively at cancer sites. *Br J Cancer* 1988;58:700.
135. Sahin U, Hartmann F, Senter P, et al. Specific activation of the prodrug mitomycin phosphate by a bispecific anti-CD30/anti-alkaline phosphatase monoclonal antibody. *Cancer Res* 1990;50:6944.
136. Burrows FJ, Watanabe Y, Thorpe PE. A murine model for antibody-directed targeting of vascular endothelial cells in solid tumors. *Cancer Res* 1992;52:5954.
137. Huang X, Molema G, King S, Watkins L, Edgington TS, Thorpe PE.Tumor infarction in mice by antibody-directed targeting of tissue factor to tumor vasculature. *Science* 1997;275:547.
138. Schiefer D, Huang X, Trieu V, et al. Enhanced expression of endoglin on blood vessels of human Hodgkin's lymphoma xenografted in SCID mice. *Ann Hematol* 1995;73(suppl 2):707a(abst).
139. Burrows F, Derbyshire EJ, Tazzari PL, et al. Up-regulation of endoglin on vascular endothelial cells in human solid tumors:implications for diagnosis and therapy. *Clin Cancer Res* 1995;1:1623.
140. Greene MI. Cellular and genetic basis of immune reactivity to tumor cells. *Contemp Top Mol Immunol* 1980;11:81.
141. Howie SM, McBride WH. Tumor-specific T-helper activity can be abrogated by two distinct suppressor-cell mechanisms. *Eur J Immunol* 1982;12:671.
142. Gause A, Pohl C, DaCosta L, et al. Clinical significance of soluble CD30 antigen in the sera of patients with Hodgkin's lymphoma. *Blood* 1991;77:1983.
143. Jerne N. Towards a network theory of the immune system. *Ann Immunol* 1974;125:373.
144. Herlyn D, Wettendorf M, Schmoll HJ, et al. Anti-idiotype immunization of cancer patients. Modulation of the immune response. *Proc Natl Acad Sci USA* 1987;84:8055.
145. Ferrone S, Chen ZJ, Yang H, et al. Active specific immunotherapy with murine anti-idiotype monoclonal antibodies which bear the internal image of the human high molecular weight melanoma-associated antigen (HMW-MAA). *Proc Am Assoc Cancer Res* 1990;31:474.
146. Hsu S-M, Ho Y-S, Hsu P-L. Effect of monoclonal antibodies anti-2H9, anti-IRac, and anti-HeFi-1 on the surface antigens of Reed-Sternberg cells. *J Natl Cancer Inst* 1987;79:1091.
147. Pohl C, Sieber M, Diehl V, Pfreundschuh M. Idiotype vaccine against Hodgkin's lymphoma: generation and characterization of an anti-idiotypic monoclonal antibody against the Hodgkin-associated (anti-CD30) monoclonal antibody HRS-3. *Anticancer Res* 1991;11: 1115.
148. Pohl C, Renner C, Schwonzen M, et al. Anti-idiotype vaccine against Hodgkin's lymphoma: induction of B- and T-cell immunity across species barriers against CD30 antigen by murine monoclonal internal image antibodies. *Int J Cancer* 1992;50:958.
149. Pohl C, Renner C, Schwonzen M, et al. CD30-specific Ab1-Ab2-Ab3 internal image antibody network: potential use as anti-idiotype vaccine against Hodgkin's lymphoma. *Int J Cancer* 1993;54:418.
150. Schober I, Renner C, Pfreundschuh M, Diehl V, Pohl C. Mimicry of the Hodgkin-associated IRac antigen by an anti-idiotype network: potential use in active immunotherapy of Hodgkin's lymphoma. *Leuk Lymph* 1994;13:429.
151. Sallusto F, Lanzavecchia A. Efficient presentation of soluble antigen by cultured human dendritic cells is maintained by granocyte/macrophage colony stimulating factor plus interleukin-4 and downregulated by tumor necrosis factor alpha. *J Exp Med* 1994;179:1109.
152. Hsu FJ, Benike C, Fangoni F, et al. Vaccination of patients with B-cell lymphoma using autologous antigen-pulsed dendritic cells. *Nature Med* 1996;2:52.
153. Hunkapiller T, Hood LE. Diversity of the immunoglobulin gene superfamily. *Adv Immunol* 1989;44:1.
154. Hombach A, Heuser C, Sircar R, et al. The anti-CD30/FcgRIII chimeric receptor mediates MHC- and CD3-ζ independent T-cell activation against Hodgkin's lymphoma cells. *Cancer Res* 1998;58:1116.
155. Lustgarten J, Eshhar Z. Specific elimination of IgE production using T cell lines expressing chimeric T-cell receptor genes. *Eur J Immunol* 1995;25:2985.
156. Hwu P, Yang J, Eshhar Z, Rosenberg S. The genetic modification of T cells for cancer therapy: preclinical and clinical studies. *Cancer Gene Ther* 1994;1:136.
157. Weijtens M, Willemsen R, Valerio D, Stam K, Bolhuis R. Single chain Ig/g gene-redirected human T-lymphocytes produce cytokines, specifically lyse tumor cells, and recycle lytic capacity. *J Immunol* 1996; 157:836.
158. Rosenberg S. The immunotherapy and gene therapy of cancer. *J Clin Oncol* 1992;10:180.
159. Weiss LM, Movahed LA, Warnke RA, Sklar J. Detection of Epstein Barr virus genomes in Reed-Sternberg cells of Hodgkin's disease. *N Engl J Med* 1989;320:502.
160. Haluska FG, Brufsky AM, Canellos GP. The cellular biology of the Reed-Sternberg cell. *Blood* 1994;89:1005.
161. Heslop HE, Brenner MK, Rooney CM, et al. Long-term restoration of immunity against Epstein-Barr virus infection by adoptive transfer of gene-modified virus specific T-lymphocytes. *Nature Med* 1996;2:551.
162. Rooney CM, Smith CA, Nab C, et al. Use of gene-modified virus-specific T lymphocytes to control Epstein-Barr virus-related lymphoproliferation. *Lancet* 1995;345:9.
163. Roskrow M, Suzuki N, Gan Y, et al. EBV-specific cytotoxic T lymphocytes for the treatment of patients with EBV-positive relapsed Hodgkin disease. *Blood* 1998;91:2925.
164. Romani N, Gruner S, Brang D, et al. Proliferating dendritic cell progenitors in human blood. *J Exp Med* 1994;180:83.
165. Roskrow MA, Suzuki N, Brenner MK, Rooney CM. Genetically modified dendritic cells generate primary and memory tumor antigen specific cytotoxic T lymphocytes. *Blood* 1996;88(suppl 1):a(abst).
166. Griffiths AD, Williams SC, Hartley O, et al. Isolation of high affinity human antibodies directly from large synthetic repertoires. *EMBO J* 1994;13:45.
167. Klimka A, Roovers RC, Barth S, et al. Human anti-CD30 phage antibody by guided selection for immunotherapy of Hodgkin's lymphoma (Abstract). *Leuk Lymphoma* 1998;29:112
168. Zewe M, Rybak SM, Dubel S, et al. Cloning and cytotoxicity of a human pancreatic RNase immunofusion. *Immunotechnology* 1997;3;127.
169. Marasco WA. Intrabodies: turning the humoral immune system outside in for intracellular immunization. *Gene Ther* 1997;4:11.
170. Richardson JH, Sodroski JG, Waldmann TA, Marasco WA. Phenotype knockout of the high-affinity human interleukin 2 receptor by intracellular single-chain antibodies against the alpha subunit of the receptor. *Proc Natl Acad Sci USA* 1995;92:3137.
171. Mulligan RC. The basic science of gene therapy. *Science* 1993;260:926.
172. Rollins BJ, Sunday ME. Suppression of tumor formation in vivo by expression of the JE gene in malignant cells. *Mol Cell Biol* 1991;11: 3125.
173. Huber BE, Richards CA, Austin EA. Virus-directed enzyme/prodrug therapy (VDEPT). Selectively engineering drug sensitivity into tumors. *Ann NY Acad Sci* 1994;716:104.
174. Mullen CA, Kilstrup R, Blaese M. Transfer of the bacterial gene for cytosine deaminase to mammalian cells confers lethal sensitivity to 5′-fluorocytosine: a negative selection system. *Proc Natl Acad Sci USA* 1992;89:33.
175. Huber BE, Austin EA, Good SS, Knick VC, Tibbels S, Richards CA. In vivo antitumor activity of 5-fluorocytosine on human colorectal carcinoma cells genetically modified to express cytosine deaminase. *Cancer Res* 1993;52:4619.
176. Yang AG, Chen SY. A new class of antigen-specific killer cells. *Nature Biotech* 1997;15:46.
177. Lim SH, Worman CP, Callaghan T, et al. Continuous intravenous infusion of high-dose recombinant interleukin-2 for advanced lymphomas. A phase II study. *Leuk Res* 1991;15:435.
178. Gisselbrecht C, Maraninchi D, Pico JL, et al. Interleukin-2 treatment in lymphoma: a phase II multicenter study. *Blood* 1994;83:2081.

SECTION VI

Selection of Treatment

Hodgkin's Disease, edited by P. M. Mauch,
J. O. Armitage, V. Diehl, R. T. Hoppe, and L. M. Weiss.
Lippincott Williams & Wilkins, Philadephia ©1999.

CHAPTER 25

Treatment of Favorable Prognosis, Stage I–II Hodgkin's Disease

Peter M. Mauch, Joseph M. Connors, Santiago Pavlovsky, and Eckhart Dühmke

Vera Peters (1), in 1950, was the first physician to present definitive evidence of the curability of early-stage Hodgkin's disease. Prior to that time Hodgkin's disease invariably had been considered a fatal illness. Treatment was mainly palliative—given to patients with advanced disease to shrink large nodes that were painful or that interfered with movement, eating, or breathing. Limited disease was not treated at all, or only with small doses of radiation.

Peters reviewed the records of 113 patients treated at the Ontario Institute of Radiotherapy from 1924 to 1942 and reported 5-year and 10-year survival rates of 88% and 79%, respectively, for patients with stage I Hodgkin's disease. The similar 5- and 10-year survival rates demonstrated that patients with limited Hodgkin's disease could be cured with an aggressive treatment approach using high doses of fractionated radiation therapy. The 10-year survival rates were only 21% and 0%, respectively, for patients with stage II and III disease; nonetheless, the results achieved in stage I led to optimism for the eventual development of techniques to cure patients with more advanced disease.

In Peters' report, patients with favorable prognosis early-stage Hodgkin's disease (i.e., those patients likely to be cured with radiation therapy) had disease limited to a single lymph node region of involvement. Over the years the definition of favorable prognosis early-stage Hodgkin's disease has been modified as a result of new classification systems for histologic subtyping (2) and staging (3), advances in radiographic and surgical staging (bipedal lymphangiography and staging laparotomy) (4,5), improvements in radiation therapy equipment that allow treatment with higher doses and larger radiation fields, and the development of effective and eventually safer multiagent chemotherapy regimens. Although clinical practice had based the amount of treatment on stage and extent of disease since the late 1960s, the concept of identifying prognostic factors, often independent of stage, to determine or modify treatment is a relatively new concept that has been employed only in the 1980s and 1990s.

This chapter discusses current approaches to the staging and treatment of favorable prognosis stage I–II Hodgkin's disease. The following chapter, by Hoppe et al., discusses current approaches to the staging and treatment of unfavorable prognosis stage I–II. Both chapters examine the role of radiation field size and dose, the use of chemotherapy alone, and approaches with combined chemotherapy and radiation therapy. Prognostic factors and their influence on treatment and outcome, factors for development of late complications, and details of ongoing clinical trials are also evaluated.

P. M. Mauch: Department of Radiation Oncology, Brigham and Women's Hospital and Dana-Farber Cancer Institute, Harvard Medical School, Boston, Massachusetts.

J. M. Connors: Division of Medical Oncology, British Columbia Cancer Agency, University of British Columbia, Vancouver, British Columbia, Canada.

S. Pavlovsky: Angelica Ocampo Hospital and Research Center-Fundaleu, Buenos Aires, Argentina.

E. Dühmke: Department of Radiation and Radiation Oncology, Ludwig-Maximilians-Universität München, München, Germany.

RANDOMIZED CLINICAL TRIALS

Significant advances in the treatment of early-stage Hodgkin's disease have been derived from information obtained from clinical trials. These trials were first organized in the 1960s. Stanford University Medical School and the European Organization for the Research and Treatment of Cancer (EORTC) pioneered some of the first approaches in treating early-stage Hodgkin's disease, and many other groups made significant contributions. Recently, Specht and colleagues (6) reported on the influence of radiation field size and separately on the impact of adjuvant chemotherapy on long-term outcome in early stage disease in a metaanalysis of 23 randomized trials involving 3,888 patients. Some of these data had been analyzed in a previous metaanalysis by Shore and colleagues (7). Early Hodgkin's disease in these trials was defined as patients with clinically or laparotomy staged I–II disease, although in some cases patients with stage III disease were included. Patients with B symptoms and patients with extensive thoracic Hodgkin's disease were also included. Thus, these trials included patients with both favorable prognosis stage I–II Hodgkin's disease (discussed further in this chapter) and unfavorable prognosis stage I–II Hodgkin's disease (discussed further in the next chapter). The randomized trials were divided into two groups: eight trials compared more extensive radiation therapy to less extensive radiation therapy (8–17), and 13 trials compared multiagent chemotherapy and radiotherapy to radiotherapy alone (8,10,17–27). Individual patient data including age, stage, date of entry, treatment allocation, date of recurrence, and date and cause of death or date last seen were collected for each patient randomized.

Metaanalysis of Studies of More-Extensive Versus Less-Extensive Radiation Therapy

Eight trials evaluated treatment with larger versus smaller radiation field sizes (6). Larger fields generally included subtotal nodal (mantle and upper abdomen) or total nodal irradiation; smaller fields included involved fields or in some cases a mantle field (see Chapter 21 for definitions of field size). Although approximately half the trials showed a significant advantage in disease-free survival with larger-field compared to smaller-field irradiation, survival differences were not seen in any of the studies. Figure 1 shows the combined risk of failure and survival by treatment in the eight trials of more-extensive versus less-extensive radiation therapy. At 10 years, the risk of recurrence was 43.4% for patients treated with less-extensive radiation therapy compared to 31.3% for those treated with more-extensive radiation therapy (p <.00001). Similar results were seen in subgroup analyses by stage, by use of staging laparotomy, by age at diagnosis (less than 20, 20 to 39, and greater than or equal to 40), and by gender. For example, for patients with stage IA Hodgkin's disease, the risk of recurrence was 36.3% with less-extensive radiation therapy compared to 24.1% with more-extensive radiation therapy (p <.05); for stage

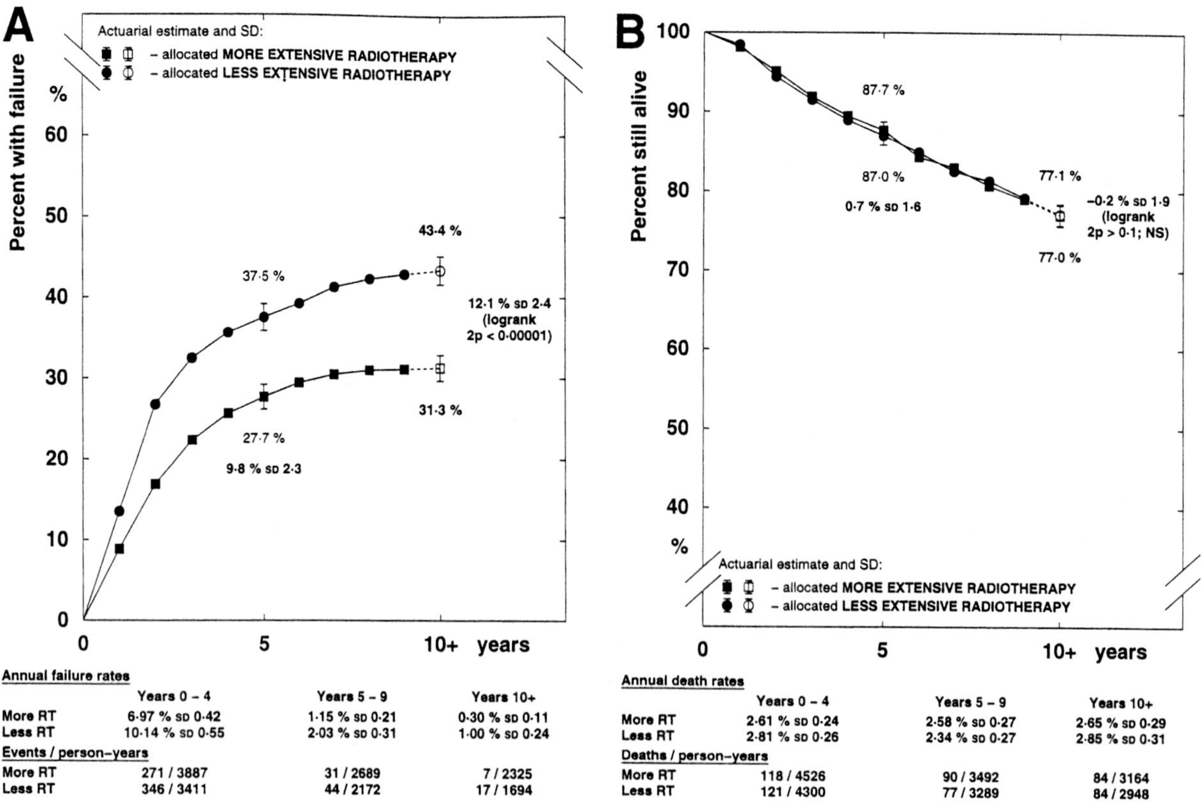

FIG. 1. The risk of failure **(A)** and survival **(B)** by treatment in the eight trials combined for more extensive versus less extensive radiation therapy. (From ref. 6, with permission.)

IIA Hodgkin's disease, the risk of recurrence was 43.5% and 33.6% for less-extensive and more-extensive radiation therapy, respectively (p <.05).

Ten-year actuarial survival rates were 77% for both groups (p >.1). The lack of a survival difference suggests that salvage chemotherapy for relapse after initial radiation therapy is effective enough to minimize the impact of any increase in relapse on survival. In addition, increased mortality from recurrent Hodgkin's disease in patients receiving smaller field irradiation appeared to be balanced by increased mortality from treatment-related causes (cardiac, second tumors) in patients receiving more extensive radiation therapy. Data from the metaanalysis supported this premise; the annual death rate for patients who died of causes other than Hodgkin's disease was 1.18% in the more-extensive radiation group compared to 0.89% in the less-extensive radiation group.

Metaanalysis of Studies of Multiagent Chemotherapy and Radiotherapy Versus Radiotherapy Alone

Thirteen trials compared treatment with multiagent chemotherapy and radiotherapy to radiotherapy alone for early stage Hodgkin's disease (6). Approximately half the individual trials showed a significant advantage in disease-free survival with combined chemotherapy and radiation therapy compared to radiation therapy alone; survival differences were not seen in any of the individual 13 studies. Figure 2 shows the combined risk of failure and survival by treatment for the 13 trials for multiagent chemotherapy and radiotherapy versus radiotherapy alone. At 10 years, the risk of recurrence was 32.7% for patients treated with radiation therapy alone and 15.8% for those treated with chemotherapy and radiation therapy (p <.00001). Similar results were seen by subgroup analysis. For stage IA Hodgkin's disease, the risk of recurrence was 20.4% for patients treated with radiation therapy alone compared to 11% for those treated with chemotherapy and radiation therapy; for stage IIA, the risk of recurrence was 27.9% with radiation therapy alone and 14.9% with chemotherapy and radiation therapy. For the population as a whole, the 10-year actuarial survival rates were 76.5% for patients treated with radiation therapy alone and 79.4% for those treated with chemotherapy and radiation therapy (p >.1). Cause-specific survival rates (i.e., only scoring death from Hodgkin's disease) were 84.6% at 10 years for patients treated with radiation therapy alone and 87.7% for those treated with chemotherapy and radiation therapy (p = .07). As in the trials of radiation field size, salvage chemotherapy for relapse after initial radiation therapy appeared to minimize the impact of any increase in relapse on survival. In addition, increased mortality from recurrent Hodgkin's

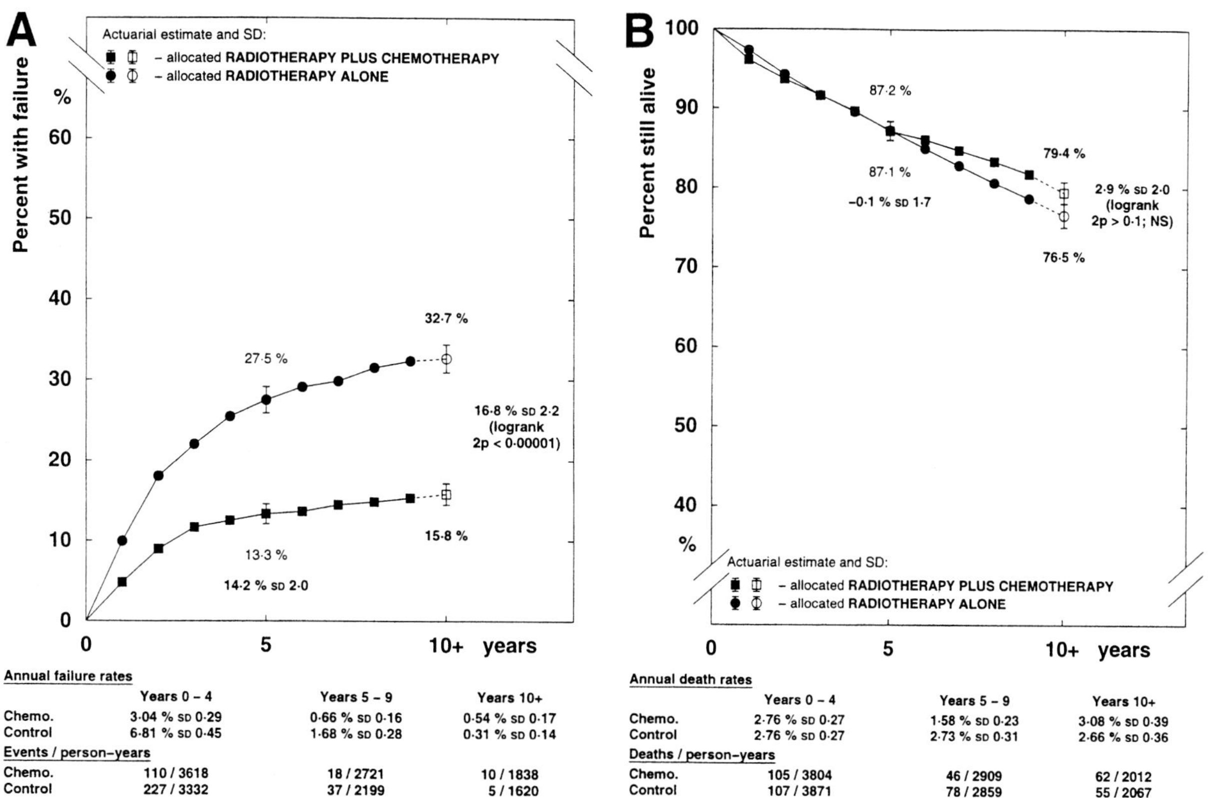

Annual failure rates	Years 0 – 4	Years 5 – 9	Years 10+
Chemo.	3·04 % SD 0·29	0·66 % SD 0·16	0·54 % SD 0·17
Control	6·81 % SD 0·45	1·68 % SD 0·28	0·31 % SD 0·14
Events / person–years			
Chemo.	110 / 3618	18 / 2721	10 / 1838
Control	227 / 3332	37 / 2199	5 / 1620

Annual death rates	Years 0 – 4	Years 5 – 9	Years 10+
Chemo.	2·76 % SD 0·27	1·58 % SD 0·23	3·08 % SD 0·39
Control	2·76 % SD 0·27	2·73 % SD 0·31	2·66 % SD 0·36
Deaths / person–years			
Chemo.	105 / 3804	46 / 2909	62 / 2012
Control	107 / 3871	78 / 2859	55 / 2067

FIG. 2. The risk of failure **(A)** and survival **(B)** by treatment for the 13 trials combined for multiagent chemotherapy and radiotherapy versus radiotherapy alone. (From ref. 6, with permission.)

disease in patients receiving radiation therapy alone was offset by increased mortality from treatment-related causes (cardiac, second tumors) in patients receiving initial radiation therapy and chemotherapy.

Most patients received alkylating agent chemotherapy [usually MOPP—mechlorethamine, Oncovin (vincristine), procarbazine, prednisone—or an equivalent] in the trials analyzed in the metaanalysis by Specht. Thus, these results may not always apply to current practice in which MOPP has been replaced by more effective treatment regimens such as ABVD (Adriamycin [doxorubicin], bleomycin, vinblastine, dacarbazine). However, longer follow-up is needed to determine the late efficacy and toxicity of ABVD and involved field irradiation in stage I–II Hodgkin's disease; early results suggest that it may be more efficacious and less toxic than alkylating agent regimens and radiation therapy.

There are a number of potential criticisms of the metaanalysis format. The quality of the data, including the details of cause of death and the length of follow-up, varies from center to center. In addition, definitions were not always consistent between studies. For example, in the more-extensive versus less-extensive radiation therapy studies, the size of the radiation therapy field varied greatly in both groups. In addition, the extent of staging differed (i.e., laparotomy versus no laparotomy), patients with more advanced stage (IIB–III) were included in some studies but not in others, and there was no randomization for bulk disease. Therefore, the influence of prognostic factors (i.e., dose, age, stage, bulk of disease, number of sites of disease) on outcome cannot be addressed by the metaanalysis. However, the analysis is a powerful and important tool in addressing the general question of how extent of treatment affects the disease-free and overall survival of patients. In all these trials, there is one consistent observation: more extensive treatment results in fewer recurrences, but does not affect long-term survival in stage I–II Hodgkin's disease.

PROGNOSTIC FACTORS

Prognostic factors such as age, size of nodal involvement, and presence of systemic symptoms help determine initial treatment strategies (see Chapter 19 for a more comprehensive review). Patients with stage I–II Hodgkin's disease with favorable prognostic factors are candidates for radiation therapy alone or for modified radiation therapy and chemotherapy (see subsequent discussion on clinical trials). Patients with unfavorable prognostic factors should receive chemotherapy and radiation therapy as initial treatment (see Chapter 26). Although many of the factors that have been identified have lost significance as more intensive combined radiation therapy and chemotherapy regimens have been used, these factors continue to be extremely important in the design of clinical trials that evaluate reduction of radiation therapy and chemotherapy for early-stage Hodgkin's disease.

Prognostic Factors in Laparotomy (Pathologically) Staged (PS) I–II Patients

Prognostic factors have been identified for stage I–II Hodgkin's disease that predict a higher risk of relapse or a lower rate of survival. Many factors predict recurrence after treatment with radiation therapy alone; fewer predict relapse after chemotherapy and radiation therapy. Only older age at diagnosis has been consistently reported as a significant adverse factor for survival, both after radiation therapy alone and after combined radiation therapy and chemotherapy (28).

Prognostic factors for patients with stage I–II Hodgkin's disease, identified in retrospective studies and adjusted for other factors, are listed in Tables 1 and 2. Table 1 lists results from three studies that have identified prognostic factors for laparotomy staged I–II patients (29–31). These studies present an analysis of significance adjusted for other factors. The first two studies evaluate PS IA–IIA patients treated with subtotal or total nodal irradiation alone. The study from the Danish National Study Group analyzed PS IA–IIB patients treated with either radiation therapy or combined chemotherapy and radiation therapy. All three studies report large mediastinal adenopathy or large tumor burden as the major factor predicting an increased risk of relapse. In neither the Stanford University nor the Harvard University (Joint Center for Radiation Therapy, JCRT) study did large mediastinal adenopathy predict a lower survival rate (29,30); patients with a large tumor burden had a lower survival rate in the Danish study (31). Age over 40 years was associated with a worse survival in the Harvard JCRT and Danish studies (30,31).

Retrospective studies also have consistently identified large mediastinal adenopathy as an adverse prognostic factor for relapse in PS IA–IIB patients treated with radiation therapy alone (29,32–41). The majority of recurrences in patients with extensive thoracic Hodgkin's disease are in lymph nodes or extranodal sites above the diaphragm (32,34–39,41,42). Routine thoracic computed axial tomographic scanning and gallium scanning have aided in determining initial treatment of patients with large mediastinal adenopathy (35,43–49). Patients with pericardial nodes, extensive pericardial involvement, bulky axillary disease, or significant involvement of the pleura or lung on radiographic evaluation have a high risk of relapse after radiation therapy alone. The potential toxicity associated with the large radiation volumes needed to treat extensive thoracic Hodgkin's disease argues for treatment with combination chemotherapy followed by involved-field or mantle irradiation (see chapter by Hoppe et al.). This approach eliminates the need for abdominal irradiation, allows for reduction of the field size and dose of radiation therapy,

TABLE 1. *Prognostic factors in PS I–II patients (p values adjusted for other factors)*

Study	Stage	Adverse factor	FFR	Survival
Stanford University (29) (109 patients, RT alone)	PS IA–IIA	LMA	$p = 0.002$	$p =$ NS
		STLI (vs. TLI)	$p = 0.04$	$p =$ NS
		No. of sites ≥4	$p =$ NS	$p =$ NS
Harvard University (JCRT) (30) (315 patients, RT alone)	PS IA–IIA	LMA	$p < 0.0001$	$p =$ NS
		Age ≥40	$p =$ NS	$p = 0.008$
		No. of sites	$p =$ NS	$p =$ NS
		Male sex	$p =$ NS	$p =$ NS
		MC/LD histology	$p =$ NS	$p = 0.001$
Danish National Study Group (31) (290 patients, RT or CMT)	PS I–II	Tumor burden	$p < .0001$	$p = 0.001$
		Age ≥40	$p =$ NS	$p = 0.04$
		RT alone	$p < .0001$	$p =$ NS
		MC/LD histology	—	$p =$ NS
		B symptoms	$p =$ NS	$p =$ NS
		Male sex	$p = 0.01$	$p =$ NS
		ESR ≥40	$p =$ NS	$p =$ NS
		No. of sites	$p =$ NS	$p =$ NS

PS, pathologic stage; RT, radiation therapy; FFR, freedom from relapse, also freedom from progression, or disease-free survival in some studies; CMT, combined radiation therapy and chemotherapy; LMA, large mediastinal adenopathy; STLI, subtotal nodal irradiation; TLI, total nodal irradiation; MC, mixed-cellularity histology; LD, lymphocyte-depletion histology; ESR, erythrocyte sedimentation rate; NS, no significant difference.
From ref. 28, with permission.

and results in a much improved freedom from recurrence compared to radiation therapy alone (41).

Patients 40 years of age or older appear to have a lower survival rate (but not a higher recurrence rate) than younger patients, both because older patients appear to be less successfully treated at relapse (50–53), and because they have a greater absolute excess risk of mortality from causes other than Hodgkin's disease, such as second tumors and cardiac disease (53–56). This argues for treatment strategies that minimize both the risk of recurrence and the risk of long-term complications in this group of patients. This may not be feasible until new, less toxic and more effective treatment approaches are developed.

Most reports also have identified B symptoms as an important factor for recurrence and survival. A large retrospective study combining data from PS IB–IIB patients treated at Stanford University Medical School and the Harvard JCRT suggested that patients with night sweats without other B symptoms treated with radiation therapy alone had a prognosis similar to that of patients with PS IA–IIA disease. However, the presence of fevers, weight loss, and large mediastinal adenopathy, and age 40 or older, all independently predicted an increased risk of

TABLE 2. *Prognostic factors in CS I–II patients (p values adjusted for other factors)*

Study	Stage	Adverse factor	FFR	Survival
EORTC (58) (1,392 patients, RT or CMT)	CS I–II	Male sex	$p = 0.006$	$p = 0.01$
		Age ≥40	$p =$ NS	$p < 0.0001$
		ESR ≥50(A) or ≥30(B)	$p < 0.0001$	$p =$ NS
		MC/LD histology	$p =$ NS	$p = 0.0006$
		No. of sites ≥4	$p < 0.0001$	$p = 0.005$
Princess Margaret Hospital (59) (250 patients, RT or CMT)	CS I–II	Age ≥50	$p = 0.0005$	$p = 0.0005$
		MC/LD histology	$p = 0.004$	$p = 0.08$
		No. of sites	$p =$ NS	$p =$ NS
		Male sex	$p =$ NS	$p =$ NS
		IF RT (vs. M/STLI)	$p = 0.024$	$p =$ NS
		ESR ≥40	$p = 0.001$	$p = 0.03$
Fundaleu (60) (277 patients, CT or CMT)	CS I–II	LMA	$p = 0.005$	$p < 0.001$
		Age ≥45	$p < 0.001$	$p < 0.001$
		No. of sites ≥3	$p < 0.001$	$p =$ NS

CS, clinical stage; RT, radiation therapy; FFR, freedom from relapse, also freedom from progression, or disease-free survival in some studies; CMT, combined radiation therapy and chemotherapy; LMA, large mediastinal adenopathy; STLI, subtotal nodal irradiation; M, mantle irradiation; MC, mixed-cellularity histology; LD, lymphocyte-depletion histology; ESR, erythrocyte sedimentation rate; NS, no significant difference.
From ref. 28, with permission.

relapse, and survival was impaired in patients who had both fevers and weight loss (57).

Thus, from studies of laparotomy-staged patients, tumor size, age, and systemic symptoms are all unfavorable prognostic factors for stage I–II Hodgkin's disease.

Prognostic Factors in Clinically Staged (CS) I–II Patients

The EORTC clinical trials and trials from the Princess Margaret Hospital and the Fundaleu have contributed greatly to our understanding of prognostic factors in clinically staged patients. Table 2 lists representative studies that have evaluated prognostic factors adjusted for other factors in clinically staged patients (58–60). Two of the three studies evaluated patients treated with either radiation therapy or combined radiation therapy and chemotherapy, and the third analyzed data from patients treated with chemotherapy or combined radiation therapy and chemotherapy. Adverse factors for relapse in these patients included male sex, large number of sites involved, age, high erythrocyte sedimentation rate (ESR), mixed-cellularity histology, involved field radiation therapy, and large mediastinal adenopathy. Other studies have also identified these adverse prognostic factors (61–63). Many of the factors, including B symptoms (similar to ESR), male sex, number of sites of involvement, and, to a lesser extent, age, also predict an increased risk of occult abdominal involvement in CS I–II patients (64,65). This may in part explain why some of these factors are identified for clinically staged, but not for laparotomy staged, patients.

Prognostic Factors Determine Treatment in Clinical Trials

Cooperative groups identify favorable (or very favorable) and unfavorable prognostic groups for different clinical trials. These prognostic factors predict likelihood of occult disease in the abdomen, and the effectiveness of treatment (usually radiation therapy alone) in maintaining a high level of freedom from recurrence (66). Prognostic factors for three large cohorts of patients from the Princess Margaret Hospital, the EORTC, and the combined Argentine Group for Treatment of Acute Leukemia (GATLA), and the Latin American Group for Treatment of Malignant Hemoplasias (GLATHEM) are discussed below.

Table 3 shows the prognostic factors for the Princess Margaret Hospital and the EORTC cohorts. At the Princess

TABLE 3. *Modern classification systems for clinically staged patients*

Institution	Prognostic features	Percentage of total patients
EORTC: *n* = 1,641 from H_1, H_2, H_5, and H_6 trials (58)	Very favorable CS I female Age <40 years No B symptoms ESR <50 mm LP or nodular sclerosis histology No bulky mediastinal involvement	6% of CS I and II supradiaphagmatic Hodgkin's disease
	Unfavorable Age >50 years No B symptoms with ESR >50, or B symptoms with ESR >30 Four or more involved sites Bulky mediastinal involvement, i.e., (M/T ratio >0.35)	40%
	Favorable All patients not in the previous two groups	54%
Princess Margaret Hospital: *n* = 250; retrospective experience >20 years of patients treated with radiation alone (59,67)	Favorable (group 2) No B symptoms Age ≤50 years ESR ≤40 Nodular sclerosis/LP histology No large mediastinal adenopathy (≥10 cm)	84% of CS I and II supradiaphagmatic Hodgkin's disease treated with radiation alone
	Very favorable (group 1) Favorable features and isolated upper cervical stage IA disease	10%
	Unfavorable (group 3) All patients not in the previous two groups	6%

ESR, erythrocyte sedimentation rate.
From ref. 66, with permission.

Margaret Hospital, patients with very favorable Hodgkin's disease, defined as stage I disease isolated to the upper cervical region, received limited radiation therapy alone (59,67). Patients with favorable disease (50 years old or younger, no B symptoms, an ESR of 40 or under, nodular sclerosis or lymphocyte-predominance histology, and without large mediastinal adenopathy) were treated with extended-field and splenic radiation therapy. Patients with unfavorable Hodgkin's disease (large mediastinal adenopathy, B symptoms, mixed-cellularity histology, age over 50, or an ESR over 40) received combined chemotherapy and radiation therapy.

Similar prognostic factors developed in the EORTC H_1, H_2, H_5, and H_6 trials have been used with some modification for treatment of patients in the H_7 and H_8 trials and in the design of the H_9 trial (68). A very favorable prognostic group consisted of CS IA female patients less than 40 years of age with an ESR under 50, no B symptoms, no large mediastinal adenopathy, and nodular sclerosis or lymphocyte-predominance histology. This group of patients, expected to have a very low risk of occult abdominal involvement (5%), was treated on a single arm prospective trial with mantle irradiation alone without a staging laparotomy in both the H_7 and H_8 trials (results are discussed below).

Favorable prognosis patients (defined in the EORTC H_7 and H_8 trials as age 50 or under, without large mediastinal adenopathy, with an ESR of less than 50 and no B symptoms or an ESR of less than 30 with B symptoms, and with disease limited to one to three regions of involvement) were treated either with modified chemotherapy and radiation therapy or with extended-field radiation therapy alone. In the EORTC H_7F trial, CS I–II patients in the favorable group were randomized to receive either six cycles of modified chemotherapy (EBVP II; epirubicin, bleomycin, vinblastine, and prednisone) (69) followed by involved-field irradiation or subtotal nodal (mantle and paraaortic fields) and splenic irradiation. In the H_8F trial, patients in the favorable group were randomized to receive either three cycles of hybrid MOPP/ABV and involved-field irradiation or subtotal nodal and splenic irradiation. Both these trials evaluated reduction of treatment (either modified chemotherapy or reduced number of cycles) in favorable prognosis patients.

Unfavorable prognosis patients (defined in the H_7 and H_8 trials as those having any one of the following features: large mediastinal adenopathy, four or more sites of involvement, B symptoms and an ESR over 30, an ESR over 50 without B symptoms, or age over 50) in the EORTC H_7UF trial were randomized to receive either six cycles of MOPP/ABV (70) followed by involved-field irradiation, or six cycles of EBVP and involved-field irradiation. In the EORTC H_8UF trial CS I–II patients were randomized to receive six cycles of hybrid MOPP/ABV and involved-field irradiation, or four cycles of hybrid MOPP/ABV and involved-field irradiation, or four cycles of hybrid MOPP/ABV and subtotal nodal irradiation (see chapter by Hoppe et al.).

Similar prognostic factors were defined in a combined GATLA/GLATHEM study. Two prognostic groups, treated with chemotherapy alone or chemotherapy plus radiotherapy, were analyzed using a Cox multivariate analysis. The favorable prognostic group included patients less than 46 years of age with fewer than three lymph node areas involved and no bulky adenopathy (peripheral lymph nodes less than 5 cm and mediastinal nodes less than 10 cm). The unfavorable group included patients with at least one of the following factors: older than 45 years of age, three or more lymph node regions involved, or the presence of bulky nodes (greater than 5 cm peripheral lymph nodes, greater than 10 cm mediastinal nodes, or a mediastinal mass greater than one-third of the widest thoracic diameter) (60).

RISK OF OCCULT ABDOMINAL INVOLVEMENT IN PATIENTS WITH CLINICAL STAGE I–II DISEASE

The probability of occult abdominal involvement must be factored into treatment approaches for patients with CS I–II disease. Approaches include surgical staging to rule out abdominal involvement, prophylactic upper abdominal and splenic irradiation, or sufficient combination chemotherapy to control occult abdominal involvement. About 20% to 30% of CS IA–IIA and 35% of CS IB–IIB patients with Hodgkin's disease have occult splenic or upper abdominal nodal involvement not detected by bipedal lymphangiography, computed axial tomography, magnetic resonance imaging, or gallium imaging (64,65). These radiographic studies have not been successful at visualizing Hodgkin's disease in the spleen and often miss nodal Hodgkin's disease in the upper abdomen (71), the two most common sites of involvement in patients with negative radiographic staging below the diaphragm (65) (see Chapters 17 and 18 for more detailed discussions on staging laparotomy).

Studies of the results of staging laparotomy have demonstrated that selected prognostic factors can predict the risk of occult abdominal involvement in CS I–II patients (64,65,72–74). Selected subgroups, making up approximately 20% of all CS I–II patients, including CS IA females, CS IA males with disease limited to the high neck, CS IA patients with interfollicular histology, and CS IA patients with lymphocyte-predominant histology, appear to be at lowest risk for occult abdominal involvement (4% to 6%). CS IIA females 26 years of age or younger with three or fewer regions involved, and CS IA males with mediastinal involvement also have been identified by some as having a low risk of abdominal involvement (64). The remainder of CS IIA and all CS IB–IIB patients remain at substantial risk for Hodgkin's disease in the spleen or abdominal nodes (24% to 36%) (64,65).

There have been a number of arguments for the continued use of staging laparotomy and splenectomy in the management of selected early-stage favorable prognosis patients with Hodgkin's disease. Although staging laparotomy has been abandoned in many parts of the world with the increasing use of chemotherapy in early-stage patients, staging laparotomy remains the most precise way to ascertain the presence and extent of abdominal involvement in patients with supradiaphragmatic presentations. It allows for reduction of the extent of radiation therapy and reduces the number of patients requiring chemotherapy (65). Laparotomy and splenectomy allow for the use of smaller radiation fields with less risk to the heart, lungs, and kidneys. In selected patients with early-stage disease, a negative laparotomy allows treatment with mantle field radiation alone (58,67,75–77). This approach requires only 4 to 5 weeks of treatment and provides disease-free and overall survival rates in selected patients similar to those of patients treated with more extensive radiation (58,67,75,77).

Many of the risks of routine staging laparotomy and splenectomy, including the discomfort and inconvenience of 3 to 5 days in the hospital, and the potential morbidity (subphrenic abscess, small bowel obstruction, wound infection) and mortality (postsurgical, bacterial sepsis), have been reduced with modern surgical techniques (64,65) and increasingly effective vaccines against encapsulated microorganisms (78–81). The development of polysaccharide-conjugate vaccines within the past 10 years has proven to be of great benefit to immunocompromised patients. These new vaccines produce significantly higher antibody titers postimmunization than did earlier vaccines, and vaccination prior to treatment has reduced the risk of bacterial sepsis (78–81). However, even with these improvements, neither immunization nor antibiotic prophylaxis can totally prevent the development of sepsis due to encapsulated microorganisms in splenectomized patients who have been heavily treated with combined radiation therapy and chemotherapy. Thus, although low, diagnostic laparotomy and splenectomy carry a defined morbidity and mortality risk; this must be evaluated against the risks of the more intensive treatment required without laparotomy.

One randomized trial (the EORTC H_6 trial; see Chapter 18 for a more detailed discussion) evaluated the role of staging laparotomy in favorable prognosis early-stage Hodgkin's disease in tailoring treatment to the diagnostic findings. In that trial, CS I–II patients with favorable prognostic features were randomized to receive subtotal nodal and splenic irradiation without a laparotomy, or a staging laparotomy followed by radiation therapy or radiation therapy and chemotherapy depending on the results at laparotomy. At 6 years, the cumulative treatment failure probability was slightly but not significantly higher in the no-laparotomy arm than the laparotomy arm (22% versus 17%, $p = .27$). Overall survival rates at 6 years were no different (93%, no-laparotomy versus 89%, laparotomy, $p = .24$). At 10 years there is still no difference in terms of cumulative treatment failure probability ($p = .16$); however, there is now a small overall survival advantage for the no-laparotomy arm compared to the laparotomy arm ($p = .035$) (Jean-Marc Cosset, Lymphoma Categorical Course, American Society for Therapeutic Radiology and Oncology, October, 1997). A more detailed analysis of these data is needed to determine whether this increased mortality is due to the involvement of many centers in the EORTC H_6F trial, some of which may have had limited surgical experience in Hodgkin's disease, or to other causes.

LONG-TERM OUTCOME OF TREATMENT FOR EARLY-STAGE HODGKIN'S DISEASE

Much of the long-term follow-up data (15 years or longer) for early-stage Hodgkin's disease is derived from laparotomy-staged patients treated with radiation therapy alone. Large, single institutional studies demonstrate greater than an 80% actuarial 10- to 15-year freedom from relapse and less than a 10% mortality from Hodgkin's disease following mantle and paraaortic irradiation for PS IA–IIA patients (29,30,82). These results have been achieved through careful delineation of the extent of Hodgkin's disease, precise delivery of radiation therapy (treatment simulation, individually contoured divergent blocks, equal doses from front and back, machine-generated verification films) (83,84), and the successful treatment of patients who relapse with multiagent chemotherapy (51,52).

The treatment of early-stage disease has become so successful that at 15 to 20 years posttreatment the overall mortality rate from causes other than Hodgkin's disease may exceed that seen from Hodgkin's disease (53,85–87). The 20-year freedom from recurrence and overall survival rates of 392 PS IA–IIA Hodgkin's disease patients without large mediastinal adenopathy treated with mantle and paraaortic-splenic pedicle irradiation are shown in Figure 3 (unpublished results from the Harvard JCRT). With a median follow-up time of 12 years and a minimum follow-up time of 5 years, the 10- and 20-year rates of freedom from recurrence were 84% and 81%, respectively. The 10- and 20-year survival rates were 92% and 82%, respectively. There have been 40 deaths out of 392 patients, 14 from second malignancy (35%), 13 from Hodgkin's disease (33%), 7 from cardiac disease (18%), and 6 from other causes.

Two series that include some patients with more advanced disease report similar results on mortality. Researchers from Stanford University Medical School studied 326 PS IA–IIIB patients treated on clinical trials either with radiation therapy alone or with combined radiation therapy and chemotherapy. A total of 107 of the 326 patients had died at the time of the study; of these, 41% died from Hodgkin's disease, 26% from second can-

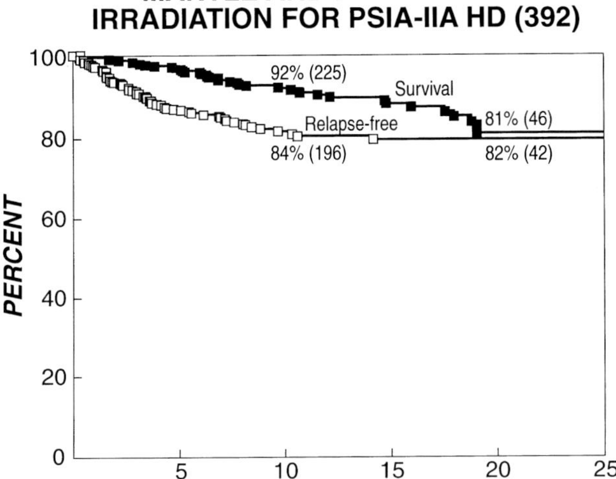

FIG. 3. With a median follow-up of 12 years and a minimum follow-up of 5 years, the 10-year and 20-year actuarial freedom from recurrence rates were 84% and 81%, respectively. The 10-year and 20-year survival rates were 92% and 82%, respectively. (Unpublished results from the Harvard Joint Center for Radiation Therapy.)

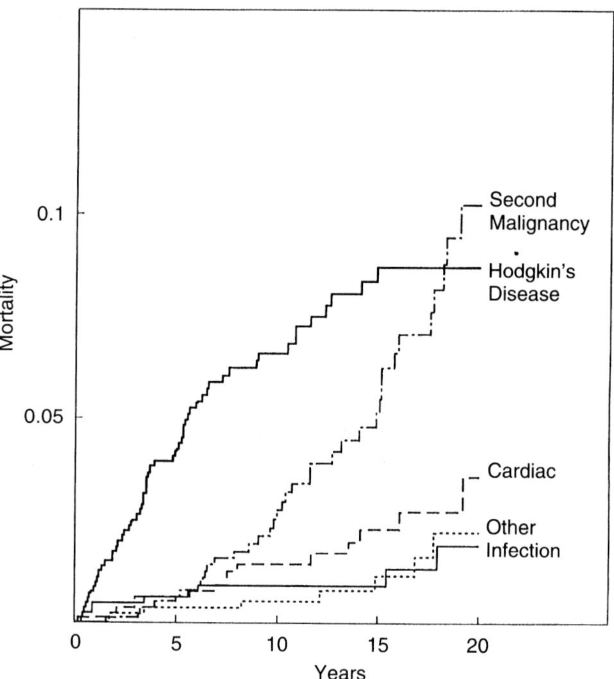

FIG. 4. Competing causes of death over time in 794 patients with Hodgkin's disease. (From ref. 53, with permission.)

cers, 16% from cardiovascular disease, and 17% from other causes (86). This data was recently updated (see Chapter 32) (88). Eighty percent of 794 PS IA–IIIB patients reported in a 1995 Harvard JCRT study had PS IA–IIA Hodgkin's disease (53). Figure 4 shows the competing causes of death for this group of patients. Between 15 and 20 years after treatment for Hodgkin's disease, cumulative mortality from second malignancy surpassed cumulative mortality from Hodgkin's disease. Deaths from Hodgkin's disease occurred most frequently in the first 5 to 10 years; causes of death other than Hodgkin's disease were most common after 5 to 10 years.

The aggressive treatment approaches developed in the 1970s and 1980s for early-stage Hodgkin's disease have resulted in high 20-year survival rates; a number of studies with long-term follow-up now report more deaths from causes other than Hodgkin's disease than from Hodgkin's disease. Table 4 shows the frequency and cause of mortality by 5-year interval after Hodgkin's disease from the Harvard JCRT study. The absolute excess risk of mortality by 5-year interval ranged from 104 to 125 per 10,000 person-years. Thus, patients had a 1.04% to 1.25% excess risk of mortality per year over the first 20 years after Hodgkin's disease. The tremendous success in treating Hodgkin's disease has led to increasing concern for the long-term effects of treatment. Understanding the causes for the excess non-Hodgkin's disease mortality should help in designing trials for early-stage disease.

The three most common causes of death after treatment for Hodgkin's disease (Hodgkin's disease, secondary malignancy, cardiac disease) are discussed briefly below and are covered in more detail later in this book (see Chapters 32, 33, and 35). Patients who develop recurrent Hodgkin's disease are more likely to be cured with combination chemotherapy if they were initially treated with radiation therapy alone as opposed to chemotherapy alone or combined radiation therapy and chemotherapy. The 10-year actuarial survival rate of patients initially treated with radiation therapy alone after relapse and treatment with multiagent chemotherapy is 57% to 62% (51,52). Most of the patients in these studies received MOPP chemotherapy for relapse; current treatment with ABVD is likely to yield an even better 10-year survival, given the advantage of ABVD over MOPP in advanced-stage Hodgkin's disease (89).

The survival rates are significantly worse for patients who relapse after chemotherapy alone or combined radiation therapy and chemotherapy, although most of the data are from patients who initially had advanced-stage Hodgkin's disease. Treatment with similar or alternative chemotherapy regimens after relapse from chemotherapy alone yields 5- to 10-year survival rates of only 20% to 32% (90–92). Because of the poor overall prognosis of patients who relapse after chemotherapy, many patients are now considered candidates for high-dose chemotherapy and autologous bone marrow rescue at first relapse. Although the results of high-dose therapy are promising, many patients with recurrent disease are not eligible for this approach due to poor tumor response, comorbid disease, or advanced age. Patients who undergo transplant and are subsequently cured of Hodgkin's disease face significant long-term treatment-related morbidity and mortality

TABLE 4. *Competing mortality with time*

Time interval	(P-Y)	AR—all causes	Dead HD	Dead, not HD	RR, not HD	AR, not HD
0–5 years	(3,723)	120.7	34	18	2.5	29.3
5–10 years	(2,627)	104.8	14	20	3.1	51.5
10–15 years	(1,575)	124.9	8	17	3.2	74.1
>15 years	(775)	110.6	0	13	2.9	110.6

P-Y, person-years; AR, absolute excess risk per 10,000 person-years; HD, Hodgkin's disease; RR, relative risk.

From ref. 53, with permission.

risks (see Chapter 29). One study reports a low rate of survival in patients with early-stage disease who relapsed after treatment with chemotherapy alone (9-year actuarial 56% survival rate) (93); these results await further confirmation. Until more data are available, current information suggests that when chemotherapy alone or combined radiation therapy and chemotherapy are used as definitive treatment for early-stage Hodgkin's disease, treatment should be designed to minimize relapse.

Many years after chemotherapy and/or radiation therapy, patients with Hodgkin's disease have an increased risk of developing acute nonlymphoblastic leukemia, non-Hodgkin's lymphoma, and second solid tumors (see Chapter 33) (94–112). This increased risk may be multifactorial, resulting both from the immune dysregulation associated with Hodgkin's disease and/or its treatment and the carcinogenic effects of radiation therapy and chemotherapy. Certain cytotoxic agents, especially those contained in the MOPP (113) and ChlVPP (chlorambucil, vinblastine, procarbazine, and prednisone) regimens (114), are associated with a marked increase in risk of developing acute nonlymphoblastic leukemia (110). The routine use of ABVD has dramatically reduced the risk of leukemogenesis, but there remains concern for secondary leukemia with alternating or hybrid regimens (110). Regimens that contain significant amounts of alkylating agents known to cause leukemia should not be used in favorable prognosis CS I–II patients.

Nearly all cases of non-Hodgkin's lymphoma occurring after Hodgkin's disease are of intermediate- or high-grade histology (98,102,112,115,116). The histologies represented are similar to lymphomas seen in patients with immunodeficiency diseases or under chronic immunosuppression for organ transplantation or autoimmune disorders. The risk is probably not treatment related, although this is still controversial, and thus should probably not be factored into the design of new trials.

The absolute excess risk of developing a solid tumor is greater than the absolute excess risk of developing leukemia or non-Hodgkin's lymphoma after treatment for Hodgkin's disease. Solid tumors constituted 55% of the second malignancies in the Tucker study, 64% in the Van Leeuwen study, and 75% in the Harvard University study (101,102,112). The relative risk of solid tumors continues to be elevated more than 20 years after Hodgkin's disease (12). Risk factors for developing a solid tumor after treatment for Hodgkin's disease include initial treatment with radiation therapy (many different solid tumors), treatment with chemotherapy (lung cancer), gender (higher for women), age at treatment, and environmental factors post-treatment (smoking and lung cancer). Volume of radiation therapy, dose of radiation therapy, and type of chemotherapy may all be independent risk factors for the development of second tumors but additional data are needed before firm recommendations for reduction of treatment can be made based on long-term risks (see Chapter 33 for more detail). However, reduction in the radiation field size will almost certainly result in a lower second tumor risk, as many of the radiation-induced tumors occur within or on the edge of the treatment field. Reduction of radiation field size should be considered as a strategy in the design of trials that use combined radiation therapy and chemotherapy. Female patients less than 25 to 30 years of age at treatment have an increased risk of breast cancer years after mantle irradiation (106,107,112,117); techniques to combine chemotherapy and radiation limited to involved fields should reduce this risk. This risk by age at treatment is shown in Table 5.

Complications related to cardiac irradiation (arrhythmias, myocardial infarction and coronary artery disease, pericarditis, myocarditis, pericardial effusion, and tamponade) have been carefully documented after radiation therapy to the mediastinum (see Chapter 35) (42,55,86, 118–127). In many of the earlier studies these complications were related to treatment techniques that resulted in a high radiation dose to the anterior mediastinum and heart (lower energy machinery, anterior weighted fields, doses per fraction of greater than 200 cGy, treatment with one field per day). Current practice, which restricts the dose to the whole heart, blocks the subcarinal region part way into treatment, delivers treatments equally from front and back, and permits lower radiation dose and volume by the use of preradiation chemotherapy, has yielded more satisfactory results. This is illustrated in a recent paper in which Boivin and colleagues (122) demonstrated a significant age-adjusted increased risk of death from myocardial infarction [relative risk (RR), 2.56; confidence interval (CI), 1.11–5.93] after mediastinal irradiation. This risk did not differ by age at treatment or time from treatment. However, when analyzed by year of diag-

TABLE 5. *Relative risk of breast cancer by age at treatment*

Age at diagnosis	(P-Y)	Observed/expected	RR (95% CI)	AR/10,000 P-Y
<15	(1,240)	3/0.007	458 (91.7–1,345)	24.1
15–24	(3,453)	5/0.21	23.3 (7.5–54.5)	13.9
25–34	(2,420)	3/0.75	4.0 (0.8–11.8)	9.3
≥35	(1,387)	2/1.02	2.0 (0.20–7.1)	7.1

P-Y, person-years; RR, relative risk; CI, confidence interval; AR/10,000 P-Y, absolute excess risk per 10,000 person-years.
From ref. 112, with permission.

nosis of Hodgkin's disease, the risk was greater for patients treated in 1966 or earlier (RR, 6.33; CI, 1.73–23.16) than for those treated in 1967 or later (RR, 1.97; CI, 0.75–5.17), suggesting that modern treatment techniques reduce the risk of cardiac complications. Similar data have been reported from Stanford University Medical School (127) (see Chapter 35). One of the advantages of using mantle irradiation alone for favorable prognosis PS IA–IIA patients without mediastinal involvement or combined chemotherapy and involved-field irradiation for clinically staged patients is the ability to place the lower border of the mediastinal field at the bottom of the hilar nodes (T7-T8). This technique covers the anterior mediastinum and the subcarinal and hilar regions, but allows blocking of the lower two-thirds to three-fourths of the heart for the entire treatment course.

REDUCTION OF STAGING OR TREATMENT: ONGOING AND RECENTLY COMPLETED STUDIES

Increasing concern for the long-term consequences of treatment has prompted many investigators to reexamine the aggressive approaches developed for the staging and treatment of early-stage Hodgkin's disease in the 1970s and 1980s. Many of the ongoing and recently completed studies were developed in an attempt to reduce the long-term complications of treatment without increasing mortality from Hodgkin's disease. These include studies that:

1. Evaluate radiation therapy alone and study reduction of radiation dose or reduction of radiation field size.
2. Evaluate combined radiation therapy and chemotherapy and attempt to identify the optimal chemotherapy regimen, identify the optimum number of cycles of chemotherapy, or determine the optimal radiation volume and dose when combined with chemotherapy.
3. Evaluate combination chemotherapy alone.

Most studies discussed below have relatively short follow-up or are ongoing and would not be expected to demonstrate survival differences. High relapse rates (i.e., greater than 30%) and significant acute toxicity are the main criteria for adverse outcome.

CLINICAL TRIALS OF RADIATION THERAPY ALONE

Evaluating Radiation Dose

Although a few studies have comprehensively reviewed dose-response data for Hodgkin's disease (128–131), only one prospective randomized study is available. This multicenter trial by the German Hodgkin's Study Group evaluated the tumoricidal doses for subclinical involvement by Hodgkin's disease (132). A total of 376 laparotomy-staged favorable prognosis stage IA–IIB patients were enrolled. Only patients without risk factors were included in the trial. Any one of the following risk factors was cause for exclusion: large mediastinal adenopathy, massive splenic involvement, extranodal disease, an ESR of >30 and B symptoms, an ESR of >50 and no B symptoms, or >3 regions of involvement. Patients were randomized to receive either 40 Gy extended-field radiation therapy or 30 Gy extended-field radiation therapy followed by an additional 10 Gy to involved lymph node regions. Recurrences were analyzed by a panel of four radiation oncologists for technique, treatment volume, and time and dose of radiation therapy and classified as in-field, marginal, or out-field recurrences (132).

The 5-year freedom from treatment failure results favored the 30 Gy extended-field plus 10 Gy arm over the 40 Gy extended-field arm (81% versus 70%, respectively, $p = .026$) (Fig. 5). The 5-year survival results also favored the 30 Gy extended-field arm (98% versus 93%, respectively, $p = .067$), although the differences were not statistically significant. These results suggest that 30 Gy is sufficient for treating subclinical involvement of Hodgkin's disease with radiotherapy alone.

Evaluating Radiation Field Size: Mantle Alone vs. Mantle plus Paraaortic-Splenic Irradiation in CS I–II Patients

The Princess Margaret Hospital has been one of the pioneers in the treatment of CS I–II Hodgkin's disease with radiation therapy alone. In a report of 250 patients with CS I–II supradiaphragmatic Hodgkin's disease treated with radiation therapy alone, the 8-year actuarial freedom from relapse rate was 71.6% with a median follow-up time of 6.3 years (59). Patients with CS I–II dis-

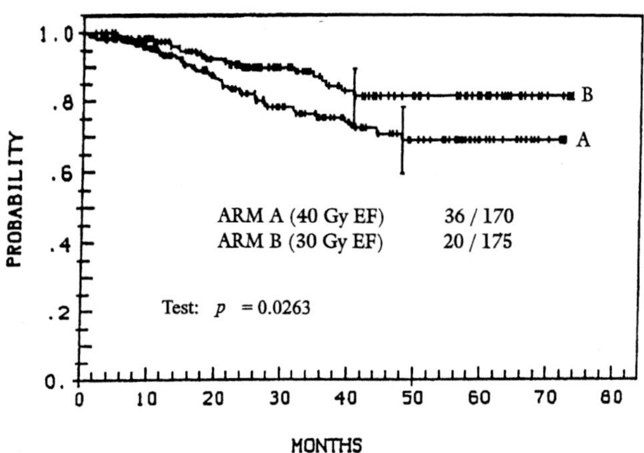

FIG. 5. Results from the German Hodgkin's Study Group trial. The 5-year freedom from treatment failure results favored the 30 Gy extended-field plus 10 Gy arm over the 40 Gy extended-field arm (81% versus 70%, respectively, p = .0263). The 5-year survival results also favored the 30 Gy extended-field arm (98% versus 93%, respectively, p = .0673), although the differences were not statistically significant. (From ref. 132, with permission.)

ease with favorable prognostic features (age <50, ESR < 40, and lymphocyte-predominance/nodular sclerosis histology) treated with mantle and paraaortic-splenic irradiation had only a 12.7% actuarial risk of relapse at 8 years.

Mantle Irradiation Alone in CS IA–IIA Patients

The use of mantle irradiation alone for early-stage Hodgkin's disease is attractive because all treatment is completed within 5 weeks, patients avoid the long-term risks of radiation to the upper abdomen (second tumors, small bowel obstruction), and the potential for salvage with combination chemotherapy is not compromised. The EORTC H_1 trial, one of the first studies to evaluate the role of chemotherapy in the treatment of early-stage Hodgkin's disease, randomized clinically staged I–II patients to receive mantle irradiation alone or combined with vinblastine chemotherapy. Prognostic factors had not been identified, and all CS I–II patients were enrolled. Fewer recurrences were seen in patients who received both mantle irradiation and vinblastine chemotherapy. However, relapse rates were high in both groups (freedom from recurrence was only 38% in the mantle alone group, the 15-year survival rate was only 58%), suggesting that mantle irradiation alone was not adequate treatment for unselected patients with CS I–II Hodgkin's disease, and that vinblastine was only partially effective in eliminating recurrences, many of which occurred below the diaphragm (58,63). Results in other retrospective studies of mantle irradiation alone for unselected CS I–II patients were also disappointing. For example, in the Toronto series the 10-year rate of freedom from recurrence was only 54% (67).

These high recurrence rates in unselected patients are not surprising, as over 20% of CS I–II patients have occult abdominal involvement, and lack of treatment of the abdomen (with radiation therapy or chemotherapy) would be expected to result in the doubling of the recurrence rates achieved with more extensive treatment. When mantle irradiation was restricted to clinically staged, asymptomatic patients with a single lymph node region involved (CS IA), better results were seen, with 10- to 15-year freedom-from-recurrence rates of 58% to 81% (67,75). Similarly, Wirth and colleagues (133) reported 81% and 71% progression-free survival rates at 5 years and 10 years, respectively, in patients with CS I disease treated with mantle irradiation alone.

What is the appropriate treatment for patients who by prognostic criteria have a very low risk (<10%) of abdominal involvement? These include female patients with CS IA nodular sclerosis Hodgkin's disease, patients with CS IA lymphocyte-predominant histology, and CS IA patients with interfollicular Hodgkin's disease (64,65). A similar subgroup of patients was defined by the EORTC (women less than 40 years of age with CS IA lymphocytic-predominance or nodular sclerosis histology, and an ESR <50 mm) and treated with mantle irradiation alone without staging laparotomy in the EORTC H_7VF (VF, very favorable) and H_8VF trials. In the H_7VF trial, 40 patients were treated according to this concept and complete remission was reached in 95%. However, 23% of patients relapsed, yielding a 6-year event-free survival rate of 66%, a relapse-free survival rate of 73%, and overall and cause-specific survival rates of 96% (134). The relapse rates were thought to be unacceptably high in this selected subgroup of stage IA patients. The very favorable subgroup is now treated according to the EORTC strategy for the favorable subgroup.

Mantle Irradiation Alone in PS IA–IIA Patients

To determine the role of prophylactic abdominal irradiation in early-stage Hodgkin's disease, the EORTC H_5 trial (1977–1982) compared the use of mantle and paraaortic-splenic pedicle irradiation to mantle irradiation alone in patients with favorable early-stage Hodgkin's disease (58,135). This study included only patients with nodular sclerosis or lymphocyte-predominance histology, age 40 or younger, PS I or PS II with mediastinal adenopathy, and an ESR of less than 70. No differences were seen in disease-free survival or overall survival between the two treatment groups. The 9-year cumulative treatment failure probability was 31% for mantle and 30% for mantle and paraaortic irradiation. The 9-year overall survival rates were 94% and 91%, respectively. A 1997 update of this trial, with 15-year follow-up, still shows no statistical difference between the two treatment arms, either for cumulative treatment failure probability (p = .62) or overall survival (p = .69). These excellent results with mantle irradiation alone have been corroborated in other retrospective studies (75,76). The large retrospective study from St. Bartholomew's Hospital in London, reported an 85% 15-year actuarial freedom from recurrence rate in PS IA patients (all histologies) treated with mantle irradiation alone (75).

In 1988, a single-arm prospective trial was initiated at the Harvard JCRT of mantle irradiation alone in laparotomy-staged IA–IIA Hodgkin's disease patients. Its objectives were to study results of mantle irradiation alone at a single institution, to identify patients most suitable for mantle irradiation alone, to establish guidelines for follow-up after treatment, to evaluate the requirement for staging laparotomy, and to provide an assessment of risk versus gain of this reduction in treatment for early-stage Hodgkin's disease. The original eligibility criteria for the study included a negative laparotomy, the absence of large mediastinal adenopathy and B symptoms, and nodular sclerosis or lymphocyte-predominance histology. In contrast to the EORTC H_5F study, patients over 40 years old and patients with a high ESR (>70) were included in the study. Later modifications in the protocol also allowed treatment of CS IA patients with lymphocyte-predominance histology (no laparotomy) and PS IA patients with mixed-cellularity histology. As guidelines for the treatment of patients with mediastinal involvement had not been reported in the EORTC H_5F trial, the JCRT trial defined parameters for eligibility and treatment of patients with mediastinal involvement. Thoracic computed axial tomographic scanning and gallium scanning were required to establish the extent of thoracic involvement, and patients with Hodgkin's disease in hilar, subcarinal, or cardiophrenic lymph node regions were not eligible for the trial. In patients without mediastinal involvement, the bottom of the mantle field extended to the bottom of T7 or T8 to include the hilar and subcarinal regions (Fig. 6A) and exclude most of the heart from the radiation field. In patients with upper mediastinal involvement, the bottom of the mantle was extended to the bottom of T10 or T11 to include the medial cardiophrenic nodes; a subcarinal block was added at 30 Gy (Fig. 6B). The mantle was treated to 30 to 36 Gy with a cone down to a total dose of 38 to 44 Gy to regions of initial involvement.

Preliminary results of the trial have been published (66,77). An update of this information is presented below. Seventy-seven patients (out of a planned 100) have been enrolled to date; the characteristics of 68 of these patients followed for a year or longer are shown in Table 6. All but three patients were laparotomy staged. The disease-free and overall survival results are shown in Figure 7. With a median follow-up time of 40 months, the 5-year actuarial rate of freedom from recurrence is 88% and the 5-year actuarial survival rate is 100%. Six patients have had recurrences, five in sites below the diaphragm (Table 7). All six patients are alive after retreatment with chemotherapy with or without radiation therapy. No significant differences in freedom from recurrence by histology (nodular sclerosis vs. lymphocyte predominance), age (39 or younger vs. 40 or older), or stage (IA vs. IIA) have been observed to date; however, accrual is incomplete and longer follow-up will be needed to ascertain the long-

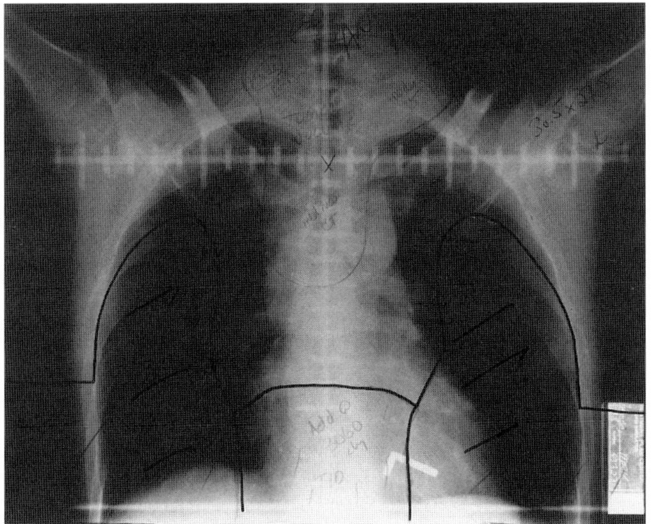

A

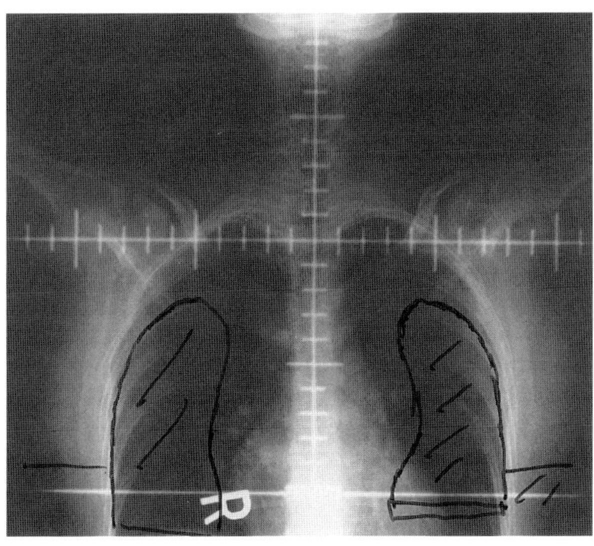

B

FIG. 6. A: Simulation film of a patient receiving mantle irradiation alone. Initial presentation revealed no evidence of mediastinal disease, allowing blocking of the lower mediastinum. **B:** Simulation film of a patient receiving mantle irradiation alone. Initial presentation revealed evidence of anterior superior mediastinal disease; the lower border of the field was set at T10-T11 to allow for treatment of the medial cardiac node.

TABLE 6. *Characteristics of patients treated with mantle radiation therapy alone at the Harvard Joint Center for Radiation Therapy*

No. of patients	68
Age (months)	
Median	28
Range	11–54
Follow-up time (months)	
Median	40
Range	12–100
Histology	
LP	16
NS	50
MC/not classified	2
Stage	
IA	37
IIA	31
No. of sites	
1	37
2	24
3	7
Age	
≤16	3
17–39	55
≥40	10

NS, nodular sclerosis histology; LP, lymphocyte-predominance histology; MC, mixed-cellularity histology; LD, lymphocyte-depletion histology.

term effects of treatment. These preliminary results are similar to those seen with treatment with mantle and paraaortic irradiation (77; Jones, unpublished data, 1996). Because of the increased risk of abdominal relapse following mantle irradiation alone, a negative staging laparotomy and splenectomy and careful radiographic follow-up with monitoring of the abdominal-pelvic nodes after treatment are essential components of the trial.

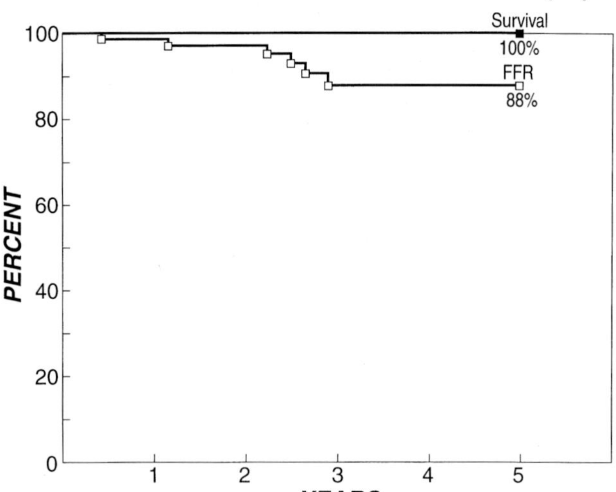

FIG. 7. Freedom from first recurrence and survival of patients enrolled in the Harvard Joint Center for Radiation Therapy prospective trial for mantle irradiation alone in selected PS IA–IIA patients (unpublished data).

TABLE 7. *Analysis of relapse in 6 of 68 patients treated with mantle radiation therapy alone*

Histology	Time to relapse (Mo.)	Site of relapse	RX	Status (Mo.)
NS	5	Retr	ABVD + IFRT	NED (10)
NS	14	Ing/ilia	ABVD	NED (61)
NS	25	Ilia	MoPP/ABV + IFRT	NED (46)
NS	27	Retr	ABVD	On CT
NS	30	Card	ABVD	NED (6)
NS	32	Ing/ilia	ABVD + IFRT	NED (29)

RX, treatment regimen, NS, nodular sclerosis; LP, lymphocyte-predominance histology; MC, mixed-cellularity histology; LD, lymphocyte-depletion histology; NED, no evident disease; IF, involved field; RT, radiation therapy; ABVD, Adriamycin (doxorubicin), vinblastine, bleomycin, dacarbazine; Retr, retroperitoneal recurrence; Ilia, iliac nodal recurrence; Card, cardiophrenic nodal recurrence; CT, chemotherapy; Ing, inguinal nodal recurrence; Mo., months.

Two questions will not be answered by this trial: (a) What is the role for this approach in patients with mixed-cellularity histology? Retrospective data from St. Bartholomew's Hospital in a limited number of patients suggest that laparotomy-staged IA patients with mixed-cellularity histology have a high rate of freedom from first recurrence after mantle irradiation alone. (b) What is the appropriate treatment for patients with lymphocyte-predominant histology? The optimal treatment of patients with lymphocyte-predominant histology is being investigated by the European Task Force on Lymphoma (see Chapter 31).

RANDOMIZED CLINICAL TRIALS OF COMBINED RADIATION THERAPY AND CHEMOTHERAPY

Favorable Prognosis Stage I–II: Identification of the Optimal Chemotherapy Combination

Recent randomized trials of combined modality therapy are based on the premise that this approach results in a very high freedom from recurrence in early-stage Hodgkin's disease, and that the efficacy of combined chemotherapy and radiation can be maintained by using chemotherapy regimens that contain less toxic drug combinations. Listed in Table 8 are recent trials of chemotherapy regimens given for four or six cycles in combination with radiation therapy. The regimens are combined with involved-field or regional (or mantle) radiation therapy with the premise that the drugs being tested will be able to control occult abdominal disease in clinically staged patients without upper abdominal and splenic irradiation. Analysis of patterns and frequency of failure will eventually provide better guidelines for such modified regimens

TABLE 8. *Recent randomized clinical trials in favorable prognosis stage I–II Hodgkin's disease: trials to identify the optimum chemotherapy combination*

Trial	Eligibility	Treatment regimens	No. of patients	Outcome
Stanford (139)	CS IA–IIA, or CS IB–IIB with only night sweats *without* Large mediastinal disease (≥1/3 maximum thoracic diameter) or two or more extranodal sites of disease	A. VBM × 6 + regional RT (36 Gy)	35	5-year freedom from disease progression: A = 88%, B = 93%, p = .60
		B. STLI(S)/TLI(S) (30–40 Gy, boost 40–44 Gy)	43	5-year survival: A = 94%, B = 98%, p = .50
EORTC H_7F(140)	CS IA–IIB *without* age >50 ESR ≥50 mm in A; ≥30 mm in B 4 or more sites of disease Large mediastinal disease (≥0.35 m/t ratio) CS IA, NS/LP, <40, ESR <50	A. EBVP × 6 + IFRT (36 Gy)	168	6-year event-free survival: A = 90%, B = 81%, p = .019
		B. STLI (S)	165	6-year relapse-free survival: A = 92%, B = 81%, p = .004; 6-year survival: A = 98%, B = 96%, p = .156
MSKCC (141)	CS IA–IIA no exclusions for age, mediastinal size, number of sites	A. MOPP × 4 + mantle (inverted Y)	61	5-year freedom from progression: A = 89%, B = 81%, p = .23
		B. TBV × 4 + mantle (inverted Y)	59	5-year survival: A = 91%, B = 91%, p = .83

VBM, vinblastine, methotrexate, bleomycin; RT, radiation therapy; STLI/TLI (S), subtotal nodal/total nodal irradiation (splenic irradiation); CS, clinical stage; EBVP II, epirubicin, bleomycin, vinblastine, and prednisone; IF, involved field; NS, nodular sclerosis histology; LP, lymphocyte-predominance histology; MOPP, mechlorethamine, Oncovin (vincristine), procarbazine, prednisone; TBV, thiotepa, bleomycin, vinblastine; ESR, erythrocyte sedimentation rate.

to control occult Hodgkin's disease not appreciated on physical examination or radiographic evaluation. If successful, these regimens should reduce treatment-related morbidity and mortality by reducing both the amount and toxicity of chemotherapy and by using smaller radiation volumes. These randomized trials compare outcome in patients receiving larger (standard) radiation fields to that of patients treated with smaller fields and chemotherapy.

Stanford Trial of Vinblastine, Methotrexate, Bleomycin, and Regional Irradiation Versus Mantle and Paraaortic-Splenic Pedicle Irradiation for CS IA–IIA Patients

With the objective of reducing acute toxicity and chronic morbidity (sterility, increased risk of leukemia), Horning and colleagues (136) developed a nontoxic chemotherapy regimen, VBM (vinblastine, methotrexate, bleomycin), which was tested in a randomized trial of PS IA–IIB and PS IIIA patients. The trial compared subtotal nodal/total nodal irradiation to involved-field irradiation (44 Gy) followed by VBM. The freedom from disease progression at 9 years favored involved-field irradiation and VBM (98%) over subtotal nodal/total nodal irradiation (78%) (p = .01). No differences were seen in overall survival (p = .09). The British National Lymphoma Investigation (BNLI) has confirmed the efficacy of VBM with involved-field irradiation, but in their experience this approach produced unacceptable pulmonary and hematologic toxicity (137). Favorable results with VBM and extended-field radiation therapy in CS IA–IIA Hodgkin's disease also have been reported by the Gruppo Italiano per lo Studio Dei Linformi (138). In that study of 50 patients, the 5-year progression-free survival rate was 82%. Eight patients in the trial experienced pulmonary toxicity.

Based on the Stanford trial results reported above, a follow-up Stanford trial has been completed (139). Patients with CS IA–IIA disease (staging laparotomy and splenectomy were eliminated) were treated either with subtotal nodal irradiation (and splenic irradiation) or two cycles of VBM, followed by regional (mantle) irradiation, followed by four additional cycles of VBM (with a reduced bleomycin dose). No differences in the 4-year freedom from disease progression or survival were noted between the two arms of the trial (Table 8).

EORTC H_7F trial (1988–1993)

The EBVP II regimen (epirubicin, bleomycin, vinblastine, and prednisone, one dose per cycle) and involved-field irradiation (n = 168) were tested versus mantle and paraaortic-splenic irradiation (n = 165) for favorable prognosis CS IA–IIA patients. EBVP II was proposed as a potentially less toxic but similarly effective regimen compared to ABVD. In the H_7F trial for patients with favorable disease, six cycles of EBVP were combined with involved-field radiation and randomly compared with subtotal nodal and splenic irradiation in favorable clinical stage I and II patients. At 6 years, the event-free survival rate was significantly higher for patients on the combined chemotherapy and radiation therapy arm than for those on the radiation therapy alone arm (90% versus

81%, respectively, p = .019); the relapse-free survival rates showed similar results (92% versus 81%, respectively, p = .004). The 6-year survival rate was excellent in both treatment arms (98% versus 96%, respectively, p = .156) (134,140). In contrast, in the H_7U trial for patients with unfavorable disease (see Chapter 26 for details), EBVP and involved-field radiation therapy was inferior to MOPP/ABV and involved-field radiation therapy, suggesting that the use of prognostic factors is crucial in selecting patients for treatment with modified chemotherapy and radiation therapy regimens.

Memorial Sloan-Kettering Cancer Center Trial of MOPP and Mantle Field Radiation Therapy Versus TBV and Mantle Field Radiation Therapy

Straus and colleagues (141) reported a randomized trial comparing four cycles of MOPP and mantle field radiation therapy to four cycles of TBV (thiotepa, 35 mg/m^2 day 1 and 15; bleomycin 2 mg/day for days 4 to 10 and 18 to 24; and vinblastine, 6 mg/m^2 for days 1 and 15) and mantle field radiation therapy for patients with CS IA–IIA disease. This trial included both favorable and unfavorable prognosis CS I–II patients as there were no exclusions for age, mediastinal size, or number of sites or involvement. With a median follow-up time of 64 months, the 5-year freedom from progression was 89% for MOPP and radiation therapy versus 81% for TBV and radiation therapy (p = .23). The 5-year actuarial survival rate was 91% for both groups. Less short-term toxicity was encountered with TBV.

Favorable Prognosis Stage I–II: Trials to Identify the Optimal Number of Cycles of Chemotherapy

The trials noted here use combination chemotherapy and radiation therapy with a limited number of chemotherapeutic agents (i.e., one or two) or with less than four cycles of chemotherapy. Although the primary goal of these trials is to evaluate the efficacy of short courses of chemotherapy, new regimens are also being tested [e.g., Stanford V, VAPEC-B (see below)]. One reason for listing these trials separately from those in Table 11 is that the optimal extent of radiation therapy needed is less certain in the short-course trials. For example, there are at least limited data that four to six cycles of chemotherapy is sufficient to control occult abdominal disease in the majority of CS I–II patients (12,35,41,142). Many of the ongoing investigations have also targeted CS I–II patients with adverse prognostic features to evaluate the volume of radiation therapy needed (see Chapter 26 for discussion of the Milan and EORTC H_8U trials). With short-course chemotherapy there are very few data on the effectiveness of different regimens to control Hodgkin's disease outside of the involved regions as defined by physical examination or radiographic evaluation. This uncertainty is reflected in some of the trial designs that use subtotal nodal and splenic radiation rather than involved-field or mantle radiation in combination with chemotherapy. Ongoing and recently completed short-course trials are listed in Table 9.

The German Hodgkin's Study Group (GHSG) HD7 and HD10 Trials

The HD7 trial (1994–1998) accrued 643 favorable prognosis CS IA–IIB Hodgkin's disease patients. The study randomized patients to subtotal nodal and splenic irradiation alone or to two courses of ABVD and the radiation therapy regimen. The first 365 patients are available for analysis. The data are preliminary (provided by Volker Diehl), but a borderline advantage in freedom from treatment failure is seen in the patients receiving ABVD × 2 and subtotal nodal and splenic irradiation (96%) compared to those treated with subtotal nodal and splenic irradiation alone (87%, p = .05) (Table 9). There are several questions raised by this study. First, with an expected long-term freedom from treatment failure in favorable prognosis CS IA–IIA disease of approximately 80% to 90% (59), is the added small benefit in freedom from treatment failure with ABVD × 2 worth the extra risk from the doxorubicin and bleomycin? Second, is it more difficult to salvage patients who recur after subtotal nodal and splenic irradiation and ABVD × 2 than after subtotal nodal and splenic irradiation alone? Do patients who relapse after combined chemotherapy and radiation therapy more frequently require high-dose chemotherapy and stem cell rescue as opposed to standard chemotherapy? These are questions that can be answered only with much longer follow-up. It might be better to devise strategies using ABVD for three to four courses and more limited or involved-field irradiation, or to test two cycles of ABVD with more limited radiation therapy. The toxicity of radiation would thus be limited, and one could determine the amount of chemotherapy needed to control occult abdominal disease. This strategy is being adapted in the GHSG HD10 trial, which opened in 1998. It has essentially the same eligibility criteria as the GHSG HD7 trial (Table 9). Patients are to be randomized to four arms: two cycles of ABVD followed by 30 Gy involved-field radiation therapy; two cycles of ABVD followed by 20 Gy involved-field radiation therapy; four cycles of ABVD followed by 30 Gy involved-field radiation therapy; four cycles of ABVD followed by 20 Gy involved-field radiation therapy. This trial should help determine the number of cycles of ABVD needed to control occult Hodgkin's disease in the abdomen, and to prevent recurrence of Hodgkin's disease in apparently uninvolved sites adjacent to known Hodgkin's disease (adjacent to the irradiated involved site). It should also help determine the dose of radiation needed to control Hodgkin's disease when combined with limited chemotherapy. Overall the

TABLE 9. *Recent randomized clinical trials in favorable prognosis stage I–II Hodgkin's disease: trials to identify the optimal number of cycles of chemotherapy*

Trial	Eligibility	Treatment regimens	No. of patients	Outcome
GHSG HD7	CS IA–IIB *without* Large mediastinal mass (≥0.33 m/t ratio) Massive splenic involvement Localized extranodal involvement ESR ≥50 mm in A; ≥30 mm in B Three or more involved areas	A. RT alone (STLI-spleen (30 Gy) + IFRT (40 Gy) B. ABVD × 2 + RT (RT regimen as in A)	180 185	22-month median FU 22-month FFTF: A = 87%, B = 96%, *p* = .05 22-month survival: A = 97%, B = 98%, NS
GHSG HD10	CS IA–IIB *without* Large mediastinal mass (≥0.33 m/t ratio) Localized extranodal involvement ESR ≥50 mm in A; ≥30 mm in B Three or more involved areas	A. ABVD × 2 + IF RT (30 Gy) B. ABVD × 2 + IF RT (20 Gy) C. ABVD × 4 + IF RT (30 Gy) D. ABVD × 4 + IF RT (20 Gy)	Open	Open
BNLI	CS IA–IIA *without* Large mediastinal disease	A. VAPEC-B × 1 + IF RT (30–40 Gy) B. Mantle RT (30–35 Gy to uninvolved nodes; 30–40 Gy to involved nodes)	Open	Open
SWOG/ CALGB	CS IA–IIA, age ≥16 *without* Large mediastinal disease Pericardial involvement	A. Doxorubicin and vinblastine × 3 and STLI (S) (36–40 Gy) B. STLI (S) (36–40 Gy) to	Open	Open
EORTC/ GELA H$_8$F (151)	CS IA–IIB *without* age ≥50 ESR ≥50 mm in A; ≥30 mm in B 4 or more sites of disease Large mediastinal disease (≥0.35 m/t ratio) CS IA, NS/LP, <40, ESR <50	A. MOPP/ABV × 3 + IF RT (36 Gy) B. STLI (S)	No report	No report
Stanford V for favorable CS IA–IIA Hodgkin's disease	CS I–II *without* B symptoms Age <16 and >60 Large mediastinal disease (≥1/3 maximum thoracic diameter) 2 or more extranodal sites of disease CS IA high neck presentations	Stanford V for 8 weeks + modified involved field radiation therapy (30 Gy to all regions of initial involvement)	Open	Open

RT, radiation therapy; STLI (S), subtotal nodal irradiation (splenic irradiation); CS, clinical stage; FFTF, freedom from treatment failure; FU, follow-up; IF, involved field; NS, nodular sclerosis histology; LP, lymphocyte-predominance histology; MOPP, mechlorethamine, Oncovin (vincristine), procarbazine, prednisone; ABVD, Adriamycin (doxorubicin), bleomycin, vinblastine, dacarbazine; Stanford V regimen, mechlorethamine, doxorubicin, vinblastine, prednisone, vincristine, bleomycin, VP-16; ESR, erythrocyte sedimentation rate; VAPEC-B, vincristine, doxorubicin, prednisolone, etoposide, cyclophosphamide, bleomycin.

trial should give physicians further guidelines for reduction of treatment in early-stage Hodgkin's disease.

Manchester Pilot Study and BNLI Trial

This trial tests VAPEC-B chemotherapy (doxorubicin, cyclophosphamide, etoposide, vincristine, bleomycin, prednisolone) for 4 weeks and involved-field irradiation versus mantle irradiation alone. Preliminary reports from the Manchester pilot study using the relatively brief 4-week VAPEC-B regimen in early-stage Hodgkin's disease provide background data for the ongoing BNLI trial. In the Manchester study, 111 CS IA–IIA patients without mediastinal bulk have been randomized since 1989 to receive either limited radiotherapy alone or VAPEC-B followed by local irradiation only to the involved regions. With a median follow-up time of 3.3 years, there have been 17 recurrences, 15 in the radiotherapy alone arm and two in the VAPEC-B plus local irradiation arm. The progression-free survival rate at 3 years is 73% for patients in the radiation therapy arm and 91% for those who received combined VAPEC-B and radiation (143). The current BNLI study has a similar design; however, the radiation therapy alone arm includes full mantle irradiation rather than a more limited field (Table 9). The interest in this trial is in the VAPEC-B and involved-field arm, as mantle irradiation alone in non–laparotomy-staged patients is associated with a high recurrence rate (approximately 30%) and is no longer felt to be sufficient treatment for favorable prognosis early-stage Hodgkin's disease based on the results of the EORTC H_7VF and H_8VF trials (see above).

SWOG/CALGB Study

The Southwest Oncology Group/Cancer and Leukemia Group B (SWOG/CALGB) study tests three cycles of adjuvant doxorubicin and vinblastine plus subtotal nodal and splenic irradiation versus to subtotal nodal and splenic irradiation alone in CS IA–IIA Hodgkin's disease patients. This study is ongoing (Table 9). As of June 1998, 284 patients have been enrolled on the study (information provided by Todd Wasserman, June 1998 CALGB update). Fifty-four patients are ineligible due to protocol violations. Eighty patients on the subtotal nodal and splenic irradiation arm and 82 patients in the doxorubicin/vinblastine and radiation arm have been evaluated for short-term toxicity. There has been one death from pneumonitis among patients on the radiation therapy alone arm. There are several questions raised by this study similar to those for the GHSG HD7 study (see above). These include the potential extra toxicity of the doxorubicin and vinblastine in a group of patients with an expected favorable prognosis for treatment with radiation therapy alone, and the overall strategy in trial design of giving enough chemotherapy to eliminate the need for abdominal irradiation.

EORTC H8F Trial (1993–1998)

This trial, activated in 1993, tests three cycles of MOPP/ABV hybrid and involved-field irradiation versus mantle and paraaortic-splenic irradiation for favorable prognosis CS IA–IIA patients. It should give answers to the following important questions: Are three cycles of standard chemotherapy sufficient to control subclinical Hodgkin's disease in favorable prognosis CS IA–IIA patients? Can patients who relapse after three cycles of MOPP/ABV and involved-field radiation therapy be cured with alternative treatment short of high-dose chemotherapy and stem cell rescue? The one concern of the trial is the use of the hybrid regimen, which confers some risk of sterility and leukemogenesis in these favorable prognosis Hodgkin's disease patients. Along this line, ABVD and EBVP without MOPP are being proposed for the H_9 trials.

Modified Stanford V Trial for Early-Stage Favorable Prognosis Patients

Stanford V is a relatively short, but intensive, chemotherapy regimen given for 12 weeks to patients with poor prognosis stage I–II disease (144). A modification of this trial has been opened for favorable prognosis CS IA–IIA patients using 8 weeks of the Stanford V regimen and modified involved-field irradiation to sites of initial involvement (identified radiographically as nodal enlargement of 1.5 cm or greater). The chemotherapy regimen includes mechlorethamine (6 mg/m^2 on weeks 1 and 5), doxorubicin (25 mg/m^2 on weeks 1, 3, 5, and 7), vinblastine (6 mg/m^2 on weeks 1, 3, 5, and 7), prednisone (40 mg/m^2 on days 1 to 36 then taper off), vincristine (1.4 mg/m^2 on weeks 2, 4, 6, and 8), bleomycin (5 U/m^2 on weeks 2, 4, 6, and 8), and VP-16 (60 mg/m^2 on days 15 and 16, and days 43 and 44). This regimen will evaluate the ability of brief but intense chemotherapy to control Hodgkin's disease outside of initially involved sites in favorable prognosis CS I–II patients.

Trials to Identify the Appropriate Radiation Volume and Dose When Combined with Chemotherapy

Completed trials evaluating radiation volume when combined with chemotherapy in poor prognosis CS I–II patients (see Chapter 26) suggest that involved-field irradiation may suffice when combined with four cycles of ABVD, but longer term follow-up is needed. Involved-field irradiation appears sufficient when combined with six cycles of chemotherapy.

Data are available suggesting that there is no difference between 20, 30, and 40 Gy to prophylactic sites (involved sites received 40 Gy in all three groups) when combined with chemotherapy in poor prognosis CS I–II patients. Two ongoing trials in favorable prognosis early-stage Hodgkin's disease are evaluating radiation dose to involved sites after chemotherapy. The GHSG initiated a trial in 1998 evaluating the number of cycles of chemotherapy and radiation dose. Patients are randomized to two or four cycles of ABVD. Patients in complete remission are then randomized to either 20 or 30 Gy involved-field radiation. Four groups of patients are being studied: ABVD × 2 and 20 Gy; ABVD × 2 and 30 Gy; ABVD × 4 and 20 Gy; ABVD × 4 and 30 Gy (see Table 9). The EORTC H_9F trial is evaluating 36 Gy, 20 Gy, or no radiation to involved sites in patients who have achieved a complete remission after six cycles of EBVP II.

RANDOMIZED CLINICAL TRIALS OF CHEMOTHERAPY ALONE

Favorable Prognosis Stage I–II: Trials of Chemotherapy Alone Versus Radiation Therapy Alone

Probably the first published experience of the use of MOPP chemotherapy alone in early stages of childhood

Hodgkin's disease came from Uganda, where no radiation therapy was available (145). Several small retrospective studies have also reported treatment with MOPP alone (146). Based on this limited experience, two randomized studies were devised to compare radiation therapy alone to MOPP chemotherapy alone in laparotomy staged patients; both studies have median follow-up times of 7.5 to 8 years (Table 10). Although both studies are now dated because of the use of the MOPP regimen and the requirement for staging laparotomy, results from these trials provide valuable information for the design of future protocols.

The American National Cancer Institute (NCI) study was initially designed to include patients with intermediate prognosis Hodgkin's disease. Although the trial included patients with favorable prognosis PS IIA disease, the most favorable patients with PS IA disease in peripheral sites were not included in the trial and were treated with radiation therapy alone, and patients with an unfavorable prognosis (B symptoms, large mediastinal adenopathy, and limited stage III disease) were included in the trial (20). Patients were randomized to 6 months of MOPP chemotherapy alone or subtotal nodal irradiation alone. After researchers recognized that patients with massive mediastinal involvement and PS IIIA disease were not optimal candidates for radiation therapy alone, the randomization criteria were changed while the study was ongoing. Table 10 shows the data for the IA (central sites), IB, IIA, and IIB patients without large mediastinal involvement. No difference in disease-free or overall survival is seen at 10 years.

The Italian prospective randomized study consists of patients with PS IA–IIA Hodgkin's disease randomized to receive either 6 months of MOPP alone or subtotal nodal irradiation alone (93). There were no differences in freedom from progression (Table 10). However, the survival rate was significantly higher in patients treated with radiation therapy alone (93%) than in those treated with chemotherapy alone (56%). The difference in survival was attributed to the inability to salvage patients relapsing after MOPP chemotherapy; these results are similar to the poor results of salvage ABVD in patients who relapsed after MOPP for advanced Hodgkin's disease (see above). Both the NCI and the Italian studies demonstrated greater acute toxicities in patients who received MOPP chemotherapy. In the Longo study, more than 50% of patients treated with MOPP had at least one hospital admission for fever and neutropenia.

The National Cancer Institute of Canada CTG HD6 study is a modification of the NCI and Italian studies with the randomization of clinically staged, rather than pathologically staged, patients and the use of ABVD as the chemotherapy regimen. Favorable prognosis patients (nodular sclerosis or lymphocyte-predominance histology, age less than 40, ESR less than 50, one to three sites of involvement) are randomized to subtotal nodal irradi-

TABLE 10. *Randomized clinical trials in favorable prognosis stage I–II Hodgkin's disease: trials of chemotherapy alone vs. radiation therapy alone*

Trial	Eligibility	Treatment regimens	No. of patients	Outcome
Italian Prospective Rand trial (93)	PS IA–IIA	A. STLI	45	8-year freedom from progression: A = 76%, B = 64%, $p > .05$
		B. MOPP × 6	44	8-year survival: A = 93%, B = 56%, $p < .001$
NCI (20)	PS IA–IIB *without* large mediastinal disease	PS IA peripheral nodes: STLI	30	30/30 FFFR; 28/30 alive
		PS IA (central), IB, IIA, IIB: A. STLI	41	10-year freedom from recurrence: A = 67%, B = 82%, $p = .27$
		B. MOPP × 6	41	10-year survival: A = 85%, B = 90%, $p = .68$
NCIC CTG HD6	CS IA–IIA *without* MC or LD histology; Age ≥40; ESR ≥50; 4 or more sites of involvement; Unilateral high neck or epitrochlear stage IA disease	A. STLI (S) or inverted-Y RT; B. ABVD × 4–6	Open	Open

RT, radiation therapy; STLI (S), subtotal nodal irradiation (splenic irradiation); CS, clinical stage; PS, pathologic stage; FFFR, freedom from first relapse; MC, mixed-cellularity histology; LD, lymphocyte-depletion histology; MOPP, mechlorethamine, Oncovin (vincristine), procarbazine, prednisone; ABVD; adriamycin (doxorubicin), bleomycin, vinblastine, dacarbazine; NCI, National Cancer Institute; NCIC, National Cancer Institute of Canada.

ation and splenic irradiation versus four cycles of ABVD alone. This study will test the efficacy of four cycles of ABVD alone in favorable prognosis early-stage Hodgkin's disease. The study is open for accrual.

Trials of Chemotherapy Alone Versus Combined Modality Therapy

The incidence of early-stage Hodgkin's disease varies in Africa, Asia, and South America and depends on the accessibility of adequate health care facilities, and the level of education and socioeconomic status of the patients. In patients with good health care, the incidence of early-stage and asymptomatic disease is similar to that seen in developed countries. However, patients with poor socioeconomic and nutritional status frequently experience a considerable delay before medical care is accessed; these patients often have signs and symptoms of advanced disease (147,148). In many large regions of developing countries, patients have no access to radiation facilities. In other regions, the radiation facilities are inadequate (147,149) due to inexperienced physicians, poor treatment techniques, inadequate machinery (<80 cm SSD or 60-Co), or the lack of treatment simulation. This is one of the principal reasons why large studies of radiation therapy alone compared to chemotherapy plus radiotherapy are lacking in South America, Asia, and Africa, and the use of chemotherapy alone is more prevalent.

In 1977, the GATLA/GLATHEM cooperative groups from Argentina and Latin America initiated a randomized study of chemotherapy with CVPP alone for six cycles (cyclophosphamide, 600 mg/m^2, and vinblastine, 6 mg/m^2, on day 1; and procarbazine, 100 mg/m^2, and prednisone, 40 mg, for days 1–14) versus CVPP plus radiation therapy consisting of 30 Gy to involved areas for patients with clinical stage I–II disease. Overall, the 7-year disease-free survival rate was 71% for chemotherapy and radiation therapy compared to 62% for chemotherapy alone (p = .01); survival rates were 89% and 81%, respectively (p = .3). In patients with favorable prognosis CS I–II Hodgkin's disease (age < 45 years, less than three lymph node areas involved, and without bulky disease), no differences were observed in the actuarial rates of disease-free survival (77% vs. 70%), or overall survival (92% vs. 91%), respectively, for CVPP and involved-field irradiation versus CVPP alone (Table 11). A criticism that has been raised of this study and the subsequent GATLA study is that nearly 50% of the patients were <16 years of age and treatment approaches with limited chemotherapy alone may be more successful in children than in adult patients (although not proven).

In a subsequent GATLA study, patients with favorable prognosis were randomized to CVPP for three cycles versus six cycles. At 5 years the actuarial event-free survival (80% vs. 84%) and overall survival (91% vs. 92%) rates

TABLE 11. *Randomized clinical trials in favorable prognosis stage I–II Hodgkin's disease: trials of chemotherapy alone vs. combined modality therapy*

Trial	Eligibility	Treatment regimens	No. of patients	Outcome
GATLA/ GLATHEM	CS I–II Age >45 *without* 3 or more regions of disease Bulky disease	A. CVPP × 6+ IF RT (30 Gy)	82	7-year disease-free survival: A = 77%, B = 70%, NS
		B. CVPP × 6	91	7-year survival: A = 92%, B = 91%, NS
GATLA	CS I–II with favorable prognostic features (see reference)	A. CVPP × 3	39	5-year event-free survival: A = 80%, B = 84%, p = .83
		B. CVPP × 6	41	5-year survival: A = 91%, B = 92%, p = .64
EORTC H9F	CS IA–IIB Age ≥50 *without* ESR ≥50 mm in A; ≥30 mm in B 4 or more sites of disease Large mediastinal disease (≥0.35 m/t ratio)	A. EBVP II × 6 + IF RT (36 Gy) B. EBVP II × 6 + IF RT (20 Gy) C. EBVP II × 6 alone	Open	Open
MSKCC	CS/PS IA–IIB, IIIA *without* Large mediastinal disease (≥1/3 maximum thoracic diameter) Peripheral or retroperitoneal nodes >10 cm	A. ABVD × 6 B. ABVD × 6 + mantle or inverted Y (36 Gy); STLI/TLI for stage IIIA	Open	Open

RT, radiation therapy; STLI/TLI (S), subtotal nodal/total nodal splenic irradiation; CS, clinical stage; PS, pathology stage; CVPP, cyclophosphamide, vincristine, procarbazine, prednisone; ABVD, Adriamycin (doxorubicin), vinblastine, bleomycin, dacarbazine; EBVP, epirubicin, bleomycin, vinblastine, prednisone; NS, not significant.

were similar for three versus six cycles, respectively (not significant) (150). This study also enrolled a high percentage of pediatric patients.

The ongoing EORTC three-armed trial (H_9F) for favorable prognosis CS I–II patients compares six cycles of the EBVP II regimen alone to the same regimen with different doses of involved-field irradiation. Patients who achieve a complete remission after the chemotherapy are randomized to 36 Gy involved-field irradiation versus 20 Gy involved-field irradiation versus no radiation therapy (see Table 11 for the trial design). This trial is designed to evaluate the role of involved-field irradiation in favorable prognosis early-stage Hodgkin's disease, and to evaluate potential differences in the dose of radiation delivered.

Memorial Sloan-Kettering Cancer Center Trial

This trial randomizes CS I–IIIA patients who have achieved a complete remission after six cycles of ABVD to either mantle irradiation (35 Gy) or no further treatment. Patients with large mediastinal adenopathy and nodes greater than 10 cm are not eligible; however, CS IIB and CS IIA patients are included. Thus, this trial is not restricted to early-stage favorable prognosis Hodgkin's disease. This trial has enrolled approximately 120 patients out of a planned total of 200 patients.

RECOMMENDATIONS AND FUTURE DIRECTIONS

Standard care currently provides a number of treatment options for patients with early-stage favorable prognosis Hodgkin's disease. These include the use of mantle irradiation alone for selected patients with negative laparotomy staging, mantle-paraaortic and splenic irradiation without laparotomy staging, and combination chemotherapy and radiation therapy, often with a modified number of cycles of chemotherapy and some modification of radiation field sizes and doses. Reasonable modification of chemotherapy off-study includes giving ABVD for four cycles. Reasonable modifications of radiation therapy off-study include involved-field doses of 36 to 40 Gy when combined with four to six cycles of chemotherapy, and mantle irradiation (for supradiaphragmatic presentations) to 25 to 30 Gy followed by a boost to 36 to 40 Gy when combined with four cycles of chemotherapy.

Current clinical trials are evaluating the use of alternative chemotherapy combinations, shortened courses of chemotherapy, chemotherapy with smaller radiation fields or lower radiation doses, and chemotherapy without radiation therapy. Fortunately, death from Hodgkin's disease in favorable prognosis early-stage patients is unusual and mortality from causes other than Hodgkin's disease occurs many years later; however, this means that survival is not a useful parameter to evaluate results in early-stage disease. Current trials must be judged by freedom-from-first-recurrence rates, acute morbidity, and by new criteria such as quality of life and perhaps cost-effectiveness (see Chapter 37). Trials with the objective of obtaining the highest freedom-from-first-recurrence rate possible ultimately may not provide the optimum treatment once long-term (10–20 year) data are available; treatment-related mortality may exceed Hodgkin's disease mortality in favorable prognosis early-stage patients as a result of this strategy. New methods in decision analysis should also help in the design of trials and in the analysis of retrospective data.

Despite the increasing availability of guidelines for the treatment of Hodgkin's disease, there must remain room for individualization of treatment. With different treatment options, some of which may result in a higher recurrence risk at the gain of less toxic initial treatment (without any difference in long-term survival), patient preferences must be assessed. In addition, treatment should be individualized when a particular treatment approach might result in a higher risk of a serious late complication, even when this complication may not influence overall survival (e.g., treatment of young female patients with large radiation fields and the risk of late breast cancer).

This is an exciting time for the development of new strategies in the treatment of early-stage Hodgkin's disease. Many of the ongoing trials ask questions that will allow us to optimize treatment for early-stage patients and minimize long-term toxicity.

REFERENCES

1. Peters M. A study in survivals in Hodgkin's disease treated radiologically. *Am J Roentgenol* 1950;63:299–311.
2. Lukes R, Butler J, Hicks E. Natural history of Hodgkin's disease as related to pathological picture. *Cancer* 1966;19:317–344.
3. Carbone P, Kaplan H, Musshoff K, Smithers D, Tubiana M. Report of the Committee on Hodgkin's Disease Staging Classification. *Cancer Res* 1971;31:1860–1861.
4. Glatstein E, Guernsey J, Rosenberg S, Kaplan H. The value of laparotomy and splenectomy in the staging of Hodgkin's disease. *Cancer* 1969;24:709–718.
5. Piro A, Hellman S, Moloney W. The influence of laparotomy on management decisions in Hodgkin's disease. *Arch Intern Med* 1972;130: 844–848.
6. Specht L, Gray R, Clarke M, Peto R. The influence of more extensive radiotherapy and adjuvant chemotherapy on long-term outcome of early stage Hodgkin's disease: a meta-analysis of 23 randomized trials involving 3888 patients. *J Clin Oncol* 1998;16:830–843.
7. Shore T, Nelson N, Weinerman B. A meta-analysis of stages I and II Hodgkin's disease. *Cancer* 1990;65:1155–1160.
8. Haybittle J, Easterling M, Bennett M, et al. Review of British National Lymphoma Investigation Studies of Hodgkin's disease and Development of Prognostic Index. *Lancet* 1985;1:967–972.
9. Hoogstraten B, Holland J, Kramer S, et al. Combination chemotherapy radiotherapy for stage III Hodgkin's disease. *Arch Intern Med* 1973;131:424–428.
10. Somers R, Tubiana M, Henry-Amar M. EORTC lymphoma cooperative group studies in clinical stage I–II Hodgkin's disease 1963–1987. *Recent Results Cancer Res* 1989;117:175–181.
11. Andrieu J, Coscas Y, Kramer P, et al. Chemotherapy plus radiotherapy in Clinical Stage IA–IIIB Hodgkin's disease. Results of the H77 trial (1977–1980). In: Cavalli F, Bonadonna G, Rozencweig M, eds. *Malignant lymphomas and Hodgkin's disease:* experimental and therapeutic advances. Martinus Nijhoff, 1985:353–361.
12. Zittoun R, Audebert A, Hoerni B, et al. Extended versus involved field

irradiation combined with MOPP chemotherapy in early clinical stages of Hodgkin's disease. *J Clin Oncol* 1985;3:207–214.
13. Tubiana M, Mathe G, Laugier A. Current clinical trials in the radiotherapy of Hodgkin's disease. *Cancer Res* 1968;26:1277–1278.
14. Nordentoft A. Radiotherapy in 50 cases of Hodgkin's disease in stages I and II. Report from the Lymphogranulomatosis Committee. *Ugeskr Laeger* 1972;134:2383–2385.
15. Johnson R, Thomsa L, Schneiderman M, et al. Preliminary experience with total nodal irradiation in Hodgkin's disease. *Radiology* 1970;96: 603–608.
16. Hutchison G, Alison R, Fuller L, et al. Collaborative study: radiotherapy of stage I and II Hodgkin's disease. *Cancer* 1984;54:1928–1942.
17. Hoppe R, Horning S, Hancock S, Rosenberg S. *Current Stanford clinical trials for Hodgkin's disease. Recent results in cancer research.* Berlin-Heidelberg: Springer-Verlag, 1989:182–190.
18. Wiernik P, Lichtenfeld J. Combined modality therapy for localized Hodgkin's disease. *Oncology* 1975;32:208–213.
19. Dutcher J, Wiernik P. Combined modality treatment of Hodgkin's disease confined to lymph nodes. *Dev Oncol* 1985;32:317–327.
20. Longo D, Glatstein E, Duffey P, et al. Radiation therapy versus combination chemotherapy in the treatment of early-stage Hodgkin's disease: seven-year results of a prospective randomized trial. *J Clin Oncol* 1991;9:906–917.
21. Bloomfield C, Pajak T, Glicksman A, et al. Chemotherapy and combined modality therapy for Hodgkin's disease: a progress report on Cancer and Leukemia Group B studies. *Cancer Treat Rep* 1982;66: 835–846.
22. Nissen N, Nordentoft A. Radiotherapy versus combined modality treatment of stage I and II Hodgkin's disease. *Cancer Treat Rep* 1982; 66:799–803.
23. Diehl V, Pfreundschuh M, Loffler M, et al. Therapiestudien der deutschen Hodgkin-Stediengruppe. Zwischenergebnisse der Studienprotokolle HD1, HD2 and HD3. *Onkologie* 1987;10:62–66.
24. Gehan E, Sullivan M, Fuller L, et al. The intergroup Hodgkin's disease study in children. *Cancer* 1990;65:1429–1437.
25. Anderson H, Crowther D, Deakin D, Ryder W, Radford J. A randomized study of adjuvant MVPP chemotherapy after mantle radiotherapy in pathologically staged IA–IIB Hodgkin's disease: 10-year follow-up. *Ann Oncol* 1991;2:49.
26. Gomez G, Sullivan M, Fuller L, et al. Large mediastinal mass in Hodgkin's disease. Results of two treatment modalities. *Am J Clin Oncol* 1984;6:65–73.
27. Coltman C, Myers J, Montague E, et al. The role of combined radiotherapy and chemotherapy in the primary management of Hodgkin's disease: Southwest Oncology Group studies. In: *Malignant lymphomas.* Academic Press, 1982:523–536.
28. Mauch P. Controversies in the management of patients with early stage Hodgkin's disease. *Blood* 1994;83:318–329.
29. Hoppe R, Coleman C, Cox R, Rosenberg S, Kaplan H. The management of stage I–II Hodgkin's disease with irradiation alone or combined modality therapy: the Stanford experience. *Blood* 1982;59:455–465.
30. Mauch P, Tarbell N, Weinstein H, et al. Stage IA and IIA supradiaphragmatic Hodgkin's disease: prognostic factors in surgically staged patients treated with mantle and paraaortic irradiation. *J Clin Oncol* 1988;6:1576–1583.
31. Specht L, Nordentoft A, Cold S, Clausen N, Nissen N. Tumor burden as the most important prognostic factor in early stage Hodgkin's disease. Relations to other prognostic factors and implications for choice of treatment. *Cancer* 1988;61:1719–1727.
32. Mauch P, Goodman R, Hellman S. The significance of mediastinal involvement in early stage Hodgkin's disease. *Cancer* 1978;42: 1039–1045.
33. Mauch P, Hellman S. Supradiaphragmatic Hodgkin's disease: Is there a role for MOPP chemotherapy in patients with bulky mediastinal disease? *Int J Radiat Oncol Biol Phys* 1980;6:947–949.
34. Mauch P, Gorshein D, Cunningham J, Hellman S. Influence of mediastinal adenopathy on site and frequency of relapse in patients with Hodgkin's disease. *Cancer Treat Rep* 1982;66:809–817.
35. Leopold K, Canellos G, Rosenthal D, Shulman L, Weinstein H, Mauch P. Stage IA–IIB Hodgkin's disease: staging and treatment of patients with large mediastinal adenopathy. *J Clin Oncol* 1989;7:1059–1065.
36. Prosnitz L, Curtis A, Knowlton A, Peters L, Farber L. Supradiaphragmatic Hodgkin's disease: significance of large mediastinal masses. *Int J Radiat Oncol Biol Phys* 1980;6:809–813.
37. Fuller L, Madoc-Jones H, Shullenberger C, et al. Further follow-up of results of treatment in 90 laparotomy-negative stage I and II Hodgkin's disease patients: significance of mediastinal and non-mediastinal presentations. *Int J Radiat Oncol Biol Phys* 1980;6:799–808.
38. Lee C, Bloomfield C, Goldman A, Levitt S. Prognostic significance of mediastinal involvement in Hodgkin's disease treated with curative radiotherapy. *Cancer* 1980;46:2403–2409.
39. Schomberg P, Evans R, O'Connell M, et al. Prognostic significance of mediastinal mass in adult Hodgkin's disease. *Cancer* 1984;53:324–328.
40. Velentjas E, Barrett A, McElwain T. Mediastinal involvement in early-stage Hodgkin's disease: response to treatment and pattern of relapse. *Eur J Cancer* 1980;16:1065–1068.
41. Hughes-Davies L, Tarbell N, Coleman C, et al. Stage IA–IIB Hodgkin's disease: management and outcome of extensive thoracic involvement. *Int J Radiat Oncol Biol Phys* 1997;39:361–369.
42. Carmel R, Kaplan H. Mantle Irradiation in Hodgkin's disease: an analysis of technique, tumor eradication, and complications. *Cancer* 1976;37:2813–2825.
43. Rostock R, Giangreco A, Wharam M, Lenhard R, Siegelman S, Order SE. CT scan modification in the treatment of mediastinal Hodgkin's disease. *Cancer* 1982;49:2267–2275.
44. Rostock R, Siegelman S, Lenhard R, Wharam M, Order S. Thoracic CT scanning for mediastinal Hodgkin's disease: results and therapeutic implications. *Int J Radiat Oncol Biol Phys* 1983;9:1451–1457.
45. Jochelson M, Balikian J, Mauch P, Liebman H. Peri- and paracardial involvement in lymphoma: a radiographic study of 11 cases. *Am J Roentgenol* 1983;140:483–488.
46. Jochelson M, Mauch P, Balikian J, Rosenthal D, Canellos G. The significance of the residual mediastinal mass in treated Hodgkin's disease. *J Clin Oncol* 1985;3:637–640.
47. Jochelson M, Herman T, Stomper P, Mauch P, Kaplan W. Planning mantle radiation therapy in patients with Hodgkin's disease: role of Gallium-67 scintigraphy. *Am J Roentgenol* 1988;151:1229–1231.
48. Hoppe R. The management of stage II Hodgkin's disease with a large mediastinal mass: a prospective program emphasizing irradiation. *Int J Radiat Oncol Biol Phys* 1985;11:349–55.
49. Radford J, Cowan R, Flanagan M, et al. The significance of residual mediastinal abnormality on the chest radiograph following treatment for Hodgkin's disease. *J Clin Oncol* 1988;6:940–946.
50. Cadman E, Bloom A, Prosnitz L, et al. The effective use of combined modality therapy for the treatment of patients with Hodgkin's disease who relapsed following radiotherapy. *Am J Clin Oncol* 1983;6:313–318.
51. Roach M, III, Brophy N, Cox R, Varghese A, Hoppe R. Prognostic factors for patients relapsing after radiotherapy for early-stage Hodgkin's disease. *J Clin Oncol* 1990;8:623–629.
52. Healey E, Tarbell N, Kalish L, et al. Prognostic factors for patients with Hodgkin's disease in first relapse. *Cancer* 1993;71:2613–2620.
53. Mauch P, Kalish L, Marcus K, et al. Long-term survival in Hodgkin's disease: relative impact of mortality, infection, second tumors, and cardiovascular disease. *Cancer J Sci Am* 1995;1:33–42.
54. Henry-Amar M. Second cancers after radiotherapy and chemotherapy for early stages of Hodgkin's disease. *J Natl Cancer Inst* 1983;71: 911–916.
55. Tarbell N, Thompson L, Mauch P. Thoracic irradiation in Hodgkin's disease: disease control and long-term complications. *Int J Radiat Oncol Biol Phys* 1990;18:275–281.
56. Pedersen-Bjergaard J, Larsen S. Incidence of acute nonlymphocytic leukemia, preleukemia and acute myeloproliferative syndrome up to 10 years after treatment of Hodgkin's disease. *N Engl J Med* 1982; 307:965–972.
57. Crnkovich M, Leopold K, Hoppe R, Mauch P. Stage I to IIB Hodgkin's disease: the combined experience at Stanford University and the Joint Center for Radiation Therapy. *J Clin Oncol* 1987;5:1041–1049.
58. Tubiana M, Henry-Amar M, Carde P, et al. Toward comprehensive management tailored to prognostic factors of patients with clinical stages I and II in Hodgkin's disease. The EORTC Lymphoma Group controlled clinical trials: 1964–1987. *Blood* 1989;73:47–56.
59. Gospodarowicz M, Sutcliffe S, Clark R, et al. Analysis of supradiaphragmatic clinical stage I and II Hodgkin's disease treated with radiation alone. *Int J Radiat Oncol Biol Phys* 1992;22:859–865.
60. Pavlovsky S, Maschio M, Santarelli M, et al. Randomized trial of chemotherapy versus chemotherapy plus radiotherapy for stage I–II Hodgkin's disease. *J Natl Cancer Inst* 1988;80:1466–1473.
61. Tubiana M, Henry-Amar M, Van Der Werf-Messing B, et al. A multi-

variate analysis of prognostic factors in early stage Hodgkin's disease. *Int J Radiat Oncol* 1985;11:23–30.
62. Henry-Amar M, Friedman S, Hayat M, et al. Erythrocyte sedimentation rate predicts early relapse and survival in early-stage Hodgkin's disease. *Ann Intern Med* 1991;114:361–365.
63. Tubiana M, Henry-Amar M, Hayat M, et al. The EORTC treatment of early stages of Hodgkin's disease: the role of radiotherapy. *Int J Radiat Oncol Biol Phys* 1984;10:197–210.
64. Leibenhaut M, Hoppe R, Efron B, Halpern J, Nelsen T, Rosenberg S. Prognostic indicators of laparotomy findings in clinical stage I–II supradiaphragmatic Hodgkin's disease. *J Clin Oncol* 1989;7:81–91.
65. Mauch P, Larson D, Osteen R, et al. Prognostic factors for positive surgical staging in patients with Hodgkin's disease. *J Clin Oncol* 1990;8:257–265.
66. Jones E, Mauch P. Limited radiation therapy for selected patients with stages IA and IIA Hodgkin's disease. *Semin Radiat Oncol* 1996;6:162–171.
67. Sutcliffe S, Gospodarowicz M, Bergsagel D, et al. Prognostic groups for management of localized Hodgkin's disease. *J Clin Oncol* 1985;3:393–401.
68. Cosset JM, Henry-Amar M, Meerwaldt J, et al. The EORTC trials for limited stage Hodgkin's disease. *Eur J Cancer* 1992;11:1847–1850.
69. Hoerni B, Orgerie MB, Eghbali H, et al. [New combination of epirubicine, bleomycin, vinblastine and prednisone (EBVP II) before radiotherapy in localized stages of Hodgkin's disease. Phase II trial in 50 patients]. *Bull Cancer* 1988;75:789–794.
70. Connors J, Klimo P. MOPP/ABV hybrid chemotherapy for advanced Hodgkin's disease. *Semin Hematol* 1987:24–35.
71. Castellino R, Dunnick N, Goffinet D, Rosenberg S, Kaplan H. Predictive value of lymphography for sites of subdiaphragmatic disease encountered at staging laparotomy in newly diagnosed Hodgkin's disease and non-Hodgkin's lymphoma. *J Clin Oncol* 1983;1:532–536.
72. Brada M, Easton D, Horwich A, et al. Clinical presentation as a predictor of laparotomy findings in supradiaphragmatic stage I and II Hodgkin's disease. *Radiother Oncol* 1986;5:15–22.
73. Rutherford C, Desforges J, Davies B, Barnett A. The decision to perform staging laparotomy in symptomatic Hodgkin's disease. *Br J Haematol* 1980;44:347–358.
74. Aragon de la Cruz G, Cardenes H, Otero J, et al. Individual risk of abdominal disease in patients with stages I and II supradiaphragmatic Hodgkin's disease. *Cancer* 1989;63:1799–1803.
75. Ganesan T, Wrigley P, Murray P, et al. Radiotherapy for stage I Hodgkin's disease: 20 years of experience at St Bartholomew's Hospital. *Br J Cancer* 1990;62:314–318.
76. Mandelli F, Anselmo A, Cartoni C, Cimino G, Enrici R, Biagini C. Evaluation of therapeutic modalities in the control of Hodgkin's disease. *Int J Radiat Oncol Biol Phys* 1986;12:1617–1620.
77. Mauch P, Canellos G, Shulman L, et al. Mantle irradiation alone for selected patients with laparotomy-staged IA to IIA Hodgkin's disease: preliminary results of a prospective trial. *J Clin Oncol* 1995;13:947–952.
78. Jakacki J, Luery N, McVerry P, Lange B. Haemophilus influenza diphtheria protein conjugate immunization after therapy in splenectomized patients with Hodgkin's disease. *Ann Intern Med* 1990;112:143.
79. Insel R, Anderson P. Response to oligosaccharide-protein conjugate vaccine against Hemophilus influenzae b in two patients with IgG2 deficiency unresponsive to capsular polysaccharide vaccine. *N Engl J Med* 1986;315:499.
80. Siber G, Priehs C, Madore D. Standardization of antibody assays for measuring the response to pneumococcal infection and immunization. *Pediatr Infect Dis J* 1989;88:584.
81. Molrine D, George S, Tarbell N, et al. Antibody responses to polysaccharide and polysaccharide-conjugate vaccines following treatment for Hodgkin's disease. *Ann Intern Med* 1995;123:824–828.
82. Farah J, Ultmann J, Griem M, Golomb H, Kalokhe U. Extended mantle radiation therapy for pathologic stage I and II Hodgkin's disease. *J Clin Oncol* 1988;6:1047–1052.
83. Kinzie J, Hanks G, Maclean C, Kramer S. Patterns of care study: Hodgkin's disease relapse rates and adequacy of portals. *Cancer* 1983;52:2223–2226.
84. Hanks G, Kinzie J, White R, Herring D, Kramer S. Patterns of care outcome studies: results of the national practice in Hodgkin's disease. *Cancer* 1983;51:569–573.
85. Cosset JM, Henry-Amar M, Meerwaldt J. Long-term toxicity of early stages of Hodgkin's disease therapy: the EORTC experience. *Ann Oncol* 1991;2:77–82.
86. Hancock S, Hoppe R, Horning S, Rosenberg S. Intercurrent death after Hodgkin disease therapy in radiotherapy and adjuvant MOPP trials. *Ann Intern Med* 1988;109:183–189.
87. Henry-Amar M, Hayat M, Meerwaldt J, et al. Causes of death after therapy for early stage Hodgkin's disease entered on EORTC protocols. *Int J Radiat Oncol Biol Phys* 1990;19:1155–1157.
88. Hoppe RT. Hodgkin's disease: complications of therapy and excess mortality. *Ann Oncol* 1997;8:S115–118.
89. Canellos G, Anderson J, Propert K, et al. Chemotherapy of advanced Hodgkin's disease with MOPP, ABVD, or MOPP alternating with ABVD. *N Engl J Med* 1992;327:1478–1484.
90. Santoro A, Bonfante V, Bonadonna G. Salvage chemotherapy with ABVD in MOPP-resistant Hodgkin's disease. *Ann Intern Med* 1982;96:139–143.
91. Harker W, Kushlan P, Rosenberg S. Combination chemotherapy for advanced Hodgkin's disease after failure of MOPP: ABVD and B-CAVe. *Ann Intern Med* 1984;101:440–46.
92. Longo D, Duffey P, Young R, et al. Conventional-dose salvage combination chemotherapy in patients relapsing with Hodgkin's disease after combination chemotherapy: the low probability for cure. *J Clin Oncol* 1992;10:210–218.
93. Biti G, Cimino G, Cartoni C, et al. Extended-field radiotherapy is superior to MOPP chemotherapy for the treatment of pathologic stage I–IIA Hodgkin's disease: eight-year update of an Italian prospective randomized study. *J Clin Oncol* 1992;10:378–382.
94. Coleman C, Williams C, Flint A, Glatstein E, Rosenberg S, Kaplan H. Hematologic neoplasia in patients treated for Hodgkin's disease. *N Engl J Med* 1977;297:1249–1252.
95. Canellos G, DeVita V, Arseneau J, Whang-Peng J, Johnson R. Second malignancies complicating Hodgkin's disease in remission. *Lancet* 1975;1:947–948.
96. Valagussa P, Santoro A, Kenda R, et al. Second malignancies in Hodgkin's disease: a complication of certain forms of treatment. *Br Med J* 1980;280:216–219.
97. Colman M, Easton D, Horwich A, Peckham M. Second malignancies and Hodgkin's disease—The Royal Marsden Hospital experience. *Radiother Oncol* 1988;11:229–238.
98. Tester W, Kinsella T, Waller B, et al. Second malignant neoplasms complicating Hodgkin's disease: the National Cancer Institute experience. *J Clin Oncol* 1984;2:762–769.
99. Armitage J, Dick F, Goeken J, Foucar K, Gingrich R. Second lymphoid malignant neoplasms occurring in patients treated for Hodgkin's disease. *Arch Intern Med* 1983;143:445–450.
100. Boivin J, Hutchison G, Lyden M, Godbold J, Chorosh J, Schottenfeld D. Second primary cancers following treatment of Hodgkin's disease. *J Natl Cancer Inst* 1984;72:233–241.
101. Tucker M, Coleman C, Cox R, Varghese A, Rosenberg S. Risk of second cancers after treatment for Hodgkin's disease. *N Engl J Med* 1988;318:76–81.
102. van Leeuwen F, Somers R, Taal B, et al. Increased risk of lung cancer, non-hodgkin's lymphoma and leukemia following Hodgkin's disease. *J Clin Oncol* 1989;7:1046–1058.
103. Andrieu J-M, Ifrah N, Payen C, Fermanian J, Coscas Y, Flandrin G. Increased risk of secondary acute nonlymphocytic leukemia after extended-field radiation combined with MOPP chemotherapy for Hodgkin's disease. *J Clin Oncol* 1990;8:1148–1154.
104. Swerdlow A, Douglas A, Vaughan Hudson G, Vaughan Hudson B, Bennett M, MacLennan K. Risk of second primary cancers after Hodgkin's disease by type of treatment: analysis of 2846 patients in the British National Lymphoma Investigation. *Br J Med* 1992;304:1137–1148.
105. Abrahamsen J, Andersen A, Hannisdal E, et al. Second malignancies after treatment of Hodgkin's disease: the influence of treatment, follow-up time, and age. *J Clin Oncol* 1993;11:255–261.
106. Hancock S, Tucker M, Hoppe R. Breast cancer after treatment for Hodgkin's disease. *J Natl Cancer Inst* 1993;85:25–31.
107. Tarbell N, Gelber R, Weinstein H, Mauch P. Sex differences in risk of second malignant tumours after Hodgkin's disease. *Lancet* 1993;341:1428–1432.
108. Tura S, Fiacchini M, Zinzani P, Brusamolino E, Gobbi P. Splenectomy and the increasing risk of secondary acute leukemia in Hodgkin's disease. *J Clin Oncol* 1993;11:925–930.

109. Van Leeuwen F, Klokman W, Hagenbeek A, et al. Second cancer risk following Hodgkin's disease: a 20-year follow-up study. *J Clin Oncol* 1994;12:312–325.
110. Van Leeuwen F, Chorus A, van den Belt-Dusebout A, et al. Leukemia risk following Hodgkin's disease: relation to cumulative dose of alkylating agents, treatment with teniposide combinations, number and episodes of chemotherapy, and bone marrow damage. *J Clin Oncol* 1994;12:1063–1073.
111. Biti G, Cellai E, Magrini S, Papi M, Ponticelli P, Boddi V. Second solid tumors and leukemia after treatment for Hodgkin's disease: an analysis of 1121 patients from a single institution. *Int J Radiat Oncol Biol Phys* 1994;29:25–31.
112. Mauch P, Kalish L, Marcus K, et al. Second malignancies after treatment for laparotomy staged IA–IIIB Hodgkin's disease: 20-year analysis of risk factors and outcome. *Blood* 1996;87:3625–3632.
113. DeVita V, Serpick A, Carbone P. Combination chemotherapy in the treatment of advanced Hodgkin's disease. *Ann Intern Med* 1970;73:881–895.
114. McKendrick J, Mead G, Sweetenham J, et al. ChlVPP chemotherapy in advanced Hodgkin's disease. *Eur J Cancer Clin Oncol* 1989;25: 557–561.
115. Krikorian J, Burke J, Rosenberg S, Kaplan H. Occurrence of non-Hodgkin's lymphoma after therapy for Hodgkin's disease. *N Engl J Med* 1979;300:452–458.
116. Jacquillat C, Khayat D, Desprez-Curely J, et al. Non-Hodgkin's lymphoma occurring after Hodgkin's disease. *Cancer* 1984;53:459–462.
117. Yahalom J, Petrek J, Biddinger PW, et al. Breast cancer in patients irradiated for Hodgkin's disease: a clinical and pathological analysis of 45 events in 37 patients. *J Clin Oncol* 1992;10:1674–1681.
118. Gomez G, Park J, Panahon A, et al. Heart size and function after radiation therapy to mediastinum in patients with Hodgkin's disease. *Cancer Treat Rep* 1983;67:1099–1103.
119. Jensen B, Carlsen N, Groth S, Nissen N. Later effects on pulmonary function of mantle-field irradiation, chemotherapy, or combined modality therapy for Hodgkin's disease. *Eur J Haematol* 1990;44: 165–171.
120. Gottdiener J, Katin M, Borer J, Bacharach S, Green M. Late cardiac effects of therapeutic mediastinal irradiation. *N Engl J Med* 1983;308: 569–588.
121. Brosius FI, Waller B, Roberts W. Radiation heart disease. *Am J Med* 1981;70:519–530.
122. Boivin J-F, Hutchison G, Lubin J, Mauch P. Coronary artery disease mortality in patients treated for Hodgkin's disease. *Cancer* 1992;69: 1241–1247.
123. Perrault D, Levy M, Herman J, et al. Echocardiographic abnormalities following cardiac radiation. *J Clin Oncol* 1985;3:546–551.
124. Mill W, Baglan R, Kurichety P, Prasad S, Lee J, Moller R. Symptomatic radiation-induced pericarditis in Hodgkin's disease. *Int J Radiat Oncol Biol Phys* 1984;10:2061–65.
125. Lagrange J-L, Darcourt J, Benoliel J, Bensadoun R-J, Migneco O. Acute cardiac effects of mediastinal irradiation: assessment by radionuclide angiography. *Int J Radiat Oncol Biol Phys* 1992;22:897–903.
126. Savage D, Constine L, Schwartz R, Rubin P. Radiation effects on left ventricular function and myocardial perfusion in long term survivors of Hodgkin's disease. *Int J Radiat Oncol Biol Phys* 1990;19:721–727.
127. Hancock S, Hoppe R. Long-term complications of treatment and causes of mortality after Hodgkin's disease. *Semin Radiat Oncol* 1996;6:225–242.
128. Schewe K, Reavis J, Kun L, Cox J. Total dose, fraction size, and tumor volume in the local control of Hodgkin's disease. *Int J Radiat Oncol Biol Phys* 1988;15:25–28.
129. Vijayakumar S, Myrianthopoulos L. An updated dose-response analysis in Hodgkin's disease. *Radiother Oncol* 1992;24:1–13.
130. Vijayakumar S, Rosenberg I, Brandt T, Spelbring D, Rubin S. Quantification of doses to mediastinal lymph nodes in Hodgkin's disease. *Med Dosimetry* 1992;17:87–94.
131. Vijayakumar S. What dose in Hodgkin's disease? A review of dose-response data. *Onkologie* 1992;15:190–196.
132. Duhmke E, Diehl V, Loeffler M, et al. Randomized trial with early-stage Hodgkin's disease testing 30 Gy vs. 40 Gy extended field radiotherapy alone. *Int J Radiat Oncol Biol Phys* 1996;36:305–310.
133. Wirth A, Byram D, Chao M, et al. Long term results of mantle irradiation alone in 261 patients with clinical stage I–II supradiaphragmatic Hodgkin's disease. *Int J Radiat Oncol Biol Phys* 1997;39:174.
134. Noordijk E, Carde P, Hagenbeek A, et al. Combination of radiotherapy and chemotherapy is advisable in all patients with clinical stage I–II Hodgkin's disease. Six-year results of the EORTC-GPMC controlled clinical trials H7-VF, H7-F, and H7-U. *Int J Radiat Oncol Biol Phys* 1997;39:173(abst).
135. Carde P, Burgers J, Henry-Amar M, et al. Clinical stages I and II Hodgkin's disease: a specifically tailored therapy according to prognostic factors. *J Clin Oncol* 1988;6:239–52.
136. Horning S, Hoppe R, Hancock S, Rosenberg S. Vinblastine, bleomycin, and methotrexate: an effective adjuvant in favorable Hodgkin's disease. *J Clin Oncol* 1988;6:1822–1831.
137. Bates N, Williams M, Bessell E, Hudson G, Hudson B. Efficacy and toxicity of vinblastine, bleomycin, and methotrexate with involved field radiotherapy in clinical stage IA and IIA Hodgkin's disease: a British National Lymphoma Investigation pilot study. *J Clin Oncol* 1994;12:288–296.
138. Gobbi P, Pieresca C, Frassoldati A, et al. Vinblastine, bleomycin, and methotrexate chemotherapy plus extended field radiotherapy in early, favorably presenting, clinically staged Hodgkin's patients: the Gruppo Italiano per lo Studio dei Linformi experience. *J Clin Oncol* 1996;14: 527–533.
139. Horning SJ, Hoppe RT, Mason J, et al. Stanford-Kaiser Permanente G1 study for clinical stage I to IIA Hodgkin's disease: subtotal lymphoid irradiation versus vinblastine, methotrexate, and bleomycin chemotherapy and regional irradiation. *J Clin Oncol* 1997;15:1736–1744.
140. Carde P, Noordijk E, Hagenbeek A, et al. Superiority of EBVP chemotherapy in combination with involved field irradiation over subtotal nodal irradiation in favorable clinical stage I–II Hodgkin's disease: the EORTC-GPMC H7F randomized trial. *Proc Am Soc Clin Oncol* 1997;16:13(abst).
141. Straus D, Yahalom J, Gaynor J, et al. Four cycles of chemotherapy and regional radiation therapy for clinical early-stage and intermediate-stage Hodgkin's disease. *Cancer* 1992;69:1052–1060.
142. Andrieu J, Bayle-Weisgerber C, Boiron M, et al. The chemotherapy-radiotherapy sequence in the management of Hodgkin's disease. Results of a clinical trial. *Eur J Cancer* 1979;48:153–161.
143. Radford J, Cowen R, Ryder W, et al. Four weeks of neo-adjuvant chemotherapy significantly reduces the progression rate in patients treated with limited field radiotherapy for clinical stage (CS IA/IIA) Hodgkin's disease. Results of a randomized pilot. *Ann Oncol* 1996;7:66.
144. Bartlett N, Rosenberg S, Hoppe R, Hancock S, Horning S. Brief chemotherapy, Stanford V, and adjuvant radiotherapy for bulky or advanced-stage Hodgkin's disease: a preliminary report. *J Clin Oncol* 1995;13:1080–1088.
145. Olweny C, Katongole-Mbidde E, Klife C, et al. Childhood Hodgkin's disease in Uganda: a 10-year experience. *Cancer* 1978;42:787–792.
146. Colonna P, Andrieu J. A suitable treatment for early stages of Hodgkin's disease? *Lancet* 1985;1:1224.
147. Ruiz-Arguelles G, Gomez-Almaguer D, Apreza-Molina M. Chemotherapy alone may be an efficient alternative in the treatment of early stage Hodgkin's disease if optimal radiotherapy is not available. *Leuk Lymph* 1997;27:179.
148. Hu E, Hufford S, Lukes R, et al. Third-world Hodgkin's disease at Los Angeles County-University of Southern California Medical Center. *J Clin Oncol* 1988;6:1285.
149. Pavlovsky S, Litvak J. Multidisciplinary consideration of cancer in Latin America. *Int J Radiat Oncol Biol Phys* 1984;10:77.
150. Pavlovsky S, Schvartzman E, Lastiri F, et al. Randomized trial of CVPP for three versus six cycles in favorable- prognosis and CVPP versus AOPE plus radiotherapy in intermediate- prognosis untreated Hodgkin's disease. *J Clin Oncol* 1997;15:2652–8.

Hodgkin's Disease, edited by P. M. Mauch, J. O. Armitage, V. Diehl, R. T. Hoppe, and L. M. Weiss. Lippincott Williams & Wilkins, Philadephia ©1999.

CHAPTER 26

Treatment of Unfavorable Prognosis, Stage I–II Hodgkin's Disease

Richard T. Hoppe, Jean-Marc Cosset, Armando Santoro, and Jürgen Wolf

The Ann Arbor staging system for Hodgkin's disease defines important prognostic subgroups of patients based on stage and the presence or absence of systemic (B) symptoms. In the years immediately following the introduction of this staging system, its stage groupings provided a reasonable means for categorizing patients in clinical trials. At that time, advances in radiation therapy techniques, including the use of high-dose extended-field irradiation, had resulted in dramatic increases in the proportion of patients with early-stage Hodgkin's disease who were being cured. The era of combination chemotherapy was still in its infancy. Although the initial clinical trials of the European Organization for the Research and Treatment of Cancer (EORTC) had utilized single-agent chemotherapy in combination with radiation therapy for early-stage disease (1,2), there was little experience utilizing combination chemotherapy in patients with stage I–II disease. It was not until the late 1960s and early 1970s, after initial favorable experience with MOPP (mechlorethamine, Oncovin, procarbazine, prednisone) in advanced-stage disease had been reported (3), that trials were introduced for patients with early-stage disease as well.

Poised with two very effective treatments for Hodgkin's disease, each of which had been demonstrated to be relatively safe, investigators began to combine extended-field irradiation and combination chemotherapy for patients with relatively limited disease. In stage I–II Hodgkin's disease, the early results of these trials, often reporting only freedom from relapse as an end point, demonstrated an improved outcome after combined modality treatment (4–6). Long-term outcome of these same studies, however, failed to demonstrate any differences in survival. A large metaanalysis of 23 randomized trials (3,888 patients) conducted by Specht et al. (7) confirmed this observation. A reason for the lack of survival differences in these trials is that patients with stage I–II disease who relapsed after treatment with radiation therapy alone were quite often salvaged successfully with combination chemotherapy (with or without additional radiation) (see Chapter 28). In addition, patients who were treated initially with combined modality therapy had a greater likelihood of mortality from treatment-related causes compared to patients treated initially with radiation therapy alone (see Chapter 32). Nevertheless, as single institutions and clinical trials groups began to evaluate the outcome of these studies in more detail, it became apparent that there were certain prognostic groups of patients who benefited from more aggressive treatment, whereas others could be treated effectively with conventional radiation therapy alone.

The decades of the 1970s and 1980s were marked by numerous analyses of clinical prognostic factors for patients with stage I–II Hodgkin's disease (8). The details of these studies, including the impact of treatment type and measured end points are discussed in great detail in Chapter 19. Based on these prognostic factors, clinical investigators have defined favorable and unfavorable (and occasionally very favorable) prognostic groups of patients with stage I–II disease in an effort to be more refined in the design of clinical trials and to tailor treatment in accordance with these prognostic factors. The challenge is to define for each prognostic group the precise amount of therapy that will achieve cure reliably, but with the least risk for long-term toxicity, i.e., to optimize

R. T. Hoppe: Department of Radiation Oncology, Stanford University, Stanford, California.

J.-M. Cosset: Department of Radiation Oncology, Institut Curie, Paris, France.

A. Santoro: Department of Medical Oncology, Istituto Clinico Humanitas, Milan, Italy.

J. Wolf: Department of Internal Medicine I, Klinik I für Innere Medizin, der Universität zu Köln, Köln, Germany.

the therapeutic ratio. Patients with unfavorable prognosis stage I–II disease have a somewhat worse underlying prognosis than patients with favorable prognosis stage I–II disease and in general they require more aggressive treatment. However, the likelihood of cure of patients with unfavorable stage I–II disease is still quite high and, therefore, consideration of long-term toxicity remains an important issue for these patients.

As noted in the analyses in Chapter 19, individual studies of prognostic factors vary in their conclusions. These differences may be explained by patient selection, subtle variations in staging and treatment policies, and even statistical quirks. Factors that have been cited as important in multiple studies and have been used to identify prognostic groups for clinical trials include the number of involved sites (9–12), the presence of bulky disease (especially in the mediastinum) (4,13–20), the presence of B symptoms (4,21,22), patient age (23–25), gender (23,24), and erythrocyte sedimentation rate (ESR) (26,27).

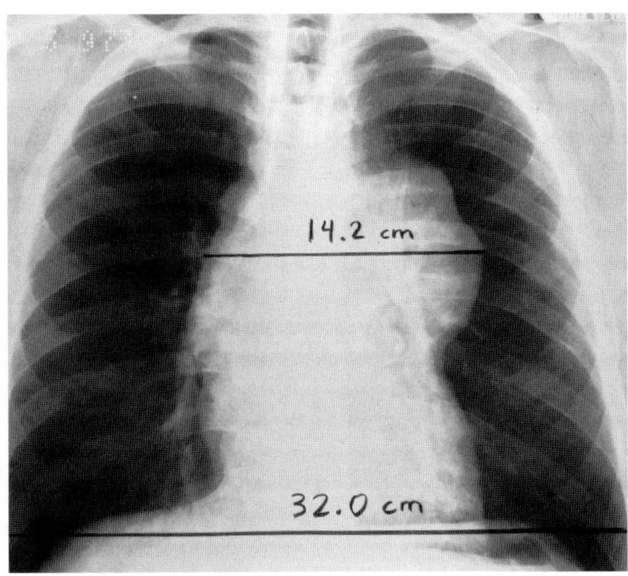

FIG. 1. An example of a large mediastinal mass. A mediastinal mass ratio (MMR) is calculated as the maximum single width of the mediastinal mass (14.2 cm) divided by the maximum intrathoracic diameter (usually at the level of the diaphragm) (32.0 cm). In this case the ratio is 0.44. A ratio >0.33 is considered unfavorable. (From ref. 88, with permission.)

BULKY DISEASE

One factor of overriding importance in stage I–II disease is the presence of bulky disease, especially in the mediastinum (4,13–20). Bulky disease has been identified as important in nearly all studies that have examined it as a potential prognostic factor in stage I–II disease. It is important to note, however, that although most series find bulky mediastinal disease to be important when freedom from relapse or event-free survival is the end point, most fail to show an impact on overall survival (4,14,15, 18–20).

The presence of mediastinal bulk is incorporated as a prognostic factor for differentiating favorable from unfavorable prognosis stage I–II Hodgkin's disease in nearly all contemporary clinical trials. Unfortunately, when the original analyses were performed evaluating the extent of mediastinal disease, multiple definitions of bulk were utilized, including absolute measurements in centimeters, surface area, volumetric calculations, and ratios of the mass size to rib cage measurements (20,28,29). As a result, the definition of mediastinal bulk in current clinical trials varies. The two most common definitions are (a) the maximum width of the mediastinal mass divided by the intrathoracic diameter at the T5-6 interspace [mediastinal tumor ratio (MTR)], with a ratio greater than 0.35 being bulky (18); and (b) the maximum width of the mediastinal mass divided by the maximum intrathoracic diameter [mediastinal mass ratio (MMR)], with a ratio greater than 0.33 being bulky (Fig. 1) (30). In fact, this difference in definition results in a marked difference in distribution of patients in favorable versus unfavorable subgroups (Fig. 2). For this reason, it is often difficult to compare the results of different clinical trials for unfavorable prognosis stage I–II disease, as the inclusion criteria may vary widely. In

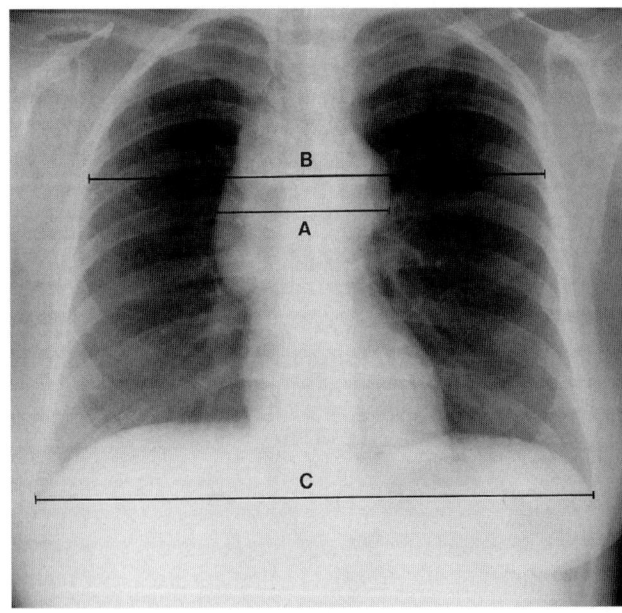

FIG. 2. Various definitions have been used to measure mediastinal bulk. The MTR is the ratio of the maximum mediastinal mass width **(A)** divided by the intrathoracic diameter at the T5-6 interspace **(B)**, with an MTR ≥0.35 generally considered to be bulky. In this example, the ratio is 9.0 cm/23.7 cm, or 0.38, so the mass is bulky. For the MMR, the maximum mediastinal mass measurement **(A)** is divided by the maximum intrathoracic diameter **(C)**. In this example, the ratio is 9.0 cm/29 cm, or 0.31, so the mass is nonbulky. (From ref. 28, with permission.)

fact, neither of these definitions is exactly consistent (although MTR is close) with the definition of mediastinal bulk according to the Cotswolds modification of the Ann Arbor staging system, which is a ratio exceeding one-third of the intrathoracic measurement at T5-6 (31).

The initial report defining mediastinal bulk and correlating bulky mediastinal disease with a worse prognosis was that of Mauch et al. (13) from the Joint Center for Radiation Therapy (JCRT). In this report, patients who had mediastinal disease less than or equal to one-third of the maximum intrathoracic diameter (MMR ≤0.33) had a relapse risk of 2% within the mediastinum, whereas patients who had mediastinal disease that exceeded one-third of the maximum intrathoracic diameter (MMR >0.33) had a relapse risk of 40% in the mediastinum. Utilizing the same definition of mediastinal bulk, Hoppe et al. (14), reporting the Stanford data, showed that patients with large mediastinal masses had a 10-year freedom from relapse of only 45% compared to 83% for patients with smaller mediastinal disease. However, the long-term survival for these two cohorts was equivalent (83% at 10 years). The freedom from relapse for patients with bulky mediastinal disease could be improved by the addition of adjuvant chemotherapy (usually MOPP). The 10-year freedom from relapse was 45% after treatment with radiation therapy alone versus 81% after combined modality treatment (Fig. 3). These general results were confirmed at a number of other centers, although varying definitions of bulky mediastinal involvement were employed, and they sometimes led to variable interpretations of the data (4,15–20,32).

The data with respect to the impact on outcome of bulk disease outside the mediastinum are limited. In fact, analysis of peripheral bulk has been completed only infrequently, likely because of the difficulty in assessing the data from medical records. In one study from the University of Florida, Mendenhall et al. (11) were able to demonstrate a higher relapse rate when peripheral nodes exceeded 6 cm in diameter. However, Bonadonna et al. (33) failed to identify an impact of peripheral bulk when disease exceeded 7 cm, despite the fact that an impact of mediastinal bulk could be demonstrated in the same series of patients. In that report, all patients were treated with chemotherapy with or without irradiation. Currently, measurement of peripheral bulk is only occasionally included as a prognostic factor to define patients as unfavorable for the purpose of clinical trials.

CONSTITUTIONAL SYMPTOMS

Constitutional symptoms (unexplained fever >38°C, drenching night sweats, and weight loss >10% in the preceding 6 months) may be correlated with other prognostic factors, such as number of sites of disease, Ann Arbor stage, total tumor burden, and ESR. However, B symptoms are usually easy to define clinically and have been associated with a worse prognosis for patients with stage I–II disease in most analyses (22,34–40). However, each B symptom does not carry equal weight. In a pooled analysis from the JCRT and Stanford University of 180 patients with pathologic stage (PS) I–IIB Hodgkin's dis-

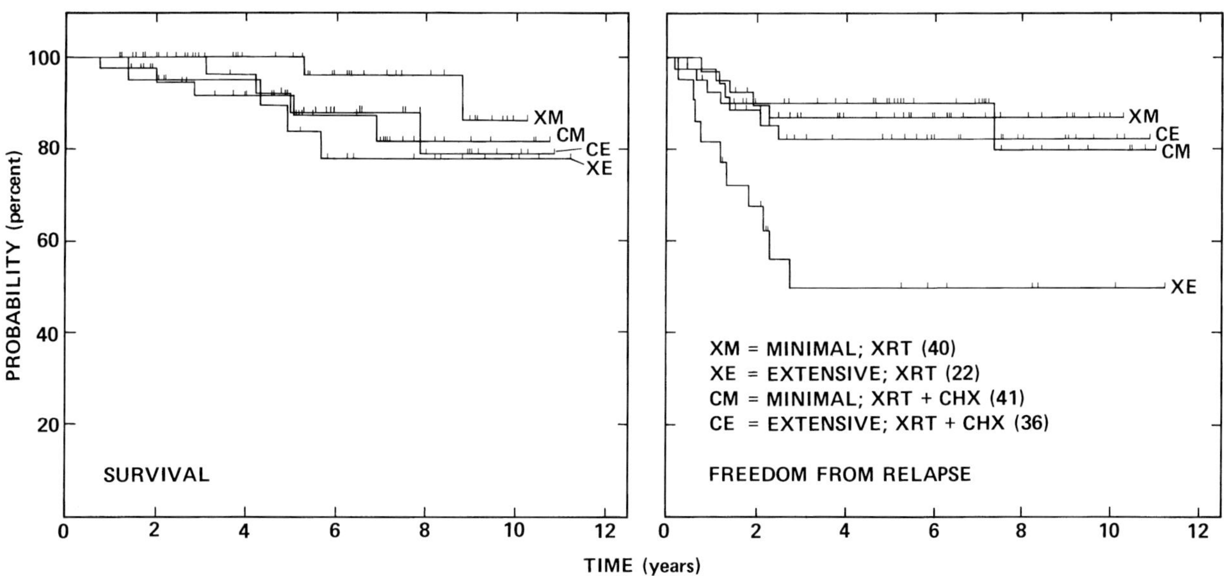

FIG. 3. The influence of bulky mediastinal disease on survival *(left)* and freedom from relapse *(right)* of 140 patients with PS I–II Hodgkin's disease treated at Stanford University with either irradiation alone (XRT) or irradiation followed by adjuvant chemotherapy (XRT + CHX). Patients with extensive mediastinal disease had a MMR >0.33. (From ref. 14, with permission.)

ease (41), the presence of night sweats alone was reported to be an inconsequential B symptom, since the freedom from relapse in that group of stage I–IIB patients was identical to that in asymptomatic stage I–IIA patients. The presence of unexplained fevers or significant weight loss each had an equivalent impact, and those patients who had both unexplained fevers and significant weight loss had an even worse prognosis, with only 48% of patients free of disease 7 years after treatment with radiation therapy alone or radiation therapy followed by adjuvant chemotherapy (Fig. 4). In a multivariate analysis of patients with single B symptoms, the relative relapse risk was 4.3 for fevers, 2.4 for weight loss, and 0.8 for night sweats.

In the total group of patients with PS I–IIB disease, the freedom from relapse was improved after treatment with combined modality therapy compared to radiation therapy alone, but the overall survival was equivalent for either management approach. This conclusion was the same as that of the randomized Stanford H2 study in which patients with PS I–IIB were randomized after laparotomy staging to treatment with total lymphoid irradiation alone or total lymphoid irradiation followed by MOPP chemotherapy. In addition, the 25-year results of the Stanford adjuvant trials for patients with PS I–IIB disease (H2, K1, and H4 trials combined) reveal no differences in survival (57% vs. 59%; $p = .5$) or freedom from relapse (71% vs. 75%; $p = .3$) for treatment with radiation therapy alone (subtotal or total lymphoid irradiation) versus the same radiation treatment followed by six cycles of MOPP (Fig. 5). It is important to remember that these patients had undergone laparotomy staging. If similar treatment approaches were used for patients after clinical staging only, substantial differences in outcome might be expected.

Another important observation in the report of Crnkovich and colleagues (41) relates to the extent of the radiation fields for patients with PS I–IIB disease. Until this publication, it was unclear whether total (including the pelvis) or subtotal (excluding the pelvis) lymphoid irradiation was the treatment of choice in PS I–IIB, for patients treated with radiation therapy alone. In this series, 69 patients were treated with total lymphoid and 34 with subtotal lymphoid irradiation alone. The 7-year survivals (87% and 88%) were similar, as were the 7-year freedom-from-relapse rates (72% and 78%). Therefore, as in supradiaphragmatic PS I–IIA disease, pelvic irradiation does not seem necessary for patients with PS I–IIB disease when the treatment is limited to irradiation.

Three other randomized clinical trials that have been reported in the literature performed subset analyses of patients with PS I–IIB disease. The Southwest Oncology Group (SWOG) 781 trial randomized patients to treatment with extended-field irradiation (mantle plus paraaortic nodes) alone versus involved-field irradiation plus six cycles of MOPP (38). The 5-year survivals were not statistically significantly different (65% versus 77%) but the 5-year relapse-free survival difference was significant (20% versus 84%; $p = .02$). It is possible that the quality control for the radiation therapy in this cooperative group trial was not sufficient (see Chapter 21), accounting for the poor outcome after treatment with irradiation alone. At the Istituto Nazionale Tumori in Milan, Italy, 69 patients with PS I–IIB disease were randomized between split-course MOPP and subtotal or total nodal irradiation versus split-course ABVD (Adriamycin, bleomycin, vinblastine, dacarbazine) plus irradiation (42). The 5-year freedom from progression was 66% versus 72% ($p = .2$). Finally, Anderson et al. (4) from Manchester reported 18 PS I–IIB patients randomized to treatment with mantle irradiation alone or mantle followed by six cycles of MVPP (mechlorethamine, vinblastine, procarbazine, and prednisone). The relapse risk was 60% after irradiation and 13% after combined modality therapy.

In a nonrandomized study, investigators from M. D. Anderson Hospital treated laparotomy-staged patients with PS I–IIB disease with combined modality therapy including mantle irradiation and only two cycles of MOPP (43). Eleven PS I–IIB patients were included, and the 4-year survival and disease-free survivals were 100%.

The current relevance of these trials is unclear, as most included laparotomy as a routine component of staging. However, the general conclusion would be that for patients with PS I–IIB disease who have undergone a staging laparotomy, either subtotal lymphoid irradiation (mantle and paraaortics) or involved field/mantle irradiation plus chemotherapy are acceptable treatment approaches. In addition, given the adverse impact of B symptoms reported in some studies, most clinical trial groups include consideration of B symptoms, either alone or in combination with ESR, in defining favorable versus unfavorable cohorts of patients with stage I–II disease.

There are no large series reporting the outcome of clinically staged patients restricted to those with I–IIB disease. In general, one must rely on studies that include multiple different adverse factors, only one of which is constitutional symptoms, to define appropriate management for clinically staged patients. For example, in a study from the Norwegian Radium Hospital, data are included for 41 patients with stage IIB Hodgkin's disease (clinical staging only) who were treated with four cycles of chemotherapy [MVPP, LVPP, ABOD, LVPP/ABVD, or EBVP (epirubicin, bleomycin, vinblastine, and prednisone)] plus mantle irradiation (44). The 10-year survival was 78% and freedom from relapse was 80%.

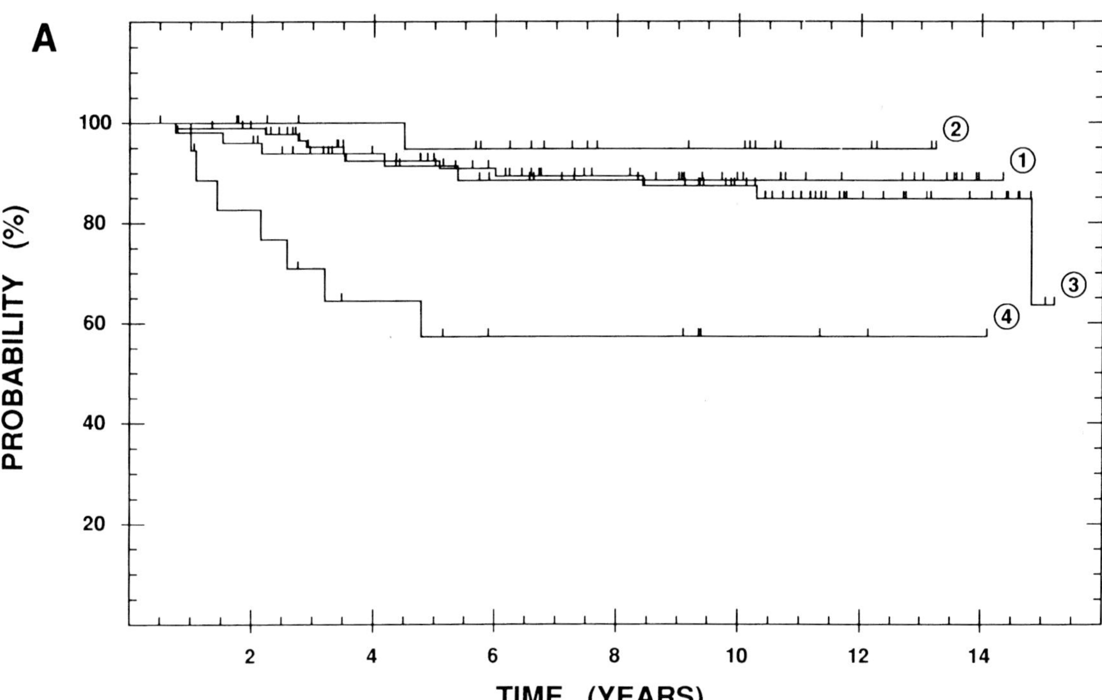

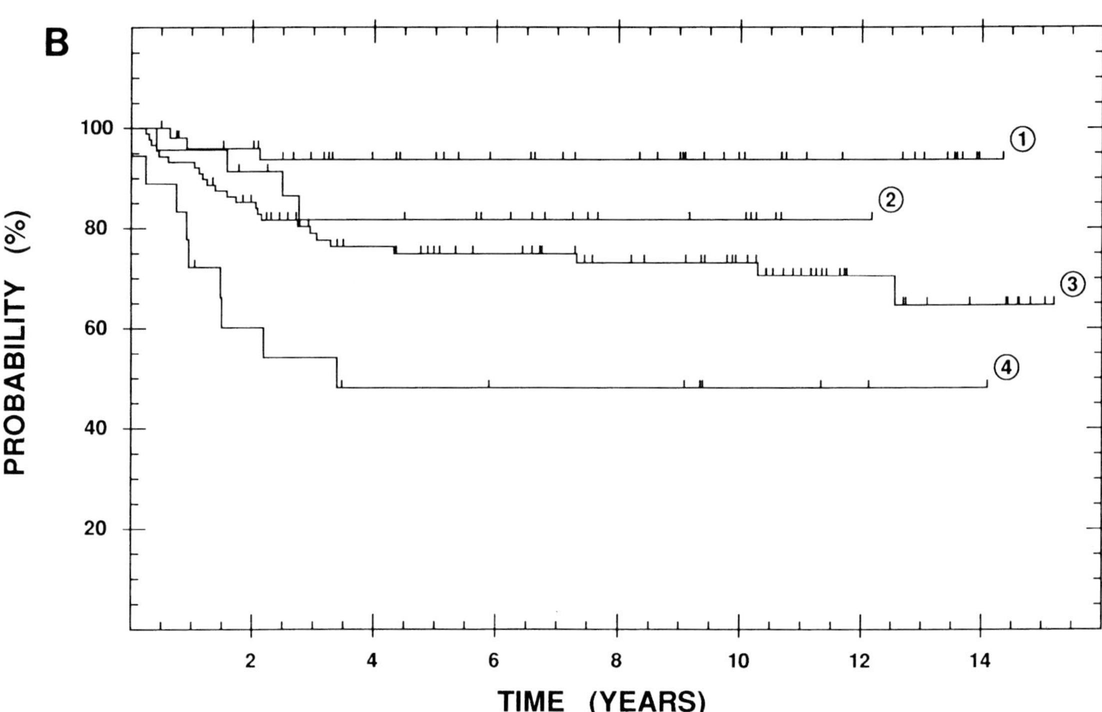

FIG. 4. **(A)** Survival and **(B)** freedom from relapse of 180 patients with PS I–IIB Hodgkin's disease treated at Stanford University or the Joint Center for Radiation Therapy, stratified according to the nature of their B symptoms. 1, night sweats only; 2, weight loss (with or without night sweats); 3, fevers (with or without night sweats); 4, both fever and weight loss present (with or without night sweats). (From ref. 41, with permission.)

A

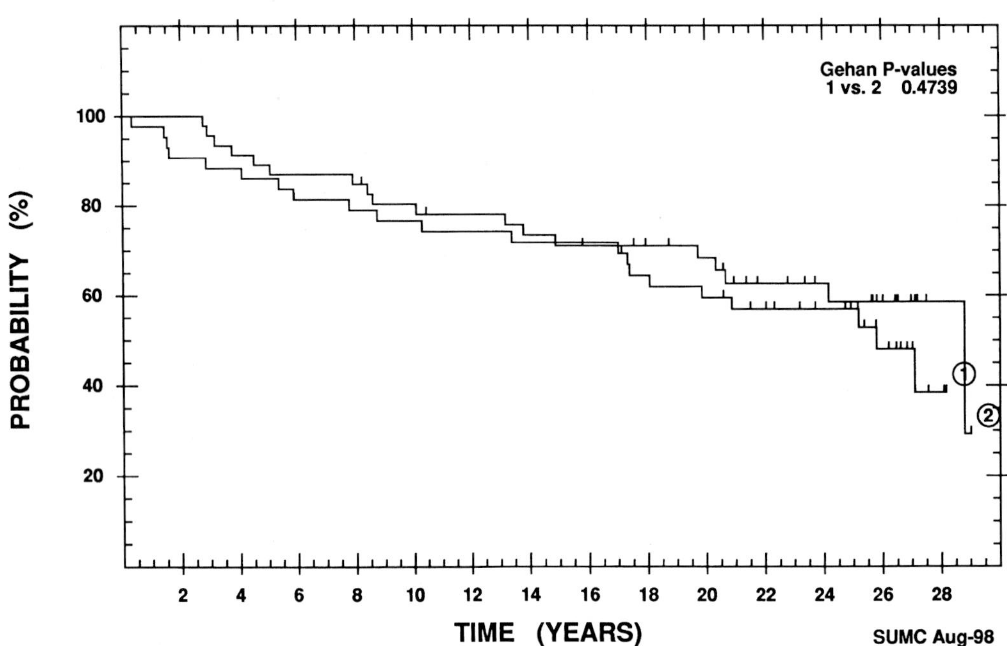

B

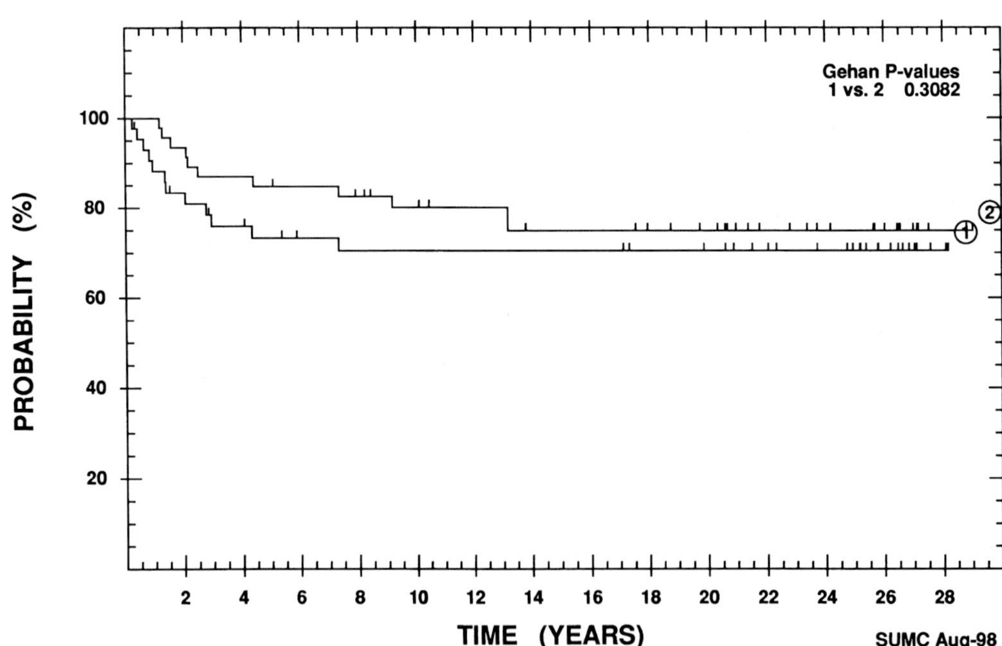

FIG. 5. (A) Survival and **(B)** freedom from relapse of 89 patients with PS I–IIB Hodgkin's disease treated on randomized clinical trials at Stanford University with either (1) radiation therapy alone (subtotal or total lymphoid irradiation) or (2) radiation followed by MOPP (mechlorethamine, Oncovin, procarbazine, prednisone) chemotherapy.

EORTC TRIALS FOR UNFAVORABLE PROGNOSIS STAGE I–II (TABLE 1)

The EORTC has made elegant use of prognostic factors in defining patient subgroups for clinical trials. However, in the very first trials (H_1 and H_2), conducted between 1964 and 1976, all patients with clinical stage (CS) I–II Hodgkin's disease were treated without distinction as to favorable or unfavorable characteristics. The long-term outcome of patients on these trials was evaluated and this led to the development of prognostic models (8). Therefore, in the H_5 trial, initiated in 1977, patients were stratified for the first time into favorable and unfavorable groups based on initial disease characteristics (45). Patients were defined as unfavorable if they had any of the following characteristics: age ≥40 years; ESR ≥70 mm (at 1 hour); mixed cellularity or lymphocyte depletion histology; or clinical stage II without mediastinal involvement. Patients with these unfavorable characteristics were assigned to the H_5U (unfavorable) trial and were randomized to treatment with total nodal radiation alone (excluding the pelvis in women younger than 40 years) or combined modality therapy. The combined modality therapy consisted of split-course MOPP and mantle, with three cycles of MOPP followed by mantle irradiation, and then another three cycles of MOPP; 296 patients were randomized. At 15 years the overall survival was 69% in both arms of the trial ($p = .36$), but the rate of treatment failure was 35% versus 16% ($p < .001$), favoring treatment with combined modality therapy (45).

In subsequent trials (H_6–H_8), the criteria for favorable and unfavorable groups were refined further. In these tri-

TABLE 1. *European Organization for Research and Treatment of Cancer (EORTC) randomized trials for unfavorable prognosis stage I–II Hodgkin's disease*

Study	Dates	Eligibility	Laparotomy	Treatment arms
H_1	1964–1971	All CS I–II	No	A. Mantle or inverted-Y (40–45 Gy) B. Mantle or inverted-Y + vinblastine weekly for 2 years
H_2	1972–1976	All CS I–II Supradiaphragmatic	Randomized	A. No laparotomy; subtotal nodal irradiation (incl. spleen) (40–45 Gy) B. Laparotomy; subtotal nodal irradiation In both arms A and B, patients with MC or LD histology received adjuvant chemotherapy (vinblastine or vinblastine plus procarbazine) for 2 years
H_5U	1977–1982	CS II with negative mediastinum *or* MC or LD histology *or* age ≥40 *or* ESR ≥70	No	A. Total nodal irradiation (40–45 Gy) B. 3 MOPP + mantle (35 Gy) + 3 MOPP
H_6U	1982–1988	≥3 regions *or* A and ESR ≥50 *or* B and ESR ≥30 *or* bulky mediastinum	No	A. 3 MOPP + mantle (35 Gy) + 3 MOPP B. 3 ABVD + mantle + 3 ABVD
H_7U	1988–1993	Age ≥50 *or* A and ESR ≥50 *or* B and ESR ≥30 *or* ≥4 sites *or* bulky mediastinum	No	A. 6 EBVP II + involved field (36–40 Gy) B. 6 MOPP/ABV + involved field
H_8U	1993–1998	Same as H_7U	No	A. 6 MOPP/ABV + involved field (36 Gy) B. 4 MOPP/ABV + involved field (36 Gy) C. 4 MOPP/ABV + subtotal nodal irradiation (36 Gy)
H_9U	1998–	Same as H_7U	No	A. 6 ABVD + involved field (30 Gy) B. 4 ABVD + involved field (30 Gy) C. 4 BEACOPP + involved field (30 Gy)

H_1 study included all CS I–II patients and H_2 study included all CS I–II patients with supradiaphragmatic disease. Retrospective analysis of prognostic factors in these trials led to definitions of "unfavorable" in subsequent EORTC trials. H_5U study also included patients from H_5F trial who were identified to be stage IIIA after laparotomy. Bulky mediastinum defined as MTR >0.35 at T5-6. H_8U and H_9U trials were in collaboration with GELA.

CS, clinical stage; LD, lymphocyte depletion; MC, mixed cellularity; ESR, erythrocyte sedimentation rate; MOPP, mechlorethamine, Oncovin, procarbazine, prednisone; ABVD, Adriamycin bleomycin, vinblastine, docarbazine; BEACOPP, bleomycin, etoposide, Adriamycin, cyclophosphamide, Oncovin, procarbazine, prednisone.

als, patients were considered unfavorable and entered into the H_6U, H_7U, and H_8U studies if they had any of the following characteristics: an ESR ≥50 mm; an ESR ≥30 mm in the presence of B symptoms; a mediastinal mass exceeding 0.35 of the intrathoracic diameter at T5-6 (MTR >0.35); or three or more sites of disease (four or more in the H_7 and H_8). In the H_6U study (no. 20822, 1982–1988), in consideration of the results of the H_5U study, which demonstrated a lower relapse risk after combined modality therapy, all patients received split-course chemotherapy and mantle irradiation. Treatment consisted of three cycles of chemotherapy, followed by mantle irradiation (35 Gy with an optional 5- to 10-Gy boost), and then three more cycles of chemotherapy. The chemotherapy was randomized between MOPP and ABVD (46). The trial included 316 patients, and at 10 years the survival in both arms was 87% (p = .5); however, the risk of treatment failure was 24% for MOPP versus 12% for ABVD (p <.01) (6) (Fig. 6). With respect to complications, there was less hematologic and late gonadal toxicity with ABVD than MOPP. However, early decrement in pulmonary vital capacity was more common after ABVD than MOPP (12% vs. 2%, p = .08) and there were two respiratory deaths in the combined modality ABVD arm (46). There were no significant differences in changes in left ventricular ejection fractions following treatment in the two different arms of the trial. In general, given the lower hematologic and gonadal toxicity, ABVD would appear to be the preferred of these two combinations in these young patients. However, careful attention must be paid to the pulmonary status of patients who receive ABVD, especially when mantle irradiation is contemplated (see Chapter 34).

In the H_7U trial (no. 20881), conducted from 1988 to 1992, combined modality therapy using two different non-MOPP combinations was compared. Treatment was with either EBVP II chemotherapy followed by involved-field irradiation (36 Gy) or six cycles of MOPP/ABV chemotherapy (47) followed by involved-field irradiation. The EBVP II combination was a less intense (and presumably safer) drug combination for early-stage Hodgkin's disease developed by Hoerni et al. (48). However, in an interim analysis at 3 years, after 316 patients had been randomized, a significant difference in failure-free survival was detected (72% vs. 88%) favoring the MOPP/ABV combination (49). At 6 years, the treatment failure rate was 31% versus 12% (p <.001) (6), the event-free survival was 68% versus 90% (p = .0001), and the overall survival was 82% versus 89% (p = .18) (50). These unexpectedly poor results for EBVP II in combined-modality programs for unfavorable early-stage disease are in contrast to the results in favorable early-stage disease, where it has become the control arm of the H9F trial (see Chapter 25).

The H_8U trial (no. 20931), a collaborative study between the EORTC and the French Adult Lymphoma Group (GELA), was a three-arm trial conducted from 1993 to 1998. Based on the H_7U results, MOPP/ABV was selected as the standard chemotherapy. A three-arm trial was designed to evaluate both the number of cycles of chemotherapy required and the extent of the radiation fields. The treatment options were MOPP/ABV × 6 plus involved-field irradiation (36 Gy), MOPP/ABV × 4 plus involved-field irradiation, and MOPP/ABV × 4 plus subtotal nodal irradiation (6). Although the results of this trial have not yet been reported, the accrual goals have been met and the trial has been closed. Given the design of the H_9U trial, it is likely that no superiority of the more extensive radiation fields has been observed in the H_8U trial thus far.

The H_9U trial is also a three-arm study, two arms of which are common with the German Hodgkin's Study Group (GHSG) HD11 trial (*vide infra*). MOPP/ABV chemotherapy has been replaced by ABVD, in part due to excessive toxicity of MOPP/ABV reported in a recent Cancer and Leukemia Group B (CALGB) trial, when com-

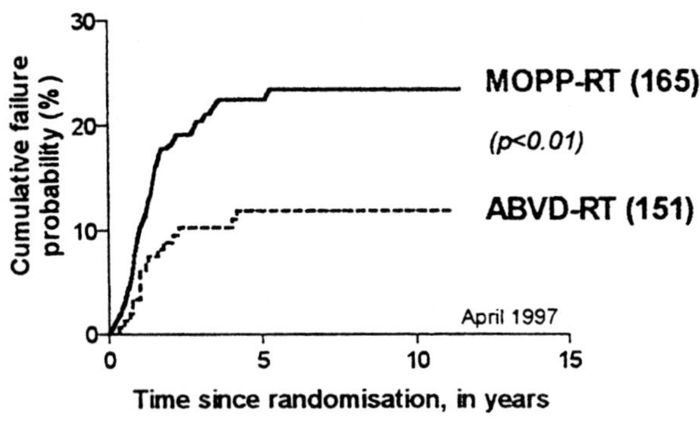

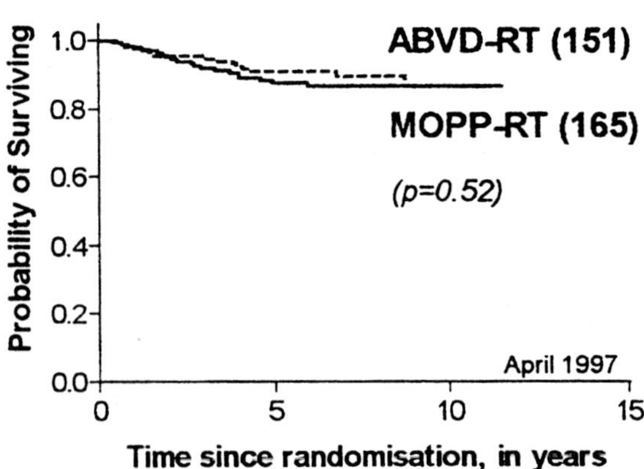

FIG. 6. Risk of failure *(left)* and overall survival *(right)* of 316 patients on the EORTC H_6U trial. Patients with CS I–II disease and unfavorable characteristics were randomized to treatment with combined-modality therapy utilizing MOPP or ABVD (Adriamycin, bleomycin, vinblastine, dacarbazine) chemotherapy sandwiched around mantle irradiation. (From ref. 6, with permission.)

pared to ABVD (51). In addition, the escalated BEACOPP [bleomycin, etoposide, Adriamycin, cyclophosphamide, Oncovin (vincristine), procarbazine and prednisone] regimen of the GHSG (52) is incorporated in one of the treatment arms. The combined modality treatments included in this trial are ABVD × 6 plus involved-field irradiation (now reduced to 30 Gy), ABVD × 4 plus involved field, and BEACOPP × 4 plus involved field (53).

GERMAN HODGKIN'S STUDY GROUP TRIALS FOR UNFAVORABLE PROGNOSIS STAGE I–II (TABLE 2)

The GHSG initiated prospective randomized clinical trials in 1983, and from the outset considered prognostic subgroupings in its assignment of patients to clinical protocols. The HD1 trial was open from 1983 to 1988 and accrued 180 patients (148 of whom were randomized). Laparotomy staging was performed routinely. Patients were considered unfavorable if they had stage I–IIA/B or IIIA disease with bulky mediastinal disease (MMR ≥0.33), extranodal involvement, or massive splenic disease (diffuse involvement or more than five nodules) (54). This was a combined modality therapy trial in which the question asked related to radiation therapy dose. All patients were treated with two cycles of COPP (cyclophosphamide, Oncovin, procarbazine, prednisone)/ABVD (4 months) followed by irradiation to extended fields. The dose was 20 Gy on one arm and 40 Gy on the other arm of the trial; however, sites of bulky disease (≥5 cm) were always treated to 40 Gy.

A separate analysis of the HD1 study has not been reported, but results have been published together with one of the arms of the HD5 trial (54). The HD5 trial, active from 1988 to 1993, included patients who had an MMR ≥0.33; an ESR ≥50 mm; B symptoms in combination with an ESR ≥30 mm; more than three sites of disease; extranodal involvement; or massive splenic disease. In addition, patients with stage IIIA in the absence of risk factors were included. The treatment randomization was between combined modality with COPP/ABVD (two double cycles) or COPP/ABV/IMEP (two triple cycles) plus extended-field irradiation (40 Gy to bulky sites, 30 Gy to nonbulky or uninvolved sites). The COPP/ABVD arm included 111 patients who had eligibility criteria identical to patients in the HD1 trial, and the results for

TABLE 2. *GHSG randomized trials for unfavorable prognosis stage I–II Hodgkin's disease*

Study	Dates	Eligibility	Laparotomy	Treatment arms
HD1	1983–1988	PS I–II with bulky mediastinal mass *or* E involvement *or* massive splenic disease	Yes	A. 2 (COPP/ABVD) + extended field (40 Gy) B. 2 (COPP/ABVD) + extended field (20 Gy) plus 20 Gy boost to initially bulky (>5 cm) sites
HD5	1988–1993	CS I–II with bulky mediastinal mass *or* A and ESR ≥50 *or* B and ESR ≥30 *or* ≥3 sites *or* E involvement *or* massive splenic disease	Yes	A. 2 (COPP/ABVD) + extended field (30 Gy) plus 10 Gy boost to initially bulky (>5 cm) sites B. 2 (COPP/ABV/IMEP) + extended field (30 Gy) plus 10 Gy boost to initially bulky (>5 cm) sites
HD8	1993–1998	CS IA–IB *or* CS IIA with bulky mediastinal mass *or* E involvement or ESR ≥50 *or* >2 sites; CS IIB with ESR ≥30 *or* >2 sites; CS IIIA without any risk factors; massive splenic disease	No	A. 2 (COPP/ABVD) + extended field (30 Gy) plus 10 Gy boost to initially bulky sites B. 2 (COPP/ABVD) + involved field (30 Gy) plus 10 Gy boost to initially bulky sites
HD9	1993–1998	CS IIB with bulky mediastinal mass *or* massive splenic disease *or* E involvement	No	A. 4 (COPP/ABVD) + limited irradiation (30 Gy to initially bulky, 40 Gy to residual) B. 8 BEACOPP + limited irradiation C. 8 BEACOPP escalated + limited irradiation
HD11	1998–	Same as HD8, except massive splenic disease no longer included; excludes stage IIIA	No	A. 4 ABVD + involved field (30 Gy) B. 4 ABVD + involved field (20 Gy) C. 4 BEACOPP + involved field (30 Gy) D. 4 BEACOPP + involved field (20 Gy)

Bulky mediastinal mass defined as MMR ≥0.33 at maximum transthoracic diameter. Massive splenic disease defined as diffuse involvement or >5 nodules. HD5 trial also included patients who were eligible for the HD4 (favorable) trial, but were found to have PS IIIA disease at the time of laparotomy.

COPP, cyclophosphamide, Oncovin, procarbazine, prednisone; IMEP, ifosfamide, methotrexate, etoposide, prednisone; MMR, ratio of mediastinal mass width to maximum intrathoracic measurement; PS, pathologic stage.

these patients were compared to the two arms of the HD1 trial. In effect, this became a comparison of combined modality therapy (2 COPP/ABVD) in which extended fields were irradiated to three different doses: 20, 30, and 40 Gy. Bulky sites (≥5 cm in any axis) were always irradiated to 40 Gy. The 4-year survivals were 93%, 94%, and 88% for 20, 30, and 40 Gy, respectively (p = .8). The corresponding survivals were 86%, 80%, and 90% (p = 0.5). This suggests that in a combined-modality program that includes the equivalent of at least 4 months of COPP/ABVD chemotherapy, as little as 20 Gy irradiation to nonbulky sites and 40 Gy to bulky sites (>5 cm) is adequate (Fig. 7) (54).

The HD8 trial, conducted between 1993 and 1998, included 1,209 patients with CS IA–B or CS IIA with any of the following risk factors: MMR >0.33, massive splenic disease, extranodal disease, ESR >50, and three or more sites of disease. It also included patients with CS IIB disease who had an ESR >30 or three or more sites of disease and patients with CS IIIA without any risk factors. Staging laparotomy was not performed. Patients with stage IIB who had an MMR ≥0.33, extranodal involvement, or massive splenic disease were treated on the HD9 study. The HD8 trial utilized the same chemotherapy as the HD1 and HD5 trials (2 COPP/ABVD) and a radiation field size question was posed. Patients were randomly assigned to involved-field (30 Gy, 40 Gy to bulky sites) or extended-field (30 Gy, 40 Gy to bulky sites) irradiation following the completion of chemotherapy. The preliminary results based on 685 evaluable patients show no difference in survival or freedom from treatment failure between the two study arms, after a median follow-up of 26 months. There was significantly greater hematopoietic and gastrointestinal toxicity in the extended-field treatment group.

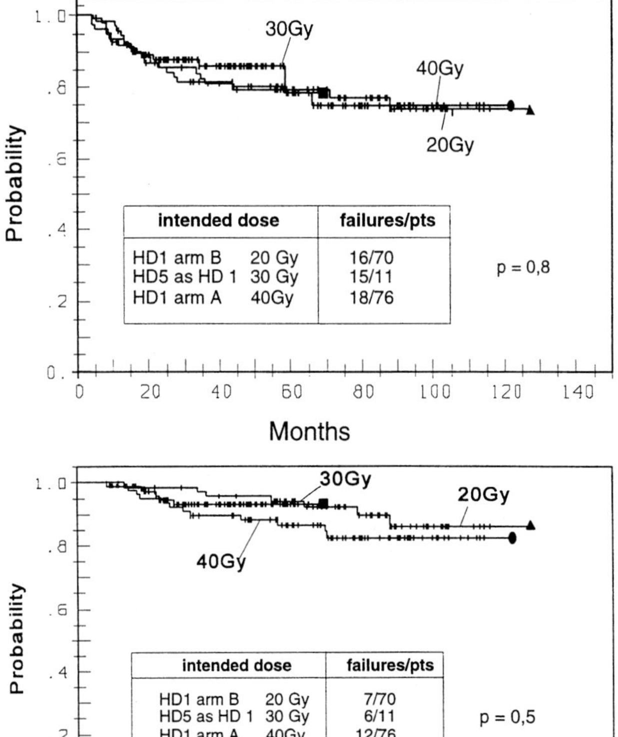

FIG. 7. Freedom from treatment failure *(top)* and overall survival *(bottom)* of 157 patients treated on the GHSG HD1 and HD5 studies. Patients with CS I–II disease and unfavorable characteristics were treated with combined-modality therapy including 40 Gy to sites of disease ≥5 cm and 20, 30, or 40 Gy to sites <5 cm. (From ref. 54, with permission.)

The HD9 trial, intended primarily for patients with advanced disease, also included patients with stage IIB disease who had an MMR ≥0.33, extranodal involvement, or massive splenic disease. This study randomized patients to three different combined modality programs. The chemotherapy was either 4 COPP/ABVD (8 months), 8 BEACOPP-baseline, or 8 BEACOPP-escalated. The GHSG developed a BEACOPP regimen as a dose-intense chemotherapy program with both higher dose and accelerated administration (see Chapter 27). Chemotherapy was followed in each instance by limited irradiation (30 Gy to initially bulky sites, 40 Gy to sites of residual disease) (52); 321 patients were accrued to this study. The complete response rate in the combined BEACOPP arms was 89%, compared to only 76% in the COPP/ABVD arm. Only 6% of the BEACOPP-treated patients progressed, versus 12% after COPP/ABVD. The freedom from treatment failure at 24 months was also significantly better for BEACOPP (85%) than for COPP/ABVD (74%). Based on these early observations, the COPP/ABVD arm was closed, and remaining patients were randomized only to the two BEACOPP schemes. Early analysis indicates a superiority of BEACOPP-escalated over BEACOPP-baseline with respect to freedom from treatment failure and progressive disease. Hematologic toxicity was greater for BEACOPP-escalated (52).

The HD11 study replaces the HD8 study, and has just opened for accrual. This is a four-arm trial of combined modality therapy, testing chemotherapy type, and radiation dose. The four arms are 4 ABVD plus involved field (30 Gy), 4 ABVD plus involved field (20 Gy), 4 BEACOPP plus involved field (30 Gy), and 4 BEACOPP plus involved field (20 Gy) (53). The first and third arms of this trial are identical to the EORTC H$_9$U trial, which was also opened recently (*vide supra*).

THE STANFORD CLINICAL TRIALS FOR UNFAVORABLE PROGNOSIS STAGE I–II (TABLE 3)

The initial Stanford clinical trial for stage I–II Hodgkin's disease (the L1 study) did not distinguish

TABLE 3. *Stanford randomized trials for unfavorable prognosis stage I–II Hodgkin's disease*

Study	Dates	Eligibility	Laparotomy	Treatment Arms
L1	1962–1967	All CS I–II	No	A. Involved field irradiation (44 Gy) B. Extended field irradiation (44 Gy/33 Gy)
H2	1968–1980	PS I–IIB (B symptoms)	Yes	A. Total lymphoid irradiation (44 Gy/35 Gy) B. Total lymphoid irradiation + 6 MOP(P)
K1	1968–1974	PS IIEA	Yes	A. Total lymphoid irradiation (44 Gy/35 Gy)
H4		PS IIEB (E lesions)		B. Total lymphoid irradiation + 6MOP(P)
S2	1974–1980	PS IIEA	Yes	A. Total lymphoid irradiation (44 Gy) + 6MOP(P)
S3		PS IIEB (E lesions)		B. Total lymphoid irradiation (44 Gy) + 6PAVe
C2	1980–1990	CS I–IIA	No	A. 3 PAVe + mantle (44 Gy) + 3 PAVe
C3		CS I–IIB (bulky mediastinum *or* multiple E lesions)		B. 3 ABVD + mantle (44 Gy) + 3 ABVD
G2	1990	CS I–II (bulky mediastinum)	No	12-week Stanford V chemotherapy plus irradiation (36 Gy) to initially bulky (>5 cm) sites

The L1 study included all patients with CS I–II disease. Radiation dose (involved/uninvolved) portions of field. Prednisone was deleted from the MOP(P) combination whenever there was prior mediastinal irradiation. Pelvic irradiation was not utilized on the K1 or S2 (PS IIEA) trials. Bulky mediastinum defined as MMR more than one-third of *maximum* intrathoracic diameter. The G2 study is nonrandomized.

PAVe, procarbazine, Alkeran, Velban.

between favorable and unfavorable presentations, and all patients were randomized to treatment with involved-field or extended-field irradiation. Based on the early results of this trial, patients with B symptoms were identified as having a worse prognosis and subsequently included in separate clinical trials. Somewhat later, other factors, including multiple sites of extranodal involvement (stage IV according to the criteria of many), and a large mediastinal mass, i.e., MMR >0.33, were identified as unfavorable prognostic signs.

The results of early clinical trials for patients with B symptoms are summarized above. In 1980, specific trials were initiated for patients with stage I–II disease and large mediastinal masses (MMR >0.33) or multiple extranodal sites of disease. Staging laparotomy was not performed. Between 1980 and 1990, patients were randomized to combined-modality therapy with either PAVe (55), a MOPP-like combination that included procarbazine, *l*-phenylalanine mustard, and vinblastine, or ABVD. The treatment was administered in a split-course fashion, i.e., three cycles (months) of chemotherapy, followed by mantle irradiation (44 Gy), followed by three more cycles of chemotherapy. At 15 years, both the survival (73% vs. 100%, $p = .06$) and freedom from relapse (56% vs. 83%, $p = .1$) were superior in the ABVD arm.

In 1990, a nonrandomized pilot study was initiated for patients with large mediastinal masses (MMR >0.33) using the Stanford V management approach, i.e., brief intensive chemotherapy followed by irradiation (at first 44 Gy, later 36 Gy) to initially bulky sites (greater than 5 cm) (see Chapter 27) (56–58); 39 patients have been treated on this protocol thus far. The 5-year survival and freedom-from-relapse rates are 100%. Based on these data, a phase III clinical trial will be initiated in the Eastern Cooperative Oncology Group (ECOG) (E2496), randomizing patients between ABVD and Stanford V chemotherapy followed in either case by 36 Gy to initially bulky sites.

TRIALS OF RADIATION THERAPY ALONE VERSUS COMBINED MODALITY THERAPY FOR UNFAVORABLE PROGNOSIS STAGE I–II (TABLE 4)

Clinical trials of radiation therapy alone versus combined modality therapy in unfavorable early-stage Hodgkin's disease are uncommon. In general, combined-modality therapy has become the treatment of choice for these patients. However, there are some older studies, conducted between 1968 and 1982, that bear on this question and, in addition, some studies that included both favorable and unfavorable prognosis patients together may be analyzed with respect to the outcome of patients with unfavorable prognostic factors. The Stanford H2 clinical trial compared total lymphoid irradiation alone with combined-modality therapy (total lymphoid irradiation plus MOPP) in the management of patients with laparotomy stage I–II disease and B symptoms. This trial demonstrated no advantage to the combined-modality approach (41). In contrast, the SWOG trial of extended-field irradiation versus involved field plus MOPP did show a significant improvement in 5-year relapse-free survival with the combined-modality approach for patients with B symptoms, although there was no signif-

TABLE 4. *Randomized clinical trials in unfavorable prognosis stage I–II Hodgkin's disease: radiation therapy vs. combined modality therapy*

Trial	Eligibility	Treatment regimens	No. of patients	Outcome
Stanford H2 1968–1980	PS I–IIB (B symptoms)	A. TLI B. TLI + 6 MOP(P)	A. 27 B. 27	25-year results: Freedom from relapse: A = 73%, B = 76%, p = .5 Survival: A = 69%, B = 55%, p = .5
SWOG* 781 1972–1978 (38)	PS IIB (B symptoms)	A. EF (35–45 Gy) B. IF + 6 MOPP	A. 17 B. 22	5-year results: Relapse-free survival: A = 20%, B = 84%, p = .02 Survival: A = 65%, B = 77%, p = NS
Manchester* 1974–1981 (4)	PS IIB (B symptoms) PS I–II MTR >0.33 (bulky mediastinum)	A. Mantle (35 Gy) B. Mantle + 6 MVPP	IIB Bulky mediastinum A. 10 A. 11 B. 8 B. 11	Relapse risk: B symptoms: A = 60%, B = 12.5% Bulky mediastinum: A = 64%, B = 18%
NCI-BCRC* 1968–1975 (61)	PS II–IIIE (extranodal disease)	A. EF (40 Gy) B. Limited RT (40 Gy) + 6 MOPP	A. 11 B. 7	Relapse risk: A = 83%, B = 14% 3-year remission duration: A = 17%, B = 85%, p < .01 4-year survival: A = 57%, B = 100%, p < .025
Stanford* Adjuvant Chemotherapy Trials 1968–1979 (60)	PS IIE–IIIAE (extranodal disease)	A. STLI/TLI B. STLI/TLI + MOP(P) or PAVe	A. 14 B. 33	10-year results: Freedom from progression: A = 71%, B = 97% Survival: A = 66%, B = 96%
Stanford* Adjuvant Chemotherapy Trials 1968–1978 (14)	PS I–II MMR>1/3 (bulky mediastinum)	A. STLI/TLI (44 Gy) B. IF/STLI/TLI + 6 MOPP or 6 PAVe	A. 14 B. 27	10-year results: Freedom from relapse A = 45%, B = 81%, p = .03 Survival A = 84%, B = 74%, p = .09
EORTC H_5U 1977–1982 (45)	CS II with uninvolved mediastinum *or* MC, LD *or* age ≥40 or ESR ≥70	A. TNI B. 3 MOPP + mantle (35 Gy) + 3 MOPP	A. 152 B. 144	15-year results: Treatment failure: A = 35%, B = 16%, p <.001 Overall survival: A = 69%, B = 69%, p = .36

*Subset analysis.

RT, radiation therapy; IF, involved field RT; EF, extended field RT; STLI, subtotal lymphoid irradiation; TLI, total lymphoid irradiation; TNI, total nodal irradiation; NS, not significant (p > .05); MTR, ratio of mediastinal mass width to intrathoracic measurement at T5-6 interspace; MMR, ratio of mediastinal mass width to maximum intrathoracic measurement.

icant difference in 5-year survival (38). As noted above, this may have been due to poor quality control of the radiation therapy in this study. The Manchester lymphoma group studied mantle irradiation alone versus mantle followed by MVPP chemotherapy, and showed a decrease in the relapse risk with combined-modality therapy (4); however, this is not surprising, as there are no data to support the use of such limited radiation fields alone in patients with stage I–IIB disease.

With respect to patients who have extensive intrathoracic disease, numerous retrospective comparisons show a significant decrease in relapse risk (or event-free survival) after treatment with combined-modality therapy compared to radiation therapy alone, but no significant improvement in survival (4,14,15,18–20) (see Fig. 2). However, in consideration of the improved freedom from relapse and the expected lower long-term toxicity, combined-modality therapy has become the treatment of choice for most of these patients.

Regarding limited extralymphatic involvement (the E lesion), the classic work of Musshoff and colleagues (59) suggested that this was not an adverse prognostic factor and that these patients could be treated adequately with irradiation alone. An analysis of the Stanford data suggested this was correct, with no significant improvement observed in either survival or freedom from relapse in these patients by the addition of chemotherapy (60). However, the trial reported from the National Cancer Institute–Baltimore

Cancer Research Center (NCI–BCRC) suggested that combined-modality therapy was superior in this setting. It is likely, however, that in this study the presence of extralymphatic disease was simply a surrogate for extensive mediastinal disease, as 15 of the 18 patients with E lesions had pulmonary parenchymal involvement and 11 of these 15 patients had "3+" mediastinal involvement ("extensive involvement, with greater than 4 cm increase in mediastinal silhouette and/or hilar involvement extending more than 2 cm beyond one or both mediastinal margins") (61). It is likely that Musshoff was correct, that patients with isolated extralymphatic disease do not have a worse prognosis.

For patients with other adverse prognostic factors, such as unfavorable histology (mixed cellularity or lymphocyte depleted), older age (≥40), and elevated ESR (≥70 mm), the most important study is the EORTC H_5U trial, which compared total lymphoid irradiation with split-course MOPP and mantle. In this trial, although the risk of relapse was markedly less with combined-modality therapy (p <.001), the survivals in the two arms were equivalent at 15 years (69%) (6).

REFINEMENTS OF COMBINED-MODALITY THERAPY FOR UNFAVORABLE PROGNOSIS STAGE I–II

Trials to Identify the Best Chemotherapy Combination (Table 5)

The evolution of studies to identify the best chemotherapy combination for unfavorable early-stage Hodgkin's disease have paralleled trials to identify the best chemotherapy in advanced Hodgkin's disease (see Chapters 22 and 27). Early trials evaluated MOPP versus MOPP-like combinations, later trials compared MOPP or MOPP-like combinations with ABVD, and the most recent trials compare novel intense chemotherapy combinations with ABVD.

The first combined modality trial to test MOPP versus ABVD in this group of patients was the Milan study conducted between 1974 and 1982, which included 69 patients with stage IIB disease (42). In this study, split-course treatment was employed, with three cycles of chemotherapy preceding and following subtotal nodal irradiation. There was no significant difference in 5-year freedom from progression. The Stanford C2-3 studies were initiated in 1980 and included patients with large mediastinal masses (MMR >0.33) or multiple E-lesions (62,63). The design was similar to the Milan study, with split-course chemotherapy; however, the extent of radiation was mantle alone. The chemotherapy randomization was between PAVe (55) and ABVD. At 15 years, the survival (73% vs. 100%; p = .06) and freedom from relapse (56% vs. 83%; p = .1) were both superior in the ABVD arm, but not at a level that reached statistical significance.

The EORTC H_6U trial (1982–1988) had a design similar to the Stanford study (split-course chemotherapy and mantle only), and compared MOPP and ABVD (6,46); 316 patients were randomized. The 10-year survival was equivalent in both arms (87%), but the treatment failure rate was worse with MOPP (23% vs. 12%; p <.01). Of concern is the fact that pulmonary toxicity in this trial was somewhat greater in the ABVD-treated patients (46). The group at Hôpital St.-Louis randomized patients to treatment with 4 months of MOP or MOP/ABVD followed by slightly extended field irradiation. The 7-year data failed to show any differences in relapse-free or overall survival (64).

In the GHSG HD5 trial (1988–1992) (54), patients with unfavorable characteristics received combined modality therapy comparing 2 × COPP/ABVD with rapidly alternating 2 × COPP/ABV/IMEP (ifosphamide, methotrexate, etoposide, and prednisone). The results of this trial have not been reported.

The failure of the ABVD-containing regimens to show convincing advantage over the MOPP or MOPP-like combinations in these studies is in contrast to the results observed in trials of chemotherapy alone for patients with advanced Hodgkin's disease (65). This may be due to two factors: (a) the studies for stage I–II patients always included irradiation, and the use of combined-modality therapy may obscure the differences that are observed after treatment with chemotherapy alone; and (b) the number of patients in these trials may have been inadequate to demonstrate a difference that truly exists.

In patients with unfavorable prognosis who receive combined-modality therapy, especially those patients with large mediastinal masses, one must consider the potential risk due to the overlapping pulmonary toxicities of bleomycin and irradiation and the potential overlapping cardiac toxicities of doxorubicin and irradiation. Careful delineation of the radiation fields is required (*vide infra*). Nevertheless, recognition of these risks has led to attempts to develop less toxic drug combinations for these patients.

The Grupo Argentino de Tratamiento de la Leucemia Aguda (GATLA) identified an unfavorable group of patients based on age, B symptoms, number of involved sites, an MMR >0.33, and peripheral nodes >5 cm. Patients were treated with split-course chemotherapy around involved-field irradiation. The chemotherapy was randomized between the MOPP-like CVPP (cyclophosphamide, vincristine, procarbazine, and prednisone) and the less intense AOPE [Adriamycin (doxorubicin), Oncovin (vincristine), prednisone, and etoposide] regimen (66); 176 patients were randomized, about one-third of whom had stage III disease. The 5-year survival (95% vs. 87%; p = .16) and event-free survival (85% vs. 66%; p = .009) were both superior in the CVPP arm. Similarly, when the EORTC attempted to reduce drug intensity in the H_7U trial, randomizing patients between six cycles of EBVP II (plus involved-field irradiation) and six cycles of MOPP/ABV (plus involved-field irradiation), the 6-

TABLE 5. *Randomized clinical trials in unfavorable prognosis stage I–II Hodgkin's disease: identification of the optimal chemotherapy combination*

Trial	Eligibility	Treatment regimens	No. of patients	Outcome
Instituto Nazionale Tumori, Milan* 1974–1982 (42)	PS IIB (B symptoms)	A. 3 MOPP + STNI/TNI + 3 MOPP B. 3 ABVD + STNI/TNI + 3 ABVD	A. 33 B. 36	5-year freedom from progression: A = 65.5%, B = 71.7%, p = .2
Stanford S2-S3 1974–1980 (62)	PS IIEA–IIEB (E involvement)	A. STLI/TLI (44 Gy) + 6 MOPP B. STLI/TLI + 6 PAVe	A. 7 B. 8	20-year results: Freedom from relapse: A = 71%, B = 100%, *p* = .1 Survival: A = 71%, B = 88%, *p* = .3
Stanford C2-C3 1980–1990 (62)	CS IIA–IIB with bulky mediastinum (MMR >1.3) or multiple E lesions	A. 3 PAVe + 3 PAVe + mantle (44 Gy) B. 3 ABVD + mantle + 3 ABVD	A. 12 B. 12	15-year results: Freedom from relapse: A = 56%, B = 83%, *p* = 0.1 Survival: A = 73%, B = 100%, *p* = .06
EORTC H_6U 1982–1988 (46)	CS I–II with ≥3 regions *or* A and ESR ≥50 *or* B and ESR ≥30 *or* bulky mediastinum (MTR >0.35 at T5-6)	A. 3 MOPP + mantle (35 Gy) + 3 MOPP B. 3 ABVD + mantle + 3 ABVD	A. 165 B. 151	10-year results: Treatment failure: A = 23%, B = 12%, *p* < .01 Survival: A = 87%, B = 87%, *p* = .52
Hôpital St. Louis* H 81 1980–1985 (64)	CS I–IIB or CS I–II with bulky mediastinal involvement (MMR >1/3 maximum intrathoracic measurement)	A. 4 MOP + local RT/EF (40 Gy) B. 2 (MOP/ABVD) + local RT/EF	A. 24 B. 19	7-year results: Relapse-free survival: A = 84%, B = 83% Overall survival: A = 91%, B = 77%
GATLA 1986–1992 (66)	"Score" of age, B symptoms, stage, no. of sites, and bulky disease (MMR >1/3 or nodes >5 cm)	A. 3 CVPP + IF (30 Gy)+ 3 CVPP B. 3 AOPE + IF + 3 AOPE	A. 92 B. 84	5-year results: Event-free survival: A = 85%, B = 66%, *p* = .009 Overall survival: A = 95%, B = 87%, *p* = .16
EORTC H_7U 1988–1992 (67)	CS I–II with age ≥50 *or* A and ESR ≥50 *or* B and ESR ≥30 *or* ≥4 sites or MTR >0.35 at T5-6	A. 6 EBVP II + IF (36 Gy) B. 6 MOPP/ABV + IF	A. 160 B. 156	6-year results: Event-free survival: A = 68%, B = 90%, *p* < .0001 Overall survival: A = 82%, B = 89%, *p* = .18
EORTC H_9U 1988– (53)	Same as H_7U	A. 6 ABVD + IF (30 Gy) B. 4 ABVD + IF C. 4 BEACOPP + IF	Open	Open
GHSG HD5 1988–1993 (54)	MMR ≥0.33 *or* A and ESR ≥50 *or* B and ESR ≥30 *or* ≥3 sites *or* E involvement *or* massive splenic disease	A. 2 (COPP/ABVD) + EF (30–40 Gy) B. 2 (COPP/ABV/ IMEP) + EF	A. 111	Not reported
GHSG HD9 1993–1998 (53)	IIB with MMR >0.33 *or* massive splenic disease *or* E involvement	A. 4 (COPP/ABVD) + limited RT (30–40 Gy) B. 8 BEACOPP baseline + limited RT C. 8 BEACOPP escalated + limited RT		Not reported separately for CS IIB patients; for all patients randomized, freedom from treatment failure in A vs. B/C (*p* = .001)
GHSG HD11 1998– (53)	CS IA–B or CS IIA with MMR ≥0.33 *or* E involvement *or* ESR ≥50 or >2 sites or CS IIB and ESR >30	A. 4 ABVD + IF (30 Gy) B. 4 ABVD + IF (20 Gy) C. 4 BEACOPP + IF (30 Gy) D. 4 BEACOPP + IF (20 Gy)	Open	Open
ECOG 2496 1998– (58)	MMR >1/3	A. 6 ABVD + RT (36 Gy) to bulky sites (>5 cm) B. 12 week Stanford V + RT to bulky sites	Open	Open

*Subset analysis.
AOPE, Adriamycin, Oncovin, prednisone, etoposide.

year survival (82% vs. 89%; $p = .18$), event-free survival (68% vs. 90%; $p = .0001$), and risk of treatment failure (31% vs. 12%; $p < .001$) were all worse in the EBVP II arm (67). Therefore, in contrast to studies for patients with favorable prognosis stage I–II Hodgkin's disease (see Chapter 25), where less toxic and less intense chemotherapy regimens have been effective in combined modality therapy programs, this does not appear to be the case for patients with unfavorable prognosis disease.

Several nonrandomized trials have evaluated alternative chemotherapy regimens. At the Fondation Bergonie, an unfavorable group of patients was identified based on age, histology, or B symptoms. Two cycles of CVPP were followed by extended-field irradiation. The disease-free survival was 80% at 10 years (68). At the M. D. Anderson Hospital, three cycles of NOVP (novantrone, vincristine, vinblastine, and prednisone) were combined with involved-field irradiation for patients with mediastinal adenopathy >7.5 cm. The 3-year freedom from progression was 89% (69). The SWOG 9051 study tested three cycles of EVA (etoposide, vinblastine, and doxorubicin) followed by subtotal lymphoid irradiation in patients with CS I–III disease. A large mediastinal mass (>9 cm) was present in 55%. The 3-year failure-free survival was only 67%, with most patients failing in sites of initial bulk, another example of less intense chemotherapy being inadequate for these patients (70). At Stanford, the Stanford V regimen (nitrogen mustard, Adriamycin, vincristine, vinblastine, etoposide, bleomycin, and prednisone), administered for 3 months, was followed by mediastinal/supraclavicular irradiation to 36 Gy in 38 patients with mediastinal mass ratios >0.33. No patients have relapsed or died (median follow-up 40 months) (58).

Largely based on trials in advanced Hodgkin's disease (65), ABVD has become the standard regimen employed in this group of patients. Therefore, current trials compare combined modality therapy utilizing ABVD with more intense, novel regimens. Both the EORTC H_9U and GHSG HD11 studies of combined modality therapy are comparing four cycles of ABVD with four cycles of BEACOPP baseline (53). In the ECOG 2496 study of combined modality therapy, six cycles of ABVD are being compared to 3 months of Stanford V (58).

Trials to Identify the Optimal Number of Cycles of Chemotherapy (Table 6)

Until recently, there was only a single randomized trial that addressed the question of how many cycles of chemotherapy are necessary to include in combined modality programs for unfavorable prognosis stage I–II Hodgkin's disease. In a trial conducted at the Hôpital St.-Louis between 1972 and 1975 (H72 02), patients with stage I–II who had B symptoms, more than two sites of disease, or extranodal involvement were assigned to management with staging laparotomy followed by three cycles of MOPP plus mantle irradiation or six cycles of MOPP followed by staging laparotomy plus mantle irradiation. Patients with large mediastinal masses were not specifically included in this trial. Among the 46 patients with B symptoms, the survival at 4 years was 100% and the disease-free survivals (among complete responders) were 93% and 96% after either three or six cycles of chemotherapy (71). The recently closed EORTC H_8U study randomized patients to combined modality therapy with four or six cycles of MOPP/ABV, but the results have not yet been reported. The new EORTC H_9U trial randomizes patients to four or six cycles of ABVD (53).

A number of nonrandomized studies also have addressed this question, evaluating outcome in patients with early-stage Hodgkin's disease who had a variety of unfavorable factors. It is logical to consider separately the results for patients with bulky mediastinal disease and patients with other unfavorable prognostic factors.

TABLE 6. *Randomized clinical trials in unfavorable prognosis stage I–II Hodgkin's disease: trials to identify the optimal number of cycles of chemotherapy*

Trial	Eligibility	Treatment regimens	No. of patients	Outcome
Hôpital St. Louis H72 02 1972–1975 (71)	CS I–II with B symptoms >2 sites *or* E involvement	A. Laparotomy + 3 MOPP + mantle (40 Gy) B. 6 MOPP + laparotomy + mantle	A. 18 B. 28	Maximum 4 years' follow-up Among patients with B symptoms: Survival A = 100%, B = 100% Disease-free survival among complete responders: A = 93%, B = 96%
EORTC H_8U 1993–1998 (6)	Age ≥50 *or* A and ESR ≥50 *or* B and ESR ≥30 *or* ≥4 sites *or* MTR >0.35	A. 6 MOPP/ABV + IF (36 Gy) B. 4 MOPP/ABV + IF C. 4 MOPP/ABV + STLI	Not reported	Not reported
EORTC H_9U 1998– (53)	Same as EORTC H_8U	A. 6 ABVD + IF (30 Gy) B. 4 ABVD + IF C. 4 BEACOPP + IF	Open	Open

Studies of Patients with Large Mediastinal Masses

In an M. D. Anderson Hospital trial incorporating only two cycles of MOPP, 14 patients with a large mediastinal mass (7.5–11.5 cm) had a disease-free survival of only 63% (43). Brusamolino and colleagues (72), from Pavia, Italy, treated patients with bulky mediastinal disease (not otherwise defined) with combined modality therapy, using three cycles of ABVD. The 10-year survival was 70% and freedom from relapse 74%.

In the Paris-Ouest-France trial 81/12, 11 patients with bulky mediastinal masses (MTR >0.45) were treated with three cycles of ABVD and methyl prednisolone followed by subtotal nodal irradiation (73). The 10-year survival was 78%, but the freedom from progression was only 63%. The Hôpital St.-Louis trial H85, conducted between 1985 and 1994, treated patients who had a variety of unfavorable prognostic factors with three cycles of ABVD (vindesine substituted for vinblastine) followed by subtotal nodal irradiation (74). Patients with large mediastinal masses (MTR >0.33) had a 5-year survival of 82%. Finally, the Milan study of four cycles of ABVD plus irradiation (involved field versus extended field) included 20% of patients with bulky disease (Table 7), which Santoro presented at European Congress of Clinical Oncology ECCO in 1997. The 4-year freedom from progression was 95%.

Miscellaneous Unfavorable Prognostic Factors

A study from Algeria (PA 80), conducted between 1980 and 1985, utilized three cycles of MOPP followed by subtotal nodal irradiation in clinically staged patients (75). Among the 20 patients with B symptoms, the 6-year survival was 88% and disease-free survival (of complete responders) was 93%. A study from the Fondation Bergonie (*vide supra*), used only two cycles of CVPP for clinically staged patients with unfavorable early-stage disease, including B symptoms, unfavorable histology, older age, and extranodal extension (68). The disease-free survival was 80% at 10 years.

Fuller et al. (43) from the M. D. Anderson Hospital analyzed outcome for a series of patients with mediastinal disease, B symptoms, or lower abdominal involvement. Patients were laparotomy staged, and treated with either two cycles of MOPP followed by mantle irradiation or mantle irradiation followed by two cycles of MOPP. Eleven patients with B symptoms had a 4-year survival and freedom from relapse of 100%. Finally, at the Norwegian Radium Hospital in Oslo, 41 patients with B symptoms were treated with 4 months of chemotherapy (several different MOPP-like and ABVD-like combinations, as well as an alternating regimen) followed by mantle irradiation (41.4 Gy) (44). The 10-year survival was 78% and freedom from relapse 80%.

Based on these retrospective data, it appears that patients with unfavorable disease by virtue of age, histology, number of sites of disease, or B symptoms may be treated adequately in combined modality programs with as little as 3 months of conventional chemotherapy. For patients with large mediastinal masses the data are less clear, and may depend somewhat on the definition of large mediastinal adenopathy; however, it appears that at least 4 months of chemotherapy is required in this group. If one looks simply at duration of chemotherapy (ignoring intensity), the Stanford V program is attractive, since the 38 patients with an MMR >0.33 who were treated with just 3 months of chemotherapy had a 4-year survival and freedom from relapse of 100% (Table 3) (58).

Trials to Identify the Optimal Timing of Chemotherapy

No randomized trials have tested the question of optimal timing of chemotherapy and irradiation for patients with unfavorable prognosis stage I–II Hodgkin's disease. The evolution of management for these patients was such that at first many patients were treated with radiation therapy followed by adjuvant chemotherapy, for example, the H_1 and H_2 studies of the EORTC, the H2, H4, and K1 Stanford studies, the SWOG 781 trial, the Manchester MVPP trial, and the NCI–BCRC study (Tables 1, 3, and 4).

Eventually, the advantages of initial treatment with chemotherapy—the opportunity to treat all involved and occult sites of disease at the outset, and the ability to use more restricted (and less toxic) radiation fields by taking advantage of tumor shrinkage secondary to chemotherapy—became apparent. Some studies, which incorporated 6 months of conventional chemotherapy, used a split-course or sandwich approach, with an initial 3 months of chemotherapy, followed by irradiation, and then completion of the chemotherapy. In addition to the advantages noted above, the use of a split-course approach meant that the delay from the start of treatment to the initiation of irradiation was never longer than 3 months. This approach was used in the EORTC H_5U and H_6U, the Stanford C2 and C3 studies, the two studies from GATLA, the French trial of involved- versus extended-field irradiation, and the Milan study of MOPP versus ABVD (Tables 1, 3, and 5).

Beginning in the 1980s, issues related to dose intensity of chemotherapy were raised and several studies noted a reduction in chemotherapy doses after irradiation was administered (42,55,76). Subsequently, especially with a reduction in the duration of chemotherapy to as few as 3 or 4 months in many trials, the majority of clinical trials now include the entire course of chemotherapy before the start of irradiation.

Trials to Identify the Appropriate Radiation Therapy Volume (Table 7)

Several randomized trials have addressed the question of radiation therapy volumes in combined modality programs.

TABLE 7. *Randomized clinical trials in unfavorable prognosis stage I–II Hodgkin's disease: trials to identify the appropriate radiation volume*

Trial	Eligibility	Treatment regimens	No. of patients	Outcome
French Cooperative 1976–1981 (77)	Age ≥40 *or* MC/LD *or* CS II without mediastinum involved *or* E involvement *or* B symptoms	A. 3 MOPP + IF 40 Gy + 3 MOPP B. 3 MOPP + EF 40 Gy + 3 MOPP	A. 109 B. 109	Six-year results: DFS A = 87%, B = 93%, $p = .15$
INT, Milan 1990– (78)	All CS I–II includes age >40, bulky disease, E involvement, >3 sites	A. 4 ABVD + STNI (36/30 Gy) B. 4 ABVD + IF (36 Gy)	A. 65 B. 68	Five-years results: FFP A = 96%, B = 93% OS A = 100%, B = 96%
EORTC/GELA H_8u 1993–1998 (6)	Age ≥50 *or* A and ESR ≥50 or B	A. 6 MOPP/ABV + IF (36 Gy) B. 4 MOPP/ABV + IF C. 4 MOPP/ABV + STLI	Not reported	Not reported
GHSG HD8 1993–1998 (53)	MT ratio ≥0.35 *or* ESR ≥50 *or* B symptoms and ESR ≥30 *or* ≥3 sites *or* E involvement *or* massive splenic involvement	A. 2 (COPP/ABVD) + EF (30 Gy, 40 Gy to bulk) B. 2 (COPP/ABVD) + IF	Not reported	Not reported

DFS, disease free survival; FFP, freedom from progression; OS, overall survival.

One of the first was a French trial reported by Zittoun et al. (77): 209 patients with stage I–II and a variety of unfavorable factors were treated with six cycles of MOPP sandwiched around involved-field (40 Gy) or extended-field (40 Gy) irradiation. The 6-year disease-free survivals were 87% and 93%, respectively ($p = .15$). The Milan study reported by Santoro et al. (78) incorporated only 4 months of chemotherapy (ABVD), followed by involved-field (36 Gy) or subtotal nodal irradiation (30–36 Gy); 133 patients were treated, 20% of whom had bulky disease. The 5-year freedom-from-progression rates were 96% and 93%.

Studies not yet reported, which bear on this issue, include the EORTC/GELA H_8U (no. 20931) trial and the GHSG HD8 trial. In the EORTC/GELA study, open from 1993 to 1998, two of the three arms were 4 × MOPP/ABV plus involved-field (36 Gy) and 4 × MOPP/ABV plus subtotal nodal irradiation. The GHSG HD8 trial, also conducted between 1993 and 1998, used two cycles (4 months) of COPP/ABVD followed by either involved-field or extended-field irradiation (30 Gy to involved or uninvolved sites, 40 Gy to initially bulky sites).

The evidence from these randomized trials, as well as numerous nonrandomized studies (44,71,79), indicates that radiation fields may be safely limited to involved regions (variably defined) in most combined modality programs.

Trials to Identify the Appropriate Radiation Therapy Dose

Initial studies of combined modality therapy for Hodgkin's disease generally utilized doses that were similar to doses used for radiation treatment alone (36–44 Gy). The GHSG HD1 tested 40 Gy versus 20 Gy extended-field irradiation (bulky sites >5 cm were always treated to 40 Gy) following two cycles (4 months) of COPP/ABVD. Because the HD5 trial used the same chemotherapy plus 30 Gy extended field (40 Gy to bulky sites), the data could be pooled for analysis, providing a comparison of 20, 30, and 40 Gy for the nonbulky and uninvolved portions of the field. Loeffler et al. (54) reported no significant differences for the three different radiation doses when employed after 4 months of conventional chemotherapy (Fig. 4).

Nonrandomized trials have infrequently utilized doses <30 Gy for these patients with unfavorable disease characteristics. However, the newest trial of the GHSG (HD11), which is a four-arm randomization, evaluates involved field doses of 30 Gy versus 20 Gy following either 4 × ABVD or 4 × BEACOPP-baseline (53). Unlike the HD1 and HD5 trials, bulky sites will no longer be boosted to 40 Gy. It will be especially important to evaluate the outcome of this trial for patients based on the presence of bulky disease.

TRIALS OF CHEMOTHERAPY ALONE VERSUS COMBINED MODALITY THERAPY FOR UNFAVORABLE PROGNOSIS STAGE I–II (TABLE 8)

Only one prospective trial of chemotherapy alone versus combined modality therapy in unfavorable prognosis stage I–II has been reported. GATLA randomized 104

TABLE 8. *Randomized clinical trials in unfavorable prognosis stage I–II Hodgkin's disease: trials of chemotherapy alone vs. combined modality therapy*

Trial	Eligibility	Treatment regimens	No. of patients	Outcome
GATLA 1977–1986 (79)	Age >45 *or* ≥3 sites *or* bulky disease (nodes >5 cm, mediastinum >10 cm, or MMR >1/3)	A. 6 CVPP B. 3 CVPP + IF(30 Gy) + 3 CVP	A. 60 B. 44	Seven-year results: DFS A = 34%, B = 75%, p = .001 OS A = 66%, B = 84%
NCI-C HD6 1993– (personal communication R. Meyer)	MC/LD *or* age ≥40 *or* ESR ≥50 *or* ≥4 sites; MMR >1/3 or nodes >10 cm *excluded*	A. 2 ABVD +extended mantle (35 Gy) or mantle + paraaortics B. 4–6 ABVD	Open	Open

CVPP, cyclophosphamide, vinblastine, procarbazine, prednisone; DFS, disease-free survival; OS, overall survival.

patients with unfavorable disease characteristics including older age, more than two sites of involvement, or bulky disease to treatment with six cycles of CVPP alone or six cycles of CVPP sandwiched around involved-field irradiation (30 Gy). The 7-year survivals were 66% and 84% and the freedom-from-relapse rates were 34% and 75% (p <.001), in both circumstances favoring the combined modality approach (80).

One ongoing trial is the National Cancer Institute of Canada (NCI-C) HD6 trial. Patients with unfavorable disease characteristics (but excluding those with MMR >0.33 or nodes >10 cm) are randomized to receive combined modality therapy with two cycles of ABVD followed by irradiation (an extended mantle plus spleen or mantle plus paraaortics and spleen) or four to six cycles (depending on the rapidity of response) of ABVD alone (R. Meyer, personal communication).

TECHNIQUES OF RADIATION THERAPY IN THE MANAGEMENT OF PATIENTS WITH UNFAVORABLE EARLY-STAGE DISEASE (LARGE MEDIASTINAL MASSES)

Radiation Alone

Although the majority of reports and the state of the art support the use of combined-modality therapy for patients with bulky mediastinal Hodgkin's disease, there may be exceptional situations where the use of radiation therapy alone is acceptable. For example, some mediastinal masses may be bulky according to standard definitions, but the location (superior mediastinum) and lack of extension to adjacent organs may permit the use of high-dose irradiation with curative intent and expectations. This may be especially so with the use of computed tomographic based treatment planning (81,82). Much of the data showing a

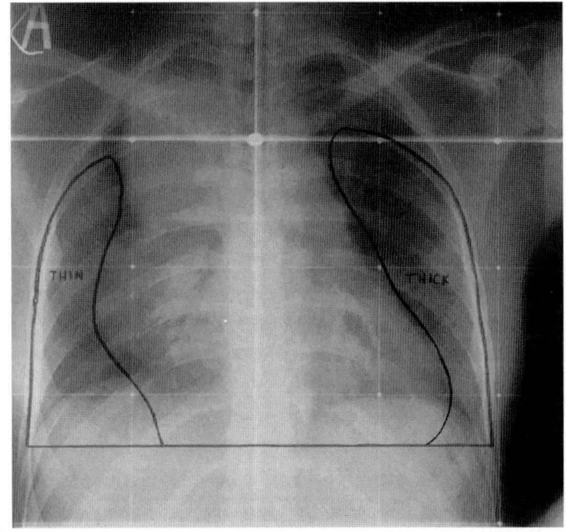

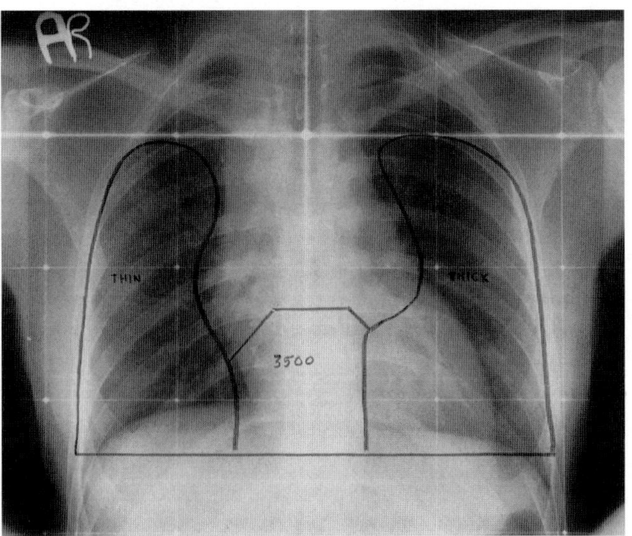

A B

FIG. 8. An example of planning films demonstrating the shrinking field technique. **A:** Initial film of a patient with a large mediastinal mass. She was treated to these fields to a dose of 15 Gy in ten fractions over 2 weeks. Treatment was then interrupted to permit tumor regression. **B:** After a break of 14 days a new mantle field could be designed incorporating larger blocks, protecting a significant proportion of the heart and lungs. The patient is alive without evidence of disease more than 20 years after treatment with irradiation alone. (From ref. 89, with permission.)

poor prognosis for patients with large mediastinal masses were based on patients who were treated in the late 1960s and early 1970s. It is likely that the extent of intrathoracic disease in many of these patients was underestimated and that inadequate radiation fields were a common cause of failure. With more careful radiographic staging and treatment, this can be avoided.

When initiating treatment to a patient with a large mediastinal mass, consideration should be given to treating the patient in a sitting (rather than supine) position (see Chapter 21). Although immobilization in the sitting position is more difficult, the lower position of the diaphragm that results generally permits more blocking of the pulmonary parenchyma (83). A shrinking field technique must be used in almost every case. Initial treatments should be fractionated at low doses (1.25–1.5 Gy) with splits or interruptions in treatment of 3 to 7 days given after 12 to 15 Gy and again at 25 to 30 Gy to permit maximum regression of mediastinal adenopathy and protection of additional lung (Fig. 8) (84,85). Not infrequently in these patients, the pulmonary hila are involved. In this setting, it is necessary to irradiate the lungs with low-dose irradiation (15–16.5 Gy), accomplished most safely by the use of partial transmission lung blocks (see Chapter 21) (86). The central mediastinal dose should be taken to 40 to 44 Gy; however, every effort should be made to limit the dose to the subcarinal portion of the heart to 30 to 36 Gy. Areas of extralymphatic extension, if present, should be treated to a full tumoricidal dose. After the completion of mantle irradiation, subdiaphragmatic irradiation (including the spleen) must follow.

Combined-Modality Therapy

After completion of a course of chemotherapy, the volume remaining to be irradiated is almost always substantially smaller than at the outset. It is important to take advantage of this tumor regression and design fields that conform to the residual disease, as this will reduce the risk of pulmonary complications related to the radiation. Treatment of the original tumor volume will lead to additional risk. For example, at the National Cancer Institute, patients were simulated to the initial tumor volume and then treated with 6 months of MOPP/ABVD. They were then irradiated to the initial treatment volume to a dose of 10 Gy, followed by radiation to a reduced volume to 35 Gy (87); 16% of patients developed symptomatic or radiographic changes of radiation pneumonitis and six required management with systemic glucocorticoids. This complication was fatal in one instance.

Ideally, radiation volumes can be reduced as a correlate to chemotherapy response. These more restricted fields will result in smaller radiation volumes and reduced risk of complications. In the Stanford V program, for example, only initially bulky sites (>5 cm) are irradiated. Commonly, this will include only the mediastinum. Even if the supraclavicular areas are treated concurrently, the volume proportional to an entire mantle is much less (Fig. 9). This may be especially beneficial, for example, in a young woman who has minimal axillary adenopathy, for whom the elimination of axillary irradiation may markedly reduce the risk for developing subsequent breast cancer.

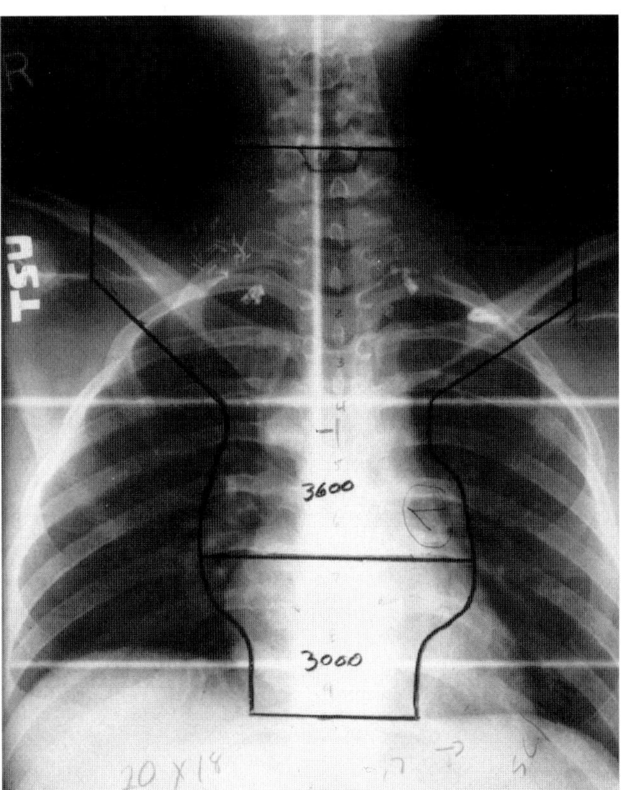

FIG. 9. A planning film of a mediastinal-supraclavicular field for consolidative radiation treatment in a patient who has completed a course of chemotherapy. The patient initially had a large mediastinal mass (MMR = 0.39) and she had an excellent response to chemotherapy. The consolidative fields incorporate only the essential mediastinal, hilar, and supraclavicular regions, including areas of residual adenopathy. The entire initial tumor volume is not treated. This permits protection of a significant proportion of the heart, lungs, and breasts. (From ref. 90, with permission.)

RECOMMENDATION AND FUTURE DIRECTIONS

The outcome of treatment for patients with unfavorable prognosis stage I–II Hodgkin's disease has improved dramatically in the past three decades. This is due primarily to the more common use of combined-modality therapy, since historically fewer than 50% of patients in the most unfavorable setting (a large mediastinal mass) were cured when radiation alone was used as the initial treatment (see Fig. 3). The introduction of the combined-modality concept in the management of these patients has permitted the following: elimination of staging laparotomy, because that procedure is most helpful when treatment with irradiation alone is contemplated; reduction of radiation field size, because the radiation oncologist can take advantage of tumor shrinkage, especially in the mediastinum (Fig. 9), and after adequate chemotherapy uninvolved regions need not be treated (EORTC H_8U and GHSG HD8 trials, Table 7); reduction in radiation dosages, especially to minimally involved regions (GHSG HD1 and HD11 trials); and a reduction of the duration of chemotherapy (EORTC H_8U and H_9U trials, Table 6).

The combined-modality approach enhances the likelihood of local tumor control and adequately addresses the problem of occult distant disease. With the effective reduction in the use of radiation, and now the reduction in duration of chemotherapy, an ideal safe combination of chemotherapy and irradiation that leads to a high likelihood of cure with minimal long-term toxicity is likely to be identified. The improved prognosis and long-term survival of these patients leads to an increased importance in monitoring late effects. For example, as far back as 30 years ago, patients with large mediastinal masses could be cured reliably with aggressive management programs that included staging laparotomy, subtotal lymphoid irradiation, and adjuvant MOPP chemotherapy (see Fig. 3). However, these patients were at risk for postsplenectomy sepsis, radiation-related cardiopulmonary problems, secondary leukemia, and secondary solid tumors, all of which led to increases in late mortality (see Chapter 32). New management programs have been tailored to reduce these risks, although large cohorts of patients will have to be followed for more than 10 years to know if we have been truly successful. Results thus far with these novel approaches suggest no compromise in the cure of Hodgkin's disease and no suggestion of late mortality. For example, among patients with large mediastinal masses treated at Stanford with programs that have excluded laparotomy, reduced radiation fields, and more recently reduced radiation dosages and chemotherapy duration, the freedom from relapse and survival (Fig. 10) are better than our historical experience using more aggressive management programs (Fig. 3).

A confusing aspect of the literature and current clinical trials is the variable definition of unfavorable prognosis. Given the common use of combined-modality therapy, rather than radiation alone, even in patients with favorable prognosis disease (see Chapter 25), it may be time to change these definitions and eligibility criteria.

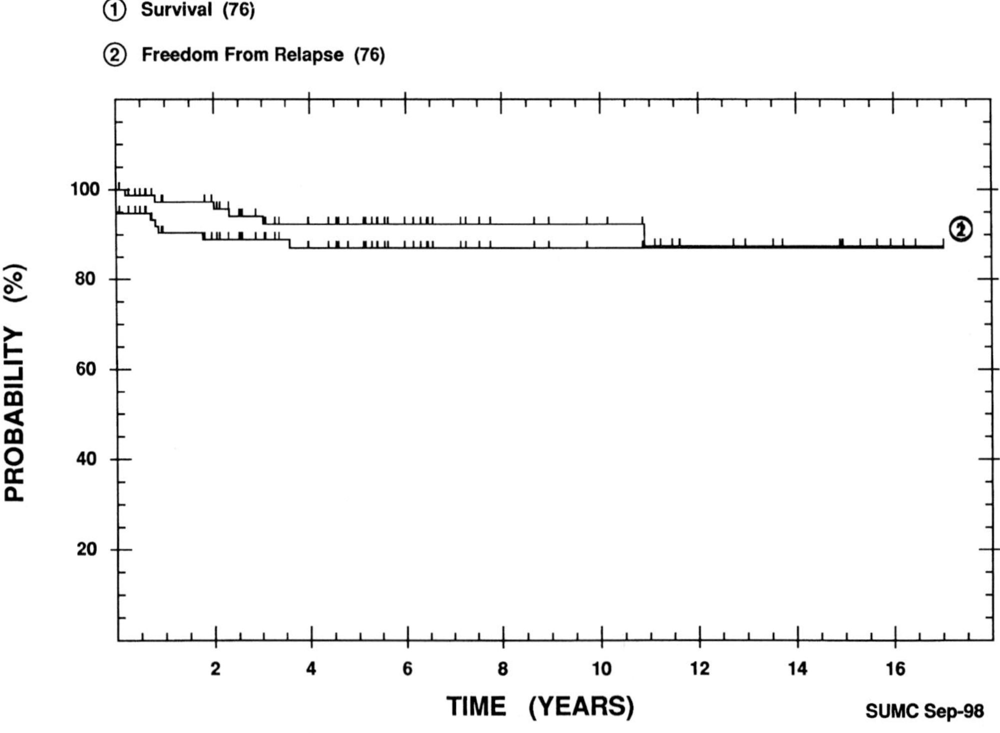

FIG. 10. Survival (92% at 10 years) and freedom from relapse (87% at 10 years) of 76 patients with CS I–II Hodgkin's disease and a large mediastinal mass (MMR >0.33) treated at Stanford University with combination chemotherapy (ABVD, PAVe, or Stanford V) and mantle or mediastinal/supraclavicular irradiation.

For example, current combined-modality management protocols for favorable prognosis disease may be entirely adequate for patients who have three sites of disease or an ESR >50, factors considered unfavorable in some clinical trials groups. Detailed analysis of completed clinical trials may permit this redefinition, which would allow these patients to be treated with even less aggressive management approaches. However, there are data to suggest that patients with large mediastinal masses (especially with MMR >0.33) are not treated adequately with some of the lower-intensity regimens used for favorable prognosis patients, and more aggressive management may always be required in this cohort.

Finally, more effective imaging studies, such as positron emission tomography (PET) scanning may prove helpful in these patients to tailor more effectively the treatment to individual patients, by reducing the duration of chemotherapy or reducing the extent of radiation treatment (or both). However, none of this should inhibit the development of new therapeutic agents that might treat this disease more effectively, and with fewer attendant complications.

REFERENCES

1. Tubiana M, Henry-Amar M, Hayat M, Breur K, van der Werf-Messing B, Burgers M. Long-term results of the E.O.R.T.C. randomized study of irradiation and vinblastine in clinical stages I and II of Hodgkin's disease. *Eur J Cancer* 1979;15:645–657.
2. Tubiana M, Henry-Amar M, Carde P, et al. Toward comprehensive management tailored to prognostic factors of patients with clinical stages I and II in Hodgkin's disease. The EORTC Lymphoma Group controlled clinical trials: 1964–1987. *Blood* 1989;73:47–56.
3. Frei EI, DeVita VJ, Moxley J Jr, Carbone P. Approaches to improving the chemotherapy of Hodgkin's disease. *Cancer Res* 1966;26:1284.
4. Anderson H, Crowther D, Deakin DP, Ryder WDJ, Radford JA. A randomized study of adjuvant MVPP chemotherapy after mantle radiotherapy in pathologically staged IA–IIB Hodgkin's disease: 10-year follow-up. *Ann Oncol* 1991;2:49.
5. Nordentoft AM. Radiotherapy in 50 cases of Hodgkin's disease in stages I and II. Report from the Lymphogranulomatosis Committee. *Ugeskr Laeger* 1972;134:2383–2385.
6. Cosset JM, Henry-Amar M, Noordijk P, Carde P. The EORTC trials for adult patients with early stage Hodgkin's disease. A 1997 update, 39th Annual Scientific Meeting of ASTRO, Orlando, FL, 1997.
7. Specht L, Gray RG, Clarke MJ, Peto R. The influence of more extensive radiotherapy and adjuvant chemotherapy on long-term outcome of early stage Hodgkin's disease: a meta-analysis of 23 randomized trials involving 3888 patients. *J Clin Oncol* 1998;16:830–843.
8. Tubiana M, Henry-Amar M, van der Werf-Messing B, et al. A multivariate analysis of prognostic factors in early stage Hodgkin's disease. *Int J Radiat Oncol Biol Phys* 1985;11:23–30.
9. Tubiana M, Henry-Amar M, Hayat M, et al. Prognostic significance of the number of involved areas in the early stages of Hodgkin's disease. *Cancer* 1984;54:885–894.
10. Lee CKK, Aeppli DM, Bloomfield CD, Levitt SH. Hodgkin's disease: a reassessment of prognostic factors following modification of radiotherapy. *Int J Radiat Oncol Biol Phys* 1987;13:983–991.
11. Mendenhall NP, Cantor AB, Barre DM, Lynch JW Jr, Million RR. The role of prognostic factors in treatment selection for early-stage Hodgkin's disease. *Am J Clin Oncol* 1994;17:189–195.
12. Barton M, Boyages J, Crennan E, et al. Radiation therapy for early stage Hodgkin's disease: Australasian patterns of care. Australasian Radiation Oncology Lymphoma Group. *Int J Radiat Oncol Biol Phys* 1995;31:227–236.
13. Mauch P, Goodman R, Hellman S. The significance of mediastinal involvement in early stage Hodgkin's disease. *Cancer* 1978;42: 1039–1045.
14. Hoppe RT, Coleman CN, Cox RS, Rosenberg SA, Kaplan HS. The management of stage I–II Hodgkin's disease with irradiation alone or combined modality therapy: the Stanford experience. *Blood* 1982;59: 455–465.
15. Prosnitz LR, Curtis AM, Knowlton AH, Peters LM, Farber LR. Supradiaphragmatic Hodgkin's disease: significance of large mediastinal masses. *Int J Radiat Oncol Biol Phys* 1980;6:809–813.
16. Fuller LM, Madoc-Jones H, Shullenberger CC, et al. Further follow-up of results of treatment in 90 laparotomy-negative stage I and II Hodgkin's disease patients: significance of mediastinal and non-mediastinal presentations. *Int J Radiat Oncol Biol Phys* 1980;6:799–808.
17. Liew KH, Easton D, Horwich A, Barrett A, Peckham MJ. Bulky mediastinal Hodgkin's disease management and prognosis. *Hematol Oncol* 1984;2:45–59.
18. Lee CKK, Bloomfield CD, Goldman AI, Levitt SH. Prognostic significance of mediastinal involvement in Hodgkin's disease treated with curative radiotherapy. *Cancer* 1980;46:2403–2409.
19. Schomberg PJ, Evans RG, O'Connell MJ, et al. Prognostic significance of mediastinal mass in adult Hodgkin's disease. *Cancer* 1984;53: 324–328.
20. Willet CG, Linggood RM, Leong JC, et al. Stage IA to IIB mediastinal Hodgkin's disease: three-dimensional volumetric assessment of response to treatment. *J Clin Oncol* 1988;6:819–824.
21. Lagarde P, Eghballi H, Bonichon F, De Mascarel I, Chauvergne J, Haerni B. Brief chemotherapy associated with extended field radiotherapy in Hodgkin's disease. Long-term results in a series of 102 patients with clinical stages I–IIIA. *Eur J Cancer Clin Oncol* 1988;24: 1191–1198.
22. Hagemeister F, Fuller L, Velasquez W, et al. Stage I and II Hodgkin's disease: involved-field radiotherapy versus extended-field radiotherapy versus involved-field radiotherapy followed by six cycles of MOPP. *Cancer Treat Rep* 1982;66:789–798.
23. Jelliffe AM, Thompson AD. The prognosis in Hodgkin's disease. *Br J Cancer* 1955;9:21–36.
24. Peters MV. A study in survivals in Hodgkin's disease treated radiologically. *Am J Roentgenol* 1950;63:299–311.
25. Bjorkholm M, Holm M, Mellstedt H. Immunologic profile in patients with cured Hodgkin's disease. *Scand J Haematol* 1977;19:361–368.
26. Henry-Amar M, Friedman S, Hayat M, et al. Erythrocyte sedimentation rate predicts early relapse and survival in early-stage Hodgkin disease. The EORTC Lymphoma Cooperative Group. *Ann Intern Med* 1991; 114:361–365.
27. Vaughan Hudson B, Maclennan KA, Bennett MH, Easterling MJ, Vaughan Hudson G, Jelliffe AM. Systemic disturbance in Hodgkin's disease and its relation to histopathology and prognosis (BNLI report no. 30). *Clin Radiol* 1987;38:257–261.
28. Hoppe RT. The management of bulky mediastinal Hodgkin's disease. *Hematol Oncol Clin North Am* 1989;3:265–276.
29. Hopper KD, Diehl LF, Lynch JC, McCauslin MA. Mediastinal bulk in Hodgkin's disease, method of measurement versus prognosis. *Invest Radiol* 1991;26:1101–1110.
30. Piro AJ, Weiss DR, Hellman S. Mediastinal Hodgkin's disease: a possible danger for intubation anesthesia. Intubation danger in Hodgkin's disease. *Int J Radiat Oncol Biol Phys* 1976;1:415–419.
31. Lister TA, Crowther D, Sutcliffe SB, et al. Report of a committee convened to discuss the evaluation and staging of patients with Hodgkin's disease: Cotswolds meeting [published erratum appears in *J Clin Oncol* 1990;8(9):1602]. *J Clin Oncol* 1989;7:1630–1636.
32. Cosset JM, Henry-Amar M, Carde PDC, Le Bourgeois JP, Tubiana M. The prognostic significance of large mediastinal masses in the treatment of Hodgkin's disease. The experience of the Institut Gustave-Roussy. *Hematol Oncol* 1984;2:33–43.
33. Bonadonna G, Valagussa P, Santoro A. Prognosis of bulky Hodgkin's disease treated with chemotherapy alone or combined with radiotherapy. *Cancer Surv* 1985;4:439–458.
34. Anderson H, Deakin D, Wagstaff J. A randomized study of adjuvant chemotherapy after mantle radiotherapy in supradiaphragmatic Hodgkin's disease PS IA–IIB: a report from the Manchester lymphoma group. *Br J Cancer* 1984;49:695–702.
35. Tubiana M, Henry-Amar M, Hayat M, et al. The EORTC treatment of early stages of Hodgkin's disease: the role of radiotherapy. *Int J Radiat Oncol Biol Phys* 1984;10:197–210.
36. Timothy AR, Sutcliffe SBJ, Stansfeld AG, Wrigleyh PFM, Jones AE. Radiotherapy in the treatment of Hodgkin's disease. *Br Med J* 1978;1: 1246–1249.

37. Mintz U, Miller JB, Golomb HM, et al. Pathologic stage I and II Hodgkin's disease, 1968–1975. Relapses and results of retreatment. *Cancer* 1979;44:72–79.
38. Coltman CA, Fuller LA, Fisher R, Frei E. Extended field radiotherapy versus involved field radiotherapy plus MOPP in stage I and II Hodgkin's disease. In: Jones S, Salmon S, eds. *Adjuvant therapy of cancer* II. New York: Grune and Stratton, 1979:129–136.
39. Stoffel TJ, Cox JD. Hodgkin's disease stage I and II. A comparison between two different treatment policies. *Cancer* 1977;40:90–97.
40. Aisenberg AC, Linggood RM, Lew RA. The changing face of Hodgkin's disease. *Am J Med* 1979;67:921–928.
41. Crnkovich MJ, Leopold K, Hoppe RT, Mauch PM. Stage I to IIB Hodgkin's disease: the combined experience at Stanford University and the Joint Center for Radiation Therapy. *J Clin Oncol* 1987;5:1041–1049.
42. Santoro A, Viviani S, Zucali R, et al. Comparative results and toxicity of MOPP vs ABVD combined with radiotherapy (RT) in PS IIB, III (A,B) Hodgkin's disease (HD). Annual Meeting American Society of Clinical Oncology, San Diego, CA, 1983.
43. Fuller LM, Hagemeister FB, North LB, McLaughlin P, Velasquez WS, Cabanillas F. The adjuvant role of two cycles of MOPP and low-dose lung irradiation in stage IA through IIB Hodgkin's disease. Preliminary results. *Int J Radiat Oncol Biol Phys* 1988;14:683–692.
44. Abrahamsen AF, Hannisdal E, Nome O, et al. Clinical stage I and II Hodgkin's disease: long-term results of therapy without laparotomy. Experience at one institution [see comments]. *Ann Oncol* 1996;7:145–150.
45. Carde P, Burgers JM, Henry-Amar M, et al. Clinical stages I and II Hodgkin's disease: a specifically tailored therapy according to prognostic factors [see comments]. *J Clin Oncol* 1988;6:239–252.
46. Carde P, Hagenbeek A, Hayat M, et al. Clinical staging versus laparotomy and combined modality with MOPP versus ABVD in early-stage Hodgkin's disease: the H6 twin randomized trials from the European Organization for Research and Treatment of Cancer Lymphoma Cooperative Group. *J Clin Oncol* 1993;11:2258–2272.
47. Klimo P, Connors JM. MOPP/ABV hybrid program: combination chemotherapy based on early introduction of seven effective drugs for advanced Hodgkin's disease. *J Clin Oncol* 1985;3:1174–1182.
48. Hoerni B, Orgerie MB, Eghbali H, et al. New combination of epirubicine, bleomycin, vinblastine and prednisone (EBVP II) before radiotherapy in localized stages of Hodgkin's disease. Phase II trial in 50 patients. *Bull Cancer* 1988;75:789–794.
49. Cosset JM, Ferme C, Noordijk EM, Dubray BM, Thirion P, Henry-Amar M. Combined modality therapy for poor prognosis stages I and II Hodgkin's disease. *Semin Radiat Oncol* 1996;6:185–195.
50. Noordijk EM, Mellink WAM, Carde P, Ferme C, Eghbali H, Henry-Amar M. Very favorable Hodgkin's disease: Does it really exist? *Leuk Lymphoma* 1998;29:49.
51. Duggan D, Petroni G, Johnson J, et al. MOPP/ABV versus ABVD for advanced Hodgkin's disease- a preliminary report of CALGB 8952 (with SWOG, ECOG, NCIC). In: Program/Proceeding of the American Society of Clinical Oncology. *Thirty-third Annual Meeting American Society of Clinical Oncology, Denver, CO,* vol. 16. 1997.
52. Tesch H, Diehl V, Latham B, et al. Interim analysis of the HD9 study of the German Hodgkin Study Group (GHSG)—BEACOPP is more effective than COPP-ABVD in advanced stage Hodgkin's disease. *Leuk Lymphoma* 1998;29:2.
53. Diehl V, Sieber M, Ruffer U, Cosset JM. Treatment of early-stage Hodgkin's disease: considerations in the use of chemotherapy. Annual Meeting of American Society of Clinical Oncology, Los Angeles, CA, 1998.
54. Loeffler M, Diehl V, Pfreundschuh M, et al. Dose-response relationship of complementary radiotherapy following four cycles of combination chemotherapy in intermediate-stage Hodgkin's disease. *J Clin Oncol* 1997;15:2275–2287.
55. Hoppe RT, Portlock CS, Glatstein E, Rosenberg SA, Kaplan HS. Alternating chemotherapy and irradiation in the treatment of advanced Hodgkin's disease. *Cancer* 1979;43:472–481.
56. Bartlett NL, Rosenberg SA, Hoppe RT, Hancock SL, Horning SJ. Brief chemotherapy, Stanford V, and adjuvant radiotherapy for bulky or advanced-stage Hodgkin's disease: a preliminary report. *J Clin Oncol* 1995;13:1080–1088.
57. Horning SJ, Rosenberg SA, Hoppe RT. Brief chemotherapy (Stanford V) and adjuvant radiotherapy for bulky or advanced Hodgkin's disease: an update. *Ann Oncol* 1996;7:S105–S108.
58. Horning SJ, Hoppe RT, Breslin S, Bartlett NL, Yuen AR, Rosenberg SA. Brief chemotherapy (CT) (Stanford V) and involved field radiotherapy (RT) are highly effective for advanced Hodgkin's disease (HD). In: Program/Proceeding of the American Society of Clinical Oncology, *Thirty-fourth Annual Meeting American Society of Clinical Oncology, Los Angeles, CA,* vol. 17. 1998.
59. Musshoff K, Boutis L. Therapy results in Hodgkin's disease. *Cancer* 1968;21:1100–1113.
60. Torti FM, Portlock CS, Rosenberg SA, Kaplan HS. Extralymphatic Hodgkin's disease. Prognosis and response to therapy. *Am J Med* 1981; 70:487–492.
61. Levi JA, Wiernik PH. Limited extranodal Hodgkin's disease. Unfavorable prognosis and therapeutic implications. *Am J Med* 1977;63: 365–372.
62. Rosenberg SA, Kaplan HS. The evolution and summary results of the Stanford randomized clinical trials of the management of Hodgkin's disease: 1962–1984. *Int J Radiat Oncol Biol Phys* 1985;11:5–22.
63. Hoppe RT, Horning SJ, Hancock SL, Rosenberg SA. Current Stanford clinical trials for Hodgkin's disease. In: Diehl V, Pfreundschuh M, Loeffler M, eds. *Recent results in cancer research, new aspects in the diagnosis and treatment of cancer.* Heidelberg: Springer-Verlag, 1989: 182–196.
64. Ferme C, Lepage E, D'Agay MF, et al. Hodgkin's disease, clinical stages I, II A–B and IIIA. Results of brief chemotherapy followed by irradiation. *Nouv Rev Fr Hematol* 1992;34:247–255.
65. Canellos GP, Anderson JR, Propert KJ, et al. Chemotherapy of advanced Hodgkin's disease with MOPP, ABVD, or MOPP alternating with ABVD. *N Engl J Med* 1992;327:1478–1484.
66. Pavlovsky S, Schvartzman E, Lastiri F, et al. Randomized trial of CVPP for three versus six cycles in favorable-prognosis and CVPP versus AOPE plus radiotherapy in intermediate-prognosis untreated Hodgkin's disease. *J Clin Oncol* 1997;15:2652–2658.
67. Noordijk EM, Carde P, Hagenbeek A, et al. Combination of radiotherapy and chemotherapy is advisable in all patients with clinical stage I–II Hodgkin's disease. Six-year results of the EORTC-GPMC controlled clinical trials H7-VF, H7-F, and H7-U. *Int J Radiat Oncol Biol Phys* 1997;39:173.
68. La Garde P, Eghbali H, Bonichon F, de Mascarel I, Chauvergne J, Hoerni B. Brief chemotherapy associated with extended field radiotherapy in Hodgkin's disease. Long-term results in a series of 102 patients with clinical stages I–IIIA. *Eur J Cancer Clin Oncol* 1988;24: 1191–1198.
69. Hagemeister FB, Purugganan R, Fuller L, et al. Treatment of early stages of Hodgkin's disease with novantrone, vincristine, vinblastine, prednisone, and radiotherapy. *Semin Hematol* 1994;31:36–43.
70. Wasserman T, Petroni GR, Millard F, et al. Etoposide, vinblastine, and doxorubicin (EVA) chemotherapy plus subtotal nodal irradiation for early stage, high risk Hodgkin's disease. In: Program/Proceeding of the American Society of Clinical Oncology. *ASCO Annual Meeting, Philadelphia, PA,* vol. 15. 1996.
71. Andrieu JM, Bayle-Weisgerber C, Boiron M, et al. The chemotherapy-radiotherapy sequence in the management of Hodgkin's disease. Results of a clinical trial. *Eur J Cancer* 1979;48:153–161.
72. Brusamolino E, Lazzarino M, Orlandi E, et al. Early-stage Hodgkin's disease: long-term results with radiotherapy alone or combined radiotherapy and chemotherapy. *Ann Oncol* 1994;5(suppl 2):101–106.
73. Colonna P, Jais JP, Desablens B, et al. Mediastinal tumor size and response to chemotherapy are the only prognostic factors in supradiaphragmatic Hodgkin's disease treated by ABVD plus radiotherapy: ten-year results of the Paris-Ouest-France 81/12 trial, including 262 patients. *J Clin Oncol* 1996;14:1928–1935.
74. Andre M, Brice P, Cazals D, et al. Results of three courses of adriamycin, bleomycin, vindesine, and dacarbazine with subtotal nodal irradiation in 189 patients with nodal Hodgkin's disease (stage I, II and IIIA). *Hematol Cell Ther* 1997;39:59–65.
75. Colonna P, Andrieu JM, Ghouadni R, et al. Hodgkin's disease, clinical stages IA to IIIB: combined modality therapy (3 MOPP followed by curative and prophylactic radiotherapy including the spleen). Six-year results. *Eur J Haematol* 1987;39:356–361.
76. Bonfante V, Santoro A, Viviani S, et al. Early stage Hodgkin's disease: ten-year results of a non-randomised study with radiotherapy alone or combined with MOPP. *Eur J Cancer* 1993;29A:24–29.
77. Zittoun R, Audebert A, Hoerni B, et al. Extended versus involved field irradiation combined with MOPP chemotherapy in early clinical stages of Hodgkin's disease. *J Clin Oncol* 1985;3:207–214.

78. Santoro A. Annual Conference of ECCO, Hamburg, Germany, 1997 (abst).
79. Preti A, Hagemeister FB, McLaughlin P, et al. Hodgkin's disease with a mediastinal mass greater than 10 cm: results of four different treatment approaches. *Ann Oncol* 1994;5:S97–S100.
80. Pavlovsky S, Maschio M, Santarelli M, et al. Randomized trial of chemotherapy versus chemotherapy plus radiotherapy for stage I–II Hodgkin's disease. *J Natl Cancer Inst* 1988;80:1466–1473.
81. Rostock RA, Siegelman SS, Lenhard RE, Wharam MD, Order SE. Thoracic CT scanning for mediastinal Hodgkin's disease: results and therapeutic implications. *Int J Radiat Oncol Biol Phys* 1983;9:1451–1457.
82. Rostock RA, Klein JL, Leichner P, Kopher KA, Order SE. Selective tumor localization in experimental hepatoma by radiolabeled antiferritin antibody. *Int J Radiat Oncol Biol Phys* 1983;9:1345–1350.
83. Marcus K, Svensson G, Rhodes L, Mauch P. Mantle irradiation in the upright position: a technique to reduce the volume of lung irradiated in patients with bulky mediastinal Hodgkin's disease. *Int J Radiat Oncol Biol Phys* 1992;23:443–447.
84. Hoppe RT. The management of stage II Hodgkin's disease with a large mediastinal mass: a prospective program emphasizing irradiation. *Int J Radiat Oncol Biol Phys* 1985;11:349–355.
85. Behar RA, Hoppe RT. Radiation therapy in the management of bulky mediastinal Hodgkin's disease. *Cancer* 1990;66:75–79.
86. Palos B, Kaplan HS, Karzmark CJ. The use of thin lung shields to deliver limited whole-lung irradiation during mantle-field treatment of Hodgkin's disease. *Radiology* 1971;101:441–442.
87. Longo DL, Glatstein E, Duffey PL, et al. Alternating MOPP and ABVD chemotherapy plus mantle-field radiation therapy in patients with massive mediastinal Hodgkin's disease. *J Clin Oncol* 1997;15:3338–3346.
88. Hoppe R. Radiation therapy in the management of Hodgkin's disease. *Semin Oncol* 1990;17:704–715.
89. Hoppe RT. Radiation therapy in the treatment of Hodgkin's disease. *Semin Oncol* 1980;7:144–154.
90. Hoppe RT. Hodgkin's Disease. In: Leibel SA, Phillips TL, eds. *Textbook of radiation oncology.* Philadelphia: WB Saunders, 1998:1079–1094.

Hodgkin's Disease, edited by P. M. Mauch, J. O. Armitage, V. Diehl, R. T. Hoppe, and L. M. Weiss. Lippincott Williams & Wilkins, Philadephia ©1999.

CHAPTER 27

Treatment of Stage III–IV Hodgkin's Disease

Sandra J. Horning, Joachim Yahalom, Hans Tesch, Richard I. Fisher, and John M. M. Raemaekers

Prior to the mid-1960s, Hodgkin's disease presenting in advanced stage was treated with single-agent chemotherapy, resulting in median survivals of approximately 1 year and less than 5% overall survival at 5 years (1). In 1964, investigators at the National Cancer Institute (NCI) developed a four-drug combination chemotherapy program, MOPP [nitrogen mustard, Oncovin (vincristine), procarbazine, and prednisone] (Table 1). This landmark study established the curability of over 50% of patients with stage III and IV disease (2). Further, the seminal observations regarding prognostic features, patterns of relapse, and toxicities have greatly influenced clinical practice and investigation to the present time.

The failure of approximately 20% of patients to enter complete remission, and the relapse of about one-third of patients following complete remission with MOPP chemotherapy, encouraged the development of strategies to decrease treatment failures through the investigation of alternate primary therapies. Patterns of failure with MOPP demonstrated the inverse relationship between tumor burden and rate of cure, and indicated that over 90% of patients failed in sites of previous, especially node-based, disease (3). Further, failure in bulky disease sites, in particular the mediastinum, was observed. These observations provided the rationale for the integration of radiation therapy in advanced-stage disease as discussed below.

S. J. Horning: Department of Medicine, Stanford University Stanford, California.

J. Yahalom: Department of Medicine, Cornell University Medical College and Department of Radiation Oncology, Memorial Sloan-Kettering Cancer Center, New York, New York.

H. Tesch: Klinik I für Innere Medizin, der Universität zu Köln, Köln, Germany.

R. I. Fisher: Cardinal Bernadin Cancer Center, Loyola University Stritch School of Medicine and Division of Hematology/Oncology, Foster G. MacGraw Hospital, Maywood, Illinois.

J. M. M. Raemaekers: Department of Medicine, Division of Hematology, University Hospital of Nijmegan, Nijmegan, The Netherlands.

Clinical studies designed to ameliorate the adverse effects of MOPP chemotherapy continue to the present time. The acute side effects, primarily gastrointestinal and neurologic toxicity, promoted the early clinical investigation of modified MOPP-like chemotherapy combinations. Late effects associated with MOPP—sterility and an increased risk of leukemia—led to the development of drug regimens in which alkylating agents were either omitted or given in lower cumulative doses (4–6).

In the 35 years since MOPP was introduced, pathologic diagnosis and radiographic techniques have become increasingly sophisticated and there have been significant advances in supportive care. These factors have resulted in the virtual disappearance of the lymphocyte-depletion histology from advanced-stage clinical series and the virtual obsolescence of laparotomy and laparoscopy as routine staging techniques. With more sensitive radiographic examination, many fewer patients enter apparent complete remission at the conclusion of therapy, even though they may be disease free, such that complete remission is no longer an important therapeutic end point. Compared with historical controls, the number and pattern of extranodal disease sites, and thus Ann Arbor staging, may be subtly altered by greater reliance on more sensitive radiographic studies in lieu of pathologic staging. The availability of potent antiemetics and the more routine use of venous access devices have changed the perception of acute chemotherapy toxicity. With the use of granulocytic growth factors to support dose intensity, deviations from optimal drug doses and schedules can be minimized. In addition, there has been a move toward the use of absolute neutrophil count over total white blood count in dose adjustment and greater tolerance of grade III and IV neutropenia. These subtleties in diagnosis, staging, and clinical practice must be considered in the interpretation of the studies discussed in this chapter, which were conducted over a period of more than three decades.

TABLE 1. *MOPP and MOPP derivative combination chemotherapy*

Drug	Dose (mg/m^2)	Route	Schedule(days)	Cycle length (days)
MOPP				21
Mechlorethamine	6	IV	1,8	
Oncovin (vincristine)	1.4	IV	1,8	
Procarbazine	100	PO	1–14	
Prednisone	40	PO	1–14	
BCVPP				28
Carmustine	100	IV	1	
Cyclophosphamide	600	IV	1	
Vinblastine	5	IV	1	
Procarbazine	50	PO	1	
	100	PO	2–10	
Prednisone	60	PO	1–10	
ChlVPP				28
Chlorambucil	6	PO	1–14	
Vinblastine	6	IV	1,8	
Procarbazine	100	PO	1–14	
Prednisone	40 total	PO	1–14	
COPP				28
Cyclophosphamide	650	IV	1,8	
Oncovin (vincristine)	1.4	IV	1,8	
Procarbazine	100	PO	1–14	
Prednisone	40	PO	1–14	
MVPP				42
Nitrogen mustard	6	IV	1,8	
Vinblastine	6	IV	1,8	
Procarbazine	100	PO	1–14	
Prednisone	40 total	PO	1–14	
LOPP				28
Chlorambucil	10 total	PO	1–10	
Oncovin (vincristine)	1.4	IV	1,8	
Procarbazine	100	PO	1–10	
Prednisone	25	PO	1–14	
CVPP				28
Lomustine	75	PO	1	
Vinblastine	4	IV	1,8	
Procarbazine	100	PO	1–14	
Prednisone	40	PO	1–14	

Some studies capped vincristine at 2 mg. Prednisone was given in cycles 1 and 4 only by some groups. Chlorambucil and vinblastine were capped at 10 mg and procarbazine was capped at 200 mg in some studies.

IV, intravenous; PO, oral.

The definition of advanced Hodgkin's disease warrants comment. In contrast to the original NCI study, recent investigations have included patients with bulky stage II or IIB disease under the rubric of "advanced" Hodgkin's disease. Clinical studies also vary with respect to the inclusion of patients with various stages who have progressed after primary radiation therapy. The NCI investigators have traditionally expressed their results as "relapse-free survival," which excluded the subset of patients who did not achieve complete remission, whereas more recent trials included all patients in their end point of "freedom from recurrence or freedom from progression." In like manner, the NCI data were expressed as "tumor-specific mortality," which excluded patients who were thought to have died from causes other than Hodgkin's disease. Currently, many lymphoma clinical investigators specify "event-free survival" or "failure-free survival," which score both relapse and death as adverse events. Comparisons across studies must consider and attempt to translate these terms.

COMBINATION CHEMOTHERAPY

MOPP

In 1964, NCI investigators administered the four-drug MOPP program, with each drug given at full dose over 2 weeks, followed by a 2-week recovery period. Patients were treated for two additional monthly cycles after a complete remission was achieved but all received a minimum of six monthly cycles unless they progressed prior to that time. Dose reductions were prospectively defined based on objective criteria, and the doses of vincristine were not capped at 2 mg. The results of the complete NCI studies were published by DeVita, et al. (2) in 1980 and have been updated subsequently (7) after a median follow-up of 14 years. Of the total of 198 patients treated,

163 had previously untreated Ann Arbor stage III and IV disease and 32 had relapsed after initial therapy with radiation. In addition, 67 patients received either maintenance chemotherapy or adjuvant radiation therapy following MOPP as part of randomized, prospective investigations. The median age at diagnosis was 32 years. The complete remission rate was 81% and the remaining 19% of patients were considered to be induction failures; 36% of the complete responders relapsed, yielding a 52% freedom from disease progression at 10 years. The overall survival was estimated at 50% at 10 years (Fig. 1). Of note, histologic reclassification of 41 cases of lymphocyte depletion Hodgkin's disease in the original series resulted in the verification of only 9 cases; 10 were reclassified as non-Hodgkin's lymphoma and 22 were thought to have other Hodgkin's disease subtypes (7).

The ability of MOPP to cure advanced Hodgkin's disease was subsequently confirmed by multiple investigators in both single institution and cooperative group trials, often as the standard arm of a randomized trial. In a small series limited to stage IV patients, some of whom had failed prior radiotherapy, Bonadonna and colleagues (8) from Milan reported a 74% complete remission rate, a 36% freedom from progression, and 64% overall survival at 8 years after MOPP chemotherapy. The Eastern Cooperative Oncology Group (ECOG) studied MOPP as one arm of a randomized trial in patients with advanced Hodgkin's disease, 45% of whom had failed prior treatment (9). The dose of vincristine in the MOPP treatment program was capped at 2 mg. The complete remission rate with MOPP was 73% and the estimated 5-year figures for freedom from progression and overall survival were 47% and 61%, respectively. More recently, Canellos et al. (10), from Cancer and Acute Leukemia Group B (CALGB), randomized 361 patients with stages $IIIA_2$ to IV, including a subgroup who had failed prior radiation therapy, to six to eight cycles of MOPP or alternative combination chemotherapy (see below). The complete remission rate for MOPP treatment was 67%. At 10 years, the failure-free survival was 38% and the overall survival was 58% among patients treated with MOPP.

In the NCI series, the treatment-related mortality associated with MOPP was 2.5% (2). Reversible bone marrow depression usually occurred by the third treatment cycle. Neurotoxicity, with no capping of vincristine, was frequent and often clinically significant, although no patients were permanently paralyzed. The acute toxicity of MOPP was generally confirmed in other studies with a 1% to 1.5% incidence of treatment-related death (8–10). Reversible bone marrow suppression was the major acute toxicity. Although hemorrhage was not observed, platelet counts <50,000 were recorded in approximately 15% of treated patients (8). The significance of this observation relates to the purported relationship of thrombocytopenia with the risk of acute leukemia (11).

Following MOPP chemotherapy, azoospermia was seen in all men, whereas amenorrhea was generally limited to women over the age of 25 years (7). The majority of women, however, experienced a premature menopause (7). Although 12 cases of acute leukemia occurred among 198 treated patients, only one of these had received MOPP alone (7). In the original report from the NCI, two additional deaths were recorded as aplastic anemia (2). Subsequent observations have shown that macrocytic anemia may be the harbinger of myelodysplasia and acute leukemia secondary to alkylating-agent treatments (12). A more complete discussion of long-term toxicity, especially second malignancies, is included in Chapters 33, 34, and 35.

NCI investigators also made important observations regarding the ability to treat patients who failed MOPP chemotherapy (13). The success of retreatment with MOPP correlated with the duration of initial remission, an observation that has been confirmed with a variety of second-line treatments (14,15). The low probability of ultimate cure with a second course of MOPP chemotherapy was largely related to relapse, but toxicity was a significant cause of failure as well, particularly second malignancy related to total doses of alkylating agents (16,17).

The development of MOPP was a milestone demonstrating that advanced-stage Hodgkin's disease could be cured. The differences in survival between historical controls and MOPP-treated patients were so dramatic that randomized clinical trials were not needed to validate this advance. Rather, the next step in the treatment of advanced Hodgkin's disease related to derivative regimens developed to address the acute adverse effects of MOPP chemotherapy.

MOPP Derivatives

Despite the relative excellence of the results with MOPP therapy, investigation of alternative regimens was motivated by the desire to obtain equivalent or improved results with less toxicity, particularly gastrointestinal and neurologic. Early studies conducted by CALGB demonstrated that omission of mechlorethamine or procarbazine from the MOPP regimen resulted in inferior complete remission rates and overall survival (18). Based on these data, chemotherapy regimens for advanced Hodgkin's disease generally have adhered to the four-drug principle established by these studies.

Table 1 illustrates the composition of established MOPP-like regimens. In several regimens, vinblastine, a vinca alkaloid with more myelosuppressive but fewer neuropathic effects, was substituted for vincristine. Alternate alkylating agents such as cyclophosphamide or chlorambucil and the nitrosourea agents lomustine and carmustine were incorporated into four or five drug regimens (9,19–24). In some cases, however, these derivative regimens also altered the doses and duration of procarbazine and prednisone.

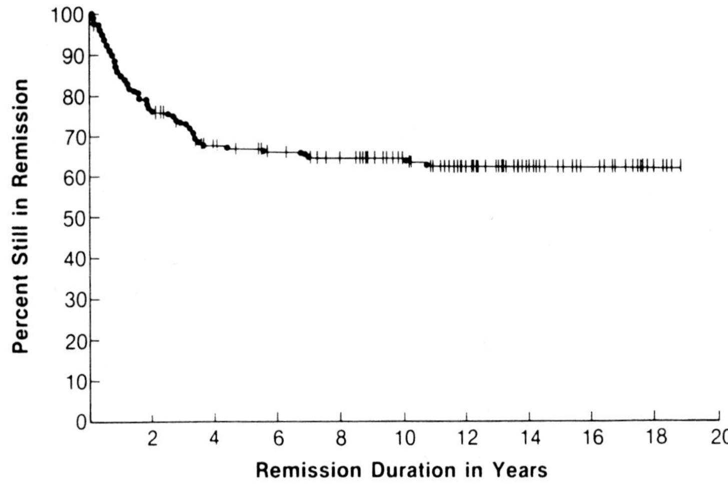

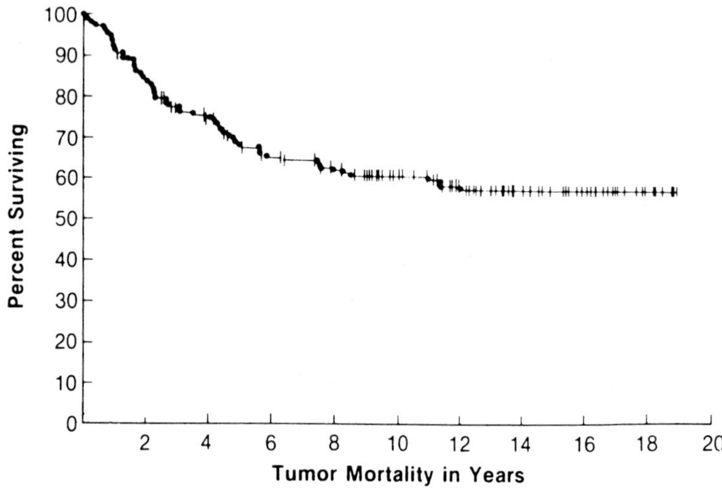

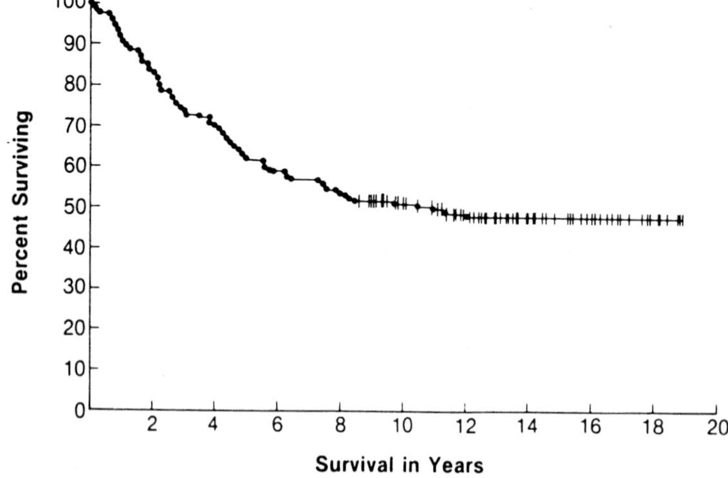

FIG. 1. Remission duration, tumor mortality, and overall survival in 188 patients with advanced Hodgkin's disease treated with MOPP combination chemotherapy at the National Cancer Institute from 1964 to 1976. Ten patients were excluded from analysis after pathology review revealed non-Hodgkin's lymphoma.

ECOG compared a five-drug regimen containing carmustine, cyclophosphamide, vinblastine, procarbazine, and prednisone (BCVPP) with MOPP chemotherapy in advanced Hodgkin's disease, including patients who had relapsed after primary irradiation (9). The freedom from progression at 5 years in previously untreated patients significantly favored the BCVPP arm over MOPP, 50% versus 33% (9). Overall survival at 5 years for previously untreated patients who achieved complete remission was 83% for BCVPP and 75% for MOPP (p = .03). As anticipated, the incidence of gastrointestinal and neurologic toxicities was significantly reduced with BCVPP. As with the NCI study, interpretation of results from this trial is complicated by the inclusion of previously treated patients and adjuvant treatments. These data, and those from other series of MOPP-treated patients, have been criticized because dose modifications for hematologic toxicity differed from the NCI series and, in most, the dose of vincristine was capped at 2 mg.

The efficacy of the MVPP (mechlorethamine, vinblastine, procarbazine, and prednisone) combination, extensively studied in the United Kingdom, was comparable to that of MOPP, with complete remission rates of 60% to 80% and 5-year survival figures of 70% to 80% (20,21). Investigators from St. Bartholomew's Hospital in London reported mature data in a series of 164 consecutive patients with stage IIIB and IV disease (25). The disease-free survival (complete responders only) was 58% and the median overall survival was 14 years.

The ChlVPP (chlorambucil, vinblastine, procarbazine, and prednisone) regimen was developed in the United Kingdom by McElwain et al. (19). Although direct comparisons with MOPP were not performed, the results obtained in several series were quite good (26–28). An international group collected data on 397 patients with stage IIIB and IV disease (29). At 10 years, the estimated failure-free survival was 45% and the overall survival was 50%. Gastrointestinal toxicity and peripheral neuropathy were far less common or severe, whereas myelosuppression was similar to that reported with MOPP chemotherapy. Of interest, the data published to date suggest that ChlVPP may be less leukemogenic or carcinogenic than MOPP (30). These data justify the conclusion that ChlVPP is an appropriate alternative to MOPP with comparable efficacy but significantly less acute toxicity.

The British National Lymphoma Investigation (BNLI) compared LOPP [chlorambucil, Oncovin (vincristine), procarbazine, and prednisone] with MOPP in 290 patients with stage III and IV Hodgkin's disease (22). The complete remission rates (38% for MOPP, 35% for LOPP) and 5-year disease-free survivals (38% for MOPP, 35% for LOPP) were low relative to those achieved at the NCI but similar in the two study arms. Overall survival figures at 5 years were 65% for MOPP and 64% for LOPP. Likewise, no significant differences in outcome were seen in 83 patients with advanced Hodgkin's disease randomized to receive MOPP or LOPP in a study conducted in Mexico (31).

In summary, multiple MOPP-like alternatives have efficacy equivalent to MOPP with less gastrointestinal and neurologic toxicity. The lower cure rates achieved with MOPP delivered outside of the NCI spurred lively debates for a number of years. Indeed, it was difficult to interpret the significance of patient selection variables (previous treatment with chemotherapy or radiotherapy, referral versus population-based practice); planned treatment variables (mandated dose reduction, vincristine capping, shortened schedules of procarbazine, maintenance therapies); and individual practice variables (dose adjustments and treatment delays based on subjective and objective toxicities). However, this phase of the quest for more optimal treatment of advanced Hodgkin's disease was ended due to two constant features: the failure of treatment in about half of advanced-stage patients, and the routine association of alkylating agent-based chemotherapy regimens with an increased risk of sterility and acute leukemia.

ABVD

In 1973 Bonadonna and colleagues (32) introduced the novel ABVD [Adriamycin (doxorubicin), bleomycin, vinblastine, and dacarbazine] regimen for patients who had failed MOPP chemotherapy (Table 2) (32). ABVD was specifically developed for MOPP resistance, incorporating four different, individually effective compounds. Vinblastine was one of the most active single agents in advanced Hodgkin's disease and lacked cross-resistance with vincristine in human tumors (33). Doxorubicin and bleomycin were also very active drugs, producing objective responses through a wide variety of treatment schedules in about 40% to 60% of patients (34–36). The single-agent activity of dacarbazine reported by Frei et al. (9) was confirmed in Milan, and, in experimental systems, dacarbazine showed synergy with doxorubicin without additional toxicity (32).

The efficacy of ABVD was initially compared with MOPP in a prospective randomized trial in previously untreated patients with stage IIB, III, and IV Hodgkin's disease or in those in first relapse after radiotherapy (32). The study design included irradiation for responding patients and a crossover design for patients failing to achieve complete remission or relapsing within 12 months. The complete remission rate favored ABVD over MOPP, 80% versus 71%. A trend at 4 years toward superior freedom from progression (53% MOPP vs. 65% ABVD) and overall survival (88% MOPP vs. 90% ABVD) was noted for ABVD. Because of the small number of patients in this study and the confounding treatment variables, the authors were able to conclude that ABVD was at least as effective as MOPP in the remission induction of advanced Hodgkin's disease, alone or with irradiation.

TABLE 2. *ABVD and ABV(D)-containing combination chemotherapy*

Drug	Dose (mg/m^2)	Route	Schedule (days)	Cycle length (days)
ABVD				28
Adriamycin (doxorubicin)	25	IV	1,15	
Bleomycin	10	IV	1,15	
Vinblastine	6	IV	1,15	
Dacarbazine	375	IV	1,15	
MOPP/ABVD alternating (Milan)				28
Alternate cycles of MOPP with ABVD				
COPP/ABVD alternating (GHSG)				28
Alternate cycles of COPP with ABVD				
MOPP → ABVD sequential (ECOG)				28
MOPP × 6–8 followed by ABVD × 3				
MOPP/ABVD hybrid (Milan)				28
Mechlorethamine	6	IV	1	
Oncovin (vincristine)	1.4*	IV	1	
Procarbazine	100	PO	1–7	
Prednisone	40	PO	1–7	
Adriamycin (doxorubicin)	25	IV	15	
Bleomycin	10	IV	15	
Vinblastine	6	IV	15	
Dacarbazine	375	IV	15	
MMOPP/ABV Hybrid (Vancouver)				28
Mechlorethamine	6	IV	1	
Oncovin (vincristine)	1.4*	IV	1	
Procarbazine	100	PO	1–7	
Prednisone	40	PO	1–14	
Adriamycin (doxorubicin)	35	IV	8	
Bleomycin	10	IV	8	
Vinblastine	6	IV	8	

*Vincristine dose capped at 2 mg.
GHSG, German Hodgkin's Study Group; ECOG, Eastern Cooperative Oncology Group; IV, intravenous; PO, oral.

Table 3 shows the 10-year results of this study, which, in retrospect, predicted the outcome of larger cooperative group studies initiated a decade or more later (32).

The Milan group followed their study in stage IV patients with a larger trial involving 232 patients with pathologic stage IIB, IIIA, and IIIB Hodgkin's disease (Table 3) (37). Patients were randomized to three cycles of MOPP or ABVD followed by subtotal or total lymphoid irradiation and three additional cycles of the same chemotherapy. Outcomes in this study at 7 years were statistically significant in favor of ABVD, with freedom from progression (63% MOPP vs. 81% ABVD, $p <.02$) and overall survival (68% MOPP vs. 77% ABVD, $p <.03$) as end points (38). This study demonstrated the difficulty in delivery of planned doses of MOPP following irradiation, a factor that led to criticism of the conclusions. Of major significance, ABVD was associated with a reduction in serious late effects (37,39).

The acute toxicities of ABVD included a higher incidence of alopecia and vomiting compared with MOPP. Prior to the current era of potent antiemetics, anticipatory nausea and vomiting complicated the delivery of ABVD. Relative to MOPP, the neurotoxicity of ABVD was mild but the administration of dacarbazine often required prolonged infusion in small peripheral vessels. Severe myelosuppression was rare when ABVD was administered alone and, therefore, ABVD could be delivered in more optimal doses in a combined-modality setting (37).

In contrast to MOPP, ABVD was not associated with a high incidence of permanent azoospermia or amenorrhea (39). Azoospermia and oligospermia were recorded with an incidence of 36% and 20% with recovery to normal values in all patients in the Milan trial (37). However, a significant proportion of patients in this combined modality trial did not receive six cycles of treatment and/or had dose modifications subsequent to irradiation. In a smaller study of ABVD alone, the incidence of azoospermia was 33% (40). Of major importance, the incidence of secondary leukemia and myelodysplasia was not increased with ABVD (41). The rate of secondary leukemia within 10 years of MOPP plus irradiation was 6.5% compared to 0 among patients treated with ABVD plus irradiation (37).

Theoretically, there is concern that ABVD may cause late cardiopulmonary toxicity, particularly in combination with mediastinal irradiation. In the Milan trial, the only adverse factor noted among ABVD recipients was an increase in pulmonary fibrosis on chest radiograph (37). However, in prospective studies conducted at Stanford and

TABLE 3. *Randomized trials with ABVD chemotherapy*

Group (reference) and treatment	No. of cycles	RT	No. of patients	Stage	% FFP (*p*)	% FFS (*p*)	% OS (*p*)	Time analyzed (years)
Milan (32)		IF	76	IIB, III, IV				10
ABVD	6				63		54	
MOPP	6				50		39	
					(NS)		(NS)	
Milan (37)		STLI	232	IIB, III				7
ABVD	6				81		77	
MOPP	6				63		68	
					(<.002)		(<.03)	
CALGB (10)		—	361	III, IV prior RT				5
ABVD	6–8					61	73	
MOPP	6–8					50	66	
MOPP/ABVD	12					65	75	
						(.03)	(NS)	
CALGB (46)		—	856	III, IV prior RT				3
ABVD	8–10					65	87	
MOPP-ABV	8–10					67	85	
						(NS)	(NS)	

RT, radiotherapy; FFP, freedom from progression; FFS, failure-free survival; OS, overall survival; IF, involved field; STLI, subtotal lymphoid irradiation; NS, not significant; CALBG, Cancer and Leukemia Group B.

the European Organization for the Research and Treatment of Cancer (EORTC), ABVD in combination with irradiation resulted in greater abnormalities on formal pulmonary function testing (42,43). Although many of these laboratory abnormalities were not clinically significant, fatal pulmonary complications related to bleomycin have occurred after ABVD alone (10,43). Children appear to be more susceptible to both the cardiotoxicity of doxorubicin and the pulmonary toxicity of bleomycin (44,45). For a full discussion of this topic, see Chapter 30.

The superior outcomes with ABVD compared with MOPP in the Milan trials set the stage for the definitive large randomized trials of chemotherapy alone in advanced Hodgkin's disease that would follow. The CALGB led a trial in advanced Hodgkin's disease comparing ABVD with MOPP and MOPP alternating with ABVD (see below) (10). The results from this study suggested that ABVD was superior to MOPP and could be substituted for MOPP/ABVD combination therapy in advanced Hodgkin's disease, eliminating a source of serious late morbidity. The efficacy of ABVD and its favorable toxicity profile, relative to that of the MOPP-ABV hybrid combination, was confirmed in a subsequent trial, also led by the CALGB, as detailed below (46). These studies have established the ABVD regimen as the current standard for advanced Hodgkin's disease.

Alternating Therapy

In 1974 the Milan group initiated a treatment strategy to alternate cycles of MOPP and ABVD in stage IV patients, based on the therapeutic limitations of MOPP and the efficacy of ABVD in patients refractory to MOPP (Table 2) (8). Patients with stage IV disease were randomized to MOPP or MOPP/ABVD, which, in the absence of disease progression, was given for 12 cycles. In this small study of 88 patients, 25 had received previous irradiation. Despite the small numbers, the results in favor of the alternating program were striking and statistically significant for freedom from progression at 8 years (36% MOPP vs. 65% MOPP/ABVD, $p < .005$). The overall survival was likewise superior for MOPP/ABVD (64% MOPP vs. 84% MOPP/ABVD) but this difference did not achieve statistical significance. An important aspect of this trial was the superiority of MOPP/ABVD in subsets considered to be prognostically unfavorable with MOPP: age over 40 years, systemic symptoms, nodular sclerosis histology, and bulky disease.

Three large cooperative group trials have confirmed the Milan results and established the superiority of combination treatment with MOPP and ABVD over treatment with MOPP or a MOPP derivative alone in advanced Hodgkin's disease. Based on their previous clinical trial and the emerging data regarding the efficacy of ABVD, ECOG randomized patients to BCVPP, BCVPP plus low-dose irradiation, or MOPP followed by ABVD (Table 2) (47). The complete remission rate was significantly higher with the sequential delivery of MOPP and ABVD, and overall survival favored the sequential regimen as well.

The Milan trial suggested the superiority of MOPP/ABVD over MOPP in stage IV patients, whereas the trials from this group testing MOPP or ABVD in combined-modality programs demonstrated an advantage for ABVD in other stages. Therefore, the CALGB designed a three-arm comparative trial to test the relative efficacy and toxicity of six to eight cycles of MOPP, six to eight cycles of ABVD, and 12 cycles of MOPP alternating with ABVD in advanced Hodgkin's disease (Table 3) (10).

Patients failing prior irradiation were eligible for this study also. A total of 361 eligible patients were randomized to MOPP (n=123), ABVD (n=115), or alternating (n=123) therapy. Figure 2 demonstrates that, at 10 years, the failure-free survival rates were 38% for MOPP, 55% for ABVD, and 50% for MOPP/ABVD, p = .02. There was a trend for superior overall survival with ABVD (68%) or MOPP/ABVD (65%) compared with MOPP alone (58%), p = .15) (Table 3).

The advantage for a doxorubicin-containing combination in the CALGB study was seen primarily among patients who were older and/or had stage IV disease with more than one extranodal site. MOPP had more severe myelosuppressive effects and was associated with greater reductions in the prescribed drug doses. Clinically important severe toxicity occurred in 6% of the ABVD group, including three fatalities. In the initial publication, two cases of secondary leukemia, one each treated with MOPP and MOPP/ABVD, were recorded.

The power of numbers in cooperative clinical trials was demonstrated in this trial. The differences in outcome mirror the Bonadonna trial of MOPP versus ABVD initiated in 1974 but the statistical significance in the CALGB trial was appropriately termed a definitive advance in the treatment of Hodgkin's disease (10).

The EORTC and the Groupe Pierre-et-Marie-Curie initiated a study in 1981 in which MOPP chemotherapy was compared with two courses of MOPP alternating with two courses of ABVD to a total of eight courses (48). Radiotherapy was given to initial nodal sites ≥5 cm in diameter or residual masses after four courses of chemotherapy. Freedom from progression data for this trial were not provided. Failure-free survival at 6 years significantly differed between the treatment arms (43% MOPP, 60% MOPP/ABVD, p = .01). There were more deaths in the MOPP arm (n = 40) compared to MOPP/ABVD (n = 29) and more patients in the MOPP arm died from Hodgkin's disease (n = 29) than in the MOPP/ABVD arm (n = 20).

Five years following the initiation of the MOPP versus MOPP/ABVD trial in Milan, Goldie and Coldman (49) proposed a mathematical model relating the drug sensitivity of tumors to their spontaneous mutation rate. The model predicted that alternation of treatments with quantitative antitumor equivalence and absence of cross-resistance would yield superior results. This hypothesis was frequently cited to support studies in advanced Hodgkin's disease, although the basic tenets of the model were rarely satisfied by the clinical designs.

A number of phase III studies using new combinations that had not been studied for equivalence with their alternating combination yielded no differences between the treatment arms (50–52). These studies included a trial at the NCI comparing MOPP with an alternating program of MOPP/CABS [lomustine, Adriamycin (doxorubicin), bleomycin and streptozotocin]; a Southeastern Cancer Study Group comparison of BCVPP-bleomycin alone or alternating with a novel combination of doxorubicin, dacarbazine, and bleomycin; and a CALGB study of CVPP, ABOS [Adriamycin (doxorubicin), bleomycin, Oncovin (vincristine), streptozocin] or CVPP alternating with ABOS. These data, together with the positive studies from ECOG and the EORTC, indicated that the true advantage of the Milan alternating program of MOPP/ABVD related to the incorporation of ABVD in the drug regimen rather than the alternating sequence.

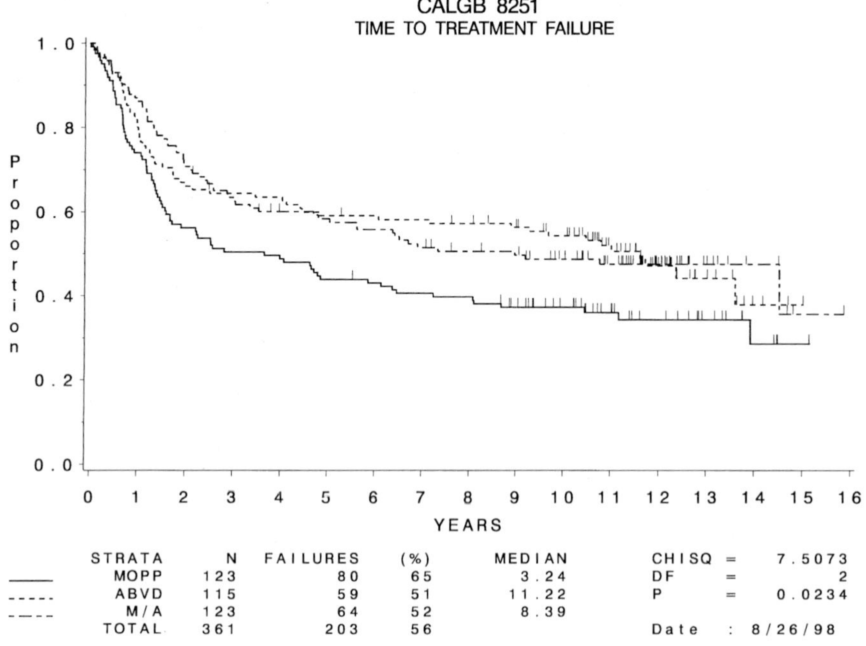

FIG. 2. Failure-free survival in 131 patients with stage III–IV Hodgkin's disease randomized in Cancer and Leukemia Group B (CALGB) study 8251 to six to eight cycles of MOPP [mechlorethamine, Oncovin (vincristine), procarbazine, and prednisone] *(solid line, n* = 123), six to eight cycles of ABVD [Adriamycin (doxorubicin), bleomycin, vinblastine, and dacarbazine] *(broken line, n* = 115) or 12 cycles of MOPP alternating with ABVD *(dotted line, n* = 123). (Data updated by George Canellos, M.D.).

Hybrid Regimens

The theoretic basis for multidrug regimens is the predicted advantage of the earliest possible introduction of all active agents to address heterogeneous tumor cell populations. The SWOG conducted one of the first clinical trials incorporating elements of MOPP with doxorubicin in a hybrid regimen (53). In the MOP-BAP regimen, doxorubicin was substituted for the day 8 mechlorethamine. A higher complete remission rate and overall survival was reported for patients with more favorable prognostic factors (absence of constitutional symptoms, absence of marrow involvement, normal hemoglobin). MOP-BAP was associated with significantly less thrombocytopenia compared to MOPP.

Working independently, the groups in Vancouver and Milan created the first true hybrids of MOPP and ABVD designed to prospectively test the Goldie-Coldman (49) hypothesis (Table 2). In 1985, Klimo and Connors (54) reported the preliminary results of a MOPP-ABV hybrid in which MOPP was given on days 1 to 7 and ABV was given on day 8. Dacarbazine was omitted and doxorubicin was increased from 25 to 35 mg/m^2. Prednisone was given for a full 14 days. Selected partial responders also received involved-field irradiation. A complete remission rate of 88% and an overall survival rate of 90% was reported at 4 years in previously untreated patients with stage IIEA, III, and IV disease.

Based on these encouraging data, the National Cancer Institute of Canada embarked on a trial comparing MOPP-ABV hybrid with alternating MOPP/ABVD in patients with IIIB or IV Hodgkin's disease or those who had previously received wide-field irradiation (Table 4) (55). Responding patients received a minimum of eight cycles of chemotherapy and those with residual disease in a localized region received irradiation between the sixth and seventh cycle. The overall survival rates at 5 years in the 301 randomized patients were similar (81% MOPP-ABV hybrid, 83% alternating MOPP/ABVD; p = .74). Failure-free survivals were also similar (71% MOPP-ABV hybrid, 67% alternating MOPP/ABVD; p = .87). The hybrid regimen proved to be more toxic with a higher incidence of febrile neutropenia and stomatitis. Of note, in planned subset analyses, the alternating regimen

TABLE 4. *Efficacy and toxicity of MOPP and ABV(D) combination chemotherapy*

Group (reference) and treatment	No. of cycles	No. of patients	Stage	% FFS (*p*)	% OS (*p*)	Time analyzed (years)	Toxicity
Canada (55)		301	III, IV prior RT				
Alternating							
MOPP/ABVD ± RT[a]	8–12			67	83	5	More febrile neutropenia and mucositis with MOPP/ABV
Hybrid							
MOPP-ABV ± RT[a]	8–12			71 (NS)	81 (NS)		No difference in toxic deaths or second malignancy
Milan (56)		427	I–IIB[b], III, IV prior RT				
Alternating							
MOPP/ABVD ± RT[c]	6–8			67[d]	74	10	6% incidence of second malignancy in all treated patients
Hybrid							
MOPP-ABVD ± RT[c]	6–8			65 (NS)	72 (NS)		
ECOG (57)		737	III, IV prior RT				
Hybrid							
MOPP-ABV	8–12			64	79	8	More neutropenia and pulmonary toxicity with hybrid; more leukemia/ MDS with sequential
Sequential							
MOPP→ABVD	9–11			54 (.01)	71 (.02)		
CALGB (46)		856	III, IV prior RT				
Hybrid							
MOPP-ABV	8–10			67	85	3	More neutropenia and pulmonary toxicity with hybrid; more leukemia/ MDS with sequential
ABVD	8–10			65 (NS)	87 (NS)		

[a]RT given for residual disease.
[b]IIA bulky also included.
[c]RT given for bulky disease.
[d]Freedom from progression.
RT, radiation therapy; FFS, failure free survival; OS, overall survival, NS, not significant; ECOG, Eastern Cooperative Oncology Group; MDS, myelodysplastic syndrome; CALGB, Cancer and Leukemia Group B.

yielded superior 5-year failure-free survival in patients with prior irradiation (73% MOPP-ABV hybrid, 94% alternating MOPP/ABVD; $p = .01$).

The hybrid regimen developed by the Milan group was initially tested in a randomized trial comparing MOPP-ABVD given in a day 1 and 15 hybrid fashion with the conventional alternating schedule (Table 2). Patients were treated for two consolidation cycles to a maximum of eight cycles. The mature data from this study were published in 1996 (Table 4) (56). A total of 427 patients with stages IB, IIA bulky, IIB, III, and IV Hodgkin's disease were enrolled. Patients relapsing after subtotal or total nodal irradiation were also eligible. Radiotherapy was planned for nodal sites of initial bulky lymphoma. At 10 years the freedom from progression rate showed no difference between the hybrid (69%) and alternating (67%) treatment arms. Similarly, the overall survival at 10 years in the two regimens was nearly identical: 72% for hybrid and 74% for alternating MOPP/ABVD. A total of 17 patients died of second malignancies, including 10 with secondary leukemia. However, 9 of these 10 patients had received salvage chemotherapy in addition to MOPP/ABVD.

ECOG led an Intergroup trial of 737 patients with advanced Hodgkin's disease or in relapse after radiotherapy (57). Patients were randomized to best response to MOPP (six to eight cycles) followed by three cycles of ABVD or MOPP-ABV hybrid as described by the Vancouver group (Table 2). At 8 years, failure-free survival significantly favored MOPP-ABV hybrid (64%) over MOPP followed by ABVD (54%), $p = .01$ (Table 4). Overall survival was statistically ($p = .02$) prolonged after MOPP-ABV. More life-threatening or fatal neutropenia and pulmonary toxicity were seen with MOPP-ABV, whereas the sequential treatment had more significant thrombocytopenia. Of note, in this study, which utilized higher cumulative doses of MOPP and no radiotherapy, the incidence of acute leukemia and myelodysplasia was greater on the sequential arm (Table 4).

The superior outcome for MOPP-ABV hybrid in the ECOG trial, together with the efficacy of ABVD in the CALGB trial, formed the basis of an Intergroup comparison of ABVD with MOPP/ABV hybrid led by CALGB. A total of 856 patients with stage III or IV Hodgkin's disease or recurrent disease following irradiation were randomized to a minimum of eight cycles of chemotherapy (Table 4) (46). An intention-to-treat analysis at 3 years showed no difference in failure-free survival for ABVD (65%) or MOPP-ABV (67%), $p = .30$. However, this study was prematurely stopped by the Data and Safety Monitoring Board due to excess treatment-related deaths and second malignancies with the hybrid regimen (Table 4). Although no difference in overall survival was seen at that time period, 87% for ABVD and 85% for MOPP-ABV ($p = .8$), hematologic and infectious toxicities were significantly greater with hybrid treatment ($p = .01$). Overall, there were 26 treatment-related deaths, 17 among patients over age 55 years. There were two second malignancies with ABVD (one non-Hodgkin's lymphoma and one thyroid adenoma) compared with 12 second cancers with MOPP-ABV, including six cases of myelodysplasia/leukemia, one non-Hodgkin's lymphoma, and five solid tumors. Based on this analysis, the study was closed and the authors concluded that ABVD was equivalent in efficacy and less toxic than hybrid treatment, particularly in older patients.

Taken together, these two CALGB studies and the groundbreaking work of Bonadonna and colleagues have established ABV(D)-containing chemotherapy as the current standard treatment of choice for advanced Hodgkin's disease to which new treatments must be compared.

Duration of Therapy

As noted previously, patients in the original studies of MOPP chemotherapy conducted by the NCI were treated for two additional monthly cycles after a complete remission was achieved (2). All received a minimum of six monthly cycles unless they progressed before that time such that the vast majority of patients received six to eight cycles of MOPP. Bonadonna lengthened the treatment to 12 cycles of MOPP such that equal time periods of chemotherapy would be compared in alternating MOPP (six cycles) and ABVD (six cycles) (8). However, the subsequent trial from the Milan group shortened the alternating program to eight cycles without apparent reduction in efficacy (56). Subsequently, the CALGB trial demonstrated that the efficacy of eight cycles of ABVD was comparable to 12 cycles of alternating MOPP/ABVD (10). A total of 8 to 12 cycles of chemotherapy was delivered in the more recent randomized phase III trials described in Table 4. It should be noted, however, that both the more recent Milan trial and the Canadian study also incorporated selective, consolidative radiotherapy.

Recently, there has been interest in utilizing fewer cycles of chemotherapy in combination with radiation therapy in early-stage Hodgkin's disease (58). Extrapolation of this approach to advanced disease is not recommended. Mathematical modeling suggests that cumulative dose as well as dose intensity may be important to the successful treatment of advanced disease (59). Although data from Stanford University indicate that a dose-intense, abbreviated chemotherapy regimen may allow lower cumulative drug doses, in combination with radiotherapy, this strategy should be tested within the context of a clinical trial as discussed below (60,61).

The interpretation of residual radiographic abnormalities and their impact on the length of therapy frequently challenge physicians. The NCI recommendation of treating patients with two cycles beyond best response is still applicable. If stable radiographic abnormalities remain, it may be extremely difficult to determine whether they represent residual disease or fibrosis. As discussed below, even though randomized trials have not been conducted, consolidation of chemotherapy-induced remissions with radiation therapy is generally accepted for patients with massive mediastinal Hodgkin's disease, regardless of stage (62,63). A positive gallium scan after the completion of therapy is highly predictive of residual disease, although false-positive studies have been reported (64–66). Conversely, a negative study has a low predictive value (66). If there is suspicion of residual disease, and the site is accessible, biopsy is recommended. Patients for whom a major surgical exploration would be required to confirm residual disease should be closely monitored, undergoing pathologic confirmation at the first sign of disease progression.

There is no role for maintenance therapy in advanced Hodgkin's disease. None of the older randomized trials that studied chemotherapy maintenance described a therapeutic benefit (67,68). Based on the available data, it is recommended that patients with stage III and IV disease be monitored for response during treatment and receive two courses of chemotherapy beyond best response, with six cycles considered to be a minimum duration.

Dose Intensity

The relationship between chemotherapy dose and tumor response has been demonstrated in a variety of animal models (69). Data supporting a relationship between actual dose received and therapeutic effect in advanced Hodgkin's disease originated from retrospective analyses of drug delivery with MOPP chemotherapy, in which patients receiving less than optimal doses had inferior outcomes (7,70,71). Patients with unfavorable prognostic factors appeared to be the primary beneficiaries of optimal dose intensity (70,71). These issues are confounded, however, by their frequent association with prognostic factors such as age, performance status, and drug delivery.

In most analyses of dose intensity, individual chemotherapy drugs have been treated as if they had equivalent antitumor effects. In retrospective analyses from Stanford University and the Netherlands, the major effects appeared to be related to mechlorethamine and procarbazine, whereas vincristine dose was found to be an independent predictor of outcome in the NCI series (7,70,71). The augmented dose of doxorubicin in MOPP-ABV was speculated to explain the superior single institution results reported by the Vancouver group (72). However, as noted above, this regimen was more toxic but not more effective in direct comparison with MOPP/ABVD in the Canadian study (55).

Until recently, no prospective randomized comparisons of dose intensity in the treatment of advanced Hodgkin's disease had been conducted. Drug delivery may be intensified by increasing individual drug dose, shortening the interval between treatments, or both. Gerhartz et al. (73) compared COPP/ABVD with a dose- and time-escalated COPP/ABVD given with growth factor support. The delivered dose intensity in the investigational arm was 1.22 compared with 0.92 in the standard arm. In preliminary analysis, the complete remission rate was higher in the intensified arm, but definitive results from this trial are pending.

The German Hodgkin's Study Group (GHSG) has recently completed an elegant series of clinical trials that address dose intensity in advanced Hodgkin's disease. A mathematical model of tumor growth and chemotherapy effects fitted to the data from 705 patients treated by the GHSG served as the basis for these studies (59). This model predicted that moderate dose escalation would increase tumor control by 10% to 15% at 5 years. The BEACOPP [bleomycin, etoposide, Adriamycin (doxorubicin), cyclophosphamide, Oncovin (vincristine), procarbazine, and prednisone] regimen (see below) was devised to serve as a standard combination for dose escalation (74). After establishing excellent tolerability as well as efficacy, a second study of escalated BEACOPP was performed in which doxorubicin was increased to a fixed level and doses of cyclophosphamide and etoposide were increased in a stepwise fashion with growth factor support (75). Maximum doses, with hematologic toxicity as an end point, were found to be 190% of cyclophosphamide and 200% of etoposide.

With the design of standard and escalated BEACOPP in place, the GHSG embarked upon a three-arm trial in which these combinations were prospectively tested together with COPP/ABVD in advanced Hodgkin's disease (75). All three arms of this randomized trial included consolidative radiotherapy for bulky or residual disease. The pooled BEACOPP arms were superior to COPP/ABVD with regard to progression rate and freedom from treatment failure in the interim analyses discussed below (75). In the most recent analyses, an advantage in freedom from treatment failure has emerged for escalated BEACOPP (H. Tesch, personal communication). As expected, the escalated BEACOPP was associated with greater hematologic toxicity (neutropenia, thrombocytopenia, and anemia) and time in hospital.

Interest in the use of hematopoietic growth factors to support optimal drug delivery or to facilitate dose escalation was stimulated by the dose-limiting neutropenia associated with most combination chemotherapy regimens for advanced Hodgkin's disease. The Stanford V regimen, detailed below, utilized granulocyte colony-stimulating factor (G-CSF) at the first occurrence of neutropenia requiring a dose reduction or delay (60,61). The escalated COPP/ABVD and BEACOPP regimens were among the first conventional combinations in which the design was dependent on the use of growth factors. Apart from these treatment programs, adherence to the guidelines of the American Society of Clinical Oncology for the use of growth factors is advised in practice (76).

Numerous phase II studies in Hodgkin's disease recurrent after primary chemotherapy have shown benefit for high-dose chemotherapy or chemoradiotherapy supported by autologous hematopoietic stem cell transplantation (77–79). Further, the superiority of high-dose BEAM (carmustine, etoposide, cytosine arabinoside, melphalan) supported by autografting compared to a lower dose "mini-BEAM" was established in a randomized trial involving patients with poor risk, recurrent Hodgkin's disease (80). Two groups have extended the concept of high-dose chemotherapy and transplantation to previously untreated patients with poor risk features. Carella et al. (81) conducted a phase II trial of myeloablative therapy and autografting among patients with poor risk features described by Straus et al. (82). Based on encouraging results in the pilot study, the European Bone Marrow Transplant Registry conducted a prospective study in poor-risk patients who were randomized to high-dose chemotherapy and autografting or additional chemotherapy after four cycles of ABVD-containing chemotherapy. Accrual to this study continues. Proctor et al. (83) have utilized their previously published model to identify patients for an ongoing study in which patients are randomized to additional chemotherapy or high-dose chemotherapy and autografting after three cycles of a hybrid regimen and radiotherapy to bulky sites.

It is imperative to identify patients who may profit most from dose intensification. Recently, an international effort involving more than 5,000 patients, led by Hasenclever and Diehl (84), identified prognostic factors in advanced Hodgkin's disease. Seven factors were recognized—stage IV, male sex, age, hemoglobin, white blood count, lymphocyte count, albumin—each of which contributed about a 7% reduction in freedom from progression at 5 years (Table 5). When five to seven adverse factors were present, one of which included age >45 years, freedom from progression at 5 years fell to 45% (84). However, this subgroup constituted only 7% of the total patient population, indicating that randomized trials would require international collaboration to evaluate new therapies in this group. At this time, the use of myeloablative therapy and transplantation should be considered investigational for patients with advanced Hodgkin's disease, regardless of prognostic features.

In clinical practice, the benefits of dose intensification, often theoretical, must be balanced against the established risks of cumulative drug doses with serious adverse effects such as second malignancies, sterility, neuropathy, and cardiopulmonary toxicity. New treatments for advanced Hodgkin's disease, discussed below, have generally focused on these issues, with the objective of increasing efficacy through dose intensification and/or the introduction of new drugs or the reduction of toxicity by lowering cumulative drug and radiation exposure, drug addition, and drug substitution.

TABLE 5. *International prognostic factors[a] for Hodgkin's disease*

No. of factors	Population (%)	Estimated freedom from disease progression at 5 years (%)
0	7	84
1	22	77
2	29	67
3	23	60
4	12	51
5+	7	42

[a]Factors: Stage IV; Male sex; Age >45 years; Hemoglobin <10.5 G/dL; WBC ≥15,000/μL; Lymphocytes <8% or <600/μL; Albumin <4 G/dL.

New Chemotherapy Regimens

The success of ABVD indicated that alkylating agents were not an essential component of curative treatment for advanced Hodgkin's disease. However, the pulmonary toxicity of bleomycin, which was more pronounced in children and in combination with mediastinal irradiation, remained a concern with ABVD (42,44,85). Meanwhile, a 20% to 60% response rate in refractory Hodgkin's disease was reported with single-agent etoposide (86). These factors led to the development of a number of new etoposide-containing drug regimens (Table 6).

Groups in Boston and the United Kingdom initially tested the EVA [etoposide, vinblastine, Adriamycin (doxorubicin)] regimen in disease recurrent after MOPP or MVPP (87). The Yale group conducted a study in 26 previously untreated patients with locally extensive, symptomatic or advanced Hodgkin's disease in which six cycles of EVA were followed by low-dose involved-field radiotherapy in responding patients (88). The estimated 2-year failure-free survival in these patients was just 44%. Results with EVA plus radiotherapy were also reported by the Boston group in bulky stage II (n = 20) and advanced (n = 20) disease (89). With a median follow-up of 15 months, the failure-free survival was 66%. A group of 66 pediatric patients with unfavorable or advanced Hodgkin's disease was enrolled in a collaborative study of VEPA [vinblastine, etoposide, prednisone, Adriamycin (doxorubicin)] and low-dose consolidative radiotherapy conducted at Stanford University, Dana-Farber Cancer Institute, and St. Jude Children's Research Hospital (90). This study was stopped when, with 15 months of follow-up, a projected failure-free survival of 66% was observed, a result inferior to historical controls.

These data suggest that etoposide-based regimens that do not include alkylating agents may be inferior treatments for advanced Hodgkin's disease. The fact that all three components in the EVA-type regimens are natural products that share the multidrug resistance phenotype may provide an explanation for these unexpected results (91). In contrast, chemotherapy combinations that incor-

TABLE 6. *Etoposide-containing combination chemotherapy*

Drug	Dose (mg/m^2)	Route	Schedule (days)	RT	Cycle/length (days)
Alkylating agent-containing					
BEACOPP (Escalated BEACOPP)				Bulky, residual	21
Bleomycin	10	IV	8		
Etoposide	100 (200)	IV	1–3		
Adriamycin (doxorubicin)	25 (35)	IV	1		
Cyclophosphamide	650 (1250)	IV	1		
Oncovin (vincristine)	1.4[a]	IV	8		
Procarbazine	100	PO	1–7		
Prednisone	40	PO	1–14		
G-CSF	–(+)	SQ	8+		
OEPA/COPP[b]				IF	28
Oncovin (vincristine)	1.5[a]	IV	1, 8, 15		
Etoposide	125	IV	3–6		
Prednisone	60	PO	1–15		
Adriamycin (doxorubicin)	40	IV	1, 15		
ChlVPP/EVA				—	28
Chlorambucil	10 total	PO	1–7		
Vinblastine	10 total	IV	1		
Procarbazine	150 total	PO	1–7		
Prednisolone	50 total	PO	1–7		
Etoposide	200	IV	8		
Vincristine	2 total	IV	8		
Adriamycin (doxorubicin)	50	IV	8		
ChlVPP/PABLOE				Bulky	50
Chlorambucil	6	PO	1–14		
Vinblastine	6	IV	1, 8		
Procarbazine	100	PO	1–14, 29–43		
Prednisolone	30	PO	1–14		
Adriamycin (doxorubicin)	40	IV	29		
Bleomycin	10	IV	29, 36		
Vincristine	1.4[a]	IV	29, 36		
Etoposide	200	PO	30–32		
Stanford V				Bulky	12 weeks
Mechlorethamine	6	IV	Wk 1, 5, 9		
Adriamycin (doxorubicin)	25	IV	Wk 1, 3, 5, 9, 11		
Vinblastine	6	IV	Wk 1, 3, 5, 9, 11		
Vincristine	1.4[a]	IV	Wk 2, 4, 6, 8, 10, 12		
Bleomycin	5	IV	Wk 2, 4, 6, 8, 10, 12		
Etoposide	60 × 2	IV	Wk 3, 7, 11		
Prednisone	40	PO	Wk 1–10 qod		
G-CSF			Dose reduction or delay		
VAPEC-B				Bulky, residual	11 weeks
Vincristine	1.4[a]	IV	Wk 2, 4, 6, 8, 10		
Adriamycin (doxorubicin)	35	IV	Wk 1, 3, 5, 7, 9, 11		
Prednisolone	50	PO	Wk 1–6		
Etoposide	75–100 × 5	PO	Wk 3, 7, 11		
Cyclophosphamide	350	IV	Wk 1, 5, 9		
Bleomycin	10	IV	Wk 2, 4, 6, 8, 10		
Non–alkylating agent-containing					
EVA				Bulky, residual	28
Etoposide	100	IV	1–3		
Vinblastine	6	IV	1		
Adriamycin (doxorubicin)	50	IV	1		
VEPA				IF	28
Vinblastine	6	IV	1, 15		
Etoposide	200	IV	1, 15		
Prednisone	40	PO	1–14		
Adriamycin (doxorobucin)	25	IV	1, 15		

[a]Vincristine dose capped at 2 mg.
[b]Two cycles of OEPA followed by 2–4 cycles COPP.
G-CSF, granulocyte colony-stimulating factor; IV, intravenous; PO, oral; SQ, subcutaneous; IF, involved field.

porate both etoposide and alkylating agents [BEACOPP, OEPA (Oncovin, etoposide, prednisone, Adriamycin)-COPP, ChlVPP/EVA, Stanford V], as described below, have been associated with superb results.

The GHSG developed the BEACOPP regimen based on mathematical modeling that suggested that modest dose intensification would yield a 10% to 20% increase in failure-free survival (59,92). With escalated BEACOPP, which is repeated at 21-day intervals, the doxorubicin dose is increased to 140%, the cyclophosphamide dose is increased to 190%, and the etoposide dose is increased to 200% of standard BEACOPP (Table 6). Figure 3 demonstrates that escalated BEACOPP provides excellent tumor control with an estimated failure-free survival of 89% at 5 years in the pilot study (H. Tesch, personal communication).

As described above, the GHSG designed a three-arm study, comparing COPP/ABVD, standard BEACOPP, and, later, escalated BEACOPP in patients with advanced Hodgkin's disease (75). Radiotherapy was prescribed for disease ≥5 cm in diameter at diagnosis or for residual disease after eight cycles of chemotherapy. Of note, about two-thirds of patients received consolidative radiotherapy. In 1996, at the time of a planned interim analysis, the COPP/ABVD arm of this trial was closed to accrual because of superior outcomes in the combined BEACOPP arms (75). In a subsequent interim analysis with 505 patients evaluated and a median follow-up of 23 months, the freedom from treatment failure was 74% for COPP/ABVD and 85% for the combined BEACOPP arms (Table 7). Further, the combined BEACOPP arms overcame the adverse prognostic variables identified in the international study (Table 5). A third interim analysis of this trial was performed recently with 698 patients evaluated (H. Tesch, personal communication). Superior freedom-from-treatment-failure results were seen with escalated BEACOPP (89%) versus BEACOPP (81%) and COPP/ABVD (72%). Of note, the incidence of induction failures was lower with escalated BEACOPP (2%) versus BEACOPP (9%) and COPP/ABVD (13%). No significant differences in overall survival among the three treatment arms were found at the time of this interim analysis. These results from a large, cooperative group trial are outstanding.

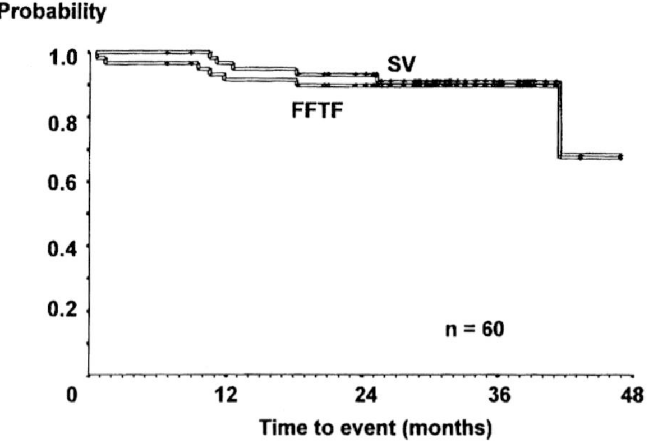

FIG. 3. Freedom from treatment failure (FFTF) and overall survival (SV) in 60 patients treated with eight cycles of escalated BEACOPP [bleomycin, etoposide, Adriamycin (doxorubicin), cyclophosphamide, Oncovin (vincristine), procarbazine, and prednisone] with or without radiotherapy to bulky or residual sites by the German Hodgkin's Study Group. (Data provided by Hans Tesch, M.D.)

As expected, escalated BEACOPP was associated with greater hematologic toxicity, including the requirement for both red blood cell and platelet transfusions (75). At the time of the first interim analysis, second malignancies, including acute leukemia, were reported with BEACOPP (Table 7). The high cumulative doses of alkylating agents and etoposide predict that both sterility and an increased risk of leukemia/myelodysplasia will complicate the use of BEACOPP. Thus, the mature data from this important study, particularly with survival as an end point, are awaited with great interest.

In boys, two cycles of the OEPA combination followed by two to four cycles of COPP and low-dose radiotherapy have been a highly successful treatment for stages IIB–IV Hodgkin's disease (93). The Central Lymphoma Group used the same drugs, with the addition of bleomycin, in a combination termed PABlOE [prednisone, Adriamycin (doxorubicin), bleomycin, Oncovin (vincristine), etoposide], which was studied in an alternating fashion with ChlVPP (94). Based on promising failure-free survival and overall survival data at 5 years, the Central Lymphoma Group and the BNLI collaborated in a randomized trial of ChlVPP/PABlOE versus PABlOE (95). Radiotherapy was not used in this trial. A marked advantage in complete remission rate was noted with the alternating regimen (79% ChlVPP/PABlOE vs. 64% PABlOE, $p = .001$). A statistically significant benefit in progression-free survival and overall survival was also seen for the alternating regimen. This study again found that an etoposide-containing combination without alkylating agents yielded disappointing results. Table 6 illustrates that there are potentially important differences with regard to drug dosing and scheduling, particularly the vinca alkaloids and etoposide, in addition to alkylating agents, that may have relevance to these findings.

The Stanford group took another approach to the concern for late toxicity in the management of Hodgkin's disease (60,61). They devised Stanford V (doxorubicin, vinblastine, mechlorethamine, bleomycin, vincristine, etoposide, prednisone), a weekly chemotherapy program given over 12 weeks for patients with locally extensive or advanced Hodgkin's disease (Table 6). Cumulative doses of doxorubicin, mechlorethamine,

TABLE 7. *BEACOPP ± RT vs. COPP/ABVD ± RT: interim analysis results of the GHSG (April 1997)*

	No. of patients	Three-year		FFP by risk factors[a] (%)		Second cancers[b]		
		% FFP	% OS	0–2	3+	NHL	AML/MDS	Other
COPP/ABVD	182	68	88	71	62	5	—	—
BEACOPP[c] and BEACOPP Escalated[d]	323	82 (p = .002)	92 (p = .04)	82	82	2	3	1

[a]International Prognostic Factors Index for Hodgkin's disease (84).
[b]At 6–40 months' follow-up duration.
[c]185 patients.
[d]138 patients.
GHSG, German Hodgkin's Study Group; FFP, freedom from progression; OS, overall survival; NHL, non-Hodgkin's lymphoma; AML, acute myelogenous leukemia; MDS, myelodysplastic syndrome.

and bleomycin were reduced over those in MOPP/ABV(D) or ABVD alone and procarbazine was omitted. An important feature of Stanford V is the application of consolidative radiotherapy to sites of disease ≥5 cm at diagnosis. At the most recent update of this clinical series, shown in Figure 4, 126 patients had been treated and followed a median of 4.5 years. The estimated 8-year freedom from progression was 89% and the overall survival was 96% (S. J. Horning, personal communication). Similar outcomes were reported in a pilot study conducted by ECOG (61). Preservation of fertility was an important objective in this study. To date, a significant proportion of both men and women have conceived offspring following treatment. An Intergroup trial of Stanford V versus ABVD is planned in selected patients with locally extensive or advanced Hodgkin's disease (Table 8).

The Manchester group also devised an abbreviated, 11-week chemotherapy program, VAPEC-B [vincristine, Adriamycin (doxorubicin), prednisone, etoposide, cyclophosphamide, bleomycin] (96). In a four-center trial VAPEC-B and ChlVPP/EVA (chlorambucil, etoposide, vincristine, procarbazine, prednisone, vinblastine, doxorubicin) were compared. ChlVPP/EVA, a hybrid regimen, was found to be well tolerated and superior to MVPP in a previous study in patients with locally extensive or symptomatic or advanced disease (97,98). Radiotherapy was given to sites of previous bulk disease or significant residual radiographic disease. After a median of 27 months, this study was stopped due to a threefold increase in the rate of progression after VAPEC-B. Another abbreviated, weekly chemotherapy program developed in the United Kingdom by the Southampton group, PACE-BOM (prednisone, doxorubicin, cyclophosphamide, etoposide, bleomycin, vincristine, methotrexate) was studied in 83 stage II–IV patients (99). Radiotherapy was applied if residual disease was demonstrable by chest x-ray. At 5 years, a 64% failure-free survival was reported.

It is hazardous to compare outcomes between studies as patient selection variables (prognostic factors) have often proved to be of greater significance than design and drug usage. However, one possible explanation for the different outcomes in the abbreviated chemotherapy pro-

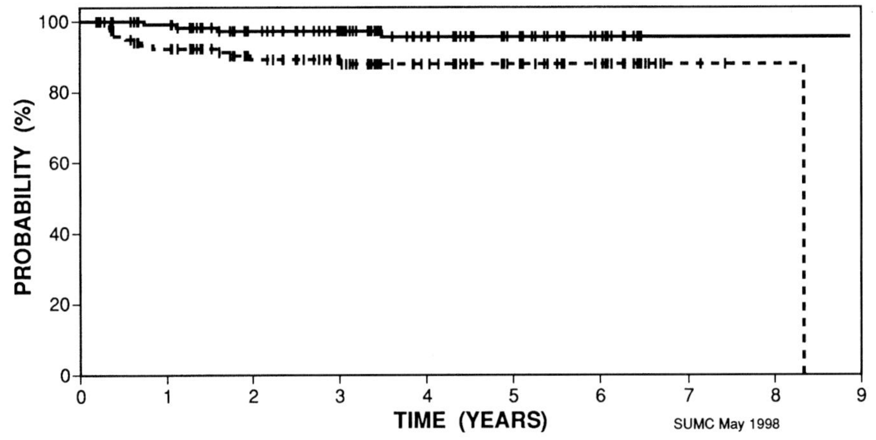

FIG. 4. Failure-free *(dotted line)* and overall *(solid line)* survival in 126 patients treated with 12 weeks of Stanford V chemotherapy with or without radiotherapy to bulky disease sites at Stanford University. (Data updated by Sandra J. Horning, M.D.)

TABLE 8. *Current and planned randomized trials in advanced Hodgkin's disease*

Group	Patients	Treatments	Objective
EORTC	III, IV	MOPP-ABV hybrid ± RT[a]	Determine contribution of RT in advanced disease
ECOG/SWOG	Bulky II, III, IV, 0–2 risk factors[b]	ABVD[c] vs. Stanford V ± RT	Compare standard (ABVD) treatment with abbreviated, dose-intense chemotherapy and selected RT
SWOG/ECOG	Bulky II, III, IV, 3+ risk factors [b]	ABVD vs. ABVD+ transplant[d]	Determine benefit and risks of myeloablative therapy in poor risk patients

[a]Randomization restricted to complete responders.
[b]Based on International Prognostic Factors.
[c]RT is included for massive mediastinal disease.
[d]Transplant includes BCNU, VP16, CY and autologous stem cells.

grams is the application of radiotherapy as a consolidation to chemotherapy, which was done in about 90% of patients treated at Stanford. The greater overall dose intensity of Stanford V, as indicated by the incidence of grade IV neutropenia and use of growth factors, the weekly administration of vinca alkaloids, or the dose of mechlorethamine in the Stanford V regimen, may also have relevance. The potential importance of dose intensity and scheduling was exemplified in a recent BNLI study in which a significant difference in outcomes was found between two regimens (LOPP/EVA hybrid and LOPP alternating with EVA that contained identical total doses) (95). The complete remission was significantly less in the hybrid arm and the trial was prematurely terminated. This outcome emphasizes the potential impact of individual drug doses and scheduling.

Randomized trials continue to be the only reliable method of determining the relative contributions of individual drugs, doses, and scheduling. As noted above, application of the international prognostic factors may serve to identify those patients who benefit most from a dose-intense approach as well as indicating those patients who may be successfully treated with less morbidity (84).

COMBINED-MODALITY THERAPY

The appropriate role of radiation therapy in advanced Hodgkin's disease has sparked lively debates and remains controversial (100–105). Confidence in the contribution of radiotherapy is evidenced by its inclusion in most of the large phase III trials discussed. The potential contribution of radiation therapy is dependent on multiple factors, including patient characteristics, the chemotherapy program, duration of chemotherapy, and response to drug therapy. Field size and dose influence both efficacy and toxicity. Radiation therapy in advanced Hodgkin's disease may be considered in three clinical settings. First, radiotherapy may be used as an adjuvant after complete remission with standard chemotherapy. Second, radiotherapy may be an integrated component of a combined-modality program, possibly with reduced or brief chemotherapy. Finally, radiotherapy can serve as a non–cross-resistant treatment for patients with partial or uncertain response after chemotherapy.

The rationale for combined-modality therapy in advanced Hodgkin's disease is based on the data discussed above, which indicated that a subset of patients treated with chemotherapy alone failed to completely respond or progressed, primarily in previously involved nodal sites. In 42 patients who relapsed after MOPP/ABVD or MOPP/ABV alternating with CAD (lomustine, melphalan, and vindesine), reported from Memorial Sloan-Kettering Cancer Center (MSKCC), 26 (62%) did so exclusively in unirradiated sites (106). Similarly, 80% of relapses after MOP-BAP chemotherapy in the SWOG study were restricted to initially involved sites (105). Although high-dose therapy and transplantation (see Chapter 29) have improved prospects for second-line cure, the success of this treatment is limited to a subset of patients and is associated with substantial cost and morbidity. Thus, there is continued interest in the selective application of radiotherapy in advanced Hodgkin's disease.

The ability of radiation therapy to provide local control in Hodgkin's disease is well established (107). Further, radiotherapy is non–cross-resistant with standard combination chemotherapy. A number of authors have reported that approximately 30% of selected patient who relapsed after chemotherapy attain durable remission with irradiation (108,109). However, the benefits of consolidative radiotherapy must be balanced against the potential for serious late effects, particularly second malignancy.

Single Institutional Experience

The Yale group reported a low rate of relapse, 16%, with a strategy of low-dose (15 to 25 Gy) involved-field irradiation following complete remission induced by MOPP chemotherapy in advanced Hodgkin's disease (110). This relapse rate and tumor mortality was lower than the figures reported for MOPP alone by the NCI. However, as noted above, 15% of patients in the NCI series received adjuvant irradiation, and another subset had failed prior treatment with radiotherapy (2).

Additional data from Duke University and MSKCC were reported in support of combined-modality therapy for advanced Hodgkin's disease. The Duke study included 154 patients who achieved a complete remission with induction chemotherapy and were then assigned to receive no further therapy or irradiation to involved areas at the discretion of the referring oncologist. At 10 years, the disease-free survival was 87% in the group receiving radiotherapy compared with 56% for those treated with chemotherapy alone (111). Overall survival was equally impressive and statistically significant: 80% for the combined-modality patients versus 50% for the chemotherapy-only patients.

The MSKCC reported on 277 patients with advanced Hodgkin's disease treated with MOPP/ABVD or MOPP/ABV/CAD (106). The treatment plan included consolidative irradiation, 20 Gy with an optional 10 Gy boost, to bulky or other critical involved sites among patients achieving complete remission. Only 56% of patients received the intended treatment; 31% were irradiated to selected nodal sites only and 13% received no irradiation. At 10 years, disease-free survival and overall survival for patients irradiated to all involved nodal sites were 89% and 94%, respectively, compared to 68% and 71% for all other patients ($p < .0001$). A proportional hazards regression analysis identified irradiation to all initial disease sites as the most significant factor predictive of disease-free and overall survival.

These studies may be criticized based on analysis of treatment delivered rather than intention to treat and the potential selection bias for irradiation based on patient characteristics. Furthermore, the application of irradiation was limited to patients achieving complete remission. Nonetheless, these studies provided the basis for subsequent randomized trials testing the hypothesis that the addition of irradiation to chemotherapy in advanced Hodgkin's disease would reduce the relapse rate and provide a survival advantage.

Randomized Trials

Table 9 details randomized trials designed to test the role of combined-modality therapy in advanced Hodgkin's disease. Following MOP-BAP chemotherapy, 322 of 530 patients (61%) who achieved complete remission were randomized to low-dose involved-field radiotherapy or to no further treatment in the SWOG study (105). No significant differences in remission duration or overall survival were seen in the intent-to-treat analysis. Subset analyses restricted to the patients who actually received irradiation (104 of 135) showed that remission duration was significantly prolonged with combined-modality treatment (85% vs. 67% disease-free survival at 5 years, $p = .002$). The rate of relapse was also linked to the quality of the irradiation received. Of the 86 patients irradiated without a major protocol violation, only seven relapses were recorded. When the analysis was confined to nodular sclerosis histology, significant differences were seen in favor of the combined-modality group (82% vs. 60% disease-free survival at 5 years, $p = .002$). There were no survival differences in this study.

The GHSG conducted a randomized multicenter study designed to evaluate the role of low-dose involved-field radiotherapy versus chemotherapy consolidation of complete remission in 288 patients with advanced Hodgkin's disease (112). After six cycles of COPP/ABVD, 59% of patients achieved complete remission and 58% of these (34% of the total accrued to study) were randomized to 20 Gy involved-field radiotherapy or two additional cycles of chemotherapy. No significant differences were noted in the study arms either for freedom from progression or overall survival. The study had sufficient power to detect a 20% difference after 7 years. The majority of relapses in both arms of this study were confined to nodal sites of disease. Of interest, the relapse rate was greatest among patients who refused further treatment on either arm of the study.

The ECOG conducted a study in which patients received six cycles of MOPP plus bleomycin followed by a randomization to 15 to 20 Gy involved-field radiother-

TABLE 9. *Randomized trials of combined-modality therapy*

Group (reference) and treatment	No. accrued	No. randomized	RT dose	RT field	% FFS	% OS	Comment
SWOG (105)	564	278	10–20 Gy	IF			CR only; RT benefit for nodular sclerosis histology and bulky disease
MOP-BAP × 6					68	86	
MOP-BAP × 6 + RT					79	79	
GHSG (112)	288	100	20 Gy	IF			CR only
COPP/ABVD × 8					76	92	
COPP/ABVD × 6 + RT					79	96	
POG (114)	183	161	21 Gy	TNI			Initial randomization
MOPP/ABVD × 8					79[a]	87	
MOPP/ABVD × 8 + RT					80[a]	96	

[a]Event-free survival.
CR, complete responders; TNI, total nodal irradiation.

apy or three cycles of ABVD (113). Both freedom from progression and overall survival favored the sequential chemotherapy arm. As described above, a second ECOG study evaluated the curative potential of BCVPP, BCVPP plus low-dose radiotherapy and sequential MOPP/ABVD (47). Outcomes in the BCVPP arms were not different and, when the data were pooled, outcome was statistically inferior to MOPP/ABVD. These studies demonstrated the superior contribution of ABVD relative to low-dose radiotherapy after MOPP-like therapy but do not address the additional benefit of irradiation to a more effective induction regimen.

This question was addressed in a recent Pediatric Oncology Group study in which children received eight cycles of MOPP alternating with ABVD followed by no further treatment or low-dose total nodal irradiation (114). It is important to note that patients were randomized at study entry. Of 186 patients accrued to the study, 161 were randomized. At 5 years, estimates for failure-free survival were no different for patients treated with radiotherapy (80%) or observation (79%). In like manner, there were no survival differences.

Unfortunately, the randomized trials have generally fallen short of the 180+ patients needed for the detection of an estimated 15% survival benefit from irradiation (102). Thus, as a group, they suffer from possible false-negative outcome (type 2 error) resulting from insufficient power. This predicament is magnified by the attrition of patients failing to achieve complete remission or refusing randomization after chemotherapy or the assigned treatment, as well as by technical errors in the prescribed irradiation.

Metaanalysis

To overcome the insufficient power of the randomized studies with too few patients to detect a statistically significant difference between combined modality and chemotherapy alone, a metaanalysis of 14 studies involving 1,740 patients included in the International Database on Hodgkin's Disease was performed by Loeffler (103). Two study designs were distinguished: the additional and the parallel. Irradiation is added to the same chemotherapy in the additional design, whereas in the parallel design, irradiation is balanced in the chemotherapy arm with either more cycles of the same chemotherapy or regimens that contain other drugs. The analysis of the additional design involved 918 patients in seven trials. The use of irradiation reduced the hazard rate by nearly 40% (relative risk 0.63) (Fig. 5A). The benefit of irradiation was more pronounced among patients with stage I–III disease, mediastinal involvement, and nodular sclerosis or lymphocyte-predominant histologies. Irradiation provided no reduction in relapse among patients with stage IV disease, and there was no survival benefit in any group.

The metaanalysis of 837 patients included in the seven trials that compared radiotherapy to enhanced chemotherapy in the parallel design showed no significant difference in disease-free survival for the whole group or any subgroup (Fig. 5B). However, overall survival was superior ($p = .045$) among patients treated with chemotherapy alone. Mortality data showed more deaths from causes other than Hodgkin's disease, including leukemia, in the combined-modality group. However, causes of death were available on only 52% of patients.

The conclusions reached in the metaanalysis should be approached cautiously for a variety of reasons. Nearly all of the chemotherapy combinations, which were primarily MOPP-based, would be considered outmoded by today's standards. Because the studies were initiated 20 or more years ago, it is likely that refinements in technique would make the radiation therapy delivered similarly dated. The extent of irradiation and dose were not considered. Randomization was based on remission in some studies and included all patients in others. The data were dominated by a few cooperative group trials with several hundred patients, whereas many of the studies had fewer than 50 patients. In addition, both adults and children were included. Unfortunately, data regarding mediastinal mass size were often missing and the definition of bulky disease varied among the studies.

The ability to extrapolate from these data is severely limited by the considerations outlined above. The most important questions today relate to the added efficacy of radiotherapy as an adjunct to modern (i.e., ABVD) chemotherapy and the added late toxicity of such an approach. Further, there is considerable interest in supplementing abbreviated but intensive chemotherapy with radiotherapy (60,61). It does not necessarily follow that the benefit for stage I–III patients or the apparent lack of benefit for stage IV patients in the metaanalysis applies to more effective chemotherapy. Likewise, the toxicity profile with regard to leukemia, cardiovascular effects, and other late toxicities may be very different. Prospective randomized trials, such as the comparison of MOPP-ABV hybrid ± consolidative radiotherapy conducted by the EORTC, are needed to address these questions (115). In this study, patients receive six cycles of chemotherapy followed by disease assessment. Those in complete remission receive two further chemotherapy cycles followed by randomization to involved-field radiotherapy or observation.

Dose and Volume

Few studies have addressed the important issues of radiation dose and volume in combination with chemotherapy for Hodgkin's disease. As a single modality, a radiation dose of 35 Gy provides local control in 95% of cases, while smaller doses of 20 to 25 Gy result in local control of 50% to 60% of involved sites (116,117). Low-dose irradiation (15–30 Gy) has been employed in many combined-modality studies in adults and children based on the hypothesis that a lower dose would suffice in the

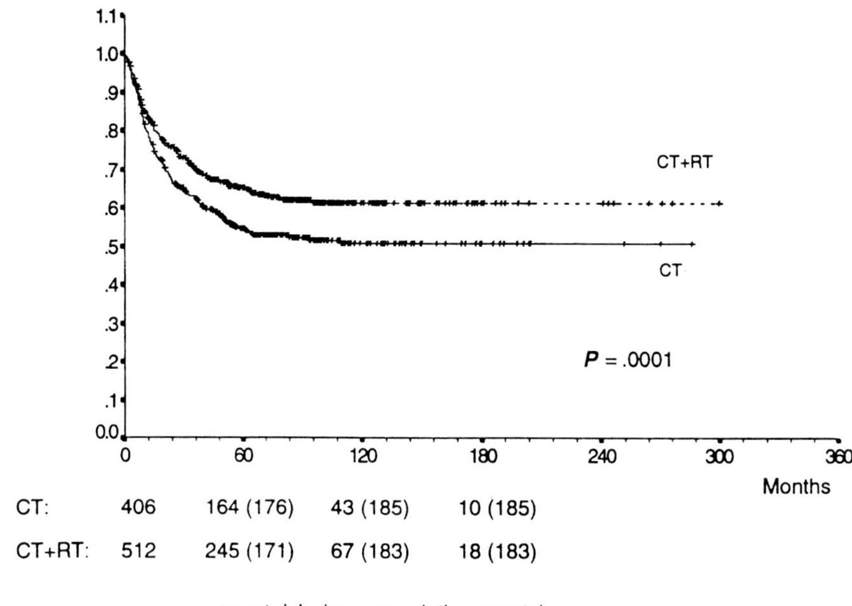

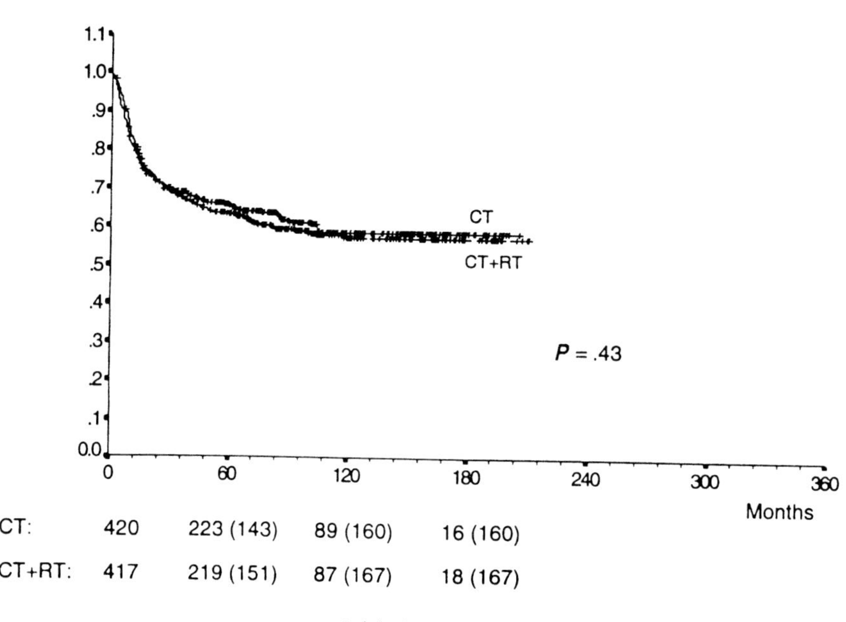

FIG. 5. A: Freedom from disease recurrence in 918 subjects considered in a meta-analysis assessing the benefit of radiation therapy added to chemotherapy. **B:** Freedom from disease recurrence in 837 subjects considered in a meta-analysis assessing the benefit of radiation therapy given in parallel to chemotherapy. (Adapted from ref. 103.)

adjuvant setting (105,118). In fact, the in-field relapse rate has generally been <10% in these studies.

Two studies have addressed the issue of dose in irradiation consolidation of chemotherapy. At the University of Pennsylvania a retrospective analysis was performed among 121 children who received low- (17.5–22.5 Gy) or high- (>32 Gy) dose irradiation following chemotherapy (119). The failure-free and overall survivals at 10 years were not significantly different. Further, the in-field failure rates in the two groups (2% high dose, 7% low dose) were similar. The GHSG evaluated the effect of 20 versus 40 Gy extended-field irradiation to nonbulky disease sites following four cycles of COPP-ABVD chemotherapy in patients with stage I–III disease (120). Patients received 40 Gy to bulky disease sites in this study. No difference in freedom from progression was seen between the two randomized groups, and most relapses occurred in sites receiving full dose irradiation. The GHSG will further explore the effect of dose in the HD9 trial for intermediate Hodgkin's disease, which is currently in progress.

Many studies have defined radiation fields as involved fields, although in most patients with advanced-stage Hodgkin's disease such a definition would require large volumes. This is an important point, because a large international collaborative effort to define prognostic factors in advanced disease confirmed that stage IV is a significant adverse factor (84). As noted above, authors of the MSKCC study concluded that it was necessary to treat all involved disease sites. In contrast, recent studies from the GHSG and Stanford University have reported promising outcomes with new chemotherapy combinations (Table 6) in combination with radiotherapy to disease sites ≥5 cm (60,61,75). The Stanford design of a 12-week chemotherapy program reflects a contemporary strategy to intensify and shorten chemotherapy, supplemented with radiotherapy, to enhance cure and concurrently lessen morbidity in advanced-stage disease.

Toxicity

A major concern in combined-modality therapy is the potential increase in risk of serious side effects, particularly second malignancy. Difficulties in quantifying the magnitude of risk include the long latency for solid tumors, the important contribution of drug combinations and cumulative doses, and the radiation variables of field size and dose.

Although the risk of second leukemia in advanced Hodgkin's disease is primarily dependent on the cumulative dose of alkylating agents, some groups have found an added risk when MOPP-like chemotherapy was combined with radiotherapy (41,121). In contrast, a large-scale epidemiologic study found no significantly increased risk with the addition of radiation (17). Some data indicate that the risk of leukemia may be larger when chemotherapy is given as salvage therapy after radiation failure or when wide-field radiotherapy is used (41,122).

The main concern regarding the additional risk of radiotherapy is the potential for induction of solid tumors. Treatment of early-stage disease with radiotherapy alone has been clearly associated with a significant and continuing risk of secondary solid tumors, particularly those involving lung, breast, gastrointestinal tract and skin (see Chapter 33). The additional impact of radiotherapy, given after induction chemotherapy, on the risk of second malignancy in advanced patients is less obvious. This is because published series have lacked a sufficient number of patients or adequate follow-up to accurately determine the risk associated with chemotherapy, usually alkylating-agent based, alone. Indeed, series that include a large number of patients treated with chemotherapy alone suggest that the risk of secondary solid tumors is as high as the risk with combined modality or radiotherapy alone (123).

The BNLI study of 2,864 patients, of whom 1,002 were treated with chemotherapy alone, showed that the relative risk for lung cancer after chemotherapy alone was 4.2 compared with 4.0 after combined-modality therapy and 3.3 after radiotherapy alone (123). A case-control study conducted by the international Hodgkin's disease registries confirmed this observation (124). In an analysis of 25,000 treated patients, the risk of lung cancer after chemotherapy alone was twice that of the risk after radiotherapy alone. In two other studies in which the relative risk of second cancers in adults and children was evaluated, no increase in relative risk for combined modality therapy was found (125,126). Again, it should be remembered that these data are primarily based on MOPP or MOPP-like chemotherapy regimens and their relevance to ABVD or new combinations is speculative. Further, there are particular clinical circumstances, such as increased risk of breast cancer in girls and women under the age of 30 treated with mantle radiotherapy, that require careful consideration in the risks and benefits of combined-modality treatment (127,128).

The use of lower doses of radiotherapy, as well as the obvious impact of limited fields, may reduce the risk of second cancers. This notion is supported by the retrospective analyses of second cancer risk in the Yale series and the Late Effects Study Group (129,130). In addition, dose may be critical in cardiac morbidity related to thoracic radiotherapy. An increased risk of cardiac-related mortality, particularly related to coronary artery disease, was documented at Stanford University in both adults and children (131). However, this risk was confined to patients receiving ≥42 Gy. Similarly, the excess risks of other causes of cardiac death, including pericarditis, valvular heart disease, and congestive heart failure, were not observed in patients receiving less than 30 Gy.

Pulmonary complications of combined-modality therapy are likewise related to volume and dose. Radiotherapy delivered in reduced dose and delivered to smaller mediastinal volumes as a consolidation to cytoreduction with chemotherapy showed no increased pulmonary complications compared to chemotherapy alone in the Duke series (111). Hirsch et al. (132) reported no significant clinical sequelae for a cohort of patients treated at MSKCC with ABVD alone or ABVD followed by mediastinal irradiation.

Selected Clinical Settings

Combined-modality treatment is currently favored for patients with massive mediastinal disease, regardless of stage, based on improved disease-free survival compared with radiotherapy or chemotherapy alone (see Chapters 25 and 26). A small retrospective study from the NCI evaluated the role of irradiation in advanced-stage Hodgkin's disease with massive mediastinal involvement (63). Thirteen of 26 patients achieving complete remission relapsed after MOPP alone compared with one of nine who received consolidative irradiation (p = .055).

Although the study was small, it provided support for combined-modality treatment.

Many patients, particularly those with massive mediastinal disease, have residual abnormalities on computed tomography scanning after chemotherapy. The Canadian study of alternating versus hybrid chemotherapy discussed above included radiotherapy for such patients (55). In this study, there was no difference in outcome for patients with a very good partial response compared to those achieving complete remission. In the EORTC study of MOPP-ABV ± radiotherapy for advanced Hodgkin's disease, a significant proportion of patients were not randomized, but rather received irradiation based on failure to achieve a complete remission (115). Outcomes for these partial-remission patients were indistinguishable from those of complete-remission patients, indicating that residual radiographic abnormalities did not represent active disease. The role of radiotherapy as a consolidation for patients with positive gallium scans after chemotherapy also remains a question (see Chapter 21). These issues, together with those discussed above, indicate that the role of adjuvant radiation therapy in advanced Hodgkin's disease requires ongoing study.

SUMMARY AND CONCLUSIONS

The goal of treatment for advanced Hodgkin's disease remains cure with no serious complications. After more than three decades of clinical research, Adriamycin-containing chemotherapy has emerged as the standard against which newer treatments must be compared. With these combinations, 60% to 70% of patients will be alive and free of disease at 5 years. ABVD is much less likely to cause severe myelotoxicity, acute leukemia, or sterility relative to treatment programs that contain significant doses of alkylating agents. Yet, there is opportunity both to improve the cure rate and lessen morbidity. The recent definition of prognostic factors by an international group identified patients who are at greatest risk for relapse with current strategies as well as those for whom less toxic approaches might be tested. Several new drug combinations hold the promise of achieving these goals, but efficacy and toxicity data must mature before their contributions can be properly analyzed. Table 8 describes current or pending multiinstitutional trials in advanced Hodgkin's disease, some of which incorporate the international prognostic factors. Today, as in the past, prospective randomized trials remain necessary for validation of single-institution results. Participation in such trials by the international community of practicing physicians is essential to achieve the objective of the least complicated cure for Hodgkin's disease. While the addition of radiotherapy improved freedom from progression in several studies, a survival benefit has not been demonstrated in randomized trials, and the role of radiotherapy remains controversial. Additional study of the selective use of radiotherapy following chemotherapy and reduction of radiation dose and volume to enhance the therapeutic ratio of the combined-modality approach is encouraged. The current challenge in advanced Hodgkin's disease is to further refine treatment to enhance cure and lessen morbidity with the selective use of chemotherapy and radiotherapy.

REFERENCES

1. DeVita VT Jr, Hubbard SM. Hodgkin's disease. *N Engl J Med* 1993; 328:560–565.
2. DeVita VT Jr, Simon RM, Hubbard SM, et al. Curability of advanced Hodgkin's disease with chemotherapy. Long-term follow-up of MOPP-treated patients at the National Cancer Institute. *Ann Intern Med* 1980;92:587–595.
3. Young RC, Canellos GP, Chabner BA, Hubbard SM, DeVita VT Jr. Patterns of relapse in advanced Hodgkin's disease treated with combination chemotherapy. *Cancer* 1978;42:1001–1007.
4. Horning SJ, Hoppe RT, Kaplan HS, Rosenberg SA. Female reproductive potential after treatment for Hodgkin's disease. *N Engl J Med* 1981;304:1377–1382.
5. Chapman RM, Sutcliffe SB, Malpas JS. Male gonadal dysfunction in Hodgkin's disease. A prospective study. *JAMA* 1981;245:1323–1328.
6. Coleman CN, Williams CJ, Flint A, Glatstein EJ, Rosenberg SA, Kaplan HS. Hematologic neoplasia in patients treated for Hodgkin's disease. *N Engl J Med* 1977;297:1249–1252.
7. Longo DL, Young RC, Wesley M, et al. Twenty years of MOPP therapy for Hodgkin's disease. *J Clin Oncol* 1986;4:1295–1306.
8. Bonadonna G, Valagussa P, Santoro A. Alternating non-cross-resistant combination chemotherapy or MOPP in stage IV Hodgkin's disease. A report of 8-year results. *Ann Intern Med* 1986;104:739–746.
9. Bakemeier RF, Anderson JR, Costello W, et al. BCVPP chemotherapy for advanced Hodgkin's disease: evidence for greater duration of complete remission, greater survival, and less toxicity than with a MOPP regimen. Results of the Eastern Cooperative Oncology Group study. *Ann Intern Med* 1984;101:447–456.
10. Canellos GP, Anderson JR, Propert KJ, et al. Chemotherapy of advanced Hodgkin's disease with MOPP, ABVD, or MOPP alternating with ABVD. *N Engl J Med* 1992;327:1478–1484.
11. van Leeuwen FE, Chorus AM, van den Belt-Dusebout AW, et al. Leukemia risk following Hodgkin's disease: relation to cumulative dose of alkylating agents, treatment with teniposide combinations, number of episodes of chemotherapy, and bone marrow damage. *J Clin Oncol* 1994;12:1063–1073.
12. de Gramont A, Louvet C, Krulik M, et al. Erythrocyte mean corpuscular volume during cytotoxic therapy is a predictive parameter of secondary leukemia in Hodgkin's disease. *Cancer* 1987;59:301–304.
13. Fisher RI, DeVita VT, Hubbard SP, Simon R, Young RC. Prolonged disease-free survival in Hodgkin's disease with MOPP reinduction after first relapse. *Ann Intern Med* 1979;90:761–763.
14. Viviani S, Santoro A, Negretti E, Bonfante V, Valagussa P, Bonadonna G. Salvage chemotherapy in Hodgkin's disease. Results in patients relapsing more than twelve months after first complete remission. *Ann Oncol* 1990;1:123–127.
15. Bonadonna G, Santoro A, Gianni AM, et al. Primary and salvage chemotherapy in advanced Hodgkin's disease: the Milan Cancer Institute experience. *Ann Oncol* 1991;1:9–16.
16. Longo DL, Duffey PL, Young RC, et al. Conventional-dose salvage combination chemotherapy in patients relapsing with Hodgkin's disease after combination chemotherapy: the low probability for cure. *J Clin Oncol* 1992;10:210–218.
17. Kaldor JM, Day NE, Clarke EA, et al. Leukemia following Hodgkin's disease. *N Engl J Med* 1990;322:7–13.
18. Nissen NI, Pajak TF, Glidewell O, et al. A comparative study of a BCNU containing 4-drug program versus MOPP versus 3-drug combinations in advanced Hodgkin's disease: a cooperative study by the Cancer and Leukemia Group B. *Cancer* 1979;43:31–40.
19. McElwain TJ, Toy J, Smith E, Peckham MJ, Austin DE. A combination of chlorambucil, vinblastine, procarbazine and prednisolone for treatment of Hodgkin's disease. *Br J Cancer* 1977;36:276–280.
20. Nicholson WM, Beard ME, Crowther D, et al. Combination chemotherapy in generalized Hodgkin's disease. *Br Med J* 1970;3:7–10.

21. Sutcliffe SB, Wrigley PF, Peto J, et al. MVPP chemotherapy regimen for advanced Hodgkin's disease. *Br Med J* 1978;1:679–683.
22. Hancock BW. Randomised study of MOPP (mustine, Oncovin, procarbazine, prednisone) against LOPP (Leukeran substituted for mustine) in advanced Hodgkin's disease. British National Lymphoma Investigation. *Radiother Oncol* 1986;7:215–221.
23. Bloomfield CD, Weiss RB, Fortuny I, Vosika G, Kennedy BJ. Combined chemotherapy with cyclophosphamide, vinblastine, procarbazine, and prednisone (CVPP) for patients with advanced Hodgkin's disease. An alternative program to MOPP. *Cancer* 1976;38:42–48.
24. Cooper MR, Pajak TF, Nissen NI, et al. A new effective four-drug combination of CCNU (1-[2-chloroethyl]-3-cyclohexyl-1-nitrosourea) (NSC-79038), vinblastine, prednisone, and procarbazine for the treatment of advanced Hodgkin's disease. *Cancer* 1980;46: 654–662.
25. Oza AM, Ganesan TS, Dorreen M, et al. Patterns of survival in patients with advanced Hodgkin's disease (HD) treated in a single centre over 20 years. *Br J Cancer* 1992;65:429–437.
26. McKendrick JJ, Mead GM, Sweetenham J, et al. ChlVPP chemotherapy in advanced Hodgkin's disease. *Eur J Cancer Clin Oncol* 1989; 25:557–561.
27. Selby P, Patel P, Milan S, et al. ChlVPP combination chemotherapy for Hodgkin's disease: long-term results. *Br J Cancer* 1990;62:279–285.
28. Vose J, Armitage J, Weisenburger D, et al. ChlVPP-an effective and well-tolerated alternative to MOPP therapy for Hodgkin's disease. *Am J Clin Oncol* 1988;11:423–426.
29. ChlVPP therapy for Hodgkin's disease: experience of 960 patients. The International ChlVPP Treatment Group. *Ann Oncol* 1995;6:167–172.
30. Swerdlow AJ, Barber JA, Horwich A, Cunningham D, Milan S, Omar RZ. Second malignancy in patients with Hodgkin's disease treated at the Royal Marsden Hospital. *Br J Cancer* 1997;75:116–123.
31. Avilés A, Díaz-Maqueo JC, García EL, Torras V, López-Vancell D. Randomized study for the treatment of advanced Hodgkin's disease: MOPP vs. LOPP. *Arch Invest Med (Mex)* 1991;22:45–50.
32. Bonadonna G, Zucali R, Monfardini S, De Lena M, Uslenghi C. Combination chemotherapy of Hodgkin's disease with Adriamycin, bleomycin, vinblastine, and imidazole carboxamide versus MOPP. *Cancer* 1975;36:252–259.
33. Carbone PP, Bono V, Frei E, Brindley CO. Clinical studies with vincristine. *Blood* 1963;21:640–647.
34. Carter SK, Livingston RB. Single-agent therapy for Hodgkin's disease. *Arch Intern Med* 1973;131:377–387.
35. Frei Ed, Luce JK, Talley RW, Vaitkevicius VK, Wilson HE. 5-(3,3-dimethyl-1-triazeno)imidazole-4-carboxamide (NSC-45388) in the treatment of lymphoma. *Cancer Chemo Rep* 1972;56(part 1): 667–670.
36. Skibba JL, Beal DD, Ramirez G, Bryan GT. N-demethylation the antineoplastic agent 4(5)-(3,3-dimethyl-1-triazeno)imidazole-5(4)-carboxamide by rats and man. *Cancer Res* 1970;30:147–150.
37. Santoro A, Bonadonna G, Valagussa P, et al. Long-term results of combined chemotherapy-radiotherapy approach in Hodgkin's disease: superiority of ABVD plus radiotherapy versus MOPP plus radiotherapy. *J Clin Oncol* 1987;5:27–37.
38. Bonfante V, Santoro A, Viviani S, Valagussa P, Bonadonna G. ABVD in the treatment of Hodgkin's disease. *Semin Oncol* 1992:38–44.
39. Viviani S, Santoro A, Ragni G, Bonfante V, Bestetti O, Bonadonna G. Gonadal toxicity after combination chemotherapy for Hodgkin's disease. Comparative results of MOPP vs ABVD. *Eur J Cancer Clin Oncol* 1985;21:601–605.
40. Anselmo AP, Cartoni C, Bellantuono P, Maurizi ER, Aboulkair N, Ermini M. Risk of infertility in patients with Hodgkin's disease treated with ABVD vs MOPP vs ABVD/MOPP. *Haematologica* 1990; 75:155–158.
41. Valagussa P, Santoro A, Fossati BF, Banfi A, Bonadonna G. Second acute leukemia and other malignancies following treatment for Hodgkin's disease. *J Clin Oncol* 1986;4:830–837.
42. Horning SJ, Adhikari A, Rizk N, Hoppe RT, Olshen RA. Effect of treatment for Hodgkin's disease on pulmonary function: results of a prospective study. *J Clin Oncol* 1994;12:297–305.
43. Carde P, Hagenbeek A, Hayat M, et al. Clinical staging versus laparotomy and combined modality with MOPP versus ABVD in early-stage Hodgkin's disease: the H6 twin randomized trials from the European Organization for Research and Treatment of Cancer Lymphoma Cooperative Group. *J Clin Oncol* 1993;11:2258–2272.
44. Mefferd JM, Donaldson SS, Link MP. Pediatric Hodgkin's disease: pulmonary, cardiac, and thyroid function following combined modality therapy. *Int J Radiat Oncol Biol Phys* 1989;16:679–685.
45. Lipshultz SE, Colan SD, Gelber RD, Perez AA, Sallan SE, Sanders SP. Late cardiac effects of doxorubicin therapy for acute lymphoblastic leukemia in childhood [see comments]. *N Engl J Med* 1991; 324:808–815.
46. Duggan D, Petroni G, Johnson J, et al. MOPP/ABV vs ABVD for advanced Hodgkin's disease: a preliminary report of CALGB 8952 (with SWOG, ECOG, NCIC). *Proc Am Soc Clin Oncol* 1997;16: 12a(abst).
47. Glick J, Tsiatis A, Chen M, Rassiga A, Mann R, O'Connell M. Radiotherapy (RT) for advanced Hodgkin's disease (HD). *Proc Am Soc Clin Oncol* 1988;7:A863(abst).
48. Somers R, Carde P, Henry-Amar M, et al. A randomized study in stage IIIB and IV Hodgkin's disease comparing eight courses of MOPP versus an alternation of MOPP with ABVD: a European Organization for Research and Treatment of Cancer Lymphoma Cooperative Group and Groupe Pierre-et-Marie-Curie controlled clinical trial. *J Clin Oncol* 1994;12:279–287.
49. Goldie JH, Coldman AJ. A mathematic model for relating the drug sensitivity of tumors to their spontaneous mutation rate. *Cancer Treat Rep* 1979;63:1727–1733.
50. Longo DL, Duffey PL, DeVita VT Jr, et al. Treatment of advanced-stage Hodgkin's disease: alternating noncrossresistant MOPP/CABS is not superior to MOPP. *J Clin Oncol* 1991;9:1409–1420.
51. Gams RA, Omura GA, Velez-Garcia E, Kellermeyer R, Raney M, Bartolucci AA. Alternating sequential combination chemotherapy in the management of advanced Hodgkin's disease. A Southeastern Cancer Study Group trial. *Cancer* 1986;58:1963–1968.
52. Vinciguerra V, Propert KJ, Coleman M, et al. Alternating cycles of combination chemotherapy for patients with recurrent Hodgkin's disease following radiotherapy. A prospectively randomized study by the Cancer and Leukemia Group B. *J Clin Oncol* 1986;4:838–846.
53. Jones SE, Haut A, Weick JK, et al. Comparison of Adriamycin-containing chemotherapy (MOP-BAP) with MOPP-bleomycin in the management of advanced Hodgkin's disease. A Southwest Oncology Group Study. *Cancer* 1983;51:1339–1347.
54. Klimo P, Connors JM. MOPP/ABV hybrid program: combination chemotherapy based on early introduction of seven effective drugs for advanced Hodgkin's disease. *J Clin Oncol* 1985;3:1174–1182.
55. Connors JM, Klimo P, Adams G, et al. Treatment of advanced Hodgkin's disease with chemotherapy—comparison of MOPP/ABV hybrid regimen with alternating courses of MOPP and ABVD: a report from the National Cancer Institute of Canada clinical trials group. *J Clin Oncol* 1997;15:1638–1645.
56. Viviani S, Bonadonna G, Santoro A, et al. Alternating versus hybrid MOPP and ABVD combinations in advanced Hodgkin's disease: ten-year results. *J Clin Oncol* 1996;14:1421–1430.
57. Glick JH, Young ML, Harrington D, et al. MOPP/ABV hybrid chemotherapy for advanced Hodgkin's disease significantly improves failure-free and overall survival: the 8-year results of the Intergroup trial. *J Clin Oncol* 1998;16:19–26.
58. Santoro A, Bonfante V, Viviani S, et al. Subtotal nodal versus involved field irradiation after four cycles of Adriamycin, bleomycin, vinblastine and dacarbazine in early stage Hodgkin's disease. *Proc Am Soc Clin Oncol* 1996;15:415(abst).
59. Hasenclever D, Loeffler M, Diehl V. Rationale for dose escalation of first line conventional chemotherapy in advanced Hodgkin's disease. German Hodgkin's Lymphoma Study Group. *Ann Oncol* 1996;7 (suppl 4):95–98.
60. Bartlett NL, Rosenberg SA, Hoppe RT, Hancock SL, Horning SJ. Brief chemotherapy, Stanford V, and adjuvant radiotherapy for bulky or advanced-stage Hodgkin's disease: a preliminary report. *J Clin Oncol* 1995;13:1080–1088.
61. Horning SJ, Bennett JM, Bartlett NL, Williams J, Neuberg D, Cassileth P. 12 weeks of chemotherapy (Stanford V) and involved field radiotherapy (RT) are highly effective for bulky and advanced stage Hodgkin's disease: a limited institution ECOG pilot study. *Blood* 1996;88:2681(abst).
62. Behar RA, Horning SJ, Hoppe RT. Hodgkin's disease with bulky mediastinal involvement: effective management with combined modality therapy [see comments]. *Int J Radiat Oncol Biol Phys* 1993;25:771–776.
63. Longo DL, Russo A, Duffey PL, et al. Treatment of advanced-stage

massive mediastinal Hodgkin's disease: the case for combined modality treatment. *J Clin Oncol* 1991;9:227–235.
64. Hagemeister FB, Purugganan R, Podoloff DA, et al. The gallium scan predicts relapse in patients with Hodgkin's disease treated with combined modality therapy. *Ann Oncol* 1994;2:59–63.
65. King SC, Reiman RJ, Prosnitz LR. Prognostic importance of restaging gallium scans following induction chemotherapy for advanced Hodgkin's disease [see comments]. *J Clin Oncol* 1994;12:306–311.
66. Salloum E, Brandt DS, Caride VJ, et al. Gallium scans in the management of patients with Hodgkin's disease: a study of 101 patients. *J Clin Oncol* 1997;15:518–527.
67. Frei E, Luce JK, Gamble JF, et al. Combination chemotherapy in advanced Hodgkin's disease. Induction and maintenance of remission. *Ann Intern Med* 1973;79:376–382.
68. Young RC, Canellos GP, Chabner BA, Schein PS, DeVita VT. Maintenance chemotherapy for advanced Hodgkin's disease in remission. *Lancet* 1973;1:1339–1343.
69. Frei E, Canellos GP. Dose: a critical factor in cancer chemotherapy. *Am J Med* 1980;69:585–594.
70. Carde P, MacKintosh FR, Rosenberg SA. A dose and time response analysis of the treatment of Hodgkin's disease with MOPP chemotherapy. *J Clin Oncol* 1983;1:146–153.
71. van Rijswijk RE, Haanen C, Dekker AW, de MA, Verbeek J. Dose intensity of MOPP chemotherapy and survival in Hodgkin's disease. *J Clin Oncol* 1989;7:1776–1782.
72. DeVita VTJ, Hubbard SM, Longo DL. The chemotherapy of lymphomas: looking back, moving forward—the Richard and Hinda Rosenthal Foundation award lecture. *Cancer Res* 1987;47:5810–5824.
73. Gerhartz HH, Schwencke H, Bazarbashi S, et al. Randomized comparison of COPP/ABVD vs. dose and time-escalated COPP/ABVD with GM-CSF support for advanced Hodgkin's disease. *Blood* 1997;90(suppl 1):389a(abst).
74. Diehl V. Dose-escalation study for the treatment of Hodgkin's disease. The German Hodgkin's Study Group (GHSG). *Ann Hematol* 1993;66: 139–140.
75. Diehl V, Tesch H, Lathan B, et al. BEACOPP, a new intensified hybrid regimen, is at least equally effective compared with COPP/ABVD in patients with advanced stage Hodgkin's disease. *Proc Am Soc Clin Oncol* 1997;16:2a(abst).
76. 1997 update of recommendations for the use of hematopoietic colony-stimulating factors: evidence-based, clinical practice guidelines. American Society of Clinical Oncology. *J Clin Oncol* 1997;15:3288.
77. Chopra R, McMillan AK, Linch DC, et al. The place of high-dose BEAM therapy and autologous bone marrow transplantation in poor-risk Hodgkin's disease. A single-center eight-year study of 155 patients. *Blood* 1993;81:1137–1145.
78. Horning SJ, Chao NJ, Negrin RS, et al. High-dose therapy and autologous hematopoietic progenitor cell transplantation for recurrent or refractory Hodgkin's disease: analysis of the Stanford University results and prognostic indices. *Blood* 1997;89:801–813.
79. Reece DE, Barnett MJ, Connors JM, et al. Intensive chemotherapy with cyclophosphamide, carmustine, and etoposide followed by autologous bone marrow transplantation for relapsed Hodgkin's disease. *J Clin Oncol* 1991;9:1871–1879.
80. Linch DC, Winfield D, Goldstone AH, et al. Dose intensification with autologous bone-marrow transplantation in relapsed and resistant Hodgkin's disease: results of a BNLI randomised trial. *Lancet* 1993; 341:1051–1054.
81. Carella AM, Carlier P, Congiu A, et al. Autologous bone marrow transplantation as adjuvant treatment for high-risk Hodgkin's disease in first complete remission after MOPP/ABVD protocol. *Bone Marrow Transplant* 1991;8:99–103.
82. Straus DJ, Gaynor JJ, Myers J, et al. Prognostic factors among 185 adults with newly diagnosed advanced Hodgkin's disease treated with alternating potentially noncross-resistant chemotherapy and intermediate-dose radiation therapy. *J Clin Oncol* 1990;8:1173–1186.
83. Proctor SJ, Taylor P, Mackie MJ, et al. A numerical prognostic index for clinical use in identification of poor-risk patients with Hodgkin's disease at diagnosis. The Scotland and Newcastle Lymphoma Group (SNLG) Therapy Working Party. *Leuk Lymphoma* 1992;7(suppl):17–20.
84. Hasenclever D, Diehl V. A prognostic score to predict freedom from progression in advanced Hodgkin's disease. *N Engl J Med* 1998; 339:1506.
85. Brice P, Tredaniel J, Monsuez JJ, et al. Cardiopulmonary toxicity after three courses of ABVD and mediastinal irradiation in favorable Hodgkin's disease. *Ann Oncol* 1991;2:73–76.
86. Schmoll H. Review of etoposide single-agent activity. *Cancer Treatment Rev* 1982;9(suppl):21–30.
87. Richards MA, Waxman JH, Man T, et al. EVA treatment for recurrent or unresponsive Hodgkin's disease. *Cancer Chemother Pharmacol* 1986;18:51–53.
88. Brizel DM, Gockerman JP, Crawford J, et al. A pilot study of etoposide, vinblastine, and doxorubicin plus involved field irradiation in advanced, previously untreated Hodgkin's disease. *Cancer* 1994;74:159–163.
89. Shulman L, Neuberg D, Gollob J, Canellos GP. Etoposide, vinblastine and doxorubicin as initial chemotherapy for patients with advanced Hodgkin's disease. *Proc Am Soc Clin Oncol* 1994;13:369(abst).
90. Link MP, Hudson M, Donaldson SS, et al. Treatment of children with unfavorable and advanced stage Hodgkin's disease with vinblastine, etoposide, prednisone and Adriamycin (VEPA) and low-dose involved field irradiation. *Proc Am Soc Clin Oncol* 1994;13:392.
91. Yuen AR, Sikic BI. Multidrug resistance in lymphomas. *J Clin Oncol* 1994;12:2453–2459.
92. Diehl V, Sieber M, Rüffer U, et al. BEACOPP: an intensified chemotherapy regimen in advanced Hodgkin's disease. The German Hodgkin's Lymphoma Study Group. *Ann Oncol* 1997;8:143–148.
93. Schellong G, Brämswig JH, Hörnig-Franz I, Schwarze EW, Pötter R, Wannenmacher M. Hodgkin's disease in children: combined modality treatment for stages IA, IB, and IIA. Results in 356 patients of the German/Austrian Pediatric Study Group. *Ann Oncol* 1994;5(suppl 2): 113–115.
94. Cullen MH, Stuart NS, Woodroffe C, et al. ChlVPP/PABlOE and radiotherapy in advanced Hodgkin's disease. The Central Lymphoma Group. *J Clin Oncol* 1994;12:779–787.
95. Gregory W, Vaughan-Hudson G, MacLennon K, et al. Alternating CHlVPP/PABlOE versus PABlOE in advanced Hodgkin's disease. *Leuk Lymphoma* 1998;29, Suppl 1:1–8 (abstract).
96. Radford JA, Whelan JS, Rohatiner AZ, et al. Weekly VAPEC-B chemotherapy for high grade non-Hodgkin's lymphoma: results of treatment in 184 patients. *Ann Oncol* 1994;5:147–151.
97. Radford JA, Crowther D, Rohatiner AZ, et al. Results of a randomized trial comparing MVPP chemotherapy with a hybrid regimen, ChlVPP/EVA, in the initial treatment of Hodgkin's disease. *J Clin Oncol* 1995;13:2379–2385.
98. Radford JA, Rohatiner AZS, Dunlop DJ, et al. Preliminary results of a four-centre randomised trial comparing weekly VAPEC-B chemotherapy with the ChlVPP/EVA hybrid regimen in previously untreated patients. *Proc Am Soc Clin Oncol* 1997;16:12a(abst 42).
99. Simmonds PD, Mead GM, Sweetenham JW, et al. PACE BOM chemotherapy: a 12-week regimen for advanced Hodgkin's disease. *Ann Oncol* 1997;8:259–266.
100. Longo DL. Chemotherapy alone in the treatment of patients with early stage Hodgkin's disease. *Ann Oncol* 1996;7(suppl 4):85–89.
101. Prosnitz LR, Wu JJ, Yahalom J. The case for adjuvant radiation therapy in advanced Hodgkin's disease. *Cancer Invest* 1996;14:361–370.
102. Hoppe RT. Hodgkin's disease—the role of radiation therapy in advanced disease. *Ann Oncol* 1996;7(suppl 4):99–103.
103. Loeffler M, Brosteanu O, Hasenclever D, et al. Meta-analysis of chemotherapy versus combined modality treatment trials in Hodgkin's disease. International Database on Hodgkin's Disease Overview Study Group [see comments]. *J Clin Oncol* 1998;16:818–829.
104. Mauch P. What is the role for adjuvant radiation therapy in advanced Hodgkin's disease. *J Clin Oncol* 1998;16:815–817.
105. Fabian CJ, Mansfield CM, Dahlberg S, et al. Low-dose involved field radiation after chemotherapy in advanced Hodgkin's disease. A Southwest Oncology Group randomized study. *Ann Intern Med* 1994;120: 903–912.
106. Yahalom J, Ryu J, Straus DJ, et al. Impact of adjuvant radiation on the patterns and rate of relapse in advanced-stage Hodgkin's disease treated with alternating chemotherapy combinations. *J Clin Oncol* 1991;9:2193–2201.
107. Kaplan HS. Evidence for a tumoricidal dose level in the radiotherapy of Hodgkin's disease. *Cancer Res* 1966;26:1221–1224.
108. Wirth A, Corry J, Laidlaw C, Matthews J, Liew KH. Salvage radiotherapy for Hodgkin's disease following chemotherapy failure [see comments]. *Int J Radiat Oncol Biol Phys* 1997;39:599–607.
109. Pezner RD, Lipsett JA, Vora N, Forman SJ. Radical radiotherapy as salvage treatment for relapse of Hodgkin's disease initially treated by

chemotherapy alone: prognostic significance of the disease-free interval. *Int J Radiat Oncol Biol Phys* 1994;30:965–970.
110. Prosnitz LR, Farber LR, Kapp DS, et al. Combined modality therapy for advanced Hodgkin's disease: 15-year follow-up data. *J Clin Oncol* 1988;6:603–612.
111. Brizel DM, Winer EP, Prosnitz LR, et al. Improved survival in advanced Hodgkin's disease with the use of combined modality therapy [see comments]. *Int J Radiat Oncol Biol Phys* 1990;19:535–542.
112. Diehl V, Loeffler M, Pfreundschuh M, et al. Further chemotherapy versus low-dose involved-field radiotherapy as consolidation of complete remission after six cycles of alternating chemotherapy in patients with advanced Hodgkin's disease. German Hodgkin's Study Group (GHSG). *Ann Oncol* 1995;6:901–910.
113. Glick J, Rubin P, Tsiatis A, Graves R, Bennett J. Hodgkin's disease stage IIIB and IV: failure of radiation consolidation to improve survival compared to B-MOPP-ABVD: an ECOG study. *Int J Radiat Biol Phys* 1987;91(suppl 1):91(abst).
114. Weiner MA, Leventhal B, Brecher ML, et al. Randomized study of intensive MOPP-ABVD with or without low-dose total-nodal radiation therapy in the treatment of stages IIB, IIIA2, IIIB, and IV Hodgkin's disease in pediatric patients: a Pediatric Oncology Group study. *J Clin Oncol* 1997;15:2769–2779.
115. Raemaekers J, Burgers M, Henry-Amar M, et al. Patients with stage III/IV Hodgkin's disease in partial remission after MOPP/ABV chemotherapy have excellent prognosis after additional involved-field radiotherapy: interim results from the ongoing EORTC-LCG and GPMC phase III trial. The EORTC Lymphoma Cooperative Group and Groupe Pierre-et-Marie-Curie. *Ann Oncol* 1997;8(suppl 1):111–114.
116. Vijayakumar S, Myrianthopoulos LC. An updated dose-response analysis in Hodgkin's disease. *Radiother Oncol* 1992;24:1–13.
117. Brincker H, Bentzen SM. A re-analysis of available dose-response and time-dose data in Hodgkin's disease. *Radiother Oncol* 1994;30: 227–230.
118. Donaldson SS, Link MP. Combined modality treatment with low-dose radiation and MOPP chemotherapy for children with Hodgkin's disease. *J Clin Oncol* 1987;5:742–749.
119. Maity A, Goldwein JW, Lange B, D'Angio GJ. Comparison of high-dose and low-dose radiation with and without chemotherapy for children with Hodgkin's disease: an analysis of the experience at the Children's Hospital of Philadelphia and the Hospital of the University of Pennsylvania. *J Clin Oncol* 1992;10:929–935.
120. Loeffler M, Diehl V, Pfreundschuh M, et al. Dose-response relationship of complementary radiotherapy following four cycles of combination chemotherapy in intermediate-stage Hodgkin's disease. *J Clin Oncol* 1997;15:2275–2287.
121. Blayney DW, Longo DL, Young RC, et al. Decreasing risk of leukemia with prolonged follow-up after chemotherapy and radiotherapy for Hodgkin's disease. *N Engl J Med* 1987;316:710–714.
122. Andrieu JM, Ifrah N, Payen C, Fermanian J, Coscas Y, Flandrin G. Increased risk of secondary acute nonlymphocytic leukemia after extended-field radiation therapy combined with MOPP chemotherapy for Hodgkin's disease [see comments]. *J Clin Oncol* 1990;8: 1148–1154.
123. Swerdlow AJ, Douglas AJ, Vaughan-Hudson GV, Vaughan-Hudson B, Bennett MH, MacLennan KA. Risk of second primary cancers after Hodgkin's disease by type of treatment: analysis of 2846 patients in the British National Lymphoma Investigation. *Br Med J* 1992;304: 1137–1143.
124. Kaldor JM, Day NE, Bell J, et al. Lung cancer following Hodgkin's disease: a case-control study. *Int J Cancer* 1992;52:677–681.
125. Lavey RS, Eby NL, Prosnitz LR. Impact on second malignancy risk of the combined use of radiation and chemotherapy for lymphomas. *Cancer* 1990;66:80–88.
126. Beaty O 3rd, Hudson MM, Greenwald C, et al. Subsequent malignancies in children and adolescents after treatment for Hodgkin's disease [see comments]. *J Clin Oncol* 1995;13:603–609.
127. Hancock SL, Tucker MA, Hoppe RT. Breast cancer after treatment of Hodgkin's disease. *J Natl Cancer Inst* 1993;85:25–31.
128. Yahalom J, Petrek JA, Biddinger PW, et al. Breast cancer in patients irradiated for Hodgkin's disease: a clinical and pathologic analysis of 45 events in 37 patients [see comments]. *J Clin Oncol* 1992;10:1674–1681.
129. Salloum E, Doria R, Schubert W, et al. Second solid tumors in patients with Hodgkin's disease cured after radiation or chemotherapy plus adjuvant low-dose radiation. *J Clin Oncol* 1996;14:2435–2443.
130. Bhatia S, Robison LL, Oberlin O, et al. Breast cancer and other second neoplasms after childhood Hodgkin's disease [see comments]. *N Engl J Med* 1996;334:745–751.
131. Hancock SL, Donaldson SS, Hoppe RT. Cardiac disease following treatment of Hodgkin's disease in children and adolescents [see comments]. *J Clin Oncol* 1993;11:1208–1215.
132. Hirsch A, Vander Els N, Straus DJ, et al. Effect of ABVD chemotherapy with and without mantle or mediastinal irradiation on pulmonary function and symptoms in early-stage Hodgkin's disease. *J Clin Oncol* 1996;14:1297–1305.

Hodgkin's Disease, edited by P. M. Mauch, J. O. Armitage, V. Diehl, R. T. Hoppe, and L. M. Weiss. Lippincott Williams & Wilkins, Philadelphia ©1999.

CHAPTER 28

Management of Recurrent Hodgkin's Disease

George P. Canellos and Alan Horwich

The problem of relapse of Hodgkin's disease following initial therapy can be appreciated from an analysis of large series of patients that include all stages and treatments. This type of global analysis shows that 10% to 15% of patients will experience a progression of disease after a satisfactory initial response, and up to another 30% of patients, especially those with more advanced disease, will suffer a relapse following initial induction of remission (1). An overall survival of nearly 75% indicates that second-line (or third-line) therapeutic measures can achieve durable responses and remissions. The unique clinical and biologic features of Hodgkin's disease that promote its sensitivity to chemotherapy and radiation apply both at the time of initial therapy and at the time of relapse. Thus, Hodgkin's disease has emerged as one of the most curable cancers.

Relapse may be defined as the reappearance of disease in sites of prior disease (recurrence) and/or in new sites (extension) after initial therapy and complete response. Progression usually refers to increasing evidence of disease after achievement of a stable partial remission. This is somewhat different from refractory disease, which is a failure to achieve a complete response or partial remission and may represent a more significant degree of radiation- or drug-resistance. Follow-up procedures to detect relapse vary somewhat from institution to institution, but they generally assume a schedule of sequential examination every 2 to 3 months for the first 2 years, followed by examination every 4 to 6 months thereafter and annually after 5 years. Retrospective reviews of follow-up procedures in patients treated for Hodgkin's disease with chemotherapy alone (2) or radiation therapy alone (3) reveal that the majority of relapses are detected during physical examination or investigation of symptoms rather than by routine blood tests or radiographs.

The clinical pattern of relapse may determine the likelihood of success in achieving a durable second remission. The rapidity of relapse may be a measure of the proliferative rate of residual or resistant disease. In the setting of late relapse, resistance to therapy is less likely to be the explanation.

Clinical judgment often enters into the decision of whether to document relapse by biopsy, but it is sound practice to obtain a tissue diagnosis. This is especially so in the setting of late relapse, as the risk for second cancers (non-Hodgkin's lymphoma or solid tumors) is significant in these patients. Early recurrence in the setting of incomplete remission, especially with persistence of constitutional symptoms or measurable radiographic abnormalities, may not demand a repetition of biopsy, although even in this setting, if the disease has been unusually resistant to therapy, a biopsy may be warranted to confirm the initial diagnosis of Hodgkin's disease. As noted below, persistent radiographic or physical abnormalities may represent residual necrosis/fibrosis.

In all cases, clinical restaging is recommended at the time of relapse, especially if there appears to be an isolated relapse. However, because most patients will receive systemic or combined-modality therapy for relapse, the restaging has more prognostic than therapeutic importance. As noted below, late isolated nodal recurrence is associated with a better prognosis than early or disseminated relapse; thus, timing and extent of failure will contribute to the definition of prognosis and selection of second-line therapy (i.e., conventional-dose or high-dose salvage treatment).

A number of restaging schemes have been proposed for relapsed Hodgkin's disease. The most straightforward simply applies the criteria of the Ann Arbor staging system to the extent of disease identified at the time of relapse and substitutes the letters RS (relapse stage) for CS (clinical stage) or PS (pathologic stage) (30).

G. P. Canellos: Department of Medicine, Harvard Medical School and Department of Adult Oncology, Dana-Farber Cancer Institute, Boston, Massachusetts.

A. Horwich: Department of Radiotherapy and Oncology, The Royal Marsden Hospital and Institute of Cancer Research, Surrey, United Kingdom.

The issue of how to define CR versus PR is vital because salvage treatments are generally intensive and potentially toxic. Clinical experience indicates that residual abnormalities persisting on computed tomography (CT) after treatment of large lymph node masses, especially in the mediastinum, may actually represent a CRu (complete remission unconfirmed) with only residual fibrosis and necrosis (4). Scanning with gallium single-photon emission computed tomography (SPECT) has been employed to evaluate residual radiographic abnormalities. A residual mass that is gallium-negative may represent only fibrosis/necrosis, and follow-up without therapy may be recommended. The majority (two-thirds) of these residual masses do not progress and may continue to regress over long periods of time, but relapse may occur in one-third despite the negative findings on gallium studies (5). Persistent gallium avidity, however, is correlated highly with residual disease activity. Experienced interpretation of the gallium scan is required, however, as a false-positive scan may be associated with rebound uptake of the isotope in normal thymus gland or with the incidental faint bilateral pulmonary hilar uptake that sometimes follows chemotherapy.

RELAPSE FOLLOWING RADIOTHERAPY: PROGNOSTIC FACTORS

The principles of radiotherapy for Hodgkin's disease are based on the concept that subclinical disease spreads to adjacent lymph node areas from clinically involved sites (6). This fact is combined with the observation of a dose response indicating that tolerable doses of radiation can completely eradicate Hodgkin's disease within the radiation field. These findings led to the use of large-field radiation techniques associated with customized blocking of normal tissues (7,8). With modern technique, recurrence within a radiation field is uncommon. The Patterns of Care Study of the American College of Radiology demonstrated 1 (1.3%) in-field recurrence within 78 nodal areas treated to a dose of 30 to 35 Gy, 13 (4%) in-field recurrences within 317 nodal areas treated to 35 to 40 Gy, and 18 (4.5%) in-field recurrences among 402 nodal areas treated to 40 to 45 Gy. These observations confirm that these dose levels achieve an in-field disease control rate of 96% to 99% (9). In addition, there is evidence from the Patterns of Care Study that outcomes vary among different centers (10). A significant proportion of mediastinal recurrences were thought to be secondary to a marginal miss rather than radiation resistance (11,12). An analysis from the M. D. Anderson Cancer Center of the pattern of failure following irradiation alone for stage I disease showed a relapse rate of 40/145 (27.6%), but only 3 in-field and 4 marginal recurrences were noted (13). Tumor burden, defined by stage and bulk of disease, remains the major prognostic factor for predicting outcome after primary treatment with radiation therapy (14).

In general, patients who have experienced a relapse are heterogeneous with respect to initial patient- and disease-related factors. Salvage treatment policies also have varied over the past 30 years. This is demonstrated in Table 1, in which data from 447 adult patients treated between 1964 and 1983 for stage I–II Hodgkin's disease at the Royal Marsden Hospital are summarized. It is clear that in the early years, most patients were staged without a laparotomy and were treated with radiotherapy alone; in the middle years, laparotomy staging was performed, and a positive study result was an indication for treatment with chemotherapy; finally, in the later years, the majority of patients were again staged clinically but treated routinely with combined chemotherapy and radiation. These changes in management philosophy influenced the timing of recurrence, as displayed in Figure 1. In the total population, the risk for relapse was 26.1% at 3 years and 37.3% at 12 years. However, if successive treatment eras are analyzed, it can be seen that the proportion of patients who relapsed within 3 years fell from 42.3% in the earliest period (1964–1969) to 8.9% in the latest period (1980–1983). Among patients treated with radiotherapy alone, the 3-year actuarial relapse rate in clinically staged patients was 42.3%, compared with 14.4% for laparotomy-staged patients.

Although the majority of relapses occur within 3 years after initial treatment, late recurrences (after more than 3 years) following radiation therapy do happen. The fact that approximately one-fourth of recurrences occur late after initial treatment emphasizes the need for prolonged follow-up. In the Royal Marsden series, late recurrence following radiation therapy was associated more frequently with stage II disease (as opposed to stage I), age over 40 years, and absence of B symptoms (15). Herman et al. (16) found late relapse to be more likely with stage I disease and the nodular sclerosing histologic subtype.

In the European Organization for Research and Treatment of Cancer (EORTC) series, late relapse (beyond 5 years) following radiation therapy of stage I–II Hodgkin's disease occurred in 3.5% of 1,082 patients. Late relapse was correlated with male sex, B symptoms, and mediastinal involvement (17).

The details of initial staging (especially whether or not laparotomy was performed) and extent of the original radi-

TABLE 1. *Changes in management of early-stage Hodgkin's disease*

Cohort	Laparotomy (%)	RT (%)	CMT (%)	CT (%)
1964–69 (n = 107)	2	85	15	0
1970–74 (n = 143)	57	85	13	2
1975–80 (n = 139)	80	57	37	6
1981–83 (n = 58)	24	40	52	8

RT, radiotherapy alone; CT, chemotherapy alone; CMT, combined chemotherapy and radiotherapy.

From ref. 15.

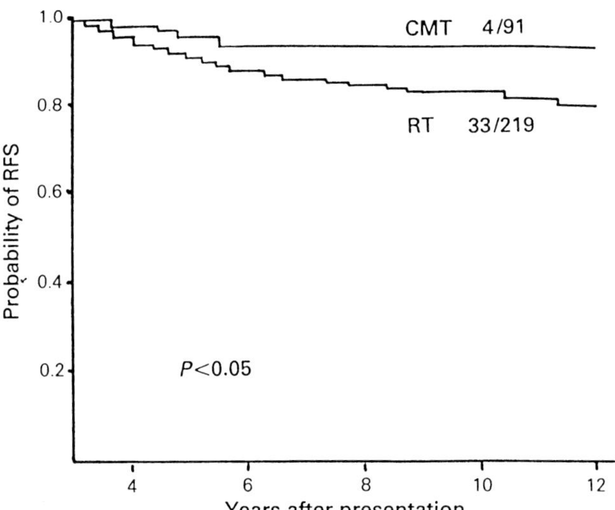

FIG. 1. Actuarial relapse-free survival of 310 patients in remission at 3 years. Patients treated with combined-modality therapy (CMT) had significantly fewer late relapses than those treated with radiotherapy alone (RT) (p <.05).

ation fields have an impact on the pattern of disease at relapse. Even in those patients staged with laparotomy, transdiaphragmatic nodal recurrence can occur (18–22). After treatment with involved-field radiotherapy, relapse of disease in adjacent, unirradiated nodes is common. Extending the radiation field can reduce the risk for recurrence (23). However, metaanalysis of clinical trials shows that the extent of the initial radiation fields does not have an impact on overall survival (24). This can be attributed to the success of salvage chemotherapy in those patients who have relapsed after initial radiation treatment.

A number of analyses of clinical factors at initial diagnosis have predicted outcome after radiotherapy for early Hodgkin's disease. In general, these factors are similar for clinically staged and laparotomy-staged patients. The data in Table 2 are derived from the International Database on Hodgkin's Disease, which contains statistics for 14,315 adult patients treated for Hodgkin's disease; of the 9,091 among them with clinical stage I–II, 3,750 were initially treated with radiotherapy alone, and 1,364 were staged without laparotomy (25). In the combined series of clinically staged and laparotomy-staged patients, there were 1,154 recurrences among 3,750 patients (31%) treated with radiotherapy alone. The factors predicting relapse included histology, number of involved sites, mediastinal involvement, systemic symptoms, an elevated erythrocyte sedimentation rate (ESR), and a low hemoglobin level (26). A review of the EORTC experience indicated that a persistent elevation (above 30 mm per hour) of the ESR was highly correlated with early relapse (27).

A metaanalysis of 2,366 patients staged with laparotomy and treated with radiotherapy alone was performed by the International Hodgkin's Disease Collaborative

TABLE 2. *Clinical stage I–II Hodgkin's disease: presentation variables and disease-free survival after radiotherapy*

Variables	No. patients	% DF at 5 y	Significance (log-rank)
Male	761	68	p >0.05
Female	603	67	
Age			
Age <25 y	375	69	p >0.05
25–39 y	472	68	
>39 y	516	66	
Histology			
LP	171	79	p <.025
NS	836	67	
MC	326	64	
LD	12	58	
No. sites involved			
1	658	72	p <.005
2	416	68	
3	170	55	
>3	67	57	
Mediastinum uninvolved	888	70	p <.05
Mediastinum involved	470	64	
Asymptomatic	1,215	70	p <.005
B symptoms present	149	52	
ESR			
<20	498	76	p <.005
20–30	253	66	
40–59	134	61	
≥60	191	53	
Hemoglobin normal[a]	903	70	p <.005
Hemoglobin below normal	109	54	

DF, disease-free; LP, lymphocyte predominance; NS, nodular sclerosis; MC, mixed cellularity; LD, lymphocyte depletion; ESR, erythrocyte sedimentation rate.

[a]≥8 mmol/L in male, ≥7 mmol/L in female patients.

Adapted from ref. 25.

Group. Among these patients, 681 (29%) relapsed, including 86 of 205 (42%) treated with involved-field radiotherapy, 213 of 741 (29%) treated with extended-field radiotherapy, and 376 of 1361 (28%) treated with total-nodal irradiation (28).

Similarly, the Harvard Joint Center for Radiation Therapy analyzed 481 patients treated initially with radiotherapy, of whom 118 (25%) relapsed, including 63 of 367 (17%) with PS IA–IIA, 11 of 35 (31%) with PS IB–IIB, 39 of 72 (54%) with PS IIIA, and 5 of 7 with PS IIIB. The site of the first relapse was nodal in 59% of these patients (29). A series from Stanford University reviewed 109 patients (19%) who relapsed after primary radiotherapy alone in a series of 565 patients with PS I–IIA, PS I–IIB, or PS IIIA Hodgkin's disease treated between 1968 and 1982. Treatment had been with total-lymphoid or subtotal-lymphoid irradiation (30). In this series, the most frequent site of relapse was the lung (primarily in patients who had presented with large mediastinal masses), which accounted for 26% of the relapses. The other sites included the axilla (23%), iliac nodes (17%), mediastinum (15%), and bone (10%), with equal percentages for hilar and paraaortic nodes and bone marrow.

RELAPSE FOLLOWING PRIMARY MANAGEMENT WITH RADIATION THERAPY: SALVAGE TREATMENT

Table 3 summarizes those series that have examined the outcome of patients treated for relapse after primary radiation therapy. The relapse rates after radiotherapy varied from 19% to 35%, the highest rates being in the series that included only clinical rather than laparotomy staging. The majority of patients in these series had salvage treatment based on MOPP (mechlorethamine, Oncovin, procarbazine, prednisone) chemotherapy or similar regimens (31). The range of 10-year survivals following salvage chemotherapy was 57% to 71%, broadly similar to the results of primary treatment with MOPP in patients presenting with more advanced disease (32). This suggests that prior radiotherapy does not cause drug resistance or a clinically significant compromise of chemotherapy dose intensity (30).

The International Database for Hodgkin's Disease showed a worse prognosis for patients older than 40 years, and for those whose relapse included an extranodal site and RS IV (Figs. 2 and 3) (25). An analysis of the Stanford University experience also found that RS (CS at relapse) was the most important prognostic factor, followed by age over 50 years (30). The Stanford series analyzed the outcome of post-irradiation salvage with chemotherapy according to three prognostic groups based on CS at relapse. The most favorable patients (RS IA) enjoyed a 10-year relapse-free survival of 88%; for the intermediate groups (RS IIA and IIIA), it was 58%; and the least favorable patients (RS I–IIIB, IV) had a 10-year relapse-free rate of 34%. In contrast to the disease-free interval after primary chemotherapy (*vide infra*), the disease-free interval after primary radiotherapy did not appear to be an important prognostic factor in salvage therapy following relapse. Horwich and colleagues (26) showed that patients with a disease-free interval of less than 1 year had a 10-year cause-specific survival of 62%, compared with 65% in 197 patients with a disease-free interval between 1 and 3 years and with 58% in 125 patients with a disease-free interval of more than 3 years (26). Both Horwich et al. (26) and Specht et al. (28) found a better prognosis for patients with nodular sclerosing or lymphocyte-predominance histology than for those with mixed-cellularity histology. In the study by Healey et al. (29), nodular sclerosis histology was also a favorable prognostic factor.

Although most of the published experiences of combination chemotherapy for salvage treatment utilized MOPP, there are sufficient data from doxorubicin-based regimens to indicate that the principles for selecting a salvage regimen are the same as the principles for selecting a primary treatment for advanced disease (see Chapter 27)—namely, maximum antitumor efficacy and minimum cumulative toxicity (33).

The extent to which prior radiation may influence tolerance for chemotherapy, including potential bone marrow or cardiac toxicity, will vary with the details of the previous radiation fields, especially the extent of bone marrow, lung, and heart irradiated. There may also be an impact of radiation dosimetry and technique. For example, historical studies analyzing the risks for myocardial infarction following mediastinal irradiation reported relative risks between 2.5 and 3.1, but no such risks have been found with the use of more modern radiation techniques. Similarly, assessments of left ventricular function after radiation report that late toxicity often is associated with anterior-field-only techniques (34–36).

The choice of chemotherapy regimen may be influenced by the risks for added toxicities. The advantage of ABVD [Adriamycin (doxorubicin), bleomycin, vinblastine, dacarbazine] over MOPP with respect to myelotoxicity may be overshadowed in certain instances by the potential risk for cardiac and pulmonary toxicity associated with Adriamycin and bleomycin, especially among patients treated previously for large mediastinal masses with generous radiation fields (37).

Despite concern that prior radiation therapy might compromise tolerance for chemotherapy, there are few data to support this concern. A recent prospective randomized trial in Canada of patients with advanced Hodgkin's disease, comparing the hybrid MOPP/ABV regimen with an alternating regimen of MOPP/ABVD, demonstrated that a higher dose intensity was achieved in the MOPP/ABV hybrid for all the drugs in this regimen (particularly doxorubicin at 7.99 mL/m^2 per week, compared with 4.22 mL/m^2 per week in the alternating regi-

TABLE 3. *Relapse after initial radiotherapy for Hodgkin's disease*

Series (ref.)	No. originally treated with RT	Stages	No. treated for relapse	Survival 10 y after relapse (%)
Roach et al., 1990 (30)	565	PS I–IIA,B, IIIB	109 (19%)	57
Healey et al., 1993 (29)	481	PS IA–IIIB	118 (24%)	62
Specht, 1996 (28)	2,366	PS IA–IIB	681 (29%)	70
Horwich et al., 1997 (26)	1,364	CS IA–IIB	473 (35%)	63

RT, radiation therapy; PS, pathologic stage; CS, clinical stage.

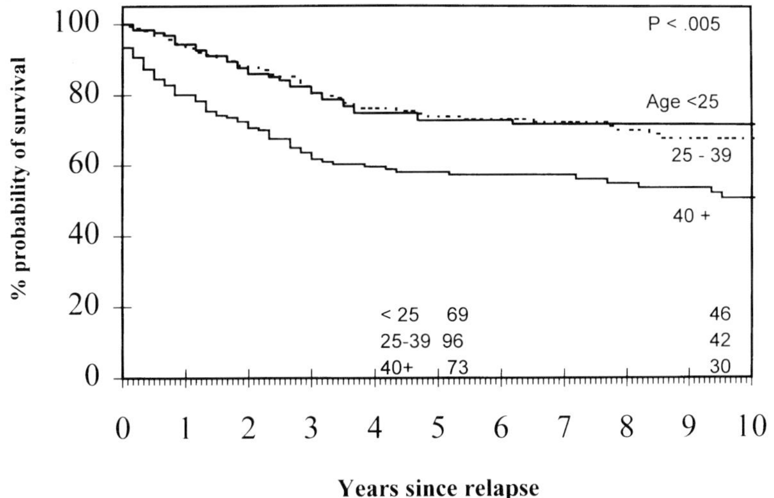

FIG. 2. Cause-specific mortality after first relapse following radiotherapy for clinical stages I and II Hodgkin's disease, comparing 375 patients less than 25 years old at presentation, 472 patients ages 25 to 39 years, and 516 patients more than 39 years old (p <.005).

men; p = .0001) (38). Despite this difference, there was no difference in outcome between the two chemotherapy regimens. Of interest, the subset of 75 patients treated for recurrence after prior radiotherapy had a better 5-year failure-free survival with the less intensive alternating MOPP/ABVD regimen than with the more intensive MOPP/ABV hybrid (94% vs. 73%; p = .017).

An additional potential toxicity that bears serious consideration when salvage treatment is planned is the risk for second malignancy. This appears to be influenced by age at the time of therapy, by the extent of the radiation fields, and by whether both radiation and chemotherapy are administered. This long-term risk for radiation-induced malignancy must be balanced by potential benefits of combined modality as a salvage program (39). However, in the salvage setting, the potential risks associated with Hodgkin's disease itself are generally much greater than the risks associated with a potential second cancer.

The rationale for using combined-modality therapy in the salvage setting is based on the same concepts applied in initial treatment—namely, there is a 30% to 40% risk for early relapse in sites of bulky disease after treatment with chemotherapy alone (40–42). Because of this, in an effort to improve response and cure rates, it has been common practice to administer adjuvant radiotherapy in addition to primary chemotherapy for advanced Hodgkin's disease. Although several prospective randomized trials have shown a disease-free survival advantage for combined-modality therapy in comparison with chemotherapy alone in patients with advanced disease, they all have failed to show (with one exception) an overall survival advantage to adjunctive low-dose (20 Gy) radiation therapy following systemic therapy. In fact, a recent meta-analysis of randomized trials confirmed the lack of a survival benefit (43). This suggests that relapse in patients who present with advanced disease may have a more "systemic" biologic component that is not affected by

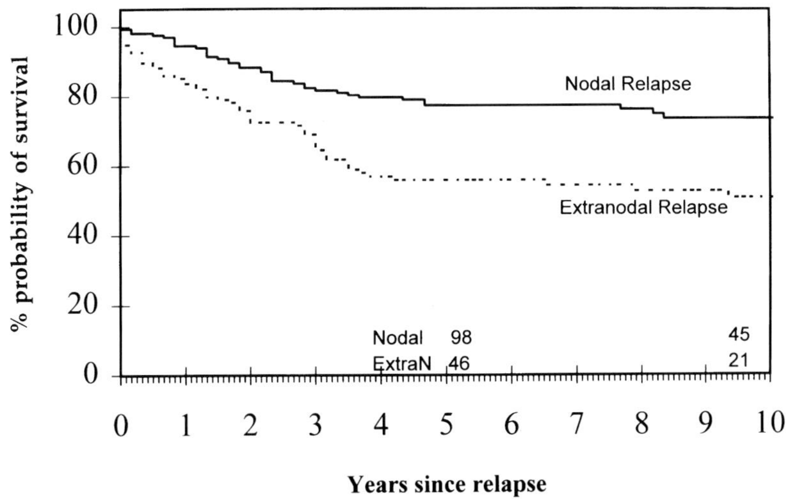

FIG. 3. Cause-specific survival after first relapse following radiotherapy for clinical stages I and II Hodgkin's disease, comparing those with only nodal relapse (n = 169) with those whose recurrence contained an extranodal component (n = 137) (p <.005).

radiation to sites of bulky disease. Alternatively, as suggested by the metaanalysis, the reduction in mortality from Hodgkin's disease associated with the use of adjuvant radiation therapy may be balanced by an increased mortality from causes other than Hodgkin's disease that are secondary to the more aggressive treatment.

Although there does not appear to be a survival benefit associated with the use of combined modality as primary therapy of advanced disease, the combined approach may be more efficacious in the salvage setting following relapse after primary radiotherapy for localized disease. In the Stanford University series referred to previously, 109 patients who relapsed after initial radiation therapy alone were analyzed with respect to salvage treatment with chemotherapy alone or combined-modality therapy (30). Patients with RS II–IV disease had a 10-year rate of freedom from second relapse of 62% after combined-modality therapy, compared with only 37% after chemotherapy alone (p = .04). Multivariate analysis showed that type of treatment for relapse was the most important predictor of outcome.

RELAPSE AFTER PRIMARY SYSTEMIC THERAPY FOR ADVANCED DISEASE: PATTERNS OF RELAPSE AND PROGNOSTIC FACTORS

Combination chemotherapy in advanced disease results in a high complete response rate (65% to 85%). The definition of complete response [confirmed (CR) or unconfirmed (CRu)] may vary because of the detection of residual abnormalities by CT, gallium scan, or magnetic resonance imaging (MRI). Salvage therapy ultimately will be necessary in about 30% to 40% of patients who present with advanced disease and relapse after primary chemotherapy (44–47).

Following treatment with chemotherapy, sites of relapse will often be in previous areas of involvement, unless complementary radiation therapy has been administered. In the latter circumstance, relapse will more likely occur in previously uninvolved nodal regions or extranodal sites (e.g., the liver or lungs). A series reported from the National Cancer Institute, in fact, showed that 75% of relapses after primary treatment with MOPP were in nodal sites and that the vast majority (92% of relapses) were in sites of prior disease (42). The central axial nodal areas and the left supraclavicular region were the most common nodal sites of relapse. New nodal sites also tended to be close to prior sites of disease. The pattern of relapse was also reported in a large series of 427 patients treated at the National Cancer Institute in Milan with chemotherapy (MOPP or ABVD) as the main treatment modality (33). Radiation therapy (30 Gy) was added to bulky and contiguous uninvolved nodal sites in 165 (38%) patients. Of the total of 373 complete responders, 85 (23%) relapsed; in those patients, 71% of the relapses were in nodal sites and the remainder in extranodal with or without nodal sites. Only 13% had recurrence in previously irradiated lymph nodes. The vast majority (80%) relapsed within 3 years of initiation of therapy. The remainder relapsed after between 3 and 10 years. The initial extent of nodal disease (more than three sites involved) was the most important factor contributing to risk for relapse. Because complementary radiation was included in the treatment program, the presence of bulky mediastinal adenopathy did not influence the likelihood of relapse.

The factors that predict relapse from complete clinical remission following chemotherapy for advanced-stage Hodgkin's disease have been reported in the series summarized in the references (28,48–51). The following features were found to be statistically significant in these relatively small series: age above 40 or 45 years, stage III versus IV disease, bulky disease, low hemoglobin or hematocrit, multiple extranodal sites, bone marrow and/or inguinal node involvement, low serum albumin, B symptoms, lymphocyte count $\leq$0.75 or 0.6 $\times$ 10^9/L, and male sex. The problem of defining a uniquely unfavorable group has been difficult. In an analysis of the Christie Hospital (Manchester, United Kingdom) experience, the authors could not identify an event-free survival in any subgroup that was less than 57% at 5 years (51). The most unfavorable group was composed of patients in stage III–IV with bulky tumor and/or B symptoms, low lymphocyte count ($\leq$0.6 $\times$ 10^9/L), or bone marrow involvement. An international prognostic factor project including 5,141 patients from 23 study groups has created an index based on the total number of unfavorable features at diagnosis. Those features were low albumin, low hemoglobin, male sex, age over 45 years, stage IV, leukocytosis, and lymphocytopenia. This analysis showed a spread in the event-free survival from 45% (five or more factors) to 80% (no factors) (52).

Persistence (as opposed to recurrence) of a mass that has regressed but does not progress may *not* represent active disease. Salvage therapy may not affect the outcome of such patients. A recent EORTC trial employed adjunctive radiation therapy (30 Gy) to sites of partial response after six monthly cycles of hybrid MOPP/ABV (53). Among these patients, 59% achieved a complete response, and their progression-free survival was 75%, numbers not significantly different from those of patients who achieved an initial complete response with MOPP/ABV alone. Although these numbers suggest a direct benefit of radiation therapy in this setting, they may be challenged in the absence of gallium nuclide scan data or pathologic confirmation. It is uncertain whether complementary radiation therapy to a residual bulky site is useful unless biopsy or gallium scan has confirmed active disease in that site. In the latter circumstance, if isolated disease is present, the real value of radiation is unconfirmed, but radiation should be considered before aggressive second-line chemotherapy is contemplated.

RELAPSE FOLLOWING CHEMOTHERAPY: SALVAGE TREATMENT

Patients with bulky or extensive stage II or III Hodgkin's disease who are treated with chemotherapy alone occasionally experience isolated nodal relapse. These patients present a strong argument for the use of combined-modality salvage therapy, including second-line conventional-dose chemotherapy and adjuvant radiation therapy.

There are relatively few instances in which radiotherapy alone would be considered the standard salvage management because the perception is that recurrence indicates disseminated disease. However, a recent report from the Peter MacCallum Cancer Institute (Melbourne, Australia) analyzed 52 patients with relapsed or refractory Hodgkin's disease treated initially with chemotherapy and treated with radiotherapy alone for relapse (54). The majority of patients had extended-field treatment. Twenty-three patients (45%) achieved a complete response following irradiation and 19 of these patients remained free of disease, for an estimated failure-free survival at 5 years of 26% and a median failure-free survival of 1.8 years. However, in this study, a retrospective subgroup analysis identified a group of 32 patients with good prognostic features (relapse confined to supradiaphragmatic nodal areas only and absence of B symptoms). In this group, the estimated 5-year failure-free survival was 36%. These figures have broadly supported previous reports of salvage radiotherapy alone for selected patients who relapse after primary systemic therapy (55–60).

Prognostic factors for event-free and overall survival following salvage systemic therapy for relapsed disease have been analyzed in a number of series. The original MOPP series from the National Cancer Institute (Bethesda) was analyzed during a long follow-up period. These data suggested that the duration of first remission was a major determinant in the achievement of a second complete response with repeated MOPP treatment (61). In that series, only age (less than 30 years) and length of first remission (more than 12 months) had a significant positive impact on survival following retreatment with MOPP. Patients whose first MOPP remission was longer than 12 months achieved a second complete response rate of 77%, with a disease-free survival of 45% at 20 years. The lower survival reflects other intervening causes of death, such as second tumors, cardiovascular events, and sepsis. Overall, only 17% of patients in the entire series of patients who relapsed were alive at 20 years. The Milan group analyzed 115 patients who relapsed after treatment with MOPP/ABV hybrid or alternating MOPP and ABVD with complementary radiation therapy (62). Patients with recurrent disease included those who had primary refractory disease (34%) and patients who relapsed after clinical CR, either within 12 months (42%) or beyond 12 months (24%). The overall survival rates of these three groups at 8 years were 8%, 28%, and 54%, respectively, following salvage systemic therapy.

The Cancer Control Agency of British Columbia analyzed a series of 80 patients who relapsed after primary systemic therapy (63). They identified three negative prognostic factors for outcome of second-line therapy. These were a duration of first remission of less than 12 months, initial stage IV disease, and B symptoms at relapse. The 5-year survival was 17% with any one of these factors, but the 5-year relapse-free survival was 82% for the group of patients who had no unfavorable factors. Overall, the second failure-free survival rate was 38%, with a median follow-up of 75 months.

The experience at Hôpital Saint-Louis (Paris) was analyzed in a series of 187 patients who relapsed following primary radiation therapy or chemotherapy for a variety of initial stages (64). Univariate analysis indicated that freedom from *second* failure was adversely affected by (a) duration of first remission of less than 12 months, (b) stage III–IV at relapse, (c) B symptoms at relapse, and (d) elevated lactate dehydrogenase (LDH). Multivariate analyses showed only two independent factors: (a) duration of first remission of less than 12 months and (b) stage III–IV at relapse. The 5-year freedom from second failure and overall survival were calculated according to the number of these negative factors: (a) none: 62% and 87%, respectively; (b) one factor: 47% and 59%, respectively; (c) two factors: 32% and 44%, respectively. The type of systemic therapy (conventional-dose therapy or high-dose therapy with stem cell support) did not influence overall outcome; however, patients with at least one factor seemed to do better with high-dose therapy. The favorable prognostic factors for response to second-line conventional-dose therapy from a number of series are summarized in Table 4.

TABLE 4. *Prognostic factors for salvage therapy in advanced Hodgkin's disease (favorable factors by multivariate analyses)*

Study	Factors	Ref.
NCI, Bethesda	Age <30 y, CR duration >12 mo	61
Istituto Nazionale, Milan	Nodal-only relapse, CR duration >12 mo, <3 nodal sites involved	62
Cancer Control Agency, British Columbia	Stage I–III at initial diagnosis, no B symptoms at relapse, CR duration >12 mo	63
Hôpital Saint-Louis, Paris	CR duration >12 months, stage I–II at relapse	64
GELA (France)	Disease status at relapse (untreated vs. refractory)	70

CR, complete response.

Second-line Regimens

Since 1990, a number of new regimens have been tested that incorporate drugs not used in the initial combination. Because most management programs employ MOPP, ABVD, combinations of both, or similar drugs as part of the primary therapy of advanced disease, new salvage regimens have been designed to anticipate resistance to these drugs in patients who have relapsed. The Milan and National Cancer Institute data suggest, however, that *late* relapse does not necessarily imply resistance, as retreatment with the initial regimen may result in significant response rates (61,62). An important goal for any retreatment or second-line regimen in late relapse is the achievement of a second complete response, as nearly 50% of second complete responses will result in prolonged progression-free survival. Failure to achieve a second complete response may require intervention with more intensive therapy. However, *early* relapse or induction failure does suggest cellular resistance to conventional doses of drugs. For the vast majority of these patients, second- or third-line chemotherapy followed by high-dose therapy, such as CVB (cyclophosphamide, etoposide, BCNU) or BEAM (BCNU, etoposide, cytosine arabinoside, melphalan), may be required.

Table 5 lists the second- and third-line regimens for Hodgkin's disease published since 1990 (65–71). A listing of earlier regimens can be found in prior reviews (72). Detailed analysis and interpretation are difficult because in some trials the numbers of patients are small, the clinical status of patients is varied, and the extent of prior therapy is not reported. A large number of these patients also received subsequent high-dose therapy with stem cell or bone marrow support. Recent second-line regimens such as EVA (etoposide, vinblastine, doxorubicin) and MINE (mitoguazone, ifosfamide, vinorelbine, etoposide) both demonstrated a better remission rate and duration in patients whose first remission was longer than 12 months than in those who had briefer initial responses (69,70). Generally, the 5-year survival for the favorable group will be approximately 50%, but some of these will be alive with active disease, reflecting the relatively indolent course with the favorable biologic and clinical features that some of these patients display.

Selection of Patients for High-dose Therapy

Induction failure and early relapse (within 12 months) from complete response are poor prognostic factors, and these patients fare poorly with conventional-dose salvage therapy. For these patients, high-dose therapy should be considered. The general value of high-dose therapy is difficult to interpret because of patient selection bias and the paucity of randomized trials. A small prospective randomized trial compared high-dose BEAM with mini-BEAM (conventional doses). This trial demonstrated an initial relapse-free benefit but no survival benefit for high-dose therapy in comparison with conventional-dose salvage (73). In an analysis of the published data, high-dose therapy for patients in first relapse resulted in an overall 5-year failure-free survival rate of about 40%. The 5-year progression-free survival following high-dose therapy ranged from 47% to 60% for patients whose initial remission exceeded 12 months to 32% for those whose remission duration was less than 12 months (74,75). In a relatively small series of 30 patients who failed to achieve an initial complete response to combined-modality therapy, the 3-year event-free survival following high-dose therapy was 34% (76). A recent report from the University College Hospital Group (London, United Kingdom) suggests that the outcome of high-dose therapy is the same when it is undertaken in first PR

TABLE 5. *Second-line (conventional-dose) salvage regimens for Hodgkin's disease published since 1990*

Regimen	No. patients	Response	Duration	Ref.
VIM-D (etoposide, ifosfamide, mitoxantrone-dexamethasone)	15	27%	2–14 mo (10 patients to ABMT)	65
CAPE/PALE (cyclophosphamide, doxorubicin, prednisolone, etoposide, CCNU)	25	52%	5 patients in CR (42+–80+ months)	66
ABDIC continuous infusion (doxorubicin, bleomycin, dacarbazine, CCNU, prednisone)	19	53% PR 11% CR	12–27 mo (7 patients to ABMT)	67
CAV (CCNU, melphalan, etoposide)	59	29% CR	18-mo median survival	68
EVA (etoposide, vinblastine, doxorubicin)	45	40% CR	11/18 CR have not relapsed, used in MOPP failures only	69
MINE (mitoguazone, ifosfamide, vinorelbine, etoposide)	100	34% CR	70% to ABMT, 40 patients NED	70
Mini-BEAM (BCNU, etoposide, cytosine arabinoside, melphalan)	44	32% CR	26 patients to ABMT	71

CR, complete response; ABMT, autologous bone marrow (or stem cell) rescue; PR, partial response; NED, no evidence of disease; CCNU, lomustine; BCNU, carmustine; MOPP, mechlorethamine, Oncovin, procarbazine, prednisone.

or in the situation of active progression after first-line therapy, with an approximate 40% progression-free survival at 4 years (77).

Matched patients were compared by the Stanford group (78) to assess the impact of high-dose versus conventional-dose salvage chemotherapy (78). Their analysis confirms that poor-risk patients (induction failures, early relapsers) have a significantly better duration of response, freedom from progression, and event-free survival after high-dose therapy than after conventional salvage therapy. Overall survival, however, was not better after high-dose therapy than after conventional-dose salvage therapy. One conclusion to be drawn is that good-risk patients who relapse may be spared high-dose therapy as an initial salvage maneuver. Pezner et al. (79) came to similar conclusions, suggesting that for patients with a long initial duration of remission, the results of conventional-dose salvage therapy may be equivalent to those of high-dose therapy. In fact, the Joint Center for Radiation Therapy identified a selected group of patients who relapsed after chemotherapy who enjoyed an 85% rate of 7-year freedom from relapse after conventional-dose second-line chemotherapy combined with radiation (55).

Patients who experience early relapse (within 12 months) after primary chemotherapy generally merit high-dose therapy. In addition, generalized systemic relapse even beyond 12 months would suggest an aggressive biologic behavior. Finally, patients in second relapse after salvage therapy should be considered candidates for high-dose therapy.

Role of Salvage Radiotherapy in Patients Receiving High-dose Therapy

Radiation therapy may have an important role in programs of high-dose chemotherapy with autologous bone marrow or peripheral stem cell support. Even after high-dose salvage chemotherapy regimens, relapse occurs in at least half of patients, often in sites of prior relapse, and this may provide a rationale for incorporating radiation into these salvage regimens (80). There are reports that radiotherapy is feasible and may be successful following failure of high-dose chemotherapy (81,82). Radiotherapy is frequently added to high-dose chemotherapy regimens, although its role has not yet been established by prospective randomized trials (80,83–87). In a series from the Princess Margaret Hospital in Toronto, 73 patients were treated with high-dose chemotherapy for relapse after conventional-dose chemotherapy. Of these, 43 underwent involved-field radiation therapy as a component of the salvage therapy, usually before high-dose therapy (85). Bulky (larger than 5 cm) sites of relapse were treated routinely. Some patients had prior radiotherapy, and it was noted that relapse in a previous field (n = 33) was an adverse prognostic factor (22% vs. 54% disease-free survival at 30 months). Univariate analysis showed that radiation therapy was associated with a significantly improved prognosis, but its independent influence was lost in multivariate analysis, probably because of linkage to "nonbulky" or disease-free status at the time of high-dose therapy.

The use of cytoreductive irradiation before transplant has the potential for altering the patterns of failure after high-dose therapy. For example, in the Stanford series (80), 18 patients received irradiation to involved sites before transplant. In subsequent follow-up, relapse was identified in only four of 67 irradiated sites in two patients. In addition, this reduction in relapse risk translated into an improved outcome. Among 49 patients with RS I–III disease who had involved-field radiation as a component of their salvage treatment (either before or after high-dose therapy), the 3-year freedom from relapse, survival, and event-free survival were 100%, 85%, and 85%, respectively, compared with only 67%, 60%, and 54%, respectively, for the 13 patients who received high-dose chemotherapy alone. The difference in freedom from relapse was statistically significant (p = .04). In the same series, an analysis was completed of patients who had no prior history of radiation therapy. Among those 14 who had involved-field irradiation included as a component of the salvage program, the 3-year freedom from relapse, survival, and event-free survival were 85%, 93%, and 79%, respectively, compared with 57%, 55%, and 52%, respectively, for the 25 patients who were treated with high-dose chemotherapy alone. The difference in survival was statistically significant (p = .02), and the difference in freedom from relapse was close to significant (p = .07). When the two criteria were combined (i.e., patients with RS I–III and no prior history of irradiation), the 3-year freedom from relapse, survival, and event-free survival were all statistically significantly better among those patients who had involved-field irradiation as a component of the high-dose therapy.

Yahalom and colleagues (86) at Memorial Hospital in New York investigated the use of involved-field radiation therapy followed by hyperfractionated total-lymphoid irradiation before high-dose therapy in 47 patients with relapsed Hodgkin's disease. Patients who had no prior history of radiation therapy underwent cytoreduction with conventional chemotherapy. They then underwent a course of irradiation including involved-field treatment to a dose of 15 Gy in 10 fractions over 5 days (two fractions daily) followed by total-lymphoid irradiation to 20 Gy in 12 fractions over 4 days (three fractions daily). This was followed by high-dose chemotherapy with a combination of etoposide and cyclophosphamide and finally autologous transplantation. In an early report (86), 47 patients had undergone transplantation. Progression was noted in 10 patients and relapse in four others. Twenty-five patients (53%) were alive and without evidence of disease. The major adverse prognostic factor was disease refractory to initial chemotherapy versus sensitive relapse. The disease-free survival was 32% for the former and 84% for the latter, with a median follow-up of 40 months. This combined-modality approach requires caution, especially because of potential lung toxicity associated with the large mediastinal fields treated so shortly before high-dose chemotherapy. Indeed, in this initial report, there were eight toxic deaths (17%). However, as experience with this regimen has increased, treatment-related mortality has decreased.

Patients who relapse systemically following high-dose therapy are in a difficult situation because of the limited bone marrow reserve; however, single-agent vinblastine has been reported to achieve significant palliation, with partial clinical remissions and control of disease activity (88).

Single-agent chemotherapy for palliation is used, but guidelines for the selection of agents do not exist. Clinical assessment of patient tolerance and the extent of prior therapy are required. Resistance, defined as failure to regress or progression on therapy, usually demands the use of agents of a differing mechanism of action. Relapse off treatment does necessarily imply true resistance. Single agents are employed in the setting of resistance to the more standard MOPP-derived and ABVD-derived regimens, including second- and third-line combinations containing etoposide. Compromised bone marrow reserve might justify the use of methyl-GAG (mitoguazone), a non-myelosuppressant used at a weekly dose of 400 to 800 mg/m^2. The latter schedule resulted in PRs in 40% of patients in one series (89). It has been a component of MIME (methyl-GAG, ifosfamide, methotrexate, etoposide), a salvage regimen for lymphoma (90).

Single-agent trials of paclitaxel, cytosine arabinoside, vinorelbine, and gemcitabine have been reported in series of patients who received at least two regimens with PRs ranging from 17% to 35% (91–94). The mean duration of response varies from 2 to 8 months. Palliation of symptoms and regression of masses can be achieved, and these agents can be used in sequence as tolerated. There is an increasing need for less myelotoxic agents, as patients usually present with a poor bone marrow reserve on relapse from high-dose therapy.

Biologic Therapy

Biologic approaches to refractory Hodgkin's disease have been limited and are outlined in Table 6 (see Chapter 24 for more details). Immunotoxins are the most common biologic therapy that has been used (95). Hodgkin's disease is a reasonable target for immunotoxin therapy because the Reed-Sternberg cells express a large number of antigens that occur only in a small fraction of normal cells. In addition, the number of tumor cells is relatively few. The two antigens that have been targeted for immunotoxin therapy are CD25 (the interleukin-2 receptor) and CD30 (the Ki-1 antigen). These biologic agents are mouse monoclonal antibodies, so that human anti-mouse antibodies (HAMAs) may be expected to develop in a considerable fraction of patients (96–98). Clinical trials have included only small numbers of patients. The use of human interleukin-2 (IL-2) in recombinant fusion to native diphtheria toxin (DAB 486 IL-2) was studied in 15 patients (99). The intent was to target the cells containing IL-2 receptor. Among these 15 patients, only a single response was observed.

Preliminary investigation of a possible adoptive immunotherapy is based on the potential to generate clones of cytotoxic T lymphocytes that are specific for Epstein-Barr virus latent membrane antigens LMP and LMP2 or Reed-Sternberg cells (100). Expanded clones of these cells may have a therapeutic role for those patients with Hodgkin's disease in which the Reed-Sternberg cells express Epstein-Barr viral antigens.

Main Principles of Salvage Therapy for Patients Who Have Failed Initial Systemic Therapy

1. The majority (80%) of relapses after initial systemic or combined-modality therapy for unfavorable-prognosis (i.e., bulky disease or constitutional symptoms) or advanced-stage Hodgkin's disease will occur within 3 years after initial therapy.

2. The majority of these relapses will occur in patients who fail to respond to initial therapy or who have a response duration of less than 12 months. About 25% of relapses will occur beyond 12 months.

3. Residual masses in previous bulky sites of disease may represent only residual necrosis or fibrosis unless gallium avidity is clearly demonstrated or disease is documented by biopsy. Complementary radiation therapy to sites of residual disease in these patients may induce a durable complete response, especially in the setting of initially bulky disease, but the overall impact on survival is debatable.

TABLE 6. *Biologic agents in the treatment of refractory Hodgkin's disease*

Biologic agent	No. patients	No. responses	Comment	Ref.
Anti-CD30 saporin	4	3 transient	antibodies made to agent	96
Anti-CD16/CD30 bi-specific antibody	15	2 (3 and 16 mo)	anti-mouse antibodies	97
Anti-CD25 ricin A immunotoxin	15	2	7/15 made antibodies	98
DAB486 IL-2 diphtheria toxin linked to IL-2	15	1 (2 yrs)		99

4. Second-line (salvage) systemic therapy is most likely to be successful in patients who relapse after a duration of initial response of more than 12 months, whose relapse is confined to limited sites, and who are without constitutional symptoms. The outcome of late progression in an isolated, previously unirradiated nodal site will be better with combined-modality therapy than with chemotherapy or radiation therapy alone.

5. Initial disease progression, failure to respond to initial therapy, and early progression from complete response or partial response merit novel and/or aggressive therapies. Currently, this entails high-dose chemotherapy or combined-modality therapy with bone marrow or peripheral stem cell support (see Chapter 29 for more details). The results of the latter approach will also be determined by clinical prognostic factors, such as bulk of residual disease, stage, constitutional symptoms, extranodal disease, and residual sensitivity to cytotoxic drugs.

REFERENCES

1. Oza AM, Ganesan TS, Leahy M, et al. Patterns of survival in patients with Hodgkin's disease: long follow-up in a single centre. *Ann Oncol* 1993;4:385.
2. Radford JA, Eardley, Woodman C, Crowther D. Follow-up policy after treatment for Hodgkin's disease: too many clinic visits and routine tests? A review of hospital records. *Br Med J* 1997:314:343.
3. Torrey MJ, Poen JC, Hoppe RT. Detection of relapse in early-stage Hodgkin's disease. Role of routine follow-up studies. *J Clin Oncol* 1997;15:1123
4. Devizzi L, Maffioli L, Bonfante V, et al. Comparison of gallium scan, computed tomography, and magnetic resonance in patients with mediastinal Hodgkin's disease. *Ann Oncol* 1997;8(Suppl 1):S53.
5. Jochelson M, Mauch P, Balikian J, Rosenthal D, Canellos GP. The significance of the residual mediastinal mass in treated Hodgkin's disease. *J Clin Oncol* 1985;3:637.
6. Gilbert R. Radiotherapy in Hodgkin's disease (malignant granulomatosis): anatomic and clinical foundations; governing principles; results. *Am J Roentgenol* 1939;41:198.
7. Peters MV. A study of survivals in Hodgkin's disease treated radiologically. *Am J Roentgenol* 1950;63:299.
8. Kaplan HS. The radical radiotherapy of regionally localized Hodgkin's disease. *Radiology* 1962;78:553.
9. Hanks GE, Kinzie JJ, White RL, Herring DF, Kramer S. Patterns of care outcome studies. Results of the national practice in Hodgkin's disease. *Cancer* 1983;51:569.
10. Kinzie JJ, Hanks GE, MacLean CJ, Kramer S. Patterns of care study: Hodgkin's disease relapse rates and adequacy of portals. *Cancer* 1983; 52:2223.
11. Farah R, Ultmann J, Griem M, et al. Extended mantle radiation therapy for pathologic stage I and II Hodgkin's disease. *J Clin Oncol* 1988;6:1047.
12. Yarnold JR, Jelliffe AM, Vaughan Hudson G. Patterns of relapse following radiotherapy for Hodgkin's disease. *Clin Radiol* 1982;33:137.
13. Vlachaki MT, Ha CS, Hagemeister FB, et al. Long-term outcome of treatment for Ann Arbor stage I Hodgkin's disease: prognostic factors for survival and freedom from progression. *Int J Radiat Oncol Biol Phys* 1997;38:593.
14. Specht L. Tumor burden as the main indicator of prognosis in Hodgkin's disease. *Eur J Cancer* 1992;28A;1982.
15. Duchesne G, Crow J, Ashley S, Brada M, Horwich A. Changing patterns of relapse in Hodgkin's disease. *Br J Cancer* 1989;60:227.
16. Herman TS, Hoppe RT, Donaldson SS, Cox RS, Rosenberg SA, Kaplan HS. Late relapse among patients treated for Hodgkin's disease. *Ann Intern Med* 1985;102:292.
17. Bodis S, Henry-Amar M, Bosq J, et al. Late relapse in early-stage Hodgkin's disease patients enrolled in European Organization for Research and Treatment of Cancer protocols. *J Clin Oncol* 1993; 11:225.
18. Hellman S, Mauch P. Role of radiation therapy in the treatment of Hodgkin's disease. *Cancer Treat Rep* 1982;66:915.
19. Hoppe RT, Coleman CN, Cox RS, Rosenberg SA, Kaplan HS. The management of stage I–II Hodgkin's disease with irradiation alone or combined modality therapy: the Stanford experience. *Blood* 1982; 59:455.
20. Verger E, Easton D, Brada M, Duschesne G, Horwich A. Radiotherapy results in laparotomy-staged early Hodgkin's disease. *Clin Radiol* 1988;39:428.
21. Tubiana M, Henry-Amar M, Carde P, et al. Toward comprehensive management tailored to prognostic factors of patients with clinical stages I and II in Hodgkin's disease. The EORTC Lymphoma Group controlled clinical trials, 1964–1987. *Blood* 1989;73:47.
22. Mauch PM, Canellos GP, Shulman LN, et al. Mantle irradiation alone for selected patients with laparotomy-staged IA to IIA Hodgkin's disease: preliminary results of a prospective trial. *J Clin Oncol* 1995; 13:947.
23. Sutcliffe SB, Gospodarowicz M, Bergsagel DE, et al. Prognostic groups for management of localized Hodgkin's disease. *J Clin Oncol* 1985;3:393.
24. Specht L, Gray RG, Clarke MJ, Peto R for the International Hodgkin's Disease Collaborative Group. Influence of more extensive radiotherapy and adjuvant chemotherapy on long-term outcome of early-stage Hodgkin's disease: a meta-analysis of 23 randomized trials involving 3,888 patients. *J Clin Oncol* 1998;16:830.
25. Mauch P, Henry-Amar M. International Database on Hodgkin's Disease: a cooperative effort to determine treatment outcome. *Ann Oncol* 1992;4:59.
26. Horwich A, Specht L, Ashley S. Survival analysis of patients with clinical stages I or II Hodgkin's disease who have relapsed after initial treatment with radiotherapy alone. *Eur J Cancer* 1997;33:848.
27. Henry-Amar M, Friedman S, Sayat M, et al. Erythrocyte sedimentation rate predicts early relapse and survival in early stage Hodgkin's disease. *Ann Intern Med* 1991;114:361.
28. Specht L. Prognostic factors in Hodgkin's disease. *Semin Radiat Oncol* 1996;6:146.
29. Healey EA, Tarbell NJ, Kalish LA, et al. Prognostic factors for patients with Hodgkin's disease in first relapse. *Cancer* 1993;71:2613.
30. Roach M, Brophy N, Cox R, Varghese A, Hoppe RT. Prognostic factors for patients relapsing after radiotherapy for early-stage Hodgkin's disease. *J Clin Oncol* 1990;8:623.
31. Olver IN, Wolf MM, Cruickshank D, et al. Nitrogen mustard, vincristine, procarbazine, and prednisolone for relapse after radiation in Hodgkin's disease. An analysis of long-term follow-up. *Cancer* 1988; 62:233.
32. Longo DL, Young RC, Wesley M, et al. Twenty years of MOPP therapy for Hodgkin's disease. *J Clin Oncol* 1986;4:1295.
33. Santoro A, Viviana S, Villarreal CJR. Salvage chemotherapy in Hodgkin's disease irradiation failures: superiority of doxorubicin-containing regimens over MOPP. *Cancer Treat Rep* 1986;70:343.
34. Corn BWS, Trock BJ, Goodman RI. Irradiation-related ischemic heart disease. *J Clin Oncol* 1990;8:741.
35. Gottdiener J, Katin M, Borer J, Bacharach S, Green M. Late cardiac effects of mediastinal irradiation. *N Engl J Med* 1983;308:569.
36. Constine LS, Schwartz RG, Savage DE, King V, Muhs A. Cardiac function, perfusion, and morbidity in irradiated long-term survivors of Hodgkin's disease. *Int J Radiat Oncol Biol Phys* 1997;39:897.
37. Hancock S, Donaldson S, Hoppe R. Cardiac disease following treatment of Hodgkin's disease in children and adolescents. *J Clin Oncol* 1993;11:1208.
38. Connors JM, Klimo P, Adams G, et al. Treatment of advanced Hodgkin's disease with chemotherapy—comparison of MOPP/ABV hybrid regimen with alternating courses of MOPP and ABVD: a report from the National Cancer Institute of Canada Clinical Trials Group. *J Clin Oncol* 1997;15:1638.
39. Henry-Amar M, Joly F. Late complications after Hodgkin's disease. *Ann Oncol* 1996;7(Suppl 4):S115.
40. Cimino G, Biti GP, Cartoni C, Magrini SM. Chemotherapy versus radiotherapy in early stage Hodgkin's disease: evidence of a more difficult rescue for patients relapsed after chemotherapy. *Eur J Cancer* 1992;28A:1853.
41. Yahalom J, Tyu J, Straus DJ, et al. Impact of adjuvant radiation on the

patterns and rate of relapse in advanced stage Hodgkin's disease treated with alternating chemotherapy combinations. *J Clin Oncol* 1991;9: 2193.
42. Young RC, Canellos GP, Chabner BA. Patterns of relapse in advanced Hodgkin's disease treated with combination chemotherapy. *Cancer* 1983;42:1001.
43. Loeffler M, Brosteanu O, Hasenclever D, et al. Meta-analysis of chemotherapy versus combined modality treatment trials in Hodgkin's disease. *J Clin Oncol* 1998;16:818.
44. Canellos GP, Anderson JR, Propert KJ, et al. Chemotherapy of advanced Hodgkin's disease with MOPP, ABVD, or MOPP alternating with ABVD. *N Engl J Med* 1992;327:1478.
45. Somers R, Carde P, Henry-Amar M, et al. A randomized study in stage IIIB and IV Hodgkin's disease comparing eight courses of MOPP versus an alternation of MOPP with ABVD: a European Organization for Research and Treatment of Cancer Lymphoma Cooperative Group and Groupe Pierre-et-Marie-Curie controlled clinical trial. *J Clin Oncol* 1994;12:279.
46. Radford JA, Crowther D, Rohatiner AZS, et al. Results of a randomized trial comparing MVPP chemotherapy with a hybrid regimen, ChlVPP/EVA, in the initial treatment of Hodgkin's disease. *J Clin Oncol* 1995;13:2379.
47. Viviani S, Bonadonna G, Santoro A, et al. Alternating versus hybrid MOPP and ABVD combinations in advanced Hodgkin's disease: ten-year results. *J Clin Oncol* 1996;14:1421.
48. Straus DJ, Gaynor JJ, Myers J, et al. Prognostic factors among 185 adults with newly diagnosed advanced Hodgkin's disease treated with alternating potentially noncross-resistant chemotherapy and intermediate-dose radiation therapy. *J Clin Oncol* 1990;8:1173.
49. Proctor SJ, Taylor P, Donnan P, et al. A numerical prognostic index for clinical use in identification of poor-risk patients with Hodgkin's disease at diagnosis. *Eur J Cancer* 1991;27:624.
50. Brusamolino E, Orlandi E, Morra E, et al. Analysis of long-term results and prognostic factors among 138 patients with advanced Hodgkin's disease treated with the alternating MOPP/ABVD chemotherapy. *Ann Oncol* 1994;5(Suppl 2):S53.
51. Lee SM, Radford JA, Ryder WDJ, Collins CD, Deakin DP, Crowther D. Prognostic factors for disease progression in advanced Hodgkin's disease: an analysis of patients aged under 60 years showing no progression in the first 6 months after starting primary chemotherapy. *Br J Cancer* 1997;75:110.
52. Hasenclever D, Diehl V for the International Prognostic Factors Project on Advanced Hodgkin's Disease. The International Prognostic Factors Project on Advanced Hodgkin's Disease: a prognostic index, but no very high risk group. *Ann Oncol* 1996;7(Suppl 3):21(abst 065).
53. Raemaekers J, Burgers M, Henry-Amar M, et al. Patients with stage III/IV Hodgkin's disease in partial remission after MOPP/ABV chemotherapy have excellent prognosis after additional involved-field radiotherapy: interim results from the ongoing EORTC-LCG and GPMC phase III trial. *Ann Oncol* 1997;8(Suppl 1):S111.
54. Wirth AJC, Corry J, Laidlaw C, Matthews J, Liew KH. Salvage radiotherapy for Hodgkin's disease following chemotherapy failure. *Int J Radiat Oncol Biol Phys* 1997;39:599.
55. Uematsu M, Tarbell NJ, Silver B, et al. Wide-field radiation therapy with or without chemotherapy for patients with Hodgkin's disease in relapse after initial combination chemotherapy. *Cancer* 1993;72:207.
56. Roach M, Kapp DS, Rosenberg SA, Hoppe RT. Radiotherapy with curative intent: an option in selected patients relapsing after chemotherapy for advanced Hodgkin's disease. *J Clin Oncol* 1987; 5:550.
57. Brada M, Eeles R, Ashley S, Nicholls J, Horwich A. Salvage radiotherapy in recurrent Hodgkin's disease. *Ann Oncol* 1992;3:131.
58. MacMillan CH, Bessell EM. The effectiveness of radiotherapy for localized relapse in patients with Hodgkin's disease (IIB–IVB) who obtained a complete response with chemotherapy alone as initial treatment. *Clin Oncol (R Coll Radiol)* 1994;6:147.
59. O'Brien PC, Parnis FX. Salvage radiotherapy following chemotherapy failure in Hodgkin's disease—what is its role? *Acta Oncol* 1995; 34:99.
60. Pezner RD, Lipsett JA, Vora N, Forman SJ. Radical radiotherapy as salvage treatment for relapse of Hodgkin's disease initially treated by chemotherapy alone: prognostic significance of the disease-free interval. *Int J Radiat Oncol Biol Phys* 1994;30:965.
61. Longo DL, Duffey PL, Young RC, et al. Conventional-dose salvage combination chemotherapy in patients relapsing with Hodgkin's disease after combination chemotherapy: the low probability for cure. *J Clin Oncol* 1992;10:210.
62. Bonfante V, Santoro A, Viviani S, et al. Outcome of patients with Hodgkin's disease failing after primary MOPP-ABVD. *J Clin Oncol* 1997;15:528.
63. Lohri A, Barnett M, Fairey RN, et al. Outcome of treatment of first relapse of Hodgkin's disease after primary chemotherapy: identification of risk factors from the British Columbia experience 1970 to 1988. *Blood* 1991;77:2292.
64. Brice P, Bastion Y, Divine M, et al. Analysis of prognostic factors after the first relapse of Hodgkin's disease in 187 patients. *Cancer* 1996;78:1293.
65. Phillips JK, Spearing RL, Davies JM, et al. VIM-D salvage chemotherapy in Hodgkin's disease. *Cancer Chemother Pharmacol* 1990;27:161.
66. Fairey AF, Mead GM, Jones HW, Sweetenham JW, Whitehouse JMA. CAPE/PALE salvage chemotherapy for Hodgkin's disease patients relapsing within 1 year of ChlVPP chemotherapy. *Ann Oncol* 1993;4: 857.
67. Smith MR, Khanuja PS, Al-Katib A, et al. Continuous infusion ABDIC therapy for relapsed or refractory Hodgkin's disease. *Cancer* 1994;73:1264.
68. Brusamolino E, Orlandi E, Canevari A, et al. Results of CAV regimen (CCNU, melphalan, and VP-16) as third-line salvage therapy for Hodgkin's disease. *Ann Oncol* 1994;5:427.
69. Canellos GP, Petroni GR, Barcos M, et al. Etoposide, vinblastine, and doxorubicin: an active regimen for the treatment of Hodgkin's disease in relapse following MOPP. *J Clin Oncol* 1995;13:2005.
70. Fermé C, Bastion Y, Lepage E, et al. The MINE regimen as intensive salvage chemotherapy for relapsed and refractory Hodgkin's disease. *Ann Oncol* 1995;6:543.
71. Colwill R, Crump M, Couture F, et al. Mini-BEAM as salvage therapy for relapsed or refractory Hodgkin's disease before intensive therapy and autologous bone marrow transplantation. *J Clin Oncol* 1995;13: 396.
72. Canellos GP. Is there an effective salvage therapy for advanced Hodgkin's disease? *Ann Oncol* 1991;2(Suppl 1):1.
73. Linch DC, Winfield D, Goldstone AH, et al. Dose intensification with autologous bone marrow transplantation in relapsed and resistant Hodgkin's disease: results of a BNLI randomised trial. *Lancet* 1993; 341:1051.
74. Bierman PJ, Anderson JR, Freeman MB, et al. High-dose chemotherapy followed by autologous hematopoietic rescue for Hodgkin's disease patients following first relapse after chemotherapy. *Ann Oncol* 1996;7:151.
75. Horning SJ, Chao NJ, Negrin RS, et al. High-dose therapy and autologous hematopoietic progenitor cell transplantation for recurrent or refractory Hodgkin's disease: analysis of the Stanford University results and prognostic indices. *Blood* 1997;89:801.
76. Prince HM, Crump M, Imrie K, et al. Intensive therapy and autotransplant for patients with an incomplete response to front-line therapy for lymphoma. *Ann Oncol* 1996;7:1043.
77. Peniket AJ, Kottaridis PD, Perry AR, et al. Outcome of BEAM autotransplantation in patients with Hodgkin's disease progressing on first-line therapy is the same as in patients transplanted in first partial remission. *Blood* 1997;10:114a.
78. Yuen AR, Rosenberg SA, Hoppe RT, Halpern JD, Horning SJ. Comparison between conventional salvage therapy and high-dose therapy with autografting for recurrent or refractory Hodgkin's disease. *Blood* 1997;89:814.
79. Pezner RD, Nademanee A, Forman SJ. High dose therapy and autologous bone marrow transplantation for Hodgkin's disease patients with relapses potentially treatable by radical radiation therapy. *Int J Radiat Oncol Biol Phys* 1995;33:189.
80. Poen JC, Hoppe RT, Horning SJ. High dose therapy and autologous bone marrow transplantation for relapsed/refractory Hodgkin's disease: the impact of involved field radiotherapy on patterns of failure and survival. *Int J Radiat Oncol Biol Phys* 1996;36:3.
81. Constine LS, Rapoport AP. Hodgkin's disease, bone marrow transplantation, and involved field radiation therapy: coming full circle from 1902 to 1996 [Editorial; Comment]. *Int J Radiat Oncol Biol Phys* 1996;36:253.
82. Prince A, Cunningham D, Horwich A, Brada M. Haematological tox-

icity of radiotherapy following high-dose chemotherapy and autologous bone marrow transplantation in patients with recurrent Hodgkin's disease. *Eur J Cancer* 1994;7:903.

83. Vose JM, Bierman PJ, Anderson JR, et al. Progressive disease after high-dose therapy and autologous transplantation for lymphoid malignancy: clinical course and patient follow-up. *Blood* 1992;80:2142.
84. Reese DE, Connors JM, Spinelli JJ, et al. Intensive therapy with cyclophosphamide, carmustine, etoposide +/- cisplatin, and autologous bone marrow transplantation for Hodgkin's disease in first relapse after combination chemotherapy. *Blood* 1994;83:1193 (*see comments*).
85. Crump M, Smith AM, Brandwein J, et al. High-dose etoposide and melphalan and autologous bone marrow transplantation for patients with advanced Hodgkin's disease: importance of disease status at transplant. *J Clin Oncol* 1993;11:704.
86. Yahalom J, Gulati SC, Toia M, et al. Accelerated hyperfractionated total lymphoid irradiation, high-dose chemotherapy, and autologous bone marrow transplantation for refractory and relapsing patients with Hodgkin's disease. *J Clin Oncol* 1993;11:1062.
87. Rapoport AP, Rowe JM, Kouides PA, et al. One hundred autotransplants for relapsed or refractory Hodgkin's disease and lymphoma: value of pretransplant disease status for predicting outcome. *J Clin Oncol* 1993;11:2351.
88. Little R, Wittes RE, Longo D, Wilson WH. Vinblastine for recurrent Hodgkin's disease following autologous bone marrow transplantation. *J Clin Oncol* 1998;16:584.
89. Warrell RP Jr, Lee BJ, Kempin SJ, et al. Effectiveness of methyl-GAG (methylglyoxal-bis[guanylhydrazone]) in patients with advanced malignant lymphoma. *Blood* 1981;57:1011.
90. Hagemeister FB, Tannir N, McLaughlin P, et al. MIME chemotherapy (methyl-GAG, ifosfamide, methotrexate, etoposide) as treatment for recurrent Hodgkin's disease. *J Clin Oncol* 1987;5:556.
91. Younes A, Cabanillas F, McLaughlin PW, et al. Preliminary experience with paclitaxel for the treatment of relapsed and refractory Hodgkin's disease. *Ann Oncol* 1996;7:1083.
92. Thomas J, de Pauw B, Hagenbeek A, et al. Phase II study of cytarabine in Hodgkin's disease. *Eur J Cancer* 1992;28A:857.
93. Devizzi L, Santoro A, Bonfante V, et al. Vinorelbine: an active drug for the management of patients with heavily pretreated Hodgkin's disease. *Ann Oncol* 1994;5:817.
94. Tesch H, Santoro A, Fiedler F, et al. Phase II study of gemcitabine in patients with multiple pretreated Hodgkin's disease. Results of a multicenter study. *Leuk Lymphoma* 1998;29(Suppl 1):P-101.
95. Barth S, Schnell R, Diehl V, Engert A. Development of immunotoxins for potential clinical use in Hodgkin's disease. *Ann Oncol* 1996;7 (Suppl 4):S135.
96. Falini B, Bolognesi A, Flenghi L, et al. Response of refractory Hodgkin's disease to monoclonal anti-CD30 immunotoxin. *Lancet* 1992;339:1195.
97. Hartmann F, Renner C, Jung W, Deisting C, et al. Treatment of refractory Hodgkin's disease with an anti-CD16/CD30 bispecific antibody. *Blood* 1997;89:2042.
98. Engert A, Diehl V, Schnell R, Radszuhn A, et al. A phase I study of an anti-CD25 ricin A-chain immunotoxin (RFT5-SMPT-dgA) in patients with refractory Hodgkin's lymphoma. *Blood* 1997;89:403.
99. Tepler I, Schwartz G, Parker K, et al. Phase I trial of an interleukin-2 fusion toxin (DAB486IL-2) in hematologic malignancies: complete response in a patient with Hodgkin's disease refractory to chemotherapy. *Cancer* 1994;73:1276.
100. Sing AP, Ambinder RF, Hong DJ, et al. Isolation of Epstein-Barr virus (EBV)-specific cytotoxic T lymphocytes that lyse Reed-Sternberg cells: implications for immune-mediated therapy of EBV- Hodgkin's disease. *Blood* 1997;89:1978.

Hodgkin's Disease, edited by P. M. Mauch,
J. O. Armitage, V. Diehl, R.T. Hoppe, and L. M. Weiss.
Lippincott Williams & Wilkins, Philadephia ©1999.

CHAPTER 29

Role of Bone Marrow Transplantation in Hodgkin's Disease

James O. Armitage, Anthony H. Goldstone, Angelo M. Carella, Norbert Schmitz, Gordon L. Phillips, and Philip J. Bierman

Hodgkin's disease is not a common illness, but it has had a disproportionate impact on our knowledge of the treatment of malignancies. The principles of staging that were developed for Hodgkin's disease have been applied to other, more common, lymphoid malignancies (1). Hodgkin's disease was one of the first malignancies for which curative, standard-field radiotherapy was widely applied and was one of the first shown to be curable with combination chemotherapy (2–4). Thus, it is not surprising that high-dose therapy with autologous bone marrow transplantation was tested in Hodgkin's disease early in the development of this procedure (5–7).

Because patients with Hodgkin's disease have a high cure rate when standard therapy is used, most of them will never be candidates for bone marrow transplantation. Unfortunately, not all patients can be cured with standard therapy. Some patients with Hodgkin's disease fail to attain an initial remission, and approximately 30% of patients with advanced disease who achieve remission with combination chemotherapy relapse (8–10).

Most patients who are not cured with radiotherapy for localized Hodgkin's disease can be salvaged with subsequent combination chemotherapy (11–14). However, the outlook for patients who do not achieve remission with combination chemotherapy is poor (15). Patients who relapse from complete remission (CR) induced by combination chemotherapy can occasionally be cured by second-line chemotherapy regimens (15–17). The chances for a good outcome are higher in patients who relapse after being in remission for longer periods of time (15,18,19). Very selected patients with localized relapse after a chemotherapy-induced remission can be cured with salvage radiotherapy or combined-modality therapy (20–23).

It has been known for many years that some patients who relapse after chemotherapy can be cured with high-dose therapy and autologous bone marrow transplantation (Table 1) (24–36). In recent years, the techniques of bone marrow transplantation have been greatly improved, both allogeneic and autologous transplantation have been tested, and the optimal timing for transplantation has been studied in numerous clinical trials.

HISTORY OF BONE MARROW TRANSPLANTATION

In common medical parlance today, bone marrow transplantation refers to the intravenous infusion of hematopoietic progenitor cells to reestablish marrow function. This treatment can be applied to patients with intrinsically defective bone marrow, but in most cases hematopoietic progenitor cells are given to patients with a malignancy to rescue them from the toxic side effects of cancer therapy. Although the origin of this procedure can be traced to the end of the last century, when patients were given bone marrow orally as a treatment for hematologic disorders (37), a more realistic starting point is 1939, when the report of a patient who had received 18 mL of marrow intravenously from his brother as a treatment for aplastic anemia was published (38). The beginning of

J. O. Armitage and P. J. Bierman: Department of Internal Medicine, Section of Oncology and Hematology, University of Nebraska, Omaha, Nebraska.

A. H. Goldstone: Department of Hematology, University College London Hospital, London, United Kingdom.

A. M. Carella: Department of Hematology, Azienda Ospedale/Università, Genova, Italy.

N. Schmitz: Department of Internal Medicine II, Christian-Albrechts-University, Kiel, Germany.

G. L. Phillips: Department of Blood and Marrow Transplant and Department of Internal Medicine, Markey Cancer Center, University of Kentucky, Lexington, Kentucky.

TABLE 1. *High-dose therapy and autologous transplantation for Hodgkin's disease*

Ref.	No. patients	Regimen	Median follow-up	Early mortality	CR	Outcome
24	155	BEAM	NA	10%	34%	50% 5-y DFS
25	128	CBV	77 mo	9%	45%	25% 4-y FFS
26	119	Various	40 mo	5%	NA	48% 4-y EFS
27	102	CBV	4.1 y	12%	NA	42% 3-y PFS
28	85	Cy + etoposide + TBI or CBV	28 mo	8%	76%	58% 2-y EFS
29	73	Etoposide + melphalan	30 mo	4%	75%	39% 4-y DFS
30	62	CBV	NA	0%	76%	38% 3-y DFS
31	58	CBV ± Plat	2.3 y	5%	NA	64% PFS
32	56	CBV	3.5 y	21%	80%	47% 5-y EFS
33	50	CBV	NA	4%	48%	12 (24%) CCR (9–32 mo)
34	47	Various	2 y	17%	NA	49% 3-y EFS
35	47	Cy + Etoposide + TLI	40 mo	17%	74%	50% DFS
36	42	BEAM	33 mo	2%	61%	74% 2-y EFS

BEAM, carmustine, etoposide, cytarabine, melphalan; NA, not available; DFS, disease-free survival; CBV, cyclophosphamide, carmustine, etoposide; FFS, failure-free survival; EFS, event-free survival; TBI, total-body irradiation; PFS, progression-free survival; CCR, continuous complete remission; TLI, total-lymphoid irradiation; BEP, carmustine, etoposide, cisplatin; MTX, methotrexate; Plat, cisplatin; Cy, cyclophosphamide.

modern bone marrow transplantation can be traced to work showing that rodents could be protected from lethal hematopoietic injury by the intravenous infusion of bone marrow cells (39). The subsequent identification of transplantation antigens, represented by the human leukocyte antigen (HLA) system in humans, and the development of cryobiologic techniques for freezing and thawing hematopoietic stem cells laid the groundwork for the difficult and time-consuming clinical trials that have brought bone marrow transplantation to its present, albeit imperfect, state. The development of bone marrow transplantation illustrates particularly clearly the close interaction that is necessary between laboratory and clinical scientists for the advancement of clinical medicine.

The first successful allogeneic bone marrow transplants for leukemia and other hematologic diseases were performed in the late 1960s (40,41), and the technique gained wide acceptance in the 1970s. Autologous bone marrow transplantation was first successfully employed in the late 1970s to cure a patient with lymphoma (42). Its use became widespread in the 1980s. Today, the total number of autologous transplants performed annually surpasses that of allogeneic transplants. Hodgkin's disease is one of the diseases for which autologous transplantation is commonly performed.

METHODS OF BONE MARROW TRANSPLANTATION

Autologous Transplantation

Autologous transplantation involves the replacement of hematopoietic stem cells that have been irreversibly injured by high doses of chemotherapy and/or radiotherapy. This can be accomplished either with bone marrow cells obtained by multiple aspirations from the posterior iliac crest under anesthesia or with blood-derived hematopoietic progenitor cells collected by apheresis. In the early reports of autologous transplantation, bone marrow-derived cells were used (5–7). However, the use of hematopoietic progenitor cells obtained from the peripheral blood has surpassed the use of bone marrow, and blood-derived cells may be used exclusively in the future (43,44). The advantages of using blood-derived cells include the avoidance of general anesthesia and more rapid hematopoietic reconstitution (45–51). In addition, blood-derived cells can be collected in patients whose pelvic marrow has been damaged by previous radiotherapy or in whom bone marrow metastases are known to be present. However, it is not certain that collections of blood progenitor cells contain fewer tumor cells than would be present in bone marrow.

If blood cells are collected at a time when the marrow is being stimulated by hematopoietic growth factors or at the time of hematopoietic recovery from a pulse of chemotherapy, very few apheresis procedures (occasionally only one) are needed to collect an adequate number of cells (i.e., 1×10^6 CD34+ cells per kilogram of recipient weight) (52). However, this may not be the case with patients who have been extensively pretreated with chemotherapy. Occasionally, adequate numbers of cells cannot be collected from such patients, regardless of the techniques used (53).

The relative merits of bone marrow-derived and blood-derived cells have been tested in prospective trials (48–50,54). Although no differences in therapeutic efficacy were observed, more rapid hematopoietic recovery was noted in patients receiving blood-derived cells. There appears to be no difference in the frequency of long-term complications, which might be related more to the high-dose regimen employed than to the rescue product.

Although it is possible to collect hematopoietic stem cells from patients whose bone marrow is involved by Hodgkin's disease, results of transplantation in these patients do not appear to be as good as in patients whose bone marrow shows no evidence of disease. In one trial, the 4-year failure-free survival was 27% for patients without a history of bone marrow involvement, but only 11% in patients with bone marrow involvement at the time cells were collected (55). This might reflect the inadvertent collection of circulating tumor cells, but more likely it simply represents the effects of an adverse prognostic factor—namely, bone marrow involvement by Hodgkin's disease. However, bone marrow involvement has not always been found to affect prognosis adversely (56).

Not all studies have shown the same outcome in patients with Hodgkin's disease who received autologous blood or bone marrow. One trial, by the European Group for Blood and Marrow Transplantation (51), found a better 4-year progression-free survival in patients who received bone marrow (52% vs. 38%; $p = .008$) despite the fact that patients who received blood-derived stem cells had a more rapid hematopoietic recovery. Because the results of the European Group for Blood and Marrow Transplantation represented a retrospective, matched-case analysis, they cannot be considered definitive. However, further studies are certainly appropriate.

Allogeneic Transplantation

The results of allogeneic bone marrow transplantation in Hodgkin's disease have been disappointing. In non-Hodgkin's lymphoma, allogeneic bone marrow transplantation has generally yielded an excellent relapse-free survival, in contrast to autologous transplantation (57–61). However, the adverse effects of graft-versus-host disease have often negated this advantage and led to an equivalent overall survival. The number of allogeneic transplants performed for Hodgkin's disease is fairly small, and the results have been disappointing (62–64). The mortality rates related to the procedure in the major series reported are surprisingly high, varying from 31% to 61%, with most series having more than 50% mortality (Table 2). The high mortality rate corresponds to a low rate of survival free from relapse.

There is no specific explanation for the high treatment-related mortality with allogeneic transplantation in Hodgkin's disease. It may be that in some patients this a reflection of excess toxicity associated with previous thoracic radiotherapy (65). However, some investigators have found a higher death rate from infection, suggesting that patients with Hodgkin's disease might have an immune defect that increases the risks associated with allogeneic transplantation. It is also possible that the poor results with allogeneic transplantation reflect a selection of higher-risk patients for this procedure (62,63,66). In any case, few physicians would suggest allogeneic transplantation for a patient in whom autologous transplantation was also feasible. If allogeneic transplantation could be performed safely, the possibility of a "graft-versus-cancer effect" in Hodgkin's disease would make further studies important (66,67).

TABLE 2. *Transplantation in HLA-identical siblings*

Ref.	No. patients	Mortality	Outcome
66	100	61%	15% 3-y DFS
62	45	31%	15% 4-y PFS
63	44	53%	26% 5-y EFS
64	21[a]	52%	56% 3-y EFS for patients in sensitive relapse

HLA, human leukocyte antigen; DFS, disease-free survival; PFS, progression-free survival; EFS, event-free survival.
[a]Includes 1 syngeneic.

High-dose Therapy Regimens

The most frequently used high-dose therapy regimens for transplantation in Hodgkin's disease are a combination of cyclophosamide, carmustine, and etoposide (often known as CBV) or a combination of carmustine, etoposide, cytosine arabinoside, and melphalan (often known as BEAM). However, even when one of these combinations is utilized in a particular center, the doses and exact timing of administration of the agents often vary. No prospective randomized trials have compared the relative merits of different regimens. Most comparisons of the outcome of transplantation between different series assume comparability of the high-dose regimens. This assumption may or may not be appropriate.

In many other diseases, high-dose regimens for bone marrow transplantation often include total-body irradiation. However, a history of prior thoracic irradiation in many patients, and early trials indicating that such patients at a high risk for fatal pulmonary toxicity after total-body irradiation (65), have reduced the use of total-body irradiation in Hodgkin's disease (26,35,38, 63). Systemic radiotherapy in the form of radiolabeled antibodies has been tried in preliminary trials in Hodgkin's disease, but the number of patients treated is not large enough for a definitive conclusion (68,69). The antibodies used in Hodgkin's disease have prolonged survival.

The wide differences in dosages of the same drugs in high-dose therapy regimens for Hodgkin's disease would seem to be an obvious place for a prospective trial, but none has been initiated. For example, in CBV, the dosage of cyclophosphamide varies between 4.8 and 7.2 mg/m^2, the dosage of carmustine varies between 300 and 800 mg/m^2, and the dosage of etoposide ranges between 750 and 2,400 mg/m^2 (25,26,31,70). In some cases, the drugs are administered in single doses, and in others, they are administered in several doses during consecutive days. Although some authors have suggested that higher-dose regimens might lead to better results, a prospective trial has not been conducted to test this hypothesis. It is certain that higher-dose regimens can lead to increased toxicity. This is particularly true for regimens with very high doses of carmustine, which are associated with a higher rate of pulmonary toxicity (63,71–74).

One area of controversy in high-dose therapy and autotransplantation in Hodgkin's disease has been the contribution of pre-transplant "debulking" therapy before administration of the high-dose regimen. Most investigators utilize this approach (75,76). Often, patients are selected for transplantation based on an excellent response to a standard-dose chemotherapy regimen, and patients who do not respond well are excluded from transplantation. It seems clear that transplant results are better in patients who undergo the procedure with minimal disease. For example, one series found a 3-year event-free survival of 70% in patients who underwent transplantation with minimal disease, in contrast to only 15% in other patients (p = .001) (34). Others studies have found similar results and suggest that patients with more advanced disease have a poorer transplant outcome (20,24,29,30).

In patients who have disease that is not bulky at the time of referral for transplantation, excellent results can be achieved with immediate transplantation. In one series, the 5-year progression-free survival in such patients was 78% (24), and in another, the 5-year overall survival was 100% (77). Investigators of the European Group for Blood and Marrow Transplantation, using a retrospective analysis, were unable to show an advantage of standard chemotherapy preceding high-dose therapy in patients treated at first relapse (78).

The value of standard-dose therapy preceding high-dose therapy remains unclear. At least one author has suggested that there may be a negative impact of standard-dose therapy before transplant (79). In other words, some patients fail standard-dose therapy and are not considered suitable candidates for transplantation. Obviously, these patients cannot be cured with a procedure they do not receive. It may be that some of them would have responded to immediate high-dose chemotherapy. Similarly, some patients who are chemotherapy-sensitive and come to transplant may have had resistance induced by the preceding therapy and fail the high-dose therapy and transplantation for this reason. This question can be resolved only by a prospective trial that takes into account all the patients referred for transplantation. Such a trial has not been initiated and may never be initiated.

At the present time, it seems logical to suggest standard-dose therapy for patients who present with bulky disease in the hope of improving their chances of benefit from the transplant. For patients who are referred for transplantation with minimal disease, it may be a superior approach to proceed immediately to the high-dose therapy regimen. In such patients treated at the University of Nebraska, the 5-year overall survival was 100% (77).

The value of adjuvant therapy following transplantation in patients who achieve remission has been studied inadequately. It may be that these patients would benefit from radiation therapy to the sites of previously bulky disease. A number of reports have used this approach (25,80–82), but its merits cannot be determined based on the available data in the absence of a prospective trial. Even so, this is a reasonable and widely applied treatment. Similarly, adjuvant therapy with biologic agents such as interferon might be an effective treatment. In one prospective trial after induction therapy, adjuvant interferon led to prolonged remission (83). Similar approaches are now being tested after bone marrow transplantation (84–86).

Outpatient Transplantation and Economic Considerations

One factor limiting the application of high-dose therapy and bone marrow transplantation for the treatment of Hodgkin's disease has been the comparatively high cost of the procedure. With increasing experience, the costs have been reduced. In one series, the mean cost decreased from $96,000 in 1987 to $55,000 in 1991, an average decrease of 10% per year (87).

Bone marrow transplantation, whether supported by bone marrow or blood-derived stem cells, was initially an inpatient procedure. In recent years, several centers have begun to perform transplants on an outpatient basis. This has become possible with the rapid hematopoietic recovery associated with hematopoietic growth factors and blood-derived progenitor cells and the effective use of prophylactic antibiotics. The use of outpatient transplantation has contributed to the steady reduction in costs (88). Successful outpatient transplantation requires a day hospital where patients can been seen many times daily if necessary, physicians are immediately available 24 hours daily for 7 days a week, and access to necessary diagnostic and therapeutic maneuvers is equivalent to that for patients who are hospitalized.

Improvement in supportive care measures and better selection of patients, along with more experience in transplant centers, also has led to a reduction in treatment-related mortality. In one series, the mortality decreased from 20% in 1987 to 0 in 1991 (87). The analysis suggested the existence of a learning curve for the transplant procedure, similar to what has been seen with other complex procedures.

IS THERE EVIDENCE THAT HIGH-DOSE THERAPY IS SUPERIOR TO STANDARD-DOSE THERAPY?

A number of phase II clinical trials have reported response rates and failure-free survival curves that appear to be superior to the results of standard salvage therapy (see Table 1). However, the history of oncology is replete with examples of phase II clinical trials that appear to represent a great advance but whose results are not confirmed in prospective randomized trials.

Only one prospective randomized trial comparing high-dose therapy with bone marrow transplantation versus standard-dose salvage chemotherapy has been completed. This was carried out within the British National Lymphoma Investigation and compared high-dose therapy with the BEAM regimen and autotransplantation versus lower doses of the same chemotherapeutic agents (88). The study was stopped early because of an event-free survival advantage for the high-dose therapy arm. Twenty patients received BEAM and 20 patients received the lower-dose regimen. The event-free survival at 3 years significantly favored the high-dose therapy arm (53% vs. 10%; $p = .025$). However, the overall survival curves were not different. This might in part be explained by the fact that patients failing in the lower-dose regimen became candidates for transplantation. Although this study shows that high-dose therapy with autotransplantation produces a better response rate than lower doses of the same agents, it does not definitively answer the question of which is the best strategy—early or delayed transplantation.

An alternative approach to comparing standard-dose therapy with high-dose therapy is to use matched, historical control patients. One such study was carried out at Stanford University (89). Sixty patients with relapsed or refractory Hodgkin's disease were compared with a matched historical control group that received salvage chemotherapy at standard doses. Survival free from progression of Hodgkin's disease was significantly better in the patients who received high-dose therapy and transplantation (62% vs. 32%; $p < .01$). However, as in the randomized trial, the overall survival did not significantly differ (54% vs. 47%).

Available data seem to confirm that high-dose therapy and transplantation produce a higher response rate in relapsed patients with Hodgkin's disease than does standard-dose therapy. However, the lack of a significant difference in overall survival rates raises the possibility that delayed transplantation in patients failing standard-dose salvage therapy might be an equally efficacious treatment strategy. The most effective way to utilize high-dose therapy and transplantation in managing patients with Hodgkin's disease remains a topic for clinical trials. The various strategies currently being studied are detailed in the next section.

STRATEGIES FOR BONE MARROW TRANSPLANTATION

In general, it can be said that the most important factor in predicting the outcome of bone marrow transplantation relates to the choice of patients undergoing the procedure. Patients with minimal and chemotherapy-responsive disease consistently have better outcomes than do patients with the opposite characteristics. Thus, the strategy utilized for the application of transplantation is vitally important. Patients might undergo transplantation as part of the initial therapy for their disease, transplantation might be reserved for patients who do not respond adequately to the initial treatment, transplantation is often used for patients who relapse from an initial remission, and transplantation could be applied to patients with multiple relapses and refractory disease (Table 3). All these approaches have been studied.

Incorporation into Primary Therapy

Bone marrow transplantation has been most effective in a variety of other illnesses when it has been incorporated into the primary treatment of high-risk patients. The treatment might be reserved for patients who have adverse prognostic factors but achieve an initial remission, or it might be incorporated early into the initial high-dose therapy regimen. In non-Hodgkin's lymphomas, a significant disease-free survival advantage resulted in one study when high-risk patients underwent transplantation during their initial remission (90). The results are much less clear when this treatment is incorporated early into the treatment of very high-risk patients before chemotherapy responsiveness has been demonstrated definitively (91,92).

Studies of early transplantation in patients with Hodgkin's disease are limited. One series from Italy has reported the results of high-dose chemotherapy and autologous transplantation in patients with high-risk Hodgkin's disease who achieved an initial remission with MOPP/ABVD (Mechlorethamine, Oncovin, procarbazine, prednisone/Adriamycin, bleomycin, vinblastine, dacarbazine) (93). In this series, 87% of the patients who underwent transplantation remained in CR at 3 years. This was in contrast to the findings in 24 similar patients

TABLE 3. *Strategies (timing) for use of bone marrow transplantation in patients with Hodgkin's disease*

As part of the primary therapy
After failure to achieve an initial remission
After first relapse from chemotherapy-induced complete remission
Second remission
No preceding conventional-dose therapy
After multiple relapses/refractory disease

who could not undergo transplantation in remission. In the latter group, only 33% of the patients continued to be alive in initial remission.

The European Group for Blood and Marrow Transplantation completed a study in conjunction with the German Hodgkin's Lymphoma Study Group comparing 56 patients transplanted in first remission with 168 patients having similar risk factors who underwent standard therapy (94). Survival free from relapse was improved in patients undergoing early transplantation, but overall survival did not differ.

The utilization of bone marrow transplantation for high-risk patients with Hodgkin's disease in first remission has been reported more frequently from Europe than from North America. Because of the comparatively small number of high-risk patients available to study, the completion of a prospective trial testing the relative merits of this approach will require a large number of cooperating centers.

Primary Treatment Failure

One of the most adverse prognostic factors in Hodgkin's disease is failure to respond to an initial chemotherapy regimen. Two studies have found a 5-year overall survival of 8% and 0 in patients who did not achieve an initial remission with MOPP/ABVD or MOPP, respectively (95,96). This would seem an obvious setting in which to test the utility of high-dose therapy and autotransplantation to improve treatment outcome.

The largest series of autotransplantation for primary refractory disease are presented in Table 4. The North American Autologous Blood and Marrow Transplant Registry reported the results in 103 patients with Hodgkin's disease transplanted after they did not achieve an initial CR with standard-dose therapy (97). Both progression-free and overall survival at 5 years was 40%. The European Group for Blood and Marrow Transplantation reported the results of transplantation in 290 patients with primary refractory Hodgkin's disease and found the 5-year progression-free survival to be 30% (98). Results from the University of Nebraska showed a 3-year progression-free survival of 22% in similar patients (102).

TABLE 4. *Results of high-dose therapy and autologous transplantation for primary refractory disease*

Ref.	No. patients	Survival free from relapse	Overall survival
98	290	30% 5-y	34% 5-y
97	103	40% 5-y	40% 5-y
24	46	33% 5-y	NA
99	42	NA	49% 4-y
100	30	42% 5-y	60% 5-y
35	28	33% 4-y	NA
101	28	31% 3-y	50% 3-y

NA, not available.

A comparison of transplant results with those in retrospectively matched patients who received standard-dose therapy after failing an initial chemotherapy regimen has been reported from Stanford University (89). Event-free survival at 4 years was 52% for transplant patients, in contrast to 10% for patients receiving conventional standard therapy. However, overall survival did not vary.

All patients who do not achieve CR promptly with standard-dose therapy for Hodgkin's disease are not equivalent. Unless a careful evaluation is performed, residual masses may be interpreted as evidence of treatment failure when in fact they contain no tumor and the patients might actually be cured. It is also true that patients with chemotherapy-responsive, minimal disease are almost certainly different from those with bulky, progressive disease after the initial treatment regimen. However, it is clear that some patients with Hodgkin's disease who fail to achieve an initial CR with a high-quality combination chemotherapy regimen can be salvaged by autotransplantation. This is probably the clearest indication for this treatment approach.

Transplantation at Relapse

The first large series of autotransplantation for Hodgkin's disease included primarily patients who had relapsed from CR (see Table 1). These patients might have been transplanted at first relapse or after multiple relapses. It seems clear at this point that the results worsen as the number of prior chemotherapy regimens increases (Fig. 1).

Patients transplanted in first relapse from CR can often be cured with high-dose therapy and autotransplantation (Table 5). However, because some patients with Hodgkin's disease who fail an initial combination chemotherapy regimen can achieve long-term disease-free survival with a second standard-dose regimen, this has been an area of controversy. At the present time, most investigators believe that patients who relapse early (i.e., within 1 year) after achieving remission with a standard-dose chemotherapy regimen are good candidates for transplantation (95,96,103,104). A report from Stanford University in which historical controls were utilized found a 4-year event-free survival of 56% for patients with a brief initial remission who underwent transplantation, in contrast to a failure-free survival of only 19% in patients who received standard-dose salvage chemotherapy (89).

The value of bone marrow transplantation in patients relapsing from a CR lasting longer than 1 year remains controversial. The results reported with transplantation have generally been superior to those reported in most series of standard chemotherapy (31,77). Event-free survival has varied from 47% to 85%. However, in the Stan-

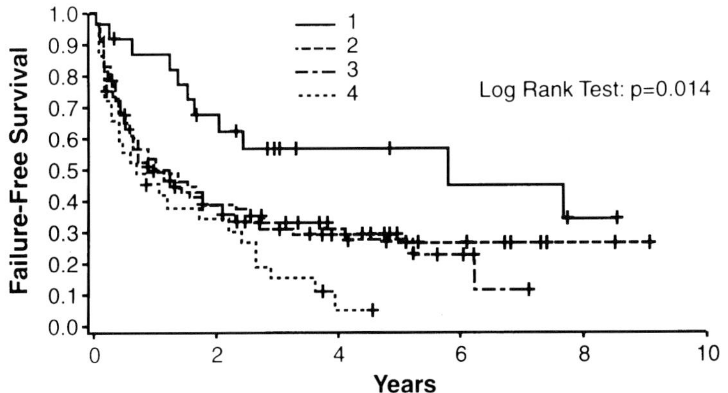

FIG. 1. Survival after increasing number of relapses. Disease-free survival in patients undergoing autotransplantation for Hodgkin's disease grouped by number of therapies failed before coming to transplant. Tick marks indicate patients alive in remission at that interval. Data from the University of Nebraska.

ford study that utilized historic controls, there was no advantage for early transplantation in patients who had long initial remissions (89). Patients with Hodgkin's disease often continue to respond to a standard-dose chemotherapy regimen after multiple relapses, but such patients are rarely cured. It may be that very long follow-up will be required to document a survival advantage after autotransplantation in patients who relapse from a CR lasting longer than 1 year. Patients who relapse from a second or third chemotherapy-induced remission have very little chance for cure with further standard chemotherapy. It is generally agreed that such patients are candidates for high-dose therapy and autotransplantation. Unfortunately, the results in this setting are not as good, with progression-free survival on the order of 10% to 30%. Better results are achieved in patients who remain chemotherapy-sensitive (24).

Multiple Treatment Failures and Resistant Relapse

Patients with disease refractory to chemotherapy who undergo high-dose therapy and autotransplantation only occasionally have prolonged disease-free survival (105). There has been considerable controversy about the advisability of this approach in patients with advanced, bulky disease that is refractory to chemotherapy. Most physicians would not recommend the treatment in this setting.

TABLE 5. *Results of high-dose therapy and transplantation in first relapse*

		Relapse-free survival			
Ref.	No. patients	All patients	CR <1 y	CR >1 y	*p*
77	85	40% 5-y	32%	47%	NS
81	58	64% 4-y	48%	85%	.016
75	52	47% 5-y	41%	57%	NS

CR, complete remission; NS, not significant.

Late Effects of Transplantation

With standard-dose therapy for Hodgkin's disease, it has become apparent that a major problem is late toxicity (10). This frequently takes the form of second malignancies related to the initial therapy, but other organ injuries, manifested as hypothyroidism, coronary artery disease, and pulmonary disease, can also result. It would be expected that similar effects might be seen in patients undergoing bone marrow transplantation for Hodgkin's disease. These patients would exhibit adverse affects of the high-dose therapy regimen in addition to those incurred during their initial, standard-dose treatment.

In one large study of late effects in patients undergoing autotransplantation for Hodgkin's disease or non-Hodgkin's lymphoma, most patients were fully functional (106). However, a number of late toxicities were seen. Hypothyroidism was found in 16% of patients. Sexual dysfunction was surprisingly frequent, being reported by approximately one-third of patients. In 24% of the patients, herpes zoster developed after the transplant.

The most significant complication of transplantation for lymphoma has been the development of myelodysplasia or acute myeloid leukemia (107–110). The actuarial frequency of this event in one series was approximately 10% in patients with Hodgkin's disease and did not vary by age (108). In patients with non-Hodgkin's lymphoma, development of secondary acute leukemia was seen only in patients who had received total-body radiotherapy, suggesting that the standard-dose chemotherapy that the patients with Hodgkin's disease had received before coming to transplant might have contributed in a significant way to their acute leukemia or myelodysplasia (108). A recent study from the European Group for Blood and Marrow Transplantation suggests that the total amount of therapy, rather than the use of transplantation, is the major factor affecting the incidence of secondary leukemia/myelodysplasia (111).

CONCLUSIONS

Autologous bone marrow or peripheral blood transplantation has become a standard therapy for patients with Hodgkin's disease who fail conventional chemotherapy regimens. There is wide agreement that patients who fail to achieve a CR or who relapse within 1 year of achieving a CR should undergo transplantation. The value of early transplantation in patients who have longer initial remissions remains controversial, but it would be recommended by many oncologists. Transplantation is better when performed early, before patients become refractory to standard-dose therapy. The place of transplantation in the primary therapy of high-risk patients remains an area for study.

REFERENCES

1. Carbone PP, Kaplan HS, Musshof K, et al. Report of the Committee on the Staging of Hodgkin's Disease. *Cancer Res* 1971;31:1860–1861.
2. Peters M. A study in survivals in Hodgkin's disease treated radiologically. *Am J Roentgenol* 1950;63:299–311.
3. Kaplan HS. The radical radiotherapy of regionally localized Hodgkin's disease. *Radiology* 1962;78:553–561.
4. DeVita VT, Serpick A, Carbone PP. Combination chemotherapy in the treatment of advanced Hodgkin's disease. *Ann Intern Med* 1970;73: 881–895.
5. Carella AM, Santini G, Santoro A, et al. Massive chemotherapy with non-frozen autologous bone marrow transplantation in 13 cases of refractory Hodgkin's disease. *Eur J Cancer* 1985;21:607–613.
6. Philip T, Dumont J, Teillet F, et al. High dose chemotherapy and autologous bone marrow transplantation in refractory Hodgkin's disease. *Br J Cancer* 1986;53:737–742.
7. Jagannath S, Dicke KA, Armitage JO, et al. High-dose cyclophosphamide, carmustine, and etoposide and autologous bone marrow transplantation for relapsed Hodgkin's disease. *Ann Intern Med* 1986;104: 163–168.
8. Urba WJ, Longo DL. Hodgkin's disease. *N Engl J Med* 1992;326: 678–687.
9. DeVita VT, Hubbard S. Hodgkin's disease. *N Engl J Med* 1993;328: 560–565.
10. Rosenberg SA. The management of Hodgkin's disease: half a century of change. *Ann Oncol* 1996;7:555–560.
11. DeVita VT, Simon RM, Hubbard SM, et al. Curability of advanced Hodgkin's disease with chemotherapy. Long-term follow-up of MOPP treated patients at the National Cancer Institute. *Ann Intern Med* 1980; 92:587–595.
12. Olver IN, Wolf MM, Cruickshank D, et al. Nitrogen mustard, vincristine, procarbazine, and prednisolone for relapse after radiation in Hodgkin's disease. An analysis of long-term follow-up. *Cancer* 1988; 62:233–239.
13. Vinciguerra V, Propert KJ, Coleman M, et al. Alternating cycles of combinational chemotherapy for patients with recurrent Hodgkin's disease following radiotherapy. A prospectively randomized study by the Cancer and Leukemia Group B. *J Clin Oncol* 1986;4:838–846.
14. Cooper MR, Pajak TF, Gottlieb AJ, et al. The effects of prior radiation therapy and age on the frequency and duration of complete remission among various four-drug treatments for advanced Hodgkin's disease. *J Clin Oncol* 1984;2:748–755.
15. Longo DL, Duffey PL, Young RC, et al. Conventional-dose salvage combination chemotherapy in patients relapsing with Hodgkin's disease after combinational chemotherapy: the low probability for cure. *J Clin Oncol* 1992;10:210–218.
16. Buzaid AC, Lippman SM, Miller TP. Salvage therapy of advanced Hodgkin's disease: critical appraisal of curative potential. *Am J Med* 1987;83:523–532.
17. Canellos GP. Is there an effective salvage therapy for advanced Hodgkin's disease? *Ann Oncol* 1991;2(Suppl 1):1–7.
18. Fisher RI, DeVita VT, Hubbard SM, et al. Prolonged disease-free survival in Hodgkin's disease with MOPP reinduction after first relapse. *Ann Intern Med* 1979;90:761–763.
19. Viviani S, Santoro A, Negretti E, et al. Salvage chemotherapy in Hodgkin's disease: results in patients relapsing more than twelve months after first complete remission. *Ann Oncol* 1990;1:123–127.
20. Fox KA, Lippman SM, Cassady JR, Heusinkveld RS, Miller TP. Radiation therapy salvage of Hodgkin's disease following chemotherapy failure. *J Clin Oncol* 1987;5:38–45.
21. Mauch P, Tarbell N, Skarin A, Rosenthal D, Weinstein H. Wide-field radiation therapy alone or with chemotherapy for Hodgkin's disease in relapse from combination chemotherapy. *J Clin Oncol* 1987;5:544–549.
22. Roach M, Kapp DS, Rosenberg SA, Hoppe RT. Radiotherapy with curative intent: an option in selected patients relapsing after chemotherapy for advanced Hodgkin's Disease. *J Clin Oncol* 1987;5:550–555.
23. Brada M, Eeles R, Ashley S, Nichols J, Horwich A. Salvage radiotherapy in recurrent Hodgkin's disease. *Ann Oncol* 1992;3:131–135.
24. Chopra R, McMillan AK, Linch DC, et al. The place of high-dose BEAM therapy and autologous bone marrow transplantation in poor-risk Hodgkin's disease. A single-center eight-year study of 155 patients. *Blood* 1993;81:1137–1145.
25. Bierman PJ, Bagin RG, Jagannath S, et al. High dose chemotherapy followed by autologous hematopoietic rescue in Hodgkin's disease: long-term follow-up in 128 patients. *Ann Oncol* 1993;4:767–773.
26. Horning SJ, Chao NJ, Negrin RS, et al. High-dose therapy and autologous hematopoietic progenitor cell transplantation for recurrent or refractory Hodgkin's disease: analysis of the Stanford University results and prognostic indices. *Blood* 1997;89:801–813.
27. Wheeler C, Eickhoff C, Elias A, et al. High-dose cyclophosphamide, carmustine, and etoposide with autologous transplantation in Hodgkin's disease: a prognostic model for treatment outcome. *Biol Blood Marrow Transplant* 1997;3:98–106.
28. Nademanee A, O'Donnell MR, Snyder DS, et al. High-dose chemotherapy with or without total body irradiation followed by autologous bone marrow and/or peripheral blood stem cell transplantation for patients with relapsed and refractory Hodgkin's disease: results in 85 patients with analysis of prognostic factors. *Blood* 1995;85:1381–1390.
29. Crump M, Smith AM, Brandwein J, et al. High-dose etoposide and melphalan, and autologous bone marrow transplantation for patients with advanced Hodgkin's disease: importance of disease status at transplant. *J Clin Oncol* 1993;11:704–711.
30. Burns LJ, Daniels KA, McGlave PB, et al. Autologous stem cell transplantation for refractory and relapsed Hodgkin's disease: factors predictive of prolonged survival. *Bone Marrow Transplant* 1995;16:13–18.
31. Reece DE, Connors JM, Spinelli JJ, et al. Intensive therapy with cyclophosphamide, carmustine, etoposide ± cisplatin, and autologous bone marrow transplantation for Hodgkin's disease in first relapse after combination chemotherapy. *Blood* 1994;83:1193–1199.
32. Reece DE, Barnett MJ, Connors JM, et al. Intensive chemotherapy with cyclophosphamide, carmustine, and etoposide followed by autologous bone marrow transplantation for relapsed Hodgkin's disease. *J Clin Oncol* 1991;9:1871–1879.
33. Carella AM, Congiu AM, Gaozza E, et al. High-dose chemotherapy with autologous bone marrow transplantation in 50 advanced resistant Hodgkin's disease patients: an Italian study group report. *J Clin Oncol* 1988;6:1411–1416.
34. Rapoport AP, Rowe JM, Kouides PA, et al. One hundred autotransplants for relapsed or refractory Hodgkin's disease and lymphoma: value of pretransplant disease status for predicting outcome. *J Clin Oncol* 1993;11:2351–2361.
35. Yahalom J, Gulati SC, Toia M, et al. Accelerated hyperfractionated total-lymphoid irradiation, high-dose chemotherapy, and autologous bone marrow transplantation for refractory and relapsing patients with Hodgkin's disease. *J Clin Oncol* 1993;11:1062–1070.
36. Lumley MA, Milligan DW, Knechtli CJC, Long SG, Billingham LJ, McDonald DF. High lactate dehydrogenase level is associated with an adverse outlook in autografting for Hodgkin's disease. *Bone Marrow Transplant* 1996;17:383–388.
37. Forkner CE. *Leukemia and allied disorders*. New York: Macmillan, 1938.
38. Osgood EE, Riddle MC, Mathews TJ. Aplastic anemia treated with daily transfusions and intravenous marrow: case report. *Ann Intern Med* 1939;13:357–367.
39. Lorenz E, Uphoff D, Reid TR, Shelton E. Modification of irradiation injury in mice and guinea pigs by bone marrow injections. *J Natl Cancer Inst* 1951;12:197–201.

40. Gatt RA, Meuwissen HJ, Allen HD, Hong R, Good RA. Immunological reconstitution of sex-linked lymphopenic immunological deficiency. *Lancet* 1968;2:1366–1369.
41. Thomas ED, Storb R, Clift RA, et al. Bone-marrow transplantation. *N Engl J Med* 1975;292:832–843,895–902.
42. Appelbaum FR, Herzig GP, Ziegler JL, Graw RG, Levine AS, Deisseroth AB. Successful engraftment of cryopreserved autologous bone marrow in patients with malignant lymphoma. *Blood* 1978;52:85–95.
43. Gratwohl A, Hermans J, Baldomero H. Blood and marrow transplantation activity in Europe 1995. *Bone Marrow Transplant* 1997;19: 407–419.
44. Passweg JK, Rowlings PA, Armitage JO, et al. Report from the International Bone Marrow Transplant Registry and Autologous Blood and Marrow Transplant Registry—North America. *Clin Transpl* 1995; 117–127.
45. Brice P, Marolleau JP, Pautier P, et al. High dose chemotherapy and autologous stem cell transplantation for advanced lymphomas: comparison of bone marrow versus peripheral blood stem cell (PBSC) in 147 patients. *Br J Haematol* 1994;87(Suppl 1):27.
46. Ager S, Scott MA, Mahendra P, et al. Peripheral blood stem cell transplantation after high-dose therapy in patients with malignant lymphoma: a retrospective comparison with autologous bone marrow transplantation. *Bone Marrow Transplant* 1995;16:79–83.
47. Brunvand MW, Bensinger WI, Soll E, et al. High-dose fractionated total-body irradiation, etoposide and cyclophosphamide for treatment of malignant lymphoma: comparison of autologous bone marrow and peripheral blood stem cells. *Bone Marrow Transplant* 1996;18: 131–141.
48. Weisdorf D, Daniels K, Miller W, et al. Bone marrow vs. peripheral blood stem cells for autologous lymphoma transplantation: a prospective randomized trial. *Blood* 1993;82(Suppl 1):444a(abst).
49. Schmitz N, Linch DC, Dreger P, et al. Randomised trial of filgrastim-mobilised peripheral blood progenitor cell transplantation versus autologous bone-marrow transplantation in lymphoma patients. *Lancet* 1996;347:353–357.
50. Smith TJ, Hillner BE, Schmitz N, et al. Economic analysis of a randomized clinical trial to compare filgrastim-mobilized peripheral-blood progenitor-cell transplantation and autologous bone marrow transplantation in patients with Hodgkin's and non-Hodgkin's lymphoma. *J Clin Oncol* 1997;15:5–10.
51. Majolino I, Pearce R, Taghipour G, Goldstone AH. Peripheral-blood stem-cell transplantation versus autologous bone marrow transplantation in Hodgkin's and non-Hodgkin's lymphomas: a new matched-pair analysis of the European Group for Blood and Marrow Transplantation Registry data. *J Clin Oncol* 1997;15:509–517.
52. Pettengell R, Morgenstern GRoll PJ, et al. Peripheral blood progenitor cell transplantation in lymphoma and leukemia using a single apheresis. *Blood* 1993;82:3770–3777.
53. Dreger P, Kloss M, Petersen B, et al. Autologous progenitor cell transplantation: prior exposure to stem cell-toxic drugs determines yield and engraftment of peripheral blood progenitor cell but not of bone marrow grafts. *Blood* 1995;86:3970–3978.
54. Beyer J, Schwella N, Zingsem J, et al. Hematopoietic rescue after high-dose chemotherapy using autologous peripheral-blood progenitor cells or bone marrow: a randomized comparison. *J Clin Oncol* 1995;13: 1328–1335.
55. Bierman P, Vose J, Anderson J, et al. Comparison of autologous bone marrow transplantation (ABMT) with peripheral stem cell transplantation (PSCT) for patients (PTS) with Hodgkin's disease (HD). *Blood* 1993;10(Suppl 1):445a(abst).
56. Munker R, Hasenclever D, Brosteanu O, et al. Bone marrow involvement in Hodgkin's disease: an analysis of 135 consecutive cases. *J Clin Oncol* 1995;13:403–409.
57. Jones RJ, Ambinder RF, Piantadosi S, Santos GW. Evidence of a graft-versus-lymphoma effect associated with allogeneic bone marrow transplantation. *Blood* 1991;77:3:649–653.
58. Chopra R, Goldstone AH, Pearce R, Philip T, Petersen F. Autologous versus allogeneic bone marrow transplantation for non-Hodgkin's lymphoma: a case-controlled analysis of the European Bone Marrow Transplant Group registry data. *J Clin Oncol* 1992;10:11:1690–1695.
59. Van Besien KW, Rakesh CM, Giralt SA, Kantarjian HM, Pugh WC. Allogeneic bone marrow transplantation for poor-prognosis lymphoma: response, toxicity, and survival depend on disease histology. *Am J Med* 1996;100:299–307.
60. Ratanatharathorn V, Uberti J, Karanes C, et al. Prospective comparative trial of autologous versus allogeneic bone marrow transplantation in patients with non-Hodgkin's lymphoma. *Blood* 1994;84:1050–1055.
61. Appelbaum FR. Treatment of aggressive non-Hodgkin's lymphoma with marrow transplantation. *Marrow Transplant Rev* 1993;3:1–16.
62. Milpied N, Fielding AK, Pearce RM, et al. Allogeneic bone marrow transplant is not better than autologous transplant for patients with relapsed Hodgkin's disease. *J Clin Oncol* 1996;14:1291–1296.
63. Anderson JE, Litzow MR, Appelbaum FR, et al. Allogeneic, syngeneic, and autologous marrow transplantation for Hodgkin's disease: the 21-year Seattle experience. *J Clin Oncol* 1993;11:2342–2350.
64. Jones RJ, Piantadosi S, Mann RB, et al. High-dose cytotoxic therapy and bone marrow transplantation for relapsed Hodgkin's disease. *J Clin Oncol* 1990;8:527–537.
65. Phillips GL, Reece DE, Barnett MJ, et al. Allogeneic marrow transplantation for refractory Hodgkin's disease. *J Clin Oncol* 1989;7: 1039–1045.
66. Gajewski JL, Phillips GL, Sobocinski KA, et al. Bone marrow transplants from HLA-identical siblings in advanced Hodgkin's disease. *J Clin Oncol* 1996;14:572–578.
67. Jones RJ, Ambinder RF, Piantadosi S, et al. Evidence of a graft-versus-lymphoma effect associated with allogeneic bone marrow transplantation. *Blood* 1991;77:649–653.
68. Press OW, Eary JF, Appelbaum FR, et al. Radiolabeled-antibody therapy of B-cell lymphoma with autologous bone marrow support. *N Engl J Med* 1993;329:1219–1224.
69. Bierman PJ, Vose JM, Leichner PK, et al. Yttrium 90-labeled antiferritin followed by high-dose chemotherapy and autologous bone marrow transplantation for poor-prognosis Hodgkin's disease. *J Clin Oncol* 1993;11:698–703.
70. Spitzer G, Dicke KA, Litam J, et al. High-dose combination chemotherapy with autologous bone marrow transplantation in adult solid tumors. *Cancer* 1980;45:3075–3085.
71. Wheeler C, Antin JH, Churchill WH, et al. Cyclophosphamide, carmustine, and etoposide with autologous bone marrow transplantation in refractory Hodgkin's disease and non-Hodgkin's lymphoma: a dose finding study. *J Clin Oncol* 1990;8:648–656.
72. Weaver CH, Appelbaum FR, Petersen FB, et al. High-dose cyclophosphamide, carmustine, and etoposide followed by autologous bone marrow transplantation in patients with lymphoid malignancies who have received dose-limiting radiation therapy. *J Clin Oncol* 1993;11: 1329–1935.
73. Ahmed T, Ciavarella D, Feldman E, et al. High-dose, potentially myeloablative chemotherapy and autologous bone marrow transplantation for patients with advanced Hodgkin's disease. *Leukemia* 1989;3: 19–22.
74. Schmitz N, Diehl V. Carmustine and the lungs. *Lancet* 1997;349: 1712–1713.
75. Brandwein JM, Callum J, Sutcliffe SB, Scott JG, Keating A. Evaluation of cytoreductive therapy prior to high dose treatment with autologous bone marrow transplantation in relapsed and refractory Hodgkin's disease. *Bone Marrow Transplant* 1990;5:99–103.
76. Colwill R, Crump M, Felix C, et al. Mini-BEAM as salvage therapy for relapsed or refractory Hodgkin's disease before intensive therapy and autologous bone marrow transplantation. *J Clin Oncol* 1995;13: 396–402.
77. Bierman PJ, Anderson JR, Freeman MB, et al. High-dose chemotherapy followed by autologous hematopoietic rescue for Hodgkin's disease patients following first relapse after chemotherapy. *Ann Oncol* 1996;7:151–156.
78. Sweetenham JW, Taghipour G, Milligan D, Goldstone AH. High dose therapy (HDT) and autologous stem cell transplantation (ASCT) for adults with Hodgkin's disease (HD) in first relapse after chemotherapy—conventional dose salvage therapy prior to ASCT has no effect on outcome: results from the EBMT. *Blood* 1996;88(Suppl 1):486a (abst).
79. Phillips GL, Reece DE, Wolff SN, Goldie JH. The use of conventional salvage chemotherapy before dose-intensive cytotoxic therapy and autologous transplantation for aggressive-histology lymphoma: a case for re-evaluation. *Leuk Lymphoma* 1997;26:507–513.
80. Moormeier JA, Williams SF, Kaminer LS, et al. Autologous bone marrow transplantation followed by involved field radiotherapy in patients with relapsed or refractory Hodgkin's disease. *Leuk Lymphoma* 1991; 5:243–248.
81. Poen JC, Hoppe RT, Horning SJ. High-dose therapy and autologous bone marrow transplantation for relapsed/refractory Hodgkin's dis-

ease: the impact of involved field radiotherapy on patterns of failure and survival. *Int J Radiat Oncol Biol Phys* 1996;36:3–12.
82. Bierman P, Freeman M, Barrios S, et al. An apparent advantage with the use of consolidative radiation therapy (XRT) following autologous transplantation for Hodgkin's disease (HD). *Proc Am Soc Blood Marrow Transplant* 1995;1:66(abst).
83. Aviles A, Diaz-Maqueo J, Talavera A, Nambo M, Garcia E. Maintenance therapy with interferon alfa 2b in Hodgkin disease. *Leuk Lymphoma* 1996;20:494–499.
84. Schenkein DP, Dixon P, Desforges JF, et al. Phase I/II study of cyclophosphamide, carboplatin, and etoposide and autologous hematopoietic stem-cell transplantation with post-transplant interferon alfa-2b for patients with lymphoma and Hodgkin's disease. *J Clin Oncol* 1994;12:2423–2431.
85. Nagler A, Ackerstein A, Or R, et al. Immunotherapy with recombinant human interleukin-2 and recombinant interferon-α in lymphoma patients postautologous marrow or stem cell transplantation. *Blood* 1997;89:3951–3959.
86. Robinson N, Benyunes MC, Thompson JA, et al. Interleukin-2 after autologous stem cell transplantation for hematologic malignancy: a phase I/II study. *Bone Marrow Transplant* 1997;19:435–442.
87. Bennett CL, Armitage JL, Armitage GO, et al. Costs of care and outcomes for high-dose therapy and autologous transplantation for lymphoid malignancies: results from the University of Nebraska 1987 through 1991. *J Clin Oncol* 1995;13:969–973.
88. Linch DC, Winfield D, Goldstone AH, et al. Dose intensification with autologous bone-marrow transplantation in relapsed and resistant Hodgkin's disease: results of a BNLI randomized trial. *Lancet* 1993; 341:1051–1054.
89. Yuen AR, Rosenberg SA, Hoppe RT, Halpern JD, Horning SJ. Comparison between conventional salvage therapy and high-dose therapy with autografting for recurrent or refractory Hodgkin's disease. *Blood* 1997;89:814–822.
90. Haioun C, Lepage E, Gisselbrecht C, Bastion Y, Coiffier B. Benefit of autologous bone marrow transplantation over sequential chemotherapy in poor-risk aggressive non-Hodgkin's lymphoma: updated results of the prospective study LNH87-2. *J Clin Oncol* 1997;15: 1131–1137.
91. Martelli M, Vignetti M, Zinzani P, Gherlinzoni F, Meloni G. High-dose chemotherapy followed by autologous bone marrow transplantation versus dexamethasone, cisplatin, and cytarabine in aggressive non-Hodgkin's lymphoma with partial response to front-line chemotherapy: a prospective randomized Italian multicenter study. *J Clin Oncol* 1996;14:534–542.
92. Verdonck LF, van Putten WLJ, Hagenbeek A, Schouten HC, Sonneveld P. Comparison of CHOP chemotherapy with autologous bone marrow transplantation for slowly responding patients with aggressive non-Hodgkin's lymphoma. *N Engl J Med* 1995;332:1045–1051.
93. Carella AM, Carlier P, Congiu A, et al. Autologous bone marrow transplantation as adjuvant treatment for high-risk Hodgkin's disease in first complete remission after MOPP/ABVD protocol. *Bone Marrow Transplant* 1991;8:99–103.
94. Schmitz N, Hasenclever D, Brosteanu O, et al. Early high-dose therapy to consolidate patients with high-risk Hodgkin's disease in first complete remission? Results of an EBMT/GHSG matched-pair analysis. *Blood* 1995;10(Suppl 1):439a(abst).
95. Longo DL, Duffey PL, Young RC, et al. Conventional-dose salvage combination chemotherapy in patients relapsing with Hodgkin's disease after combination chemotherapy: the low probability for cure. *J Clin Oncol* 1992;10:210–218.
96. Bonfante V, Santoro A, Viviani S, et al. Outcome of patients with Hodgkin's disease failing after primary MOPP-ABVD. *J Clin Oncol* 1997;15:528–534.
97. Lazarus HM, Rowlings PA, Phillips GL, et al. Autotransplants for Hodgkin's disease never in complete remission. *Proc Am Soc Clin Oncol* 1997;16:89a(abst).
98. Sweetenham JW, Taghipour G, Linch DC, Goldstone AH. Thirty percent of adult patients with primary refractory Hodgkin's disease (HD) are progression free at 5 years after high dose therapy (HDT) and autologous stem cell transplantation (ASCT): data from 290 patients reported to the EBMT. *Blood* 1996;88(Suppl 1):486a(abst).
99. Ahmed T, Lake DE, Beer M, et al. Single and double autotransplants for relapsing/refractory Hodgkin's disease: results of two consecutive trials. *Bone Marrow Transplant* 1997;19:449–454.
100. Reece DE, Barnett MJ, Sheperd JD, et al. High-dose cyclophosphamide, carmustine (BCNU), and etoposide (VP16-213) with or without cisplatin (CBV + P) and autologous transplantation for patients with Hodgkin's disease who fail to enter a complete remission after combination chemotherapy. *Blood* 1995;86:451–456.
101. Moreau P, Fleury J, Bouabdallah R, et al. Early intensive therapy with autologous stem cell transplantation (ASCT) in high-risk Hodgkin's disease (HD): report of 158 cases from the French Registry (SFGM). *Blood* 1996;88(Suppl 1):486a(abst).
102. Bierman PJ, Vose JM, Armitage JO. Autologous transplantation for Hodgkin's disease: coming of age? *Blood* 1994;83:1161–1164.
103. Gianni AM, Siena S, Bregni M, et al. High-dose sequential chemoradiotherapy with peripheral blood progenitor cell support for relapsed or refractory Hodgkin's disease—a 6-year update. *Ann Oncol* 1993;4:889–891.
104. Canellos GP, Petroni GR, Barcos M, Duggan DB, Peterson BA. Etoposide, vinblastine, and doxorubicin: an active regimen for the treatment of Hodgkin's disease in relapse following MOPP. *J Clin Oncol* 1995;13:2005–2011.
105. Jagannath S, Armitage JO, Dicke KA, et al. Prognostic factors for response and survival after high-dose cyclophosphamide, carmustine, and etoposide with autologous bone marrow transplantation for relapsed Hodgkin's disease. *J Clin Oncol* 1989;7:179–185.
106. Vose JM, Kennedy BC, Bierman PJ, Kessinger A, Armitage JO. Long-term sequelae of autologous bone marrow or peripheral stem cell transplantation for lymphoid malignancies. *Cancer* 1992;69:784–789.
107. Traweek ST, Slovak ML, Nademanee AP, Brynes RK, Niland JC, Forman SJ. Clonal karyotypic hematopoietic cell abnormalities occurring after autologous bone marrow transplantation for Hodgkin's disease and non-Hodgkin's lymphoma. *Blood* 1994;84:957–963.
108. Darrington DL, Vose JM, Anderson JR, et al. Incidence and characterization of secondary myelodysplastic syndrome and acute myelogenous leukemia following high-dose chemoradiotherapy and autologous stem-cell transplantation for lymphoid malignancies. *J Clin Oncol* 1994;12:2527–2534.
109. Miller JS, Arthur DC, Litz CE, Neglia JP, Miller WJ, Weisdorf DJ. Myelodysplastic syndrome after autologous bone marrow transplantation: an additional late complication of curative cancer therapy. *Blood* 1994;83:3780–3786.
110. Bhatia S, Ramsay N, Steinbuch M, et al. Malignant neoplasms following bone marrow transplantation. *Blood* 1995;87:3633–3639.
111. Goldstone AH. Personal communication.

Hodgkin's Disease, edited by P. M. Mauch,
J. O. Armitage, V. Diehl, R. T. Hoppe, and L. M. Weiss.
Lippincott Williams & Wilkins, Philadephia ©1999.

CHAPTER 30

Pediatric Hodgkin's Disease

Sarah S. Donaldson, Melissa Hudson, Odile Oberlin,
Jürgen H. Bramswig, and Gunther Schellong

HISTORICAL ASPECTS OF TREATMENT

Although Hodgkin's disease presenting in children is similar to the disease in adults in regard to biology and natural history, some of the features unique to Hodgkin's disease in childhood are emphasized in this chapter as a means of augmenting the general discussion of the disease. To discuss the uniqueness of the pediatric population, we must understand the historical aspects of the disease and its treatment. Thirty years ago, pediatric and adult patients with Hodgkin's disease were managed in a similar fashion. Radiation therapy was delivered in high doses and extended volumes. With radiotherapy alone, during the 1960s and early 1970s, a significant number of patients with Hodgkin's disease were cured. Although the prognosis in children was at first believed to be poorer than in adults, children were later shown to do as well as adults (1), but with a higher risk for the development of late consequences of therapy. The development of the four-drug combination of Mustargen (mechlorethamine), Oncovin (vincristine), procarbazine, and prednisone (MOPP) in the 1960s, and a better appreciation of the adverse effects of high-dose radiation therapy on musculoskeletal development, provided the cornerstone for the first investigations of combined-modality therapy in pediatric patients with Hodgkin's disease (2,3). These pediatric trials implemented in the 1970s modified treatment strategies to address the specific problems of children. They were designed to determine whether multiple cycles of chemotherapy could replace a portion of the radiation therapy in laparotomy-staged children with Hodgkin's disease (4–7). These trials served as the model for institutional and cooperative group investigations of low-dose radiation therapy and chemotherapy in the treatment of pediatric Hodgkin's disease.

Until the 1980s, the surgical staging of children in whom Hodgkin's disease had been newly diagnosed was routinely utilized because of the dependence on radiation therapy for local disease control. When treatment was based on radiation therapy alone, staging laparotomy with splenectomy was the most precise way to determine the presence and extent of subdiaphragmatic involvement in patients with supradiaphragmatic disease, and to determine appropriate radiation fields. Several factors contributed to the replacement of pathologic staging with clinical staging, including the increased use of systemic therapy in pediatric patients, advances in diagnostic imaging technology, which permitted more accurate evaluation of retroperitoneal lymph nodes, and the recognition of life-threatening sequelae, including overwhelming bacterial infections in asplenic children. Whereas precise anatomic staging was required for the design of radiation fields when the treatment plan utilized radiation therapy alone, histologic confirmation of microscopic abdominal disease became less important when systemic therapy became routinely used. Currently, surgical staging is rarely utilized in most pediatric centers.

In France, laparotomy with splenectomy has not been performed since 1975 (8). Of 60 clinically staged children treated with MOPP chemotherapy and involved-field radiation therapy, none have relapsed in a subdiaphragmatic nonirradiated area (9). In Germany, a stepwise reduction of surgical staging has been performed during successive studies. In the first German study (HD-78), all children underwent laparotomy and splenectomy. In the subsequent

S. S. Donaldson: Department of Radiation Oncology, Stanford University School of Medicine, Stanford, California.

M. Hudson: Department of Hematology and Oncology, St. Jude Children's Research Hospital, Memphis, Tennessee.

O. Oberlin: Department of Pediatrics, Institut Gustave-Roussy, Villejuif, France.

J. H. Bramswig: Department of Pediatrics, University of Münster and University Children's Hospital, Münster, Germany.

G. Schellong: Department of Hematology and Oncology, University Children's Hospital, Münster, Germany.

study (HD-82), laparotomy was performed in all patients, but splenectomy was undertaken only in those with visible abnormalities detected during intraabdominal exploration (10,11). In the German HD-85 study, laparotomy was reserved for patients with abnormalities on an abdominal ultrasonogram/computed tomogram (CT) and/or those with enlargement of the pulmonary hilus; selective splenectomy was performed according to the previously mentioned criteria. In the HD-90 study, splenectomy was abandoned (10,12,13). The Italian AIEOP study confirmed that effective chemotherapy is sufficient to eradicate occult microfoci of subdiaphragmatic involvement (14).

The development of the four-drug ABVD [Adriamycin (doxorubicin), bleomycin, vinblastine, dacarbazine] regimen and the desire to avoid MOPP-associated sequelae of infertility and secondary leukemia resulted in the use of alternating multiagent chemotherapy regimens (15,16). The ABVD combination appears not to be associated with permanent germ cell dysfunction or an increased risk for leukemogenesis, but it does produce a dose-related risk of cardiopulmonary dysfunction (15). The prototype MOPP/ABVD regimen has the theoretical advantage of enhanced antineoplastic activity, reduced MOPP-related sequelae because of the limited exposure to alkylating agent chemotherapy, and reduced ABVD-related sequelae because of the limited doses of doxorubicin and bleomycin (17). This and similar trials of alternating multidrug combinations have shown them to be uniformly efficacious and have led to subsequent pediatric trials in which radiation doses have been further reduced to 15 to 25.5 Gy and volumes reduced to involved fields (2,18–22). Monitoring of survivors treated with these regimens thus far indicates a significant reduction in life-threatening toxicity (cardiopulmonary sequelae and secondary malignancies), which has been attributed to the reduced exposure to alkylating drugs, doxorubicin, and bleomycin (18,19,23).

By the 1990s, treatment goals in pediatric Hodgkin's disease evolved to those of continuing the excellent disease-free survival rates in clinically staged children and adolescents and to improving the outcome for advanced-stage patients, especially those with extranodal disease. Pediatric trials in the early 1990s established that excellent outcomes could be achieved in favorable early-stage patients treated with fewer than six cycles of multiagent combination chemotherapy and lower radiation doses and volumes. Challenges for the future are to determine for which patients cure can be achieved with even fewer cycles of nontoxic chemotherapy and for which patients radiotherapy can be safely omitted. In addition, we are challenged to identify those patients at high risk for treatment failure who may benefit from intensification of therapy.

EPIDEMIOLOGY AND PATHOLOGY

The age incidence in Hodgkin's disease is bimodal. In industrialized countries, including the United States, the first peak occurs in young adults ages 20 to 30, and the second peak occurs in late adulthood (24). In developing countries, the first peak is seen before adolescence (25). Among children less than 15 years of age, the relative risk for Hodgkin's disease tends to increase with increasing family size, with a sibship relative risk of 1.28 reported in a Danish study summarizing a population-based database from the Danish Civil Registration system (25). The trend for birth order was 1.26 among Danish children. Among young adults older than 15 years, the risk for Hodgkin's disease decreases with increased sibship size and birth order, with significant differences in the two age groups ($p <.05$).

There is a slight overall male predominance in the incidence of Hodgkin's disease, which is most marked in the very young children. Hodgkin's disease is very rare before the age of 5 years. In children less than 10 years old, the incidence is much higher in boys than in girls, whereas among teenagers, the incidence is approximately equal between the sexes. Table 1 summarizes the age and sex distribution of children under 15 years of age in five consecutive German-Austrian pediatric Hodgkin's disease studies, confirming the marked sex difference as a function of age (26).

Although the etiology of Hodgkin's disease is unknown, it has been proposed that Hodgkin's disease diagnosed at different ages might have different causes and that infection might be involved in the development of Hodgkin's disease in young adults (27). Whereas a delayed exposure to infection might be a risk factor for Hodgkin's disease in young adults, early exposure to perhaps another infectious agent might increase the risk for Hodgkin's disease in children. Serologic and epidemio-

TABLE 1. *Age and sex distribution among 1,025 children under 15 years of age entered into five German-Austrian DAL-HD studies 1978–1995*

		Age		
	No. patients	<5 y	5–<10 y	10–<15 y
Total	1,025	82 (8.0%)	298 (29.1%)	645 (62.9%)
Boys	642	69 (10.8%)	226 (35.2%)	347 (54.0%)
Girls	383	13 (3.4%)	72 (18.8%)	298 (77.8%)
Ratio of boys to girls	1.7:1	5.3:1	3.1:1	1.2:1

From ref. 26.

logic studies raise the possibility of an association between the Epstein-Barr virus (EBV) and Hodgkin's disease. Testing for EBV within Reed-Sternberg and Hodgkin's cells among children with Hodgkin's disease from 10 different countries has shown that EBV strain type 1 is predominant in the United Kingdom, South Africa, Australia, and Greece, whereas EBV type 2 is predominant in Egypt (28,29). However, as many as 21% of cases show evidence of dual infection, supporting the possibility of an underlying immune deficiency in these cases (see Chapter 10). Molecular evidence of prior EBV infection is found less frequently in some histologic subtypes and presentations than in others (30–32). Current theories of etiology suggest that Hodgkin's disease is a rare consequence of a latent infection with EBV virus developing in the setting of a sustained host response to chronic tissue-based antigenic stimulation (33,34).

When the Rye modification of the Lukes and Butler classification of Hodgkin's disease is used, one finds differences in histologic subtypes as a function of age in the pediatric population. The lymphocyte predominant subtype is seen more commonly in children than adults, the mixed cellularity subtype is more common in children less than 10 years of age at diagnosis, and the nodular sclerosing variant is most common in adolescents (26,35). Table 2 shows the histologic subtypes by age for children less than 15 years old in the German-Austrian DAL-HD-90 study. Historically, the lymphocyte predominance and nodular sclerosis subtypes were considered the most favorable, whereas mixed cellularity and lymphocyte depletion were considered less favorable. Today, lymphocyte depletion is rarely diagnosed in children from developed countries. Children with stage I mixed cellularity Hodgkin's disease treated with local-field radiation alone without chemotherapy have a higher relapse rate than children with nodular sclerosis Hodgkin's disease in the United Kingdom Children's Cancer Study Group experience (36). With effective combined-modality therapy, as used today, differences in histologic subtypes are less apparent. On the other hand, lymphocyte predominance Hodgkin's disease, which is seen with increased frequency in children, has been considered to be a biologically indolent entity in which 90% of children present with an early clinical stage (CS I and II) and have an excellent long-term outcome irrespective of therapy (37). In the Pediatric Oncology Group experience of 26 cases of stage I–III lymphocyte predominance Hodgkin's disease, the event-free survival after 5 years was 86% (38). Immunologic evidence now suggests that the nodular variant of lymphocyte predominance Hodgkin's disease is of B-cell origin and behaves in an indolent clinical pattern, with a tendency for late recurrence (39). Despite the suggestion that nodular lymphocyte predominance Hodgkin's disease may be biologically closer to non-Hodgkin's lymphoma than to other subtypes of Hodgkin's disease, the current recommendation for children with this entity is to treat as appropriate for early-stage and favorable presentations of Hodgkin's disease, with a goal to limit the risk for serious sequelae (38).

CLINICAL PRESENTATION AND STAGING

The Ann Arbor staging system, which defines anatomic lymph node regions in adults with Hodgkin's disease, also is utilized for children. When this system is used, among laparotomy-staged children, approximately 60% present with stage I–IIA or B disease, and the remaining 40% have stage III–IV disease (35). More recently, however, an appreciation of the prognostic importance of tumor size and bulk has led investigators to redefine stages as early-stage/favorable versus advanced-stage/unfavorable; this serves as a useful guide in making treatment decisions. When one defines advanced-stage/unfavorable as CS III–IVA or B and includes CS I–II large mediastinal disease (more than one-third maximal mediastinal diameter), approximately 66% of clinically staged children are found to have advanced-stage/unfavorable disease, and approximately 33% present with early-stage/favorable disease.

In the past, detailed and precise staging procedures, including staging laparotomy, were essential to determine

TABLE 2. *Histologic subtypes of Hodgkin's disease as a function of age among children less than 15 years old entered into the German-Austrian DAL-HD-90 study*

	Age			
	<10 y		10–<15 y	
Histologic subtype	No. patients	(%)	No. patients	(%)
Lymphocyte predominance	13	(8.4)	33	(11.9)
Nodular sclerosis	62	(40.2)	201	(72.3)
Mixed cellularity	77	(50.0)	43	(15.5)
Lymphocyte depletion	1	(0.7)	1	(0.4)
Unknown	1	(0.7)		

From ref. 26.

appropriate treatment, especially when radiotherapy alone was considered for patients with early-stage disease. However, the risk for serious bacterial infections (bacteremia and meningitis) from encapsulated organisms in asplenic children (40), the need for prolonged administration of prophylactic antibiotics, and the occurrence of postsurgical complications, such as intestinal obstruction, remained serious issues, particularly in the management of children. Comparative studies investigating the risks for infection in asplenic adults versus children have not been reported. The increasing use of chemotherapy-radiotherapy treatment programs renders the precise anatomic localization of small foci of disease, obtained by laparotomy staging, less crucial. However, in the comparison of treatment results, clinically staged patients cannot be compared directly with those in whom pathologic staging has been performed.

Routine clinical staging for children today includes history and physical examination, with attention to lymph node draining areas, including Waldeyer's ring, in patients with high cervical nodal disease. Useful and important laboratory studies for the staging and management of disease in children include complete blood count with differential, erythrocyte sedimentation rate (ESR), and tests of renal and hepatic function, including alkaline phosphatase level and serum lactate dehydrogenase (LDH) level. Important radiographic studies include chest roentgenography (posteroanterior and lateral); computed tomography (CT) of the chest, abdomen, and pelvis; gallium scan; and bone marrow biopsy for children with advanced-stage/unfavorable disease. Gallium/67 scanning is particularly useful in the evaluation and follow-up of supradiaphragmatic Hodgkin's disease. In patients whose mediastinal mass has not completely regressed after therapy, persistent gallium avidity may indicate residual disease (41). The lymphangiogram continues to be considered the most reliable method to detect retroperitoneal lymph node involvement by Hodgkin's disease. The lymphangiogram is unique in its ability to display the internal architecture of lymph nodes and is superior to abdominal and pelvic CT to detect subdiaphragmatic disease in children (42). Unfortunately, fewer and fewer diagnostic radiologists today have expertise in performing and interpreting lymphangiograms, particularly in children, which limits the use of this important test to just a few reference centers. A radionuclide bone scan with corresponding plain radiographs of abnormal areas may aid in the assessment of skeletal metastases and is useful for the child who presents with bone pain or a serum alkaline phosphatase concentration elevated beyond that expected for age. Magnetic resonance imaging (MRI) may also be useful in the assessment of subdiaphragmatic sites and aids in the evaluation of fat-encased retroperitoneal lymph nodes (43). The value of positron emission tomography (PET) in the staging of Hodgkin's disease is currently being studied.

PROGNOSTIC FACTORS

Early reports of the results of treatment for Hodgkin's disease suggested that the youngest patients had the worst prognosis (44). However, in an analysis of more than 2,200 patients with Hodgkin's disease treated and followed at Stanford University during the 30 years between 1961 and 1991, a very young age was shown to be a favorable prognostic factor (45). Patients less than 10 years of age had a significantly improved freedom from relapse and survival in comparison with adolescents 11 to 16 years of age, and a highly significantly improved outcome compared with patients more than 17 years of age (Fig. 1). The differences were also apparent in comparisons of children with Ann Arbor stage I and II disease across various age groups, and in those with Ann Arbor stage III and IV disease. Age, stage, and treatment modality were important prognostic factors for freedom from relapse and survival by multivariate analyses (45). However, the German-Austrian studies have challenged these observations. From 1978 to 1995, 1,181 children throughout Germany and Austria were treated with uniform combined-modality protocols in five consecutive multicenter studies (DAL-HD-78, HD-82, HD-85, HD-87, HD-90) (10,12,46). The disease-free survival rates of children less than 10 years of age (n = 382) and of those between 10 and less than 16 years of age (n = 799) were nearly identical for the groups considered as a whole and according to stage (Fig. 2A). However, the survival was significantly worse in children less than 10 years of age because of the higher rate of fatal

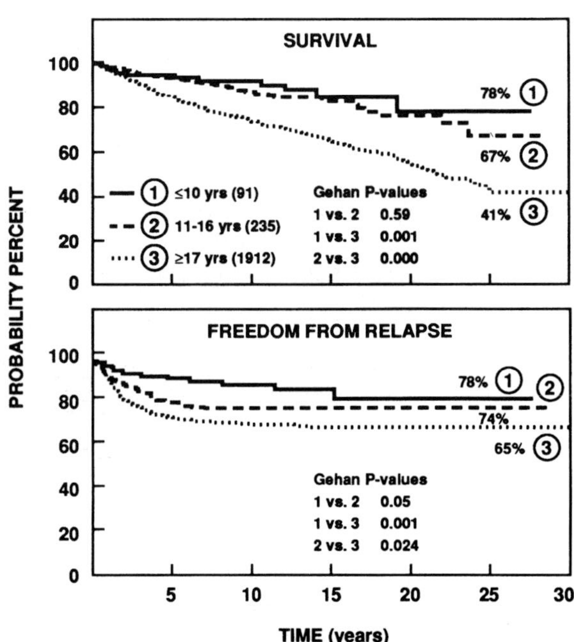

FIG. 1. Actuarial survival and freedom from relapse for patients with Hodgkin's disease from Stanford ages less than 10 years, 11 to 16 years, and more than 17 years. (From ref. 45, with permission from Elsevier Science.)

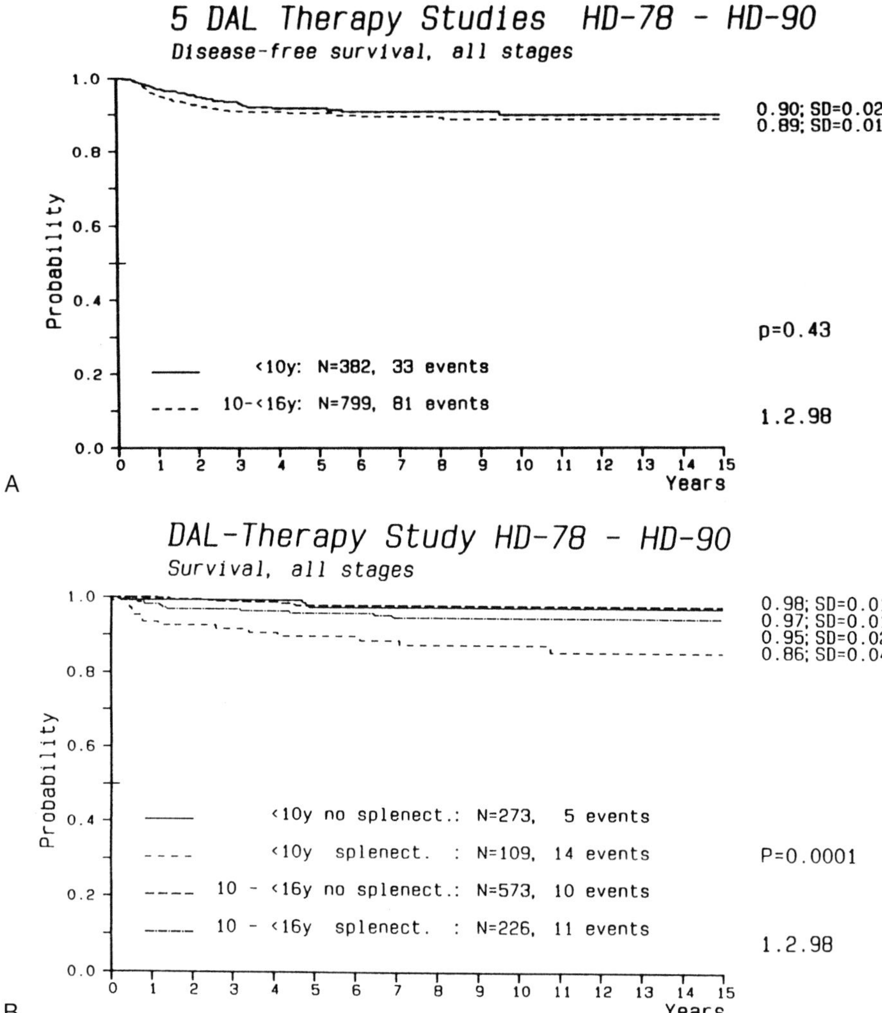

FIG. 2. A: Actuarial disease-free survival by age among children less than 16 years old entered into five consecutive German-Austrian studies. **B:** Actuarial survival by age and splenectomy among children less than 16 years old entered into five consecutive German-Austrian studies. (From ref. 12, with permission from Harcourt Brace.)

infectious episodes among splenectomized children (Fig. 2B). In the HD-90 study, splenectomy was omitted. A comparative analysis of children less than 10 years old, between 10 and less than 15 years old, and between 15 and less than 18 years old reveals no significant differences in disease-free survival and survival (Fig. 3). These differences are best explained by noting that the HD-90 analysis was limited to patients less than 18 years of age and employed uniform therapy, while the Stanford study evaluated age as a prognostic indicator across pediatric and adult age groups during time periods in which treatment recommendations varied. Unfortunately, we lack studies in which children, adolescents, and adults have been concurrently treated with uniform therapy.

AGE-RELATED TOXICITY OF TREATMENT

An appreciation of the manifestation of late effects of the disease and its treatment has become possible with improvements in long-term disease-free survival of children and adolescents with Hodgkin's disease. Because children have such a high likelihood of cure, and because they then have many years of life after Hodgkin's disease, much attention has been paid to potential late effects among this young age group. However, some of the serious sequelae of treatment are most pronounced in the youngest of patients, in whom growth and development are particularly active when therapy is administered (47). In addition, cardiac toxicity appears to be age-related, with younger patients at highest risk (48,49), and risk continues to evolve as the treated patients age. In this section, we discuss age-related toxicity, which has a significant impact on children and adolescents with Hodgkin's disease. The definition of a "pediatric" age group largely depends on treatment-related toxicity. An upper age limit of less than 16 years is appropriate for studies of youngsters and adolescents of immature skeletal growth, for whom less than standard doses of radiation are recommended. An upper age limit of 18 to 21 is commonly used for treatment protocols focused on reducing overall therapy and minimizing late organ toxicity. Avoidance of the toxicities mentioned here has become the focus of current

A

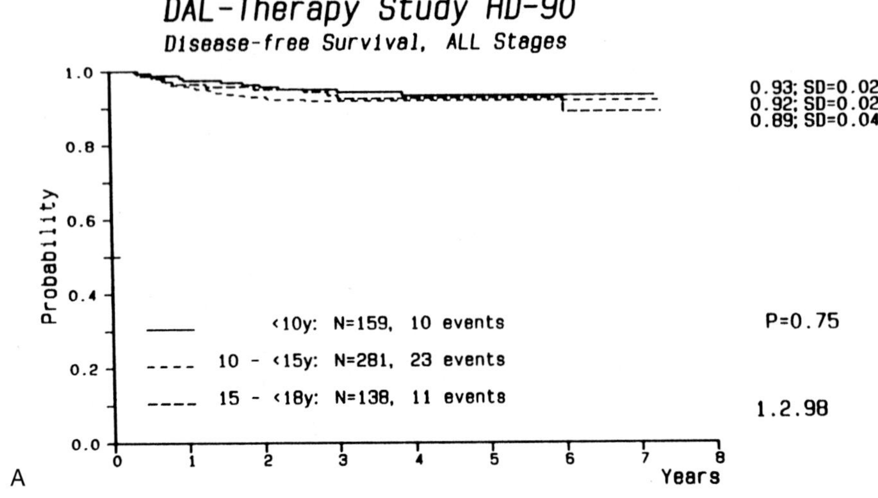

B

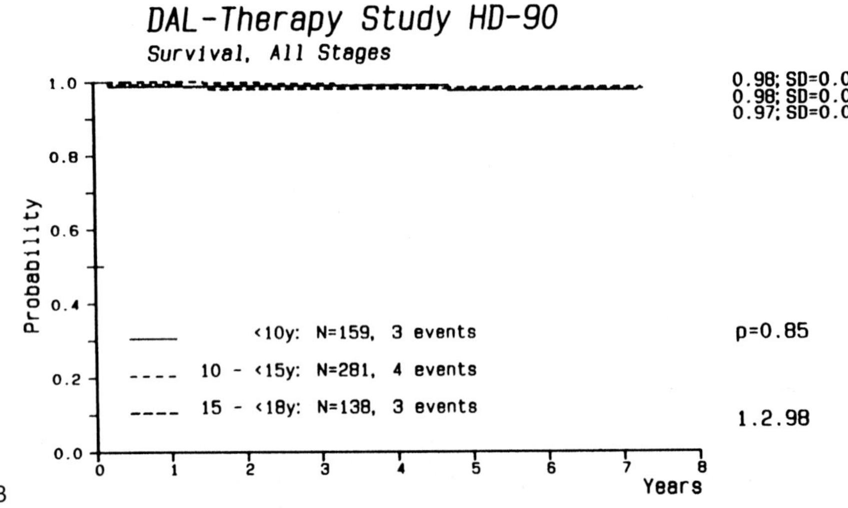

FIG. 3. Actuarial disease-free survival **(A)** and survival by age group **(B)** among children less than 18 years old in the German-Austrian DAL-HD-90 study. (From ref. 12, with permission from Harcourt Brace.)

protocol therapies. Thus, it is important to realize that current therapy is directed toward avoiding the toxicities observed after prior treatment programs.

Infertility after Treatment of Hodgkin's Disease

Chemotherapy and radiotherapy can cause severe testicular and ovarian dysfunction. Both treatment modalities can affect the production of testicular and ovarian hormones and/or cause infertility (50–63). In addition, ionizing radiation to the testes or ovaries may affect gonadal function following direct or scattered gonadal irradiation (56,62,64). Testicular and ovarian function can be damaged from exposure to the drugs mechlorethamine, procarbazine, chlorambucil, and cyclophosphamide, all frequently used in the treatment of Hodgkin's disease (52, 60,65).

Testicular dysfunction has been described in boys and men treated for Hodgkin's disease (51,52,54,58–60,66). Similar changes are seen in boys receiving chemotherapy with or without pelvic irradiation (52,60). Thus, cytotoxic drugs, especially the alkylating agents, have been incriminated in damage to the male gonads. Germinal aplasia, documented by testicular biopsy, high levels of follicle-stimulating hormone (FSH), and gynecomastia, has long been recognized following MOPP chemotherapy (65). Azoospermia has been demonstrated in 80% to 90% of male patients receiving 6 to 8 cycles of MOPP chemotherapy in several subsequent studies (51,61). Recovery of spermatogenesis is rare but has been reported in boys ages 10 to 15 years after documented azoospermia following 6 cycles of MOPP in childhood (60), and in adult men following 2 to 3 cycles of MOPP chemotherapy (67).

The ChlVPP regimen (chlorambucil, vinblastine, procarbazine, and prednisolone) was developed from the MOPP program in attempt to reduce chemotherapy-related toxicity. However, testicular function is also severely impaired with this therapeutic regimen, as demonstrated by elevated FSH levels and azoospermia in 80% to 90% of male patients (53,58). These data confirm earlier results documenting a complete loss of the germinal cell line in adult men receiving more than 400 mg of chlorambucil (59). Thus, the ChlVPP and MOPP regimens have similar detrimental effects on germinal epithelial function.

A high and apparently dose-related incidence of testicular dysfunction is also seen in pediatric patients treated without mechlorethamine and chlorambucil, but with OPPA or OPPA/COPP chemotherapy [Oncovin (vincristine), prednisone, procarbazine, Adriamycin (doxorubicin), cyclophosphamide] (52). The incidence of elevated FSH levels is directly related to the cumulative doses of chemotherapy. Basal FSH levels are increased after 2 cycles of OPPA, 2 OPPA/2 COPP, and 2 OPPA/4–6 COPP at a frequency of 28.9%, 45.5%, 62.5%, respectively. Pubertal development and testosterone levels are normal, although elevated basal and stimulated luteinizing hormone levels are found in 24% and 87.8% of boys, indicating subclinical Leydig cell damage. It is unknown whether Leydig cell function will return to normal or if premature Leydig cell failure with low testosterone values will develop.

Testicular function has also been studied in boys treated without mechlorethamine, chlorambucil, and procarbazine. They have received OPA/COMP chemotherapy [Oncovin (vincristine), prednisone, Adriamycin (doxorubicin), cyclophosphamide, methotrexate] (68). Procarbazine, a major gonadotoxic agent, was omitted from OPPA in the German-Austrian HD-85 protocol and replaced by methotrexate in COMP. This study yielded normal gonadal function in 16 patients treated with 2 cycles of OPA and in nine patients treated with 2 OPA and 2 or 4 cycles of COMP chemotherapy. The mean total doses of cyclophosphamide (with 2,004 or 3,720 mg/m^2 in 2 or 4 COMP cycles of chemotherapy) were similar to the cyclophosphamide doses received by patients with 2 or 4 cycles of COPP chemotherapy. These results indicate that the dose-dependent testicular damage observed in the previous OPPA/COPP study was the result of the gonadotoxic agent procarbazine (68).

Anthracycline-based therapeutic regimens such as ABVD are associated with a lower incidence of severe testicular damage. Azoospermia is documented in only 36% of patients treated with ABVD (51,61). The azoospermia appears transitory, and full recovery of spermatogenesis can be expected following therapy.

Similar results have been reported in a phase II study with VEEP chemotherapy (vincristine, epirubicin, etoposide, and prednisolone) (69). Sperm counts were normal in 23 of 25 adult patients (93%) who consented to have a sperm count performed after treatment. Two further patients fathered children 2 and 14 months after the final course of VEEP.

The incidence of testicular dysfunction is greatly reduced among adult men with advanced-stage Hodgkin's disease treated with the 12-week Stanford V protocol (doxorubicin, vinblastine, mechlorethamine, vincristine, bleomycin, etoposide, and prednisone). Sixteen of 17 tested adult men are normospermic/oligospermic following treatment, and posttreatment offspring are normal (70). The Stanford V regimen has not yet been used in children.

Recently, the German authors have investigated the effects of another etoposide-based therapeutic regimen on testicular function. Two courses of OEPA chemotherapy [Oncovin (vincristine), etoposide, prednisone, and Adriamycin (doxorubicin)] have been used in the treatment of pediatric patients with stage I–IIA Hodgkin's disease (66). Testicular function has been normal among 27 boys. However, basal FSH levels were outside the normal range when the patients received 2 cycles of OEPA in combination with 2 or 4 cycles of COPP (37.5% and 36.4%, respectively). Thus, the combination chemotherapy containing cyclophosphamide and procarbazine again is highly gonadotoxic. This toxicity is thought to be a consequence of the effects of procarbazine, although an additional effect of etoposide and cyclophosphamide cannot be excluded. Data from these studies (66,69) and the Stanford V protocol (70), with the lower incidence of testicular dysfunction, make these regimens attractive therapeutic alternatives to other, highly gonadotoxic combinations of chemotherapy.

With respect to radiation therapy, aggressive testicular shielding should be attempted when pelvic irradiation is administered to boys. Unfortunately, this is often difficult to achieve, technically, with the prepubertal testes. With adequate testicular shielding, high-dose pelvic radiation may be associated with a transient oligospermia or azoospermia; however, recovery of function is common (71). Testicular damage is a severe long-term sequela in boys treated with chemotherapy for Hodgkin's disease. Germinal epithelial dysfunction is much more frequently observed than is Leydig cell failure, although subclinical Leydig cell insufficiency warrants careful long-term evaluation so that testosterone replacement therapy can be initiated if Leydig cell failure is documented. Because many male survivors of childhood Hodgkin's disease will be infertile after treatment with most of the presently available chemotherapy regimens, alternative therapeutic strategies should be developed to reduce the unacceptable high rates of azoospermia. In addition, cryopreservation of semen should be considered as an option for adolescent boys who face the risk of sterility (72).

Ovarian dysfunction has been described in girls treated for Hodgkin's disease (53,58). However, in general, ovarian toxicity is more marked in older women than in young girls (50,55,63). The effects of chemotherapy appear to be proportional to the age of the patient at treatment. Fertility is usually not permanently impaired in prepubertal and pubertal girls exposed to chemotherapy alone (58,60). For female patients treated before the age of 20 to 30, the likelihood of retaining regular menses or resuming regular ovarian function after a short period of amenorrhea is high (50,55,62).

Female patients with Hodgkin's disease exposed to pelvic nodal irradiation may experience ovarian dysfunction. Direct ovarian radiation to total doses of 20 to 35 Gy will cause ovarian failure. However, radiation to fields including the mantle, spleen, and paraaortic lymph nodes, but excluding the pelvic lymph nodes, does not alter normal menstrual function and does not produce premature menopause (73). Lateral or midline oophoropexy can be performed to reduce the dose delivered to the ovaries (74,75). Amenorrhea can be avoided and ovarian function preserved in most patients when the involved nodal regions are irradiated following oophoropexy. Normal offspring have been produced by women after midline oophoropexy. The reduction in the incidence of amenorrhea may be more than 50% (74). To protect the ovaries from radiation, they should be localized, with a radiopaque clip placed at the time of ovarian transposition. The position of the ovaries can subsequently be confirmed by ultrasound or CT before irradiation. A customized pelvic block should be used for ovarian shielding (74).

Several studies have documented the outcome of pregnancies among cancer survivors. These include a large cohort of children from patients previously treated for Hodgkin's disease (60,74,76–80). No increase in risk for congenital abnormalities has been detected in the offspring. In a case-control study of 54 mothers and 61 fathers who have had cancer, the RR of congenital anomalies was 1.04 (95% CI, 0.7–1.5) among mothers and 0.9 (95% CI, 0.7–1.4) among fathers, no higher than that in the general population (80,81). In several other studies, similar results have been obtained. Thus, no increased incidence of congenital abnormalities is expected in children of long-term survivors of childhood malignancy.

The complications of chemotherapy in the treatment of Hodgkin's disease are age-dependent and thus affect children and adolescents to a lesser extent than adult women when similar cancer treatment is used. In an individual patient with primary or secondary ovarian failure, hormonal replacement therapy is recommended to allow normal pubertal and sexual development in young women and to prevent osteoporosis in older woman. In addition, long-term follow-up is needed to document the outcome of all pregnancies and the development of the offspring.

Growth, Height, and Musculoskeletal Effects

Impaired growth and diminished adult height are serious late effects in children treated with radiotherapy and chemotherapy. They have most frequently been demonstrated following treatment for tumors of the brain, head, and neck and for leukemia (82–90). Only limited information is available concerning the effects of radiation and chemotherapy on growth patterns and ultimate adult height among children treated for Hodgkin's disease (91,92). Chronologic age (and thus growth potential at the time of treatment), total radiation dose, dose per fraction, beam energy, treatment sites, symmetry of treatment volumes, homogeneity of growth plate irradiation, surgery, and chemotherapy are major factors influencing growth and causing musculoskeletal changes (93,94).

High doses of radiation delivered to the axial skeleton in patients with medulloblastoma, leukemia, and Hodgkin's disease can cause disproportionate growth (95). The changes are most marked for those children who receive doses of spinal irradiation in excess of 35 Gy, and who are irradiated before the age of 6 years or during the pubertal growth spurt. Others have shown that combined-modality therapy (chemotherapy and radiotherapy) is more injurious to final height and sex-adjusted growth than are chemotherapy or radiotherapy alone (92).

Adult height has been measured in 124 children treated for Hodgkin's disease with high or low doses of radiation (91). The relative loss of height, based on pretreatment measurements of height, was 7.7% or 13 cm when radiation doses larger than 33 Gy were administered to the entire spine to prepubertal children (Fig. 4). No disproportionate height was noted when standing height was compared with sitting height. A smaller and clinically insignificant impairment of growth was seen in pubertal and postpubertal patients given high-dose, large-volume treatment, and no clinically significant impairment was noted in children receiving lower doses of radiation (91,92). Thus, current protocols appear not to cause clinically significant growth retardation when doses of spinal radiation of 25 Gy or less are used.

Adult standing height has been measured in 183 of 273 (67.5%) children treated according to the German DAL-HD-78 and DAL-HD-82 studies. In DAL-HD-78, children received 36 to 40 Gy of extended-field radiation and chemotherapy, and in DAL-HD-82 they received 25 to 35 Gy of involved-field radiation and chemotherapy. All patients were older than 18 years and free of disease at the time of evaluation. Mean adult height was 177.8 cm in boys and 166.9 cm in girls (Table 3). This is only slightly below normal standards in German men, and compares favorably with the standards in German women (96). Clinically relevant differences in height were not observed between the two patient groups, although higher-dose, extended-field irradiation was used in HD-78 and lower-

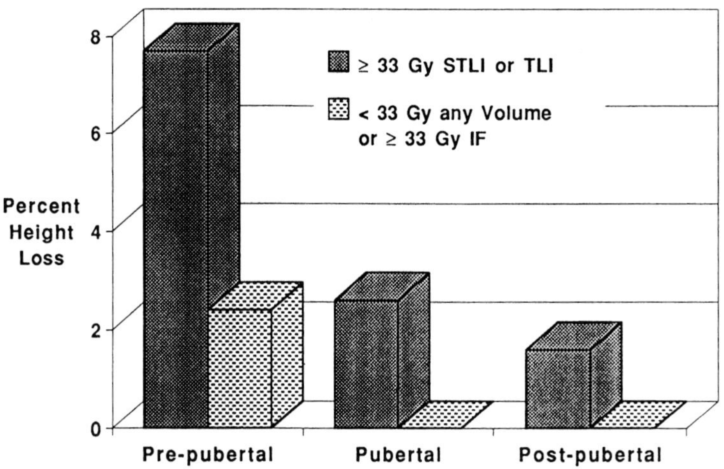

FIG. 4. Height impairment in children from Stanford with Hodgkin's disease as a function of pubertal status at the time of treatment and the intensity of treatment administered. (From ref. 91, with permission from Elsevier Science.)

dose, involved-field irradiation was used in the HD-82 study. Thus, higher doses of radiation may not necessarily affect adult height. In addition, these investigators were unable to demonstrate that chronologic age at the time of therapy is an important predictor of ultimate adult height, as in their studies the final adult height was similar whether children were treated before or after the age of 10 (Fig. 5).

Combined-modality therapy (chemotherapy and radiation therapy) may be more detrimental to ultimate adult height than chemotherapy or radiation therapy alone (92). Newer treatment regimens with lower doses of radiation are most probably not associated with clinically significant growth retardation. The current treatment recommendations with better-quality, lower-dose, and smaller-volume radiation will likely improve growth patterns and final height in most children treated for Hodgkin's disease. Adult height should preferably be compared with expected height and, when possible, with the adult height of siblings to obtain additional information if patients have reached their genetic height potential (83).

However, based on observations of patients treated many years ago, it is apparent that the ultimate impact of the effects of radiation therapy may not be realized for many years; thus, long-term follow-up is essential, particularly regarding musculoskeletal effects. Major side effects of radiation therapy include narrowing of the thoracic apex, intraclavicular narrowing with symmetric shortening of the clavicles, and atrophy of the soft tissues of the neck. These changes are commonly observed in patients treated many years ago with radiation doses and techniques considered standard at that time (Fig. 6). They are particularly prominent in young patients treated with high-dose and large-volume irradiation. Unfortunately, standard measurements are not available to quantify soft-tissue atrophy and intraclavicular or sternal length.

Rare late musculoskeletal sequelae include retroperitoneal fibrosis and brachial plexopathy (97,98). Avascular necrosis of the femoral head is another complication of corticosteroid use in combination chemotherapy, although high-dose radiation may also be a contributing factor (99,100). The current treatment regimens with lower doses and smaller volumes of radiation are designed to lessen and/or eliminate altogether the marked changes seen in young patients treated in the past with high-dose radiation.

TABLE 3. *Adult standing height in the German-Austrian DAL-HD-78 and DAL-HD-82 studies of Hodgkin's disease*[a]

	Boys		Girls	
Study	Patients	Controls	Patients	Controls
DAL-HD-78	n = 50 176.1 ± 8.3	n = 73 179.9 ± 6.4	n = 33 166.1 ± 7.6	n = 70 167.0 ± 5.1
DAL-HD-82	n = 60 179.1 ± 7.6		n = 42 167.7 ± 7.0	
Total	n = 110 177.8 ± 8.1		n = 75 167.0 ± 7.3	

[a]Data in centimeters, mean ± standard deviation.

Cardiovascular Sequelae

Both radiation therapy and chemotherapy used in the treatment of Hodgkin's disease may have toxic effects on the heart and blood vessels, although symptomatic sequelae are uncommon (Table 4). Reduction of anthracycline chemotherapy doses and radiation doses and volumes in contemporary pediatric regimens has diminished the frequency of acute toxicity. However, delayed subclinical cardiovascular injury and its effect on the progression of degenerative cardiovascular disease is just now becoming apparent as survivors of pediatric Hodgkin's disease enter their third and fourth decades (see Chapter 35 for further details).

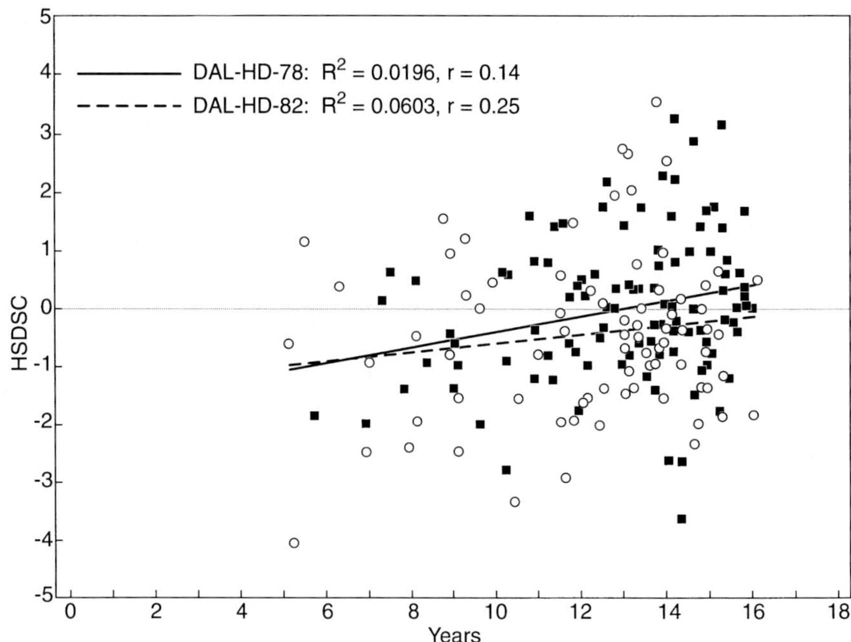

FIG. 5. Correlation and linear regression analysis between chronologic age before therapy and adult height in patients with Hodgkin's disease in the DAL-HD-78 and DAL-HD-82 studies.

Radiation Injury

External-beam irradiation may affect any of the cardiovascular tissues. The most problematic cardiovascular sequelae observed in patients with Hodgkin's disease treated during childhood are premature coronary artery disease, myocardial infarction, and chronic constrictive pericarditis. Radiation-induced tissue fibrosis and necrosis of the vascular endothelium lead to ischemic damage by impairment of microcirculation of the pericardium and coronary arteries. Because this injury may not become clinically significant until many years after therapy (101), the true risk for cardiac injury in children treated with radiation is not yet defined. The frequency of radiation-related cardiovascular injury is related to the total and fractional doses, volume and specific region of the heart treated, and the relative weighting of the radiation portals (102). Higher rates of pericardial and coronary artery disease have been observed in patients irradiated by techniques considered unacceptable by contemporary radiation oncologists. Techniques and treatment that are not acceptable today include anteriorly weighted ports, tumor doses greater than 40 Gy,

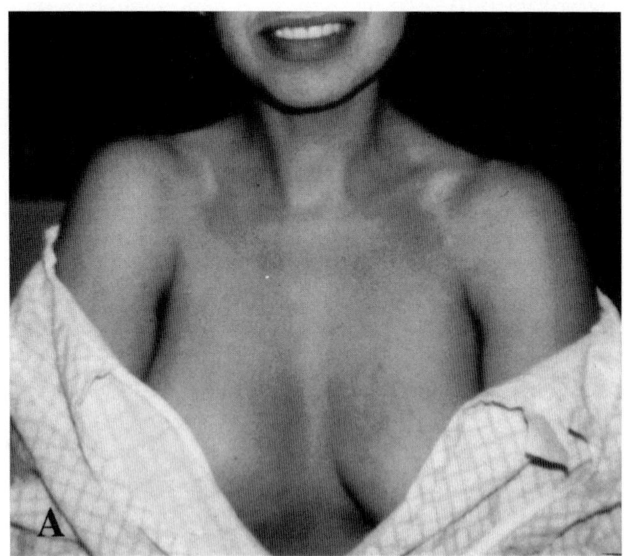

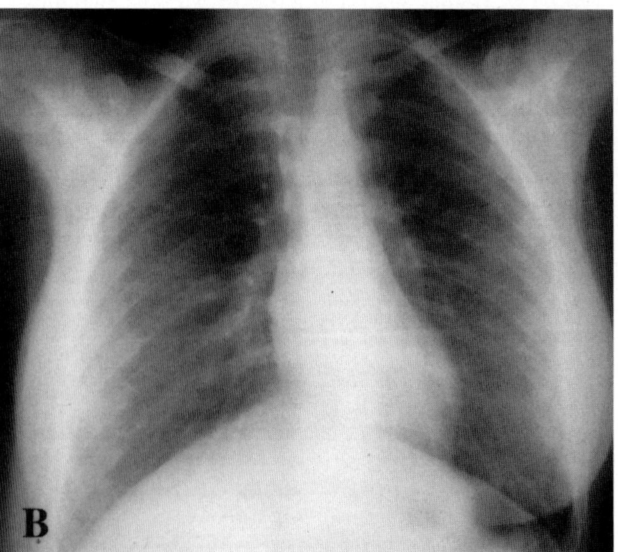

FIG. 6. Clinical **(A)** and radiographic **(B)** 25-year follow-up demonstrating narrowing of the thoracic apex, symmetric shortening of the clavicles, and atrophy of the neck tissues in a woman treated with 40 Gy of total-lymphoid irradiation at age 5. (From ref. 93, with permission of Wiley-Liss.)

TABLE 4. *Cardiopulmonary complications after Hodgkin's disease*

Cardiovascular sequelae
Cardiomyopathy with congestive heart failure
Acute pericarditis
Pericardial effusion
Chronic constrictive pericarditis
Coronary artery disease with myocardial infarction
Conducting system abnormalities, e.g., complete heart or bundle branch block, ventricular arrhythmia
Valvular dysfunction
Peripheral vascular disease
Pulmonary sequelae
Radiation pneumonitis
Pulmonary fibrosis
Spontaneous pneumothorax
Veno-occlusive disease

daily fraction doses greater than 2 Gy, and multiple courses of radiation. Clinically apparent cardiac disease occurs infrequently in survivors of Hodgkin's disease treated during childhood or adolescence with modern radiation therapy techniques (103,104). However, morphologic abnormalities of screening echocardiograms observed in high frequency in some pediatric cohorts emphasize the importance of longitudinal follow-up to determine the incidence of clinically significant pericardial disease and myocardial dysfunction as this group ages (103–105).

The clinical manifestations of radiation-related cardiovascular injury include pericarditis, cardiomyopathy, coronary artery disease with myocardial infarction, conduction system disease, valvular disease, and peripheral vascular disease. Pericardial injury from radiation may present as acute pericarditis during mediastinal radiation, delayed acute pericarditis, chronic pericardial effusions, or chronic constrictive pericarditis (102,106). In a Stanford series of survivors of childhood Hodgkin's disease, the actuarial risk of cardiac disease requiring pericardiectomy was 4% at 17 years (107). Patients with severe pericardial complications received little or no cardiac blocking, and most were irradiated before the introduction of subcarinal blocking. The recognition of radiation-induced pericardial diseases described in this and other series has resulted in the modification of irradiation techniques to reduce the dose of radiation to the heart (105,108). Incidence rates of acute pericarditis or asymptomatic effusions have declined in later cohorts who received partial cardiac shielding and subcarinal blocking (109), suggesting that the risk for clinically significant pericardial disease is related to the total cardiac dose and volume.

Results of studies of adult survivors of Hodgkin's disease implicating mediastinal radiation therapy in the acceleration of ischemic coronary artery disease were conflicting and difficult to interpret because of the presence of coexisting clinical and familial risk factors for the development of atherosclerosis (102,106,110–113). Subsequent reports in survivors of pediatric Hodgkin's disease suggested that they were at risk for premature coronary artery disease and acute myocardial infarction (107,114,115). Younger age at diagnosis increases the risk. Hancock et al. (48) observed a 45-fold excess risk of death from acute myocardial infarction in patients who received mediastinal irradiation in doses exceeding 30 Gy before 20 years of age. An increased risk for a fatal cardiac event after Hodgkin's disease in patients in their cohort was associated with irradiation with high mediastinal doses, minimal protective cardiac blocking, young age at irradiation, and increasing duration of follow-up. This and other studies of survivors of adult and pediatric Hodgkin's disease did not suggest an association between use of chemotherapy, with or without mediastinal irradiation, and an increased risk for premature coronary artery disease (116). The potential contribution of chemotherapy to radiation-related cardiac injury may be difficult to determine, as combined-modality treatment plans now prescribe lower doses and volumes of mediastinal radiation and protective cardiac shielding. Follow-up of the Stanford cohort indicates that none of the 192 children treated with combined therapy have died of a myocardial infarction (107).

Radiation injury to the cardiovascular microcirculation has been implicated in other sequelae involving the myocardium, conducting system, valves, and peripheral blood vessels. The more prevalent use of noninvasive cardiac imaging has facilitated the diagnosis of myocardial injury, which may range from asymptomatic ventricular dysfunction to severe exercise intolerance, dyspnea, and edema. Conducting system abnormalities are well-documented sequelae of high-dose mediastinal radiation therapy. Conducting system disease may result from diffuse fibrosis extending from the myocardium or limitation of the arterial supply to the conduction pathways. Clinical manifestations of ischemia of the conducting system observed in survivors of Hodgkin's disease include complete heart and bundle branch blocks (106,114,117,118). Valvular disease has seldom been observed after radiation therapy, despite earlier reports of thickened valvular endocardium in autopsy specimens of patients heavily irradiated before 27 years of age. Fatal cardiac events have been attributed to valvular dysfunction in several series of pediatric patients with Hodgkin's disease (105,106). Their infrequent occurrence, however, has led to the conclusion that radiation-induced valvular injury is rarely clinically significant. Finally, radiation therapy has been implicated in peripheral vascular abnormalities, including fibrosis, inflammation, atherosclerosis, narrowing, occlusion, thrombosis, and necrosis (101). These pathologic changes have been associated with clinical syndromes of chronic peripheral vascular disease, stroke, and vessel rupture.

Sequelae of Chemotherapy

The most common chemotherapeutic agents implicated in the development of cardiovascular complications in patients with Hodgkin's disease include the Vinca alkaloids, alkylating agents, and anthracyclines. Raynaud's syndrome is an uncommon toxicity observed in some patients. This phenomenon appears to be caused by irreversible microvascular injury in patients treated with the combination of vinblastine and bleomycin. Rarely, myocardial infarctions in Hodgkin's patients have been attributed to Vinca alkaloid therapy. Proposed mechanisms for this complication include ischemia resulting from coronary artery spasm or hypercoagulability.

Adverse effects of cyclophosphamide on the myocardium are observed primarily when high cumulative doses are administered in the setting of high-dose preparatory regimens for hematopoietic stem cell transplantation in adults (119,120). There are no studies of cyclophosphamide-related cardiac sequelae unique to the pediatric population, and so age-related toxicity remains unclear. Conventional doses of cyclophosphamide are generally well tolerated but may exacerbate anthracycline- or radiation-induced cardiac injury. Cardiac complications reported in association with cyclophosphamide include acute myocarditis, congestive heart failure, QRS voltage abnormalities, left ventricular dysfunction, pericardial effusions, fibrinous pericarditis, myocardial fibrosis, and hemorrhage. Cyclophosphamide cardiotoxicity has been attributed to myocardial endothelial damage, resulting in extravasation of blood containing high levels of the drug.

Cardiac dysfunction in survivors of Hodgkin's disease treated with chemotherapy is most commonly related to anthracycline chemotherapy, particularly with doxorubicin. Clinical manifestations of cardiac injury observed after doxorubicin therapy range from minor rhythm disturbances to life-threatening congestive heart failure. Acute toxicities observed during doxorubicin infusions are relatively common and include sinus and supraventricular tachycardias and premature ventricular complexes. More serious arrhythmias uncommonly occur, including complete heart block, ventricular tachycardia, and sudden death, which have no relationship to the development of chronic cardiomyopathy. Rarely, acute toxicity is manifested by the onset of congestive heart failure associated with pericardial effusions and diffuse myocardial injury (121). Chronic toxic effects of anthracycline are manifested as a rapidly progressive biventricular congestive heart failure that is associated with a 50% to 60% early mortality.

Several clinical parameters have been associated with an increased risk for doxorubicin-induced cardiomyopathy. The incidence of congestive heart failure begins to increase logarithmically when cumulative doses of doxorubicin exceed 550 mg/m^2 (122). Studies of survivors of childhood leukemia indicate that young children may be more sensitive to anthracycline injury because of its adverse effect on cardiac myocyte growth (49). Children show a high frequency of abnormalities of afterload and contractility at lower cumulative doses of anthracyclines in follow-up of long-term survivors (49). These abnormalities correlate with an increased risk for congestive heart failure. Concomitant treatment exposures (e.g., mediastinal radiation therapy and other chemotherapeutic agents, including cyclophosphamide, ifosfamide, actinomycin D, mitomycin C, and dacarbazine) may intensify the cardiotoxic effects of anthracyclines and lower the threshold cumulative dose to approximately 350 to 400 mg/m^2 (123,124). The schedule of doxorubicin administration may also have a significant impact on the risk for development of congestive heart failure. Several studies have indicated that patients treated with smaller doses on a weekly schedule or by continuous infusion have a lower incidence of congestive failure than patients receiving larger doses every 3 weeks (125–127). Thus, the occurrence of chemotherapy induced cardiac dysfunction is rare with contemporary regimens that limit cumulative doses of anthracycline-containing chemotherapy programs.

Noninvasive diagnostic imaging modalities have permitted the assessment of ventricular function during and after anthracycline therapy. A decline in resting left ventricular function, manifested by fractional shortening on echocardiography or shortened ejection fraction on radionuclear angiography (128), is useful in predicting impending cardiac failure in patients on therapy. The QT_c interval, prolongation of which is predictive of impending cardiomyopathy during anthracycline therapy and the potential for sudden death from dysrhythmia, may also be a useful parameter to follow in patients during and after anthracycline therapy (129,130). The more costly and invasive procedures of endomyocardial biopsy and cardiac catheterization provide the most accurate assessment of ventricular function, but these are typically reserved for symptomatic patients.

Clinically significant anthracycline-related cardiotoxicity may be acute (beginning within 6 months of completion of therapy) or late in onset. The risk for late cardiac decompensation is greatest in patients with abnormal cardiac function at the end of therapy (131). Late-onset anthracycline-induced cardiomyopathy may present as congestive heart failure, conduction abnormalities, and ventricular dysrhythmia (132). Factors precipitating late cardiac decompensation are childbirth (131,133), viral infections (118), isometric exercise (132), alcohol and cocaine ingestion (132), and growth hormone-induced growth spurts (134).

Treatment of anthracycline-induced cardiomyopathy includes withdrawal of the drug and conventional treatment for congestive heart failure. Patients with progressive deterioration may be candidates for cardiac transplantation. The best management is prevention of cardiac injury by restricting the cumulative dose of anthracycline. Preliminary investigations of newly developed intracellular iron-chelating agents indicate that anthracycline-induced cardiotoxicity as well as bleomycin-induced pulmonary fibrosis can be prevented by protecting cardiopulmonary tissues from damaging free radicals. Further evaluation of these agents is under way to ensure that the cytotoxic effects of these drugs are not compromised.

Pulmonary Sequelae

Several acute and chronic pulmonary complications have been reported following therapy for Hodgkin's disease, including radiation pneumonitis, pulmonary fibrosis, spontaneous pneumothorax, and veno-occlusive disease of the lung, although symptomatic sequelae are uncommon among pediatric patients (Table 4). Many early studies describing pulmonary sequelae after Hodgkin's therapy reflect toxicity caused by treatment practices that have been significantly modified as a result of greater appreciation of late effects and advances in radiation technology. Recent studies of pediatric patients with Hodgkin's disease indicate a significant incidence of asymptomatic pulmonary dysfunction after treatment with combined-modality regimens that include radiation therapy and ABVD (18,19,135). Sequential evaluations after completion of therapy show improvement in pulmonary function in some pediatric cohorts (136). However, the impact of residual subclinical pulmonary injury remains to be determined as this population ages (see Chapter 34 for further details).

Radiation pneumonitis and pulmonary fibrosis are the most frequent pulmonary complications observed following mantle irradiation. The degree of pulmonary injury from irradiation is related to the total radiation dose, daily fraction size, and treatment volume (137,138). Mediastinal radiation therapy unavoidably results in irradiation of nearby pulmonary tissues, which can be substantial if extensive nodal involvement is present. Signs and symptoms of radiation pneumonitis develop in up to 20% of patients who receive mantle irradiation. The majority of these patients are asymptomatic, and only 25% require treatment. The use of lung blocks and the administration of chemotherapy in patients with bulky mediastinal disease has reduced the incidence of symptomatic pulmonary dysfunction to less than 5%.

Radiation-related lung damage is characterized by an early inflammatory phase that develops 1 to 8 months after irradiation, followed by a late fibrotic phase. Pulmonary dysfunction observed in the early phase has been reported to remit partly or completely, unless fibrosis develops. The volume of lung irradiated appears to be the most important factor in the development of pulmonary fibrosis; the type of chemotherapy prescribed in combined-modality regimens is also significant. Minor restrictive ventilatory defects (reduction in vital capacity and total lung compliance) observed after mediastinal irradiation are increased in patients treated with combined-modality regimens that include ABVD chemotherapy (15,139). ABVD-related pulmonary toxicity may result from fibrosis induced by bleomycin or "radiation recall" pneumonitis related to administration of doxorubicin (140).

Less commonly reported complications after Hodgkin's disease include spontaneous pneumothorax and pulmonary veno-occlusive disease. An increased frequency of spontaneous pneumothorax has been observed in patients receiving standard-dose mantle irradiation for Hodgkin's disease (141,142). This complication tends to recur and is seen most commonly in patients with radiographic evidence of pulmonary fibrosis. Reexpansion is often spontaneous, but occasionally tube thoracostomy or rarely pleurectomy is necessary.

Pulmonary veno-occlusive disease has been rarely reported in patients with Hodgkin's disease (143). In most cases, this complication has been attributed to chemotherapeutic agents, particularly bleomycin. Other predisposing treatments include cytoreductive agents used in hematopoietic stem cell transplantation (high-dose cyclophosphamide and busulfan) and possibly radiation therapy. The damage to the venous system is confined to the radiation therapy portal and is typified by hypertensive pulmonary arterial changes and thrombotic veno-occlusive lesions in the pulmonary veins. The incidence of veno-occlusive disease may be underreported because some cases are misdiagnosed as pulmonary fibrosis.

Second Malignant Tumors

The development of a second malignancy is the most serious late treatment complication to occur in survivors of Hodgkin's disease. The most common risk factors to be considered, particularly in patients treated during childhood, are potential genetic influences and the type of treatment received. Newly acquired knowledge of genetic predisposition and secondary carcinogenesis related to tumor suppressor genes such as Rb and p53 has greatly augmented our understanding of cancers in both children and adults. However, among survivors of Hodgkin's disease, the association of malignancies with treatment has been given more attention than the genetic influences predisposing survivors to a second malignancy. Possible genetic influences are of particular importance in the light of the recent discovery of BRCA1 and BRCA2 genes associated with breast, ovarian, and prostate cancers. In addition, Hodgkin's disease is known to be accompanied by defective cellular immunity, which may leave a patient at risk for the development of other malignancies. Finally, in assessing the severity and impact of a second cancer in survivors of Hodgkin's disease, it is important to consider all causes of mortality in children and adolescents in whom Hodgkin's disease has been previously diagnosed. In the Stanford experience of 694 children and teenagers followed for up to 31 years after treatment for Hodgkin's disease and analyzed for causes of death, recurrent Hodgkin's disease accounted for more than half of all deaths, accidents or other causes for one-fourth, and secondary cancers for one-fifth (144) (Fig. 7).

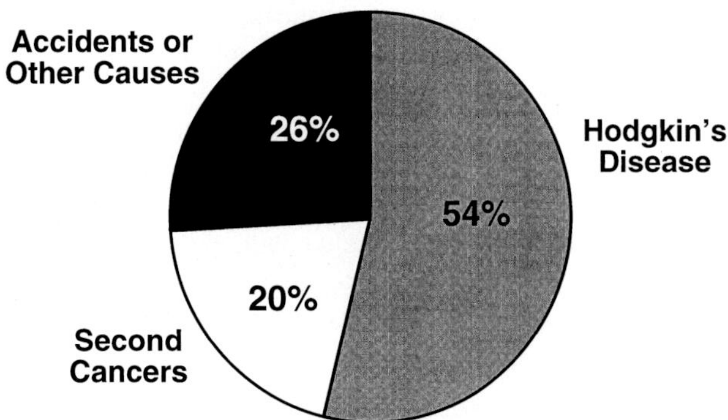

FIG. 7. Causes of mortality among children with Hodgkin's disease. (From ref. 144, with permission of WB Saunders.)

In the early 1970s, it became apparent that chemotherapy with alkylating agents, such as were administered in the MOPP combination, could cause second malignancies. This sequela has since been documented in both adults and children (145–147). These malignancies present as acute myeloid leukemia or myelodysplastic syndrome and have a poor prognosis. The main risk for these leukemias is the cumulative dose of alkylating agent received, particularly mechlorethamine (nitrogen mustard) (148,149), although cyclophosphamide is also a likely leukemogen (150). A standardized incidence ratio (calculated as the ratio of observed to expected cases, or relative risk) for any leukemia of 78.8 (95% CI, 56.6–123.2) and a standard incidence ratio of 321.3 (95% CI, 207.5–76.1) for acute myeloid leukemia/myelodysplastic syndrome were reported from the Late Effects Study Group (LESG) for children less than 16 years of age treated with chemotherapy (151). The standard incidence ratio was reduced to 122 (95% CI, 36–254) with lower cumulative doses of alkylating agents and the omission of mechlorethamine in the German-Austrian OPPA (or OPA)/COPP (or COMP) studies of pediatric Hodgkin's disease (23). The use of ABVD in lieu of MOPP greatly reduces this risk (149). The epipodophyllotoxins and nitrosoureas have also contributed to the development of secondary acute nonlymphocytic leukemia (152). Acute lymphoblastic leukemia and chronic myelogenous leukemia have been reported in patients with Hodgkin's disease, but their incidence does not exceed that expected on the basis of chance. The leukemia risk following radiation alone is extremely low (zero probability in the LESG experience).

The highest risk for secondary leukemia is within the first 5 years of follow-up. It is extraordinarily rare for leukemia to occur after 15 years of follow-up (98,144,151). The risk for leukemia as a function of prior splenectomy or splenic radiotherapy varies. The Institut Gustave-Roussy investigators found an increased relative risk (RR) for leukemia following splenectomy (RR, 2.54; $p = .018$) and prior splenic irradiation (RR, 3.67; $p = .003$) among adults with Hodgkin's disease (153). However, other large series of children and adolescents have not confirmed an increased incidence of leukemia associated with splenectomy among children treated for Hodgkin's disease (see Chapter 33 for further details) (144,151).

The risk for non-Hodgkin's lymphoma is also increased following treatment, with a standard incidence ratio of 20.9 (95% CI, 7.7–42) in the LESG experience (children were less than 16 years of age) (15) and a standard incidence ratio of 15 (95% CI, 4.9–35) in the five Nordic countries (Denmark, Finland, Iceland, Norway, and Sweden) (children were less than 20 years of age) (154). As well as being associated with treatment administered, this risk may be related to overall immunosuppression associated with the disease and its treatment. Several authors have reported the risks for non-Hodgkin's lymphoma combined with the risk for acute nonlymphocytic leukemia in pediatric Hodgkin's disease. When the two entities are combined, acute nonlymphocytic leukemia and non-Hodgkin's lymphoma are seen more commonly in adolescents than in patients less than 10 years of age (155).

The standard incidence ratio of a solid tumor that arises after treatment for Hodgkin's disease is 11.8 (95% CI, 8.7–15.4) in the LESG study (151). The most common solid tumors in that report were of the breast (SIR, 75.3; CI, 44.9–118.4), thyroid (SIR, 32.7; CI, 15.3–55.3), bone (SIR, 24.6; CI, 6.4–54.5), brain (SIR, 10.5; CI, 2.7–23.4), colorectum (SIR, 38.9; CI, 7.3–95.3), and stomach (SIR, 12.3; CI, 11.4–145.2). Similarly, the Stanford experience in children (less than 21 years of age) revealed significantly increased but differing risks for such solid tumors as sarcoma (RR, 81.9; CI, 43.6–140.1), melanoma (RR, 8.7; CI, 2.7–21.1), and cancers of the breast (RR, 26.2; CI, 15.0–42.6), lung (RR, 29.9; CI, 9.4–72.3), thyroid (RR, 9.7; CI, 2.4–26.4), salivary gland (RR, 24.4; CI, 6.1–66.6), and stomach (RR, 55.6; CI, 9.2–183.6) (144). Non-melanomatous skin cancers, including basal cell carcinomas, are also common. Figure 8 reveals the actuarial risk for any second malignancy, solid tumor, or hematologic malignancy among 372 pediatric patients from the St. Jude Children's Research Hospital with 27-year follow-up.

The latency period for the development of solid tumors is much longer than that for the development of leukemia, with solid tumors appearing more than 10 years after treatment; the incidence rises with increasing follow-up (144,151). The incidence of solid tumors is related to the treatment administered and is most common following radiotherapy and chemotherapy. The 15-year cumulative probability of induction of solid tumors in the LESG experience was as follows: radiation, 3.3 (CI, 2.9–3.7); chemotherapy, 2.9 (CI, 2.3–3.5); and radiation plus chemotherapy, 4.6 (CI, 4.4–4.8). Many of the secondary solid tumors are effectively treated. Among 56 patients in the LESG experience with solid tumors, 17 died, 10 of second neoplasms (8%) and seven as the result of acci-

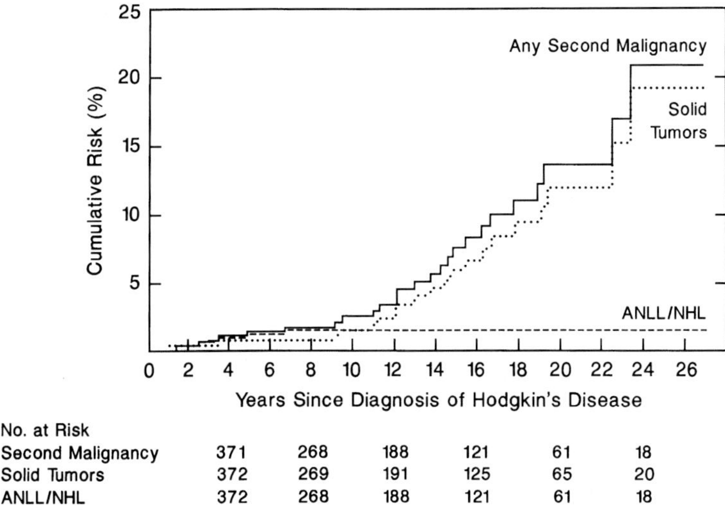

FIG. 8. Cumulative risk for second malignancy, second solid tumor, or second ANLL/NHL (acute nonlymphocytic leukemia/non-Hodgkin's lymphoma) following therapy for Hodgkin's disease in childhood. (From ref. 155, with permission of WB Saunders.)

dents (11%), whereas 39 (70%) were alive 12.5 months after diagnosis (151).

In the Stanford experience, of the tumors that developed in irradiated patients, 90% were within or at the margin of a radiotherapy portal (144). All sarcomas were within radiotherapy ports. The mean radiation dose was 45.8 Gy in this series. In contrast, however, thyroid tumors may occur after low doses of radiation doses (9.8–25 Gy) in the Stanford experience (144).

Much attention has been given to the increasing awareness of the significant risk for breast cancer after treatment for Hodgkin's disease. Although early reports showed only a modestly increased risk among women treated with radiation and MOPP chemotherapy, the dramatic increase in risk became apparent when patients were followed longer than 15 years after Hodgkin's disease therapy (156). The relative risk for the development of invasive breast cancer among Hodgkin's disease survivors was 4.1 (95% CI, 2.5–5.7) in 885 women (ages 4 to 81 years; mean, 28 years) from Stanford followed for an average of 10 years, or 8,832 person-years of observation (156). The risk was highest for those who received irradiation before the age of 15 years: the relative risk was 136 (95% CI, 34–371) and the absolute risk was 38.4. The relative risk declines with age but remains elevated in female patients less than 30 years of age at the time of irradiation. No increased risk was detected for women older than 30 years at the time of treatment. Similarly, the absolute risk is elevated in these groups until age 30 (Table 5) (156). In a follow-up analysis of 694 children with Hodgkin's disease, the relative risk for breast cancer was 26.2, with 3,741 person-years at risk. All cases were in female patients; no male breast cancers have been reported. Other investigators have attributed the increased risk in female patients for induction of a second malignant tumor after treatment to the increased incidence of breast cancer among those in the adolescent age group when treated (151,154,157,158).

Breast cancer is related to radiation exposure, although chemotherapy with alkylating agents also increases the risk (151,156). A high dose of radiation is a risk factor, with most breast cancers arising after 40 to 46 Gy of

TABLE 5. *Breast cancer risk after treatment of Hodgkin's disease*

Group	No. at risk	Person-years at risk	Observed/ expected events	RR[a]	95% CIs	Absolute risk[b]
All patients	885	8,759	25/6.13	4.1	2.5–5.7	21.5
Age (y)						
<15	76	776	3/0.02	136.0	34–371	38.4
15–19	156	1,696	3/0.16	19.0	4.7–51	16.7
20–24	180	1,807	9/0.47	19.0	9.3–35	47.2
25–29	173	1,853	7/0.96	7.3	3.2–14	32.6
30–39	177	1,651	1/1.75	0.6	0.0–2.8	—
40–49	51	502	1/1.08	0.9	0.0–4.6	—
≥50	72	474	1/1.69	0.6	0.0–2.9	—

[a]Relative risk (RR) calculated as ratio of observed to expected events, with 95% confidence intervals (CIs).
[b]Absolute risk expressed as excess numbers of cases per 10,000 person-years.
From ref. 156.

mantle irradiation, although some reported cases also received 12 to 16 Gy of lung irradiation on the side of the breast cancer (156). In the Stanford pediatric experience, no breast cancers have occurred in any girls who received a radiation dose of less than 40 Gy (144).

The impact of genetics on breast cancer (patients receiving combined-modality treatment may carry the BRCA1 or BRCA2 gene) has not yet been evaluated.

Treatment for second solid tumors, particularly breast cancer, must be individualized. However, most oncologists today recommend mastectomy as opposed to breast-conserving therapy with lumpectomy and breast radiation for a patient previously irradiated for Hodgkin's disease.

Sex is a factor influencing the risk for a second cancer; female patients have a hazard ratio of 1.8 in comparison with male patients, explained by their increased incidence of breast cancer. However, the strongest predictor for development of a second malignancy is relapse of Hodgkin's disease, for which the hazard ratio is 2.6 (p <0.001) (144). Additionally, exposure to chemotherapeutic regimens containing alkylating agents correlates with the development of leukemia, with a hazard ratio 10.7 (p = .03). These observations serve as a guide to the management of children in whom Hodgkin's disease has been newly diagnosed. Thus, new protocols must be designed with the following goals kept in mind:

1. Initial treatment should be administered with a curative intent so to minimize the likelihood of relapse of disease and the aggressive salvage therapy that is mandated by relapse.
2. High doses of irradiation, particularly to the axilla and mediastinum, should be avoided in women younger than 30 years at the time of treatment. Current protocols for pediatric Hodgkin's disease in which low-dose involved-field radiotherapy and chemotherapy are used meet this goal.

Guidelines for follow-up of previously treated patients at high risk for the development of second malignant tumors include the following:

1. The complete blood count should be monitored for at least 10 years after administration of chemotherapy to evaluate for leukemia and myelodysplastic syndrome.
2. A follow-up examination should be performed annually by an oncologist, who inspects and images areas irradiated more than 10 years previously and looks for solid tumors.
3. Breast self-examination and mammography, beginning 10 years after treatment and continued annually, are mandatory for any woman who was 30 years or younger when irradiated for Hodgkin's disease.
4. A careful examination of the skin, with a search for lesions, should be performed annually.

TABLE 6. *Risk for a second cancer following childhood Hodgkin's disease*

	After 15 y	After 30 y
Any cancer	7.0%	14.4%
Solid tumor	4.1%	8.2%

From refs. 151 and 159.

5. The patient should undergo a routine physical examination and general surveillance annually, with special attention given to the thyroid examination.
6. Specific signs or symptoms in a patient previously treated for Hodgkin's disease that could possibly suggest a new primary tumor (i.e., bone pain, dysphagia, cough, pigmented skin lesion) should be evaluated.

Current pediatric protocols, which comprise clinical staging and combined-modality treatment with a limited number of cycles of chemotherapy, thereby minimizing exposure to alkylating agents, and low-dose involved-field radiotherapy, are designed to decrease or eliminate altogether the risk for second malignant tumors.

Reports of second malignant tumors in Hodgkin's disease reveal widely differing estimates of risk and raise issues about the best way to estimate these risks. The results of standard incidence ratio or relative risk tests of observed events compared with expected events in a population are markedly elevated because of the rarity of events in the comparable general population at similar ages. Actuarial or cumulative risks are high when a single event develops late in the course of follow-up. The actuarial or cumulative analysis is also magnified when data are censored at early follow-up intervals or patients are lost to follow-up, and a late adverse event is more likely to be reported—in other words, "bad news travels fast." In addition, actuarial risks are derived from treatments given several decades ago and may be a poor predictor for outcome of more modern therapy. The assessment of absolute risk provides a method of quantifying magnitude of risk. The absolute risk of a secondary cancer in the LESG assessment is 17.7 excess cancers or 27.5 excess solid tumors per 10,000 person-years of observation (159). At 15 years after exposure, this predicts a 7% risk for a secondary cancer and a 4.1% risk for a solid tumor (159). By 30 years after exposure, the likelihood of a second cancer is 14.4%, and for a solid tumor it is 8.2% (Table 6). Thus, with current therapy for children who have Hodgkin's disease, in which chemotherapy containing alkylating agents is limited or omitted altogether, the risk for a second cancer should be much less than 5% at 15 years after treatment. However, because the number of deaths caused by Hodgkin's disease far surpasses the number caused by a complication of therapy, protocols to provide high cure rates remain the highest priority for treatment.

CURRENT TRIALS

Combined-modality Therapy

In the 1970s, several pediatric institutions and cooperative groups initiated clinical trials evaluating combined-modality therapy for pediatric patients with Hodgkin's disease. Late sequelae of treatment, identified during long-term follow-up of survivors of childhood disease, guided the development of protocol therapy. The early trials used the novel concept of combined-modality therapy as a means to improve cure rates in patients with advanced-stage disease and reduce impairment of musculoskeletal growth caused by standard-dose radiation therapy. In the 1980s, with long-term follow-up demonstrating the feasibility and efficacy of combination chemotherapy in pediatric Hodgkin's disease, study objectives were focused specifically on further improving cure rates for patients with advanced-stage disease and reducing the MOPP-related sequelae of infertility and secondary leukemia. During this era, the use of standard-dose radiation therapy was eventually limited to adolescents with localized disease who had completed their growth. Radiation was reduced in combined-modality regimens to lower doses and involved fields. As combined-modality therapy became the standard for most pediatric patients with Hodgkin's disease, staging laparotomy was abandoned at most centers because of potential acute toxicity and concern about infectious, gastrointestinal, and neoplastic complications of splenectomy. By the end of the era, 6 cycles of combination therapy had evolved as the standard. Follow-up of survivors treated with multiagent chemotherapy regimens has indicated excellent sustained, disease-free survival and reduced incidence of chemotherapy-induced cardiopulmonary, gonadal, and neoplastic complications; however, much longer follow-up periods are required to assess late effects.

The desire to avoid the secondary development of radiation-related solid tumors observed in long-term survivors of Hodgkin's disease has been the driving force behind protocols developed in the 1990s. Ongoing trials are evaluating the efficacy of regimens that further limit chemotherapy and radiation therapy exposures in clinically staged patients. Novel intensive and abbreviated regimens are also under investigation in patients with advanced-stage disease; these are anticipated to improve outcome, particularly for patients with extranodal disease. Tables 7, 8, and 9 summarize the results of selected series of combined-modality therapy in pediatric Hodgkin's disease.

A major objective of the use of chemotherapy in pediatric protocols was to replace prophylactic irradiation in children with localized disease. At the time of the randomized American Intergroup Hodgkin's Disease Study (162), a separate study was conducted in France in which MOPP chemotherapy and involved-field high-dose radiation therapy were used. Among 37 children with CS IA–IIA disease, no infradiaphragmatic recurrence was observed (9). The second cooperative study of the German-Austria Study Group, HD-82, demonstrated that effective chemotherapy makes it possible to limit the radiation fields to involved areas (10,13). The same radiation fields were used in the first French MDH82 cooperative study and in the Polish study with excellent results (20,167). These studies have repeatedly demonstrated excellent outcome with involved-field radiation and multiagent chemotherapy. Failures have been rare, and specific patterns of failure are not apparent.

Reduction of radiation doses was another objective of the combined-modality approach. Investigators at Stanford and at the Princess Margaret Hospital in Toronto were the first to initiate combined-modality protocols uniquely designed for children with Hodgkin's disease (2,168). In the first Stanford study, laparotomy-staged children received low doses of radiation therapy in conjunction with 6 cycles of MOPP chemotherapy (4). The Princess Margaret investigators extended this approach of using low-dose radiation and 6 cycles of MOPP chemotherapy in clinically staged children, thus avoiding staging laparotomy (163). The actuarial and freedom-from-relapse rates achieved with this combination demonstrated that undesirable growth alterations could be avoided by using low-dose radiation therapy without compromising local control. MOPP was the first widely used chemotherapy combination, but it was associated with male infertility and secondary leukemias among survivors. The 10-year risk of 6.5% for the development of secondary leukemia observed during follow-up of the Stanford children influenced the subsequent Stanford study, which investigated 6 months of alternating ABVD/MOPP and low-dose involved-field irradiation (18). This regimen produced excellent overall and event-free survival rates and was not associated with the development of secondary leukemia. Further, symptomatic cardiac, pulmonary, or thyroid disease did not develop in any of the patients. However, subclinical abnormalities of pulmonary function were detected in 32% of children, and chemical hypothyroidism was found in 16% of children treated with this program.

Simultaneously, the European groups confirmed the efficacy of low doses of radiation with chemotherapy among larger groups of patients. The French MDH82 study tailored radiation according to the response to primary chemotherapy. At the end of chemotherapy, patients who had achieved a good response (at least 70% regression of initially measurable disease) received 20 Gy of involved-field radiation. Only 5% of patients who did not achieve this good response were given 40 Gy. The updated results show that overall survival and disease-free survival rates are, respectively, 93% and 86% at 5 years (20). In the Italian AIEOP study, the radiation dose was 20 or 25 Gy (according to the age of the patient) (14). The results were similar to those in the French experience and validated the safety of 20 Gy of radiotherapy after

TABLE 7. *European-South American combined-modality trials in pediatric Hodgkin's disease*

Institution or group (ref.)	Stage	Chemotherapy	Radiation therapy	No. patients	Outcome (years)			
					EFS	DFS	FFS	Survival (y)
Institut Gustave-Roussy (9)	All stages	6 MOPP	40 Gy, IF	40	86% (15)			93% (15)
		3 MOPP	40 Gy, IF	20				
SFOP MDH-82 (20)	I–IIA	4 ABVD	20–40 Gy, IF	79		90% (6)		
		2 MOPP/2 ABVD	20–40 Gy, IF	67		87% (6)		
	I–IIB	3 MOPP/3 ABVD	20–40 Gy, EF	31				92% (6)
	III	3 MOPP/3 ABVD	20–40 Gy, EF	40		82% (6)		
	IV	3 MOPP/3 ABVD	20–40 Gy, EF	21		62% (6)		
Germany-Austria HD-82 (13)	IA-B–IIA	2 OPPA	35 Gy, IF	100	98% (9)			100% (9)
	IIB–IIIA	2 OPPA/2 COPP	30 Gy, IF	53	94%			96%
	IIIB–IV	2 OPPA/4 COPP	25 Gy, IF	50	86%			85%
HD-85 (13)	IA-B–IIA	2 OPA	35 Gy, IF	53	85% (6)			98% (6)
	IIB–IIIA	2 OPA/2 COMP	30 Gy, IF	21	55%			95%
	IIIB–IV	2 OPA/4 COMP	25 Gy, IF	24	49%			100%
HD-90 (12)	IA-B	2 OEPA/OPPA	25 Gy, IF	274	93/96% (5)			100/100% (5)
	IIB–IIIA	2 OEPA/OPPA + 2 COPP	25 Gy, IF	123	90/96%			100/97%
	IIIB–IV	2 OEPA/OPPA + 4 COPP	20 Gy, IF	178	83/91%			98/89%
AEIOP MH-83 (14)	IA	3 ABVD	20–40 Gy, IF	83			95% (7)	
	IIA (M/T <0.33)	3 ABVD	20–40 Gy, R					
	IIA (M/T ≥0.33)	3 MOPP/3 ABVD	20–40 Gy, R	132			81%	86%
	IIIA	3 MOPP/3 ABVD	20–40 Gy, EF					
	IIIB–IV	5 MOPP/5 ABVD	20–40 Gy, EF				60%	
AIEOP MH'89 (160)	I–IIA (M/T ≥0.33)	3 ABVD	20 Gy, IF	100			91% (7)	
	IB, IEA-B, I–IIA (M/T ≥0.33), IIEA, IIEB, IIB	2 MOPP/2 ABVD	20 Gy, IF	107			79%	94%
	IIIA-IIIEA	4 MOPP/4 ABVD	20 Gy, IF					
	IIIB–IV	2 OPPA/4 COPP	20–36 Gy, IF	50				83%
UKCCSG (36)	I	—	35 Gy, IF	99			70% (10)	92%
	II	6–10 ChlVPP	35 Gy, IF	125			85%	92%
	III		(MMR >1/3)	80			73%	84%
	IV			27			38%	71%
Argentina (161)	I–IV	6 CVPP	30–40 Gy, IF	64	87% (5)			—
	Intermediate prognostic group[a]	6 AOPE	30–40 Gy, IF		67% (5)			—

EFS, event-free survival; DFS, disease-free survival; FFP, freedom from progression; MOPP, Mustargen, Oncovin, procarbazine, prednisone; ABVD, Adriamycin, bleomycin, vinblastine, dacarbazine; OPPA, Oncovin, prednisone, procarbazine, Adriamycin; COPP, cyclophosphamide, Oncovin, procarbazine, prednisone; COMP, cyclophosphamide, Oncovin, methotrexate, prednisone; OEPA, Oncovin, etoposide, prednisone, Adriamycin; ChlVPP, chlorambucil, vinblastine, procarbazine, prednisolone; OPA, Oncovin, prednisone, Adriamycin; CVPP, cyclophosphamide, vincristine, prednisone, procarbazine; AOPE, Adriamycin, Oncovin, prednisone, etopside; IF, involved field; EF, extended field; R, regional; MMR, mediastinal mass rates; M/T, mediastinal mass/thorax rates.

[a]Intermediate prognostic group determined on the basis of age, symptoms, stage and number of nodal regions.

TABLE 8. *North American combined-modality trials in early-stage and favorable pediatric Hodgkin's disease*

Institution or group (ref.)	Stage	Chemotherapy	Radiation therapy	No. patients	Outcome (years)			
					EFS	DFS	RFS	Survival (y)
Stanford (18)	CS/PS I–III	3 MOPP/3 ABVD	15–25 Gy, IF	44	100% (10)			100% (10)
Toronto (22)	CS I–III	3 MOPP/3 ABVD	15 Gy, EF				92% (5)	96% (5)
St. Jude (19)	CS I–IIB	4–5 COP(P)/3–4 ABVD	20 Gy, IF	28		96% (5)		96% (5)
Intergroup Hodgkin's (162)	PS I–II	6 MOPP	≥35 Gy, IF	97			95% (5)	90% (5)
Toronto (163)	CS I–II	6 MOPP	20–30 Gy, EF	22			89% (5)	
Stanford (4)	PS I–II	6 MOPP	15–25 Gy, IF	27			96% (5)	100% (5)
Pediatric Oncology Group (164)	PS I, IIA, IIIA	2 MOPP/2 ABVD	25 Gy, IF	85		84% (4)		—

CS, clinical stage; PS, pathologic stage; MOPP, Mustargen, Oncovin, procarbazine, prednisone; ABVD, Adriamycin, bleomycin, vinblastine, dacarbazine; COP(P), cyclophosphamide, Oncovin, procarbazine, prednisone; IF, involved field; EF, extended field; EFS, event-free survival; DFS, disease-free survival; RFS, relapse-free survival.

effective primary chemotherapy. In addition, the German-Austrian studies demonstrated that 25 and 20 Gy with chemotherapy were effective in their HD-90 study.

Combinations other than MOPP were brought into use to limit exposure to alkylating agents. The ABVD combination is associated with less leukemia induction and less sterility. In Europe, the French group evaluated the results of treatment with 4 cycles of ABVD versus 4 alternating months of MOPP and ABVD in CS IA–IIA disease in the randomized MDH82 study. Disease control in the ABVD arm appeared comparable with that in the MOPP/ABVD arm (20). In a nonrandomized study, the Italian pediatric group confirmed the efficacy of 3 courses of ABVD combined with limited-field radiation in CS IA and IIA patients who did not have large areas of mediastinal disease (14).

The German-Austrian group, which has not used mechlorethamine since the beginning of their studies in 1978, tried to reduce the risk for testicular damage by eliminating procarbazine from the chemotherapy program. Building from their prior OPPA/COPP experience, in their HD-85 study they changed the OPPA cycles to OPA and replaced procarbazine with methotrexate in COPP, producing COMP. The study was stopped prematurely because of disappointing results, confirming the need for an effective agent to replace procarbazine (10,13). This led to the HD-90 study, in which girls received the same OPPA/COPP chemotherapy that had been given in the HD-82 study because no ovarian damage had resulted from this chemotherapy. In boys, etoposide was substituted for procarbazine in the initial OPPA cycles, so that they received OEPA. After 5 years, there appeared to be no difference in the results between the boys and girls (26). Simultaneously, the German-Austrian investigators reduced the radiation doses to 20 to 25 Gy in the HD-90 study.

The St. Jude investigators initiated a similar series of combined-modality trials with the objectives of improving

TABLE 9. *North American combined-modality trials in advanced-stage and unfavorable pediatric Hodgkin's disease*

Institution or group (ref.)	Stage	Chemotherapy	Radiation therapy	No. patients	Outcome (years)			
					EFS	DFS	RFS	Survival (y)
CCG (165)	PS III–IV	6 ABVD	21 Gy, IF, EF, or TLI	54	87% (4)			90% (4)
Stanford (18)	CS/PS IV	3 MOPP/3 ABVD	15–25 Gy, IF	13	69% (10)			85% (10)
St. Jude (19)	CS III–IV	4–5 COP(P)/3–4 ABVD	20 Gy, IF	57		93% (5)		93% (5)
POG (21)	PS III–IV	4 MOPP/4 ABVD	21 Gy, TLI	80	80% (5)			87% (5)
Toronto (5)	CS IV	6 MOPP	25–35 Gy, EF	15			82% (5)	80% (5)
CCG (166)	PS III–IV	12 ABVD	21 Gy, R	65	87% (3)			89% (3)
Stanford (4)	PS III–IV	6 MOPP	15–25 Gy, IF	28			84% (5)	78% (5)

CCG, Children's Cancer Group; POG, Pediatric Oncology Group; PS, pathologic stage; CS, clinical stage; ABVD, Adriamycin, bleomycin, vinblastine, dacarbazine; COP(P), cyclophosphamide, Oncovin, procarbazine, prednisone; MOPP, Mustargen, Oncovin, procarbazine, prednisone; IF, involved field; EF, extended field; TLF, total lymphoid irradiation; EFS, event-free survival; DFS, disease-free survival; RFS, relapse-free survival.

cure rates and reducing late treatment sequelae in children and adolescents with Hodgkin's disease. They substituted cyclophosphamide for mechlorethamine in the MOPP combination. Previous combined-modality trials with COPP [cyclophosphamide, Oncovin (vincristine), procarbazine, and prednisone] and low-dose (20-Gy) radiation therapy showed that in comparison with MOPP, COPP had similar efficacy, produced less gonadal damage, and was associated with fewer acute toxic effects, such as emesis, phlebitis, and myelosuppression. In the 1980s, the St. Jude investigators used COP(P)/ABVD in combination with low-dose, involved-field radiation therapy in predominantly clinically staged patients. The 5-year actuarial disease-free survival for children in this cohort (93% +/– 5% for all patients and 85% +/– 7% for stage IV patients) was maintained during subsequent follow-up (19). Symptomatic cardiopulmonary dysfunction rarely occurred. Thyroid abnormalities occurred in approximately one-third of patients, of which subclinical hypothyroidism was the most common. Asymptomatic abnormalities of pulmonary function were evident in 25% of patients tested at least 1 year after completion of therapy. No cases of secondary leukemia were observed in this cohort. However, subsequent follow-up has disclosed one case of secondary breast cancer that developed 9 years after 20 Gy of mantle radiation therapy.

The pediatric cooperative groups established the feasibility and efficacy of combined-modality treatment programs in the multi-institutional setting. Investigators from the Children's Cancer Study Group (CCG) evaluated the efficacy and toxicity of 12 cycles of ABVD chemotherapy followed by low-dose regional irradiation (21 Gy) in advanced-stage Hodgkin's disease. Event-free and overall survival indicated efficacy of this combination in advanced-stage pediatric Hodgkin's disease, but the 9% incidence of acute pulmonary toxicity has limited its application in subsequent trials (166). The Pediatric Oncology Group (POG) investigators initially demonstrated the short-term safety of the alternating non–cross-resistant regimen MOPP/ABVD in conjunction with 21 Gy of total-nodal or modified total-nodal radiation therapy (21). This study has served as the basis for randomized trials in early-stage and advanced-stage pediatric Hodgkin's disease. Surgically staged patients with localized disease had equivalent outcomes when treated with 3 cycles of MOPP alternating with ABVD or 2 cycles of MOPP alternating with ABVD followed by 25 Gy of radiation therapy to involved fields, or with standard-dose radiation therapy alone. A companion study investigated the benefits of low-dose radiation therapy added to 8 cycles of MOPP/ABVD chemotherapy in patients with advanced-stage disease (169).

The goal of all these pediatric combined-modality trials is improved outcome with less short- and long-term toxicity. Although efficacy in terms of event-free survival can be estimated within 5 years of study entry, toxicity issues require many more years of careful assessment. Today, most investigators of pediatric Hodgkin's disease believe that combined-modality therapy is optimal treatment for most children in that it offers the possibility of clinical staging, lower doses and smaller volumes of radiation, and fewer cycles of less toxic chemotherapy in comparison with single-modality therapy. These combined-modality programs now emphasize chemotherapy regimens that limit the cumulative doses of alkylating agents, anthracyclines, and bleomycin, and they use low-dose, involved-field radiation therapy to reduce the frequency and severity of treatment sequelae. However, some unsuccessful modifications of therapy have been associated with inferior disease control, which underscore the caution with which investigators must proceed when attempting to reduce late effects of treatment.

Chemotherapy Alone versus Combined-modality Therapy

Several investigators have demonstrated disease-free survival rates in children with Hodgkin's disease treated with chemotherapy alone that are comparable with those observed after combined-modality therapy. Chemotherapy-alone protocols have several advantages: (a) single-modality treatment with chemotherapy can be utilized in developing countries, where radiation equipment and trained personnel may be lacking; (b) precise surgical or clinical staging, which may be difficult to accomplish in some centers, is not needed; and (c) long-term growth and neoplastic complications associated with radiation therapy are avoided with chemotherapy alone. The potential disadvantages of chemotherapy-alone regimens include (a) higher exposure to alkylating drugs (compared with exposures in combined-modality regimens) and (b) increased morbidity from myelosuppression, gonadal injury, and secondary leukemia.

Early trials reported satisfactory outcomes in children treated with MOPP and similar therapies containing alkylating agents (170–173). Acute hematologic and infectious toxicity was acceptable and manageable in centers with limited resources. As anticipated, the limited reports describing long-term gonadal toxicity indicated a high incidence of irreversible sterility and possibly germinal epithelial damage in boys treated with 6 or more cycles of combination chemotherapy containing alkylating agents, regardless of their pubertal status (174). Long-term toxicity has not been thoroughly evaluated, and it may be underestimated because of the difficulty or unwillingness of patients to return for follow-up evaluations after completion of therapy.

Later chemotherapy-only trials in pediatric patients with Hodgkin's disease sought to improve cure rates and reduce treatment sequelae related to alkylating agent chemotherapy by using alternating non–cross-resistant regimens (MOPP/ABVD, COPP/ABV hybrid, CVPP/EBO [cyclophosphamide, vinblastine, procarbazine, prednisone/Epirubicine, bleomycin, vincristine (Oncovin)]) (164,175–

177) or by using combinations without alkylating agents, such as ABVD or EVAP/ABV (etoposide, vinblastine, cytosine arabinoside, *cis*-platinum, doxorubicin, bleomycin, and vincristine) (178,179). Most of these trials comprised small cohorts of clinically staged patients with early-stage Hodgkin's disease; some trials specifically excluded patients with "bulky" disease. Results indicate that treatment with 6 cycles of alternating chemotherapy programs can produce disease-free survival rates comparable in short-term follow-up with those achieved with combined-modality regimens of fewer than 6 cycles of chemotherapy plus low-dose, involved-field radiation (Table 10). Acute toxicity related to these regimens appears to be acceptable; however, long-term follow-up is not available to evaluate long-term morbidity.

More than 25 years ago, because of the lack of radiation facilities in Uganda, children were treated with 6 cycles of MOPP chemotherapy alone. Among the 48 treated children, 42 entered complete remission (11 of 11 stages I and II, 21 of 23 stage III, and 10 of 14 stage IV) and 11 (26%) relapsed. Overall survival was 75% for stages I and II and 60% for stages III and IV (180). With this background, several pediatric teams opted for programs of chemotherapy alone to avoid the late consequences of radiation therapy. In Australia, children with stages I and II disease received 6 cycles of MOPP, and children with more advanced disease received from 6 to 12 cycles (172). In a subsequent study, in an attempt to reduce the risk for sterility and secondary leukemias, depending on the bulk of disease, the same investigators used 3 to 6 cycles of the EVAP/ABV combination. This regimen achieved long-lasting remission in only 60% of the patients. The patients who relapsed were often salvaged with MOPP or ChlVPP chemotherapy. This therapy was considered by the authors to be suboptimal

TABLE 10. *Treatment results in pediatric Hodgkin's disease with chemotherapy alone*

Institution or group (ref.)	Stage	Chemotherapy	No. patients	Outcome (years) EFS	DFS	RFS	TFF	Survival
POG (169)	CS IIB, IIIA2 IIIB, IV	4 MOPP/4 ABVD	81	79% (5)				96% (5)
Argentina (161)	CS IA, IIA	3 CVPP	10	86% (6.7)				—
	CS IB, IIB	6 CVPP	16	87% (6.7)				
The Netherlands (175)	CS I–IV (lymph nodes <4 cm)	6 MOPP	21	91% (10)				10% (10)
		6 ABVD	17	70% (10)				94%
	CS I–IV	6 ABVD/MOPP	21	91% (10)				91%
POG (164)	PSI, IIA, IIIA	3 MOPP/3 ABVD	83		84% (4)			—
The Netherlands (179)	CS I–IV	6 ABVD	17		71% (8)			92% (8)
Nicaragua (180)	CS I, IIA	6 COPP	14	100% (3)				100% (3)
	CS IIB, III, IV	8–10 COPP-ABV	34	75% (3)				
Madras, India (176)	CS I–IIA	6 COPP-ABV	10	89% (5)				—
	CS IIB–IVB		43	90% (5)				—
Costa Rica (177)	CS IA–IIIA	6 CVPP	52			90% (5)		100% (5)
	CS IIIB, IV	6 CVPP/6 EBO	24			60% (5)		81% (5)
Australia-New Zealand (178)	CS IA–IVA	3 EVAP/ABV	25				60% (3.5)	100%
Australia-New) Zealand (167	CS I–IIB	6–8 MOPP or 6 ChlVPP	38				92% (4)	94% (4)
The Netherlands (173)	CS I–II	6 MOPP (<4 cm lymph node)	21		100% (5)			100% (5)
		6 MOPP (≥4 cm lymph node)	16		92% (5)			—
Uganda (170)	CS I–IIIA	6 MOPP	38		75% (5)			—
	CS IIIB–IV	6 MOPP	10		60% (5)			—

EFS, Event-free survival; DFS, disease-free survival; RFS, relapse-free survival; TFF, treatment failure-free; CS, clinical stage; PS, pathologic stage; POG, Pediatric Oncology Group; MOPP, Mustargen, Oncovin, procarbazine, prednisone; ABVD, Adriamycin, bleomycin, vinblastine, dacarbazine; COPP, cyclophopshamide, Oncovin, procarbazine, prednisone; CVPP, cyclophosphamide, vincristine, procarbazine, prednisone; EBO, Epirubicine, bleomycin, Oncovin; EVAP, etoposide, vinblastine, cytosine arabinoside, cis-platium; ChlVPP, vinblastine, procarbazine, prednisone.

mal (178). In Amsterdam, 59 children have been treated with chemotherapy alone since 1975; the first 21, who had no disease greater than 4 cm, received 6 cycles of MOPP (173). The next 17 children received 6 cycles of ABVD; however, the outcome was considered unacceptable, and in a subsequent study, 21 patients received 6 alternating cycles of MOPP and ABVD. The event-free survival and overall survival in this last group was 91%. The authors conclude that this last therapy yields a high cure rate in all children with Hodgkin's disease; however, only six patients had stage III or IV disease, and the number of patients with bulky disease is unknown (175). In the United Kingdom, from 1982 to 1992, patients with stages of disease beyond IA were treated with 6 to 10 cycles of ChlVPP, depending on the time to achieve complete remission. Children with bulky mediastinal disease also were given 35 Gy of consolidative radiotherapy to the mediastinum. The 10-year progression-free survival was 85% for those with stage II disease, 73% for those with stage III disease, and 38% for those with stage IV disease. The overall survival rates were 92%, 84%, and 71%, respectively (36). In a recent study performed in Nicaragua, children with localized disease (IA–IIA) received 6 courses of COPP. Patients with more advanced disease (IB–IIB–III) received 8 cycles of hybrid COPP/ABV, and patients with stage IV received 10 cycles of chemotherapy. Event-free survival was 100% at 3 years for patients with localized disease and 75% for patients with advanced disease (181). These results are comparable with those of other studies of combined-modality therapy. Among the long-term survivors of the studies in which at least 6 cycles of chemotherapy including alkylating agents and procarbazine (MOPP or ChlVPP) were used, there is an increased risk for secondary leukemia, and sterility can be anticipated in more than 90% of the boys.

There are few randomized trials comparing chemotherapy alone with combined-modality treatment in children. The Grupo Argentino de Tratamiento de Leucemia Aguda (GATLA) compared chemotherapy with CVPP alone (CVPP is a modification of MOPP in which cyclophosphamide and vinblastine are substituted for the mechlorethamine and vincristine of MOPP) versus CVPP plus involved-field radiotherapy (30–40 Gy) in patients with CS I–IV. In patients with stage I and II disease, CVPP alone produced event-free survival and overall survival rates similar to those produced by CVPP plus radiotherapy. However, patients with stage I and II disease and unfavorable characteristics (more than two nodal areas, lymph nodes larger than 5 cm, or bulky mediastinal disease) treated with CVPP plus radiotherapy had a superior disease-free survival and overall survival than did similar patients treated with CVPP alone. Also, among patients with CS III and IV, the combined-modality (CVPP plus radiotherapy) group had better disease-free survival rates than did the group treated with CVPP alone (182). In a second GATLA study, a prognostic index was designed that took into account the number of involved nodes, systemic symptoms, and the presence of bulky mediastinal disease at the time of diagnosis. In the favorable group, patients were randomized to receive 3 or 6 cycles of CVPP without radiotherapy. It was concluded that in the favorable-risk group, 3 cycles of CVPP without radiotherapy are equally as effective as 6 cycles (161).

Because of the known late effects of chemotherapy, the option of treatment with radiation therapy alone was offered by the CCG to patients with very limited CS IA disease, who were treated with 35 Gy of involved-field radiation only. Twenty-eight of 99 children relapsed. All but two recurrences were outside the treatment field. Their 10-year progression-free survival was 70%, and their overall survival was 92%. This large difference between progression-free survival and overall survival is a result of effective salvage after relapse with additional radiotherapy and multiagent chemotherapy; however, 30% of the stage I patients were subjected to a salvage treatment program, and the complications of salvage therapy may exceed those observed when combined-modality therapy with low-dose radiation therapy and short-duration chemotherapy are given initially (36). These poor results in a very favorable group of patients may relate to the absence of surgical staging, which is the only way to ascertain the absence of abdominal disease. Moreover, even in patients with early-stage Hodgkin's disease confirmed by laparotomy, the classic approach of radiotherapy alone for adults includes an entire mantle field. Even in these adult patients, for whom late effects linked to growth do not occur, the choice between radiation therapy alone or radiotherapy combined with chemotherapy for favorable cases continues to be a point of controversy (see Chapter 25). In the previously mentioned British study, histology appeared to influence outcome. The 10-year progression free survival rates for the individual histologic subtype were as follows: 77% for lymphocyte predominance, 80% for nodular sclerosis, 48% for mixed cellularity, and 67% for unclassified patients. Patients with stage I MC disease treated with radiation therapy alone had the highest relapse rate, which confirms that these patients are more likely to have occult disease; they require an approach combining chemotherapy and radiation therapy (36). Such a combined-modality approach is the only way to decrease the dose intensity of both chemotherapy and radiation therapy so as to provide treatment with a reduced risk for late complications.

A recent POG study was one of the largest to investigate combined-modality therapy versus MOPP/ABVD chemotherapy alone in advanced-stage pediatric Hodgkin's disease (169). Of 161 patients in remission after completion of 8 cycles of alternating MOPP/ABVD, 81 were randomized to observation and 80 to receive low-dose total-nodal or subtotal-nodal radiation therapy. Event-free survival and overall survival (based on treatment intent) were not significantly improved by the addi-

iting that may be seen with repeated cycles of chemotherapy, may cause a teen ager to resist or refuse potentially life-saving therapy.

Changes in body image and loss of self-esteem occur in nearly one-half (49%) of patients interviewed from 1 to 21 years after treatment for Hodgkin's disease (median, 9 years) (196). Loss of body image correlates with symptoms of depression and stage of disease. The perception of change in body image may correlate directly with physical alterations that can be attributed to treatment administered during childhood, particularly impairment of musculoskeletal growth and development. Although such impairment is often difficult to quantify, it is not uncommon for male survivors to attempt body building to augment the atrophy and muscular wasting that may follow high-dose irradiation administered to a prepubertal child. Other physical complaints reported among pediatric survivors of Hodgkin's disease include disfigurement (30%), neurologic problems (30%), dyspnea (15%), and easy fatigability (5%) (195). With modern treatment approaches, including newer radiation techniques, lower radiation doses to more restricted fields, and less toxic chemotherapy protocols, these problems will likely be less severe for those most recently treated.

Sexual problems have been reported in 22% to 37% of survivors of Hodgkin's disease (196–198). The issues relate to problems of future longevity, possible sterility, and reproductive dysfunction, whether they were treated when children or adults. However, this concern is of particular relevance to adolescents and/or young adults, who face developmental aspects of intimacy and child rearing. No differences in psychosocial adaptation or function have been seen among survivors of Hodgkin's disease treated with MOPP, ABVD, or MOPP alternating with ABVD, although the ABVD combination is reported to have fewer adverse effects on male fertility (198).

As a rule, Hodgkin's disease survivors are less likely to marry than persons without cancer, and if they do marry, they tend to do so at a later age. A higher rate of divorce among male Hodgkin's disease survivors has been reported in comparison with age and race-specific statistics for the United States (23% vs. 5.4%; $p = .002$) (195). On the other hand, other investigators have found that survivors of Hodgkin's disease have closer marital relationships, with increased support and communication during and after the illness (199).

Education and employment issues require long-term adjustments following therapy. In one review, 17% of children dropped out of school, citing cancer therapy as a reason (195). In another report, 42% of employed survivors of Hodgkin's disease cited problems in the work place (196). The perception of job discrimination as a result of having had Hodgkin's disease has been reported in 11% of patients, with assertions of being encouraged to leave a job or being fired or demoted (200). Overall, 36% of survivors of Hodgkin's disease perceive negative social and economic effects related to employment, income, and education (200).

Discrimination in the military has also been reported for both young patients and adults. In studies in which discrimination is not reported, it is generally because of failure to reveal a cancer history on an application form. Today, the Department of Defense Directive No. 6130, March 31, 1986, "Physical Standards for Enlistment, Appointment, and Induction," makes it possible for survivors of childhood cancer to serve in the Armed Forces, military reserves, and Reserved Officers Training Core. By this directive, persons with a history of childhood cancer who have not received therapy for 5 years and are free of cancer will be considered fit for acceptance into the Armed Forces on a case-by-case basis (201).

Survivors of Hodgkin's disease continue to report difficulties in obtaining insurance because their risk for dying of Hodgkin's disease or of treatment-related causes is higher than that of the normal population. Health insurance was denied to 22% of patients in one study, and 15% had no health insurance in another (200,202). Health coverage concerns may affect vocational advancement, as some survivors feel they cannot accept a better position for fear of losing group health coverage. In North Carolina, survivors of childhood cancer were found to be more likely to be denied health insurance than their siblings, with an odds ratio of 15.1. In addition, the health insurance policies of these persons excluded care for preexisting medical conditions more often than did those of their siblings, with an odds ratio of 5.5. The cancer survivors reported problems in obtaining health insurance more frequently than did their siblings, with an odds ratio of 22.8 (203). Similarly, life insurance may be denied outright, or survivors may have to purchase policies with restrictive clauses. Life insurance problems are reported in 11% to 31% of disease-free survivors of Hodgkin's disease (196,198). Terms of insurance policies and contracts are constantly changing. Cancer survivors who have problems with insurance should seek help from hospital insurance departments, local independent insurance agents, state insurance commission offices, patient support groups, and community agencies. Pediatric protocol therapy, coordinated by the cooperative clinical trials groups, has evolved as the standard of care for children with cancer. This standard has resulted in the development of safe and effective therapy for the majority of children with malignancies. Denial of payment still can be expected for investigational or experimental (phase I) therapy. However, Childhood Cooperative Group phase II and III clinical trials should be routinely reimbursed (201). Patients are encouraged to appeal claims denied for treatment prescribed by a therapeutic trial.

The significance of quality-of-life effects among survivors of childhood Hodgkin's disease is probably underestimated, as only recently has research funding become available to study these important issues. Although investigators report that Hodgkin's disease survivors seem to have learned to cope with problems related to their disease and treatment (204), others caution that the impact of the disease and treatment can still be felt 10 to 18 years after treatment (205). Continued attention to these important issues is essential if the stigmata and sequelae suffered by survivors of Hodgkin's disease are to be reversed.

Children in whom Hodgkin's disease is diagnosed require continuous follow-up and assessment throughout their lives. During the childhood years, they should be managed by a multidisciplinary team concerned with the disease and its late effects. The issue arises regarding who should provide follow-up when a child reaches adulthood. Ideally, such persons will be followed by an internist or family practice physician for general medical concerns, and by a multidisciplinary oncology team concerned with late effects. With this dual management approach, long-term survivors have the greatest likelihood of having all late effects recognized and optimally managed.

THE FUTURE

The next step in reducing the late effects of therapy while maintaining excellent survival rates is to try to reduce, as much as possible, chemotherapy and/or radiation therapy in patients with favorable-prognosis stage I–II disease. To date, curative regimens prescribing chemotherapy alone have relied heavily on combinations with high cumulative doses of alkylating agents. These regimens have been preferred in developing countries because of a lack of adequate equipment to administer radiation therapy, a lack of trained pediatric radiation oncologists, and the difficulty of performing accurate clinical staging. However, the late sequelae of infertility and secondary leukemia associated with aggressive chemotherapy regimens have led to a reduction in their use by other investigators, who have preferred to accept potential morbidity related to low-dose involved-field radiation therapy. In every cooperative group and institution, the common denominator of the different approaches has been to limit the cumulative doses of the most toxic drugs and to reduce the dose and volume of radiotherapy. In the HD-90 study, the German-Austrian group used 2 cycles of OPPA for girls [Oncovin (vincristine), procarbazine, prednisone, Adriamycin (doxorubicin)] and 2 cycles of OEPA for boys (etoposide substituted for procarbazine) in an attempt to reduce the risk for sterility (12). In the Italian MH89 study, patients with stages IA–IIA disease without mediastinal involvement were given 3 cycles of ABVD (160). In the French study, patients with stages IA–IIA, regardless of the size of mediastinal disease, received 4 cycles of VBVP (vinblastine, bleomycin, VP-16 (etoposide) and prednisone) (206). In the Stanford, Dana-Farber, and St. Jude (SDS) study of stage I–II favorable disease, patients received 4 cycles of VAMP (vinblastine, Adriamycin, methotrexate, prednisone) (207). Table 12 shows the cumulative doses of chemotherapy agents applied to similar patients within these studies. In all four trials, involved-field irradiation was given at a dose of 15 to 25 Gy. It is obviously difficult to predict the late effects of these four regimens, which contain low cumulative doses of all drugs.

In a further attempt to decrease the treatment intensity in selected favorable cases, the German group has initiated the HD-95 study, which is aimed at omitting radiation therapy in patients who achieve complete remission after chemotherapy without intensification or prolongation of the regimen: 2 cycles of OPPA or OEPA for favorable-prognosis CS I–IIA and 2 cycles of OPPA or OEPA plus 2 or 4 cycles of COPP for intermediate and advanced stages, respectively (208) (see Table 13 for current studies).

In 1990, investigators from Stanford University, St. Jude, and the Dana-Farber Cancer Institute collaboratively developed pediatric Hodgkin's studies with the long-term objectives of reducing cardiopulmonary, gonadal, and neoplastic treatment sequelae by the use of multiple chemotherapy agents that did not include alkylating agents

TABLE 12. *Cumulative doses of chemotherapy (mg/m^2) and radiation (Gy) in four pediatric trials for patients with stages I–II*

	Italian MH 89 study (160) 3 ABVD	German-Austrian HD-90 study (12)		French MDH90 study (206) 4 VBVP	Stanford, Dana-Farber, St. Jude (SDS) study (207) 4 VAMP
		2 OPPA (girls)	2 OEPA (boys)		
Adriamycin	150	160	160	—	200
Bleomycin	60	—	—	40	—
Dacarbazine	2,250	—	—	—	—
Procarbazine	—	3,000	—	—	—
Etoposide	—	—	1,000	2,000	—
Vinblastine	36	—	—	48	48
Vincristine	—	9	9	—	—
Prednisone	—	1,800	1,800	1,120	160
Methotrexate	—	—	—	—	160
Duration	12 wk	8 wk	8 wk	12 wk	16 wk
Involved-field radiation	20 Gy	20 Gy	20 Gy	20 Gy	15–25.5 Gy

ABVD, Adriamycin, bleomycin, vinblastine, dacarbazine; OPPA, Oncovin, prednisone, procarbazine, Adriamycin; OEPA, Oncovin, etoposide, prednisone, Adriamycin; VBVP, VP16, bleomycin, vinblastine, prednisone; VAMP, vinblastine, Adriamycin, methotrexate, prednisone.

TABLE 13. *Ongoing studies in pediatric Hodgkin's disease*

Institution or group	Stage	Therapy
SFOP MDH90 (France)	I–II	4 VBVP if regression >75%: RT 20 Gy if regression <75% OPPA if regression >75%: RT 20 Gy if regression <75%: RT 40 Gy
	III	2 MOPP + 2 ABVD + RT 20 Gy
	IV	2 OPPA + 4 COPP + IF RT 20 Gy
HD-95 (Germany-Austria)	IA/IB–IIA	2 OEPA/OPPA + if no CR IF RT 20 Gy
	IIB–IIIA	2 OEPA/OPPA + 2 COPP + if no CR IF RT 20 Gy
	IIIB–IV	2 OEPA/OPPA + 4 COPP + if no CR IF RT 20 Gy
SEOP 95 (Spain)	IA–IIA no mediastinal disease	2 OPPA + 2 COM(P) RT 20 Gy if CR
	IIB–III–IV any stage with mediastinal disease	2 OPPA + 4 COM(P) RT 20 Gy if CR
POG (pediatric oncology group) (U.S.)	IA–IIA–IIIA IB–IIB IIIA1–IIIA2 IIIB–IV large mediastinal disease	2 DBVE + DZR if CR IF RT 25.5 Gy if PR 2 DBVE + DZR + IF RT 25.5 Gy 3 DBVE-PC + DZR if CR RT 21 Gy if PR 2 DBVE - PC + DZR + RT 21 Gy
CCG (children's cancer group) (U.S.)	IA–IB–IIA favorable (no bulk disease, no hilar disease, <4-cm nodal size)	4 COPP/ABV if CR +/- RT 21 Gy if PR RT 21 Gy
	I–II unfavorable, III	6 COPP/ABV if CR +/- RT 21 Gy if PR RT 21 Gy
	IV	2 Ara-C/VP16 + COPP/ABV + CHOP if CR +/- RT 21 Gy if PR RT 21 Gy
SDS (Stanford, Dana Farber, St. Jude) (U.S.)	I–IIA favorable (mediastinal mass ratio <1/3, peripheral nodal size <6 cm)	4 VAMP if CR after 2 cycles IF RT 15 Gy if PR after 2 cycles IF RT 25.5 Gy
	I–IIB unfavorable or III–IV	3 VAMP/3 COP if CR after 2 cycles IF RT 15 Gy if PR after 2 cycles or bulky disease IF RT 25.5 Gy

VBVP, vinblastine, bleomycin, VP-16 (etoposide) , prednisone; MOPP/ABVD, Mustargen, Oncovin, procarbazine, prednisone/Adriamycin, bleomycin, vinblastine, dacarbazine; OPPA/COPP, Oncovin, prednisone, procarbazine, Adriamycin/cyclophosphamide, Oncovin, procarbazine, prednisone; OEPA/OPPA, Oncovin, etoposide, prednisone, Adriamycin/Oncovin, procarbazine, prednisone, Adriamycin; OPPA/COMP, Oncovin, procarbazine, prednisone, Adriamycin/cyclophosphamide, Oncovin, methotrexate, prednisone; DBVE-PC/DZR, doxorubicin, bleomycin, vincristine, etoposide, prednisone, cyclophosphamide/dexrazoxane; COPP/ABV, cyclophosphamide, Oncovin, procarbazine, prednisone/Adriamycin, bleomycin, vinblastine; Ara-C/VP16, cytarabine/etoposide; CHOP, cyclophosphamide, Adriamycin, Oncovin, prednisone; VAMP/COP, vinblastine, Adriamycin, methotrexate, prednisone/cyclophosphamide, Oncovin, procarbazine; IF, involved field; RT, radiotherapy; CR, complete response; PR, partial response.

or bleomycin. Patients with favorable (peripheral nodal disease under 6 cm or ratio of mediastinal mass to thoracic cavity of less than 33% by chest radiography) localized disease received 4 cycles of VAMP (vinblastine, Adriamycin, methotrexate, and prednisone) chemotherapy. Patients with unfavorable or advanced disease received six cycles of VEPA (vinblastine, etoposide, prednisone, and Adriamycin). All patients received involved-field radiation with the prescribed dose based on disease response after two cycles of chemotherapy. Patients with a complete response received 15 Gy; those with a partial response or bulky disease at presentation received 25.5 Gy. Preliminary results among the first 91 patients entered indicate a 5-year event-free survival of 89% with the regimen of VAMP plus radiotherapy (207). However, accrual to the advanced-stage regimen was discontinued in 1993 because of the inferior event-free survival of patients treated with VEPA plus radiotherapy (209). These early results suggested that disease control in pediatric patients with advanced-stage Hodgkin's disease was compromised when they were treated with regimens that did not contain alkylating agent chemotherapy. The current advanced-stage study prescribes alternating cycles of VAMP and COP chemotherapy plus low-dose, involved-field radiation therapy. Preliminary results indicate disease-free survival rates equivalent to those reported with other combined-modality regimens. A lower frequency of late treatment sequelae is anticipated because of the elimination of bleomycin and the reduction in anthracycline and alkylating agent chemotherapy and radiation doses and volumes.

Both U.S. pediatric cooperative groups have ongoing trials that are evaluating reduced therapy in early-stage and intensified therapy in advanced-stage pediatric Hodgkin's disease. The CCG trial prescribes COPP/ABV hybrid chemotherapy for all patients. Patients with favorable (no bulky disease, fewer than four nodal regions of disease, no hilar adenopathy) localized disease are randomized to observation or low-dose (21 Gy), involved-field radiation therapy if they achieve a complete remission after 4 cycles of COPP/ABV hybrid. Patients with unfavorable or advanced-stage disease are randomized after 6 courses of COPP/ABV hybrid. Stage IV patients are randomized after 6 cycles of intensive chemotherapy with cytarabine/etoposide, COPP/ABV hybrid, and CHOP (cyclophosphamide, doxorubicine (adriamycin, Oncovin, prednisone).

The POG early-stage trial is evaluating the efficacy of response-dependent therapy (2 vs. 4 cycles) with DBVE (doxorubicin, bleomycin, vinblastine, and etoposide) chemotherapy and low-dose (21 Gy), involved-field radiotherapy in patients with early-stage Hodgkin's disease. The advanced-stage protocol prescribes 3 to 4 cycles of a dose-intensive chemotherapy regimen comprised of DBVE with prednisone and cyclophosphamide followed by low-dose (21 Gy) consolidative radiation therapy. Both protocols include a randomization that evaluates the efficacy of dexrazoxane (Zinecard) in reducing pulmonary and cardiac toxicity of DBVE-based therapy and its effect on disease control.

The improvement of treatment efficacy for patients with advanced-stage disease remains problematic. More aggressive treatment approaches are clearly needed for some patients with advanced-stage disease; however, identification of patients at risk for treatment failure remains difficult. Prognostic data currently available have failed to distinguish a specific group of patients who would clearly benefit from early intensification of treatment (210). The excellent cure rates accomplished with contemporary conventional regimens has limited the use of more intensive therapies, such as hematopoietic stem cell transplantation, to the setting of salvage therapy.

Recent trials have investigated regimens of early intensive or abbreviated dose-intensive chemotherapy and consolidative radiation therapy. In the MOPP/ABV hybrid combination, exposure to seven different chemotherapeutic agents is provided earlier than in the traditional alternating MOPP/ABVD regimens. Treatment results indicate the feasibility and efficacy of this regimen in clinically staged pediatric patients. The Stanford V regimen uses a shortened duration of dose-intensive chemotherapy and consolidative radiation therapy to sites of bulky disease (211). The advantages of these approaches include reduced duration of therapy and lower cumulative doses of individual drugs, which should reduce the risks for second malignancies and infertility. These regimens have served as the basis for ongoing cooperative group and institutional trials of dose-intensive therapy in advanced-stage patients.

Contemporary treatment planning for pediatric patients with Hodgkin's disease involves a multidisciplinary approach from the time of diagnosis. Factors that should be considered when therapy is designed include the age and physical maturity of the patient, disease stage and bulk, and potential treatment sequelae. Recommended therapy should provide the best opportunity for long-term disease-free survival with the lowest risk for severe treatment toxicity. In particular, efforts should be made to reduce or eliminate treatment exposures that increase the risk for serious treatment sequelae and so influence early mortality. With this approach, investigators have pioneered the effort to provide safe and effective treatment for pediatric patients with Hodgkin's disease and other childhood cancers.

REFERENCES

1. Teillet F, Schweisguth O. Hodgkin's disease in children. Notes on diagnosis and prognosis based on experiences with 72 cases in children. *Clin Pediatr* 1969;8:698.
2. Donaldson SS. Pediatric Hodgkin's disease—focus on the future. In: Van Eys J, Sullivan MP, eds. *Status of the curability of childhood cancers*. New York: Raven Press, 1980:235.
3. DeVita VT Jr, Serpick A, Carbone PP. Combination chemotherapy in the treatment of advanced Hodgkin's disease. *Ann Intern Med* 1970; 73:881.
4. Donaldson SS, Link MP. Combined modality trials with low-dose radiation therapy and MOPP chemotherapy for children with Hodgkin's disease. *J Clin Oncol* 1987;5:742.
5. Jenkin D, Chan H, Freedman M, et al. Hodgkin's disease in children: treatment results with MOPP and low-dose, extended-field irradiation. *Cancer Treat Rep* 1982;66:949.
6. Maity A, Goldwein JW, Lange B, et al. Comparison of high-dose and low-dose radiation with and without chemotherapy for children with Hodgkin's disease: an analysis of the experience at the Children's Hospital of Philadelphia and the Hospital of the University of Pennsylvania. *J Clin Oncol* 1992;10:929.
7. Wilimas J, Thompson E, Smith KL. Long-term results of treatment of children and adolescents with Hodgkin's disease. *Cancer* 1980;46:2123.
8. Cramer P, Andrieu J-M. Hodgkin's disease in childhood and adolescence: results of chemotherapy-radiotherapy in clinical stages IA–IIB. *J Clin Oncol* 1985;3:1495.
9. Oberlin O, Boilletot A, Leverger G, et al. Clinical staging, primary chemotherapy and involved field radiotherapy in childhood Hodgkin's disease. *Eur Paediatr Haematol Oncol* 1985;2:65.
10. Bramswig JH, Hornig-Franz I, Riepenhausen M, et al. The challenge of pediatric Hodgkin's disease—where is the balance between cure and long-term toxicity? A report of the West German Multicenter Studies DAL-HD-78, DAL- HD-82, DAL-HD-85. *Leuk Lymphoma* 1990;2:183.
11. Schellong G, Waubke-Landwehr AK, Langermann HJ, et al. Prediction of splenic involvement in children with Hodgkin's disease. Significance of clinical and intraoperative findings. A retrospective statistical analysis of 154 patients in the German Therapy Study DAL-HD-78. *Cancer* 1986;57:2049.
12. Schellong G. Treatment of children and adolescents with Hodgkin's disease: the experience of the German-Austrian Pediatric Study Group. *Baillieres Clin Haematol* 1996;9:619.
13. Schellong G, Bramswig JH, Hornig-Franz I. Treatment of children with Hodgkin's disease. Results of the German Pediatric Oncology Group. *Ann Oncol* 1992;3:S73.

14. Vecchi V, Pileri S, Burnelli R, et al. Treatment of pediatric Hodgkin's disease tailored to stage, mediastinal mass, and age: an Italian (AIEOP) multicenter study on 215 patients. *Cancer* 1993;72:2049.
15. Santoro A, Bonadonna G, Bonfante V, et al. Alternating drug combinations in the treatment of advanced Hodgkin's disease. *J Clin Oncol* 1982;306:770.
16. Klimo P, Conners JM. MOPP/ABV hybrid program: combination chemotherapy based on early introduction of seven effective drugs for advanced stage Hodgkin's disease. *J Clin Oncol* 1985;3:1174.
17. Santoro A, Bonadonna G, Valagussa P, et al. Long-term results of combined chemotherapy-radiotherapy approach in Hodgkin's disease: superiority of ABVD plus radiotherapy versus MOPP plus radiotherapy. *J Clin Oncol* 1987;5:27.
18. Hunger SP, Link MP, Donaldson SS. ABVD/MOPP and low-dose involved-field radiotherapy in pediatric Hodgkin's disease: the Stanford experience. *J Clin Oncol* 1994;12:2160.
19. Hudson MM, Greenwald C, Thompson E, et al. Efficacy and toxicity of multiagent chemotherapy and low-dose involved-field radiotherapy in children and adolescents with Hodgkin's disease. *J Clin Oncol* 1993;11:100.
20. Oberlin O, Leverger G, Pacquement H, et al. Low-dose radiation therapy and reduced chemotherapy in childhood Hodgkin's disease: the experience of the French Society of Pediatric Oncology. *J Clin Oncol* 1992;10:1602.
21. Weiner MA, Leventhal BG, Marcus R, et al. Intensive chemotherapy and low-dose radiotherapy for the treatment of advanced-stage Hodgkin's disease in pediatric patients: a Pediatric Oncology Group study. *J Clin Oncol* 1991;9:1591.
22. Jenkin D, Greenberg M. Hodgkin's disease in childhood. Early treatment results in clinically staged patients utilizing MOPP/ABV (3 cycles) and extended field radiation treatment (1500 cGy). *Med Pediatr Oncol* 1993;21:542(abst).
23. Schellong G, Riepenhausen M, Creutzig U, et al. Low risk of secondary leukemias after chemotherapy without mechlorethamine in childhood Hodgkin's disease. *J Clin Oncol* 1997;15:2247.
24. Grufferman SL, Delzell E. Epidemiology of Hodgkin's disease. *Epidemiol Rev* 1984;6:76.
25. Westergaard T, Melbye M, Pederson JB, et al. Birth order, sibship size and risk of Hodgkin's disease in children and young adults: a population-based study of 31 million person-years. *Int J Cancer* 1997;72:977.
26. Schellong G. Personal communication. Presented at the Symposium on Childhood Hodgkin's Disease, Istanbul, November 13–15, 1996.
27. MacMahon B. Epidemiology of Hodgkin's disease. *Cancer Res* 1966;26:1189.
28. Weinreb M, Day PJR, Niggli F, et al. The consistent association between Epstein-Barr Virus and Hodgkin's disease in children in Kenya. *Blood* 1996;87:382.
29. Weinreb M, Day PJR, Niggli F, et al. The role of Epstein-Barr virus in Hodgkin's disease from different geographical areas. *Arch Dis Child* 1996;74:27.
30. Weiss LM. Epstein-Barr virus and Hodgkin's disease. A correlative *in situ* hybridization and polymerase chain reaction study. *Am J Pathol* 1991;139:1269.
31. Jarrett RF, Gallagher A, Jones DB, et al. Detection of Epstein-Barr virus genomes in Hodgkin's disease: relation to age. *J Clin Pathol* 1991;44:844.
32. Preciado MV, De Matteo E, Diez B, et al. Epstein-Barr virus (EBV). Latent membrane protein (LMP) in tumor cells and Hodgkin's disease in pediatric patients. *Med Pediatr Oncol* 1995;24:1.
33. Mueller N. An epidemiologist's view of the new molecular biology findings in Hodgkin's disease. *Ann Oncol* 1991;2(Suppl 2):23.
34. Glaser SL, Lin RJ, Stewart SL, et al. Epstein-Barr virus associated Hodgkin's disease: epidemiologic characteristics in international data. *Int J Cancer* 1997;70:375.
35. Leventhal BG, Donaldson SS. Hodgkin's disease. In: Pizzo PA, Poplack DG, eds. *Principles and practice of pediatric oncology*, 2nd ed. Philadelphia: JB Lippincott Co, 1993:577.
36. Shankar AG, Ashley S, Radford M, et al. Does histology influence outcome in childhood Hodgkin's disease? Results from the United Kingdom Children's Cancer Study Group. *J Clin Oncol* 1997;15:2622.
37. Russell KJ, Hoppe RT, Burns BF, et al. Lymphocyte predominant Hodgkin's disease: clinical presentation and results of treatment. *Radiother Oncol* 1989;1:197.
38. Karayalcin G, Behm FG, Geiser PW, et al. Lymphocyte predominant Hodgkin's disease: clinico-pathologic features and results of treatment—the Pediatric Oncology Group experience. *Med Pediatr Oncol* 1997;29:519.
39. Regula DP, Hoppe RT, Weiss LM. Nodular and diffuse types of lymphocyte predominance Hodgkin's disease. *N Engl J Med* 1988; 318:214.
40. Donaldson SS, Glatstein E, Vosti KL. Bacterial infections in pediatric Hodgkin's disease: relationship to radiotherapy, chemotherapy, and splenectomy. *Cancer* 1978;41:1949.
41. Weiner MA, Leventhal BG, Cantor A, et al. Gallium-67 scans as an adjunct to CT scans for the assessment of a residual mediastinal mass in pediatric patients with Hodgkin's disease: a Pediatric Oncology Group study. *Cancer* 1996;68:2478.
42. Baker LL, Parker BR, Donaldson SS, et al. Staging of Hodgkin's disease in children: comparison of CT and lymphography with laparotomy. *Am J Roentgenol* 1990;154:1251.
43. Hanna SL, Fletcher BD, Boulden TF, et al. MR imaging of infradiaphragmatic lymphadenopathy in children and adolescents with Hodgkin disease: comparisons with lymphography and CT. *J Magn Reson Imaging* 1993;3:461.
44. Young RC, DeVita VT, Johnson RE. Hodgkin's disease in childhood. *Blood* 1973;42:163.
45. Cleary SF, Link MP, Donaldson SS. Hodgkin's disease in the very young. *Int J Radiat Oncol Biol Phys* 1993;28:77.
46. Schellong G, Hornig-Franz I, Roth B, et al. Reduction of radiation dosage to 20–30 Gy in the frame-work of a combined chemo-/radiotherapy in childhood Hodgkin's disease—a report of the Cooperative Therapy Study DAL-HD-87. *Klin Padiatr* 1994;206:253.
47. Donaldson SS, Kaplan HS. Complications of treatment of Hodgkin's disease in children. *Cancer Treat Rep* 1982;66:977.
48. Hancock SL, Tucker MA, Hoppe RT. Factors affecting late mortality from heart disease after treatment of Hodgkin's disease. *JAMA* 1993;270:1949.
49. Lipshultz SE. Late cardiac effects of doxorubicin therapy for acute lymphoblastic leukemia in childhood. *N Engl J Med* 1991;324:808.
50. Andrieu JM, Ochoa-Molina ME. Menstrual cycle, pregnancies and offspring before and after MOPP therapy for Hodgkin's disease. *Cancer* 1983;52:435.
51. Anselmo AP, Cartoni C, Bellantuono P, et al. Risk of infertility in patients with Hodgkin's disease treated with ABVD vs MOPP vs ABVD/MOPP. *Haematologica* 1990;75:155.
52. Bramswig JH, Heimes U, Heiermann E, et al. The effects of different cumulative doses of chemotherapy on testicular function. Results in 75 patients treated for Hodgkin's disease during childhood and adolescence. *Cancer* 1990;65:1298.
53. Clark ST, Radford JA, Crowther D, Swindell R, Shalet SM. Gonadal function following chemotherapy for Hodgkin's disease: a comparative study of MVPP and a seven-drug hybrid regimen. *J Clin Oncol* 1995;13:134.
54. Green DM, Brecher ML, Lindsay AN, et al. Gonadal function in pediatric patients following treatment for Hodgkin's disease. *Med Pediatr Oncol* 1981;9:235.
55. Horning SJ, Hoppe RT, Kaplan HS, et al. Female reproductive potential after treatment for Hodgkin's disease. *N Engl J Med* 1981;304: 1377.
56. Leiper AD, Grant DB, Chessells JM. Gonadal function after testicular irradiation for acute lymphoblastic leukemia. *Arch Dis Child* 1986; 61:53.
57. Leventhal BG, Halperin EC, Torano AE. The testes. In: Schwartz CL, Hobbie WL, Constine LS, Ruccione KS, eds. *Survivors of childhood cancer. Assessment and management*. St. Louis: Mosby, 1994:225.
58. Mackie EJ, Radford M, Shalet SM. Gonadal function following chemotherapy for childhood Hodgkin's disease. *Med Pediatr Oncol* 1996;27:74.
59. Richter P, Calamera JC, Morgenfield MC, et al. Effect of chlorambucil on spermatogenesis in the human with malignant lymphoma. *Cancer* 1970;25:1026.
60. Ortin TT, Shostak CA, Donaldson SS. Gonadal status and reproductive function following treatment for Hodgkin's disease in childhood: the Stanford experience. *Int J Radiat Oncol Biol Phys* 1990;19:873.
61. Viviani S, Santoro A, Ragni G, et al. Gonadal toxicity after combination chemotherapy for Hodgkin's disease. Comparative results of MOPP vs ABVD. *Eur J Cancer Clin Oncol* 1985;5:601.
62. Wallace WHB, Shalet SM, Hendry JH, et al. Ovarian failure follow-

ing abdominal irradiation in childhood: the radiosensitivity of the human oocyte. *Br J Radiol* 1989;62:995.
63. Whitehead E, Shalet SM, Blackledge G, et al. The effect of combination chemotherapy on ovarian function in women treated for Hodgkin's disease. *Cancer* 1983;52:988.
64. Hamre MR, Robison LL, Nesbit ME, et al. Effects of radiation on ovarian function in long-term survivors of childhood leukemia. *J Clin Oncol* 1987;5:1759.
65. Sherins RJ, Olweny CLM, Ziegler JL. Gynecomastia and gonadal dysfunction in adolescent boys treated with combination chemotherapy for Hodgkin's disease. *N Engl J Med* 1978;299:12.
66. Gerres L, Bramswig JH, Schlegel W, et al. The effects of etoposide on testicular function in boys treated for Hodgkin's disease. *Cancer* 1998;83:2217.
67. DaCunha MF, Meistrich ML, Fuller LM, et al. Recovery of spermatogenesis after treatment for Hodgkin's disease: limiting dose of MOPP chemotherapy. *J Clin Oncol* 1984;2:571.
68. Hassel J-U, Bramswig JH, Schlegel W, et al. Testicular function following OPA/COMP chemotherapy in pubertal boys treated for Hodgkin's disease—results in 25 patients of the West-German therapy study DAL-HD-85 not receiving procarbazine. *Klin Padiatr* 1991;203:268.
69. Hill M, Milan S, Cunningham D, et al. Evaluation of the efficacy of the VEEP regimen in adult Hodgkin's disease with assessment of gonadal and cardiac toxicity. *J Clin Oncol* 1995;13:387.
70. Horning SJ, Hoppe RT, Breslin S, et al. Brief chemotherapy (CT) (Stanford V) and involved field radiotherapy (RT) are highly effective for advanced Hodgkin's disease (HD). *Proc Am Soc Clin Oncol* 1998;17:16a(abst).
71. Pedrick TJ, Hoppe RT. Recovery of spermatogenesis following pelvic irradiation for Hodgkin's disease. *Int J Radiat Oncol Biol Phys* 1986;12:117.
72. Kliesch S, Behre HM, Jurgens H, et al. Cryopreservation of semen from adolescent patients with malignancies. *Med Pediatr Oncol* 1996;26:20.
73. Madsen BL, Giudice L, Donaldson SS. Radiation-induced premature menopause: a misconception. *Int J Radiat Oncol Biol Phys* 1995;32:1461.
74. LeFloch O, Donaldson SS, Kaplan HS. Pregnancy following oophoropexy and total nodal irradiation in women with Hodgkin's disease. *Cancer* 1976;38:2263.
75. Hadar H, Loven D, Herskovitz P, et al. An evaluation of lateral and medial transportation of the ovaries out of radiation fields. *Cancer* 1994;74:774.
76. Holmes GE, Holmes F. Pregnancy outcome in patients treated for Hodgkin's disease. A controlled study. *Cancer* 1978;41:1317.
77. Li FP, Fine W, Jaffe N, et al. Offspring of patients treated for cancer in childhood. *J Natl Cancer Inst* 1979;62:1193.
78. Mulvihill JJ, McKeen EA, Rosner F, et al. Pregnancy outcome in cancer patients. Experience in a large cooperative group. *Cancer* 1987;60:1143.
79. Shalet SM. Endocrine sequelae of cancer therapy. *Eur J Endocrinol* 1996;135:135.
80. Nuggard R, Clausen N, Siimes MA, et al. Reproduction following treatment for childhood leukemia: a population-based prospective cohort study of fertility and offspring. *Med Pediatr Oncol* 1991;19:459.
81. Dodds L, Marrett LD, Tomkins DJ, et al. Case-control study of congenital anomalies in children of cancer patients. *Br Med J* 1993;307:164.
82. Bramswig JH, Wegele M, von Lenger KE, et al. The effect of the number of fractions of cranial irradiation on growth in children with acute lymphoblastic leukaemia. *Acta Paediatr Scand* 1989;78:269.
83. Bramswig JH, Zielinski G, Schellong G. Adult height, target height and siblings' adult height in 107 patients treated for acute lymphoblastic leukemia (ALL). Comparison of the effects of 4 different chemotherapeutic regimens and different doses of cranial irradiation. *Horm Res* 1990;33:32.
84. Didcock E, Davies HA, Didi M, et al. Pubertal growth in young adult survivors of childhood leukemia. *J Clin Oncol* 1995;13:2503.
85. Kirk JA, Stevens MM, Menser MA, et al. Growth failure and growth hormone deficiency after treatment for acute lymphoblastic leukemia. *Lancet* 1987;1:190.
86. Mohnike K, Dorffel W, Timme J, et al. Final height and puberty in 40 patients after antileukaemic treatment during childhood. *Eur J Pediatr* 1997;156:272.
87. Littley MD, Shalet SM, Beardwell CG, et al. Radiation-induced hypopituitarism is dose dependent. *Clin Endocrinol* 1989;31:363.
88. Ogilvy-Stuart AL, Shalet SM. Growth and puberty after growth hormone treatment after irradiation for brain tumors. *Arch Dis Child* 1995;73:141.
89. Bajorunas DR, Ghavimi F, Jereb B, et al. Endocrine sequelae of antineoplastic therapy in childhood head and neck malignancies. *J Clin Endocrinol Metab* 1980;50:329.
90. Schriok EA, Schell MJ, Carter M, et al. Abnormal growth patterns and adult short stature in 115 long-term survivors of childhood leukemia. *J Clin Oncol* 1991;9:400.
91. Willman KY, Cox SR, Donaldson SS. Radiation induced height impairment in pediatric Hodgkin's disease. *Int J Radiat Oncol Biol Phys* 1993;28:85.
92. Papadakis V, Tan C, Heller G, et al. Growth and final height for childhood Hodgkin's disease. *J Pediatr Hematol Oncol* 1996;18:272.
93. Donaldson SS. Effects of irradiation on skeletal growth and development. In: Green DM, D'Angio GJ, eds. *Late effects of treatment for childhood cancer*. New York: Wiley-Liss, 1992:63.
94. Eifel PJ, Donaldson SS, Thomas PRM. Response of growing bone to irradiation: a proposed late effects scoring system. *Int J Radiat Oncol Biol Phys* 1995;31:1301.
95. Probert JC, Parker BR. The effects of radiation therapy on bone growth. *Radiology* 1975;114:155.
96. Reinken L, van Oost G. Physical growth in normal German children from birth to 18 years: longitudinal study of height, weight, height velocity. *Klin Padiatr* 1992;204:129.
97. Chao N, Levine J, Horning SJ. Retroperitoneal fibrosis following treatment for Hodgkin's disease. *J Clin Oncol* 1987;5:231.
98. Hancock SL, Hoppe RT. Long-term complications of treatment and causes of mortality after Hodgkin's disease. *Semin Radiat Oncol* 1996;6:225.
99. Prosnitz LR, Lawson JP, Friedlaender GE, et al. Avascular necrosis of bone in Hodgkin's disease patients treated with combined modality therapy. *Cancer* 1981;47:2793.
100. Rossleigh MA, Smith J, Straus DJ. Osteonecrosis in patients with malignant lymphoma: a review of 31 cases. *Cancer* 1986;58:1112.
101. Gerling B, Gottdiener J, Borer JS. Cardiovascular complications of the treatment of Hodgkin's disease. In: Lacher MJ, Redman JR, eds. *Hodgkin's disease: the consequences of survival*. Philadelphia: Lea & Febiger, 1990:267.
102. Stewart JR, Cohn HE, Fajardo LF, et al. Radiation-induced heart disease. *Radiology* 1967;89:302.
103. Green DM, Gingell RL, Pearce J, et al. The effect of mediastinal irradiation on cardiac function of patients treated during childhood and adolescence for Hodgkin's disease. *J Clin Oncol* 1987;5:239.
104. Kadota RP, Burgert EO, Driscoll DJ, et al. Cardiopulmonary function in long-term survivors of childhood Hodgkin's lymphoma: a pilot study. *Mayo Clin Proc* 1988;63:362.
105. Brosius FC, Waller BF, Roberts WC. Radiation heart disease: analysis of 16 young (age 15 to 33 years) necropsy patients who received over 3500 rads to the heart. *Am J Med* 1981;70:519.
106. Cohn KE, Stewart JR, Fajardo LF, et al. Heart disease following radiation. *Medicine* 1967;46:281.
107. Hancock SL, Donaldson SS, Hoppe RT. Cardiac disease following treatment of Hodgkin's disease in children and adolescents. *J Clin Oncol* 1993;11:1208.
108. Greenwood RD, Rosenthal A, Cassady R, et al. Constrictive pericarditis in childhood due to mediastinal irradiation. *Circulation* 1972;50:1033.
109. Carmel RJ, Kaplan HS. Mantle irradiation in Hodgkin's disease: an analysis of technique, tumor eradication, and complications. *Cancer* 1976;37:2813.
110. Josensuu H. Myocardial infarction after irradiation in Hodgkin's disease: a review. *Recent Results Cancer Res* 1993;130:157.
111. Huff H, Sanders EM. Coronary artery occlusion after radiation. *N Engl J Med* 1972;286:780.
112. Prentice RTW. Myocardial infarction following radiation. *Lancet* 1965;1:388.
113. Dollinger MR, Lavine DM, Foye LV Jr. Myocardial infarction following radiation. *Lancet* 1965;1:246.
114. Cohen SI, Bharati S, Glass J, Lev M. Radiotherapy as a cause of complete atrioventricular block in Hodgkin's disease. *Arch Intern Med* 1981;141:676.

115. Scholz KH, Herrmann C, Tebbe U, et al. Myocardial infarction in young people with Hodgkin's disease—potential pathogenic role of radiotherapy, chemotherapy, and splenectomy. *Clin Invest* 1993;71:57.
116. Boivin JF, Hutchison GB, Lubin JH, et al. Coronary artery disease mortality in patients treated for Hodgkin's disease. *Cancer* 1992;69:1241.
117. Rubin E, Camara J, Gravyzel DM, et al. Radiation-induced cardiac fibrosis. *Am J Med* 1963;34:71.
118. Ali MK, Kahlil KG, Fuller LM, et al. Radiation-related myocardial injury. *Cancer* 1976;38:1941.
119. Mills BA, Roberts RW. Cyclophosphamide-induced cardiomyopathy. *Cancer* 1979;43:223.
120. O'Connell TX, Berenbaum MC. Cardiac and pulmonary effects of high doses of cyclophosphamide and ifosfamide. *Cancer Res* 1974;34:1586.
121. Bristow MR, Thompson PD, Martin RP, et al. Early anthracycline cardiotoxicity. *Am J Med* 1978;65:823.
122. Von Hoff DD, Layard MW, Basa P, et al. Risk factors for doxorubicin-induced congestive heart failure. *Ann Intern Med* 1979;9:710.
123. Minow RA, Benjamin RS, Lee ET, et al. Adriamycin cardiomyopathy-risk factors. *Cancer* 1977;39:1397.
124. Oberlin O, Habrand J-L, Zucker JM, et al. No benefit of ifosfamide in Ewing's sarcoma: a nonrandomized study of the French Society of Pediatric Oncology. *J Clin Oncol* 1992;10:1407.
125. Weiss AJ, Manthel RW. Experience with the use of Adriamycin in combination with other anticancer agents using a weekly schedule with particular reference to lack of cardiac toxicity. *Cancer* 1977;40:2046.
126. Torti FM, Bristow MR, Howes AE, et al. Reduced cardiotoxicity of doxorubicin delivered on a weekly schedule. Assessment by endomyocardial biopsy. *Ann Intern Med* 1983;99:745.
127. Legha SS, Benjamin RS, Mackay B, et al. Reduction of doxorubicin cardiotoxicity by prolonged continuous infusion. *Ann Intern Med* 1982;96:133.
128. Gottdiener JS, Katin MJ, Borer JS, et al. Late cardiac effects of therapeutic mediastinal irradiation. *N Engl J Med* 1983;308:569.
129. Bender KS, Shematek JP, Leventhal BG, et al. QT interval prolongation associated with anthracycline cardiotoxicity. *J Pediatr* 1984;105:442.
130. Phillips J, Ichinose H. Clinical and pathologic studies in the hereditary syndrome of a long QT interval, syncopal spells and sudden death. *Chest* 1970;58:236.
131. Goorin AM, Borow KM, Goldman A, et al. Congestive heart failure due to Adriamycin cardiotoxicity: its natural history in children. *Cancer* 1981;47:2810.
132. Steinherz LJ, Steinherz PG, Tan CTC, et al. Cardiac toxicity 4 to 20 years after completing anthracycline therapy. *JAMA* 1991;266:1672.
133. Freter CE, Lee TC, Billingham ME, et al. Doxorubicin cardiac toxicity manifesting seven years after treatment. *Am J Med* 1986;80:483.
134. Lipshultz S, Colan SD, Sanders SP, et al. Cardiac mechanics after growth hormone therapy in pediatric Adriamycin recipients. *Proc Am Soc Clin Oncol* 1989;8:296 (abst).
135. Bossi G, Cerveri I, Volpini E, et al. Long-term pulmonary sequelae after treatment of childhood Hodgkin's disease. *Ann Oncol* 1997;8:S19.
136. Marina NM, Greenwald CA, Fairclough DL, et al. Serial pulmonary function studies in children treated for newly diagnosed Hodgkin's disease with mantle radiotherapy plus cycles of cyclophosphamide, vincristine, and procarbazine alternating with cycles of doxorubicin, bleomycin, vinblastine, and dacarbazine. *Cancer* 1995;75:1706.
137. Kaplan HS, Stewart JR, Bissinger PA. Complications of intensive megavoltage radiotherapy for Hodgkin's disease. *Natl Cancer Inst Monogr* 1973;36:439.
138. Dubray B, Henry-Amar M, Meerwaldt JH, et al. Radiation-induced lung damage after thoracic irradiation for Hodgkin's disease: the role of fractionation. *Radiother Oncol* 1995;36:211.
139. Gustavsson A, Eskilsson J, Landberg T, et al. Long-term effects on pulmonary function of mantle radiotherapy in patients with Hodgkin's disease. *Ann Oncol* 1992;3:455.
140. Young RC, Bookman MA, Longo DL. Late complications of Hodgkin's disease management. *Natl Cancer Inst Monogr* 1990;10:55.
141. Libshitz HI, Banner MP. Spontaneous pneumothorax as a complication of radiation therapy to the thorax. *Radiology* 1974;112:199.
142. Rowinsky EK, Abeloff MD, Wharam MD. Spontaneous pneumothorax following thoracic irradiation. *Chest* 1985;88:703.
143. Pollack A. Late therapy-induced cardiac and pulmonary complications in cured patients with Hodgkin's disease treated with conventional combination chemo-radiotherapy. *Leuk Lymphoma* 1995;15:7.
144. Wolden SL, Lamborn KR, Cleary SF, et al. Second cancers following pediatric Hodgkin's disease. *J Clin Oncol* 1997;16:536.
145. Meadows AT, Baum E, Fossati-Bellani F, et al. Second malignant neoplasms in children: an update from the Late Effects Study Group. *J Clin Oncol* 1985;3:532.
146. Meadows AT, Obringer AL, Marrero O, et al. Second malignant neoplasms following childhood Hodgkin's disease: treatment and splenectomy as risk factors. *Med Pediatr Oncol* 1989;17:477.
147. Kushner BH, Zauber A, Tan CTC. Second malignancies after childhood Hodgkin's disease. The Memorial Sloan-Kettering Cancer Center experience. *Cancer* 1988;62:1364.
148. Rodriguez MA, Fuller LM, Zimmerman SO, et al. Hodgkin's disease: study of treatment intensities and incidences of second malignancies. *Ann Oncol* 1993;4:125.
149. Cimino G, Papa G, Tura S, et al. Second primary cancer following Hodgkin's disease: updated results of an Italian multicentric study. *J Clin Oncol* 1991;9:432.
150. Coleman CN. Secondary malignancies after treatment of Hodgkin's disease: an evolving picture. *J Clin Oncol* 1986;4:821.
151. Bhatia S, Robinson L, Oberlin O, et al. Breast cancer and other second neoplasms after childhood Hodgkin's disease. *N Engl J Med* 1996;12:745.
152. van Leeuwen FE, Chorus AMJ, van den Belt-Dusebout AW, et al. Leukemia risk following Hodgkin's disease. *J Clin Oncol* 1994;12:1063.
153. Dietrich P-Y, Henry-Amar M, Cosset J-M, et al. Second primary cancers in patients continuously disease-free from Hodgkin's disease: a protective role for the spleen? *Blood* 1994;84:1209.
154. Sankila R, Garwicz S, Olsen JH, et al. Risk of subsequent malignant neoplasms among 1641 Hodgkin's disease patients diagnosed in childhood and adolescence: a population-based cohort study in the five Nordic countries. *J Clin Oncol* 1996;14:1442.
155. Beaty O, Hudson MM, Greenwald C, et al. Subsequent malignancies in children and adolescents after treatment for Hodgkin's disease. *J Clin Oncol* 1995;13:603.
156. Hancock, SL, Tucker MA, Hoppe RT. Breast cancer after treatment of Hodgkin's disease. *J Natl Cancer Inst* 1993;85:25.
157. Tarbell NJ, Gelber RD, Weinstein HJ, Mauch P. Sex differences in risk of second malignant tumours after Hodgkin's disease in childhood. *Lancet* 1993;341:1428.
158. Mauch PM, Kalish LA, Marcus KC, et al. Second malignancies after treatment for laparotomy staged IA–IIIB Hodgkin's disease: long-term analysis of risk factors and outcome. *Blood* 1996;87:3625.
159. Donaldson SS, Hancock SL. Second cancers after Hodgkin's disease in childhood. *N Engl J Med* 1996;12:792.
160. Vecchi V, Burnelli R, Di Fabio F, et al. Childhood Hodgkin's disease: results of the Italian muticentric study AIEOP-MH 89-CNR. *Med Pediatr Oncol* 1997;29:434(abst).
161. Sackmann-Muriel F, Zubizarreta P, Gallo G, et al. Hodgkin disease in children: results of a prospective randomized trial in a single institution in Argentina. *Med Pediatr Oncol* 1997;29:544.
162. Gehan EA, Sullivan MP, Fuller LM, et al. The intergroup Hodgkin's disease in children. A study of stages I and II. *Cancer* 1990;65:1429.
163. Jenkin D, Doyle J, Berry M, et al. Hodgkin's disease in children: treatment with MOPP and low-dose, extended field irradiation without laparotomy: late results and toxicity. *Med Pediatr Oncol* 1990;18:265.
164. Kung FH, Behm FG, Cantor A, et al. Abbreviated chemotherapy vs. chemoradiotherapy in early stage Hodgkin's disease of childhood. *Proc Am Soc Clin Oncol* 1991;9:1591(abst).
165. Hutchinson RJ, Fryer CJH, Davis PC, et al. MOPP or radiation in addition to ABVD in the treatment of pathologically staged advanced Hodgkin's disease in children: results of the Children's Cancer Group phase III trial. *J Clin Oncol* 1998;16:897.
166. Fryer CJ, Hutchinson RJ, Krailo M, et al. Efficacy and toxicity of 12 courses of ABVD chemotherapy followed by low-dose regional radiation in advanced Hodgkin's disease in children: a report from the Children's Cancer Study Group. *J Clin Oncol* 1990;8:1971.
167. Balwierz W, Armata J, Moryl-Bujakowska A, et al. Chemotherapy combined with involved field radiotherapy for 177 children with Hodgkin's disease treated in 1983–1987. *Acta Paediatr Jpn* 1991;33:703.
168. Jenkin RD, Berry MP. Hodgkin's disease in children. *Semin Oncol* 1980;7:202.

169. Weiner MA, Leventhal B, Brecher ML, et al. Randomized study of intensive MOPP-ABVD with or without low-dose total-nodal radiation therapy in the treatment of stages IIB, IIIA2, IIIB, and IV Hodgkin's disease in pediatric patients: a Pediatric Oncology Group study. *J Clin Oncol* 1997;5:2769.
170. Olweny CLM, Katongole-Mbidde E, Kiire C, et al. Childhood Hodgkin's disease in Uganda. *Cancer* 1978;42:787.
171. Jacobs P, King HS, Karabus C, et al. Hodgkin's disease in children: a ten-year experience in South Africa. *Cancer* 1984;53:210.
172. Ekert H, Waters KD, Smith PJ, et al. Treatment with MOPP or ChlVPP chemotherapy only for all stages of childhood Hodgkin's disease. *J Clin Oncol* 1988;6:1845.
173. Behrendt H, Van Bunningen BNFR, Van Leeuwen EF. Treatment of Hodgkin's disease in children with or without radiotherapy. *Cancer* 1987;59:1870.
174. Ekert H, Waters KD. Results of treatment of 18 children with Hodgkin's disease with MOPP chemotherapy as the only treatment modality. *Med Pediatr Oncol* 1983;11:322.
175. van den Berg H, Zsiros J, Behrendt H. Treatment of childhood Hodgkin's disease without radiotherapy. *Ann Oncol* 1997;8(Suppl 1):15.
176. Sripada PVSS, Tenali SG, Vasudevan M, et al. Hybrid (COPP/ABV) therapy in childhood Hodgkin's disease: a study of 53 cases during 1989–1993 at the Cancer Institute, Madras. *Pediatr Hematol Oncol* 1995;12:333.
177. Lobo-Sanahuja F, Garcia I, Barrantes JC, et al. Pediatric Hodgkin's disease in Costa Rica: twelve years' experience of primary treatment by chemotherapy alone, without staging laparotomy. *Med Pediatr Oncol* 1994;22:398.
178. Ekert H, Fok T, Dalla-Pozza L, et al. A pilot study of EVAP/ABV chemotherapy in 25 newly diagnosed children with Hodgkin's disease. *Br J Cancer* 1993;67:159.
179. Behrendt H, Brinkhuis M, Van Leeuwen EF. Treatment of childhood Hodgkin's disease with ABVD without radiotherapy. *Med Pediatr Oncol* 1996;26:244.
180. Olweny CL, Katongole-Mbidde E, Kiire C, Lwanga SK, Magrath I, Ziegler JL. Childhood Hodgkin's disease in Uganda. *Cancer* 1971; 27:1295.
181. Baez F, Ocampo E, Conter V, et al. Treatment of childhood Hodgkin's disease with COPP or COPP-ABV (hybrid) without radiotherapy in Nicaragua. *Ann Oncol* 1997;8:247.
182. Sackmann-Muriel F, Bonesana AC, Pavlovsky S, et al. Hodgkin's disease in childhood: therapy results in Argentina. *Am J Pediatr Hematol Oncol* 1981;3:247.
183. Marcus RB, Weiner MA, Chauvenet AR. Radiation in pediatrics Hodgkin's disease [In Reply]. *J Clin Oncol* 1998;16:392.
184. Donaldson SS, Lamborn KR. Radiation in pediatric Hodgkin's disease [To the Editor]. *J Clin Oncol* 1998;16:391.
185. Schellong G, Oberlin O, Ripenhausen M, et al. Stage IV Hodgkin's disease: updated results of the SIOP Collaborative Study. *Med Pediatr Oncol* 1997;29:332(abst).
186. Williams CD, Goldstone AH, Pearce R, et al. Autologous bone marrow transplantation for pediatric Hodgkin's disease: a case-matched comparison with adult patients by the European Bone Marrow Transplant Group Lymphoma Registry. *J Clin Oncol* 1993;11:2243.
187. Hudson MM, Donaldson SS. Hodgkin's disease. In: Pizzo PA, Poplack DG, eds. Principles and practice of pediatric oncology, 3rd ed. Philadelphia: JB Lippincott Co, 1997:523.
188. Ferrell BR, Dow KH. Quality of life among long-term cancer survivors. *Oncology* 1997;11:565.
189. Gill TM, Feinstein AR. A critical appraisal of the quality of quality-of-life measurements. *JAMA* 1994;272:619.
190. Karnofsky DA, Burchenal JH. The clinical evaluation of chemotherapeutic agents in cancer. In: Macleod CM, ed. *Evaluation of chemotherapeutic agents*. New York: Columbia University Press, 1949:191.
191. Jenney MEM, Kane RL, Lurie N. Developing a measure of health outcomes in survivors of childhood cancer: a review on the issues. *Med Pediatr Oncol* 1995;24:145.
192. Lansky LL, List MA, Lansky SB, et al. Toward the development of a Play Performance Scale for Children (PPSC). *Cancer* 1985;56:1837.
193. Yellen SB, Cella DF, Bonomi A. Quality of life in people with Hodgkin's disease. *Oncology* 1993;7:41.
194. Hoerni B, Eghbali H. Quality of life during and after treatment of Hodgkin's disease. *Recent Results Cancer Res* 1989;117:257.
195. Wasserman AL, Thompson EI, Wilimas JA, Fairclough DL. The psychological status of survivors of childhood/adolescent Hodgkin's disease. *Am J Dis Child* 1987;141:626.
196. Fobair P, Hoppe RT, Bloom J, et al. Psychosocial problems among survivors of Hodgkin's disease. *J Clin Oncol* 1986;4:805.
197. Bloom JR, Fobair P, Gritz E, et al. Psychosocial outcomes of cancer: a comparative analysis of Hodgkin's disease and testicular cancer. *J Clin Oncol* 1993;11:979.
198. Kornblith AB, Anderson J, Cella DF, et al. Comparison of psychosocial adaptation and sexual function of survivors of advanced Hodgkin disease treated by MOPP, ABVD, or MOPP alternating with ABVD. *Cancer* 1992;70:2508.
199. Hannah MT, Gritz ER, Wellisch DK, et al. Changes in marital and sexual functioning in long-term survivors and their spouses: testicular cancer versus Hodgkin's disease. *Psychosocial Oncol* 1992;1:89.
200. Kornblith AB, Anderson J, Cella DI, et al. Hodgkin disease survivors at increased risk for problems in psychosocial adaptation. *Cancer* 1992;70:2214.
201. Monaco GP. Pediatric cancer: advocacy, legal, insurance, and employment issues. In: Pizzo PA, Poplack DG, eds. *Principles and practice of pediatric oncology*, 2nd ed. Philadelphia, JB Lippincott Co, 1993:1203.
202. Hubbard SM, Longo DL. Treatment-related morbidity in patients with lymphoma. *Curr Opin Oncol* 1991;3:852.
203. Vann JCJ, Biddle AK, Daeschner CW, et al. Health insurance access to young adult survivors of childhood cancer in North Carolina. *Med Pediatr Oncol* 1995;25:389.
204. Joly F, Henry-Amar M, Arveux P, et al. Late psychosocial sequelae in Hodgkin's disease survivors: a French population-based case-control study. *J Clin Oncol* 1996;14:2444.
205. van Tulder MW, Aaronson NK, Bruning PF. The quality of life of long-term survivors of Hodgkin's disease. *Ann Oncol* 1994;5:153.
206. Landmann-Parker J, Oberlin O, Pacquement H, et al. Localized childhood Hodgkin's disease: response adapted treatment by chemotherapy regimen with VP16, bleomycin, vinblastine, prednisone (VBVP) before low-dose radiation therapy. A study by the French Society of Pediatric Oncology. *Med Pediatr Oncol* 1997;29:355(abst).
207. Donaldson SS, Hudson MM, Link MP, et al. Treatment of children with early stage and favorable Hodgkin's disease: a model of success. *Proc Am Soc Clin Oncol* 1995;14:408(abst).
208. Dorffel W, Luders H, Marciniak H, et al. Therapiestudie fur den Morbus Hodgkin bei Kindern und Jugendlichen GPOH-HD-95: Design und Interims-report nach z Jahren. *Mschr Kinderheilk* 1997;145:1261.
209. Link MP, Hudson MM, Donaldson SS, et al. Treatment of children with unfavorable and advanced stage Hodgkin's disease with vinblastine, etoposide, prednisone, and Adriamcyin (VEPA) and low-dose, involved field irradiation. *Proc Am Soc Clin Oncol* 1994;13:392(abst).
210. Faguet GB. Hodgkin's disease: basing treatment decisions on prognostic factors. *Leuk Lymphoma* 1995;17:223.
211. Horning SJ, Rosenberg SA, Hoppe RT. Brief chemotherapy (Stanford V) and adjuvant radiotherapy for bulky or advanced Hodgkin's disease: an update. *Ann Oncol* 1996;7:5105.

Hodgkin's Disease, edited by P. M. Mauch,
J. O. Armitage, V. Diehl, R. T. Hoppe, and L. M. Weiss.
Lippincott Williams & Wilkins, Philadelphia ©1999.

CHAPTER 31

Clinical Presentation and Treatment of Lymphocyte Predominance Hodgkin's Disease*

Volker Diehl, Jeremy Franklin, Michael Sextro, and Peter M. Mauch

There have long been controversies on the nature and appropriate treatment of lymphocyte predominance Hodgkin's disease. Patients with lymphocyte predominance Hodgkin's disease usually present with early clinical stage, cervical or inguinal involvement, and few if any adverse prognostic factors. Patients are predominantly male and most frequently in the 25- to 45-year age group. Lymphocyte predominance Hodgkin's disease may be associated with progressively transformed germinal centers, which it morphologically resembles. The disease progresses slowly, with fairly frequent relapses, which are rarely fatal. Nonetheless, cases with advanced stage and deaths from Hodgkin's disease have been observed in lymphocyte predominance Hodgkin's disease. At present, instead of the former Rye-subtype lymphocyte predominance, two subtypes are recognized: lymphocyte predominance Hodgkin's disease and lymphocyte-rich classical Hodgkin's disease. This chapter aims to compare the clinical characteristics, prognosis, and management of lymphocyte predominance Hodgkin's disease and lymphocyte-rich classical Hodgkin's disease with the classical Hodgkin's disease subtypes, with special consideration being given to the question of reducing primary treatment for early-stage lymphocyte predominance Hodgkin's disease patients.

For more than half a century, efforts have been made to classify Hodgkin's disease pathologically. The aim was to establish reproducible and clinically useful categories and to understand better the underlying pathology of the disease.

A lucid and comprehensive understanding of the so-called lymphocyte predominance Hodgkin's disease or "nodular paragranuloma" has been hampered by several factors, including the rarity of this diagnosis with only occasional referrals to major centers. Therefore, published reports included few patients, and histologic subclassifications often diverged substantially, mainly because of ignorance of the origin and nature of the tumor cells. The unique biological and immunologic processes responsible for the cellular architecture of the tumor lesion, the clinical presentation, and the prognosis of this disease were also largely unknown.

An indolent form of Hodgkin's disease morphologically characterized by a lymphocytic and histiocytic background was first distinguished from other types in 1937 with use of the terms "early Hodgkin's" and later (1944) "paragranuloma" (1) (Table 1). In 1966 it was renamed Hodgkin's disease of the lymphocytic and histiocytic (L&H) type and subdivided into a nodular and a diffuse form (2). For practical reasons, these two infrequent subforms were combined at the Rye conference (3) into lymphocyte predominance Hodgkin's disease. In the last decade a large body of evidence has accumulated that lymphocyte predominance Hodgkin's disease is a distinct type of B-cell lymphoma (4). Accordingly, the International Lymphoma Study Group proposed in the Revised European American Lymphoma (REAL) classification (5) to separate lymphocyte predominance Hodgkin's disease from the other subtypes of Hodgkin's disease as a clinicopathologic entity by subsuming these under the term "classical Hodgkin's disease."

The merging of nodular and diffuse forms at the Rye conference was not unanimously accepted because of conflicting study results. This question became more complex when several authors described T-cell–rich B-cell lymphomas, which morphologically resemble diffuse lymphocyte predominance Hodgkin's disease but progress aggres-

V. Diehl, J. Franklin, and M. Sextro: Department of Internal Medicine, Klinik I für Innere Medizin, der Universität zu Köln, Köln,, Germany.

P. M. Mauch: Joint Center for Radiation Therapy, Harvard Medical School, Boston, Massachusetts.

*For the European Task Force on Lymphoma project for lymphocyte predominance Hodgkin's disease.

TABLE 1. *Historical development of the classification and nomenclature of lymphocyte predominance Hodgkin's disease*

Year of publication	Authors	Lymphocyte Predominance	Other Hodgkin's disease
1944	Jackson and Parker	Paragranuloma	Granuloma, sarcoma
1966	Lukes and Butler	Lymphohistiocytic nodular Lymphohistiocytic diffuse Diffuse fibrosis reticular	Nodular sclerosis Mixed cellularity
1966	Rye conference	Lymphocyte predominance	Nodular sclerosis Mixed cellularity Lymphocyte depletion
1974	Lennert and Mohri	Nodular paragranuloma Diffuse paragranuloma LP (others) Partial involvement	
1994	REAL (ILSG)	Lymphocyte predominance Lymphocyte-rich classical	Nodular sclerosis Mixed cellularity Lymphocyte depletion

sively. Furthermore, over the last 3 years, it became evident that within classical Hodgkin's disease there are two lymphocyte-rich forms that are often confused with lymphocyte predominance Hodgkin's disease: (a) the diffuse lymphocyte-rich classical Hodgkin's disease, as described in the REAL classification, and (b) a nodular B-cell–rich form recognized at the Toledo workshop in 1994 and subsequently referred to as follicular Hodgkin's disease.

Westling (6) provides a useful overview of the relationship between histologic type and prognosis in the early development of the study of Hodgkin's disease. As early as 1936, Rosenthal (7), using a histopathologic subdivision similar to that of Jackson and Parker, recognized that longer expected survival was associated with a predominance of lymphocytes. Jackson and Parker found that many paragranuloma patients remained disease-free for many years or had further localized recurrences of paragranuloma that did not progress, in stark contrast to the short life expectancy of most Hodgkin's disease patients. Others (about 20%) suffered a transformation to granuloma, whereupon their prognosis worsened to that seen for primary granuloma. This was the only transformation among their three subtypes that was at all frequently observed. In a monograph (8) they describe four case histories of paragranuloma showing typical features: initial appearance of painless enlarged lymph nodes, which often remained untreated but stable for several years; long symptom-free periods following excision (sometimes with local irradiation); later histologic progression to granuloma and subsequent death.

In 1954, Lennert and Hippchen (9) confirmed the prognostic relevance of predominance of lymphocytes as opposed to predominance of reticulum cells, which they saw as a continuous scale between two extremes rather than as two discrete subtypes. Westling (6), Harrison (10), Wright (11), and others confirmed the features of paragranuloma already described: good survival, nonprogressive relapses, and transformation to granuloma. Table 2 lists 5-year survival rates from various studies according to Jackson and Parker's classification (11–14). However, the results of other investigators cast some doubt on the prognostic value of histopathology. Peters in 1950 (12) classified 113 patients according to both histologic subtype (a modification of Jackson and Parker's scheme) and extent of disease (using three clinical stages). The results demonstrate that clinical stage is a stronger prognostic factor than histologic subtype and that within a given clinical stage prognosis shows little or no dependence on histology. All patients received intensive involved-field or extended-field irradiation; this may well explain the generally good results and the reduced effect of histology on prognosis, which is representative of the trends in later years. Early studies based on the Rye classification (15–19) still suggested that patients with lymphocyte predominance Hodgkin's disease had a better prognosis than other histologic subtypes (Table 3). Recent studies with modern treatment strategies, however, have indicated a reduced impact of histology on overall and tumor-free survival in Hodgkin's disease (20–22).

TABLE 2. *Survival rates of histiologic subtypes in the Jackson and Parker classification*[a]

Year of publication	Authors (citation)	Paragranuloma	Granuloma	Sarcoma
1944	Jackson and Parker (8)	(28) 53%	(136) 13%	(32) 0%
1956	Smetana and Cohen (13)	(35) 77%	(308) 27%	(5) 0%
1960	Wright (11)	(19) 95%	(157) 27%	(10) 10%
1964	Hanson (14)	(16) 94%	(176) 37%	(8) 0%

[a]Data are shown as number of cases (in parentheses) followed by 5-year survival percentage.

TABLE 3. *Survival rates of histiologic subtypes in the Rye classification (1967–1976)*[a]

Year of publication	Authors [citation]	LP	NS	MC	LD
1967	Franssila et al. (15)	(9) 55%	(45) 47%	(32) 3%	(11) 0%
1968	Keller (16)[b]	(9) 89%	(92) 70%	(65) 36%	(10) 38%
1969	Landsberg and Larsson (17)	(18) 50%	(31) 55%	(80) 21%	(20) 5%
1970	Gough (18)[b]	(19) 58%	(14) 45%	(28) 18%	(35) 8%
1976	Kaplan (19)[b]	90%	87%	71%	45%

[a]Data are shown as number of cases (in parentheses) followed by 5-year survival percentage.
[b]Actuarial survival.

In spite of the diminishing difference in clinical outcome between lymphocyte predominance Hodgkin's disease and the other forms of classical Hodgkin's disease, there is mounting evidence by morphologic, immunologic, and, above all, molecular-genetic data that nodular lymphocyte predominance Hodgkin's disease is a distinct disease entity, different from the classical Hodgkin's disease types, in some respects more closely ressembling the indolent follicular non-Hodgkin's lymphomas than classical Hodgkin's disease (23,24) (Table 4).

Because lymphocyte predominance Hodgkin's disease accounts for only about 5% of all Hodgkin's disease cases, conclusive studies concerning pathogenetic, morphologic, and clinical aspects are lacking. Therefore, in 1994, an international group of clinicians and pathologists under the auspices of the European Task Force on Lymphomas (ETFL) started a multicenter effort to collect pathologic and clinical material from patients primarily diagnosed as lymphocyte predominance Hodgkin's disease, in order to understand better this rare disease (25). In particular, the study aimed to answer the following questions:

1. What is the initial clinical presentation for lymphocyte predominance Hodgkin's disease?
2. What is the clinical course (response to therapy, relapse rate, and survival)?
3. Can lymphocyte predominance Hodgkin's disease, T-cell–rich B-cell lymphoma, and the new provisional entity lymphocyte-rich classical Hodgkin's disease be distinguished clinically?
4. How can one discriminate clinically between lymphocyte predominance Hodgkin's disease and the other types of classical Hodgkin's disease?
5. Is there clinical evidence for a close relationship to non-Hodgkin's lymphomas?
6. What kind of clinical management can be recommended?

The clinical results of this project are described below, and a detailed analysis of the pathologic results is given in Chapter 11.

The crucial question for the practicing pathologist and oncologist is whether these morphologic subtypes can be discriminated by purely morphologic criteria and whether they bear therapeutic and prognostic consequences. Concerning the first question, the hematopathologists in the ETFL study were of the opinion that the subtle discrimination between these subtypes necessitates immunohisto-

TABLE 4. *Morphologic and molecular-genetic characteristics of the indolent germinal center lymphomas compared with classical Hodgkin's disease*

	Classical Hodgkin's disease	Lymphocyte predomiannce Hodgkin's disease	Follicular Lymphoma
Tumor cells	H-RS	L&H	Centroblasts/centrocytes
Clonal Ig rearrangements	Yes	Yes	Yes
Mutated V genes	Yes	Yes	Yes
Ongoing mutations	No	Detected in about 50% of cases	Yes
Follicular dendritic cells[a]	Rare/absent	Present	Present
CD57-positive T cells[a]	Rare/absent	Present	Present
Ig protein expression	Rare/absent	In some cases	In most cases
IgM RNA	No	Often detected	Yes
Precursor cell	Crippled B cell	Mutating germinal center B cell	Mutating germinal center B-cell
B-cell marker (CD20) expression	Usually no	Yes	Yes
CD30, CD15 expression	Yes	No	No
bcl-2 expression	Yes	No	In 70–80% of cases

[a]Normal cellular constituents of the germinal center.

logic methods and extensive experience. The second question was answered at least partially by the clinical results of the ETFL study (see next section).

RESULTS FROM THE ETFL PROJECT AND OTHER MAJOR STUDIES

The aim of this section is to summarize information on clinical aspects of lymphocyte predominance Hodgkin's disease arising mainly from two sources: a recent large collaborative study and other major studies reported since 1984.

Sources of Data

The European Task Force on Lymphoma Project on Lymphocyte Predominance

This international, multicenter, retrospective study was initiated in 1994. Its purpose was to investigate the clinical characteristics and course of patients diagnosed with lymphocyte predominance Hodgkin's disease and lymphocyte-rich classical Hodgkin's disease, classified by morphologic and immunophenotypic criteria. The Revised European-American classification of lymphoma neoplasms (5) formed the basis for the histopathologic classification.

Clinical data and biopsy material (paraffin blocks) of all available cases diagnosed initially as lymphocyte predominance Hodgkin's disease (lymphocyte predominance-Rye) were collected from 17 European and American centers (listed in the Appendix). Clinical data were obtained on stage, age, sex, laparotomy, B symptoms, E stage, mediastinal tumor, bulky disease, type of organ involvement, survival, relapse, number of relapses, death, causes of death, and therapy. Seven patients who were not treated or had surgery only, and patients younger than 16 years, were excluded from the analysis. Cases were newly classified, without prior knowledge of any corresponding clinical data, by a team of expert pathologists (see Chapter 11) according to a modified REAL classification using morphologic and immunohistochemical criteria. The following categories were used: lymphocyte predominance Hodgkin's disease (n = 219 cases; 51%), lymphocyte-rich classical Hodgkin's disease (n = 115; 27%), non-Hodgkin's lymphoma (n = 12; 3%), classical Hodgkin's disease (n = 19; 5%), reactive lesions (n = 14; 3%), and technically inadequate sample (n = 47; 11%) (Fig. 1). Originally, lymphocyte predominance Hodgkin's disease was subdivided according to lymph node architecture into nodular (n = 189), diffuse (n = 9), and nodular and diffuse (n = 19) cases, but because no significant differences between these categories in clinical characteristics or prognosis were seen, they were pooled for subsequent analysis (see section on Nodular and Diffuse lymphocyte predominance Hodgkin's disease). For purposes of comparison, data were drawn from all evaluable patients in the multicenter trials of the German Hodgkin's Lymphoma Study Group (GHSG) recruiting from 1988 to 1992 (26) who were classified by the GHSG pathology panel as nodular sclerosis Hodgkin's disease or mixed cellularity Hodgkin's disease (27).

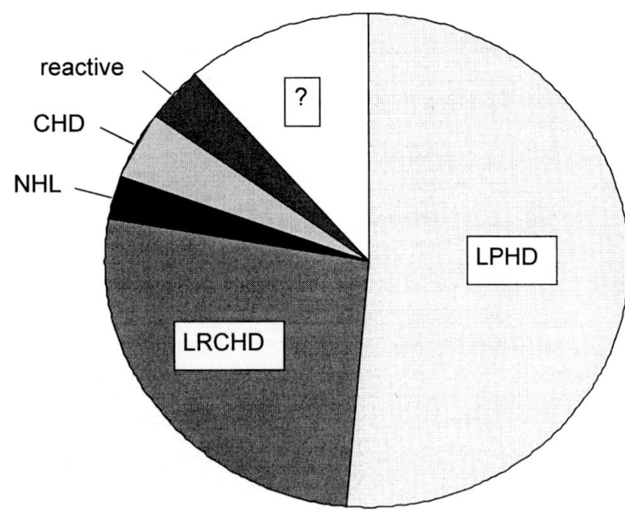

FIG. 1. ETFL project: Histopathologic reclassification of the evaluable cases by the project review panel. LPHD, lymphocyte predominance Hodgkin's disease (51%); LRCHD, lymphocyte-rich classical Hodgkin's disease (27%); CHD, classical Hodgkin's disease (NS, MC, LD, UC) (5%); NHL, non-Hodgkin's lymphoma (3%); reactive (3%); unclassifiable (11%).

Other Major Studies

We found nine publications since 1984 reporting (retrospectively) clinical characteristics and/or treatment results of at least 50 cases of lymphocyte predominance Hodgkin's disease. In all reports before or shortly after the announcement of the REAL classification in 1994, the cases included were selected according to the definition "lymphohistiocytic nodular" of Lukes and Butler or "lymphocyte predominance" of the Rye conference. For simplicity, these subsets are referred to as "nodular lymphocyte predominance" and "lymphocyte predominance," respectively. In only two studies (G and H) were the selected cases representative of the REAL category "lymphocyte predominance Hodgkin's disease " The category lymphocyte-rich classical Hodgkin's disease as such is not represented in the literature. The studies are now briefly described in chronological order.

Miettinen et al. (28) (1983) reclassified 51 cases as nodular lymphocyte predominance from a review of all material diagnosed in Finland as malignant lymphoma (1961 to 1964: nine cases), atypical hyperplasia with suspected malignant lymphoma (1963 to 1978: 34 cases), or toxoplasmosis (1963 to 1978: eight cases). The diagnostic criteria of Lukes and Butler were employed. Thirty-one patients received surgical treatment only, while 20 received limited treatment, mostly involving field irradiation and/or single cytostatic agents. The implications of the observed course of disease for the untreated patients are discussed later in this chapter.

Hansmann et al. (29) (1984) describe clinical aspects of 145 cases of nodular lymphocyte predominance, selected as those cases with adequate clinical information from 206 originally diagnosed as "nodular paragranuloma" in the Lymph Node Registry in Kiel, Germany. Treatment varied widely: no treatment except excision of the lymph node was given to 24 stage I patients (see section on Treatment Results); most patients received radiotherapy, mainly involved-field, whereas stage III or IV patients had polychemotherapy.

Regula et al. (23) (1988) confirmed 73 of 101 cases of lymphocyte predominance treated at Stanford University Medical Center (1963 to 1985). Rye criteria were used, without immunophenotyping. Treatment was mainly radiotherapy, including 21 cases given only "limited irradiation."

Borg-Grech et al. (30) (1989) reviewed all cases of lymphocyte predominance and unspecified Hodgkin's disease in the histopathology files of Christie Hospital, Manchester, England. By use of conventional staining methods, 110 cases were confirmed as lymphocyte predominance Hodgkin's disease. All patients were treated according to the Manchester Lymphoma Group protocols.

Crennan et al. (31) (1995) reviewed the 64 cases where pathologic material was available from 75 lymphocyte predominance patients treated at the Peter MacCallum Cancer Institute, Melbourne, Australia between 1969 and 1989. Conventional stains were reviewed. B-cell markers were present in 19 of the 36 cases in which immunophenotyping could be performed (this characteristic did not correlate with nodularity or with prognosis). Patients had received standard treatment: 81% extended-field RT, 8% involved-field RT, and 11% chemotherapy or combined modality.

Pappa et al. (32) (1995) reviewed 90 cases initially diagnosed as lymphocyte predominance at St. Bartholomew's Hospital, London from 1971 to 1992 and confirmed 50 as nodular lymphocyte predominance (no purely diffuse lymphocyte predominance Hodgkin's disease cases were found; the remainder were mostly mixed cellularity). The criteria of Lukes and Butler were applied. The nodular lymphocyte predominance subtype thus represents 7% of all Hodgkin's disease in this patient population. Seventy-eight percent of these patients were treated with radiotherapy alone, whereas most advanced-stage patients received chemotherapy alone.

Von Wasielewski et al. (33) (1997) used immunostaining techniques (CD15, CD20, CD30, CD57) to reinvestigate 208 cases in which lymphocyte predominance-Rye had been suggested as the original diagnosis and confirmed 92 of these as immunophenotypically lymphocyte predominance Hodgkin's disease. Approximately one-third of cases previously reviewed without immunophenotyping as lymphocyte predominance Hodgkin's disease turned out to display a classical type of marker profile; cases of lymphocyte-rich classical Hodgkin's disease could well form a considerable part of this group. Treatment was according to the protocols of the German Hodgkin's Lymphoma Study Group (1984 to 1993) (26).

Bodis et al. (34) (1997) requested slides for all 97 lymphocyte predominance Hodgkin's disease diagnoses out of 1,533 patients seen at the Joint Center for Radiation Therapy (JCRT), Boston, Massachussetts from 1969 to 1973. Seventy-five of 89 evaluable cases were confirmed as lymphocyte predominance Hodgkin's disease using REAL criteria, and six cases were rediagnosed as lymphocyte-rich classical Hodgkin's disease (lymphocyte-rich nodular sclerosis-Hodgkin's disease). The majority of lymphocyte predominance Hodgkin's disease cases were subclassifiable as nodular ($n = 55$) or diffuse ($n = 14$). For calculation of treatment results, only the 71 patients treated at JCRT were included. Most of them received extended-field radiotherapy of 30 to 40 Gy with the exception of ten patients who received five to eight cycles of modern polychemotherapy with or without irradiation.

Orlandi et al. (35) (1997) investigated 68 consecutive cases of nodular lymphocyte predominance (Rye) diagnosed in the Policlinico S. Matteo, Pavia, Italy between 1975 and 1994, which represented 8% of all Hodgkin's disease patients seen in this period. Routine techniques were augmented by a palette of immunohistochemical stainings. Early-stage patients mostly received radiotherapy or combined modality; advanced-stage patients had chemotherapy or combined modality, using modern polychemotherapy regimens.

Table 5 summarizes the statistical results concerning clinical characteristics and course in all nine studies, which are discussed in the following sections.

Clinical Presentation of Lymphocyte Predominance Hodgkin's Disease and Lymphocyte-Rich Classical Hodgkin's disease

Where results are averaged over the nine major studies in the literature, the mean value has been weighted according to the number of cases in each study.

Age and Gender

The age distributions of ETFL project lymphocyte predominance Hodgkin's disease and lymphocyte-rich classical Hodgkin's disease and of German classical Hodgkin's disease cases are compared in Figure 2. The lymphocyte predominance Hodgkin's disease has a similar age distribution (median 35 years) to classical Hodgkin's disease, especially mixed-cellularity Hodgkin's disease, whereas lymphocyte-rich classical Hodgkin's disease patients are on average markedly older, with a median age of 43 years. Approximately 70% of lymphocyte predominance Hodgkin's disease and of lymphocyte-rich classical Hodgkin's disease cases were male (Table 6), similar to mixed cellularity Hodgkin's disease and differ-

TABLE 5. *Major studies with clinical data on at least 50 patients[a]*

Author/source/ (no. of cases)	Age	Sex (male)	Stage	B symptoms	RF organs	Prognosis (years)	Second neoplasia
Bodis JCRT, Harvard, USA (75)		80%	I + II 88%		Mediast. 7% Spleen 15% (of 66 lap. pts.)	SV(10) 93% RFS (10) 80%	NHL 0
Borg-Grech Manchester, UK (110)	Median 39 (range 3–80)	75%	I 59% II 11% III 21% IV 9%	12%	Bulk 25% Mediast./hili 12%	SV(5) 80% RFS (5) 88%	
Hansmann + Zwingers Germany (145) (nod)		73%	I 50% II 21% III 22% IV 7%	10%	Mediast. 3% Liver 3% B.marrow 1%	SV(5) 90%	AML 0
Pappa St. Barts, UK (50) (nod)	Median 36	86%	I 52% B 6% II 26% III 16% IV 6%		Liver 4% B.marrow 2%	SV(4) 92% SV(12) 82% RFS (4) 100% RFS (12) 81%	ALL 1 hgB NHL 2 Ca 3
Miettinen Finland 1961-4 (51) (nod)	Median 42 (range 11–76)	69%				SV(5) 88%	NHL 5
Wasielewski GHSG, Germany 1984–93 (92)		67%	I 34% II 32% III 26% IV 8%			SV(4) 98%	
Regula Stanford, USA (73)	Median 29 (range 5–62)	84%	I 40% II 36% III 23% IV 1%		Liver 1% B.marrow 0 (nod), 92% (dif)	SV(10) 82% RFS(10) 60% Ca 4	AML 3 NHL 2
Crennan MacCallum CI Melbourne, Aus. (64)	Median 29 (range 9–70)	81% 81%	I 55% II 27% III 17% IV 1%	9%	Mediast. 9% Liver + b.marrow 1%	SV(10) 85% FFP(10) 74%	diff.LCL 1 Ca 2
Orlandi Pavia, Italy (68) (nod)	Median 35 (range 14–86)	68%	I 51% II 24% III 13% IV 12%	15%	Mediast. 15% Liver 7% Spleen 15% B. marrow 4%	SV(10) 71% FFP(10) 45%	NHL 5

[a]NHL, non-Hodgkin's lymphoma; AML, acute myeloid leukemia; ALL, acute lymphocytic leukemia; hg, high grade; LCL, large-cell lymphoma; Ca, carcinoma; nod, nodular; dif, diffuse; RFS, relapse-free survival; FFP, freedom from progression; SV, survival.

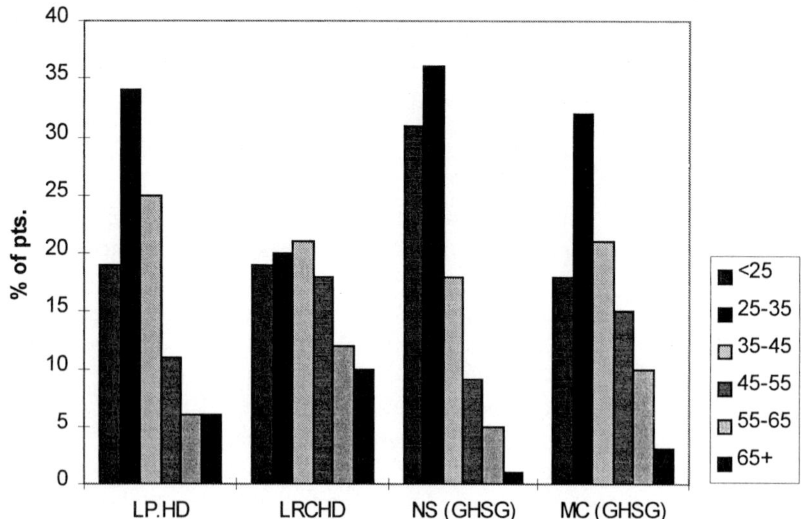

FIG. 2. ETFL project: Age distribution of lymphocyte predominance Hodgkin's disease and lymphocyte-rich Hodgkin's disease cases compared with nodular sclerosis and mixed-cellularity cases of the German Hodgkin's Lymphoma Study Group (GHSG).

TABLE 6. *ETFL project: Patient characteristics*

	LPHD (*n* = 219)	LRCHD (*n* = 115)	NS (GHSG) (*n* = 599)	MC (GHSG) (*n* = 174)
Age (median)	35 yr[a]	41 yr[a]	28 yr	35 yr
Sex (male)	74%	69%	49%	73%
Stage I	53%	46%	10%	21%
II	28%	24%	47%	32%
III	14%	24%	29%	35%
IV	6%	6%	14%	13%
B symptoms	10%	11%	42%	35%

LPHD, lymphocyte predominance Hodgkin's disease; LRCHD, lymphocyte-rich classical Hodgkin's disease; NS, nodular sclerosis; MC, mixed cellularity.

[a]For comparability with the GHSG trials, where entry is restricted to patients under 75 years of age, patients 75 or older were excluded in calculating these medians. Unrestricted values are 35 years for LPHD and 43 years for LRCHD.

ent from the approximately equal gender balance for nodular sclerosis Hodgkin's disease.

In the other major studies, median age varied between 29 (Regula, range 5 to 62) and 42 (Miettinen, range 11 to 76). Clearly, the median value depends on age inclusion criteria, especially on whether or not pediatric patients are included. All studies consistently report a strong male predominance with a mean value of 76%.

Stage and Systemic Symptoms

Table 6 shows that both lymphocyte predominance Hodgkin's disease and lymphocyte-rich classical Hodgkin's disease cases (ETFL project) are predominantly early-stage patients: 53% of lymphocyte predominance Hodgkin's disease and 46% of lymphocyte-rich classical Hodgkin's disease patients had stage I and only 6% of each group had stage IV. This contrasts markedly with the classical Hodgkin's disease cases. B symptoms were rare in both lymphocyte predominance Hodgkin's disease (10%) and in lymphocyte-rich classical Hodgkin's disease (11%), in contrast to 42% for nodular sclerosis patients in the German trials.

Seven of the other major studies report their stage distributions. Stage I accounted for between 34% and 59%, and stage IV for between 1% and 12%. Thus, the proportion of early stages is consistently high in comparison with classical Hodgkin's disease, and stage IV is consistently, but not negligibly, rare. B symptoms were present in between 6% and 15% of cases. The average distribution of stages was as follows: stage I, 49%; stage II, 24%; stage III, 20%; stage IV, 7%; B symptoms, 11%.

Organ Involvement and Other Negative Prognostic Factors

Table 7 shows that site-specific organ involvement occurred with similar low frequency in lymphocyte predominance Hodgkin's disease and lymphocyte-rich classical Hodgkin's disease in ETFL project cases. It is chiefly lung involvement in nodular sclerosis Hodgkin's disease and bone marrow involvement in mixed cellularity Hodgkin's disease that account for the higher fractions of stage IV cases among the classical Hodgkin's disease cases of the GHSG. The prognostic factors bulky disease and mediastinal involvement are both comparatively rare in lymphocyte predominance Hodgkin's disease and in lymphocyte-rich classical Hodgkin's disease; mediastinal disease occurred in only 7% of lymphocyte predominance case and 15% of lymphocyte-rich classical Hodgkin's disease cases (p = .04). A small but fairly consistent percentage (1% to 4%) of patients with liver involvement is described in all four other major studies for which organ involvement rates are reported. In five articles, bone marrow involvement between zero and 4% are mentioned. Mediastinal involvement rates between 3% and 15% were found.

For a reliable comparison of the frequencies of involvement in various nodal sites between lymphocyte predominance Hodgkin's disease and other Hodgkin's disease subtypes (these data were not collected in the ETFL project),

TABLE 7. *ETFL project: patient characteristics*

Type of involvement	LPHD (*n* = 219)	LRCHD (*n* = 115)	NS (GHSG) (*n* = 599)	MC (GHSG) (*n* = 174)
Bulky	13%	11%	54%	40%
Mediastinal	7%	15%	80%	40%
Spleen	8%	15%	10%	22%
Bone marrow	1%	1%	3%	10%
Liver	3%	3%	3%	5%
Lung	1%	4%	10%	1%
Skeletal	1%	0%	6%	3%
Other organ	2%	3%	8%	1%

LPHD, lymphocyte predominance Hodgkin's disease; LRCHD, lymphocyte-rich classical Hodgkin's disease; NS, nodular sclerosis; MC, mixed cellularity.

the analysis by Mauch et al. (36) of 719 patients uniformly staged using laparotomy and splenectomy is particularly suitable. Table 8 shows the prevalence of involvement of sites of lymphocyte predominance, nodular sclerosis, and mixed cellularity/lymphocyte depletion. Lymphocyte predominance Hodgkin's disease seems to favor the peripheral sites, such as upper neck, epitrochlear, and inguinal nodes, and to occur relatively seldom in central sites such as mediastinum, lung hili, lower neck, and upper abdomen.

Treatment Results

Current Treatment Concepts for Lymphocyte Predominance Hodgkin's Disease

State-of-the-art treatment for Hodgkin's disease employs stage and other clinical prognostic factors for the determination of treatment but usually treats all histologic subtypes alike. Nearly all large cooperative clinical trial groups around the world have included patients with lymphocyte predominance Hodgkin's disease in their treatment protocols designed for the majority of Hodgkin's disease patients, that is, the classical Hodgkin's disease subtypes nodular sclerosis and mixed cellularity. In nearly all studies, patients with lymphocyte predominance Hodgkin's disease were treated according to anatomic spread and prognostic factors as described above. A notable exception is the EORTC Lymphoma Cooperative Group, which treats supradiaphragmatic stage I nodular lymphocyte predominance Hodgkin's disease (previously together with comparable non-Hodgkin's lymphoma patients) separately using involved-field radiation alone (37,38).

Evidence for Comparatively Good Survival of Untreated Lymphocyte Predominance Hodgkin's Disease Cases

In the set of 51 nodular lymphocyte predominance cases reported by Miettinen, 31 were given no treatment except possibly surgical removal of the tumor because malignant disease was not suspected. With a median follow-up of 7 years for the whole set, only seven of the untreated patients died, one from Hodgkin's disease, two from non-Hodgkin's lymphoma, two from a carcinoma, and two from other causes. There were 14 Hodgkin's disease relapses in the entire set ($n = 51$), which implies a moderately high relapse rate (27%). These results suggest that the survival of lymphocyte predominance Hodgkin's disease cases is good despite relapses, even without treatment. However, it must be remembered that the chosen cases are not necessarily representative of nodular lymphocyte predominance as a whole. Because the majority (42/51) were not originally diagnosed as malignant lymphoma, it seems likely that especially mild examples would predominate in this sample. It can nevertheless be concluded that some patients with histologically confirmed, untreated lymphocyte predominance Hodgkin's disease enjoy long-term survival.

The publication by Hansmann et al. (1984) includes 24 stage I lymphocyte predominance Hodgkin's disease patients who received no therapy beyond excision of the involved node with or without the surrounding tissue. Fifteen of these relapsed, but the other nine remained free of relapse and symptoms for up to 14 years.

In 1961, Dawson et al. (39) described 44 cases of benign Hodgkin's disease in the sense of Harrison (10). Local excision was the only initial treatment in 15 cases, which had a median follow-up of about 9 years. Despite recurrence in 10 of these cases, only two died, following late recurrence of benign and classical Hodgkin's disease, respectively.

In summary, there is some evidence to support the hypothesis that certain lymphocyte predominance Hodgkin's disease patients do well without any therapy beyond excision. This would seem to represent a real difference in clinical characteristics compared with classical Hodgkin's disease. The problem remains that all available data are retrospective: the good clinical course of a not clearly defined subset of past lymphocyte predominance patients does not allow us to infer favorable prognosis for a given newly diagnosed lymphocyte predominance patient. Apart from the ETFL project results, no data are yet available for the recently defined category lymphocyte-rich classical Hodgkin's disease on this question.

Treatment Given

Tables 9 and 10 give details about treatment by stage and type of chemotherapy given to cases included in the ETFL project. Therapy on the whole was considered to be

TABLE 8. *Prevalence (%) of involvement in nodal sites and spleen according to histologic subtype*[a]

Involved site	LP (n = 63)	NS (n = 433)	MC/LD (n = 223)	p value
Upper neck	14	4	4	.006
Side of neck (L,R)	41, 46	62, 55	53, 60	.002 (L)
Axilla (L,R)	14, 13	15, 11	14, 16	NS
Mediastinum	8	73	46	<.0001
Lung hilum (L,R)	5, 3	15, 14	8, 9	.006
Upper abdomen	5	13	18	.01
Lower abdomen	8	8	17	.002
Inguinal (L,R)	10, 10	1, 1	3, 3	.001

LP, lymphocyte predominance; NS, nocular sclerosis; MC/LD, mixed cellularity/lymphocyte depletion
[a]Based on 719 laparotomy-staged patients reported by Mauch et al. (36).

TABLE 9. *ETFL project: Treatment of ETFL project cases (LPHD and LRCHD combined)*

	Radiotherapy	Chemotherapy	Combined modality	*n* (100%)
Stage I	87%	1%	12%	168
Stage II	57%	6%	37%	88
Stage III	18%	41%	41%	59
Stage IV	5%	63%	32%	19

LPHD, lymphocyte predominance Hodgkin's disease; LRCHD lymphocyte-rich classical Hodgkin's disease.

adequate for stage: 99% of stage I and 94% of stage II patients received radiotherapy or combined-modality treatment; 82% of stage III and 95% of stage IV patients received chemotherapy or chemotherapy plus radiotherapy. There were no significant differences in primary treatment between lymphocyte predominance Hodgkin's disease and lymphocyte-rich classical Hodgkin's disease (data not shown). If chemotherapy alone was given, 93% of patients received MOPP-like, ABVD-like, or MOPP/ABVD-like regimens (Table 10).

Prognosis After Primary Therapy

Primary treatment results in the two major histopathologic groups of the ETFL project were identical, with 96% complete remission for both lymphocyte predominance Hodgkin's disease and lymphocyte-rich classical Hodgkin's disease, somewhat higher than for the classical Hodgkin's disease cases of the GHSG (ndoular sclerosis, 89%; mixed cellularity, 93%). There were slightly more relapses in the lymphocyte predominance Hodgkin's disease group (21% vs. 17%).

Survival and failure-free survival were analyzed using Hodgkin's-specific measures because therapy-related or other nonlymphoma deaths are not relevant here. Figures 3 and 4 show Hodgkin's disease–specific survivial and failure-free survivalfor four ETFL histopathologic groups: lymphocyte predominance Hodgkin's disease, lymphocyte-rich classical Hodgkin's disease, classical Hodgkin's disease, and non-Hodgkin's lymphoma. Both survival and failure-free survival are markedly and significantly worse for those cases originally diagnosed as lymphocyte predominance Hodgkin's disease that were reclassified as classical Hodgkin's disease (n = 19) or as non-Hodgkin's lymphoma (n = 12) by the ETFL review panel. It is therefore apparent that the review process has separated out a

TABLE 10. *ETFL project: Type of chemotherapy (lymphocyte predominant Hodgkin's disease and lymphocyte-rich classical Hodgkin's disease combined)*

	CT alone	Combined Modality
MOPP–ABVD-like	36%	36%
ABVD-like	2%	5%
MOPP-like	55%	43%
Other	7%	16%
n (=100%)	42	88

small fraction of cases with poor prognosis that do not belong to the lymphocyte predominance Hodgkin's disease or lymphocyte-rich classical Hodgkin's disease groups. The classical Hodgkin's disease group is, however, not necessarily representative of classical Hodgkin's disease in general because all these cases had originally been classified as lymphocyte predominance. Surprisingly, older patients predominate in both classical Hodgkin's disease and non-Hodgkin's lymphoma groups (47% and 58%, respectively, were over 50 years old at diagnosis).

Figures 5 and 6 compare the survival and failure-free survival of the ETFL groups lymphocyte predominance Hodgkin's disease and lymphocyte-rich classical Hodgkin's disease with classical Hodgkin's disease cases from the GHSG. At 8 years the estimated rates are for lymphocyte predominance Hodgkin's disease 95% (survival) and 74% (failure-free survival), and for lymphocyte-rich classical Hodgkin's disease 87% (survival) and 75% (failure-free survival). Nonspecific survival was 89% for lymphocyte predominance Hodgkin's disease and 74% for lymphocyte-rich classical Hodgkin's disease at 8 years. Although survival is slightly worse for lymphocyte-rich classical Hodgkin's disease, no significant difference was observed between these two groups ($p = .067$ for survival; $p = .57$ for failure-free survival). Nor is the course of the lymphocyte predominance Hodgkin's disease or lymphocyte-rich classical Hodgkin's disease cases significantly different from that of the ndoular sclerosis and mixed cellularity cases of the GHSG. There is a trend toward better failure-free survival, but this, even if it is real, would be directly accounted for by the preponderance of early-stage cases in lymphocyte predominance Hodgkin's disease and lymphocyte-rich classical Hodgkin's disease (Table 6). Table 11 makes a stage-specific comparison between the 8-year Kaplan-Meier estimates for failure-free survival and survival in lymphocyte predominance Hodgkin's disease and lymphocyte-rich classical Hodgkin's disease, respectively. There were no statistically significant differences in survival or failure-free survival between the two cohorts in the analysis stratified for stage. Early-stage patients in both groups had a good to excellent survival, but treatment failures were common in both groups.

Other major studies gave largely similar results for lymphocyte predominance Hodgkin's disease. The (nonspecific) survival varied between 98% at 4 years and 71% at 10 years; failure-free survival or a similar measure,

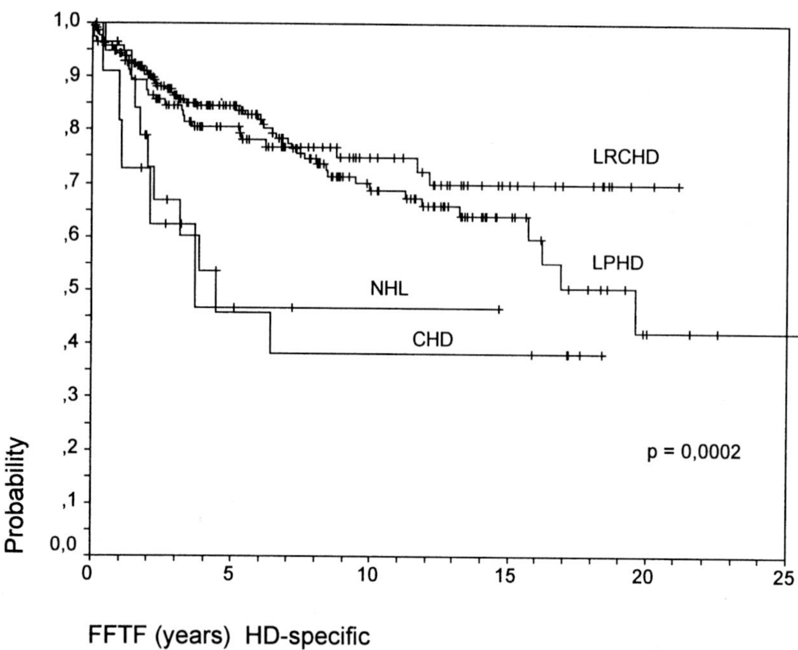

FIG. 3. ETFL project: Failure-free survival of lymphocyte predominance Hodgkin's disease (LPH), lymphocyte-rich classical Hodgkin's disease (LRCHD), classical Hodgkin's disease (CHD), and non-Hodgkin's lymphoma (NHL) cases.

usually the Hodgkin's disease–specific measure relapse-free survival, varied between 88% (5 years) and 45% (10 years). These results were in most studies achieved using modern therapy protocols, mainly radiotherapy, the main exception being the 50 cases of Miettinen (see above). Borg-Grech compared the course of stage I to III cases classified as lymphocyte predominance, nodular sclerosis, and mixed cellularity (n = 86, 51, and 59, respectively) treated at the same institution during a similar time period and found no significant difference in either relapse-free or overall survival between lymphocyte predominance and classical subtypes. Von Wasielewski observed a significantly better survival for immunophenotypically confirmed lymphocyte predominance Hodgkin's disease compared with cases showing a classical immunophenotype.

The indolent course with frequent but nonaggressive recurrences has long been regarded as typical of paragranuloma/lymphocyte predominance Hodgkin's disease. The ETFL project results show a tendency (not statistically significant) to more frequent late relapses and better long-term survival in lymphocyte predominance Hodgkin's disease compared with lymphocyte-rich classical Hodgkin's

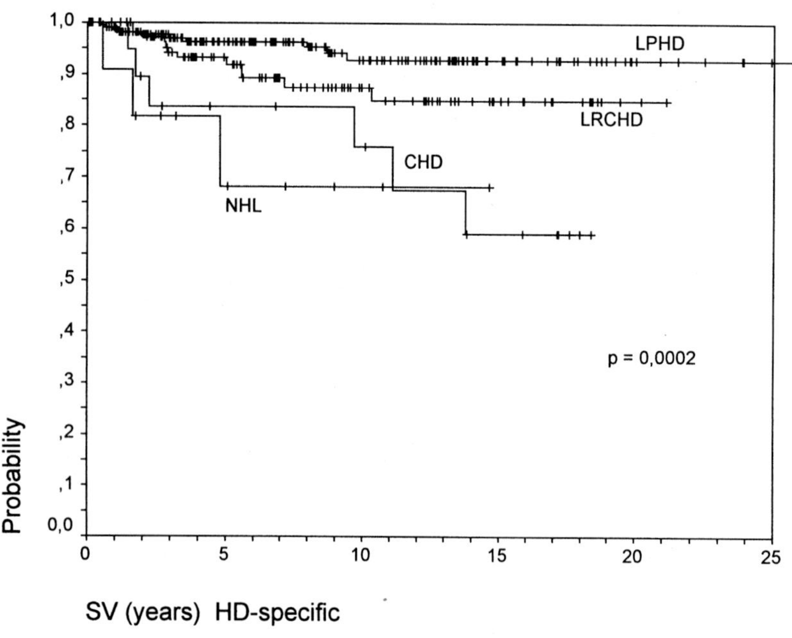

FIG. 4. ETFL project: survival (SV) of lymphocyte predominance Hodkgin's disease (LPHD), lymphocyte-rich classical Hodgkin's disease (LRCHD), classical Hodgkin's disease (CHD), and non-Hodgkin's lymphoma (NHL) cases.

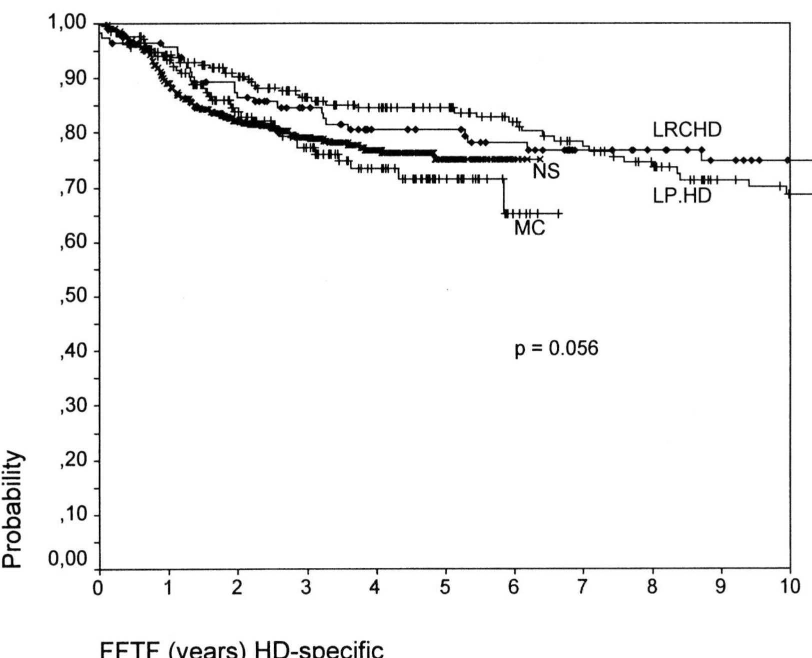

FIG. 5. ETFL project: Failure-free survival (FFS) of lymphocyte predominance Hodgkin's disease (LPHD), lymphocyte-rich classical Hodgkin's disease (LRCHD) cases compared with nodular sclerosis (NS) and mixed cellularity (MC) cases of the German Hodgkin's Lymphoma Study Group (GHSG).

disease or classical Hodgkin's disease. Orlandi observed a constant pattern of recurrence over 10 or more years, even for the early-stage patients: with a freedom-from-progression rate of only 45% after 10 years, much poorer than comparable rates for the other major studies, relapses were indeed frequent. In general, the literature does not substantiate the assertion that lymphocyte predominance Hodgkin's disease patients experience a late recurrence (after 10 years or more) more frequently than other Hodgkin's disease subtypes; however, long-term follow-up data for lymphocyte predominance Hodgkin's disease are sparce.

Prognosis After Relapse

In the ETFL study, most first recurrences (76%) after an initial diagnosis of lymphocyte predominance Hodgkin's disease were reported to be again lymphocyte predominance Hodgkin's disease (diagnoses not reviewed), but 14% could not be definitely identifed as Hodgkin's disease, and 10% were classified as other Hodgkin's disease. In contrast, more than half of first recurrences after lymphocyte-rich classical Hodgkin's disease were diagnosed as classical or unclassifiable Hodgkin's disease.

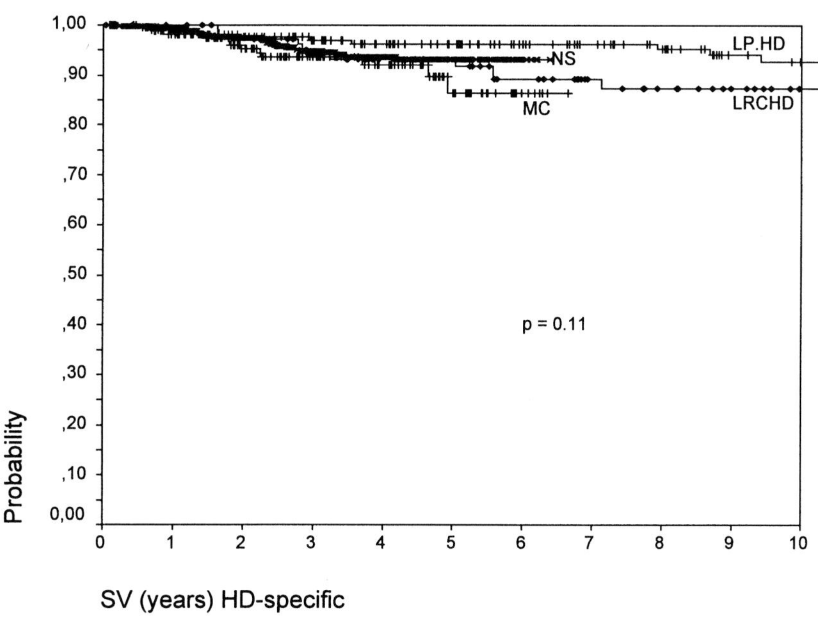

FIG. 6. ETFL project: Survival (SV) of lymphocyte predominance Hodgkin's disease (LPHD), lymphocyte-rich classical Hodgkin's disease (LRCHD) cases compared with nodular sclerosis (NS) and mixed cellularity (MC) cases of the German Hodgkin's Lymphoma Study Group (GHSG).

TABLE 11. *ETFL project: Failure-free survival (FFS) and survival (SV) at 8 years*

	Stage	LPHD	SE[a]	LRCHD	SE[a]
FFS	I	85%	4.3	81%	6.1
	II	71%	7.3	76%	8.7
	III	62%	9.8	74%	8.5
	IV	24%	18	57%	19
SV	I	99%	1.2	91%	5.1
	II	94%	2.9	86%	7.6
	III	94%	4.4	88%	6.4
	IV	41%	30	67%	19

LPHD, lymphocyte predominance Hodgkin's disease; LRCHD, lymphocyte-rich classical Hodgkin's disease.
[a]SE, standard error (%).

Patients with lymphocyte-rich classical Hodgkin's disease had a worse prognosis than lymphocyte predominance Hodgkin's disease patients ($p = .024$) after relapse (Fig. 7). Further analysis revealed that this difference could partly be explained by the higher average age of lymphocyte-rich classical Hodgkin's disease patients (Fig. 2). Nevertheless, subgroup analysis of patients younger than 45 years also revealed a favorable prognosis after relapse for lymphocyte predominance Hodgkin's disease patients (Fig. 8). lymphocyte predominance Hodgkin's disease patients also showed a tendency to more favorable survival after relapse than classical Hodgkin's disease patients in the GHSG ($p = .050$). This, however, should be interpreted with caution because the lymphocyte predominance Hodgkin's disease patients more often had early stage at first diagnosis and therefore received less intensive first-line therapy on average.

Multiple relapses were observed in 12 of 45 relapsing patients (27%) of the lymphocyte predominance Hodgkin's disease group but only one of 19 relapsed patients (5%) with initial lymphocyte-rich classical Hodgkin's disease ($p = .044$). Information on the sequence of relapse diagnoses was very incomplete but suggests (Table 12) that transformation to classical Hodgkin's disease is rare. This contrasts with the early observations of Jackson and Parker (8).

Information on multiple relapses is given in four of the eight major studies. Hansmann observed 17 with multiple relapses among the 52 relapsing patients, whereas Pappa reported that no multiple relapses were seen (six relapses out of 50 patients) despite very long follow-up. In the other studies, three of 13 and five of 14 relapses, respectively, had a second recurrence.

Nodular and Diffuse Lymphocyte Predominance Hodgkin's Disease : Clinical Differences

Nodular lymphocyte predominance Hodgkin's disease is considered by many investigators to be a distinct disorder within the spectrum of Hodgkin's disease, with a better prognosis than the classical types of Hodgkin's disease. There are conflicting data, however, about the nature and prognosis of the diffuse and mixed variants of lymphocyte predominance Hodgkin's disease. Hansmann et al. (40) claim that these variants differ mainly in follicular dendritic cell meshwork pattern but not in origin and nature of the tumor cells.

As stated above, in the ETFL project data no significant (or even suggestive) prognostic differences were observed between cases with nodular, diffuse, and nodular-plus-diffuse architecture. Neither were any differences in patient or disease characteristics visible. However, because there were only nine purely diffuse cases (4%), the project data are inconclusive on these points.

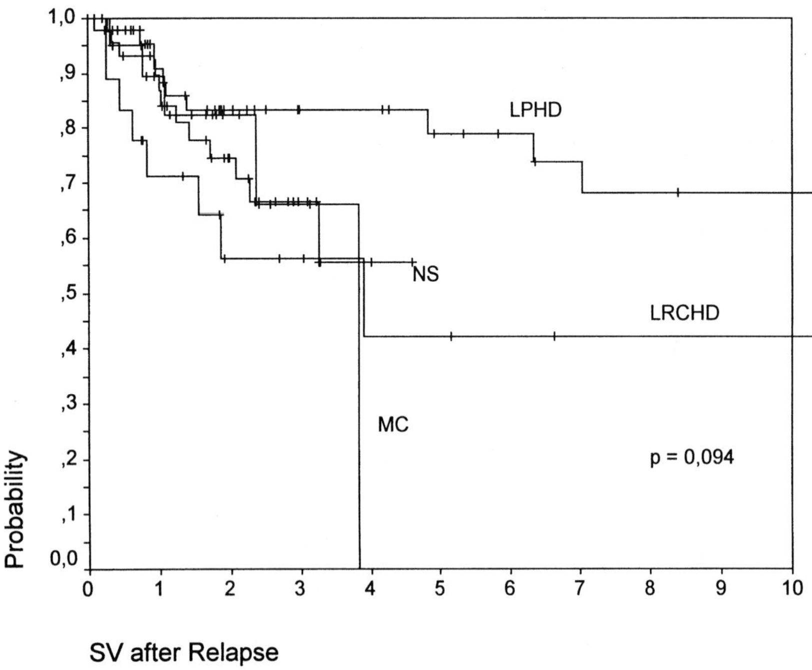

FIG. 7. ETFL project: Survival (SV) after relapse of lymphocyte predominance Hodgkin's disease (LPHD), lymphocyte-rich classical Hodgkin's disease (LRCHD) cases compared with nodular sclerosis (NS) and mixed cellularity (MC) cases of the German Hodgkin's Lymphoma Study Group (GHSG).

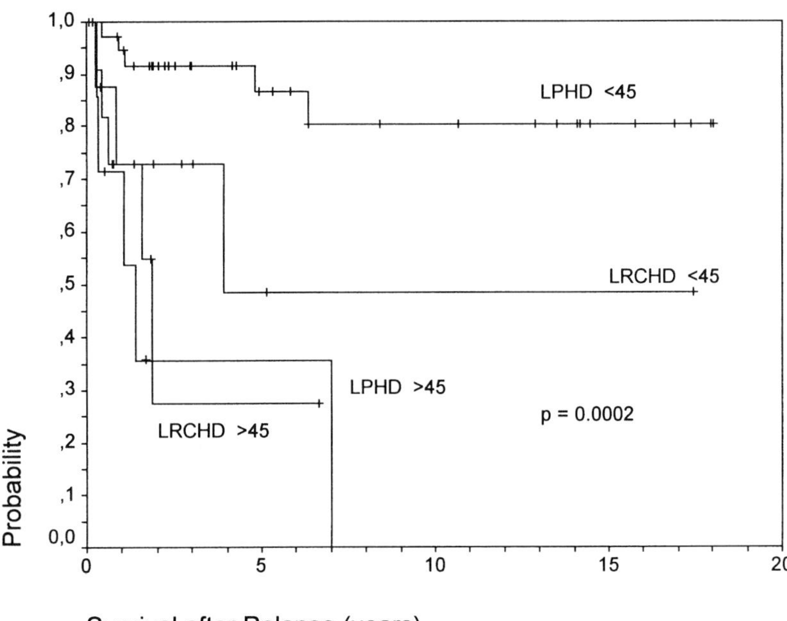

FIG. 8. ETFL project: Survival after relapse of lymphocyte predominance Hodgkin's disease (LPHD), lymphocyte-rich classical Hodgkin's disease (LRCHD) cases, subdivided according to age above or below 45 years.

Clinical comparisons between nodular and diffuse forms were reported in four of the other major studies, and the results are summarized in Table 13. Two studies (Borg-Grech, Crennan) revealed no prognostic differences between nodular and diffuse lymphocyte predominance Hodgkin's disease , whereas two (Regula, Bodis) showed superior relapse-free survival for diffuse cases, albeit with only borderline significance (p = .05 and .06, respectively) and without any sign of survival differences. The proportion of cases classified as diffuse varied widely from 22% to 56% (indeed, Pappa did not find any purely diffuse cases among 50 lymphocyte predominances), suggesting that the methods or criteria employed in this classification may not be consistent. Divergent proportions of 22% and 56% were both reported in studies showing a significant prognostic difference between nodular and diffuse variants.

Difficulties can occur in the differential diagnosis between diffuse lymphocyte predominance Hodgkin's disease and both lymphocyte-rich classical Hodgkin's disease and T-cell–rich B-cell Lymphoma (41–43). The inclusion of a few borderline cases in the diffuse lymphocyte predominance Hodgkin's disease samples could explain the apparently worse prognosis in some reports. Moreover, the small proportion of diffuse cases diagnosed in the ETFL study, which had shrunk as further efforts were made to detect nodularity, casts doubt on the clinical relevance of this subdivision.

Relationship to Other Lymph Node Disorders

Progressively Transformed Germinal Centers

Those alterations of the lymph node structure termed progressively transformed germinal centers are frequently found in patients with certain nonmalignant lymphatic disorders (44–46). They closely resemble the nodules of nodular lymphocyte predominance Hodgkin's disease with the exception that no L&H cells are present; indeed, Poppema (41) has proposed that lymphocyte predominance Hodgkin's disease develops from progressively transformed germinal centers. Progressively transformed germinal centers may occur before, after, or together with nodular lymphocyte predominance Hodgkin's disease.

TABLE 12. *ETFL project: Multiple-relapse cases after LPHD with information on sequence of relapse histology*[a]

Case	Initial diagnosis	First relapse	Second relapse	Third relapse	Fourth relapse
LE105	LPHD	LP	LP	Interfollic. HD	LP
LE109	LPHD	LP	??	??	NHL
LE110	LPHD	MC/LP	nLP	nLP	LP + MC?
LE114	LPHD	LP	LP		
HE011	LPHD	nLP	nLP	nLP	
HE101	LPHD	nLP	nLP		
HE006	LPHD	??	nLP		
ST008	LPHD	NHL	??		

LPHD, lymphocyte predominance Hodgkin's disease; LP, lymphocyte predominance; MC, mixed cellularity; nLP, nodular lymphocyte predominance; NHL, non-Hodgkin's lymphoma; no biopsy or not available.

TABLE 13. *Major studies comparing nodular and diffuse forms of LPHD*

Study	*n*	Proportion nodular	Prognostic differences
Bodis	75	78%	RFS: D > N (p=.05)
Borg-Grech	110	68%	no
ETFL			no
Pappa	50	100%	—
Regula	73	44%	RFS: D > N (p=.06)
Crennan	64	48%	no

LPHD, lymphocyte predominance Hodgkin's disease; RFS, relapse-free survival.

The following questions are clinically relevant:

1. How should progressively transformed germinal centers and lymphocyte predominance Hodgkin's disease be reliably distinguished?
2. Does progressively transformed germinal centers predict lymphocyte predominance?
3. Does the occurrence of progressively transformed germinal centers simultaneously with lymphocyte predominance Hodgkin's disease have prognostic significance?

In response to these questions:

1. Burns et al. (44) recommended the examination of three or four cross-sections of the lymph node showing progressively transformed germinal centers for L&H cells to ensure that a diagnosis of lymphocyte predominance Hodgkin's disease is not missed. Conversely, they recommend histologic confirmation of all apparent relapses of lymphocyte predominance Hodgkin's disease to exclude the possibility that it is merely a progressively transformed germinal centers.
2. Despite the many observed cases where progressively transformed germinal centers precedes nodular lymphocyte predominance Hodgkin's disease , no study has convincingly shown that detection of progressively transformed germinal centers implies an increased risk of developing lymphocyte predominance Hodgkin's disease (41,45,46). Most studies have collected cases partly or wholly from diagnoses of classical Hodgkin's disease or lymphocyte predominance Hodgkin's disease and therefore do not allow the relative risk to be estimated.
3. In the ETFL project, 91% of samples reviewed as lymphocyte predominance Hodgkin's disease and evaluable for estimation of resemblance to progressively transformed germinal centers were judged to be "progressively transformed germinal centers-like"; the corresponding percentage for lymphocyte-rich classical Hodgkin's disease cases was 11%. This factor did not show any prognostic significance within the lymphocyte predominance Hodgkin's disease cases. Among lymphocyte predominance Hodgkin's disease and lymphocyte-rich classical Hodgkin's disease cases together, Hodgkin's disease–specific survival was somewhat (though not significantly) better for progressively transformed germinal centers-like cases, reflecting its association with lymphocyte predominance Hodgkin's disease.

Composite Lymphoma

Only a few cases of composite (i.e., simultaneous in the same lymph node or organ) lymphocyte predominance Hodgkin's disease with a large-cell lymphoma have been reported. Sundeen (47) described seven such cases: after various treatment regimens, mostly radiotherapy, none of these patients developed disseminated large-cell lymphoma, and six were in continuing complete remission. This contrasts with the usually poor prognosis of large-cell lymphoma. Similarly, Hansmann et al. (48)

TABLE 14. *ETFL project: Fatal secondary malignancies*

Diagnosis	Cause of death	Age at death (years)	Primary therapy	HD Relapse
LPHD	Leukemia/MDS	77	CMT	No
LPHD	Leukemia/MDS	62	RX	Yes
LPHD	Leukemia/MDS	66	RX	No
LPHD	Leukemia/MDS	34	CT	Yes
LPHD	Leukemia/MDS	75	RX	No
LPHD	NHL	57	CT	No
LPHD	NHL	51	RX	No
LPHD	Solid tumor	67	RX	No
LPHD	Solid tumor	79	CT	Yes
LPHD	Solid tumor	83	RX	No
LRCHD	Leukemia/MDS	36	CMT	No
LRCHD	NHL	72	CT	No
LRCHD	NHL	45	RX	Yes
LRCHD	Solid tumor	82	RX	No

LPHD, lymphocyte predominance Hodkgin's disease; MDS, myelodysplastic syndrome; CMT, combined modality treatment; RX, radiotherapy; CT, chemotherapy alone; NHL, non-Hodgkin's lymphoma; LRCHD lymphocyte-rich classical Hodgkin's disease.

found 11 large-cell lymphoma composites among 537 cases of nodular lymphocyte predominance Hodgkin's disease, at least nine of whom were alive between 1 and 10 years after diagnosis. In view of the rarity of such composite lymphomas, the clinical relevance would seem to be limited. However, Sundeen recommends that these patients be regarded clinically as Hodgkin's disease rather than non-Hodgkin's lymphoma.

Secondary Non-Hodgkin's Lymphoma After Lymphocyte predominance Hodgkin's disease

The possibility of occurrence of a non-Hodgkin's lymphoma after primary lymphocyte predominance Hodgkin's disease is clinically important because of the following considerations: (a) choice of monitoring strategy after primary treatment and of diagnostic measures in the event of a malignancy, (b) choice of primary treatment to destroy the seed of a potential concomitant non-Hodgkin's lymphoma, and (c) choice of primary treatment to avoid treatment-related non-Hodgkin's lymphoma.

In the ETFL project, complete data on occurrence of second malignancies after lymphocyte predominance were not collected, but all deaths from a second malignancy were recorded (Table 14). There were two fatal non-Hodgkin's lymphomas following lymphocyte predominance Hodgkin's disease ($n = 219$) and two following lymphocyte-rich classical Hodgkin's disease ($n = 115$). Median follow-up was 6.8 years for lymphocyte predominance Hodgkin's disease and 8.2 years for lymphocyte-rich classical Hodgkin's disease. Four further nonfatal occurrences of secondary non-Hodgkin's lymphoma were documented, two directly following primary lymphocyte predominance Hodgkin's disease and two after one or more relapses of lymphocyte predominance Hodgkin's disease, giving a total of at least six non-Hodgkin's lymphomas after 219 cases of primary lymphocyte predominance Hodgkin's disease (2.9%).

Seven of the other eight major studies give information on secondary non-Hodgkin's lymphoma, although in one publication only the fatal cases are given. Median follow-up ranged from 7 to 11 years. They report a total of 15 non-Hodgkin's lymphoma cases among 567 lymphocyte predominance patients (2.6%). These rates can be compared with those for Hodgkin's disease as a whole from the International Database on Hodgkin's Disease (IDHD) (49). Of 12,411 Hodgkin's disease patients, 106 developed a secondary non-Hodgkin's lymphoma (0.9%), and the cumulative incidence rate for non-Hodgkin's lymphoma was estimated as 1.0% after 10 years. A significantly higher risk for secondary non-Hodgkin's lymphoma, increased by a factor 1.8, was found for lymphocyte predominance patients compared with nodular sclerosis and mixed cellularity ($p < .01$). On the basis of this evidence, an approximately two- to threefold higher rate of secondary non-Hodgkin's lymphoma following lymphocyte predominance Hodgkin's disease compared with classical Hodgkin's disease is indicated.

Regarding the causal role of treatment for secondary non-Hodgkin's lymphoma, in the report of Miettinen four of the five secondary non-Hodgkin's lymphomas occurred in untreated patients. In the above-mentioned IDHD analysis, combined-modality therapy was associated with increased risk in univariate analysis but not in multivariate analysis.

In summary, there is evidence that non-Hodgkin's lymphomas are more likely following lymphocyte predominance Hodgkin's disease than following other subtypes of Hodgkin's disease. Treatment seems to play at most a minor role in causing secondary non-Hodgkin's lymphoma.

PERSPECTIVES FOR FUTURE TREATMENT

Lymphocyte predominant Hodgkin's disease is considered to have the best prognosis of all histologic subtypes of Hodgkin's disease. The disease even resembles a recurrent reactive process in view of the excellent survival rate in spite of frequent relapses. Most studies report a survival rate for lymphocyte predominance Hodgkin's disease of more than 80% irrespective of the kind of treatment (21,23,30); even without radiotherapy or chemotherapy, the prognosis is good (28,29). It is noteworthy, however, that the prognosis for the treated lymphocyte predominance Hodgkin's disease patients in the reviewed cohort of the ETFL study was no better than that for stage-matched classical Hodgkin's disease (nodular sclerosis and mixed cellularity cases from the GHSG study, Figs. 3 and 4). From these data alone, there is no rationale for a less intensive treatment of lymphocyte predominance Hodgkin's disease compared with classical Hodgkin's disease. However, the observed causes of death should be considered. Only 4% of patients in the ETFL series (Table 15), as well as in the report by Regula, died of Hodgkin's disease; more

TABLE 15. *ETFL project: Causes of death*

	LPHD		LRCHD	
HD	8	3.7%	10	8.7%
Therapy				
Primary	0		3	2.6%
Salvage	1	0.5%	1	0.9%
Cardiovascular	4	1.8%	7	6.1%
Secondary tumors				
Acute leukemia	5	2.3%	1	0.9%
NHL	2	0.9%	2	1.7%
Solid tumor	3	1.4%	1	0.9%
Other				
Known	6	2.7%	2	1.7%
Unknown	1	0.5%	1	0.9%
Unknown, in CR	1	0.5%	2	1.7%
Total deaths	31	14%	30	26%
Total patients	219	100%	115	100%

LPHD, lymphocyte predominance Hodgkin's disease; LRCHD lymphocyte-rich classical Hodgkin's disease; NHL, non-Hodgkin's lymphoma.

patients died of fatal secondary tumors (5% in the ETFL series and 10% in the series of Regula). These numbers suggest that current treatment strategies might be too intensive, particularly when late effects such as secondary malignancies and cardiac and pulmonary complications are taken into account. However, secondary non-Hodgkin's lymphomas seem to be disease-related rather than treatment-related (see above), and their relatively high frequency (about 3%) speaks for the retention rather than reduction of an effective primary therapy.

A watch-and-wait treatment strategy, in which patients are monitored without treatment until the disease shows signs of progression, has been advocated for lymphocyte predominance Hodgkin's disease and for other indolent lymphomas (29,50). However, most authors report only anecdotal cases, and prospective randomized trials do not exist. Miettinen (28) described 31 of 51 cases with lymphocyte predominance Hodgkin's disease who remained untreated because the original histologic diagnosis was not malignant. The survival for these 31 patients, mostly in stage IA, was 93% at 5 years and 80% at 10 years. Five of the 51 untreated patients developed a diffuse large-cell non-Hodgkin's lymphoma 4 to 11 years after the onset of the primary nodular lymphocyte predominance Hodgkin's disease. In the series of Hansmann (29), nine of 24 patients with nodular lymphocyte predominance Hodgkin's disease in stage IA who were not treated after lymph node biopsy remained free of disease even after 7 to 14 years. A prospective trial with explicit inclusion criteria is required in order to assess the feasibility, risks, and benefits of a watch-and-wait strategy.

It is important to notice that about 20% to 25% of the patients with lymphocyte predominance Hodgkin's disease are diagnosed in stage III or IV. This implies that thorough staging is still needed irrespective of histologic subtype because overall survival and tumor-free survival were substantially worse for patients with advanced-stage lymphocyte predominance Hodgkin's disease as compared to patients with early-stage disease. In the ETFL series, stage was a significant prognostic factor for lymphocyte predominance Hodgkin's disease cases with respect to both survival and failure-free survival. The 8-year survival estimates for stage III were 94%, and for stage IV approximately 40%, following adequate polychemotherapy in most cases. The 8-year failure-free survival estimates for stage III were 62% and for stage IV about 25% (see Table 11). These data imply that the outcome for advanced lymphocyte predominance Hodgkin's disease patients is not better than for patients with advanced disease of the classical Hodgkin's disease type. The conclusion from these data is to treat patients with lymphocyte predominance Hodgkin's disease stages III and IV like patients with classical Hodgkin's disease of the same stages.

A potential new avenue for clinical research in lymphocyte predominance Hodgkin's disease is the use of immunotherapy, for instance immunotoxins, bispecific antibodies, or the monoclonal antibody Rituximab. The latter antibody is directed against the B-cell restricted CD20 antigen; this antigen is expressed by the L&H cells of lymphocyte predominance Hodgkin's disease but rarely by the Hodgkin and Reed-Sternberg cells of classical Hodgkin's disease. First experiences with indolent follicular B-cell lymphomas have shown unexpectedly good results, with about 55% overall responses even in relapsing patients (51–53). Relapses occur up to 20 years after primary diagnosis of lymphocyte predominance Hodgkin's disease, in the ETFL study in about 50% of cases. Further, 27% of patients relapsing after lymphocyte predominance Hodgkin's disease suffered multiple recurrences, mostly again nodular lymphocyte predominance Hodgkin's disease lesions, which are rarely fatal. Survival after lymphocyte predominance Hodgkin's disease relapses is more than 70% after 10 years in the ETFL study (Fig. 5). This favorable course implies that immunotherapy could turn out to be a realistic strategy even for relapsing lymphocyte predominance Hodgkin's disease patients.

CONCLUSIONS

The REAL classification replaced the previous (Rye) category lymphocyte predominance Hodgkin's disease with lymphocyte predominance Hodgkin's disease and the provisional entity lymphocyte-rich classical Hodgkin's disease on the basis of the morphologic and immunmophenotypic characteristics of the tumor cells and the pattern of the reactive environment.

Despite the clear separation of lymphocyte-rich classical Hodgkin's disease from lymphocyte predominance Hodgkin's disease on this histopathologic basis, the clinical features of these two subtypes are similar. They are diagnosed typically in male patients with a median age around 35 years as early-stage disease without systemic symptoms or other adverse prognostic factors. However, advanced-stage cases do occur. The two subtypes do not differ markedly in clinical characteristics except for the greater average age of the lymphocyte-rich classical Hodgkin's disease cases. These clinical features distinguish lymphocyte predominance Hodgkin's disease and lymphocyte-rich classical Hodgkin's disease clearly from classical Hodgkin's disease of the nodular sclerosis and mixed cellularity types, which in general occur with more advanced stage and more systemic symptoms and other adverse prognostic factors.

The lymphocyte predominance Hodgkin's disease patients in earlier studies have tended to have a better prognosis than classical Hodgkin's disease patients, but under modern protocol treatment, this advantage seems to be minimal or absent. When patients of the same stage are compared, no significant differences in survival or failure-free survival were seen for lymphocyte predominance Hodgkin's disease or lymphocyte-rich classical Hodgkin's disease as compared to classical Hodgkin's disease cases from the GHSG. Lymphocyte predominance Hodgkin's disease patients tend to relapse frequently, but they survive these predominantly late relapses better than classical or lymphocyte-rich classical Hodgkin's disease patients. This gives rise to a relatively large proportion of multiple recurrences in lymphocyte predominance Hodgkin's disease.

There is no conclusive evidence for clinical or prognostic differences between the nodular, diffuse or mixed forms of lymphocyte predominance Hodgkin's disease. Studies differ widely in the proportion of diffuse cases; in the ETFL cohort only 4% of lymphocyte predominance Hodgkin's disease cases were purely diffuse. This division does not seem to be clinically relevant.

Lymphocyte predominant Hodgkin's disease is sometimes preceded by a reactive enlargement of the lymph node termed "progressively transformed germinal center" progressively transformed germinal center, which closely resembles lymphocyte predominance Hodgkin's disease. However, progressively transformed germinal center has not conclusively been shown to be a risk factor for later development of lymphocyte predominance Hodgkin's disease; progressively transformed germinal center can also occur after lymphocyte predominance Hodgkin's disease, so a careful differential diagnosis is necessary when a relapse of lymphocyte predominance Hodgkin's disease is suspected.

Secondary low-grade non-Hodgkin's lymphomas occur more frequently after lymphocyte predominance Hodgkin's disease than after classical Hodgkin's disease. They seem to be disease-related rather than treatment-induced.

Their resemblance to nonneoplastic disorders, capability for ongoing mutation of the tumor cells, favorable clinical presentation, and good survival rates (even after relapse) all suggest that the optimal primary treatment strategy might be less intensive for lymphocyte predominance Hodgkin's disease than for classical Hodgkin's disease. Late toxicities, which contribute considerably to the death rate, could thus be reduced. The long survival of several early-stage lymphocyte predominance Hodgkin's disease patients without any treatment beyond lymph node excision could favor a watch-and-wait strategy, albeit only after rigorous staging. New experimental therapy techniques such as immunotherapy might also be suitable. These possibilities must first be tested in a large-scale prospective study.

APPENDIX: PARTICIPANTS IN THE ETFL PROJECT ON LYMPHOCYTE PREDOMINANCE HODGKIN'S DISEASE

In addition to the authors of this chapter the following persons contributed to the project:

Pathology Review Panel

I. Anagnostopoulos
K. Franssila
M. Harris
N.L. Harris
M.-L. Hansmann
E. Jaffe
T.Marafioti
H. Stein
J.H.J.R. van Krieken

Contributors of Cases

Institution	Clinician	Pathologist
Christie Hospital, Manchester, UK	D. Crowther, J. Radford	M. Harris
Helsinki University , Central Hospital Helsinki, Finland	L. Teerenhovi	K. Franssila
German Hodgkin's Lymphoma Study Group, Cologne, Germany		A. Georgii
Istituto Nazionale per lo Studio e la Cura deiTumori, Milan, Italy	V. Bonfante, A. Gianni	S. Pilotti
Swedish National Health Care Programme, Uppsala, Sweden	B. Glimelius	M. Dictor
Mayo Clinic, Rochester, Minnesota, USA	T. Haberman	P. Kurtin
Rigshospitalet, University of Copenhagen, Copenhagen, Denmark	L. Specht	K. Hou-Jensen
Royal Victoria Infirmary, Newcastle-upon-Tyne, UK	P. Taylor, S. Proctor	B. Angus
St. Bartholomew's Hospital, London, UK	T.A. Lister	A. Norton
Akademisch Ziekenhuis Leiden, Leiden, The Netherlands	E. Noordijk	J. van Krieken, P. Kluin
M. D. Anderson Cancer Center, Houston, Texas, USA	F. Hagemeister	J. McBride, W. Pugh
Institut Bergonié, Bordeaux, France	H. Eghbali	I. Soubeyran
Karolinska Hospital, Stockholm, Sweden	U. Axdorph, M. Björkholm	A. MacDonald, A. Öst

Hospital Gregorio Marañón, Madrid, Spain		J. Menarguez
Università degli Studie "La Sapienza," Rome, Italy	A. Anselmo, F. Mandelli	C. Baroni
Centre Hospitalier Lyon-Sud, Lyon, France	B. Coiffier	F. Berger

REFERENCES

1. Jackson H, Parker F. Hodgkin's disease; II, pathology. *N Engl J Med* 1944;231:35.
2. Lukes RJ, Butler JJ. The pathology and nomenclature of Hodgkin's disease. *Cancer Res* 1966;26:1063.
3. Lukes RJ, Butler JJ, Hicks EB. Natural history of Hodgkin's disease as related to its pathologic picture. *Cancer* 1966;19:317.
4. Chittal SM, Alard C, Rossi JF, et al. Further phenotypic evidence that nodular, lymphocytic predominance Hodgkin's disease is a large B-cell lymphoma in evolution. *Am J Surg Pathol* 1990;14:1024.
5. Harris NL, Jaffe ES, Stein H, et al. A revised European-American classification of lymphoid neoplasms: a proposal from the International Lymphoma Study Group. *Blood* 1994;84:1361.
6. Westling P. Studies of the prognosis in Hodgkin's disease. *Acta Radiol* 1965;245(Suppl):5.
7. Rosenthal SR. Significance of tissue lymphocytes in the prognosis of lymphogranulomatosis. *Arch Pathol* 1936;21:628.
8. Jackson H, Parker F. *Hodgkin's disease and allied disorders*. New York: Oxford University Press, 1947.
9. Lennert K, Hippchen AM. Zur Prognose der Lymphogranulomatose. Abhängigkeit von histologischem Bild, Alter und Geschlecht. *Frankfurt Z Pathol* 1954;65:378.
10. Harrison CV. Benign Hodgkin's disease (Hodgkin's granuloma). *J Pathol Bacteriol* 1952;64:513.
11. Wright CJE. The "benign" form of Hodgkin's disease (Hodgkin's paragranuloma). *J Pathol Bacteriol* 1960;80:157.
12. Peters MV. A study of survivals in Hodgkin's disease treated radiologically. *Am J Roentgenol* 1950;63:299.
13. Smetana HF, Cohen BM. Mortality in relation to histiologic subtype in Hodgkin's disease. *Blood* 1956;11:211.
14. Hanson TAS. Histological classification and survival in Hodgkin's disease. A study of 251 cases with special reference to nodular sclerosis Hodgkin's disease. *Cancer* 1964;17:1595.
15. Franssila KO, Heiskala MK, Heiskala HJ. Epidemiology and histopathology of Hodgkin's disease in Finland. *Cancer* 1977;39:1280.
16. Keller AR, Kaplan HS, Lukes RJ, Rappaport H. Correlation of histopathology with other prognostic indicators in Hodgkin's disease. *Cancer* 1968;22:487.
17. Landsberg T, Larsson L-E. Hodgkin's disease retrospective clinicopathologic study in 149 patients. *Acta Radiol* 1969;8:390.
18. Gough J. Hodgkin's disease: a correlation of histopathology with survival. *Int J Cancer* 1970;5:273.
19. Kaplan HS. Hodgkin's disease and other human malignant lymphomas: advances and prospects. G.H.A. Clowes Memorial Lecture. *Cancer Res* 1976;36:3863.
20. Culine S, Henry-Amar M, Diebold J, et al. Relationship of histological subtypes to prognosis in early stage Hodgkin's disease: a review of 312 cases in a controlled clinical trial. *Eur J Cancer Clin Oncol* 1989;25:551.
21. Bennett MH, MacLennan KA, Vaughan Hudson B, Vaughan Hudson G. The clinical and prognostic relevance of histopathologic classification in Hodgkin's disease. *Prog Surg Pathol* 1990;10:127.
22. Shankar AG, Ashley S, Radford M, Barrett A, Wright D, Pinkerton CR. Does histology influence outcome in childhood Hodgkin's disease? Results from the United Kingdom Children's Cancer Study Group. *J Clin Oncol* 1997;15:2262.
23. Regula DP, Hoppe RT, Weiss LM. Nodular and diffuse types of lymphocyte predominance Hodgkin's disease. *N Engl J Med* 1988;318:214.
24. Jaffe ES, Zarate-Osorno A, Medeiros J. The interrelationship of Hodgkin's disease and non-Hodgkin's lymphomas—Lessons learned from composite and sequential malignancies. *Semin Diag Pathol* 1992;9:297.
25. Diehl V, Sextro M, Franklin J et al. Clinical presentation, course and prognostic factors in lymphocyte-predominant Hodgkin's disease and lymphocyte-rich classical Hodgkin's disease: report from the European Task Force on Lymphoma project on lymphocate predominant Hodgkin's disease. *J Clin Oncol* 1999,17:XX
26. Loeffler M, Pfreundschuh M, Rühl U, et al. Risk factor adapted treatment of Hodgkin's lymphoma: strategies and perspectives. *Recent Results Cancer Res* 1989;117:142.
27. Georgii A, Fischer R, Hübner K, et al. Classification of Hodgkin's disease biopsies by a panel of four histopathologists. Report of 1140 patients from the German national trial. *Leuk Lymphoma* 1993;9:365.
28. Miettinen M, Franssila KO, Saxen E. Hodgkin's disease, lymphocyte predominance nodular. Increased risk of subsequent non-Hodgkin's lymphoma. *Cancer* 1983;51:2293.
29. Hansmann M-L, Zwingers T, Boeske A, Loeffler H, Lennert K. Clinical features of nodular paragranuloma (Hodgkin's disease, lymphocyte predominance type, nodular). *J Cancer Res Clin Oncol* 1984;108:321.
30. Borg-Grech A, Radford JA, Crowther D, Swindell R, Harris M. A comparative study of the nodular and diffuse variants of lymphocyte-predominant Hodgkin's disease. *J Clin Oncol* 1989;7:1303.
31. Crennan E, D'Costa I, Liew KH, et al. Lymphocyte predominant Hodgkin's disease: a clinicopathologic comparative study study of histologic and immunophenotypic subtypes. *Int J Radiat Oncol Biol Phys* 1995;31:337.
32. Pappa I, Norton AJ, Gupta RK, Wilson AM, Rohatiner AZ, Lister TA. Nodular type of lymphocyte predominance Hodgkin's disease. *Ann Oncol* 1995;6:559.
33. von Wasielewski R, Werner M, Fischer R, et al. Lymphocyte predominant Hodgkin's disease. An immunohistochemical analysis of 208 reviewed Hodgkin's disease cases from the German Hodgkin Study Group. *Am J Pathol* 1997;150:793.
34. Bodis S, Kraus MD, Pinkus G, et al. Clinical presentation and outcome in lymphocyte-predominant Hodgkin's disease. *J Clin Oncol* 1997; 15:3060.
35. Orlandi E, Lazzarino M, Brusamolino E, et al. Nodular lymphocyte predominance Hodgkin's disease: long-term observation reveals a continuous pattern of recurrence. *Leuk Lymphoma* 1997;26:359.
36. Mauch PM, Kalish LA, Kadin M, Coleman CN, Osteen RO, Hellman S. Patterns of presentation of Hodgkin's disease. Implications for etiology and prognosis. *Cancer* 1993;71:2062.
37. Carde P, Burgers JMV, Henry-Amar M, et al. Clinical stages I and II Hodgkin's disease: a specifically tailored therapy according to prognostic factors. *J Clin Oncol* 1988;6:329.
38. Noordijk EM, Carde P, Mandard A-M, et al. Preliminary results of the EORTC-GPMC controlled clinical trial H7 in early-stage Hodgkin's disease. *Ann Oncol* 1994;5(suppl 2):107.
39. Dawson PJ, Harrison CV. A clinicopathological study of benign Hodgkin's disease. *J Clin Pathol* 1961;14:219.
40. Hansmann M-L, Gödde-Salz E, Hui P-K, Müller-Hermelink H-K, Lennert K. Cytogenetic findings in nodular paragranuloma (Hodgkin's disease with lymphocytic predominance; nodular) and in progressively transformed germinal centers. *Cancer Genet Cytogenet* 1986;21:319.
41. Poppema S. Lymphocyte-predominance Hodgkin's disease. *Semin Diag Pathol* 1992;9:257.
42. Hansmann M-L, Stein H, Dallenbach F, Fellbaum C. Diffuse lymphocyte-predominant Hodgkin's disease (diffuse paragranuloma). A variant of the B-cell-derived nodular type. *Am J Pathol* 1991;138:29.
43. Schmidt U, Metz KA, Leder L-D. T-cell-rich B-cell lymphoma and lymphocyte predominant Hodgkin's disease: two closely related entities? *Br J Haematol* 1995;90:398.
44. Burns BF, Colby TV, Dorfman RF. Differential diagnostic features of nodular L&H Hodgkin's disease, including progressive transformation of germinal centers. *Am J Surg Pathol* 1984;8:253.
45. Poppema S, Kaiserling E, Lennert K. Hodgkin's disease with lymphocytic predominace, nodular type (nodular paragranuloma) and progressively transformed germinal centres—a cytohistological study. *Histopathology* 1979;3:295.
46. Osborne BM, Butler JJ. Clinical implications of progressive transformation of germinal centers. *Am J Surg Pathol* 1984;8:725.
47. Sundeen JT, Cossman J, Jaffe ES. Lymphocyte predominant Hodgkin's disease nodular subtype with coexistent "large cell lymphoma." Histological progression or composite malignancy? *Am J Surg Pathol* 1988;12:599.
48. Hansmann ML, Stein H, Fellbaum C, et al. Nodular paragranuloma can

transform into high-grade malignant lymphoma of B type. *Hum Pathol* 1989;20:1169.
49. Henry-Amar M. Second cancer after the treatment of Hodgkin's disease: a report from the International Database on Hodgkin's disease. *Ann Oncol* 1992;3(suppl 4):117.
50. Soubeyran P, Eghbali H, Trojani M, Bonichon F, Richaud P, Hoerni B. Is there any place for a wait-and-see policy in stage I.0 follicular lymphoma. A study of 43 consecutive patients in a single center. *Ann Oncol* 1996;7:713.
51. Czuczmann M, Grillo-Lopez AJ, White CA, et al. IDEC-C2B8/Chop chemotherapy in patients with low grade lymphoma: clinical and bcl-2 (PCR) results (abstract). *J Mol Med* 1997;75:7.
52. Maloney DG, Grillo-Lopez AJ, Bodkin DJ. et al. IDEC-C2B8: results of a phase I multiple-dose trial in patients with relapsed non-Hodgkin's Lymphoma. *J Clin Oncol* 1997;15:3266.
53. Coiffier B, Haioun C, Ketterer N, et al. Rituximab (anti-CD20 monoclonal antibody) for the treatment of patients with relapsing or refractory aggressive lymphoma: a multicenter phase II study. *Blood* 1998;92:1927.

SUGGESTED READINGS

Historical

Peters MV, Hasselback R, Brown TC. The natural history of the lymphomas related to the clinical classification. In: Zarafonetis CJD, ed. *Proceedings of the International Conference on Leukemia-Lymphoma.* Philadelphia: Lea & Febiger, 1968:357.

Rappaport H, Berard CW, Butler JJ, Dorfman RF, Lukes RJ, Thomas LB. Report of the committee on histopathological criteria contributing to the staging of Hodgkin's disease. *Cancer Res* 1971;31:1864.

Rappaport H, Winter WJ, Hicks EB. Follicular lymphoma. A reevaluation of its position in the scheme of malignant lymphoma, based on a survey of 253 cases. *Cancer* 1956;9:792.

Robb-Smith AHG. The lymph node biopsy. In Dyke SC, ed. *Recent advances in clinical pathology,* London: J. and A. Churchill, 1947:350.

Symmers WStC. XX. In: Raven RW, ed. *Cancer,* vol 2. London: Butterworth, 1958:478.

Nature of Lymphocyte Predominance Hodgkin's Disease

Algara P, Martinez P, Sanchez L, et al. Lymphocyte predominance Hodgkin's disease (nodular paragranuloma)—a *bcl-2* negative germinal centre lymphoma. *Histopathology* 1991;19:69.

Ashton-Key M, Thorpe PA, Allen JP, Isaacson PG. Follicular Hodgkin's disease. *Am J Surg Pathol* 1995;19:1294.

Bräuninger A, Küppers R, Strickler JG, Wacker H-H, Rajewsky K, Hansmann M-L. Hodgkin and Reed-Sternberg cells in lymphocyte predominance Hodgkin's disease represent clonal populations of germinal center-derived tumor cells. *Proc Natl Acad Sci USA* 1997;94:9337.

Delabie J, Tierens A, Wu G, Weisenberger DD, Chan WC. Lymphocyte predominance Hodgkin's disease: lineage and clonality determination using a single-cell assay. *Blood* 1994;84:3291.

Hansmann M-L, Fellbaum C, Hui PK, Zwingers T. Correlation of content of B cells and Leu7-positive cells with subtype and stage in lymphocyte predominance type Hodgkin's disease. *J Cancer Res Clin Oncol* 1988; 114:405.

Hansmann M-L, Gödde-Salz E, Hui P-K, Müller-Hermelink H-K, Lennert K. Cytogenetic findings in nodular paragranuloma (Hodgkin's disease with lymphocytic predominance; nodular) and in progressively transformed germinal centers. *Cancer Genet Cytogenet* 1986;21:319.

Hansmann M-L, Wacker H-H, Radzun HJ. Paragranuloma is a variant of Hodgkin's disease with predominance of B-cells. *Virchows Arch (Pathol Anat)* 1986;409:171.

Küppers R, Zhao M, Hansmann ML, Rajewsky K. Tracing B cell development in human germinal centres by molecular analysis of single cells picked from histological sections. *EMBO J* 1993;12:4955.

Marafioti T, Hummel M, Anagnostopoulos I, et al. Origin of nodular lymphocyte-predominant Hodgkin's disease from a clonal expansion of highly mutated germinal-center B cells. *N Engl J Med* 1997;337:453.

Mason DY, Banks PM, Chan J, et al. Nodular lymphocyte predominance Hodgkin's disease. A distinct clinicopathological entity. *Am J Surg Pathol* 1994;18:526.

Ohno T, Stribley JA, Wu G, Hinrichs SH, Weisenburger DD, Chan WC. Clonality in nodular lymphocyte-predominant Hodgkin's disease. *N Engl J Med* 1997;337:495.

Poppema S. Lymphocyte-predominance Hodgkin's disease. *Int Rev Exp Pathol* 1992;13:53.

Poppema S, Kaiserling E, Lennert K. Epidemiology of nodular paragranuloma (Hodgkin's disease with lymphocytic predominace, nodular). *J Cancer Res Clin Oncol* 1979;95:57.

Poppema S, Kaiserling E, Lennert K. Hodgkin's disease with lymphocytic predominace, nodular type (nodular paragranuloma) and progressively transformed germinal centres—a cytohistological study . *Histopathology* 1979;3:295.

Timens W, Visser L, Poppema S. Nodular lymphocyte predominance type of Hodgkin's disease is a germinal center lymphoma. *Lab Invest* 1986;54:457.

Wright DH. Lymphocyte predominance Hodgkin's disease (letter). *N Engl J Med* 1988;319:246.

Clinical Aspects

Molina T, Diebold J. Paragranulome nodulaire Hodgkinien (maladie de Hodgkin nodulaire, avec predominance lymphocytaire): A propos de 29 cas. *Bull Cancer* 1987;74:463.

Rohde D, Niedermeyer H, Fellbaum C, et al. Nodulares Paragranulom und Epstein-Barr-Virus: Häufigkeit von EBV-DNA und klinische Relevanz. *Verh Dtsch Ges Pathol* 1992;76:177.

Russell KJ, Hoppe RT, Colby TV, Burns BF, Cox RS, Kaplan HS. Lymphocyte predominant Hodgkin's disease: clinical presentation and results of treatment. *Radiother Oncol* 1984;1:197.

Tefferi A, Zellers RA, Banks PM, Therneau TM, Colgan JP. Clinical correlates of distinct immunophenotypic and histologic subcategories of lymphocyte-predominance Hodgkin's disease. *J Clin Oncol* 1990;8:1959.

Related Lymphomas

Baddoura FK, Chan WC, Masih AS, Mitchell D, Sun NCJ, Weisenburger DD. T-cell–rich B-cell lymphoma. A clinicopathologic study of eight cases. *Am J Clin Pathol* 1995;103:65.

Banks PM. The distinction of Hodgkin's disease from T-cell lymphoma. *Semin Diag Pathol* 1992;9:279.

Banks P. The interrelationship of Hodgkin's disease and non-Hodgkin's lymphomas. Introduction. *Semin Diag Pathol* 1992;9:249.

Bernhards J, Fischer R, Werner M, Hübner K, Schwarze EW, Georgii A. Grenzfälle zwischen Hodgkin- und Non-Hodgkin-Lymphomen mit ungünstigem klinischen Verlauf: klinische, histologische und immunchemische Analyse von 33 innerhalb der Deutschen Hodgkin-Studie beobachteten Fällen. *Verh Dtsch Ges Path* 1992;76:159.

De Wolf-Peeters C, Pittalunga S. T-cell–rich B-cell lymphoma: a morphological variant of a variety of non-Hodgkin's lymphomas or a clinicopathological entity? *Histopathology* 1995;26:383.

Delabie J, Vandenberghe E, Kennes C, et al. Histiocyte-rich B-cell lymphoma. A distinct clinicopathologic entity possibly related to lymphocyte predominant Hodgkin's disease, paragranuloma subtype. *Am J Surg Pathol* 1992;16:37.

Farhi DC. T-cell–rich B-cell lymphoma. Reflections on changes in hematopathology (editorial). *Am J Clin Pathol* 1995;103:4.

Greer JP, Macon WR, Lamar RE, et al. T-cell–rich B-cell lymphomas: diagnosis and response to therapy in 44 patients. *J Clin Oncol* 1995;13:1742.

Hansmann ML, Küppers R. Pathology and "molecular histology" of Hodgkin's disease and the border to non-Hodgkin's lymphomas. *Baillieres Clin Haematol* 1996;9:459.

Harris NL. The relationship between Hodgkin's disease and non-Hodgkin's lymphoma. *Semin Diag Pathol* 1992;9:304.

Harris NL. Principles of the European-American lymphoma classification (for the International Lymphoma Study Group). *Ann Oncol* 1997;8:11.

Jaffe ES, Zarate-Osorno A, Kingma DW, Raffeld M, Medeiros J. The interrelationship of Hodgkin's disease and Non-Hodgkin's lymphomas. *Ann Oncol* 1994;5(Suppl 1):7.

Krishnan J, Wallberg K, Frizzera G. T-cell–rich large B-cell lymphoma. A study of 30 cases, supporting its histologic heterogeneity and lack of clinical distinctiveness. *Am J Surg Pathol* 1994;18:455.

Lennert K, Mohri N, Stein H, Kaiserling E. The histopathology of malignant lymphoma. *Br J Haematol* 1975;31(Suppl):193.

Macon WR, Williams ME, Greer JP, Stein RS, Collins RD, Cousar JB. T-cell–rich B-cell lymphomas. A clinicopathologic study of 19 cases. *Am J Surg Pathol* 1992;16:351.

Pileri S, for the Hematopathology Study Group of the Societa Italiana di Anatomia Pathologica. Controversies on Hodgkin's disease and anaplastic large cell lymphoma. *Haematologica* 1994;79:299.

Pileri S, Bocchia M, Baroni CD, et al. Anaplastic large cell lymphoma ($CD30^+/Ki1^+$): results of a prospective clinico-pathological study of 69 cases. *Br J Haematol* 1994;86:513.

Rodriguez J, Pugh WC, Cabanillas F. T-cell–rich B-cell lymphoma. *Blood* 1993;82:1586.

Rosenberg SA. The low-grade non-Hodgkin's lymphomas: challenges and opportunities. *J Clin Oncol* 1985;3:299.

Rosso R, Paulli M, Magrini U, et al. Anaplastic large cell lymphoma, CD30/Ki-1 positive, expressing the CD15/Leu-M1 antigen. Immunohistochemical and morphological relationships to Hodgkin's disease. *Virchows Arch A (Pathol Anat)* 1990;416:229.

Warnke RA. The distinction of Hodgkin's disease from B cell lymphoma. *Semin Diag Pathol* 1992;9:284.

Zinzani PL, Bendandi M, Martelli M. Anaplastic large cell lymphoma: clinical and prognostic evaluation of 90 adult patients. *J Clin Oncol* 1996; 14:955.

Composite Lymphoma

Gonzalez CL, Medeiros LJ, Jaffe ES. Composite lymphoma. A clinicopathologic analysis of nine patients with Hodgkin's disease and B-cell non-Hodgkin's lymphoma. *Am J Clin Pathol* 1991;96:81.

Grossman DM, Hanson CA, Schnitzer B. Simultaneous lymphocyte predominant Hodgkin's disease and large-cell lymphoma. *Am J Surg Pathol* 1991;15:668.

Guarner J, del Rio C, Hendrix L, Unger ER. Composite Hodgkin's and non-Hodgkin's lymphoma in a patient with aquired immune deficiency syndrome. *In-situ* demonstration of Epstein-Barr virus. *Cancer* 1990;66: 796.

Hansmann ML, Fellbaum C, Hui PK, Lennert K. Morphological and immunohistochemical investigation of non-Hodgkin's lymphoma combined with Hodgkin's disease. *Histopathology* 1989;15:35.

Jaffe ES, Zarate-Osorno A, Medeiros J. The interrelationship of Hodgkin's disease and non-Hodgkin's lymphomas—Lessons learned from composite and sequential malignancies. *Semin Diag Pathol* 1992;9:297.

Kim H, Hendrickson MR, Dorfman RF. Composite lymphoma. *Cancer* 1977;40:959.

Kim H. Composite lymphoma and related disorders. *Am J Clin Pathol* 1993;99:445.

Toner GC, Sinclair RA, Sutherland RC, Schwarz MA. Composite lymphoma. *Am J Clin Pathol* 1986;86:375.

Non-Hodgkin's Lymphoma After Hodgkin's Disease

Bennett MH, MacLennan KA, Vaughan Hudson G, Vaughan Hudson B, from the British National Lymphoma Investigation. Non-Hodgkin's lymphoma arising in patients treated for Hodgkin's disease in the BNLI: a 20 year experience. *Ann Oncol* 1991;2(Suppl 2):83.

Björkholm M, Holm G, Mellstedt H, Johansson B, Askergen J, Söderberg G. Prognostic factors in Hodgkin's disease. I. Analysis of histopathology, stage distribution and results of therapy. *Scand J Haematol* 1977;19:487.

Casey TT, Cousar JB, Mangum M, et al. Monomorphic lymphomas arising in patients with Hodgkin's disease. Correlation of morphologic, immunophenotypic and molecular genetic findings in 12 cases. *Am J Pathol* 1990;136:81.

Greiner TC. Nodular Lymphocyte-predominant Hodgkin's disease associated with large-cell lymphoma: analysis of Ig gene rearrangements by V-J polymerase chain reaction. *Blood* 1996;88:657.

Hansmann M-L, Stein H, Fellbaum C, Hui PK, Parwaresch MR, Lennert K. Nodular paragranuloma can transform into high-grade malignant lymphoma of B type. *Hum Pathol* 1989;20:1169.

Krikorian JG, Burke JS, Rosenberg SA, Kaplan HS. Occurrence of non-Hodgkin's lymphoma after therapy for Hodgkin's disease. *N Engl J Med* 1979;300:452.

Wickert RS, Weisenburger DD, Tierens A, Greiner TC, Chan WC. Clonal relationship between lymphocytic predominance Hodgkin's disease and concurrent or subsequent large-cell lymphoma of B-lineage. *Blood* 1995; 86:2312.

Progressively Transformed Germinal Centers

Ferry JA, Zukerberg LR, Harris NL. Florid progressive transformation of germinal centers. A syndrome affecting young men, without early progression to nodular lymphocyte predominance Hodgkin's disease. *Am J Surg Pathol* 1992;16:252.

Hansmann M-L, Fellbaum C, Hui PK, Moubayed P. Progressive transformation of germinal centers with and without association to Hodgkin's disease. *Am J Clin Pathol* 1990;93:219.

Osborne BM, Butler JJ, Gresik MV. Progressive transformation of germinal centers: comparison of 23 pediatric patients to the adult population. *Mod Pathol* 1992;5:135.

Poppema S, Kaiserling E, Lennert K. Nodular paragranuloma and progressively transformed germinal centers. *Virchows Arch B (Cell Pathol)* 1979;31:211.

Clinical Relevance of Histologic Subtype

Bennett MH, Tu A, Vaughan Hudson G. Analysis of grade 1 Hodgkin's disease (report no 6). Part 1. Lymphocyte predominant Hodgkin's disease in the BNLI—a histological review. Part 2. Nodular sclerotic Hodgkin's disease. Cellular subtypes related to prognosis. *Clin Radiol* 1981;32(suppl 2):491.

Dorfman RF. Relationship of histology to site in Hodgkin's disease. *Cancer Res* 1971;31:1786.

Dorfman RF, Colby TV. The pathologist's role in management of patients with Hodgkin's disease. *Cancer Treat Rep* 1982;66:675.

Grogran TM, Berard CW, Steinhorn SC, et al. Changing patterns of Hodgkin's disease at autopsy: a 25-year experience at the National Cancer Institute, 1953–1978. *Cancer Treat Rep* 1982;66:653.

Kadin ME, Glatstein E, Dorfman RF. Clinico-pathologic studies of 117 untreated patients subjected to laparotomy for the staging of Hodgkin's disease. *Cancer* 1971;27:1277.

Treatment Options Relevant to Lymphocyte Predominance Hodgkin's Disease

Aster JC. Lymphocyte-predominant Hodgkin's disease: how little therapy is enough? *J Clin Oncol* 1999;17:XX.

Cannellos GP. Current strategies for early Hodgkin's disease. *Ann Oncol* 1996;7:91.

Lister TA. Follicular lymphoma: grounds for optimism. *Ann Oncol* 1997;8:89.

Mauch PM, Canellos GP, Shulman LN, et al. Mantle irradiation alone for selected patients with laparotomy-staged IA to IIA Hodgkin's disease: preliminary results of a prospective trial. *J Clin Oncol* 1995;13:947.

Specht L, Horwich A, Ashley S. Salvage of relapse of patients with Hodgkin's disease in clinical stages I or II who were staged with laparotomy and initially treated with radiotherapy alone. A report from the International Database on Hodgkin's Disease. *Int J Radiat Oncol Biol Phys* 1994;30:805.

SECTION VII

Late Effects

Hodgkin's Disease, edited by P. M. Mauch,
J. O. Armitage, V. Diehl, R. T. Hoppe, and L. M. Weiss.
Lippincott Williams & Wilkins, Philadelphia ©1999.

CHAPTER 32

Life Expectancy of Patients with Hodgkin's Disease

Andrea K. Ng, Richard T. Hoppe, and Peter M. Mauch

In the last three decades, as a result of advances in staging techniques and the successful development of effective therapeutic regimens, Hodgkin's disease, a previously fatal malignancy, has become highly curable. It is estimated that approximately three-quarters of all patients with Hodgkin's disease will be cured of their disease. As the number of patients who have survived Hodgkin's disease increases, and as they are followed over a longer period of time, however, it is becoming evident that their average survival does not revert completely to that of the age-matched general population (1–7). The excessive mortality that patients face after they are cured of their Hodgkin's disease is largely a result of the long-term effects from management of their disease. A number of investigators have independently demonstrated that although the cumulative Hodgkin's disease-specific mortality levels off over time, intercurrent deaths continue to rise with time, and with long enough follow-up, combinations of treatment-related mortality including second malignancies, cardiac diseases, and infections begin to exceed mortality as a result of Hodgkin's disease (2,5–7).

The various causes of intercurrent death over time after Hodgkin's disease therapy deserve special attention and close examination, especially as data on the late effects of the treatment of Hodgkin's disease accumulate. The long life expectancy after treatment and the young age of the majority of patients affected with Hodgkin's disease suggest that many patients may live to experience late complications related to their disease or treatments. Patients with a history of Hodgkin's disease, in addition to having to face the prospect of late relapses and treatment-related complications, are confronted with negative psychosocial and economic consequences (8–12). It has been shown that survivors of Hodgkin's disease are more frequently denied life and health insurance (8,9), conceivably because of their continuous excessive morbidity and mortality risks. As a result of their shorter life expectancy compared with other young people in the general population, survivors of Hodgkin's disease may face other barriers in society, such as lower employment opportunities and decreased chance of adoption of children (9,10,12).

Although there are other types of malignancies that affect the young population and at the same time have a high cure rate, the extensive documentation and substantial evidence of increased mortality risks over time from causes other than the original malignancy appear to be unique to Hodgkin's disease. For instance, childhood acute lymphoblastic leukemia, the single most common childhood malignancy, has a long-term cure rate of 60% to 70% (13). However, the leading cause of death over time remains relapsed leukemia, and second malignant neoplasms appear thus far to be rare (14). The unique pattern of mortality risks in survivors of Hodgkin's disease may be a result of the types of interventions and therapy they receive as well as the inherent immune deficits associated with Hodgkin's disease.

Detailed knowledge and comprehensive understanding of the timing and distribution of mortality causes among survivors of Hodgkin's disease are crucial for physicians involved in their follow-up care. They may also help clarify the expectations for the overall prognosis of the affected patients and their families. Identification of factors that influence the long-term survival of patients with Hodgkin's disease may facilitate development of strategies that can help to prolong their life expectancy as well as improve their quality of life. Potential approaches include fine-tuning of initial staging and treatment,

A. K. Ng and P. M. Mauch: Department of Radiation Oncology, Brigham and Women's Hospital and Dana-Farber Cancer Institute, Harvard Medical School, Boston, Massachusetts.

R. T. Hoppe: Department of Radiation Oncology, Stanford University Stanford, California.

design of follow-up guidelines that extend long after a patient has been treated and is considered to be disease-free, devising more rigorous preventive measures and screening programs, and encouraging patient behavioral modifications.

In this chapter, we summarize the data on the major causes of excessive deaths over time in patients who had been treated for Hodgkin's disease, and factors that affect Hodgkin's disease–specific mortality, intercurrent mortality, and overall mortality. In addition, based on available information, we propose ways that may improve the overall survival of patients successfully treated for Hodgkin's disease and minimize the negative medical and psychosocial sequelae associated with their diagnosis and treatments.

LONG-TERM RELATIVE CAUSES OF MORTALITY AFTER TREATMENT OF HODGKIN'S DISEASE

A number of studies have evaluated the long-term outcomes of patients who have survived Hodgkin's disease (1–7,15–18). However, only a few of them have comprehensively examined the relative causes of mortality after treatment. The distribution of the causes of mortality is highly dependent on the length of follow-up of the individual studies. Studies with inadequate follow-up time will capture only short-term causes of mortality such as death as a result of refractory or relapsing disease and death related to immediate treatment toxicity. There is substantial evidence that survivors of Hodgkin's disease are faced with various late effects of interventions and treatments, and in order to capture events with protracted latency and to have a more accurate sense of the long-term causes of death, an adequate follow-up period is essential. In addition, because most of these fatal events are rare occurrences, a sufficiently large number of patients is necessary to reliably assess the relative magnitude of these different causes of death. Table 1 summarizes the results of studies that reported causes of mortality among patients treated for Hodgkin's disease. It is difficult to compare the results of these studies, as the follow-up lengths and grouping of mortality causes vary from study to study. Also, different investigators may define intercurrent and treatment-related deaths differently. For instance, in the study by the International Database on Hodgkin's Disease, intercurrent deaths included deaths from cardiac causes or infections but did not include deaths from second malignancies (2). Nevertheless, it is apparent that in studies with relatively short follow-up, Hodgkin's disease death has by far the greatest impact on mortality (1–3), but for studies with longer follow-up time (5–7), other causes of death, especially second malignancies and cardiac toxicities, increasingly contribute to the overall mortality.

Three of the studies were of adequate duration to include the period of time when deaths from Hodgkin's disease begin to be exceeded by deaths from other causes (2,5,7). At the Joint Center for Radiation Therapy (JCRT), deaths from second malignancies and cardiac toxicities combined exceeded deaths from Hodgkin's disease after 15 years of follow-up (5). At 20 years after treatment, deaths from second cancers had the greatest impact on mortality (Fig. 1). Data from Stanford University revealed that the curves for the actuarial probability of death from Hodgkin's disease and death from other causes (including cardiovascular, secondary cancer, infection, pulmonary, gastrointestinal, accident/suicide, unknown causes) intersect at 15 years after treatment (7). The risk of dying from Hodgkin's disease beyond 15 years rose only slightly, whereas the risk of death from other causes increased sharply after 15 years (Fig. 2). Results on the survival outcome of patients from the International Database on Hodgkin's Disease demonstrated that the cumulative incidence of Hodgkin's disease death and other causes of death overlap each other at about 19 years (Fig. 3) (2).

It is clear that patients who enjoy long-term survival after treatment for Hodgkin's disease continue to face a markedly increased mortality risk. As illustrated by data from the JCRT (5), the absolute excess risk for all causes of deaths remained at a constant, elevated level even more than 15 years after initial diagnosis, when patients are no longer at risk for deaths from Hodgkin's disease (Table 2). Absolute excess risk can be calculated as follows, expressed as absolute excess risk per 10,000 person-years:

$$\frac{\text{(observed events—expected events)}}{\text{number of person-years of follow-up}} \times 10{,}000$$

The persistently increased risk of death emphasizes the importance of life-long follow-up care. Only time will tell whether the excessive mortality in these patients will plateau or continue to rise and when, if ever, their overall survival rate will return to that of the general population. In the interim, we need to continue to meticulously gather information and document events on these patients as they carry through life in order broaden our knowledge base on the lifetime clinical course of these cancer survivors. In the following section, we describe each of the major causes of death in patients treated for Hodgkin's disease, their relative impact on overall mortality over time, and possible ways to minimize these fatal events, including therapeutic changes.

HODGKIN'S DISEASE MORTALITY

Impact of Hodgkin's Disease on Overall Survival

Only very few studies, in reporting their overall survival results, clearly separate Hodgkin's disease mortality from mortality from causes other than Hodgkin's disease

TABLE 1. *Long-term causes of death in Hodgkin's disease*

Institution	Sample size	Stages I–II	Mean or median follow-up	Number dead at follow-up	Distribution of mortality
The Netherlands (1)	340	52.4%	76.6 mo (mean)	113	HD 67.3% Leukemia 5.3% Solid tumor 7.1% Cardiac 7.1% Infection 4.4% Others 6.2%
IDHD (2)	14,225	63.6%	87.6 mo (mean)	4,139	HD 67.1% Treatment-related 5.6% SM 10% Other intercurrent (including cardiac, infections) 13.9% Unspecified 3.4%
EORTC (4)	1,660	100%	Not stated	320	HD 52.8% Treatment-related 8.1% SM 14.4% Cardiac 7.5% Intercurrent death 10% Unspecified 7.2%
BNLI (3)	1,057	Not stated	80 months (median)	43[a]	SM 30.2% Cardiac 14.0% Infection 30.2% Accident/suicide 7.0% Other 18.6%
JCRT (5)	794	77%	10.7 years (mean)	124	HD 45.2% SM 29.0% Cardiac 12.1% Infection 7.3% Miscellaneous 6.5%
Stanford (7)	2,498	59%	Not stated	754	HD 44% Other cancers 21% Cardiovascular 16% Pulmonary 7% Infection 4% Accidental 2% Hematologic 1% Gastrointestinal 1% Other, multiple 2% Unknown 3%
Specht et al. (17)[b]	3,888	Majority	Not stated	360[a]	SST 26% SL 3.9% NHL 2.8% Cardiac 33.0% Pulmonary/iatrogenic 6.1% Infection 8.6% Other known cause 4.7% Unknown causes 11.7%

[a]Cause of death excluded HD.
[b]Metaanalysis of 23 randomized trials on early-stage patients.
Abbreviations: MO, months; HD, Hodgkin's disease; NHL, non-Hodgkin's lymphoma; IDHD, International Data Base on Hodgkin's Disease; SM, second malignancy; EORTC, European Organization for Research and Treatment of Cancer Lymphoma Cooperative Group; BNLI, British National Lymphoma Investigation; JCRT, Joint Center for Radiation Therapy; SST, secondary solid tumors; SL, secondary leukemia.

(1,5,19). Because deaths from Hodgkin's disease occur in the first few years after treatment, whereas other causes of deaths tend to occur much later, only large studies with mature, long-term follow-up results will offer useful information on various cause-specific survival rates over time. Dividing survival outcomes into Hodgkin's disease–specific and other causes is especially important in an attempt to identify factors or means to minimize these different causes of mortality that may be significant at different times.

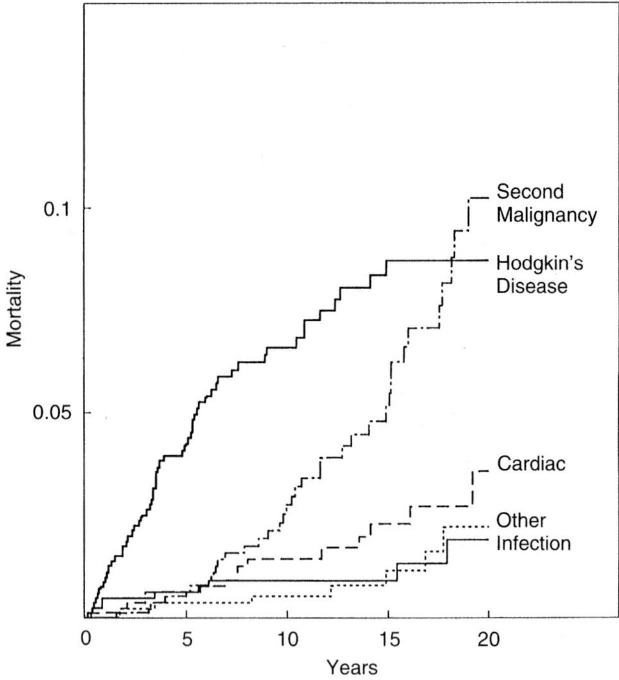

FIG. 1. Data from JCRT on causes of mortality over time. (Adapted from ref. 5.)

Various factors have been associated with the risk of dying from Hodgkin's disease. Development of relapse clearly leads to increased chance of death from Hodgkin's disease, and a number of predictors for relapse have been identified (4,17,18,20–27). Other factors that affect Hodgkin's disease–specific survival include stage at presentation, patient age at diagnosis, tumor histology and salvage potential after relapse (see Chapter 19) (1,6,17,26).

Hodgkin's Disease Relapse

The most obvious factor influencing Hodgkin's disease mortality is the development of relapse. A number of host-related and treatment-related factors have been identified to predict for Hodgkin's disease relapse (4,17,18,20–27). However, interestingly, only a minority of them are also predictive of Hodgkin's disease–specific survival and overall survival. As illustrated in Table 3, a number of tumor-related factors including large mediastinal adenopathy (20,22–24,27), number of sites of disease (4,20,23), and systemic symptoms of fever and weight loss have been associated with increased relapse risk (22). However, their association with Hodgkin's disease–specific survival and overall survival is not as clear. The main reason for the observation is likely the availability of effective salvage therapy for recurrent Hodgkin's disease so that the increased relapse rate does not lead to excessive Hodgkin's disease–specific and overall mortality.

Several factors associated with treatment extent have also been shown to affect the chance of relapse but to have little impact on Hodgkin's disease–specific survival and overall survival. These include smaller versus larger radiation fields (17,26) and radiation therapy alone versus combined-modality therapy (17,21,22,26). The lack of influence of less aggressive treatment on Hodgkin's disease–specific survival despite the higher relapse rate is likely related to better chance of successful salvage with less extensive initial treatment. The lack of effect on overall survival with less treatment is a result of better salvage potential and fewer competing causes of death as a result of exposure to a lower amount of toxic therapy. This subject matter is well illustrated by results of the metaanalysis by Specht et al. on early-stage Hodgkin's disease (17). The authors found that the addition of chemotherapy to radia-

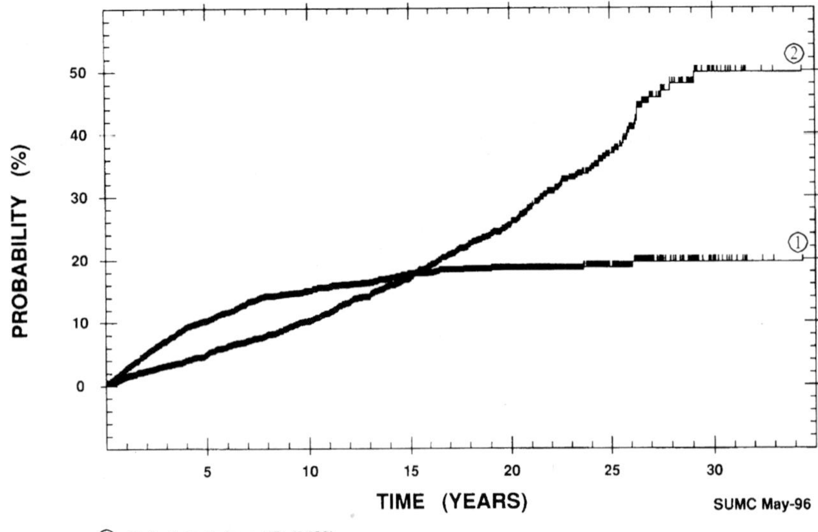

FIG. 2. Data from Stanford on causes of mortality over time. (Adapted from ref. 7.)

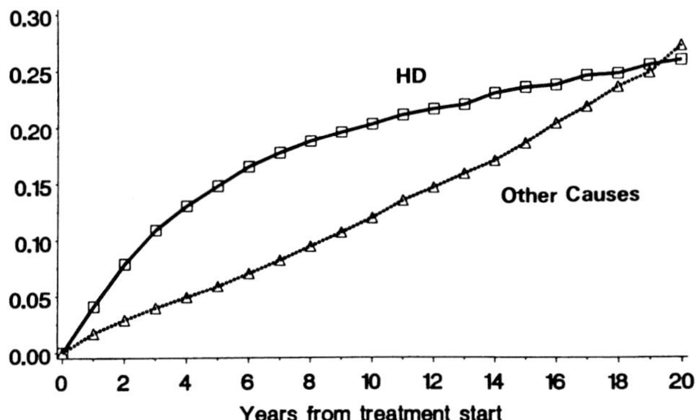

FIG. 3. Data from International Data Base on Hodgkin's Disease on causes of mortality over time. (Adapted from ref. 2.)

tion therapy halved the relapse rate, leading to a higher Hodgkin's disease–specific survival of borderline significance (p = .07) in the combined-modality therapy arm. However, they observed a 9% increase in the odds of death from known causes other than Hodgkin's disease in the combined-modality therapy group, and 11% if unknown causes are included with the deaths from other causes. Even though the elevated mortality from other causes was not statistically significant in the combined-modality therapy group, it was sufficient to counterbalance the borderline significantly higher Hodgkin's disease–specific survival in patients who received combined-modality therapy, such that no overall survival differences were observed between the two arms.

Despite the numerous reports in the literature demonstrating that differences in relapse rates generally do not translate into survival differences, there is evidence that with a large enough difference in relapse rate between two therapeutic approaches, a significant survival difference may emerge. For instance, in the EORTC H_1 trial, clinical stage I and II patients were randomized to mantle radiation therapy versus mantle radiation therapy followed by 2 years of vinblastine. According to Dr. J.-M. Cosset (*personal communication,* October, 1997), a significant survival difference has now appeared between the two treatment arms favoring combined-modality treatment. Similarly, the markedly higher relapse rate in stage III1A patients treated with radiation therapy alone, compared with treatment with combined-modality therapy, has led to a significant difference in overall survival rate (28,29). The findings suggest that with a sufficiently large difference in disease control rate between two treatment designs, the excessive Hodgkin's disease death from recurrent disease overpowers the effect of better salvage potential and lower treatment-related mortality with the less aggressive treatment approach.

Age

As shown in Table 3, patient age at diagnosis is one of the most consistently reported factors affecting Hodgkin's disease survival and overall survival (1,2,4,5,21,23–25). The association between age and Hodgkin's disease–specific survival is not as well documented because only very few studies specifically isolated deaths as a result of Hodgkin's disease from all causes of deaths in assessing the relationship between age and survival (4,5,25). At the JCRT, it was noted that, although there was no significant difference in relapse rate between older and younger patients, patients who were 40 or older at the time of diagnosis were significantly more likely to die from Hodgkin's disease (as well as other causes) (5). Similar observations were made in the EORTC trials in that patients older than 40 years of age had a lower survival because of both Hodgkin's disease progression and more frequent unrelated deaths (4,25). These findings suggest that older patients may have similar chance of initial disease control as younger patients but that, once they relapse, they are not as easily salvaged, and that older patients are more vulnerable to fatal treatment-related complications. Indeed, in a study from the Netherlands on 340 patients with Hodgkin's disease, older age did not affect risk of dying from Hodgkin's disease, but the 10-year actuarial risk of dying from other causes was significantly higher in patients age 40 or older (32.7% vs. 4.9%) (1). Causes of death other than Hodgkin's disease are reviewed in greater detail in a later section.

TABLE 2. *Data from JCRT showing competing mortality over time*

			Not Hodgkin's disease		
Time interval[a]	AR all causes (per 10,000 person-years)	Dead of Hodgkin's disease	Dead	RR	AR
0–5 yrs (3,725)	120.7	34	18	2.5	29.3
5–10 yrs (2,627)	104.7	14	20	3.1	51.5
10–15 yrs (1,575)	124.9	8	17	3.2	74.1
>15 yrs (775)	110.6	0	13	2.9	110.6

[a]Numbers in parentheses indicate total person-years.
Abbreviations: RR, relative risk; AR, absolute excess risk.
Adapted from ref. 5.

TABLE 3. *Factors identified to be associated with Hodgkin's disease recurrence, Hodgkin's disease mortality, other causes of mortality, and overall mortality*[f]

Prognostic factors	HD recurrence	HD mortality	Other causes of mortality	Overall mortality
Age (older vs. younger)	Fundaleu (20) (≥45, $p < .001$) Princess Margaret (21) (≥50, $p = .0005$) Combined Harvard/ Stanford (22) (≥40, $p = .04$)	JCRT (5) (AR of ≥40: 130.2; AR of 17–39: 61.6; AR of <17: 37.6) EORTC (25) (>50, $p = .002$)	JCRT (5) (AR ≥40, 141.3; AR of 17–39, 36.5) Netherlands, van Rijswijk (1) (10-year act. risk ≥40, 32.7%;<40, 4.9%) IDHD (2) (≥50, 20% SM death, 40% intercurrent death; <50, 3% and 5%, respectively) EORTC (25) (>50, $p = .001$)	Harvard (24) (≥40, $p = .008$) Danish (23) (≥40, $p = .04$) Princess Margaret (21) (≥50, $p = .0005$) EORTC (25) (≥50, $p = .001$) JCRT (5) (20-year survival: >40, 46%; <40, 78%)
Gender	EORTC (4) (male worse, $p = .006$) Danish (23) (male worse, $p = .012$)	—	—	IDHD (2) (female, SMR = 9.21; male, SMR = 7.09) EORTC (4) (male worse,) $p = .01$
MC/LD histology	Princess Margaret (21) ($p = .004$) Danish (23) ($p = .0084$)	Netherlands, van Rijswijk (1) ($p < .001$)	—	JCRT (5) (20-year survival: MC/LD, 68%; NS/LP, 75%) Princess Margaret (21) ($p = .08$)
LMA	Stanford (27) ($p = .002$) Harvard (24) ($p < .0001$) Fundaleu (20) ($p = .005$) Combined Harvard/ Stanford (22) ($p = .01$)	—	—	Fundaleu (20) ($p < .001$)
Sites ≥4	EORTC (4) ($p < .0001$) Fundaleu (20) ($p < .001$)	—	—	EORTC (4) ($p = .005$)
Tumor burden (combination of tumor size and number of sites)	Danish (23) ($p < .0001$)	—	—	Danish (23) ($p = .0014$)
B symptoms (fever and weight loss)	Combined Harvard/ Stanford (22) ($p < .0001$)	—	—	—
Stage at diagnosis	—	Netherlands, van Rijswijk (1) ($p < .001$)	—	JCRT (5) (20-year survival: stage III, 60%; stage I–II, 78%) IDHD (2) (SMR: advanced stages,11.22; early stages, 5.68)
Lap vs. no lap	Shore (26)[a] (lap better, $p < .01$)	—	—	Shore (26)[a] (lap better, $p < .01$) EORTC H6F (18,79) (no lap better, $p = .035$)
Extensive RT vs. limited RT	Shore (26)[a] ($p < .01$) Specht (17)[b] ($p < .00001$)	—	—	—
CMT vs. RT alone	Specht (17)[c] ($p < .00001$) Danish (23) ($p < .0001$) Combined Harvard/ Stanford (22) ($p = .03$)	Specht (17)[c] ($p = .07$)	JCRT (5) (AR: CMT-85.7 RT alone- 40.4)	—
CMT vs. chemo alone (additional RT design)	Loeffler (18)[d] ($p < .001$)	—	—	—
CMT vs. additional chemotherapy (parallel design)	—	—	—	Loeffler (18)[d] (additional chemotherapy better, $p = .045$)
Salvage chemo vs. CMT vs. RT vs. chemo	—	Netherlands, van Rijswijk (1) ($p < .001$)	—	—
Treatment era	—	—	Stanford (6) (Act. probability of death:[e] 1962–80, 24%; 1980–95, 6%) see Table 7 IDHD (2) Excess of deaths/100 person-years: 1960, 69, 0.83; 1970–79, 0.52; 1980+, 0.46)	Cancer statistics 1998 (138) (5-year survival in Caucasian: 1960–63, 40%; 1970–73, 67%; 1974–76, 72%; 1980–82, 75%; 1986–93, 82%; African-American: 1974–76, 69%; 1980–82, 72%; 1986–93, 74%)

[a]A metaanalysis on early-stage patients from six randomized trials.
[b]A metaanalysis on early-stage patients from eight randomized trials.
[c]A metaanalysis on early-stage patients from 12 randomized trials.
[d]A metaanalysis on advanced-stage patients from seven randomized trials.
[e]Estimated from curves.

Abbreviations: HD, Hodgkin's disease; JCRT, Joint Center for Radiation Therapy; AR, absolute risk; IDHD, International Database on Hodgkin's Disease; SM, secondary malignancy; EORTC, European Organization for Research and Treatment of Cancer; MC, mixed cellularity; LD, lymphocyte depleted; NS, nodular sclerosing; LP, lymphocyte predominant; LMA, large mediastinal adenopathy; lap, laparotomy; RT, radiation therapy; CMT, combined modality therapy.

Stage

Another factor that should naturally affect Hodgkin's disease–specific survival is disease stage at diagnosis. Again, because of the paucity of studies that break out Hodgkin's disease–specific survival from overall survival, there has been only limited documentation on the effect of disease stage on Hodgkin's disease mortality. A study from the Netherlands by van Rijswijk et al. (1) looked at the relative impact of prognostic factors on Hodgkin's disease death and found disease stage to be one of the significant determinants of risk of dying of Hodgkin's disease ($p < .001$). There is evidence from the literature that in general, a greater proportion of advanced-stage patients die of Hodgkin's disease, whereas patients with early-stage disease have a relatively lower Hodgkin's disease mortality. From the International Database on Hodgkin's Disease, Henry-Amar et al. reported that deaths not directly related to Hodgkin's disease accounted for 37% of the overall deaths in early-stage patients but for only 19% in advanced-stage patients, in whom the predominant cause of death was Hodgkin's disease progression (2).

Histology

A factor that has been shown by some investigators, but not others, to be associated with Hodgkin's disease–specific survival is tumor histology. Van Rijswijk et al. identified mixed-cellularity/lymphocyte-depleted histology to be associated with increased risk of death from Hodgkin's disease (1). At the JCRT, although mixed-cellularity/lymphocyte-depleted histology did not affect relapse risk, it was found to be associated with inferior overall survival compared with nodular sclerosis/lymphocyte predominant histology (84% vs. 97%, $p = .001$) (24). Although the effect was not specifically on Hodgkin's disease–specific survival, the poorer overall survival was attributed to the tendency of mixed-cellularity/lymphocyte-depleted histology to relapse transdiaphragmatically. Infradiaphragmatic relapse is often bulky and not as easily salvaged, which in turn may lead to higher risk of death from Hodgkin's disease.

Salvage Potential After Relapse

In assessing Hodgkin's disease–specific survival, in addition to evaluating primary disease control, the salvage potential after relapse is an important consideration. One of the main influences on survival after a relapse is the extent of prior therapy. Patients who relapse after radiotherapy alone have a better than 60% chance of achieving durable second remissions (30,31), compared with patients who relapse after chemotherapy or combined-modality therapy, in which the chances are only 20% to 30% (32–36). The differences in prognosis based on the type of initial treatment received were well depicted by the randomized study by Biti et al. comparing mechlorethamine, vincristine, procarbazine, and prednisone (MOPP) chemotherapy with radiation therapy in pathological stage (PS) I to IIA patients (37). At 80 months, the actuarial survival rates of patients who relapsed after mantle and paraaortic radiotherapy and MOPP chemotherapy were 85% and 15%, respectively ($p = .02$). In recent years, reports of high-dose therapy and bone marrow or stem-cell rescue for selected patients who have relapsed after treatment with chemotherapy or combined-modality therapy have shown promising results (38–46). In the practical setting, however, a certain proportion of patients will not be eligible for the procedure for medical or nonmedical reasons (38). In addition to the long-term toxicity of high-dose therapy in these young patients, the high cost of this procedure is another potential hindrance to its routine use.

Other factors that affect survival outcome after relapse include age at relapse (32), extent of relapse as reflected by relapse stage, nodal versus extranodal relapse, and number of involved sites at relapse (33,36,47–50). The length of first complete remission appears to have significant prognostic influence on patients relapsing after chemotherapy or combined-modality therapy, with better outcome in those who have a time to relapse longer than 12 months (32–34,47,49).

Minimizing Hodgkin's Disease Mortality: Clinical Implications

The dilemma confronting physicians in deciding on the optimal management approach for patients with Hodgkin's disease is to balance between the goals of maximizing Hodgkin's disease–specific survival by comprehensive staging and adequate treatment and attempting to limit the extent of intervention to reduce long-term mortality from treatment-related causes. Current focus in the management of patients with Hodgkin's disease has been to explore ways to limit treatment extent without overly compromising initial disease control. One rationale for curtailing treatment extent is to maintain salvage ability. A slightly higher relapse rate is usually tolerated in patients treated with radiation therapy alone, whereas for patients receiving chemotherapy or combined-modality therapy as initial treatment, maximizing up-front disease control rate is important because of the poor salvage ability after relapse. Another reason for limiting treatment is the growing evidence that the gain in Hodgkin's disease–specific survival associated with aggressive initial treatment may eventually be offset by the excessive deaths from other causes (17,51). However, there have been findings to suggest that significantly curtailed treatment may be associated with such a high relapse rate that in time it may lead to a significantly inferior Hodgkin's disease–specific as well as overall survival. Therefore, protocols that are designed purely to reduce treatment but are associated with a potentially high relapse risk should be avoided.

TABLE 4. *Data from Stanford and JCRT showing absolute excess risk[a] of death from causes other than Hodgkin's disease according to follow-up interval*

	Stanford (7)				
Follow-up interval	Stage I–II (1962–1980)	Stage I–II (1980–1996)	Stage III–IV (1962–1980)	Stage III–IV (1980–1996)	JCRT (5), all pts (1969–1988)
0–5 yrs	45	17	130	70	29.3
5–10 yrs	84	16	132	72	51.5
10–15 yrs	106	44	158	219	74.1
15–20 yrs	156	—	222	—	110.6
≥ 20 yrs	296	—	383	—	—

[a]Expressed per 10,000 person-years.

INTERCURRENT MORTALITY

Unlike Hodgkin's disease–specific deaths, which tend to take place in the initial part of the follow-up period and have been relatively well documented, other causes of death in survivors of Hodgkin's disease occur later, and their effect on long-term survival is still being defined. Of particular concern is the evidence of rising risk of death from other causes with increasing follow-up time. As illustrated in Table 4, data from both Stanford (7) and the JCRT (5) showed increasing absolute excess risk of death from causes other than Hodgkin's disease at increasing follow-up intervals.

In evaluating the impact of various events on overall survival, one approach is to compare the median time from diagnosis of Hodgkin's disease to development of the event, and the median time to death as a result of the event. At the JCRT, the median time to Hodgkin's disease relapse was estimated to be 28 months (24). From the long-term survival data, the median time to Hodgkin's disease–specific death was 5 to 9 years (5). The observed time gap of 3 to 7 years between Hodgkin's disease relapse and death indicates that recurrent or progressive Hodgkin's disease is not immediately fatal. This is in contrast to other events that contribute to the long-term mortality of Hodgkin's disease survivors, in which the interval between onset of the event and subsequent death is on average measured in months. For instance, in a study from the Netherlands on causes of death in patients treated for Hodgkin's disease (1), the interval from Hodgkin's disease diagnosis to event and to death from the event were carefully documented for each patient. The average length of time between diagnosis of a second malignancy and resulting death was only 6 months. With respect to cardiac events, the majority were immediately fatal, with an average interval between diagnosis of the cardiac complication and subsequent death of only 3 months. The seemingly greater lethality associated with causes of death other than Hodgkin's disease, and their increasing contribution to overall mortality over time, suggest that a better understanding of intercurrent deaths and ways to minimize their occurrences are imperative in the follow-up care of patients who have been successfully treated for Hodgkin's disease.

TABLE 5. *Data from Stanford and JCRT showing relative and absolute excess risks of second malignancy and cardiac deaths in Hodgkin's disease survivors*

	Stanford (7)	JCRT (5)
O/E[a] number of second malignancy deaths	104/16.6	36/5.2
RR of second malignancy death	6.3	6.8
AR of second malignancy death	43.5	35.3
O/E number of cardiac deaths	88/28.8	15/6.8
RR of cardiac death	3.1	2.2
AR of cardiac death	28	9.3

[a]Abbreviations: *O/E,* observed to expected; RR, relative risk; AR, absolute excess risk.

The two major causes of deaths other than Hodgkin's disease in the long-term survivors are second malignancies and cardiac diseases. Table 5 shows the results from Stanford (7) and the JCRT (5) on the relative risk and absolute excess risk of death from second cancer and cardiac diseases. Other main causes of deaths in survivors of Hodgkin's disease include infection and pulmonary toxicities.

SECOND MALIGNANCIES

Development of second malignancies is a long-term complication that has received increasing attention since the early 1970s and has been a growing contribution to the long-term mortality of patients treated for Hodgkin's disease. The elevated risk for second tumors in patients with Hodgkin's disease has been attributed to several factors, including direct leukemogenic or carcinogenic effects of the treatments, an impaired immune system related to treatments or the disease itself, and underlying genetic susceptibility to environmental carcinogens. Second malignancies after Hodgkin's disease can be divided into three main categories: leukemia, non-Hodgkin's lymphoma, and solid tumors. The relative impact of each type of second malignancy on overall mortality depends on the timing and frequency of its occurrence and the survival outcome after its development.

Leukemia

Impact of Secondary Leukemia on Overall Survival

Leukemia contributes to less than 5% of all mortality in patients with Hodgkin's disease (1,17). This is because of the overall rarity of leukemia among Hodgkin's disease survivors, with an estimated long-term cumulative risk of only 1% to 4% (52,53). Its risk is likely to decline with the diminishing use of alkylating-agent chemotherapy. Despite its relatively modest impact on overall survival, understanding its development and the associated contributing factors are important because of the dismal prognosis in patients who develop leukemia after Hodgkin's disease therapy.

Leukemia after Hodgkin's disease is almost uniformly fatal. In a study from the International Database on Hodgkin's Disease, among the 158 patients with secondary acute leukemia or myelodysplastic syndrome, the 2-year survival rate was 10%, and the 5-year survival rate was less than 5% (53). At the JCRT, all eight patients with secondary leukemia died of disease (54). Results from several studies suggest that treatment-related secondary leukemia may carry a worse prognosis than primary leukemia, with a median survival ranging from 2 to 5 months (55–57). In recent years, the use of high-dose therapy and bone marrow transplantation has led to promising outcomes in some patients with secondary leukemia, in both response to treatment and disease-free survival (58). Given the high mortality rate associated with secondary leukemia, it is important to minimize leukemia risk by targeting factors related to its development.

Factors Associated with Risks of Secondary Leukemia

A number of factors are associated with an increased risk for development of acute leukemia after Hodgkin's disease therapy. Exposure to alkylating-agent chemotherapy has clearly been identified by a number of series as the main culprit for secondary acute nonlymphocytic leukemia, the predominant form of leukemia after Hodgkin's disease (59–62). Other factors that have been implicated include radiation therapy (53,56,59), splenectomy (53,59,63,64), advanced stage (59), older age (52–55), and female gender (59,62), although the findings have not been uniform.

The most comprehensive study on leukemia risk following Hodgkin's disease treatment with respect to chemotherapy history is a case-control study by van Leeuwen et al. from the Netherlands Cancer Institute (60). Detailed information was obtained for 44 cases of leukemia and compared against 124 matched controls. The cumulative dose of mechlorethamine was identified as the most important factor in determining leukemia risk. A significantly elevated risk was particularly seen for patients who received a cumulative dose greater than 110 mg. A study from the same group reported that leukemia risk in patients treated with chemotherapy before 1980, compared with patients treated after 1980, was approximately threefold higher. Patients treated in the earlier period received predominantly MOPP chemotherapy, whereas the more recently treated patients received mainly alternating MOPP/ABVD (adriamycin, bleomycin, vinblastine, and dacarbazine), in which the total dose of alkylating chemotherapy agents is lower (52). The results again demonstrated the association between mechlorethamine-based chemotherapy and secondary leukemia. The leukemogenic potential of ABVD alone is likely to be substantially lower, as demonstrated by the data available thus far (52,65).

Data on the relationship between leukemia and radiation exposure are mostly in low-dose ranges of under 10 Gy and in patients who are exposed to total-body irradiation or in whom a large amount of bone marrow is treated (66–70). There is little evidence that patients who received therapeutic doses to a limited field are at excessive risk for secondary leukemia, and most studies found leukemia risk after radiotherapy alone for Hodgkin's disease to be negligible (19,55,59,71–74). Whether the addition of radiation therapy increases the leukemia risk in patients treated with chemotherapy is controversial, and the results vary from study to study, with some reporting a significantly elevated risk after combined-modality therapy compared with chemotherapy alone (53,56,59), although other studies did not detect a significant difference in risk (19,52,59,60,62,71,75). The main difficulty is the differences in types and doses of chemotherapy and in the radiotherapy doses and extent used in the studies. In one large case-control study from a collaborative study group (59), 163 cases of leukemia following treatment for Hodgkin's disease were reviewed. The results demonstrated that when the number of cycles of chemotherapy was held constant, addition of radiotherapy did not increase the risk of leukemia above that produced by the use of chemotherapy alone.

The association between splenectomy and secondary leukemia was first reported by van Leeuwen et al. in 1987 (63). Their findings were confirmed by a number of subsequent studies, some of which controlled for the amount of chemotherapy received (53,59,63,64), although others have not been able to come to the same conclusion (56,75,76). Similar elevated risk has not been observed in patients who were splenectomized for other reasons, such as trauma (77), implying that cancer risk after a splenectomy may be influenced by a patient's baseline immune status.

The case-control study by van Leeuwen et al. is the only one to report an elevated leukemia risk associated with thrombocytopenia. Patients who had a greater than 70% decrease in platelet count in response to treatment, or low platelet counts under 75×10^6/mL for more than 1 year after treatment, were at increased risk for this complication (60). The observation suggests that the extent of bone marrow damage, which is reflected by platelet counts, may be associated with development of secondary leukemia, and response of platelet counts to initial Hodgkin's disease therapy may be a potential way to identify patients at increased leukemia risk.

Minimizing Secondary Leukemia Mortality: Clinical Implications

Given the overwhelming evidence of the association between alkylating agents and leukemia risk, the most effective way to minimize leukemia deaths is to decrease the use of alkylating agents. A number of studies have demonstrated the superiority of ABVD or ABVD alternating with MOPP over MOPP alone in tumor control rate, and for these reasons (78–81), MOPP chemotherapy alone should no longer be used for primary treatment. Trials are also under way, including the EORTC H_8 study, investigating the feasibility of decreased number of cycles of chemotherapy (78). In the interim, it is crucial that patients treated with the modern, predominantly nonalkylating chemotherapy regimen be carefully followed in order to determine if an elevated leukemia risk exists.

The avoidance of alkylating agents may be particularly important in patients over the age of 40, as some of the study results indicate a higher leukemia risk and associated mortality among the older patient population (52–55). In addition, as discussed in the previous section, patients aged 40 or older are at higher risk for dying of causes not directly related to Hodgkin's disease (1,2,5,25), and presumably second malignancy is one of the main causes of intercurrent deaths in the older age group, again stressing the importance of avoiding needlessly extensive treatment in older patients.

The suggestion that the addition of radiotherapy to chemotherapy increases secondary leukemia risk is debatable (59). It is important to keep in mind that, compared to Hodgkin's disease death, secondary leukemia death contributes only a very small proportion of overall mortality (1,17). It may therefore be unreasonable to risk disease control by eliminating radiotherapy as part of treatment in order to reduce the small leukemia risk. Similarly, avoiding staging laparotomy simply to decrease the potential risk of leukemia associated with splenectomy may be illogical, as the chance of tailored treatment is sacrificed. In addition, the increased relapse rate associated with inadequate treatment or staging would mean a need for more salvage therapy, in which employment of alkylating agents may be inevitable.

Non-Hodgkin's Lymphoma

Impact of Non-Hodgkin's Lymphoma on Overall Survival

The long-term cumulative risk of non-Hodgkin's lymphoma after Hodgkin's disease is only 1% to 2%, and its reported absolute excess risk ranges from 2.5 to 14 per 10,000 person-years (19,52–54,71,76). The risk of non-Hodgkin's lymphoma is slightly lower than the risk of secondary leukemia, and the associated prognosis is better than that for patients with leukemia. Its contribution to the overall mortality of Hodgkin's disease survivors is therefore quite small, less than 5% (17,18).

Only limited data are available on the survival outcome of patients who develop non-Hodgkin's lymphoma after treatment of Hodgkin's disease. In the International Database on Hodgkin's Disease, Henry-Amar et al. observed 5-year and 10-year survival rates of 30% and 22%, respectively, for patients with non-Hodgkin's lymphoma (53). Tucker et al. reported that 45% of cases of non-Hodgkin's lymphoma cases were fatal, with a mean follow-up of 2.1 years (71). At the JCRT, four of ten patients who developed non-Hodgkin's lymphoma died of disease (54). Although there has been no direct comparison between prognosis of patients with primary versus secondary non-Hodgkin's lymphoma, outcomes of non-Hodgkin's lymphoma after Hodgkin's disease are comparable to those observed in stage III or IV aggressive primary non-Hodgkin's lymphoma, in which the 5-year overall survival rates range between 30% and 40% (82). Indeed, secondary non-Hodgkin's lymphomas are typically of intermediate or high grade and, at least in the older series, tend to be relatively resistant to treatment (52,83). On the other hand, there is evidence that a high remission rate can be achieved when appropriate combination chemotherapy is given (84). Finally, age at Hodgkin's disease diagnosis may have an impact on non-Hodgkin's lymphoma mortality. At the JCRT, patients treated for Hodgkin's disease at age 40 or older were at significantly higher risk of dying of a second tumor, including non-Hodgkin's lymphoma (54).

Factors Associated with Risks of Non-Hodgkin's Lymphoma

The risk of developing non-Hodgkin's lymphoma after Hodgkin's disease appears to be relatively independent of the time from completion of treatment or type of initial treatment received (19,71,76). Results from several larger series suggested that there may be an elevated risk after more extensive treatment (52,53). Other factors that have been associated with increased risk for non-Hodgkin's lymphoma include older age at diagnosis (54) and lymphocyte predominant histology (19,53). Overall, however, there appears to be a lack of consistent pattern on risk factors for subsequent development of non-Hodgkin's lymphoma. It may partly reflect pathologic misclassification in some of the studies or differences in diagnostic criteria for Hodgkin's disease and non-Hodgkin's lymphoma. Development of non-Hodgkin's lymphoma after Hodgkin's disease treatment may be multifactorial. It may be directly treatment-induced, or it could be part of the natural course of Hodgkin's disease, especially for the lymphocyte predominant subtype (83,85). The excessive risk could also be a result of the immunosuppressed status of Hodgkin's disease patients, similar to the increased non-Hodgkin's lymphoma risk in other groups of immunocompromised patients such as transplant patients or patients infected with the human immunodeficiency virus (86).

Minimizing Non-Hodgkin's Lymphoma Mortality: Clinical Implications

The possible association between treatment extent and non-Hodgkin's lymphoma risk suggested by some of the larger series (52,53) and evidence that patients in the older age group may be more susceptible to secondary non-Hodgkin's lymphoma death, again stress the importance of tailored treatment and minimizing overtreatment, especially in patients aged 40 or older. Although the overall prognosis of patients with non-Hodgkin's lymphoma after Hodgkin's disease is only fair, they do respond to standard lymphoma treatment (84), suggesting that early detection of secondary non-Hodgkin's lymphoma and timely delivery of treatment may improve survival outcome. Finally, careful pathologic review and confirmation at the time of initial Hodgkin's disease diagnosis, suspected disease recurrence, or diagnosis of subsequent non-Hodgkin's lymphoma are crucial. In addition to ensuring that proper therapy is given, a better understanding of the pathogenesis and relationship between Hodgkin's disease and second malignancies can be established.

Solid Tumors

Impact of Solid Tumors on Overall Survival

In contrast to leukemia, which rarely occurs beyond 10 to 15 years after therapy for Hodgkin's disease, the risk of developing solid tumor continues to increase beyond 15 years (52–54,75,76,87–89), and in some series, solid tumors have constituted over half of all cases of second malignancies (19,52,54). With sufficient follow-up, solid tumors may represent the most serious threat to the survival of patients who have been cured of their Hodgkin's disease. Other than the relative incidence over time, the impact of various secondary solid tumors on overall survival will also depend on the prognosis of the individual types of tumors, disease stage, and presence or absence of other associated prognostic factors at presentation.

Lung cancer was initially recognized as the most common solid tumor in patients treated for Hodgkin's disease (19,52,62,71). In the series from the British National Lymphoma Investigation group, lung cancer represented one-third of all second cancers (19). However, in recent years, breast cancer, which typically has a latency of 15 years or longer, has emerged as one of the predominant forms of solid tumors after treatment for Hodgkin's disease, especially in women irradiated at a young age (75,87). Overall, it appears that lung cancer and breast cancer, which is rapidly gaining in significance, are the two major contributors to mortality from solid tumors.

Given the long latency between Hodgkin's disease therapy and subsequent solid tumor, data on survival after diagnosis are relatively scarce. At the JCRT, 25 of 53 patients with subsequent solid tumors died of disease (54). At Stanford, Tucker et al. reported that 55% of solid tumor cases were fatal at a mean follow up of 1.6 years (75). Among the 367 patients with solid tumors found in the International Database on Hodgkin's Disease study, the 5- and 10-year survival rates were noted to be 34% and 25%, respectively (53). However, these numbers have somewhat limited meaning, as individual prognosis largely depends on the type, stage, and other prognostic characteristics of the solid malignancy.

Among the various solid tumors, data on survival in patients who developed breast cancer following Hodgkin's disease are probably the best-documented. A study from the Memorial Sloan-Kettering Cancer Center was the only one thus far that directly compared breast cancer after Hodgkin's disease with primary breast cancer (90). The clinical and pathologic features of breast cancers in 37 women previously treated for Hodgkin's disease were reviewed, and it was found that their histopathologic characteristics were very similar to those of primary breast cancers. The 6-year disease-free survival rates for node-negative and node-positive breast cancers were 85% and 33%, respectively, and were noted to be similar to the survival outcomes of patients presenting with primary breast cancers seen and treated at the Memorial Sloan-Kettering Cancer Center. At Stanford, the relapse-free survival and overall survival of 26 women with breast cancer following Hodgkin's disease were 50% and 60%, respectively (87). At the JCRT, among the 13 patients with secondary breast cancer, 11 were alive at the time of last follow-up (54). However, with the short follow-up and small number of patients, it is hard to draw conclusions on how the prognosis of these patients compares with that of patients presenting with primary breast cancer. For lung cancer following Hodgkin's disease, survival outcome is poor, similar to primary lung cancer. In the series reported by Valagussa et al. (55), among the ten cases of lung cancer, eight patients died within 18 months of diagnosis. At the JCRT (54), only two patients were alive at the time of last follow-up among the eight patients with lung cancer.

Solid tumors are a late-developing complication that will play an increasing part in negatively affecting the survival of patients who have been successfully treated for Hodgkin's disease. Understanding their pattern of development and factors that influence it may help in finding ways to diminish their risks or to improve their survival outcomes (e.g., through early detection and treatment).

Factors Associated with Risks of Secondary Solid Tumors

Time Interval from Hodgkin's Disease Therapy

The reported time from Hodgkin's disease diagnosis to solid-tumor development ranges from a mean of 5.8 years to a median of 16 years (52,54,76,87,91–100). In most studies with long enough follow-up, the median time to solid tumors is over 10 years (54,87,96,98).

In addition to a long latency, there is also evidence that the risks for solid tumors increase with increasing time from completion of Hodgkin's disease therapy. Several studies have reviewed risks over increasing time after treatment for Hodgkin's disease, and their results are summarized in Table 6 (52–54,71,75,76,87,89,101). The increasing risks over time are more apparent in the first 10 years but become less obvious after 15 years. This may be because the number of patients with long enough follow-up is still small.

Radiation Field Size

The relationship between radiation field extent and subsequent solid-tumor risks has not been established definitively. Most studies were able to detect only a nonsignificant trend of increased risk of subsequent solid cancer with extended-field radiotherapy (19,53,93,95). One possible source of indirect evidence of association between solid-tumor risks and radiation field size is to look at tumor location in relation to the radiotherapy fields. Studies that reported on the proportion of solid tumors found within or at the edge of prior radiation fields showed that the majority of solid cancers arise within or in close vicinity to the previous radiotherapy fields (52,54,55,71,74–76,87,89,91–94,96,98,102–104).

Radiation Dose (Low Scattered Dose Range)

Data on the dose–response relationship for solid-tumor development after Hodgkin's disease are limited because of the narrow distribution of radiation doses in most studies and the lack of precise dosimetry at the site of the cancer. The effect of low-dose versus high-dose radiation therapy on solid cancer risk is controversial. Doria et al. reported a significantly elevated solid-tumor risk in patients who received salvage therapy for relapse after primary full-dose radiation therapy compared with patients with previously untreated Hodgkin's disease who received chemotherapy and low-dose irradiation (101). The results led the authors to the conclusion that the higher cumulative radiation dose may explain the elevated solid-tumor risks. However, the group of patients who were salvaged after recurrent disease had a longer follow-up period of 212 months, compared with 153 months in the other group of patients. The difference in follow-up length alone may explain the difference in risks between the two groups of patients. Two other studies demonstrated increasing risk of solid tumor development with increasing radiation dose (105,106). However, the excessive risks were limited to doses within low scattered dose ranges of under 10 Gy.

Chemotherapy

Conflicting data exist on whether the addition of chemotherapy to radiotherapy increases the risk of solid tumors (53,54,71,87,88,93,95,107). Results from Stanford University did suggest that alkylating agents may have enhanced the breast-cancer risk in the first 15 years after treatment (87). The risks of solid tumors after chemotherapy alone are yet to be defined, as relatively few patients have been treated with chemotherapy alone, and their follow-up time tends to be shorter than that of patients treated with radiation therapy. One study that included the largest number of patients treated with chemotherapy alone was the British National Lymphoma Investigation Study in which results on 987 patients treated with alkylating chemotherapy were reported (19). Despite a relatively short average follow-up of 4.7 years, the relative risk for lung cancer was elevated at 4.2 (95% C.I. 2.2 to 7.3), and the relative risk for all other solid

TABLE 6. *Relative risks of solid tumors over increasing time period after completion of HD treatments*

Institution	Relative risks			
	1–4 years	5–9 years	≥ 10 years	≥ 15 years
IDHD (53) (male patients)	1.18	1.86	2.33	1.73 (> 20 years: RR = 1.33)
IDHD (53) (female patients)	0.71	1.99	2.33	3.6 (> 20 years: RR = 6.25)
Stanford (71)	1.9	4.9	6.3	not stated
Norway (76)	1.1	1.8	1.6	not stated
Stanford (87)	0.5	2.9	2.7	1.5
Netherlands (52)	1.9	2.6	2.8	4.2
Yale (101)	5.1	5.9	12	15.1
JCRT (54)	3.7 (AR = 23.7)	2.8 (AR = 22.7)	5.9 (AR = 87.2)	7.4 (AR = 193.3)
LESG (75)	9	7	14	7 (> 20 years: RR = 10)
Yale (89)	1	—	6.5	—

Abbreviations: HD, Hodgkin's disease; IDHD, International Data base on Hodgkin's Disease; JCRT, Joint Center for Radiation Therapy; LESG, Late Effect Study Group; RR, relative risk; AR, absolute excess risk.

cancer was 1.5 (95% C.I. 0.8 to 2.4). Moreover, it was found that the pattern of relative risk of solid tumors by time after chemotherapy was similar to that in patients exposed to radiation, with a substantially higher risk at 10 years or more after completion of the chemotherapy.

Age

Different studies on the relationship between age at diagnosis and solid-tumor risks have yielded varying results (53,54,87,95), likely because the age distribution of the initial study population, length of follow-up time, and the ways the risks (relative risk versus absolute excess risk) are measured are different among the studies.

One of the most consistent findings is the positive relationship between radiation treatment at a young age and breast-cancer risk in women, reflecting the greater sensitivity of developing breast tissue to ionizing radiation. Hancock et al. at Stanford reported a significantly elevated risk for breast cancer in women treated under the age of 30 (87). However, women who were treated after age 30 did not appear to be at excessive risk for developing breast cancer. Van Leeuwen et al. at the Netherlands Cancer Institute found that in women who received treatment at age 30 or younger, the relative risk for breast cancer was 11.4, whereas that for women treated at age 20 or younger was 41.9 (52). At the JCRT, the relative risks for breast cancer in patients treated at age under 15, 15 to 24, 25 to 34, and over 34 were 458 (95% C.I. 91.7 to 1,345), 23.3 (95% C.I. 7.5 to 54.5), 4.0 (95% C.I. 0.8 to 11.8), and 2.0 (95% C.I. 0.20 to 7.1), respectively (54).

Gender

Tarbell et al. at the JCRT were the first to report a female predominance among patients with solid tumors (98). A review of a larger pediatric patient population at St. Jude confirmed that second malignancies were more common in female patients, even when those with breast cancer were excluded (99). The Late Effect Study Group found, on multivariate analysis, that female sex was an independent predictor for secondary solid tumors, with a relative risk of 2.9 (95% C.I 1.5 to 5.4) (75).

Patient Habits: Tobacco Use

The relationship between smoking history, Hodgkin's disease, and subsequent lung cancer is hard to establish. A detailed smoking history including the amount smoked and period of tobacco use in relation to the time of diagnosis of Hodgkin's disease and lung cancer is difficult to obtain for all patients retrospectively. Also, the smoking habits of patients who did not develop lung cancers are invariably not as well documented.

Two case-control studies reviewed the risk of lung cancer following Hodgkin's disease treatment in relationship to tobacco use (105,106). A significant increase in the relative risk for lung cancer with increasing number of pack-years of smoking after the diagnosis of Hodgkin's disease was found by van Leeuwen et al. However, the effect of the number of pack-years smoked at diagnosis or total amount ever smoked was not significant. For patients who smoked one or more pack-years after the diagnosis and treatment of Hodgkin's disease, the risk of lung cancer increased significantly with increasing radiation dose, whereas no such trend was observed among patients who had smoked less, suggesting a possible positive interaction between the carcinogenic effects of smoking and radiation.

Predisposing Genetic Factors

Among the six patients who developed malignant melanoma in a report from Stanford, five had precursor nevi in the specimen on pathology review or had clinical characteristics of dysplastic nevus syndrome (92). It was hypothesized that immune deficits in Hodgkin's disease patients, when exacerbated by their treatment, may allow the transformation of precursor nevi to cutaneous melanoma, similar to that observed in renal transplant patients. The authors also observed that these patients appeared to have unusual responses to radiation therapy, with significant atrophy, neurologic deficits, pulmonary fibrosis, and retroperitoneal fibrosis, raising the possibility of an inherently increased tissue sensitivity to ionizing radiation.

Splenectomy/Splenic Irradiation

An association between splenectomy or splenic irradiation and solid tumor risk was reported by Dietrich et al. from the Institut Gustave Roussy (107). Potential explanations for their findings include higher blood counts after splenectomy, thus allowing higher doses of chemotherapy, or the larger radiation field size associated with splenic irradiation. However, according to the authors, no adjustment in chemotherapy doses was made. Also, on multivariate analysis, splenectomy or splenic radiotherapy was an independent risk factor for development of solid cancers.

Minimizing Secondary Solid Tumor Mortality: Clinical Implications

Given direct and indirect evidence of association between solid tumors and field size, careful selection of patients for treatment based on clinical characteristics and/or pathologic staging should allow for irradiation of the smallest possible volume as one way to decrease subsequent solid-tumor risk. Limiting radiation field size may be especially important in patients who also are receiving chemotherapy, as demonstrated by the study by Biti et al., in which the cumulative probability of solid tumor was significantly higher in patients treated with chemotherapy in addition to subtotal or total nodal irradiation (95).

Although a dose–response relationship has been demonstrated for solid-tumor development (105,106), this relationship appears to be limited to the dose range under 10 Gy, suggesting that protocols that use reduced doses of radiation in combination with chemotherapy may not significantly alter the second-tumor risks because the radiation doses are still in the 15- to 20-Gy range.

The contribution of chemotherapy alone to solid-tumor development after Hodgkin's disease remains unclear. From the limited data available, the risk after chemotherapy alone appears to be elevated (19). Use of chemotherapy alone in place of radiotherapy in early-stage patients may potentially result in sacrifice of disease control rate and salvage ability. Therefore, employing chemotherapy alone in order to lower secondary solid-tumor risk in early-stage patients is probably best conducted in a protocol setting in which patients can be followed closely and the treatment efficacy and toxicity can be carefully documented.

Data on solid tumors after Hodgkin's disease have helped identify when the excessive risks appear and what patient groups are at increased risk for various types of cancer, thereby providing useful insights to the timing and frequency of cancer-screening tests and the patient population to be targeted. An illustrative example is breast cancer in survivors of Hodgkin's disease, in which women irradiated at a young age have been shown to be at particularly high risk after a latency of at least 10 years. In the study by Yahalom et al. on breast cancer after Hodgkin's disease, mammograms were reviewed in 32 cases, and as many as 81% were read as abnormal (90), leading the authors to the recommendation that routine mammogram screening begin as early as eight years after Hodgkin's disease treatment. Another argument for rigorous screening in these patients is that there does not appear to be a marked difference between mortality from breast cancer that developed after Hodgkin's disease and primary breast cancer, suggesting that early detection may help in increasing long-term survival. A prospective screening protocol in young female survivors of Hodgkin's disease is under way at the Dana-Farber Cancer Institute, and the results may shed light on the impact of screening on morbidity and mortality, and the optimal screening schedule, after taking into account other breast cancer risk factors.

Finally, data on the possible interaction between other environmental carcinogens and Hodgkin's disease treatment and its impact on future cancer risks suggest that counseling for behavioral changes such as smoking cessation and avoidance of sun exposure may be an important part of follow-up care of patients with Hodgkin's disease (92,105,106).

CARDIAC MORTALITY

Impact of Cardiac Diseases on Overall Mortality

After Hodgkin's disease and second malignancies, cardiovascular disease is a distant third cause of death following treatment for Hodgkin's disease, contributing to approximately 10% to 15% of all causes of mortality thus far (1,3–5). A wide spectrum of cardiac complications has been observed after Hodgkin's disease treatment, including pericarditis, pancarditis, pericardial effusions, pericardial fibrosis, congestive heart failure, valvular defects, conduction defects, and coronary artery disease (1,3–5, 108–115). The most common fatal cardiovascular complication after Hodgkin's disease therapy, however, is acute myocardial infarction secondary to coronary artery disease. At Stanford University, results on 2,232 patients treated for Hodgkin's disease were reported, in which 88 patients died of cardiac diseases. Over 60% of the cardiac deaths were from acute myocardial infarction (113). The absolute excess risk for acute myocardial infarction deaths increased from 6.4 to 70.6 per 10,000 person-years, and the relative risk increased from 2.0 to 5.6, within 5 years of Hodgkin's disease diagnosis and at greater than 20 years from diagnosis, respectively. The absolute excess risk for other cardiac causes increased from 11.3 at 5 to 9 years from diagnosis to 76.1 at more than 20 years from diagnosis. The corresponding relative risks were 3.2 and 8.8, respectively. The results suggest that the impact of cardiac deaths on overall mortality increases with follow-up time and remains elevated even 20 years after completion of therapy. However, there are also data to suggest that treatment modification, in particular, improvements in radiotherapy techniques in recent years, may have reduced the incidence of cardiovascular mortality (111,113).

Mediastinal Irradiation and Risk of Cardiac Death

A number of studies have documented an association between mediastinal irradiation and risk of fatal cardiovascular complications. Boivin et al. reported results on 957 patients treated for Hodgkin's disease and found that the standardized mortality ratio of death from coronary artery disease was significantly elevated at 2.1 (95% C.I. 1 to 3.9, $p < .05$) in patients who received mediastinal radiation therapy, whereas the risk was not increased in patients who were not irradiated (115). In a collaborative study from 11 cancer treatment centers that included 4,665 patients with Hodgkin's disease, a significantly elevated relative risk of 2.56 of death from myocardial infarction (C.I. 1.11 to 5.93) was observed after mediastinal irradiation but not after chemotherapy (108). Cosset et al. found that among the 499 patients who received mantle-field irradiation, there was a 3.9% cumulative incidence at 10 years of acute myocardial infarction, but in the 138 patients who did not receive mediastinal irradiation, no acute myocardial infarction was observed (109). In the Stanford series, among the 171 patients who received no mediastinal irradiation or less than 30 Gy to the mediastinum, no significantly increased risk of heart-disease death was observed (113). In their pediatric and adolescent population, 85% of the acute myocardial infarction deaths occurred in patients who had received mediastinal doses of 36 Gy or more (112).

At Stanford, cardiac and subcarinal blocking was introduced in 1972, resulting in a decline in relative risk for non–myocardial-infarction cardiac death from 5.3 to 1.4 in subsequent years (111). However, the implementation of the blocking did not affect the risk of death from acute myocardial infarction, likely because the blocks did not adequately shield the proximal coronary arteries.

Treatment techniques used in the earlier years with cobalt or orthovoltage equipment, anterior field weighting, daily fractions larger than 2 Gy, and lack of cardiac blocking, all resulted in higher cardiac doses. In the multiinstitutional study by Boivin et al., the relative risk for fatal myocardial infarction after mediastinal irradiation was associated with the time period of Hodgkin's disease therapy. Patients treated from 1940 to 1966, which is during the era when orthovoltage irradiation and anterior or predominantly anterior techniques were employed, had a higher relative risk of acute myocardial infarction death than patients treated from 1967 to 1985 (6.33 vs. 1.97), although the difference did not achieve statistical significance. At the University of Rochester, cardiac evaluations were performed on 50 patients with Hodgkin's disease treated predominantly with modern techniques using megavoltage radiation therapy, subcarinal blocking, and dose fraction under 2 Gy, and 86% of the patients were treated with equally weighted parallel opposed AP–PA mantle fields daily (110). With an average follow up of 13.5 years, other than some modest abnormalities in a minority of patients, most had ejection fraction and myocardial perfusion that were within normal limits, suggesting intact cardiac function in most patients irradiated for Hodgkin's disease with modern techniques.

Minimizing Cardiac Mortality: Clinical Implications

Most of the changes in the technique of radiation in the past 10 to 20 years, including use of megavoltage machines, cardiac and subcarinal blocks, equal radiation beam weighting, and smaller fraction size, have contributed to the decrease in cardiac death after Hodgkin's disease (108,110). In pediatric patients, low-dose involved-field irradiation in combination with chemotherapy will probably reduce the chance of cardiac complications as well (116,117) by lowering the radiation dose received by the heart. However, the long-term toxicities of chemotherapeutic agents known to have dose-related cardiotoxicity, and their potential synergistic effects with radiotherapy, remain unknown. Also, the magnitude of the impact of the above technique modifications on late cardiovascular effects is still not entirely clear. Physicians taking care of survivors of Hodgkin's disease need to be aware of the increased risk of cardiac deaths that may persist years after treatment. Long-term monitoring of cardiac functions will be crucial in assessing the true risks of various cardiac sequelae.

As part of long-term follow-up care of patients with Hodgkin's disease, the role of different screening tests such as electrocardiogram, echocardiogram, and exercise tolerance tests in asymptomatic patients remains to be defined. Cardiac disease screening may have some influence on mortality, considering that some of the cases of cardiac deaths are unexpected deaths in young patients. The potential survival advantage from early detection and timely intervention to manage cardiac sequelae, however, needs to be balanced against the possible unwarranted anxiety evoked by the tests on asymptomatic patients, effect of the test results on their insurance eligibility, and the costs associated with the procedures. The role of screening, along with other unresolved questions including the subgroup of patients to be targeted, which of the tests should be used for routine screening, and how frequently the tests are to be conducted are probably best addressed by prospective studies on survivors of Hodgkin's disease.

Because of the retrospective nature of long-term studies on Hodgkin's disease and the young age of most of the patients, little data exist on the association between other known cardiac risk factors and Hodgkin's disease treatment in contributing to cardiac mortality. Given the clear evidence that patients after Hodgkin's disease therapy are at excessive risk for cardiac disease, and that cardiac death is one of the main causes of death in long-term survivors, efforts should be made to minimize other cardiac risk factors by, for example, smoking cessation counseling, diet modification, encouraging regular exercise, routine screening, and proper therapeutic interventions for hypercholesterolemia and hypertension.

INFECTIOUS MORTALITY

After cardiac complications, infection is the next most common cause of death in patients treated for Hodgkin's disease. In most series, infection accounts for under 10% of all deaths (1,5,6,17). In studies with shorter follow-up, infection may have a higher contribution to overall mortality, as serious infectious complications tend to occur during or immediately following treatment. Increased infection risks are secondary to the immunologic defects associated with Hodgkin's disease, which are further aggravated by various diagnostic and therapeutic interventions, including chemotherapy, radiation therapy, splenectomy, or splenic irradiation.

Herpes zoster is the most commonly identified infectious complication following Hodgkin's disease therapy, occurring in about 15% to 20% of the patients (114,115).

However, the associated mortality is relatively low, and especially with the widespread use of prompt antiviral therapy, the risk of disseminated disease, which can be fatal, has decreased.

Of all infectious complications, the most serious and life-threatening one is overwhelming sepsis (118–121), seen predominantly in postsplenectomy patients, with a crude overall incidence estimated to be 2% to 3%. In addition to the high associated mortality rate of up to 66%, the clinical course is rapid, and death can ensue within hours of onset of the infection (120). Although most of these highly fatal bacterial sepses occur around or shortly after treatment, fatal overwhelming sepsis has been described up to 47 years after a splenectomy (119).

A number of changes in the management of patients with Hodgkin's disease, however, have resulted in a decline in infectious mortality after Hodgkin's disease therapy. These include use of less myelosuppressive chemotherapeutic agents, decreased performance of staging laparotomy and splenectomy, routine administration of prelaparotomy vaccination (122–126), and increased awareness of the danger of overwhelming sepsis and importance of prompt antibiotic therapy. At Stanford, the crude incidence of fatal infection among patients treated for Hodgkin's disease who were disease-free at the time of death decreased from 0.96% during the period from 1962 to 1980 to 0.38% during the period from 1980 to the present (111). On the other hand, increasing use of bone marrow transplantation for salvage therapy may increase the incidence of infectious mortality in patients with Hodgkin's disease. However, better supportive care and routine use of colony-stimulating factors as part of high-dose therapy have substantially reduced the risk of fatal infections in the peritransplant period.

Minimizing Infectious Mortality: Clinical Implications

Although infectious mortality has had a finite contribution to the overall mortality of patients treated for Hodgkin's disease, many of the recent changes in practice described above have reduced the risks of fatal infections, and it is likely that the incidence will continue to decline with time.

Despite the diminishing risk of infectious death, given the high fatality associated with overwhelming sepsis and its persistent risks over time, it is important to continue to reinforce education in asplenic patients or patients who have received splenic radiotherapy of the potential grave consequences of febrile illnesses. Health care providers should know to act promptly when fever is reported, as early detection and aggressive treatment of bacterial sepsis can lower the mortality risk. In addition, clinical features that predict a very low risk of occult abdominal disease (e.g., CS IA female patients, or CS IA patients with LP histology) have been recognized (127), and other studies have identified patients who are at high risk of relapse for whom up-front combined-modality therapy is indicated (e.g., patients with large mediastinal adenopathy) (20,22,24,25). Therefore, there are subgroups of patients who will be unlikely to benefit from staging laparotomy, and in whom splenectomy can be avoided.

PULMONARY MORTALITY

Pulmonary toxicities after Hodgkin's disease treatment are well documented and range from acute interstitial pneumonitis to chronic lung injury such as pulmonary fibrosis and recurrent pleural effusions (128–133). Several series have found symptomatic diminished lung capacity in up to a third of the patients treated for Hodgkin's disease (48,131,134). Deaths as a result of lung injury following Hodgkin's disease therapy, on the other hand, have not been systematically analyzed, likely because it is infrequently fatal. Although pulmonary deaths contribute to only a very small proportion of mortality in patients treated for Hodgkin's disease, it may be gaining in significance for patients treated in recent years. This is because of the increasing use of bleomycin-based regimens, which, especially when combined with mediastinal radiotherapy, have led to pulmonary deaths. In an NCI study, 80 patients with Hodgkin's disease presenting with large mediastinal disease were treated with MOPP alternated with ABVD chemotherapy, followed by mantle radiation therapy (135). The radiation fields were shaped to conform to the prechemotherapy tumor volume. Treatment-related pneumonitis developed in 16%, and some pulmonary reaction was noted in 21% of the patients. One 51-year-old patient died of treatment-related pneumonitis. In the EORTC H_6U trial, two patients in the ABVD-and-radiotherapy arm died from lung toxicity (79). Both were patients with bulky mediastinal disease, and one of the patients received a daily fraction of 2.5 Gy. In an Italian study on 50 early-stage Hodgkin's disease patients treated with vinblastine, bleomycin, methotrexate and radiotherapy, one 70-year-old developed grade 4 pulmonary toxicity and subsequently died of respiratory failure (136). A similar regimen used in a British National Lymphoma Investigation study resulted in stopping of the trial because of unexpected severity of pulmonary toxicity in 47% of the patients, although no deaths were reported (137). In the CALGB study, Canellos et al. reported fatal lung toxicity in three relatively older patients, aged 42, 69, and 72, respectively, among the 115 advanced-stage patients treated with ABVD (81). Although one of the patients did receive prior irradiation, the results suggest that chemotherapy alone can lead to pulmonary deaths.

The gaining popularity of high-dose therapy for salvage of refractory or recurrent disease has also contributed to pulmonary mortality in patients with Hodgkin's disease. A significant fraction of transplant-related deaths have been attributed to interstitial pneumonitis. As illustrated in Table 7, lung toxicities account for over 50% of all peritransplant mortality (38–46).

TABLE 7. *Contribution of pulmonary deaths to peritransplant mortality*

Institution	Number of peritransplant deaths	Number of pulmonary deaths
Johns Hopkins (46)	17	10 interstitial pneumonitis (59%)
Toronto (44)	7	3 interstitial pneumonitis (43%)
London (43)	16	4 interstitial pneumonitis 4 fungal pneumonitis (50%)
M.D. Anderson (42)	11	7 interstitial pneumonitis/alveolar hemorrhage (64%)
British Columbia (41)	5	2 acute lung toxicity (40%)
Fred Hutchison (40)	51	16 idiopathic pneumonitis 12 infectious pneumonitis (55%)
MSKCC (39)	8	5 pulmonary decompensation (63%)
Stanford (38)	6	2 interstitial pneumonitis 2 respiratory failure 1 *Legionella* pneumonitis (83%)

Minimizing Pulmonary Mortality: Clinical Implications

Possible ways to minimize pulmonary morbidity and mortality include exploring regimens that allow a lower cumulative dose of bleomycin, especially when given in combination with radiotherapy. The high rate of pulmonary toxicity observed in the NCI study emphasizes the importance of limiting radiation therapy fields following chemotherapy to the postchemotherapy tumor volume (135). Data from the JCRT demonstrated significantly increased risk of pneumonitis with whole-lung radiation therapy as well as when chemotherapy is combined with the radiation treatment (128). The results again support the importance of limiting radiation field size, especially when it is given in conjunction with chemotherapy. Further work needs to be done in determining the effect of modification of the treatment sequence and the time interval between chemotherapy and radiation therapy on the risk of pulmonary morbidity and mortality. From the limited available data, there are some indications that older patients may be more susceptible to fatal treatment-related pulmonary complications (81,135,136), suggesting the importance of carefully monitoring the pulmonary function of these patients during treatment and attenuating the treatment as necessary. Smoking-cessation counseling may also have a significant role in minimizing pulmonary complications in patients treated for Hodgkin's disease.

The main cause of pulmonary deaths in the peritransplant period is interstitial pneumonitis, which may be related to various drugs and/or radiation therapy given or to infection. Improved supportive care and avoidance of mediastinal or lung irradiation before transplantation may decrease the risk of pulmonary complications.

FACTORS AFFECTING OVERALL MORTALITY

We have reviewed the leading causes of death in patients treated for Hodgkin's disease. The following summarizes the factors that have a major influence on long-term survival. Because of the excellent overall prognosis of Hodgkin's disease, there are only a limited number of factors that correlate with long-term survival.

Older age at diagnosis (cutoffs ranging from 40 to 50 or older) has uniformly been identified as a significant predictor of lower overall survival (5,21,22,24,25). The increased risk of death is a combination of higher Hodgkin's disease–specific mortality secondary to poor salvage ability (5,25) and elevated probability of dying from other causes, including second malignancies or cardiac, infectious, and pulmonary complications (1,2,5,25). The strong associations between age and various causes of death have been reviewed in the above sections. Overall, one needs to be mindful of the excess mortality risk in the older age group and be especially stringent in the selection of their treatment design as well as in monitoring them during and after their treatments.

Disease stage is a tumor-specific predictor of overall survival (2,5), with most of the effect likely secondary to higher risk of death from Hodgkin's disease in the more advanced-stage patients. Proportionally, patients with advanced-stage Hodgkin's disease have fewer deaths from other causes, as they may not live long enough to experience the treatment-related long-term side effects. On the other hand, for those patients with advanced-stage disease who do survive, because they have been more heavily treated, their absolute incidence of long-term complications and treatment-related mortality should be expected to increase with longer follow-up time.

The EORTC H_6F trial is the only randomized trial that addressed the question of the role of staging laparotomy and tailored treatment in early-stage Hodgkin's disease patients (79). In their recently updated results, at 10 years of follow-up, a significant difference in overall survival emerged, favoring the no-laparotomy arm (78). The excess mortality in the laparotomy group was attributed to laparotomy-related toxicities. In interpreting the results of this trial, one needs to be aware of the rarity of postlaparotomy mortality in the modern era, given the new development and routine administration of vaccinations and decreased use of myelosuppressive agents (122–126).

From the 1998 Cancer Statistics, there is a clear trend of improvement of survival outcome in Hodgkin's disease patients treated in the modern era (138). The difference in survival rates between 1974 to 1976 and 1986 to 1993, at least in the Caucasian population, was statistically significant (72% vs. 82%, $p < .05$). Data from Stanford and the International Database on Hodgkin's Disease showed that reduction in causes of death other than Hodgkin's disease in the more recent years is at least partly responsible for the decrease in mortality rates over time (2,6,7). At Stanford, the absolute excess risk of death from causes other than Hodgkin's disease in patients treated during the period of 1962 to 1980 was compared with that of patients treated during the period of 1980 to 1996 (7) (Table 4). For patients with stage I or II disease, there was a clear decrease in absolute risk of death in patients treated in the more recent time period. Patients with stage III or IV disease treated more recently also had a decreased risk of death from other causes in the first 10 years of follow-up. The findings are encouraging and suggest that modifications of management approaches over the years have decreased treatment-related complications and improved overall survival.

USE OF MARKOV MODELING TO ESTIMATE LIFE EXPECTANCY

Although extensive data exist indicating that survivors of Hodgkin's disease face an excess risk of death from various causes, the magnitude of the decrease in life expectancy in patients who have been treated for Hodgkin's disease is difficult to quantify. Techniques of Markov modeling (139) can predict life expectancy of patients, which is a measure of average survival. For example, a Markov state-transition model designed to model the lifetime events of patients with Hodgkin's disease may consist of health states including remission, refractory disease, relapse, second malignancy, and cardiac disease. The probabilities of transition from one health state to another will be conditional on the patient and disease characteristics and the type of treatment received. Estimates of these transition probabilities can be extrapolated from data in the literature. Patients in each of the different health states face different risks of death. The model is allowed to run until the entire cohort has entered the death state. The life expectancy of the cohort of patients can then be calculated by summing up the time spent in the various alive health states. Using such modeling technique, one can not only estimate the life expectancy of patients affected by Hodgkin's disease but also compare the survival of patients who received different types of intervention. It is analogous to a computer-simulated trial in which small survival differences can be detected, and there is no limitation by inadequate sample size, noncompliance, loss to follow-up, or insufficient follow-up time.

CONCLUSIONS

Survivors of Hodgkin's disease do not enjoy the same life expectancy as the general population, even after they have been rendered disease-free, because they have an excess risk of death from other causes. As these delayed and potentially life-threatening events are being recognized, and as more is learned about them, therapeutic modifications have been made to limit their likelihood. So far, preliminary data appear to indicate that the changes have been reasonably effective in reducing the risks of secondary leukemia, cardiac toxicities, and infectious complications. However, not many patients have lived for longer than 15 years following introduction of these treatment modifications. It is therefore prudent that patients successfully treated continue to be closely followed so that the true long-term risk can be documented, and improvements in management approaches can continue to be made.

Perhaps the most alarming observation is the rising incidence of solid cancer in survivors of Hodgkin's disease. Given the relatively long latency of most solid tumors, their actual incidence over time and effect on overall survival are evolving and remain to be determined. There are few data on the impact of therapeutic modifications and implementation of screening programs on solid-tumor risks and the associated mortality. This again underscores the importance of continuing to monitor patients who have been treated for Hodgkin's disease, even many years after treatment. In this way, we can determine if the excess risks persist throughout a patient's remaining lifetime.

Finally, it is important to recognize that not all of the unwanted late effects in the survivors are entirely iatrogenic. The disease itself, patient genetic predisposition, and their interactions with some of the ubiquitous environmental factors may at least partially account for the late changes. It is therefore possible that the excess morbidity and mortality risks faced by survivors of Hodgkin's disease may not ever be completely eliminated, although at least for now, there is undoubtedly room for improvement.

REFERENCES

1. Van Rijswijk R, Verbeek J, Haanen C, et al. Major complications and causes of death in patients treated for Hodgkin's disease. *J Clin Oncol* 1987;5:1624–1633.
2. Henry-Amar M, Somers R. Survival outcome after Hodgkin's disease: A report from the International Data Base on Hodgkin's disease. *Semin Oncol* 1990;17:758–768.
3. Vaughan Hudson B, Vaughan Hudson G, Linch D, et al. Late mortality in young British National Lymphoma Investigation patients cured of Hodgkin's disease. *Ann Oncol* 1994;5:565–566.
4. Cosset J-M, Henry-Amar M, Meerwaldt J. Long-term toxicity of early stage of Hodgkin's disease therapy: The EORTC experience. *Ann Oncol* 1991;2(Suppl 2):77–82.
5. Mauch P, Kalish L, Marcus K, et al. Long-term survival in Hodgkin's disease: Relative impact of mortality, second tumors, infection and cardiovascular disease. *Cancer J Sci Am* 1995;1:33–42.
6. Hancock S, Hoppe R. Long-term complications of treatment and

causes of mortality after Hodgkin's disease. *Semin Radiat Oncol* 1996;6:225–242.

7. Hoppe R. Hodgkin's disease: Complications of therapy and excess mortality. *Ann Oncol* 1997;8(Suppl 1):S115–S118.
8. Joly F, Henry-Amar M, Arveux P, et al. Late psychosocial sequelae in Hodgkin's disease survivors. *J Clin Oncol* 1996;14:2444–2453.
9. Kornblith A, Anderson J, Cella D, et al. Hodgkin's disease survivors at increased risk for problems in psychosocial adaptations. *Cancer* 1992; 70:2244–2224.
10. Fabian P, Hoppe R, Bloom J, et al. Psychosocial problems among survivors of Hodgkin's disease. *J Clin Oncol* 1986;4:805–814.
11. Cella D, Tross S. Psychological adjustment to survival for Hodgkin's disease. *J Consult Clin Psychol* 1986;54:616–622.
12. Siegel K, Christ G. *Psychosocial consequences in Hodgkin's disease: the consequences of survival.* Philadelphia: Lea & Febiger, 1990: 383–399.
13. Gurney J, Severson R, Davis S, et al. Incidence of cancer in children in the United States: Sex-, race-, and one-year age-specific rates by histological type. *Cancer* 1995;75:2186–2195.
14. Gaynon P, Qu R, Chappell R, et al. Survival after relapse childhood acute lymphoblastic leukemia: Impact of site and time to first relapse—The Children's Cancer Group experience. *Cancer* 1998;82:1387–1395.
15. Hancock S, Hoppe R, Horning S, et al. Intercurrent death after Hodgkin's disease therapy in radiotherapy and adjuvant MOPP trials. *Ann Intern Med* 1988;109:183–189.
16. Vlachake M, Ha C, Hagemeister F, et al. Long-term outcome of treatment for Ann Arbor stage I Hodgkin's disease: Patterns of failure, late toxicity and second malignancies. *Int J Radiat Oncol Biol Phys* 1997; 39:609–616.
17. Specht L, Gray K, Clarke M, et al. Influence of more extensive radiotherapy and adjuvant chemotherapy on long-term outcome of early-stage Hodgkin's disease: A metaanalysis of 23 randomized trials involving 3,888 patients. *J Clin Oncol* 1998;16:830–843.
18. Loeffler M, Brosteanu O, Hasenclever D, et al. Meta-analysis of chemotherapy versus combined modality therapy trials in Hodgkin's disease. *J Clin Oncol* 1998;16:818–829.
19. Swerdlow A, Douglas A, Vaughan Hudson G, et al. Risk of second primary cancer after Hodgkin's disease in patients in the British National Lymphoma Investigation: Relationships to host factors, histology and stage of Hodgkin's disease, and splenectomy. *Br J Cancer* 1993;68: 1006–1011.
20. Pavlovsky S, Maschio M, Santarelli M, et al. Randomized trial of chemotherapy versus chemotherapy plus radiotherapy for stage I–II Hodgkin's disease. *J Natl Cancer Inst* 1988;80:1466–1473.
21. Gospodarowicz M, Sutcliffe S, Clark R, et al. Analysis of supradiaphragmatic clinical stages I and II Hodgkin's disease treated with radiation alone. *Int J Radiat Oncol Biol Phys* 1992;22:859–865.
22. Crnkovich M, Leopold K, Hoppe R, et al. Stage I to IIB Hodgkin's disease: The combined experience at Stanford University and the Joint Center for Radiation Therapy. *J Clin Oncol* 1987;5:1041–1049.
23. Specht L, Nordentoft A, Cold S, et al. Tumor burden as the most important prognostic factor in early stage Hodgkin's disease. Relations to other prognostic factors in early-stage Hodgkin's disease and implications for choice of treatment. *Cancer* 1988;61:1719–1727.
24. Mauch P, Tarbell N, Weinstein H, et al. Stage IA and IIA supradiaphragmatic Hodgkin's disease: Prognostic factors in surgically staged patients treated with mantle and paraaortic irradiation. *J Clin Oncol* 1988;6:1576–1583.
25. Henry-Amar M, Tirelli U, Dupoy N. Age less than 50 versus greater than 50 years as a prognostic factor in 1624 patients with stage I–II Hodgkin's disease entered in EORTC clinical trials since 1964 (abstract). *Ann Oncol* 1990;1(Suppl):3.
26. Shore T, Nelson N, Weinerman B. A meta-analysis of stages I and II Hodgkin's disease. *Cancer* 1990;65:1155–1160.
27. Hoppe R, Coleman C, Cox R, et al. The management of stage I–II Hodgkin's disease with irradiation alone or combined modality therapy: The Stanford experience. *Blood* 1982;59:455–465.
28. Marcus K, Kalish L, Coleman C, et al. Improved survival in patients with limited stage IIIA Hodgkin's disease treated with combined radiation therapy and chemotherapy. *J Clin Oncol* 1994;12:2567–2572.
29. Mauch P, Goffman T, Rosenthal D, et al. Stage III Hodgkin's disease: Improved survival with combined modality therapy as compared with radiation therapy alone. *J Clin Oncol* 1985;3:1166–1173.
30. Specht L, Horwich A, Ashley S. Salvage of relapse of patients with Hodgkin's disease in clinical stages I or II who were staged with laparotomy and initially treated with radiotherapy alone: A report from the International Data Base on Hodgkin's Disease. *Int J Radiat Oncol Biol Phys* 1994;30:805–811.
31. Healey E, Tarbell N, Kalish L, et al. Prognostic factors for patients with Hodgkin's disease in first relapse. *Cancer* 1993;71:2613–2620.
32. Longo D, Duffey P, Young R, et al. Conventional-dose salvage combination chemotherapy in patients relapsing with Hodgkin's disease after combination chemotherapy: The low probability after cure. *J Clin Oncol* 1992;10:210–218.
33. Salvagno L, Sarorau M, Aversa S, et al. Late relapses in Hodgkin's disease: Outcomes of patients relapsing more than 12 months after primary chemotherapy. *Ann Oncol* 1993;4:657–662.
34. Canellos G, Petroni G, Bareos M, et al. Etoposide, vinblastine, and doxorubicin: An active regimen for the treatment of Hodgkin's disease in relapse following MOPP. *J Clin Oncol* 1995;13:2005–2011.
35. Fairey A, Mead G, Jones H, et al. CAPE/AALE salvage chemotherapy for Hodgkin's disease patients relapsing within 1 year of ChlVPP chemotherapy. *Ann Oncol* 1993;4:857–860.
36. Lohri A, Barnett M, Fairey R, et al. Outcome of treatment of first relapse of Hodgkin's disease after primary chemotherapy: Identification of risk factors from the British Columbia experience 1970 to 1988. *Blood* 1991;77:2292–2298.
37. Biti G, Cimino G, Cartoni C, et al. Extended-field radiotherapy is superior to MOPP chemotherapy for the treatment of pathologic stage I–IIA Hodgkin's disease: Eight-year update of an Italian prospective randomized study. *J Clin Oncol* 1992;10:378–382.
38. Horning S, Chao N, Negrin R, et al. High-dose therapy and autologous hematopoietic progenitor cell transplantation from recurrent or refractory Hodgkin's disease: Analysis of the Stanford University results and prognostic indices. *Blood* 1997;89:801–813.
39. Yahalom J, Gulati S, Toia M, et al. Accelerated hyperfractionated total lymphoid irradiation, high-dose chemotherapy, and autologous bone marrow transplantation for refractory and relapsing patients with Hodgkin's disease. *J Clin Oncol* 1993;16:1062–1070.
40. Anderson J, Litzow M, Appelbaum F, et al. Allogeneic, synergistic, and autologous marrow transplantation for Hodgkin's disease: The 21-year Seattle experience. *J Clin Oncol* 1993;11:2342–2350.
41. Reece D, Barnett M, Shepard J, et al. High-dose cyclophosphamide, carmustine (BCNU), and etoposide (VP16-213) with or without cisplatin (CBV +/– P) and autologous transplantation for patients with Hodgkin's disease who fail to enter a complete remission after combination chemotherapy. *Blood* 1985;86:451–456.
42. Bierman P, Bagin R, Jagannath S, et al. High-dose chemotherapy followed by autologous hematopoietic rescue in Hodgkin's disease. *Ann Oncol* 1993;4:767–773.
43. Chopra R, McMillan A, Linch D, et al. The place of high-dose BEAM therapy and autologous bone marrow transplantation in poor-risk Hodgkin's disease. A single-center eight-year study of 155 patients. *Blood* 1993;81:1137–1145.
44. Linch D, Winfield D, Goldstone A, et al. Dose intensification with autologous bone marrow transplantation in relapsed and resistant Hodgkin's disease: Results of a BNLI randomised trial. *Lancet* 1993; 341:1051–1054.
45. Jones R, Piantadosi S, Mann R, et al. High-dose cytotoxic therapy and bone marrow transplantation for relapsed Hodgkin's disease. *J Clin Oncol* 1990;8:527–537.
46. Crump M, Smith A, Brandwein J, et al. High-dose etoposide and melphalan, and autologous bone marrow transplantation for patients with advanced Hodgkin's disease: Importance of disease status at transplant. *J Clin Oncol* 1993;11:704–711.
47. Hagemeister F, Tannir N, McLaughlin P, et al. MIME chemotherapy (Methyl–GAG, ifosfamide, methotrexate, etoposide) as treatment for recurrent Hodgkin's disease. *J Clin Oncol* 1987;5:556–561.
48. Santoro A, Bonfante U, Bonadonna G. Salvage chemotherapy with ABVD in MOPP-resistant Hodkgin's disease. *Ann Intern Med* 1982; 96:139–143.
49. Viviani S, Santoro A, Negretti E, et al. Salvage chemotherapy in Hodgkin's disease. *Ann Oncol* 1990;1:123–127.
50. Perren T, Selby P, Milan S, et al. Etoposide and Adriamycin containing combination chemotherapy (HOPE-Bleo) for relapsed Hodgkin's disease. *Br J Cancer* 1990;61:919–923.
51. Fabian C, Mansfield C, Dahlberg S, et al. Low-dose involved field radiation after chemotherapy in advanced Hodgkin's disease: A South-

west Oncology Group randomized study. *Ann Intern Med* 1994;120: 903–912.

52. Van Leeuwen F, Klokman W, Hagenbeek A, et al. Second cancer risk following Hodgkin's disease: A 20-year follow-up study. *J Clin Oncol* 1994;12:312–325.
53. Henry-Amar M. Second cancer after the treatment for Hodgkin's disease: A report from the International Data Base on Hodgkin's Disease. *Ann Oncol* 1992;3(Suppl 4):117–128.
54. Mauch P, Kalish L, Marcus K, et al. Second malignancies after treatment for laparotomy-staged IA–IIIB Hodgkin's disease: Long-term analysis of risk factors and outcome. *Blood* 1996;87:3625–3632.
55. Valagussa P, Santoro A, Fossati-Bellani F, et al. Second acute leukemia and other malignancies following treatment for Hodgkin's disease. *J Clin Oncol* 1986;4:830–837.
56. Andrieu J, Ifrah N, Payen C, et al. Increased risk of secondary acute nonlymphocytic leukemia after extended-field radiation therapy combined with MOPP chemotherapy for Hodgkin's disease. *J Clin Oncol* 1990;8:1148–1154.
57. Michels S, McKenna R, Arthur D, et al. Therapy-related acute myeloid leukemia and myelodysplastic syndrome: A clinical and morphological study of 65 cases. *Blood* 1985;65:1364–1372.
58. Longmore G, Guinan E, Weinstein H, et al. Bone marrow transplantation for myelodysplasia and secondary acute nonlymphoblastic leukemia. *J Clin Oncol* 1990;8:1707–1714.
59. Kaldor J, Day N, Clarke E, et al. Leukemia following Hodgkin's disease. *N Engl J Med* 1990;322:7–13.
60. Van Leeuwen F, Chorus A, van den Belt-Dusebout A, et al. Leukemia risk following Hodgkin's disease: Relation to cumulative dose of alkylating agents, treatment with teniposide combinations, number of episodes of chemotherapy, and bone marrow damage. *J Clin Oncol* 1994;12:1063–1073.
61. Tucker M, Meadows A, Boice J, et al. Leukemia after therapy with alkylating agents for childhood cancer. *J Natl Cancer Inst* 1987;78: 459–464.
62. Swerdlow A, Barber J, Horwich A, et al. Second malignancy in patients with Hodgkin's disease treated at the Royal Marsden Hospital. *Br J Cancer* 1997;75:116–123.
63. Van Leeuwen F, Somers R, Hart A. Splenectomy in Hodgkin's disease and second leukaemias (letter). *Lancet* 1987;2:210–211.
64. Tura S, Fiacchini M, Zinzani P, et al. Splenectomy and the increased risk of secondary acute leukemia in Hodgkin's disease. *J Clin Oncol* 1993;11:925–930.
65. Bonfante V, Santoro A, Viviani S, et al. ABVD in the treatment of Hodgkin's disease. *Semin Oncol* 1992;19(2 Suppl 5):38–44.
66. Boice J, Blettner M, Kleinerman R, et al. Radiation dose and leukemia risk in patients treated for cancer of the cervix. *J Natl Cancer Inst* 1987;79:1295–1311.
67. Preston D, Kasumi S, Tomonaga M, et al. Cancer incidence in atomic bomb survivors. Part III. Leukemia, lymphoma and multiple myeloma. 1960–1987. *Radiat Res* 1994;137(2 Suppl):S68–S97.
68. Boice J. Carcinogenesis—A synopsis of human experience with external exposure in medicine (review). *Health Phys* 1988;55:621–630.
69. Travis L, Weeks J, Curtis R, et al. Leukemia following low-dose total body irradiation and chemotherapy for non-Hodgkin's lymphoma. *J Clin Oncol* 1996;14:565–571.
70. Greene M, Young R, Merrill J, et al. Evidence of a treatment dose response in acute nonlymphocytic leukemias which occur after therapy of non-Hodgkin's lymphoma. *Cancer Res* 1983;43:1891–1898.
71. Tucker M, Coleman C, Cox R, et al. Risk of second cancers after treatment for Hodgkin's disease. *N Engl J Med* 1988;318:76–81.
72. Pedersen-Bjergaard J, Specht L, Lansen S, et al. Risk of therapy-related leukaemia and pre-leukaemia after Hodgkin's disease. Relation to age, cumulative dose of alkylating agents and time from chemotherapy. *Lancet* 1987;2:83–88.
73. Coleman M, Easton D, Horwich A, et al. Second malignancies and Hodgkin's disease—The Royal Marsden Hospital experience. *Radiother Oncol* 1988;11:229–238.
74. Van Leeuwen F, Somers R, Taal B, et al. Increased risk of lung cancer, non-Hodgkin's lymphoma, and leukemia following Hodgkin's disease. *J Clin Oncol* 1989;7:1046–1058.
75. Bhatia S, Robison L, Oberlin O, et al. Breast cancer and other second neoplasms after childhood Hodgkin's disease. *N Engl J Med* 1996; 334:745–751.
76. Abrahamsen J, Andersen A, Hannisdal E, et al. Second malignancies after treatment of Hodgkin's disease: The influence of treatment, follow-up time, and age. *J Clin Oncol* 1993;11:255–261.
77. Robinette C, Fraumeni J. Splenectomy and subsequent mortality in veterans of the 1939–45 war. *Lancet* 1977;2:127–129.
78. Cosset J-M, Henry-Amar M, Noordyk E, et al. The EORTC trials for adult patients with early-stage Hodgkin's disease. A 1997 update. *American Society for Therapeutic Radiology and Oncology Syllabus,* 1997 (Reston, VA).
79. Carde P, Hagenbeek A, Hayat M, et al. Clinical staging versus laparotomy and combined modality with MOPP versus ABVD in early-stage Hodgkin's disease: The H6 twin randomized trials for the European Organization for Research and Treatment of Cancer Lymphoma Cooperative Group. *J Clin Oncol* 1993;11:2258–2272.
80. Santoro A, Bonadonna G, Valagussa P, et al. Long-term results of combined modality therapy approach in Hodgkin's disease: Superiority of ABVD plus radiotherapy versus MOPP plus radiotherapy. *J Clin Oncol* 1987;5:27–37.
81. Canellos G, Anderson J, Propert K, et al. Chemotherapy of advanced Hodgkin's disease with MOPP, ABVD or MOPP alternating with ABVD. *N Engl J Med* 1992;327:1478–1484.
82. Fisher R, Gaynor E, Dahlberg S, et al. Comparison of a standard regimen (CHOP) with 3 intensive chemotherapy regimens for advanced non-Hodgkin's lymphoma. *N Engl J Med* 1993;328:1002–1006.
83. Bennett M, MacLennan K, Vaughan Hudson G, et al. Non-Hodgkin's lymphoma arising in patients treated for Hodgkin's disease in the BNLI: A 20-year experience. British National Lymphoma Investigation. *Ann Oncol* 1991;2(Suppl 2):83–92.
84. Zarate-Osorno A, Medeiros L, Longos D, et al. Non-Hodgkin's lymphoma arising in patients successfully treated for Hodgkin's disease. A clinical, histologic, and immunophenotypic study of 14 cases. *Am J Surg Pathol* 1992;16:885–895.
85. Kim H, Zelman R, Fox M, et al. Pathology panel for lymphoma clinical studies: A comprehensive analysis of cases accumulated since its inception. *J Natl Cancer Inst* 1982;68:43–67.
86. Penn I. Cancers complicating organ transplantation. *N Engl J Med* 1990;323:1767–1769.
87. Hancock S, Tucker M, Hoppe R. Breast cancer after treatment of Hodgkin's disease. *J Natl Cancer Inst* 1993;85:25–31.
88. Boivin J, Hutchison G, Zaxber A, et al. Incidence of second cancers in patients treated for Hodgkin's disease. *J Natl Cancer Inst* 1995;87: 732–741.
89. Salboum E, Doria R, Schubert W, et al. Second solid tumors in patients with Hodgkin's disease cured after radiation or chemotherapy plus adjuvant low-dose radiation. *J Clin Oncol* 1996;14:2435–2443.
90. Yahalom J, Petrek J, Biddinger P, et al. Breast cancer in patients irradiated for Hodgkin's disease: A clinical and pathological analysis of 45 events in 37 patients. *J Clin Oncol* 1992;10:1674–1681.
91. List A, Doll C, Greco F. Lung cancer in Hodgkin's disease: Association with previous radiotherapy. *J Clin Oncol* 1985;3.
92. Tucker M, Misfeldt D, Coleman N, et al. Cutaneous malignant melanoma after Hodgkin's disease. *Ann Intern Med* 1985;102:37–41.
93. Kushner B, Zauker A, Tan C. Second malignancies after childhood Hodgkin's disease. *Cancer* 1988;62:1364–1370.
94. Meadows A, Obringer A, Merrero O, et al. Second malignant neoplasms following childhood Hodgkin's disease: Treatment and splenectomy as risk factors. *Med Pediatr Oncol* 1989;17:477–484.
95. Biti G, Cellai E, Magrini S, et al. Second solid tumors and leukemia after treatment for Hodgkin's disease: An analysis of 1121 patients from a single institution. *Int J Radiat Oncol Biol Phys* 1994;29: 25–31.
96. Cimino G, Papa G, Tura S, et al. Second primary cancer following Hodgkin's disease: Updated results of an Italian multicentric study. *J Clin Oncol* 1991;9:432–437.
97. Hancock S, Cox R, McDougall I. Thyroid disease after treatment of Hodgkin's disease. *N Engl J Med* 1991;325:599–605.
98. Tarbell N, Gelber R, Weinstein H, et al. Sex differences in risk of second malignant tumors after Hodgkin's disease in childhood. *Lancet* 1993;341:1428–1432.
99. Beaty O III, Hudson M, Greenwald C, et al. Subsequent malignancies in children and adolescents after treatment for Hodgkin's disease. *J Clin Oncol* 1995;13:603–609.
100. Kaletsky A, Bertino J, Farber L, et al. Second neoplasms in patients

with Hodgkin's disease following combined modality therapy– The Yale experience. *J Clin Oncol* 1986;4:311–317.
101. Doria R, Holford T, Farber L, et al. Second solid malignancies after combined modality therapy for Hodgkin's disease. *J Clin Oncol* 1995;13:2016–2022.
102. Tester W, Kinsella T, Waller B, et al. Second malignant neoplasms complicating Hodgkin's disease: The National Cancer Institute experience. *J Clin Oncol* 1984;2:762–768.
103. Weissmann L, Corson J, Neugut A, et al. Malignant mesothelioma following treatment for Hodgkin's disease. *J Clin Oncol* 1996;14: 2098–2100.
104. Sankila R, Garwicz S, Olsen J, et al. Risk of subsequent malignant neoplasms among 1,641 Hodgkin's disease patients diagnosed in childhood and adolescence: A population-based cohort study in the 5 Nordic countries. *J Clin Oncol* 1996;14:1442–1446.
105. Van Leeuwen F, Klokman W, Stovall M, et al. Roles of radiotherapy and smoking in lung cancer following Hodgkin's disease. *J Natl Cancer Inst* 1995;87:1530–1537.
106. Kaldor J, Day N, Bell J, et al. Lung cancer following Hodgkin's disease: A case-control study. *Br J Cancer* 1992;52:677–681.
107. Dietrich P, Henry-Amar M, Cosset J-M, et al. Second primary cancers in patients continuously disease-free from Hodgkin's disease: A protective role for the spleen? *Blood* 1994;84:1209–1215.
108. Boivin J, Hutchison G, Lubin J, et al. Coronary artery disease mortality in patients treated for Hodgkin's disease. *Cancer* 1992;69: 1241–1247.
109. Cosset J-M, Henry-Amar M, Pallae-Cosset B, et al. Pericarditis and myocardial infarctions after Hodgkin's disease therapy. *Int J Radiat Oncol Biol Phys* 1991;21:447–449.
110. Constine L, Schwartz R, Savage D, et al. Cardiac function, perfusion and morbidity in irradiated long-term survivors of Hodgkin's disease. *Int J Radiat Oncol Biol Phys* 1997;39:897–906.
111. Hancock S, Hoppe R. Long-term complications of treatment and cancer mortality after Hodgkin's disease. *Semin Radiat Oncol* 1996;6:225–242.
112. Hancock S, Donaldson S, Hoppe R. Cardiac disease following treatment of Hodgkin's diseases children and adolescents. *J Clin Oncol* 1993;11:1208–1215.
113. Hancock S, Tucker M, Hoppe R. Factors affecting late mortality from heart disease after treatment of Hodgkin's disease. *JAMA* 1993;270: 1949–1955.
114. Cameron J, Oesterle S, Baldwin J, et al. The etiologic spectrum of constrictive pericarditis. *Am Heart J* 1987;113:354–360.
115. Boivin J, Hutchison G. Coronary heart disease mortality after irradiation for Hodgkin's disease. *Cancer* 1982;49:2470–2475.
116. Hunger S, Link M, Donaldson S. ABVD/MOPP and low-dose involved field radiotherapy in pediatric Hodgkin's disease: The Stanford experience. *J Clin Oncol* 1994;12:2160–2166.
117. Donaldson. Treatment of children with early stage and favorable Hodgkin's disease—a model of success (abstract). *Proc ASCO* 1995;14:A1289.
118. Donaldson S, Glatstein E, Vosti K. Bacterial infections in pediatric Hodgkin's disease. Relationship to radiotherapy, chemotherapy and splenectomy. *Cancer* 1978;41:1949–1958.
119. Waldron D, Harding B, Duigran J. Overwhelming infection occurring in the immediate post-splenectomy period. *Br J Clin Pract* 1989; 43:421–422.
120. Frezzato M, Castaman G, Rodeghiero F. Fulminant sepsis in adults splenectomized for Hodgkin's disease. *Haematologica* 1993;78(Suppl 2):73–77.
121. Bookman M, Longo D, Young R. Late complications of curative treatment in Hodgkin's disease. *JAMA* 1988;260:680–683.
122. Jockovich M, Mendenhall NP, Sombeck MD, et al. Long-term complications of laparotomy in Hodgkin's disease. *Ann Surg* 1994;219: 615–624.
123. Chan C, Molrine D, George S, et al. Pneumococcal conjugate vaccine primes for antibody response to polysaccharide pneumococcal vaccine following treatment of Hodgkin's disease. *J Infect Dis* 1996;173: 256–258.
124. Molrine D, George S, Tarbell N, et al. Antibody responses to polysaccharide and polysaccharide-conjugate vaccines following treatment for Hodgkin's disease. *Ann Intern Med* 1995;123:824–828.
125. Grimfors G, Soderquist M, Holar G, et al. A longitudinal study of class and subclass of antibody response to pneumococcal vaccination in splenectomized individuals with special reference to patients with Hodgkin's disease. *Eur J Haematol* 1990;45:101–108.
126. Siber G, Gorham C, Martin P, et al. Antibody response to pretreatment immunization and post-treatment boosting with bacterial polysaccharide vaccines in patients with Hodgkin's disease. *Ann Intern Med* 1986;104:467–475.
127. Mauch P, Larson D, Young R. Prognostic factors for positive surgical staging in patients with Hodgkin's disease. *J Clin Oncol* 1990;8: 257–265.
128. Tarbell N, Thompson L, Mauch P. Thoracic irradiation in Hodgkin's disease: Disease control and long-term complications. *Int J Radiat Oncol Biol Phys* 1990;18:275–281.
129. Smith L, Mendenhall N, Cicale M, et al. Results of a prospective study evaluating the effects of mantle irradiation on pulmonary function. *Int J Radiat Oncol Biol Phys* 1989;1:79–84.
130. Shapiro S, Shapiro S, Mill W, et al. Prospective study of long-term pulmonary manifestation of mantle irradiation. *Int J Radiat Oncol Biol Phys* 1990;3:707–714.
131. Horning S, Adhikari A, Rizk N, et al. Effects of treatment for Hodgkin's disease on pulmonary function: Results of a prospective study. *J Clin Oncol* 1994;2:297–305.
132. Rodriguez-Garcia J, Fraile G, Moreno M, et al. Recurrent massive pleural effusions as a late complication of radiotherapy in Hodgkin's disease. *Chest* 1991;4:1165–1166.
133. Morrone N, Ganae Silva Volope V, Dourado A, et al. Bilateral pleural effusion due to mediastinal fibrosis induced by radiotherapy. *Chest* 1993;4:1276–1278.
134. Lund M, Kongerud J, Nome O, et al. Lung function impairment in long-term survivors of Hodgkin's disease. *Ann Oncol* 1995;6:495–501.
135. Longo D, Glatstein E, Duffey P, et al. Alternating MOPP and ABVD chemotherapy plus mantle-field radiation therapy in patients with massive mediastinal Hodgkin's disease. *J Clin Oncol* 1997;15:3338–3346.
136. Gobbi P, Pieresca C, Frassoldate A, et al. Vinblastine, bleomycin and methotrexate chemotherapy plus extended field radiotherapy in early, favorably presenting, clinically staged Hodgkin's disease: The Gruppo Italiano per lo Studio dei Linfomi experience. *J Clin Oncol* 1996; 14:527–533.
137. Bates N, Williams M, Bessell E, et al. Efficacy and toxicity of vinblastine, bleomycin and methotrexate with involved-field radiotherapy in CS IA and IIA Hodgkin's disease: A British National Lymphoma Investigation pilot study. *J Clin Oncol* 1994;12:288–296.
138. Landis S, Murray T, Bolden S, et al. Cancer Statistics, 1998. *Ca J Clinicians* 1998;48:6–29.
139. Sonnenberg FA, Beck JR. Markov models in medical decision making: a practical guide. *Med Decis Making* 1993;13:322–338.

Hodgkin's Disease, edited by P. M. Mauch,
J. O. Armitage, V. Diehl, R. T. Hoppe, and L. M. Weiss.
Published by Lippincott Williams & Wilkins, Philadephia 1999.

CHAPTER 33

Second Cancers After Treatment of Hodgkin's Disease

Flora E. van Leeuwen, Anthony J. Swerdlow, Pinuccia Valagussa, and Margaret A. Tucker

Now that the majority of patients with Hodgkin's disease have such a favorable prognosis, it has become increasingly important to evaluate the long-term complications of treatment. Paradoxically, research conducted over the last two decades has clearly demonstrated that some treatments used to control cancer have the potential to induce new (second) primary malignancies. Of all late complications of treatment, second malignancies are generally considered to be the most serious because they cause not only substantial morbidity but also considerable mortality. For example, most second leukemias are resistant to therapy. Increased risk of second cancers has been observed after both radiotherapy and chemotherapy.

In any discussion of treatment-related second malignancies, it is of primary importance to remember that not all second cancers are caused by treatment. The occurrence of two primary malignancies in the same individual may have several causes. It may represent a chance occurrence, it may result from host susceptibility factors (e.g., genetic predisposition or immunodeficiency), it may be linked to common carcinogenic influences or a clustering of different risk factors in the same individual, or it may represent an association with treatment for the first tumor (1). In view of the high prevalence of cancer in the general population and the increasing incidence of most cancers with age, chance alone is likely to be responsible for a substantial proportion of second cancers, especially in older populations. To exclude the role of chance, comparison with cancer incidence in the general population is imperative in all studies of second cancer risk. If a second malignancy has been demonstrated to occur in excess, the contributions of other risk factors and the role of host susceptibility factors need to be ruled out convincingly before the risk increase can be attributed to treatment. The evaluation of the carcinogenic effects of therapy is further complicated by the fact that therapeutic agents are frequently given in combination. Appropriate epidemiologic and statistical methods are required to quantify the excess risk and to unravel treatment factors responsible for it.

Whenever one is interpreting results of second cancer studies, it must be kept in mind that the problem of treatment-induced malignancies has arisen by virtue of the successes of cancer treatment. As more becomes known about the effects of various treatment factors on second cancer risk, therapies may be modified to decrease second cancer risk while maintaining equal levels of therapeutic effectiveness.

This chapter addresses major aspects of second malignancy risk following treatment for Hodgkin's disease. After a brief overview of the carcinogenic effects of radiotherapy and chemotherapy, we first discuss the methods used for assessing second cancer risk. Subsequently, a review is given of the risks of leukemia, non-Hodgkin's lymphoma, and selected solid tumors in patients treated for Hodgkin's disease. Emphasis is on large studies that were published recently. Clinical implications of the most important findings are discussed, and, finally, we give some directions for future research.

F. E. van Leeuwen: Department of Epidemiology, Netherlands Cancer Institute, Amsterdam, The Netherlands.

A. J. Swerdlow: Department of Epidemiology and Population Health, London School of Hygiene and Tropical Medicine, London, United Kingdom.

P. Valagussa: Department of Biostatistics, Istituto Nazionale Tumori, Milan, Italy.

M. A. Tucker: Genetic Epidemiology Branch, National Cancer Institute, Rockville, Maryland.

CARCINOGENIC PROPERTIES OF RADIATION AND CYTOTOXIC DRUGS

Radiation

There is an abundance of literature demonstrating the carcinogenic potential of various exposures to ionizing radiation. The ability of radiation to produce malignancies, particularly squamous cell carcinomas of the skin, sarcomas, and leukemia, was already recognized more than half a century ago (2–4). Comprehensive reviews of the carcinogenic effects of radiation have been published recently (5–7). Most knowledge about radiation effects in humans has come from epidemiologic studies of the atomic bomb survivors in Japan (8–12), occupationally irradiated workers (13,14), patients exposed to large amounts of diagnostic radiation (15,16), and patients treated with radiation for malignant (17–21) and nonmalignant diseases (22–26). Almost all types of cancer can be caused by exposure to ionizing radiation, with the probable exception of chronic lymphocytic leukemia (5,6,10,27). Certain sites, such as the thyroid, the female breast, and the bone marrow, appear to be more radiosensitive than others.

The excess risk of leukemia attributable to radiation is observed within a few years of exposure, with a peak after 5 to 9 years, and declines slowly thereafter (7,10,17,22,23).

Increased risk of solid tumors has been shown to take much longer to emerge. Although increased risks have been reported in the 5- to 9-year period following irradiation (18,23,28–31), most solid tumors do not occur in excess until 10 years after radiation exposure, and for some cancers (e.g., breast and bladder), excess risks emerge only 15 years or even longer following irradiation. Generally, radiation-induced solid cancers do not occur until the ages are reached at which they normally occur. Thus, in children exposed to radiation, excess risks may take much longer to emerge than in adults with similar exposures. In some cohorts of childhood cancer survivors, however, increased risk of solid tumors was observed at unusually young ages (19,32).

After a minimum induction period of 5 to 10 years, solid tumor risk appears to follow a time-response model consistent with a multiplicative relationship with the underlying incidence in the population; that is, risk after exposure is proportional to the background incidence of cancer over time (7,9,23). It is not known at the present time whether the relative risk remains elevated throughout life. Studies in the atomic bomb survivors (11) and in women treated for benign gynecologic disorders (23,33) have shown that the excess relative risk per Gray tends to be fairly stable over time for at least 30 years following radiation. However, a recent update of the mortality experience of ankylosing spondylitis patients showed that, 25 years after irradiation, risk had decreased for a number of malignancies, particularly lung cancer (22). In studies of second cancer risk following high-dose radiation therapy for malignant disease, follow-up has rarely exceeded 20 years, and no decrease of risk has been observed in that period. A recent cancer incidence report on the atomic bomb survivors, with 42 years of follow-up, indicated that the excess relative risk decreased with time for the younger-age-at-exposure groups but remained virtually constant for the older cohorts (11).

An important part of our knowledge of radiation carcinogenesis derives from populations exposed to relatively low levels of radiation, such as the atomic bomb survivors. Extrapolation of radiation effects from low doses to the high dose ranges used therapeutically cannot be done with certainty (5) because of the possibility of cell killing at high doses (see below). Therefore, recent studies of second cancer risk have focused on the shape of the radiation dose–response curve in the high-dose range.

For leukemia, data from most low-dose studies are compatible with a linear trend in risk for doses below 1.5 to 2 Gy (10,17,27). There is consistent evidence that the excess risk of leukemia per unit radiation dose to the active bone marrow is much higher at low doses than at the high doses administered for the treatment of malignant disease (10,17,27). This phenomenon has been attributed to cell killing or inactivation of potentially leukemic cells at the higher radiation doses (7,17). Many studies in cancer patients have shown that high radiation doses to limited fields, such as commonly used in the treatment of Hodgkin's disease, confer very little or no increased risk of leukemia (34–37). In contrast, a significant risk of leukemia (6%) has been observed in non-Hodgkin's lymphoma patients receiving total-body irradiation with low doses of radiation to large volumes of bone marrow (38,39). Both in the atomic bomb survivors and in patients who received radiotherapy for cervical cancer, leukemia risk appeared to increase with increasing average dose to the bone marrow until about 4 Gy, above which leukemia risk was progressively reduced with increasing dose (5,9,17). However, a recent study of leukemia risk in survivors of uterine cancer showed little evidence for such a clear downturn in risk (27). More research is needed to investigate how dose fractionation and portion of bone marrow irradiated affect leukemia risk.

With regard to solid tumors, studies in populations exposed to relatively low levels of radiation have convincingly shown that the risk increases linearly with radiation dose in the lower dose ranges (up to about 5 Gy) (11,15,22). Very few studies have examined whether linear dose–response extends to the higher dose ranges used therapeutically. Long-term survivors of Hodgkin's disease who received breast doses between 4 and 45 Gy from mantle field irradiation were found to have an approximately 40-fold increased risk of breast cancer when irradiated before age 20 (21,28). Per unit dose, their excess risk of breast cancer is of the same magnitude as that seen in populations exposed to much lower radiation levels (15), indicating that breast carcinogenic response to dose may not be affected much by cell killing at doses as high as 20 to 40 Gy.

With respect to lung cancer risk after high-dose radiation, recent studies in survivors of Hodgkin's disease (20) and breast cancer (40) suggested that the risk levels off at doses higher than 9 to 10 Gy. A similar leveling of risk at doses of 10 Gy or more has been observed for radiation-induced thyroid cancer (41,42). However, even at thyroid doses up to 60 Gy, the risk of thyroid cancer did not decrease (42). The radiation dose–response relationship for bone sarcoma was addressed in survivors of childhood cancer (19). There was no evidence of increased risk for doses below 10 Gy to the site of the bone tumor. Beyond 10 Gy, risk for bone sarcoma rose sharply with increasing dose, reaching 40-fold excess at doses of 60 Gy or more.

Young age at radiation exposure has been found to be a particular risk factor for the development of various radiation-associated solid cancers. For example, in atomic bomb survivors who were less than 10 years old at the time of bombing, the excess relative risk of breast cancer per Gray was five times that of women who were over 40 years old when exposed (12). Irradiation may thus affect cells of the mammary ducts before full organ development begins. A strong trend of increasing breast cancer risk with decreasing age at exposure was also observed in patients irradiated for Hodgkin's disease (21,28). For thyroid cancer and bone sarcoma, the excess risks from radiation are also much greater for children than for adults (11,31,41–43).

The carcinogenic effects of therapeutic irradiation deserve much more study. Issues to be clarified include the shape of the radiation dose–response curve in the higher dose range, the duration of radiation-induced cancer risk, the effects of dose fractionation and age at exposure, and, importantly, the interaction of radiotherapy with environmental carcinogens (e.g., smoking, chemotherapy) and genetic susceptibility. Because the mechanisms underlying the carcinogenic effects of radiation are still poorly understood, research should also focus on the identification of specific (somatic) gene alterations associated with the development of radiation-induced cancer (44,45). Recent studies have suggested that the mutational spectrum of the p53 tumor suppressor gene in radiation-induced lung cancer may differ from that observed in smoking-related lung cancer (46–48).

Chemotherapy

The carcinogenic potential of chemotherapy was recognized much later than that of ionizing radiation. This obviously has to do with the fact that chemotherapeutic agents were not introduced in cancer control until the late 1940s (49), and modern multiagent combination chemotherapy, which is now known to have the strongest carcinogenic potential, was not used until the 1960s. Until the introduction of combination chemotherapy, patients treated with antineoplastic agents did not live long enough for an increased risk of second malignancies from treatment to become manifest. A review of the literature indicates that, generally, it takes 5 to 20 years from the introduction of a drug into clinical practice before a carcinogenic effect of the agent becomes evident (49–51). Evidence of the carcinogenicity of chemotherapeutic agents has come not only from clinical observations of second malignancies in patients treated with these drugs but also, to a great extent, from *in vivo* and *in vitro* laboratory studies. Pioneering work in this field was conducted before clinical studies had shown increased risk of second malignancies following chemotherapy (52–54).

The predominant malignancy associated with chemotherapy is acute nonlymphocytic leukemia. The leukemogenicity of chemotherapy in man was first discovered in patients treated for multiple myeloma. The first report suggesting a role of alkylating agents was published in 1970 (55), and the association was confirmed in a number of subsequent studies (56,57). The increased leukemia incidence in myeloma patients followed the introduction of melphalan and other alkylating agents in 1962. MOPP combination chemotherapy for Hodgkin's disease (consisting of mechlorethamine, vincristine, procarbazine, and prednisone) was introduced in 1967; the leukemogenic potential of this regimen became evident in reports published in 1973, 1975, and 1977 (58–60). After the early recognition of increased risk of acute nonlymphocytic leukemia in survivors of Hodgkin's disease and multiple myeloma, strongly increased risks have now also been demonstrated following combination-alkylating agent chemotherapy for a large number of other malignancies, such as ovarian, lung, and breast cancer and non-Hodgkin's lymphoma (61). Because no evidence was found of increased leukemia risk in patients treated with surgery and/or radiotherapy alone, the excess leukemia risk could be attributed to treatment with alkylating agents rather than to immunosuppression related to the primary malignancy. In recent years it has become evident that there are at least two different syndromes of treatment-related leukemia (62–64): "classical" alkylating agent–induced acute nonlymphocytic leukemia and acute nonlymphocytic leukemia related to the topoisomerase II inhibitors.

Alkylating agents with known leukemogenic effects in humans are mechlorethamine, chlorambucil, cyclophosphamide, melphalan, semustine, lomustine, carmustine, prednimustine, busulfan, and dihydroxybusulfan (61,64). The relative leukemogenicity of these drugs is not completely known, and studies in this field are surrounded by methodologic problems. First, chemotherapeutic drugs are commonly given in combination, which renders it difficult to disentangle their effects. Second, the leukemogenic potency of drugs can be compared in different ways: in terms of absolute (cumulative) drug dose (in grams, or grams/m^2) or in terms of units of equal therapeutic or clinical effect (35,65). Convincing evidence has accumulated that, with both definitions, cyclophosphamide is substantially less leukemogenic than melphalan, mechlorethamine, chlorambucil, lomustine, and thiotepa (34–36,66–69). There is general agreement that cumulative cyclophosphamide doses below 20 g do not confer an appreciable increase of leukemia risk (36,66,67). Only few studies have compared the leukemogenic potency of alkylating agents other than cyclophosphamide.

There is abundant evidence that the risk of alkylating agent–related acute nonlymphocytic leukemia rises with increasing cumulative dose. The few studies that attempted to disentangle the effects of cumulative dose, duration of use, and dose intensity, reported that cumulative dose appeared to be the strongest determinant of risk (36,66). Although age and gender do not seem to have an important modifying effect on alkylating agent–related acute nonlymphocytic leukemia (discussed later in the section on leukemia risk), other host-related factors may play a role. Van Leeuwen and co-workers (66) found significantly increased risk of acute nonlymphocytic leukemia among patients with low platelet counts, both in response to initial therapy and during follow-up. Furthermore, platelet counts at the time of transplant were found to be predictive of subsequent acute nonlymphocytic leukemia risk in non-Hodgkin's lymphoma patients who underwent autologous bone marrow transplantation after intensive chemotherapy (70). These observations might be explained by large interpatient variability in the pharmacokinetics and metabolism of alkylating drugs. Severe thrombocytopenia may indicate greater bioavailability of or greater individual sensitivity to these agents, which would enhance leukemia risk.

Risk of alkylating agent–related leukemia begins to increase 2 years after start of chemotherapy, peaks in the 5- to 10-year follow-up period, and seems to decrease afterwards (28,34,35,71). Even in large patient series, the number of patients has been too small to determine whether 15 to 20 years posttreatment the risk of leukemia returns to the background level of the population (28). More than 50% of leukemias following alkylating-agent therapy present initially as myelodysplasia, whereas *de novo* acute nonlymphocytic leukemia is preceded by myelodysplastic syndrome much less frequently (61). Most cases of myelodysplastic syndrome progress to acute nonlymphocytic leukemia within a year (61,72). Cytogenetic studies of alkylating agent–related acute nonlymphocytic leukemia/myelodysplastic syndrome have shown unbalanced chromosome aberrations, primarily with loss of whole chromosomes 5 and/or 7 or various parts of the long arms of these chromosomes (72,73). Morphologically, alkylating agent–related acute nonlymphocytic leukemia is most commonly of French-American-British (FAB) subtypes M1 and M2, but all subtypes except M3 have been observed (61).

In recent years, the topoisomerase II inhibitors, especially the epipodophyllotoxins, have been implicated in the development of a clinically and cytogenetically distinct type of acute nonlymphocytic leukemia. As compared to "classical" alkylating agent–induced acute nonlymphocytic leukemia, epipodophyllotoxin-related acute nonlymphocytic leukemia has a shorter induction period (median 2 to 3 years following treatment), and it generally lacks a preceding phase of myelodysplastic syndrome. Further, this type of acute nonlymphocytic leukemia appears to be characterized by balanced translocations involving chromosome bands 11q23 and 21q22. These chromosome aberrations are more frequently associated with the development of acute monoblastic or myelomonocytic leukemia (M4 or M5 according to the FAB criteria) (64,74,75). Very recently, evidence has accumulated that the anthracyclines doxorubicin and 4-epidoxorubicin, which are intercalating topoisomerase II inhibitors, may induce a similar type of acute nonlymphocytic leukemia as the one related to epipodophyllotoxin treatment (35,76,77).

To date, the causal link between cyclophosphamide and bladder cancer represents the only established relationship between a specific cytostatic drug and a solid tumor (78–80). Risk of bladder cancer rises significantly with increasing cumulative dose of cyclophosphamide, with 15-fold excess risk among patients receiving doses of 50 g or more. Increased risks of bone sarcomas (19) and, in some studies, lung cancer (29,81,82) have also been reported after chemotherapy alone. Many chemotherapeutic agents are known mutagens and animal carcinogens (83), and the induction period of solid tumors may be longer than the observation period available in published research. Therefore, prolonged follow-up studies are warranted to determine whether chemotherapy affects solid tumor risk.

METHODS OF ASSESSING SECOND CANCER RISK

The *cohort study* and the *nested case-control study* are the epidemiologic study designs generally used in second cancer research (30). Case reports have an important role in the early recognition of associations between different malignancies (55,56). However, because of lack of information on the underlying population at risk, they are not useful in quantifying risks.

In a cohort study of second cancer risk, a large group of patients (the cohort) with a specified first malignancy is followed up for a number of years to determine the incidence of second (and subsequent) malignancies. In nearly all studies of second cancer risk, the cohorts have been defined retrospectively from existing data sources. Useful sources for the identification of such cohorts are population-based cancer registries, hospital-based tumor registries, or clinical trial databases (see below). Because most cohort studies of second cancer risk have been conducted retrospectively, follow-up of all patients in such studies is completed up to some point in the recent past. In order to evaluate whether second cancer risk in the cohort is increased as compared to cancer risk in the general population, the observed number of second cancers in the cohort is compared with the number expected on the basis of cancer incidence rates in the general population. This can be done in a so-called "person-years" type of analysis. In this approach, adjustment is made for the distribution of the cohort according to age, sex, and calendar period, while the observation period of individual patients (person-years at risk) is also taken into account. The expected number of second primary cancers in the cohort is derived by multiplying the person-years by age-, sex-, and calendar period–specific incidence rates of cancers of all selected sites from a population-based cancer registry. Ideally, the cancer incidence rates used to calculate the expected numbers are derived from the same source population as that from which the cohort has been drawn. The *relative risk* of developing a second cancer is estimated by the ratio of the observed number of second cancer cases in the cohort to the number expected. In epidemiologic terminology, the observed-to-expected ratio is sometimes called standardized incidence ratio.

A disadvantage of the person-years method as applied in its simplest form is that it assumes the risk of second cancer development to be constant over time; that is, it assumes the second cancer experience of 1,000 patients followed for 1 year to be comparable to that of 100 patients followed for 10 years. When this assumption is inappropriate (as with treatment-related cancers developing after an induction period), it is more informative to calculate relative risks within specified posttreatment intervals (usually 5-year periods) (84,85). Such a procedure highlights situations in which an inadequate number of patients are followed sufficiently long to evaluate the long-term carcinogenic risk of treatment.

When the observed-to-expected ratio is increased, the question arises whether the risk increase is caused by the treatment. This can be evaluated by comparing relative risks between treatment groups, preferably with a reference group of patients not treated with radiotherapy or chemotherapy. Such a comparison group is available when second cancer risk is examined in patients with breast or testicular cancer but, unfortunately, not for patients with Hodgkin's disease. When the observation period (or survival rate) differs between treatments, their overall observed-to-expected ratios cannot be validly compared. In such cases, treatment-specific relative risks must be calculated by interval after start of therapy. When too few patients are left for observation in one treatment group, comparisons of second cancer risk between treatments are not appropriate beyond that observation period.

Second cancer risk in the cohort (and in different treatment groups) can also be expressed by the *cumulative* (actuarial estimated) risk (86), which gives the proportion of patients expected to develop a second malignancy by time t (e.g., 5 years from diagnosis) if they do not die before then. When the cohort's death rate from causes other than second malignancy is high, the assumptions underlying the actuarial method may not be valid, and competing-risk techniques should be used to estimate cumulative risk (87–89). Unfortunately, most studies reporting cumulative risks make no comparison with cancer risk in the general population. Yet, the population-expected cumulative risks over time can be easily calculated on the basis of cancer incidence rates from a population-based registry (90). In comparing estimates of cumulative risk across studies, it is important to keep in mind that this measure of absolute risk depends very strongly on the age distribution of a specific cohort; because of the low background incidence of cancer at young ages, cohorts of Hodgkin's disease patients that include patients treated as children will report much lower cumulative risks than cohorts including adults only.

Because many treatment-related cancers are rare in the general population (e.g., leukemia, sarcoma), a high relative risk (compared to the population) may still translate into a rather low cumulative risk. *Absolute excess risk,* which estimates the excess number of second malignancies per 10,000 patients per year (beyond those expected from rates in the general population), perhaps best reflects the second cancer burden in a cohort. This risk measure is also the most appropriate one to judge which second malignancies contribute most to the excess risk.

The calculation of observed-to-expected ratios on the basis of person-years analysis, and the calculation of cumulative risks using life table analysis, involve rather simple statistical methods, which have a strong intuitive appeal. Besides these elementary methods, statistical modeling with Cox proportional hazards model and Poisson regression techniques is increasingly being used to refine the quantification of second cancer risk (e.g., by estimating dose– and time–response relationships) and to examine the interplay between treatment variables and other factors (91,92).

Each of the data sources used to constitute a cohort has its own specific advantages and disadvantages. Population-based cancer registries have large numbers of patients available, which allows the detection of even small excess risks of second cancers (1,93,94). An additional advantage is that the observed and expected numbers of cancers come from the same reference population. Disadvantages include limited availability of treatment data, underreporting of second cancers (1,34,95) (in particular hematologic malignancies and bilateral cancers in paired organs), and inconsistent diagnostic criteria for second cancers. Population-based registries differ greatly in these aspects and hence in their usefulness for second cancer studies. If treatment data are not available, it is impossible to be sure whether excess risk for a second malignancy is related to treatment or to shared etiology with the first cancer. Underreporting of second cancers clearly leads to an underestimation of second cancer risk. Far higher risks of second leukemia following Hodgkin's disease have been found in hospital series (28,31) than in population-based studies (34,93). Part of this difference, however, may be attributable to the more intensive treatments administered in large treatment centers (34). Despite their disadvantages, population-based registries are well suited to evaluate broadly which second cancers occur in excess following a wide spectrum of different first primary malignancies. They are also a valuable starting point for case-control studies that evaluate treatment effects in detail (see below).

A major advantage of clinical trial databases is that detailed treatment data on all patients are available. Comparison of second cancer risk between the treatment arms of the trial controls for any intrinsic risk for a second malignancy associated with the first cancer. However, a limitation of most trials is the small number of patients involved. This disadvantage becomes more serious when the second cancer of interest has a low background incidence rate (e.g., leukemia). Although this problem can be overcome by combining data from a number of trials, multicenter trial series pose other problems, such as difficult access of the investigator to the medical records and the histologic slides of patients in individual centers. Furthermore, the endpoints of interest in the majority of clinical trials are treatment response and survival, not the development of second cancers. Therefore, many clinical trials do not routinely collect information on second malignancies, and some do not collect any data beyond 5 years. Routine reporting and assessment of second malignancy risk should become an integral part of clinical trial research (96).

Many large cancer treatment centers maintain registries of all admitted patients. Most of these registries have been in existence for decades and collect extensive data on treatment and follow-up. They share the advantages of clinical trial databases without having their disadvantages. Investigators using hospital tumor registries have easy access to the medical records; often a review of the histologic slides of the first and the second malignancy can also be arranged easily. An additional advantage is that, as compared with trial data, hospital registries provide a wider variety of treatments and dose levels, which may yield important information on drug and radiation carcinogenesis. Most studies of second cancer risk following Hodgkin's disease have been based on hospital registries (28,31,60,82,97,98).

The cohort study is not an efficient study design for examining detailed treatment factors (e.g., cumulative dose of alkylating agents) in relation to second cancer risk. Most cohorts are fairly large (in order to yield stable estimates of second cancer risk), rendering the collection of detailed treatment data time consuming and costly. In such cases, the so-called "nested" case-control study within an existing cohort is the preferred approach. The case group consists of all patients identified with the second cancer of interest, and the controls are a random sample of all patients in the cohort who did not develop the cancer concerned, although they experienced the same amount of follow-up time. To achieve maximum statistical power, most case-control studies of second cancer risk use a design in which three to four controls are individually matched to the second cancer "case." Matching factors employed in most studies include gender, year of birth, and year at diagnosis of the first primary cancer. The most important criterion for control selection is that each control must have survived, without developing the second cancer of interest, for at least as long as the interval between the diagnosis of the first and the second malignancy of the corresponding case. Even if the control group is 3 times as large as the case group, detailed treatment data need be collected for only a small proportion of the total cohort. In each case-control study it is critical to the validity of the study results that the controls are truly representative of all patients who did not contract the second cancer of interest. For example, biased results may be obtained when controls with untraceable records are replaced by controls with traceable records.

In the data analysis of a case-control study of second cancer risk, treatment factors are compared between cases and controls. Treatments that have been administered more often, for a longer duration, or with a higher dose to the case group than to the controls are associated with increased risk of developing the second malignancy of interest. It is important to understand that in a nested case-control study, the risk associated with specific treatments is estimated relative to the risk in patients receiving other treatment and not relative to the risk in the general population. The cumulative risk of developing a second malignancy cannot be derived from a case-control study. Estimates of the absolute excess risks associated with specific treatments can be derived, however, if the case-control study follows a cohort analysis in which observed-to-expected ratios were calculated for broad treatment groups. Although case-control methodology has only recently come into use for the investigation of second cancer risk (39,99), several landmark studies have already demonstrated its strengths (17,19,34–37,78,100).

INCIDENCE AND RISK FACTORS OF SELECTED SECOND CANCERS

General

Since the first reports of increased second cancer risk in Hodgkin's disease patients in the early 1970s

(58,59,101), many treatment centers have reported on second cancer risk in their patients. An excess of acute nonlymphocytic leukemia in chemotherapy-treated patients and an increased risk of solid tumors in radiotherapy-treated patients have been reported consistently in the literature. For 11 recent large cohort studies, the overall relative risks of selected second malignancies compared with the general population are given in Tables 1 and 2.

The greatest relative risk (ten- to 80-fold) is observed for leukemia, followed by a three- to 35-fold risk increase for non-Hodgkin's lymphoma. Moderately elevated risks (over twofold) are observed for a number of solid tumors, such as cancers of the lung, breast, bone, connective tissue, stomach, colon, thyroid, and melanoma. Leukemia and non-Hodgkin's lymphoma are diseases with a low incidence in the general population, which implies that even a high relative risk compared to the population may translate into a rather low cumulative (actuarial) risk. The cumulative risk picture for one of the studies (28) included in Table 1 shows that, during the entire follow-up period, the cumulative risk of solid tumors is much higher than that of leukemia or non-Hodgkin's lymphoma. Absolute excess risk is the best measure to judge which malignancies contribute most to the increased second cancer risk (see Methods above). Table 3 gives absolute excess risks from five recent large studies, showing that, compared with the general population, Hodgkin's disease patients experience an excess of 40 to 70 malignancies per 10,000 patients per year. Solid tumors contribute most to this excess, followed by leukemia and non-Hodgkin's lymphoma.

Table 4 compares relative and absolute excess risks of selected second malignancies overall and in 10-year survivors, on the basis of a combined analysis of three large studies that included a total of 6,292 patients (28,29,31). Because the relative risks of leukemia, non-Hodgkin's lymphoma, and solid tumors each show a distinctive pattern with time since first treatment, the relative and absolute excess risks in 10-year survivors differ greatly from those observed in the entire patient population (Table 4). With longer follow-up, the relative risks of solid tumors increase, while leukemia risk decreases, resulting in an increasingly large contribution of solid tumors to the excess second malignancy risk over time. In the period of 10 years or more after first treatment, lung cancer contributes most to the absolute excess risk, with 34 excess cases per 10,000 Hodgkin's disease patients per year, followed by non-Hodgkin's lymphoma (28/10,000/year) and leukemia (10/10,000/year). In women, breast cancer accounts for the largest absolute excess risk (40/10,000/year) in 10-year survivors. Below we report in more detail on the magnitude of the risk increases for leukemia, non-Hodgkin's lymphoma, and selected solid tumors. In addition, we discuss treatment and other factors associated with the excess risk.

Risk of Leukemia

The risk of second leukemias following Hodgkin's disease has been actively studied since the early 1970s. Leukemia was the second cancer after treatment for Hodgkin's disease that was first systematically noticed, probably because of the relatively short latency and the rarity of acute nonlymphocytic leukemia in the general population. Most large treatment centers have reported their experience with second leukemias. Overall, risks compared with the general population have been reported

TABLE 1. *Relative risks of second malignancy of selected sites in recent large-cohort studies of patients with Hodgkin's disease, predominantly adults*

	Kaldor (93) (International, all ages; N=28,462)[a]		Tucker (31) (US, all ages; N=1,507)[a]	Henry-Amar (71) (International, ages ≥ 15; N=12,411)[a]		Swerdlow (29) (Britain, ages ≥ 10; N=2,846)[a]	Abrahamsen (103) (Norway, ages ≥ 15; N=1,152)[a]	van Leeuwen (Netherlands, (28) all ages; N=1,939)[a]
Site	♂RR (n)[e]	♀RR (n)[e]	RR (n)[e]	♂RR (n)[e]	♀RR (n)[e]	RR (n)[e]	RR (n)[e]	RR (n)[e]
Stomach	1.5 (28)	0.5 (4)	10.0 (4)[b]	1.7 (14)	0.8 (2)	1.3 (3)	2.0 (5)	1.6 (4)
Colon	1.3 (23)	1.1 (16)	3.5 (4)	1.9 (18)[b]	0.9 (5)	3.2 (8)[b]	–[c]	2.5 (8)
Lung	1.9 (89)[b]	2.2 (17)[b]	7.7 (14)[b]	2.2 (68)[b]	4.6 (27)[b]	3.8 (32)[b]	3.3 (11)[b]	3.7 (31)[b]
Bone	1.3 (1)	10.6 (4)[b]	31.0 (2)[b]	6.2 (4)[b]	6.5 (2)	15.2 (2)[b]	–(0)	– (0)
Soft tissue	0.7 (1)	3.6 (3)	15.0 (2)[b]	2.8 (3)	1.6 (1)	–[c]	–[c] (1)	8.8 (3)[b]
Melanoma	2.4 (9)[b]	1.3 (5)	8.9 (4)[b]	1.9 (7)	1.2 (4)	–[c]	3.6 (5)[b]	4.9 (5)[b]
Breast	–	1.4 (62)[b]	1.7 (3)	–[c]	1.5 (39)[b]	1.6 (6)	1.2 (4)	1.3 (8)
Cervix	–	2.1 (23)[b]	–[c] (1)	–	1.4 (9)	1.9 (2)	2.2 (2)	5.9 (4)[b]
Thyroid	2.8 (3)	2.2 (5)	–[c] (1)	5.1 (5)[b]	1.5 (3)	9.4 (2)[b]	– (0)	– (0)
NHL	3.0 (15)[b]	3.1 (9)[b]	18.0 (9)[b]	35.6 (79)[b]	24.2 (27)[b]	16.8 (17)[b]	8.4 (8)[b]	20.6 (23)[b]
Leukemia	10.3 (69)[b]	10.9 (37)[b]	66.0 (28)[b]	28.6 (102)	25.7 (56)[b]	16.0 (16)[b]	24.3 (9)[b]	34.7 (31)[b]
All sites	1.8 (430)[b]	1.7 (281)[b]	5.2 (83)[bd]	3.0 (410)[b]	2.6 (221)[b]	2.7 (113)[b]	1.9 (68)[bd]	3.5 (146)[bd]

NHL, non-Hodgkin's lymphoma; ♂, male; ♀, female; RR, relative risk.
[a]Number of Hodgkin's disease patients included in study.
[b]Significantly raised ($p < 0.05$).
[c]Data not published.
[d]Excluding nonmelanoma skin cancer.
[e]Observed number of second cancers

TABLE 2. *Relative risks of second malignancy of selected sites in recent large-cohort studies of patients with Hodgkin's disease*

	Predominantly adults			Children	
	Boivin (104) (U.S. and Canada, all ages; N=10,472)[a]	Mauch (106) (U.S., all ages; N=749)[a]	Swerdlow (82) (England, all ages; N=1,039)[a]	Bhatia (135) (U.S., ages < 16; N=1,380)[a]	Sankila (107) (Scandinavia, ages < 20; N=1,641)[a]
Stomach	–[c]	–[c]	4.0 (4)[b]	121.3 (2)	– (0)
Colon	–[c]	–[c]	1.4 (2)	–[c]	3.6 (1)
Lung	–[c]	4.5 (8)[b]	3.8 (15)[b]	– (0)	– (0)
Bone			26.5 (2)[b]	24.6 (4)[b]	
Bone and soft tissue	12.0 (24)[b]	44.5 (6)[b]			10.0 (3)
Soft tissue			16.9 (2)[b]	–[c]	
Melanoma	2.2 (15)[b]	4.1 (3)	4.0 (2)	– (0)	2.7 (2)
Breast	1.4 (39)	6.5 (13)[b]	1.8 (5)	75.3 (17)[a]	17.0 (16)[b]
Cervix	–[c]	–[c]	–[c] (1)	–[c]	– (0)
Thyroid	4.5 (13)[b]	–[c]	8.2 (1)	32.7 (10)	33.0 (9)[b]
NHL	5.6 (35)[b]	18.4 (10)[b]	4.6 (3)[b]	20.9 (6)[b]	15.0 (5)[b]
Leukemia	23.9 (122)[b]	66.2 (8)[b]	23.5 (13)[b]	78.8 (26)[b]	17.0 (7)[b]
All sites	2.7 (521)[a]	5.6 (72)[b]	3.3 (67)[bd]	18.1 (79)[bd]	7.7 (62)[g]

NHL, non-Hodgkin's lymphoma.
[a]Number of Hodgkin's disease patients included in the study
[b]Significantly raised (p<0.05).
[c]Data not published.
[d]Excluding nonmelanoma skin cancers.
[e]Observed number of second cancers.
[f]Unclear whether nonmelanoma skin cancer is included.
[g]Partially includes nonmelanoma skin cancers

to be ten- to 80-fold increased (Tables 1 and 2). Nearly all studies show that the relative risk of leukemia is higher than that of non-Hodgkin's lymphoma and much greater than that of solid tumors (Tables 1 and 2). Because the background risk of leukemia in the population is low, this strongly increased relative risk translates into a relatively low cumulative risk, ranging between 1.4% and 4.1% at 15 years (28,29,31,32,37,71,102). Overall, absolute excess risk has varied between 9 and 30 excess cases per 10,000 patients per year (Table 3).

Although the relative risks of leukemia are quite elevated, leukemia is a rare outcome, and any one series has limited ability to examine all of the suspected cofactors in the development of leukemia. This review focuses primarily on the current questions that are being addressed in large studies. The major areas of active research include the relationship with specific treatments, the timing of onset of leukemia, the association with splenectomy, and the variation in risk by age at treatment for Hodgkin's disease.

TABLE 3. *Absolute excess risks of second malignancy of selected sites (per 10,000 Hodgkin's disease patients per year) in recent large-cohort studies of patients with Hodgkin's disease*

Site	Tucker (31)	Swerdlow (29)	van Leeuwen (28)	Mauch (106)	Swerdlow (82)
Stomach	3.9	0.4	0.9	–[a]	3.2
Colon	–[a]	3.2	2.8	–[a]	0.6
Lung	13.2	13.6	13.6	7.3	11.6
Bone	2.1	1.1	–[b]		2.0
Bone and soft tissue				6.9	
Soft tissue	2.0	–[a]	1.6		2.0
Melanoma	3.8	–[a]	2.4	2.7	1.6
Breast	–[a]	1.2	1.1	13.0	2.4
Cervix	–[a]	1.5	2.0	–[a]	–[a]
Thyroid	–[a]	1.0	–[b]	–[a]	0.9
NHL	9.2	9.2	13.1	11.1	2.5
Leukemia	29.9	8.7	18.1	9.3	13.1
All sites	72.6	41.4	62.5	69.6	49.2

[a] No data published for this site.
[b]No cases of this site

TABLE 4. *Relative risk of second cancers after Hodgkin's disease: combined results from three large studies in 6,292 patients*

Site or type	Observed cases	Expected cases	Relative risk (O/E cases) (95% confidence interval)	Absolute excess risk per 10,000 patients per year	Relative risk (O[a]/E cases) in 10-year survivors (95% confidence interval)	Absolute excess risk in 10-year survivors, per 10,000 patients per year
All cancers	342	99.1	3.5 (3.1–3.8)	56.2	4.7 (3.8–5.7)	111.7
Leukemia	75	2.3	32.4 (25.5–40.6)	16.8	16.2 (6.5–33.3)	9.9
Acute nonlymphocytic leukemia	68	1.0	70.8 (55.0–89.8)	15.5		
Non-Hodgkin's lymphoma	49	2.6	18.6 (13.8–24.6)	10.7	32.7 (19.7–51.1)	27.8
Solid tumors	219	92.4	2.4 (2.1–2.7)	29.3	3.6 (2.8–4.6)	74.4
Lung	77	18.5	4.2 (3.3–5.2)	13.5	7.3 (4.7–10.6)	33.8
Female breast[b]	42	16.9	2.5 (1.8–3.4)	11.3	4.6 (3.0–6.6)	39.5
All solid tumors except lung cancer	142	73.9	1.9 (1.6–2.3)	15.8	2.8 (2.0–3.8)	40.6

o, observed; e, expected.
[a]Based on the following numbers of observed cases: all cancers, 94; leukemia, 7; NHL, 19; solid tumors, 68; lung cancer, 26; breast cancer, 28; all solid tumors except lung, 42.
[b]With Stanford data based on extended follow-up (21).
Data from refs. 28, 29, and 31.

Most leukemias that occur after Hodgkin's disease are acute nonlymphocytic leukemias related to alkylating agent exposure (29,31,34,37,66,71,82,102–104). The relative risk increase associated with irradiation alone is comparatively small or even nonexistent (see below). The actuarial risks at 15 years vary substantially with treatment categories, from 0 to 0.6% among those receiving only radiation therapy to as high as 16.5% at 15 years in heavily treated groups (28,31,32,102,105). The relative risks of leukemia associated with specific treatment categories also vary widely, depending on the referent category and the types of leukemia considered. The relative risks in chemotherapy-treated patients tend to be over 20-fold increased in cohort analyses that use population-based comparisons of all leukemia risks, over 50-fold increased with population-based estimates of acute nonlymphocytic leukemia risks, and less in case-control analyses, where the referent category usually consisted of patients treated with radiotherapy alone (28,31,32,34, 66,82,106,107).

Overall, whether considering cumulative or relative risks, there appears to be a modest risk, usually not statistically significant, associated with radiation therapy alone in comparison with population rates (28,29, 31,105,108). There does not appear to be a consistent relationship with extent of radiation therapy among all investigations, but in the larger studies, there are suggestions that the risk may be higher in patients receiving extended-field radiotherapy (34,71,104). Among patients treated with radiation therapy alone who received a total radiation dose to the bone marrow greater than 20 Gy, the risk of leukemia was eightfold higher than among those who received less than 10 Gy (34).

There are several difficulties in estimating risk of leukemia according to specific chemotherapy drugs and doses. Successful treatment of more advanced stages of Hodgkin's disease is in large part with combination chemotherapy, and patients frequently receive more than one combination, especially if they are treated for relapse. Given the number of different combinations of drugs used over different geographic areas and calendar-year periods, it is difficult to compare the regimens and doses. This becomes particularly crucial when several trials or series are combined to accrue sufficient numbers of leukemias to analyze risk factors. Where exposure has been quantified, risk appears to be most related to total dose of alkylating agents or nitrosoureas (32,34,37,66,82). Exposure has usually been characterized as number of chemotherapy cycles (34,66), but the number of cycles does not take into consideration the individual doses of drugs, which can vary substantially according to individual toxicity. Despite this limitation, an increased number (more than six) of cycles of MOPP or MOPP-like regimens is associated with a very high risk of leukemia, ranging from 20- to over 60-fold increased in comparison with patients treated with radiation alone and three- to fivefold increased compared with patients treated with six or fewer cycles (34,66). Total dose of alkylators and nitrosoureas is likely the explanation of the reports of higher risk associated with salvage chemotherapy or maintenance chemotherapy (66,71,109), but there is evidence that retreatment may be a factor in risk (29,32,66,110). The risk associated with specific alkylators and nitrosoureas varies; the risks appear highest after MOPP treatment (28,29,31,32,34,37,66,102). Mechlorethamine and procarbazine are usually given in combination, so it is difficult to disentangle the effects of each. Among those treated with variations of MOPP that substitute chlorambucil for mechlorethamine, the risks appear similar, but with melphalan or cyclophosphamide in place of mechlorethamine, the risks are lower (31,66,82,103,104). From studies of leukemia following ovarian cancer, single-agent melphalan is a more potent leukemogen than cyclophosphamide (69). The lower risk associated with melphalan-containing combinations may result from the lower dose of melphalan given orally with variable absorption than of mechlorethamine given intravenously (31). In addition, the cumulative risk of leukemia following treatment without mechlorethamine, but including procarbazine, appears lower than with MOPP-like regimens (111). One study, in which the cumulative doses of individual cytostatic drugs were available, and in which mechlorethamine and procarbazine doses were not highly correlated, showed that mechlorethamine rather than procarbazine had the strongest effect on leukemia risk (66). These data suggest that mechlorethamine plays a larger role in leukemia risk than procarbazine. It is also important to note that because of the efficacy of MOPP in treatment of advanced stages of Hodgkin's disease, more long-term survivors have been observed for longer periods of time so that we have the most information about long-term toxicities associated with MOPP and its variants.

The risk of leukemia is much lower following treatment with doxorubicin, vinblastine, bleomycin, and dacarbazine (ABVD) than following MOPP and MOPP-like combinations (102,112). Van Leeuwen and colleagues reported a decrease in leukemia risk among those treated for Hodgkin's disease after 1980, when treatment with MOPP/ABVD largely replaced MOPP-like combinations (28). This finding is extremely promising in that the risks of leukemia in the future will be substantially lower than they have been in the past. Many of the newer regimens have been designed to minimize the risk of sterility and leukemia without compromising the efficacy of proven modalities of treatment (see other chapters in this volume) by minimizing total doses of alkylating agents. There is, however, also concern about the role of anthracyclines and epipodophyllotoxins (both of which are topoisomerase II inhibitors) in the risk of leukemia. Limited evidence suggests that doxorubicin in combination with higher doses of alkylating agents may have a synergistic effect in the risk of acute nonlymphocytic leukemia (37). This initial observation has not been systematically confirmed or refuted, but some supportive data are emerging (66,77,111,113). With the increasing number of patients who are currently receiving hybrid combinations of alkylating agents and anthracyclines, this issue is likely to be addressed shortly (113,114). Recently, the risk of leukemia associated with epipodophyllotoxins has been evaluated, again in combination with alkylating agents (including nitrosoureas) and/or anthracyclines (66,113). Again, because multiple drugs are given in combination, it is difficult to tease out individual effects. Although the leukemogenic potential of epipodophyllotoxin-containing chemotherapy has been clearly demonstrated, the risk has not been quantified well, and the data are much more limited than for MOPP and MOPP-related combinations.

A very important question is whether radiotherapy adds to the leukemia risk from chemotherapy. Evidence that combined-modality treatment produces greater risk than chemotherapy alone comes from a number of reports (71,102,115–117), although other large series find the risk of acute nonlymphocytic leukemia after combined treatment to be comparable to that after chemotherapy alone (28,29,31,32,34,66,82). These inconsistent results may be partly related to differences in treatment regimens between studies, but also to lack of adjustment for type and amount of chemotherapy in some reports. The interaction between radiotherapy and chemotherapy could be examined best in the large case-control study by Kaldor and associates (34), which estimated the total radiation dose delivered to the active bone marrow. When the combined effects of radiation dose and number of mechlorethamine-procarbazine containing cycles were examined, it was found that in each category of radiation dose (<10, 10 to 20, >20 Gy to the marrow), leukemia risk increased with a larger number of chemotherapy cycles. In contrast, among patients with a given number of chemotherapy cycles, risk of leukemia did not consistently increase with increasing radiation dose. Among patients who did not have any radiotherapy, and among those in the highest radiation dose category (>20 Gy), the increased risks of leukemia from chemotherapy were of similar magnitude. Both in patients who had received up to six cycles and in those who had more than six cycles, leukemia risk tended to be somewhat higher at intermediate radiation dose levels (10 to 20 Gy). Taking together the results of the various studies, the preponderance of data does not support the notion that the combination of chemotherapy and radiotherapy, in particular extended-field irradiation, confers higher risk of leukemia than chemotherapy alone. Because this important issue remains controversial, new studies are needed. Such studies should be large and be capable of investigating the effects of extent of radiotherapy, while also considering amount of chemotherapy.

Most groups reporting risks of leukemia have also examined the latency of leukemia after chemotherapy treatment. After initial reports that the excess risk of leukemia was limited to the first 10 years after treatment (118), subsequent studies with longer follow-up have shown a smaller risk increase of leukemia that persists after 10 years (28,29,71,93,109,119). In a 20-year follow-up study of 11,241 patients continuously disease-free after treatment for Hodgkin's disease, leukemia risk reached a plateau after 15 years (71,105). Even in large patient series, the number of patients has been too small to determine whether 15 to 20 years posttreatment the risk of leukemia returns to the background level of the population. It is clear, however, that the highest risks and the greatest number of cases do occur between 5 and 10 years after initiation of treatment, usually with alkylating agents. Some of the larger studies do not evaluate time since initiation of chemotherapy, but time since start of all treatment. In cases in which a patient is treated for relapse after initial radiation therapy, this would overestimate latency, since the time at maximum risk begins with initiation of alkylating-agent chemotherapy.

The role of splenectomy in the etiology of treatment-related leukemia remains somewhat controversial. Since the initial report of the association in 1987 (120), most large groups have evaluated their data. The most recent update of the Dutch data reveals a persistent threefold risk associated with splenectomy, controlled for type and dose of chemotherapy (66). In this group of patients, there was no increased risk of leukemia in those who received splenic irradiation and therefore had functional hyposplenism. The effect of splenectomy has also been found in independent groups (34,71,102,104,119,121), most of which demonstrate risks of the order of twofold increased. In a large metaanalysis, however, splenectomy was not a significant risk factor for leukemia (71). Other separate groups with smaller numbers have also not found splenectomy to be a risk factor (32,103,111,117). The biologic plausibility of the relationship is not completely clear. An alteration in immune status by splenectomy has been postulated (120). Another hypothesis could be higher delivered doses of chemotherapy because of higher circulating white cell and platelet counts in those who had splenectomy. Adjusting for type and amount of chemotherapy, however, did not alter risks in the Dutch patients (66). The reported finding of a (non-significantly) higher risk among patients whose platelet and white counts showed a stronger response to splenectomy is consistent with this hypothesis, however.

Age over 40 years at treatment has been reported to be a significant risk factor for leukemia in some studies (28,71,106) but not in others (31,82,97,103). Part of the discrepancy could result from analytic differences between studies or differential intensity of treatment of differing age groups. Another important part of the variance could well be the limited numbers of older affected individuals in any single study. When interpreting the results of these studies, it must be kept in mind that the effect of age is strongly dependent on the type of risk measure used. The higher cumulative risks of acute nonlymphocytic leukemia in Hodgkin's disease patients diagnosed over age 40 as compared to younger ones may simply reflect the higher baseline (general population) incidence of the disease in older persons. Real differences in the magnitude of treatment-related acute nonlymphocytic leukemia risk between age groups can only be assessed after adjustment for age-specific differences in acute nonlymphocytic leukemia incidence in the general population. In the few studies that analyzed relative risk of leukemia by age, based on comparisons to the general population expectations, no differences between age groups were observed (31) or the relative risk of acute nonlymphocytic leukemia was even significantly greater at younger ages than at older (122). Two case-control studies also suggested a greater increase of treatment-related acute nonlymphocytic leukemia risk in patients who were younger at Hodgkin's disease diagnosis (34,123). Very few studies specifically examined whether there is a difference in relative risk of leukemia between children and adults. According to a recent study, the relative risk of leukemia following treatment of childhood or adolescent Hodgkin's disease was approximately 80-fold increased, but over 300-fold increased for acute myelogenous leukemia (32), compared with the adult risks of 66-fold increased overall and 115-fold increased for acute nonlymphocytic leukemia (28,31,106). However, because of the different treatments used in the adult and childhood Hodgkin's disease studies, it is not possible to compare directly risks associated with specific treatments in the differing age categories (32,34,66). In summary, there is not much evidence that age at treatment has an important modifying effect on chemotherapy-associated leukemia risk. Few studies have examined the modifying effect of gender on leukemia risk. A greater risk for women than for men was found in two studies (34,122) but not in another large series (71).

Despite all of the work that has been done evaluating the causes of secondary leukemia after Hodgkin's disease, there remain many unanswered questions. Van Leeuwen and colleagues have made initial observations that may give clues to the interindividual variation in leukemia risk among patients treated with alkylating agents. They reported that patients with prolonged thrombocytopenia were at increased risk of developing leukemia and postulated that this may be a marker of increased bioavailability of drug (66). In support of these findings, a study of leukemia risk after autologous bone marrow transplantation found that low platelet counts at the time of transplant were predictive for myelodysplastic syndrome/acute nonlymphocytic leukemia development in non-Hodgkin's lymphoma patients who had received intensive pretransplant chemotherapy (70). These important observations need to be repeated in other populations. With the previously collected patient groups, one should be able to assess level of thrombocytopenia in relation to delivered drug doses. It is not a trivial task to collect the information on the number of patients necessary, but it would be extremely useful. Thrombocytopenia might well be an informative bioassay for predicting leukemia risk until the time when pharmacogenetic phenotyping or genotyping is feasible. More work to clarify the metabolic pathways of the alkylating agents and to isolate the genes of the necessary enzymes needs to be done to be able to predict toxicity before administering chemotherapy. The issues of splenectomy need to be studied further with more precise drug information to assess whether individuals with splenectomy receive higher total delivered doses. The preliminary evidence that the chemotherapy regimens currently used appear to be associated with lower leukemia risk (28) is extremely encouraging and needs to be repeated in other populations.

Risk of Non-Hodgkin's Lymphoma

The first observation on the occurrence of non-Hodgkin's lymphoma in patients previously treated for Hodgkin's disease dates back to the early 1970s (124) and was soon followed by other case reports. However, Krikorian et al. were the first to demonstrate a clearly elevated cumulative risk, which amounted to 4.4% at 10 years in patients given both irradiation and chemotherapy (125). Subsequently, other investigators confirmed that patients with Hodgkin's disease are at risk of developing non-Hodgkin's lymphoma (28,29,31,71,102,103,106). In most studies, the person-year analysis shows that, compared with the risk in the general population, the relative risk for non-Hodgkin's lymphoma ranks soon after that for leukemia and before the overall relative risk for solid tumors, ranging between 8 and 36 (Tables 1, 2, and 5). Because the background risk of non-Hodgkin's lymphoma in the general population is low, this fairly high relative risk translates into a relatively low cumulative risk, ranging between 1.2% and 2.1% at 15 years in the larger studies (28,29,31,71,102,103,106). Absolute excess risk in these studies has varied between 9.2 and 14 excess non-Hodgkin's lymphoma cases per 10,000 patients per year (Table 5).

Analyses aimed at assessing the relative risk of non-Hodgkin's lymphoma by treatment modality and follow-up interval have generated different findings. In the studies by Tucker, Swerdlow, and Abrahamsen, there were no apparent differences in risk among patients treated with chemotherapy alone, radiotherapy alone, or a combination of radiotherapy and chemotherapy (29,31,103). In addition, the relative risk remained relatively constant throughout the observation period, the only exception being greater risk among 10-year survivors in the study by Tucker (RR 38; 95% C.I. 7.5 to 109.6) (31). Other studies, however, did report differences in non-Hodgkin's lymphoma risk according to treatment modality and follow-up time (28,71,125). Henry-Amar reported findings from the International Database on Hodgkin's Disease that gathered data from 12,411 patients, some of whom were also included in other studies reported in Table 5 (71). In this very large series, in which 106 cases of non-Hodgkin's lymphoma were observed, there was a continuous increase in relative risk of non-Hodgkin's lymphoma with follow-up time in men (from 28.2 during the 5- to 9-year period to 120 during the 15- to 19-year period), whereas in women the risk increase was confined to the first 15 years, with a peak (RR 45.4) during the 5- to 9-year observation period. A multivariate Cox model analysis showed that some types of combined-modality treatment and treatment for relapse (any type) were associated with increased risk of non-Hodgkin's lymphoma (RRs in the order of 2.2 to 4.5). Van Leeuwen et al. reported that, despite the fact that the overall risk of non-Hodgkin's lymphoma did not vary significantly among types of treatment, in each follow-up interval the highest risk appeared to occur in patients who had received initial combined-modality treatment followed by salvage therapy for Hodgkin's disease relapse. In this treatment group, non-Hodgkin's lymphoma risk increased steadily with duration of follow-up. The increased risk associated with salvage treatment was confirmed in a multivariate analysis. Regardless of treatment modality, the RR of non-Hodgkin's lymphoma was

TABLE 5. *Risk of non-Hodgkin's lymphomas after Hodgkin's disease*

	Tucker (31)	Swerdlow (29)	Henry-Amar (71) M	F	Abrahamsen (103)	van Leeuwen (28)	Mauch (106)
Total case series	1,507	2,846	12,411		1,152	1,939	794
Observed NHL	9	17	79	27	8	23	10
Expected NHL	0.5	1.0	2.2	1.1	0.9	1.1	0.5
Relative risk (95% Confidence Interval)	18.0 (8.1–33.5)	16.8 (9.8–26.9)	35.6	24.2	8.4 (3.6–16.6)	20.6 (13.1–30.9)	18.4 (8.6–33.8)
Relative risk by							
Treatment modality							
Radiotherapy only	21	15.0	NR[a]	NR	7.9	9.9	NR
Chemotherapy only	—	18.5	NR	NR	9.1	29.2	—
Combined	22	17.6	NR	NR	8.8	35.0	NR
Follow-up interval							
<5 yr	13	13.2	28.2	21.4	9.4	6.5	5.8
5–9 yr	10	21.9	31.9	45.4	6.9	22.3	38.3
10–14 yr	38*	18.6*	44.7	13.6	8.8*	53.2	15.9
≥ 15 yr	38	18.6	120	0	8.8	14.9	11.1
Absolute excess risk per 10,000 patients per year	9.2	9.2	14	7	9.3	13.1	11.1

M, male; F, female; NR, not reported; NHL, non-Hodgkin's lymphoma.
*Numbers represent a combined estimate for the 10–14 year and ≥15 year follow-up periods.

exceptionally high in the first year following start of treatment for Hodgkin's disease (RR 18.4), declined during the subsequent 4 years, and then sharply increased to reach a 53-fold excess in the 10- to 14-year period of observation (Table 5) (28). Swerdlow et al. reported no differences in non-Hodgkin's lymphoma risk according to broad treatment categories (radiotherapy, chemotherapy, combined treatment) (29). However, when patients receiving extensive or local irradiation were considered separately, the relative risk in patients given local radiotherapy was significantly higher than that in patients treated with extensive irradiation (RR 33.8 vs. 3.9) (29). The relative risk of non-Hodgkin's lymphoma was also significantly higher after treatment with multiple alkylating agents compared to treatment with a single alkylating agent (RR 53.3 vs. 14.2), and the risk was nonsignificantly greater after multiple treatment courses than after one course of treatment. Mauch et al. documented fairly similar absolute excess risks for patients given radiotherapy alone and those receiving combined treatment (10.6 and 16.1 excess cases per 10,000 person-years, respectively) (106). In their study, the relative risk of non-Hodgkin's lymphoma by 5-year intervals of follow-up did not significantly increase with time from treatment, but it increased to 38.3 in the 5- to 9-year interval to decline to less than half that risk in the subsequent follow-up intervals (Table 5).

Attempts at assessing host-related factors predictive for the development of non-Hodgkin's lymphoma also generated discordant findings. In the study by Mauch et al., the relative risk (compared with the general population) did not differ significantly by gender or age at treatment (106). The absolute excess risk was highest for patients 40 years or older at starting treatment (28 excess cases per 10,000 per year) compared with 11.8/10,000/year for younger adults and 0.2/10,000/year for children and adolescents. The absolute excess risk in male patients was higher than in women (15.6 vs. 5.1 per 10,000 per year, respectively). Henry-Amar reported fairly similar relative risks of non-Hodgkin's lymphoma for male and female patients with Hodgkin's disease (RR 35.6 and 24.2, respectively) (71). Swerdlow et al. also found that relative risks for non-Hodgkin's lymphoma as compared with the general population did not differ significantly by gender (male 20.4 vs. female 7.3) (122). Furthermore, they did not observe an association with age at treatment, stage of Hodgkin's disease, or splenectomy. By contrast, relative risks were significantly related to histology of the original Hodgkin's disease, with the greatest risk occurring in patients with the lymphocyte predominance subtype (55.6; 95% C.I. 18.0 to 129.7), and the lowest risk associated with nodular sclerosis (RR 9.8) (122). Henry-Amar also reported that lymphocyte predominance Hodgkin's disease was more strongly associated with increased risk of non-Hodgkin's lymphoma than other histologic types (71). However, this association was only very weak in the study by van Leeuwen et al. (28). This issue is complicated in that lymphocyte predominance Hodgkin's disease is a different entity and may be related to B-cell non-Hodgkin's lymphoma.

It is possible that the differences between studies in reported risk factors for non-Hodgkin's lymphoma mainly reflect differences between patient populations examined. For example, some investigators included only adult patients (71,103), whereas others included the whole age spectrum. Furthermore, the proportion of patients who received multiple treatment courses because of a relapse of their Hodgkin's disease varied substantially among the three studies reporting on it (11% to 22%) (28,31,106) and was not mentioned in the remaining ones. Inconsistencies in the literature regarding the overall risk increase of non-Hodgkin's lymphoma may, at least in part, be attributed to diagnostic misclassification; that is, recurrences of Hodgkin's disease might have been misdiagnosed as non-Hodgkin's lymphoma, or, more likely, the initial primary lymphoma may have been misdiagnosed as Hodgkin's disease although it would be considered non-Hodgkin's lymphoma or a composite lymphoma according to present views regarding lymphoma pathology. For this reason, it is desirable that in studies of second cancer risk, all slides of the second non-Hodgkin's lymphoma and the original Hodgkin's disease diagnosis are reviewed by an expert pathologist. So far, such a slide review has been undertaken in only two studies (28,29).

The cause of the excess risk of non-Hodgkin's lymphoma in patients treated for Hodgkin's disease is still controversial. There exists some evidence indicating that the transformation to non-Hodgkin's lymphoma may be part of the natural history of the lymphocyte predominant subtype of Hodgkin's disease (126,127), and this would explain the association observed in the International Database on Hodgkin's Disease (71) and the British National Lymphoma Investigation (122). Some investigators argue that the high risk of non-Hodgkin's lymphoma may be attributed to Hodgkin's disease itself because increased risk of non-Hodgkin's lymphoma is known to occur in immunosuppressed patients such as transplant recipients (128) and because Hodgkin's disease itself may be accompanied by immunosuppression (129). In support of this hypothesis, investigators from the National Cancer Institute reported a detailed study on 14 patients who developed non-Hodgkin's lymphoma within a median of 136 months from the diagnosis of Hodgkin's disease (130). Twelve patients had the nodular sclerosis subtype, one had mixed cellularity Hodgkin's disease, and one was not further classified. The original treatment for Hodgkin's disease consisted of radiation alone in two patients, chemotherapy alone in four patients, and combined modality in the remaining eight cases. Immunophenotypic studies in nine cases showed that the Reed-Sternberg and Hodgkin's cells were $CD15^{+}$, $CD45^{-}$. Second non-Hodgkin's lymphoma usually arose in extranodal sites (79%), with frequent presentation as abdominal masses, and a high proportion (86%) were classified as either intermediate- or high-grade lymphomas according to the Working Formulation. All 14 neoplasms had an immunophenotype typical of non-Hodgkin's lymphoma of B-cell lineage and were CD15$^-$. The authors concluded that the clinical, histologic, and immunophenotypic findings of non-Hodgkin's lymphoma in these patients were analogous to those of non-Hodgkin's lymphoma arising in immunosuppressed patients, suggesting that immunodeficiency plays a role in the pathogenesis of second non-Hodgkin's lymphoma in patients treated for Hodgkin's disease (130). However, despite the above intriguing findings, the literature suggests that intensive combined-modality treatment may also contribute to the excess risk. Likely, more than one of the above mechanisms operates in the development of non-Hodgkin's lymphoma following treatment for Hodgkin's disease.

Risk of Solid Cancers

Despite the large relative risks of leukemia and non-Hodgkin's lymphoma in the early years after treatment of Hodgkin's disease, in the longer term most of the excess risk of second malignancy is from solid cancers (Table 4). In recent studies with 15 years or more of follow-up, about half (28,29) to two-thirds (106) of second malignancies have been solid cancers. The risk of solid tumor development depends greatly on age at treatment, follow-up interval, and treatments given for Hodgkin's disease.

The relative risk for solid cancer overall, compared with general population expectations, is about 1.5 to 4.5 in long-term follow-up of studies of predominantly adult patients (28,31,71,97,103,106,131–133) but much larger, around 12, in children (Tables 1 and 2) (32). This latter finding reflects a general trend toward greater relative risks of solid cancer at younger ages rather than a dichotomy between children and adults (82,122). The cumulative risk in adults[1] has been 8.5% to 13% at 15 years (29,31,134) and 8% to 13% at 18 to 20 years (28,71,82,103,109,133) and, in patients treated as children, has been 4% at 15 years and 27% at 30 years (135). The absolute excess risk of solid cancer in adults (28,29,31,82,106) or children (135) with Hodgkin's disease has ranged from 23 to 49 excess cases per 10,000 Hodgkin's disease patients per year in large studies (Table 3). The variation in absolute excess risks with age is less clear than the pattern for relative risks: in one study they increased with age (122), but in another they decreased (106).

Results of studies differ on whether solid cancer risks have been greater in men or women. The relative risks of solid tumors were slightly greater for men in three studies of (predominantly) adult patients (71,82,122) but were much greater for women in two studies of patients treated in childhood (32,136). Absolute excess risks after adult treatment have been found to be substantially greater in men (122) or women (106) or to be similar between the sexes (82). Where data for breast cancer were available separately, the studies finding excess tumors in females still did so after excluding this tumor.

Unlike the pattern for leukemia, solid-tumor relative-risks do not reach a peak in the early years after first treatment but rather continue to rise for 15 and perhaps more years (Table 4) (28,31,32,71,106). Typically, the risk is raised little if at all in the first 5 years but substantially, severalfold, raised thereafter. In one large study in children, however, the risk has been found large (RR 12) in the first 5 years after treatment, with no consistent variation thereafter (32). It should be noted that the large relative risks at young ages, when background (general population) cancer rates are low, equate with relatively low absolute risks of cancer. However, if the same magnitude of relative risk persists as the patients grow older, then very large absolute risks of second malignancy will occur.

The risk of solid cancer overall (28,29,31,82,131), and of several specific solid malignancies (see below), is raised after radiotherapy, unsurprisingly because there is widespread evidence of the carcinogenicity of ionizing radiation (5). It is far more uncertain, however, whether chemotherapy for Hodgkin's disease can cause solid malignancies, and if so, of which site(s). Certain studies have found raised risk (not always significantly) for solid cancers overall (29,82,133,134,136) or for solid cancers plus non-Hodgkin's lymphoma (104), but others have not (28,31,98,103). In single studies, not yet replicated, risk of solid malignancy in relation to chemotherapy has been found highly significantly increased with duration since first treatment (29), significantly tenfold increased in patients receiving chemotherapy as children (104),[2] significantly raised for patients treated with a group of rarely used drugs (104), and significantly reduced after hormone treatment, a category including prednisone, other corticosteroids, and adrenocorticotropic hormone (104). One study has reported significantly raised risks of solid tumors if splenectomy or splenic irradiation had been performed (97), but another found no relation to splenectomy (122). There have been few data on risk in relation to number of cycles or courses of treatment, and inconsistent results (29,134).

It would be expected from the general epidemiology of cancer that if there is an effect of chemotherapy on solid cancer risk, it would be site-specific rather than for all

[1]It has varied among studies whether nonmelanoma skin cancer has been included or excluded and whether the data included or did not include a small portion of patients treated as children.

[2]When the results of this study (104) are considered, it should be taken into account that solid tumors and NHL were combined in the analysis and that some uncertainties have been raised about the completeness of data collection (157).

sites, and it would, at least to some extent, be agent-specific. Thus, results on the relation of solid tumors overall to chemotherapy overall provide a poor test of the solid-tumor carcinogenicity of this treatment, and the critical test comes from site-specific data, discussed below. Similarly, other aspects of the risk of solid malignancy are also often site-specific, and therefore, the following sections consider site-specific risks. Large-cohort studies of patients with Hodgkin's disease have fairly consistently shown raised risks of lung cancer, breast cancer, gastrointestinal cancers considered in aggregate, melanoma (although often not significantly), nonmelanoma skin cancer, bone and soft tissue cancers, and thyroid cancer (28,29,31,32,42,71,82,93,103,104,106,107,137–139). In the largest studies, elevated risk of salivary gland cancer was also observed (71,93). There have also been, less consistently, significantly raised risks in some studies for cancers of the mouth, tongue and pharynx, stomach, small intestine, colon, rectum, pancreas, pleura, cervix, ovary, and urogenital cancers overall (28,29,31,32,71,82, 93,103,104,106,107,139), and in children for cancers of the esophagus and brain (32,107).

Lung Cancer

In most large-cohort studies with 15 or more years of follow-up, the site accounting for the largest excess of solid malignancy after Hodgkin's disease is the lung (Table 4) (28,29,31,82). In Britain, a third of all excess malignancies were lung cancers (29); in a recent U.S. study, however, only 10% of excess second malignancies were lung cancers, and breast was the most common site (106). The relative risk of lung cancer is slightly if at all raised in the initial 5 years after first treatment, with larger relative risks, usually around 5 or greater, thereafter until at least 20 years (28,29,31,71,82,93,103). Relative risks of lung cancer have tended, but not entirely consistently, to be greater for patients treated at young than at older ages (82,122), but absolute excess risks have been found to rise with age at first treatment (82,122). There has been a tendency (71,82,93), although not in all studies (20,28,122), toward greater relative risks in female than male patients, a pattern seen in the general literature on radiation risks (5). The absolute excess risks by sex have been inconsistent (82,122).

Risk of lung cancer is substantially raised in Hodgkin's disease patients treated with radiotherapy (with or without chemotherapy) (20,28,29,82,103). One study found no significant trend in relation to dose to the lung overall (81), but another, which investigated dose to the affected area of lung, found a strong dose–response relationship between radiation dose and risk of lung cancer. There was a relative risk of 9.6 for a dose of ≥9 Gy compared with <1 Gy, although with a possible downturn in risk for doses of 15 Gy or greater (20). The decrease in risk for the highest doses is supported by similar results for lung cancer risk after radiotherapy for breast cancer (40). Risk after Hodgkin's disease was not related to number of episodes of radiotherapy (20).

Whereas the raised risk of lung cancer from radiotherapy is undoubted, it is an important unresolved question whether chemotherapy alone is etiologic; several studies have found a raised risk, sometimes significantly (29,81, 82,104,131), but others did not (20,28,103). These analyses have often been based on relatively small numbers, and the relation is uncertain. In one study, risks were particularly large and highly significant after treatments including mustine and after treatment with multiple alkylating agents (29). In another (20), there was no relation to several specific agents, including mustine, and the only positive relation was a borderline significant risk with teniposide. Where the relationship to dose of chemotherapy has been examined (20,81), no increase in risk with greater dose has been present. In studies where relative risks after combined-modality treatment (i.e., chemotherapy plus radiotherapy) have been examined, these risks have been similar to those after radiotherapy alone (28,29,81,82,103,131). Several cytostatic agents including mustine and chlorambucil have been shown to cause lung tumors in experimental animals (83). Clearly, the relation of chemotherapy to risk of lung cancer needs further exploration.

Although several studies have noted a large proportion of smokers among Hodgkin's disease patients who develop lung cancer (31,98,103,106), only two have examined risks in relation to smoking. Kaldor et al. (81) found a relative risk of 13 for ever-smokers compared with never-smokers, and van Leeuwen et al. (20) found a nonsignificant relation for cumulative pack-years ever smoked and a significantly raised risk in relation to amount smoked after diagnosis of Hodgkin's disease (but not amount smoked before diagnosis), which remained after adjustment for radiation dose. In van Leeuwen's study a significant rise in risk with radiation dose occurred for patients who smoked after treatment, but there was no significant trend for those who had not smoked (or had smoked little), and there was evidence for a more than multiplicative relation between smoking-related and radiation-related risks (i.e., the relative risk for smoking plus radiotherapy was greater than would be obtained by multiplying the separate relative risks for these exposures).

In summary, the above data suggest that patients with Hodgkin's disease who smoke will have a considerably greater risk of lung cancer after chest radiotherapy than those who do not smoke, and this accords with experience in other radiation-exposed groups (5). Thus, the smoking status of the patient should be taken into account when chest radiotherapy is under consideration. Furthermore, although the data from van Leeuwen (20) are the only ones available on risks in relation to smoking after treatment, and the study was not large (30 cases), so that the issue cannot be regarded as completely resolved, the evidence suggests that continued smoking is hazardous and that smokers who have received chest radiotherapy should be particularly strongly advised to cease smoking.

Breast Cancer

The relative risk of breast cancer in women treated for Hodgkin's disease has generally been only slightly raised in all-age studies—about 1.5 in most investigations (28,29,31,71,82,93,103,104), but larger in two recent U.S. studies (Tables 1 and 2) (21,106). Absolute excess risks for all ages have been around one to two per 10,000 Hodgkin's disease patients per year (28,29,82), again with a greater risk (13 per 10,000 per year) in recent U.S. data (Table 3) (106). In women treated at young ages and followed for long durations, however, the picture is very different. It has emerged in recent years that breast cancer is one of the most serious long-term sequelae of radiotherapy in women with Hodgkin's disease treated under about age 25. The relative risk of breast cancer after treatment at ages under 16 has ranged from 17 to 458 (106,107), with other studies showing relative risks around 100 (21,32,140). For female survivors of Hodgkin's disease treated at Stanford University, Table 6 gives relative and absolute excess risks of breast cancer by age at treatment, follow-up interval, and treatment modality. The relative risk of developing breast cancer increased strongly with decreasing age at diagnosis. The risks were highest among women with 15 or more years of follow-up, with relative risks of 38, 17, and 4.4 in this follow-up period for women irradiated before age 20, at ages 20 to 29, and above 30 years of age, respectively.

One study reported the relative risk of breast cancer to be significantly greater for treatment at ages 10 to 16 than at ages younger than this (32). At ages beyond childhood, the relative risk has decreased steeply with age at first treatment, and from ages 25 or 30 onward, it has generally been little if at all raised (21,28,82,106,140,141). Absolute excess risks, however, have shown no consistent variation by age of treatment among women treated under age 30 (21), with values around 15 to 45 per 10,000 person-years. A strong trend of increasing relative risk of breast cancer with decreasing age at exposure has also been observed in other radiation-exposed cohorts (12,15,142).

The raised risk of breast cancer develops late and is typically far larger at 15 or more years after first treatment than previously (21,28). In patients treated as children, however, large and highly significant risks have been seen earlier, after 5 (140) or 10 (107) years, or even in the first 5 years after treatment (32). Actuarial risk for those treated at young ages has been estimated as 34% at 25 years after first treatment for women treated at ages under 20 (141) and 42% at 30 years of follow-up for those treated under age 16 (135) in two studies in the United States. The risks were somewhat lower, however, in a study in the Nordic countries—12% at 30 years after treatment at ages under 20 (107). Differences in risk estimates between studies are likely to be caused by differences in patterns of treatment, the age composition of the patient populations, and also the degree of completeness of follow-up. Losses to follow-up [as in the study by Bhatia and colleagues (32)] could exaggerate the risks if, as seems likely, those who remain well tend to lose contact with clinical follow-up while those with second cancer come to attention because of this (143). Bilateral breast cancer and tumors in the medial half of the breast occur

TABLE 6. *Relative risk of breast cancer following Hodgkin's disease by age at diagnosis, follow-up interval, and treatment*

	Observed	Relative risk (95% CI)	Absolute excess risk[a]
Age at diagnosis of HD			
<20	6	33.0 (12–73)	23.5
20–24	9	19.0 (9–35)	47.2
25–29	7	7.3 (3.2–14)	32.6
≥30	3	0.7 (0.1–1.9)	—
Duration since first treatment (yrs)			
<5	1	0.5 (0.0–2.7)	—
5–9	5	2.9 (1.1–6.5)	12.9
10–14	4	2.7 (0.9–6.6)	16.7
15–19	12	15.0 (97.9–25)	169.0
≥20	3	11.0 (2.8–30)	155.0
Treatment			
Radiation alone	12	3.5 (1.9–5.8)	18.8
<15 yrs	2	0.8 (1.1–2.5)	—
≥15 yrs	10	13.0 (6.6–23)	164.0
Radiation + MOPP	12	7.3 (4.0–12)	35.3
<15 yrs	9	6.3 (3.1–12)	27.4
≥15 yrs	3	15.0 (3.7–40)	163.0

CI, confidence interval; HD, Hodgkin's disease; MOPP, mechlorethamine, Oncovin, procorbazine, prednisone.
[a]Per 10,000 female patients per year.
Adapted from ref. 21.

more frequently among cases after Hodgkin's disease than among primary breast cancers (144).

The main cause of the large risk of breast cancer after Hodgkin's disease is mantle radiotherapy.[3] Although stable estimates of the relative risk for this treatment compared with other treatments have not been published, in several cohort studies almost all cases of breast cancer after Hodgkin's disease have been in or at the margin of the radiation field: for instance, 16 of 16 cases (107), 16 of 17 (32), and 22 of 26 (21) in three recent publications. In studies of the relation of risk to dose of radiotherapy, all but two of 25 cases reported by Hancock et al. had received a mantle dose of 40 Gy or greater (21), whereas Bhatia et al. found a significant dose–response relationship for patients treated in childhood, with a relative risk of 23.7 for more than 40 Gy compared with less than 20 Gy (32).

There is some evidence suggesting greater risk of breast cancer in patients treated with MOPP plus radiotherapy than in those treated with radiotherapy alone (21,141), and of increased risk in relation to splenectomy or splenic irradiation (32,97), but these factors are not established. There are no data yet available on the effects of reproductive history, hormone supplementation, family history of breast cancer, or genotype on the radiotherapy-related risks.

In summary, mantle radiotherapy at young ages is associated with a very large risk of breast cancer 15 years and more later, and this hazard needs to be borne in mind both when selecting treatment for girls and young women with Hodgkin's disease and when following up patients treated in this way. From studies examining other radiation exposures, it is well established that, in the low-dose range, breast-cancer risk increases linearly with radiation dose. In discussing the possibility of dose reductions in mantle radiotherapy, an important question is whether linear dose–response extends to the high-dose range used for Hodgkin's disease treatment. New studies should focus on radiation dosimetry and examine breast-cancer risk in relation to the radiation dose administered to the area in the breast where the tumor developed.

Bone and Soft Tissues

Although it accounts for only a small proportion of the absolute excess risk of second malignancy after Hodgkin's disease (about 5% to 10%, Table 3) (29,31,106), the relative risks of bone and soft tissue cancers tend to be large, generally greater for bone than for soft tissue tumors (Tables 1 and 2) (31,71,82,93). There is little information on the relation of the bone and soft tissue tumor risks to age. One study found a relative risk of 106 for bone cancer in patients treated in childhood (19), and another a relative risk of 85 in patients treated under age 20 (145), but others have found relative risks for bone tumors (32) or sarcomas overall (107) in patients treated in childhood that were well within the range of findings in studies of predominantly adult patients (28,29,31,71,82,93,104,106). There have been no analyses published of variation in risk by age within adults, and no substantial data on the time course of bone and soft tissue cancer risks after Hodgkin's disease. In the largest study (93), cases occurred throughout follow-up from 1 to 4 to 20 years and more after treatment, but with too few cases to assess variation in risk over time. In children treated for cancer generally, relative risks of bone cancer continue to rise from 2 to 4 to over 20 years after first treatment, with a relative risk of several hundred at 20 years or more of follow-up (19). On this basis, very large relative risks can be expected in Hodgkin's disease patients treated in childhood, as longer follow-up becomes available.

Bone and soft tissue tumor risks are greatly increased after radiotherapy (131), as would be expected from experience of radiation exposure in other circumstances (5,19). A study in childhood cancer survivors showed that, beyond 10 Gy, risk of bone sarcoma rose sharply with increasing radiation dose, reaching a 40-fold excess at doses of 60 Gy or more (19). There is also intriguing evidence, however, that chemotherapy may be etiologic for these malignancies. A large U.S. study found a significant sixfold relative risk in relation to chemotherapy, with significant risks at each of 0 to 4, 5 to 9, and 10 years and more after first treatment (104). When specific drug treatments (categorized into 13 groups) were considered, there were significant associations with procarbazine, vincristine, doxorubicin, bleomycin, and other rare drugs (104). The possibility that alkylating chemotherapy may cause these tumors would accord with a significantly raised risk associated with this treatment in a study of bone cancers in childhood cancer survivors generally (19).

Thyroid Cancer

Thyroid cancers are an uncommon sequel of Hodgkin's disease treatment, with an absolute excess risk of about one to three per 10,000 patients per year (Table 3) (29,82,138), about 2% of the excess risk of second cancers overall (29,82). The relative risks, however, are large, particularly after treatment in childhood; relative risks of 33 to 67 have been found after childhood Hodgkin's disease (32,42,107), whereas risks have been much lower than this—9 at most—in all-age studies (Tables 1 and 2) (28,29,71,82,93,103,104). Among ages at first treatment under 20, risks are greater for younger ages at treatment, with a relative risk of 790 (95% C.I. 9.5 to 2,800) found

[3]The risks cited above were generally for breast cancer patients overall rather than specifically those treated with chest radiotherapy [an exception is seen in the results of Aisenberg et al. (141)], so that the risks would presumably be larger for patients treated with mantle radiotherapy, considered separately.

for treatment at ages 0 to 4 (107). Data on other radiation-exposed cohorts suggest that absolute excess risks are similar for treatments at any childhood age (42) and that there is little risk from treatment over age 20 (41). Risks after Hodgkin's disease appear to be raised throughout follow-up to 20 and more years, without a trend with time in one study (32) and with uneven evidence for increasing relative risks with time in another (93), based on small numbers. From studies in other radiation-exposed cohorts (41,42), one would expect a higher relative risk of thyroid cancer with a longer observation period.

Radiotherapy is likely to be the main cause of thyroid cancers after Hodgkin's disease because the thyroid is known to be a highly radiosensitive organ, particularly in children (5,42). There is little information on this specifically for Hodgkin's disease patients. In one study (107), eight of eight thyroid cancers for whom data were available, and in another study six of six (138), occurred within radiotherapy fields. From experience of thyroid cancer after childhood radiation exposure in other circumstances, the absolute excess risk per Gray has been calculated at about three to four per 10,000 patients per year, and greater in female than male patients; risk was found to increase with dose up to 10 Gy, but beyond this it appears to level off or even decrease (41,42).

There have also been suggestions, as yet unconfirmed, of a possible link of thyroid-cancer risk to chemotherapy: in a study examining risks of nine solid tumor sites after Hodgkin's disease in relation to 13 categories of drugs, a significantly raised risk of thyroid cancer was found after lomustine and after "other alkylating agents" (104); the greatest risk of thyroid cancer in relation to chemotherapy was in the first 5 years after treatment.

Malignant Melanoma

Risk of malignant melanoma has been increased in the great majority of large-cohort studies of patients with Hodgkin's disease, although often not significantly, based on small numbers (Tables 1 and 2). Relative risks have generally been around two to five (28,31,32,71,82,93, 103,104,106,107) and have not been larger in patients treated in childhood (32,107) than in those treated as adults or at all ages (28,31,71,82,93,103,104,106). Absolute excess rates have been two to four per 10,000 Hodgkin's disease patients per year (Table 3) (28,31, 82,106). In one study that examined the time course of this risk (31,137), most cases occurred in the first 5 years of follow-up, two of six patients had more than one primary melanoma, and five of six patients had biopsy or clinical evidence of dysplastic nevus syndrome (137), implying that patients with this syndrome may particularly be at risk. The melanomas in this study were mostly bulky, deeply invasive lesions at diagnosis, so it seems unlikely that the raised risk was a biased consequence of increased surveillance of Hodgkin's disease patients compared with the general population (137). There has been some evidence of raised risk in association with radiotherapy (131), although this is not a relationship that would be expected from the radiation literature generally. It is possible that the melanoma risk is not caused by a carcinogenic effect of treatment; melanoma rates are raised in several immunosuppressed groups.

Gastrointestinal Cancers

Gastrointestinal cancers account for about 10% of the excess risk of cancer after Hodgkin's disease, with an absolute excess risk of about six per 10,000 Hodgkin's disease patients per year (Table 3) (28,139). Relative and absolute excess risks have tended to be greater in male than female patients (71,139). Studies have varied as to whether they examined gastrointestinal-cancer risks in aggregate or separately by cancer site (Tables 1 and 2). In aggregate, risks have generally been found raised from 5 years onward (28,71), but not before this, and a recent study found relative risks continuing to rise through 20 years after first treatment (139). Data on the time course of risk for individual gastrointestinal sites have been few and inconsistent (28,31,93).

Much greater risks of esophageal (107), colorectal (32,107), and stomach (32,106) cancers have been found in patients treated as children (or under age 20) than those treated at older ages, and relative risk of gastrointestinal cancers overall has been found to decrease with increasing age in adults (139), as would be expected, especially for stomach cancers, from other experience of the effects of radiation (11).

There is little information on the relation of gastrointestinal-cancer risks to type of treatment, although from other epidemiologic findings one would expect raised risks of most gastrointestinal sites after radiotherapy (5). A recent study found risks in Hodgkin's disease patients significantly raised after combined-modality treatment and near-significantly raised after radiotherapy alone (with few subjects receiving only chemotherapy) (139). There have been unconfirmed findings of significantly raised risk of digestive and peritoneal cancers after doxorubicin treatment and significantly reduced risk of these cancers after hormonal treatments (a category including corticosteroids and adrenocorticotropic hormone) (104).

Other Solid Cancer Sites

Although there is relatively little evidence on the risks of other solid cancer sites after Hodgkin's disease (104,131), it is likely on the basis of radiation epidemiology generally (5) that risks of several other tumors, including salivary gland tumors, nonmelanoma skin cancer, and bladder cancer will prove to be raised after radiotherapy for Hodgkin's disease. One study (104), unconfirmed, has found significantly raised risks of tumors of the female genital system in relation to chemotherapy with vincristine and with other "rare drugs" and a significantly diminished risk of these tumors after hormonal treatments.

SURVIVAL AFTER SECOND CANCER DIAGNOSIS

Despite a multitude of reports on the magnitude of second cancer risk in patients treated for Hodgkin's disease, data on survival after such a diagnosis are somewhat scanty. In their 20-year follow-up study of patients treated from 1966 onward, van Leeuwen and co-workers reported that the cumulative risk of dying from Hodgkin's disease or acute treatment toxicity was 33%, while the risk of dying from a second cancer was 14% and that from all other causes was 20% (28). The International Database on Hodgkin's Disease, by far the largest study of second cancer risk conducted, found that, at 20 years, the overall probability of survival in 14,315 patients with Hodgkin's disease was 50% (71). Seventy-three percent of deaths were directly related to Hodgkin's disease (including deaths from acute treatment toxicity). Second cancer deaths accounted for 10% of all deaths following Hodgkin's disease and for 37% of deaths from causes unrelated to Hodgkin's disease. They comprised 413 of the 631 patients in whom a second cancer was documented. The impact of second cancer on long-term overall survival was substantial, as evidenced by the increase in the 20-year survival rate from 50% to 61% when second cancer deaths were removed (censored in analysis). Survival was extremely poor for patients who developed an acute leukemia or a myelodysplastic syndrome (2-year survival rate of 10%), whereas in patients who developed a second non-Hodgkin's lymphoma or a second solid tumor, the 5- and 10-year survival rates were approximately 32% and 23%, respectively. Similar findings were also reported in the study by Mauch and colleagues; the median survival from diagnosis of second tumor was approximately 42 months and was especially poor in patients developing a second cancer following a Hodgkin's disease diagnosis at the age of 40 years or older (median survival approximately 1 year) (106). The above figures suggest that the development of a second malignancy in patients with Hodgkin's disease is almost always associated with a dismal prognosis.

However, solid tumors are usually documented after prolonged follow-up and present with a variety of types and prognostic features, which makes it difficult to give an overall estimate of long-term survival after their diagnosis. In the following paragraphs we summarize the literature on the prognosis of selected second cancers.

Acute Leukemias and Myelodysplastic Syndromes

For many years, supportive therapy has been considered the standard care in patients with therapy-related acute nonlymphocytic leukemia and myelodysplastic syndromes. Subsequently, early reports in patients treated with chemotherapy found that only 10% of these patients were able to achieve a complete remission (146). In reviewing 65 patients with secondary acute nonlymphocytic leukemia/myelodysplastic syndrome, Michels et al. reported that the overall median survival was only 4 months. In this study, no survival difference was found between patients who received chemotherapy and those who were given supportive therapy alone (72).

Scattered reports of remission rates up to 70% after aggressive chemotherapy have been published in more recent years. The majority of these studies included patients with both primary and second acute nonlymphocytic leukemia/myelodysplastic syndrome, and fewer than half of the patients had therapy-related disease. Table 7 summarizes the most important findings achieved in therapy-related and, when available, *de novo* leukemias treated with the same regimens.

It should be noted that not all second acute nonlymphocytic leukemia occurred in patients with a first Hodgkin's disease, but in all cases the patients had been treated with multiple chemotherapeutic agents. In sum-

TABLE 7. *Chemotherapy results in therapy-related and de novo acute myelogenous leukemia: representative case series*

Authors	Drugs used	Therapy-related				*De novo*			
		No. Pts	Median age (yr)	% CR[a]	Median survival (mos)	No. Pts	Median age (yr)	% CR	Median survival (mos)
De Witte et al. (147)	DNR Ara-C	7	47	62	7	126	44	67	10
Hoyle et al. (148)	DNR Ara-C 6-TG	20	54	25	4	688	NR	66	11
Vaughan et al. 1983 (148a)	DNR HD Ara-C	8	64	50	6	—	—	—	—
Priesler et al. (149)	HD Ara-C	11	54	73	4	—	—	—	—

[a]CR, complete remission; DNR, daunorubicin; Ara-C, cytarabine; 6-TG, 6-thioguanine; HD Ara-C, high-dose cytarabine; NR, not reported, but younger than in therapy-related leukemia.

mary, in one study there was no significant difference in remission rate between primary and therapy-related acute nonlymphocytic leukemia, but median survival duration was 3 months shorter in patients with therapy-related acute nonlymphocytic leukemia, and only 8% of the patients who achieved complete remission were alive at 4 years (147). In the series by Hoyle et al., only 25% of the patients with therapy-related acute nonlymphocytic leukemia entered complete remission, and the overall median survival was 4 months (Table 7); in these patients, treatment outcome was significantly worse compared with patients with primary acute nonlymphocytic leukemia, of whom 66% achieved a complete remission (148). In contrast, median duration of remission appeared to be similar in both groups (12 and 13 months, respectively), and, after stratification for age, the difference in overall survival was not statistically significant. In an attempt to assess potential prognostic indicators in patients with therapy-related acute nonlymphocytic leukemia, Hoyle and co-workers reported that the only characteristic correlating with improved prognosis was the presence of Auer rods, which were detected in four of the five cases who achieved a complete remission, compared with three of 15 who did not have a complete remission. High-dose cytarabine, alone or combined with daunorubicin, was delivered in two case series and was able to induce complete remissions in 50% and 73% of patients, respectively (Table 7). Despite a fairly high remission rate in the series by Preisler et al., median overall survival was only 4 months. In this series, no characteristics could be identified that correlated with prognosis (149).

Promising results have been reported with the use of bone-marrow transplantation in patients with therapy-related acute nonlymphocytic leukemia/myelodysplastic syndrome, with a 27% disease-free survival at 5 years (150). However, these results require some caution in that they were achieved in a very small patient group, the vast majority was subjected to allogenic transplantation. A special concern in this heavily pretreated patient population is the risk of regimen-related toxicity; other problems remain infection, graft-versus-host disease, and leukemia recurrence.

A consistent result from all studies discussed above is that the outcome of therapy-related acute nonlymphocytic leukemia/myelodysplastic syndrome is almost always fatal. For this reason, their impact is generally considered to be deleterious to the overall survival of patients with Hodgkin's disease. However, it must be remembered that the cumulative incidence of acute nonlymphocytic leukemia/myelodysplastic syndrome is rather low in most studies (<4% at 10 years) and should decrease further with modern, less leukemogenic chemotherapy regimens. As previously mentioned, the International Database on Hodgkin's Disease investigated the issue of causes of deaths in detail and reported that deaths related to acute nonlymphocytic leukemia/myelodysplastic syndrome accounted for 4% of all deaths recorded, and their impact on the overall survival rate of Hodgkin's disease patients was very limited, less than 1% at 20 years (71). When patients who never relapsed after an initial complete remission were considered, it was estimated that the impact of therapy-related acute nonlymphocytic leukemia/myelodysplastic syndrome on the 20-year overall survival rate accounted for a deficit of approximately 3%.

Non-Hodgkin's Lymphoma

Little is known about the prognosis of non-Hodgkin's lymphoma following a diagnosis of Hodgkin's disease. Initial publications have reported poor outcomes following the diagnosis of this second malignancy (125,151). More recent data, however, suggest that these patients may be curable with aggressive multiagent chemotherapy.

In the detailed report by Zarate-Osorno et al. on 14 cases of second non-Hodgkin's lymphoma, all patients but one were treated with chemotherapy, although not in a uniform manner, and complete remission was achieved in seven patients (50%). Five patients were alive without disease after a mean of 3.1 years (130). Other case series have reported that the majority of non-Hodgkin's lymphoma arising in patients with a first Hodgkin's disease appeared to be diffuse lymphoma of intermediate- or high-grade malignancy (28,127), histologic subtypes that, when appropriately treated, can achieve high remission rates. Of the 106 patients with secondary non-Hodgkin's lymphoma documented in the International Database on Hodgkin's Disease, 45 were alive at the time of the report, with a 5-year probability of survival of 30% (71). Two smaller case series reported that more than half of their patients were effectively treated (98,106), but a longer follow-up is needed to fully assess final outcome. Unfortunately, none of the above studies compared the characteristics and prognosis of non-Hodgkin's lymphoma in patients treated for Hodgkin's disease with those of a large series of primary non-Hodgkin's lymphoma cases.

In summary, it appears that secondary non-Hodgkin's lymphoma is responsive to combination chemotherapy and that, as in primary non-Hodgkin's lymphoma, achievement and duration of complete remission are important prognostic factors.

Breast Cancer

To characterize the clinical and pathologic features of patients who developed breast cancer after treatment for Hodgkin's disease, Yahalom and co-workers analyzed 45 events occurring in 37 patients diagnosed at the Memorial Sloan-Kettering Cancer Center in New York (144). Compared with patients with primary breast cancer, women who developed a second breast cancer after Hodgkin's disease were more likely to be young, to develop bilateral disease (eight of 37; four had synchronous bilateral tumors), and to have breast tumors that involved the medial half of the breast. By contrast, no significant differences in nuclear and histologic grade, lymphocytic reaction, and lymphatic invasion were detected between second and first primary tumors. Apparently, all patients received locoregional treatment only, and prognosis strongly depended on the axillary nodal status. The 6-year disease-free survival rates were 85% for patients with node-negative tumors and 33% for patients with axillary involvement. According to the authors, these survival rates were similar to those of patients with primary breast cancer seen at the Memorial Sloan-Kettering Cancer Center.

Four studies specifically focused on the risk of breast cancer in women previously treated for Hodgkin's disease (21,32,141,152). Unfortunately, none of them reported details on pathologic characteristics and treatments for second cancers, but some data are available on survival. Hancock et al. reported that the women who developed invasive breast cancer averaged 40 years of age at diagnosis of breast cancer (range 22 to 75 years) (21). In the vast majority of breast cancers (22 of 26, 87%), pathology specimens showed infiltrating ductal carcinoma; eight tumors were poorly differentiated. At the time of the report, breast cancer had recurred in ten of 26 patients, and seven patients had died of disease progression. Relapse-free and overall survival rates 5 years after the diagnosis of second cancer were 50% and 60%, respectively. The Late Effects Study Group documented 17 patients with breast cancer in a large cohort of female patients treated for childhood Hodgkin's disease (32). The median age at the time of diagnosis of breast cancer was very young (31.5 years; range 16 to 42), and five patients presented with bilateral tumors. At the end of follow-up, 12 patients were alive (eight with recurrent disease after a median follow-up time of 10 months; four without disease after a median survival of 4.5 years), and three patients had died of their breast cancer after a median survival of 3 years (the status of two patients was unknown). Aisenberg and co-workers reported 14 cases of breast cancer in a series of 111 women younger than 60 years at the time of diagnosis of Hodgkin's disease (141). Axillary lymph nodes were involved in four of 11 cases, and two patients developed asynchronous bilateral carcinoma. Only one patient died of breast cancer, but the median follow-up was very short (slightly longer than 1 year, with only three patients followed for more than 5 years). Finally, Chung et al. observed 11 cases of breast cancer in a series of 136 patients (152). One patient died of breast cancer, and eight were alive without evidence of disease after a median follow-up of approximately 2 years (the status of two patients was unknown).

From the above reported data, it appears that the prognosis of breast cancers arising in patients treated for Hodgkin's disease is not strikingly different from that of primary breast cancers. However, because only one study directly compared the characteristics and prognosis of breast cancers following Hodgkin's disease with those arising in patients without a previous malignancy, no firm conclusion on this issue can be drawn. It should be emphasized that treatment strategies in primary operable breast cancer have changed during the last two decades and that adjuvant systemic treatment has been demonstrated to decrease significantly the risk of both recurrence and death (153). Thus, in addition to an early detection program for female patients treated with mantle or mediastinal irradiation, appropriate multimodality treatment strategies should be applied once a second breast cancer has been diagnosed. Because of the very high risk of breast cancer in women irradiated for Hodgkin's disease at a young age (21,32), early diagnosis and optimal treatment of this second malignancy may have considerable impact on the ultimate survival of female patients cured from Hodgkin's disease.

CLINICAL IMPLICATIONS

The occurrence of treatment-related cancers is a major problem in survivors of Hodgkin's disease. Therefore, the results discussed in this chapter have multiple clinical implications.

First, increased knowledge of treatment factors responsible for the occurrence of second cancers is of crucial importance for the development of new treatment strategies. Clinical research should focus on the development of therapeutic regimens with lesser carcinogenic potential, without compromising the excellent cure rates that have been achieved. Despite the strongly increased risks observed for several cancer sites, the issue of treatment-induced second cancers must always be viewed in relation to the dramatic increase in survival rates of patients with Hodgkin's disease. When a specific treatment is the best way to cure the patient, the treatment should obviously not be abandoned because of its carcinogenic effects. The short- and long-term risks of second malignancy (and other complications) that are associated with a specific treatment regimen should be weighed carefully against the consequences of not using such treatment. The arbitrary alteration of a therapy successful against a particular malignancy in order to mitigate second cancer risk is unwarranted. Hence, it is of the utmost importance that changes in therapy to reduce the risk of late complications be made only in the context of carefully designed clinical trials that can evaluate whether the overall efficacy of treatment is maintained.

The replacement of high-dose MOPP chemotherapy with the far less leukemogenic ABV-based regimens introduced in the 1980s has shown that it is indeed possible to reduce second cancer risk while maintaining equal levels of therapeutic effectiveness. It is to be hoped that the reduction of dose and fields of irradiation, as applied in several recent Hodgkin's disease trials, will result in a lower risk of solid tumors.

Knowledge of risk factors for second malignancy has also made it possible to identify patient groups at high risk of developing second cancers as a result of treatments that they have received in the past. Whenever effective screening methods are available, these should be implemented in the patients' follow-up program to improve their survival from a second primary malignancy. In some cases, preventive strategies (e.g., smoking cessation) may substantially reduce the risk of developing a treatment-related cancer.

Patients with Hodgkin's disease who have been disease-free for more than 5 years are often told that they are cured; as a result, they are sometimes discharged from further routine follow-up by their treating physicians. Yet, paradoxically, after 5 years, the risk of developing a solid cancer is increasing rapidly. Treating physicians, family physicians, and also the patients themselves must be made aware of this potential risk in order to increase motivation for lifelong medical surveillance. The risk of a particular second malignancy depends on the treatment administered for Hodgkin's disease but also on various patient characteristics, such as age and gender. This implies that advice to the patient, and additional screening methods during follow-up, may vary among different patient groups.

In all patients with Hodgkin's disease, special attention should be given throughout follow-up to new clinical signs or symptoms of lymphoma. The greatly increased risk of non-Hodgkin's lymphoma demonstrates the importance of performing biopsies to discriminate between recurrent Hodgkin's disease and non-Hodgkin's lymphoma. Because smokers experience a significantly greater risk of lung cancer in relation to radiotherapy than nonsmokers, physicians should make a special effort to dissuade Hodgkin's disease patients from smoking even before treatment starts, and also in the course of follow-up. If the treating physician succeeds in getting this message across, the excess risk of lung cancer following Hodgkin's disease may decrease substantially in the future. The usefulness of screening for lung cancer in survivors of Hodgkin's disease is questionable. Women treated with mantle field irradiation before age 30 are at greatly increased risk of breast cancer. The importance of regular breast examinations should be explained to them, and they should be taught breast self-examination. From 5 to 10 years after irradiation, the follow-up program of these women should include yearly breast palpation and mammography. The diagnostic process of the breast tumors in two Hodgkin's disease series illustrates that routine mammography alone has only limited value in this young patient group (21,28). Physicians should also be alert to the higher risk of gastrointestinal cancers in patients treated with paraaortic and pelvic radiation fields. Thorough examination of gastrointestinal complaints is indicated.

In regard to the clinical implications of the findings discussed in this chapter, it is important to keep in mind that, over the past decades, there has been a continuous evolution of new therapies aimed at increasing treatment efficacy and/or, more recently, decreasing the risk of acute and late complications. Thus, the results presented in this chapter reflect the risks associated with treatments used 5 to 20 years ago. This fact, which is inherent to the study of late effects, implies that the risks observed cannot always be extrapolated directly to patient populations currently being treated. Whereas some treatments have changed little, or not al all, there has been a general tendency in radiotherapy to minimize radiation dose to surrounding normal tissues and, recently, also to decrease the tumor dose. With regard to chemotherapy, the total dose of alkylating agents has been reduced while new cytostatic agents have been introduced, the long-term effects of which are not yet known (e.g., the epipodophyllotoxins). In most cases it is very difficult, if not impossible, to predict the effect of these treatment alterations on second cancer risk. It is only through large, well-designed, and long-term follow-up studies that the effects of such new treatments on second-cancer risk can be evaluated.

DIRECTIONS FOR FUTURE RESEARCH

In this final section we give some directions for future research with respect to second-cancer risk following Hodgkin's disease.

First, more data are needed with regard to the evolution of second cancer risk over prolonged follow-up periods. The risks of developing second malignancies more than 20 years following treatment of Hodgkin's disease are not known. It is not clear whether the radiation-related increased relative risks of solid tumors observed in the 10- to 20-year follow-up interval will continue to increase further with more prolonged follow-up or will level off or decrease at some point in time. This question is of great importance in view of the fact that, even with constant relative risks over time, the aging of a cohort of Hodgkin's disease survivors with more prolonged follow-up will result in greatly increased absolute excess risks of second malignancy. In view of existing data showing that the risk of some solid tumors increases with decreasing age at first treatment, it is important to carefully consider age at treatment in future studies.

Another question of major importance is whether chemotherapy contributes to the increased risk of solid tumors (and non-Hodgkin's lymphoma), as suggested by some recent studies. Because the findings are inconsistent so far, large and long-term follow-up studies are needed to examine whether chemotherapy, possibly in interaction with radiotherapy, affects the risk of certain solid tumors (and non-Hodgkin's lymphoma). Effects of chemotherapy on solid-cancer risk are likely to be site-specific as well as agent-specific, so there is a need for detailed (case-control) studies of the risk of selected solid tumors in relation to the cumulative dose of various cytostatic drugs.

With regard to the radiation-related risk of solid tumors, an important issue to be clarified is the shape of the radiation dose–response curve in the high dose range used therapeutically. It is not clear whether at high doses the risks of specific solid tumors (e.g., cancers of the breast, lung, and gastrointestinal tract) increase linearly with increasing radiation dose. Thus, it is not known whether the lower radiation doses currently applied in several trials will indeed result in reduced risk of solid malignancies. Studies examining radiation dose–response relationships for selected solid tumors should perform accurate radiation dosimetry to estimate the radiation dose administered to the specific site where the second tumor developed.

Furthermore, little is known so far about possible interaction between treatment effects (radiotherapy, chemotherapy) on the one hand and environmental carcinogens (e.g., smoking) or hormonal risk factors on the other. For example, it would be of interest to examine whether reproductive risk factors and hormone treatment following chemotherapy-induced premature menopause affect radiation-related breast cancer in young female survivors of Hodgkin's disease.

Genetic susceptibility may also play a role in the pathogenesis of treatment-related second malignancies. An intriguing research question regarding genetic predisposition relates to the known radiation sensitivity of heterozygous carriers of the mutated ataxia telangiectasia gene. With the recent identification of the ataxia telangiectasia gene (154), it will be possible to examine whether ataxia telangiectasia heterozygotes (about 1.0% of the population) have an increased risk of radiation-induced cancer, specifically breast cancer (155,156). Because the mechanisms underlying the carcinogenic effects of radiation are still poorly understood, research should also focus on the identification of specific (somatic) gene alterations associated with the development of radiation-induced cancer (44,45). Recent studies have suggested that the mutational spectrum of the p53 tumor suppressor gene in radiation-induced lung cancer may differ from that observed in smoking-related lung cancer (46–48). With the rapid advances in molecular biology, our understanding of radiation carcinogenesis at the molecular level is likely to increase significantly in the years to come.

New cohorts should be assembled to evaluate the extent of second-cancer risk (leukemia, non-Hodgkin's lymphoma, solid tumors) associated with treatments introduced in the 1990s (in particular, new chemotherapy regimens). It is only through future long-term follow-up studies that the late effects of such treatments can be evaluated.

Finally, it is of great importance to evaluate the benefits as well as possible adverse effects of screening and lifelong medical surveillance in survivors of Hodgkin's disease.

Although knowledge about the carcinogenic effects of Hodgkin's disease treatments has increased substantially over the last decade, it is clear that many important questions remain to be answered. The long induction period of many carcinogenic agents, including radiation, as well as the continuous evolution of new therapies necessitate the evaluation of the risk of second malignancy for many years to come. Proper and innovative epidemiologic methods, preferably incorporating biological measurements, are needed to quantify the risk, to identify treatment factors responsible for such risk, and to shed light on the mechanisms of therapy-induced carcinogenesis.

REFERENCES

1. Boice JD Jr, Storm HH, Curtis RE, et al. Introduction to the study of multiple primary cancers. *Natl Cancer Inst Monogr* 1985;68:3.
2. Court-Brown WM, Doll R. *Leukaemia and aplastic anaemia in patients irradiated for ankylosing spondylitis.* London: Her Majesty's Stationery Office, 1957.
3. Upton AC. Physical carcinogenesis: radiation, history and sources. In: Becker FF, ed. *Cancer: a comprehensive treatise.* New York: Plenum Press, 1975:387.
4. Martland HS. The occurrence of malignancy in radioactive persons: a general review of data gathered in the study of the radium dial painters, with special reference to the occurrence of osteogenic sarcoma and the interrelationship of certain blood diseases. *Am J Cancer* 1931;15:2435.
5. National Research Council. *Health effects of exposure to low levels of ionizing radiation (BEIR V).* Washington, DC: National Academy Press, 1990.
6. United Nations Scientific Committee on the Effects of Atomic Radiation. *Sources and effects of ionizing radiation: UNSCEAR 1994 report to the general assembly with scientific annexes.* New York: United Nations, 1994.
7. Boice JD Jr. Carcinogenesis—a synopsis of human experience with external exposure in medicine (Review). *Health Phys* 1988;55:621.
8. Heyssel R, Brill AB, Woodbury L, et al. Leukemia in Hiroshima atomic bomb survivors. *Blood* 1960;15:313.
9. Shimizu Y, Kato H, Schull WJ. Studies of the mortality of A-bomb survivors. 9. Mortality, 1950–1985: Part 2. Cancer mortality based on the recently revised doses (DS86). *Radiat Res* 1990;121:120.
10. Preston DL, Kusumi S, Tomonaga M, et al. Cancer incidence in atomic bomb survivors. Part III. Leukemia, lymphoma and multiple myeloma, 1950–1987. *Radiat Res* 1994;137:S68. Published erratum appears in *Radiat Res* 1994;139(1):129.
11. Thompson DE, Mabuchi K, Ron E, et al. Cancer incidence in atomic bomb survivors. Part II: Solid tumors, 1958–1987. *Radiat Res* 1994; 137:S17. Published erratum appears in *Radiat Res* 1994;139(1):129.
12. Tokunaga M, Land CE, Tokuoka S, Nishimori I, Soda M, Akiba S. Incidence of female breast cancer among atomic bomb survivors, 1950–1985. *Radiat Res* 1994;138:209.
13. Smith PG, Doll R. Mortality from cancer and all causes among British radiologists. *Br J Radiol* 1981;54:187.
14. Wang JX, Inskip PD, Boice JD Jr, Li BX, Zhang JY, Fraumeni JF Jr. Cancer incidence among medical diagnostic x-ray workers in China, 1950 to 1985. *Int J Cancer* 1990;45:889.
15. Boice JD Jr, Preston D, Davis FG, Monson RR. Frequent chest x-ray fluoroscopy and breast cancer incidence among tuberculosis patients in Massachusetts. *Radiat Res* 1991;125:214.

16. Miller AB, Howe GR, Sherman GJ, et al. Mortality from breast cancer after irradiation during fluoroscopic examinations in patients being treated for tuberculosis. *N Engl J Med* 1989;321:1285.
17. Boice JD Jr, Blettner M, Kleinerman RA, et al. Radiation dose and leukemia risk in patients treated for cancer of the cervix. *J Natl Cancer Inst* 1987;79:1295.
18. Boice JD Jr, Engholm G, Kleinerman RA, et al. Radiation dose and second cancer risk in patients treated for cancer of the cervix. *Radiat Res* 1988;116:3.
19. Tucker MA, D'Angio GJ, Boice JD Jr, et al. Bone sarcomas linked to radiotherapy and chemotherapy in children. *N Engl J Med* 1987; 317:588.
20. van Leeuwen FE, Klokman WJ, Stovall M, et al. Roles of radiotherapy and smoking in lung cancer following Hodgkin's disease. *J Natl Cancer Inst* 1995;87:1530.
21. Hancock SL, Tucker MA, Hoppe RT. Breast cancer after treatment of Hodgkin's disease. *J Natl Cancer Inst* 1993;85:25.
22. Weiss HA, Darby SC, Doll R. Cancer mortality following x-ray treatment for ankylosing spondylitis. *Int J Cancer* 1994;59:327.
23. Darby SC, Reeves G, Key T, Doll R, Stovall M. Mortality in a cohort of women given x-ray therapy for metropathia haemorrhagica. *Int J Cancer* 1994;56:793.
24. Ron E, Modan B, Boice JD Jr. Mortality after radiotherapy for ringworm of the scalp. *Am J Epidemiol* 1988;127:713.
25. Hildreth NG, Shore RE, Hempelmann LH, Rosenstein M. Risk of extrathyroid tumors following radiation treatment in infancy for thymic enlargement. *Radiat Res* 1985;102:378.
26. Shore RE, Hildreth N, Woodard E, Dvoretsky P, Hempelmann L, Pasternack B. Breast cancer among women given x-ray therapy for acute postpartum mastitis. *J Natl Cancer Inst* 1986;77:689.
27. Curtis RE, Boice JD Jr, Stovall M, et al. Relationship of leukemia risk to radiation dose following cancer of the uterine corpus. *J Natl Cancer Inst* 1994;86:1315.
28. van Leeuwen FE, Klokman WJ, Hagenbeek A, et al. Second cancer risk following Hodgkin's disease: a 20-year follow-up study. *J Clin Oncol* 1994;12:312.
29. Swerdlow AJ, Douglas AJ, Vaughan Hudson G, Vaughan Hudson B, Bennett MH, MacLennan KA. Risk of second primary cancers after Hodgkin's disease by type of treatment: analysis of 2846 patients in the British National Lymphoma Investigation. *Br Med J* 1992;304:1137.
30. Kaldor JM, Day NE, Shiboski S. Epidemiological studies of anticancer drug carcinogenicity. In: Schmäl D, Kaldor JM, eds. *Carcinogenicity of alkylating cytostatic drugs: proceedings of a symposium by IARC and the German Cancer Research Centre.* IARC Science Publications no. 78. Lyons, France: International Agency for Research on Cancer, 1986;189.
31. Tucker MA, Coleman CN, Cox RS, Varghese A, Rosenberg SA. Risk of second cancers after treatment for Hodgkin's disease. *N Engl J Med* 1988;318:76.
32. Bhatia S, Robison LL, Oberlin O, et al. Breast cancer and other second neoplasms after childhood Hodgkin's disease. *N Engl J Med* 1996;334:745.
33. Inskip PD, Monson RR, Wagoner JK, et al. Cancer mortality following radium treatment for uterine bleeding. *Radiat Res* 1990;123:331. Published erratum appears in *Radiat Res* 1991;128(3):326.
34. Kaldor JM, Day NE, Clarke EA, et al. Leukemia following Hodgkin's disease [see comments]. *N Engl J Med* 1990;322:7.
35. Kaldor JM, Day NE, Pettersson F, et al. Leukemia following chemotherapy for ovarian cancer [see comments]. *N Engl J Med* 1990;322:1.
36. Curtis RE, Boice JD Jr, Stovall M, et al. Risk of leukemia after chemotherapy and radiation treatment for breast cancer [see comments]. *N Engl J Med* 1992;326:1745.
37. Tucker MA, Meadows AT, Boice JD Jr, et al. Leukemia after therapy with alkylating agents for childhood cancer. *J Natl Cancer Inst* 1987; 78:459.
38. Travis LB, Weeks J, Curtis RE, et al. Leukemia following low-dose total body irradiation and chemotherapy for non-Hodgkin's lymphoma. *J Clin Oncol* 1996;14:565.
39. Greene MH, Young RC, Merrill JM, DeVita VT. Evidence of a treatment dose response in acute nonlymphocytic leukemias which occur after therapy of non-Hodgkin's lymphoma. *Cancer Res* 1983;43:1891.
40. Inskip PD, Stovall M, Flannery JT. Lung cancer risk and radiation dose among women treated for breast cancer. *J Natl Cancer Inst* 1994;86:983.
41. Ron E, Lubin JH, Shore RE, et al. Thyroid cancer after exposure to external radiation: a pooled analysis of seven studies. *Radiat Res* 1995;141:259.
42. Tucker MA, Jones PH, Boice JD Jr, et al. Therapeutic radiation at a young age is linked to secondary thyroid cancer. The Late Effects Study Group. *Cancer Res* 1991;51:2885.
43. Tucker MA, Meadows AT, Boice JD Jr, Hoover RN, Fraumeni JF Jr. Cancer risk following treatment of childhood cancer. In: Boice JD, Fraumeni JF, eds. *Radiation carcinogenesis: epidemiology and biological significance.* New York: Raven Press, 1984:211.
44. Sankaranarayanan K, Chakraborty R. Cancer predisposition, radiosensitivity and the risk of radiation-induced cancers. I. Background. *Radiat Res* 1995;143:121.
45. Greenblatt MS, Bennett WP, Hollstein M, Harris CC. Mutations in the p53 tumor suppressor gene: clues to cancer etiology and molecular pathogenesis (review). *Cancer Res* 1994;54:4855.
46. Vahakangas KH, Samet JM, Metcalf RA, et al. Mutations of p53 and *ras* genes in radon-associated lung cancer from uranium miners. *Lancet* 1992;339:576.
47. Taylor JA, Watson MA, Devereux TR, Michels RY, Saccomanno G, Anderson M. p53 mutation hotspot in radon-associated lung cancer [see comments]. *Lancet* 1994;343:86.
48. De Benedetti VMG, Travis LB, Welsh JA, et al. p53 mutations in lung cancer following radiation therapy for Hodgkin's disease. *Cancer Epidemiol, Biomarkers and Prevention* 1996;5:93.
49. Rieche K. Carcinogenicity of antineoplastic agents in man (review). *Cancer Treat Rev* 1984;11:39.
50. Sieber SM, Adamson RH. Toxicity of antineoplastic agents in man, chromosomal aberrations antifertility effects, congenital malformations, and carcinogenic potential. *Adv Cancer Res* 1975;22:57.
51. Stolley PD, Hibberd PL. Drugs. In: Schottenfeld D, Fraumeni JF, eds. *Cancer epidemiology and prevention.* Philadelphia: WB Saunders, 1982:304.
52. Haddow A, Harris R, Kon GAR. The growth-inhibitory and carcinogenic properties of 4-aminostilbene and derivatives. *Phil Trans R Soc* 1948;241(Ser A):247.
53. Shimkin B, Weisburger JH, Weisburger EK. Bioassay of 29 alkylating chemicals by the pulmonary-tumor response in strain A mice. *J Natl Cancer Inst* 1966;36:915.
54. Schmähl D, Thomas C, Auer R. *Iatrogenic carcinogenesis.* Berlin: Springer Verlag, 1977.
55. Kyle RA, Pierre RV, Bayrd ED. Multiple myeloma and acute myelomonocytic leukemia. *N Engl J Med* 1970;283:1121.
56. Rosner F, Grunwald H. Multiple myeloma terminating in acute leukemia. Report of 12 cases and review of the literature. *Am J Med* 1974;57:927.
57. Bergsagel DE, Bailey AJ, Langley GR, MacDonald RN, White DF, Miller AB. The chemotherapy on plasma-cell myeloma and the incidence of acute leukemia. *N Engl J Med* 1979;301:743.
58. Bonadonna G, De Lena M, Banfi A, Lattuada A. Secondary neoplasms in malignant lymphomas after intensive therapy. *N Engl J Med* 1973;288:1242.
59. Canellos GP, Arseneau JC, DeVita VT, Whang-Peng J, Johnson RE. Second malignancies complicating Hodgkin's disease in remission. *Lancet* 1975;1:947.
60. Coleman CN, Williams CJ, Flint A, Glatstein EJ, Rosenberg SA, Kaplan HS. Hematologic neoplasia in patients treated for Hodgkin's disease. *N Engl J Med* 1977;297:1249.
61. Levine EG, Bloomfield CD. Leukemias and myelodysplastic syndromes secondary to drug, radiation, and environmental exposure. *Semin Oncol* 1992;19:47.
62. Smith MA, Rubinstein L, Ungerleider RS. Therapy-related acute myeloid leukemia following treatment with epipodophyllotoxins: estimating the risks (review). *Med Pediatr Oncol* 1994;23:86.
63. Pedersen-Bjergaard J, Philip P, Larsen SO, et al. Therapy-related myelodysplasia and acute myeloid leukemia. Cytogenetic characteristics of 115 consecutive cases and risk in seven cohorts of patients treated intensively for malignant diseases in the Copenhagen series. *Leukemia* 1993;7:1975.
64. Pedersen-Bjergaard J, Rowley JD. The balanced and the unbalanced chromosome aberrations of acute myeloid leukemia may develop in different ways and may contribute differently to malignant transformation (review). *Blood* 1994;83:2780.
65. Kaldor JM, Day NE, Hemminki K. Quantifying the carcinogenicity of antineoplastic drugs. *Eur J Cancer Clin Oncol* 1988;24:703.

66. van Leeuwen FE, Chorus AM, van den Belt-Dusebout AW, et al. Leukemia risk following Hodgkin's disease: relation to cumulative dose of alkylating agents, treatment with teniposide combinations, number of episodes of chemotherapy, and bone marrow damage. *J Clin Oncol* 1994;12:1063.
67. Travis LB, Curtis RE, Stovall M, et al. Risk of leukemia following treatment for non-Hodgkin's lymphoma. *J Natl Cancer Inst* 1994;86:1450.
68. Cuzick J, Erskine S, Edelman D, Galton DA. A comparison of the incidence of the myelodysplastic syndrome and acute myeloid leukaemia following melphalan and cyclophosphamide treatment for myelomatosis. A report to the Medical Research Council's working party on leukaemia in adults. *Br J Cancer* 1987;55:523.
69. Greene MH, Harris EL, Gershenson DM, et al. Melphalan may be a more potent leukemogen than cyclophosphamide. *Ann Intern Med* 1986;105:360.
70. Stone RM, Neuberg D, Soiffer R, et al. Myelodysplastic syndrome as a late complication following autologous bone marrow transplantation for non-Hodgkin's lymphoma. *J Clin Oncol* 1994;12:2535.
71. Henry-Amar M. Second cancer after the treatment for Hodgkin's disease: a report from the International Database on Hodgkin's Disease. *Ann Oncol* 1992;3(Suppl 4):117.
72. Michels SD, McKenna RW, Arthur DC, Brunning RD. Therapy-related acute myeloid leukemia and myelodysplastic syndrome: a clinical and morphologic study of 65 cases. *Blood* 1985;65:1364.
73. Pedersen-Bjergaard J, Philip P, Larsen SO, Jensen G, Byrsting K. Chromosome aberrations and prognostic factors in therapy-related myelodysplasia and acute nonlymphocytic leukemia. *Blood* 1990; 76:1083.
74. Pedersen-Bjergaard J, Philip P. Balanced translocations involving chromosome bands 11q23 and 21q22 are highly characteristic of myelodysplasia and leukemia following therapy with cytostatic agents targeting at DNA-topoisomerase II (letter). *Blood* 1991;78:1147.
75. Rubin CM, Arthur DC, Woods WG, et al. Therapy-related myelodysplastic syndrome and acute myeloid leukemia in children: correlation between chromosomal abnormalities and prior therapy. *Blood* 1991; 78:2982.
76. Pedersen-Bjergaard J, Sigsgaard TC, Nielsen D, et al. Acute monocytic or myelomonocytic leukemia with balanced chromosome translocations to band 11q23 after therapy with 4-epi-doxorubicin and cisplatin or cyclophosphamide for breast cancer [see comments]. *J Clin Oncol* 1992;10:1444.
77. Sandoval C, Pui CH, Bowman LC, et al. Secondary acute myeloid leukemia in children previously treated with alkylating agents, intercalating topoisomerase II inhibitors, and irradiation. *J Clin Oncol* 1993;11:1039.
78. Travis LB, Curtis RE, Glimelius B, et al. Bladder and kidney cancer following cyclophosphamide therapy for non-Hodgkin's lymphoma. *J Natl Cancer Inst* 1995;87:524.
79. Pedersen-Bjergaard J, Ersboll J, Hansen VL, et al. Carcinoma of the urinary bladder after treatment with cyclophosphamide for non-Hodgkin's lymphoma. *N Engl J Med* 1988;318:1028.
80. Kaldor JM, Day NE, Kittelmann B, et al. Bladder tumours following chemotherapy and radiotherapy for ovarian cancer: a case-control study. *Int J Cancer* 1996;63:1.
81. Kaldor JM, Day NE, Bell J, et al. Lung cancer following Hodgkin's disease: a case-control study. *Int J Cancer* 1992;52:677.
82. Swerdlow AJ, Barber JA, Horwich A, Cunningham D, Milan S, Omar RZ. Second malignancy in patients with Hodgkin's disease treated at the Royal Marsden Hospital. *Br J Cancer* 1997;75:116.
83. Anonymous. Overall evaluations of carcinogenicity: an updating of IARC Monographs volumes 1 to 42. *IARC Monogr Eval Carcinog Risks Hum Suppl* 1987;7:1.
84. Schoenberg BS, Myers MH. Statistical methods for studying multiple primary malignant neoplasms. *Cancer* 1977;40:1892.
85. Makuch R, Simon R. Recommendations for the analysis of the effect of treatment on the development of second malignancies. *Cancer* 1979;44:250.
86. Kaplan EL, Meier P. Non-parametric estimation from incomplete observations. *J Am Stat Assoc* 1958;53:457.
87. Pepe MS, Mori M. Kaplan-Meier, marginal or conditional probability curves in summarizing competing risks failure time data? *Stat Med* 1993;12:737.
88. Darrington DL, Vose JM, Anderson JR, et al. Incidence and characterization of secondary myelodysplastic syndrome and acute myelogenous leukemia following high-dose chemoradiotherapy and autologous stem-cell transplantation for lymphoid malignancies. *J Clin Oncol* 1994;12:2527.
89. Mauch PM, Kalish LA, Marcus KC, et al. Long-term survival in Hodgkin's disease: relative impact of mortality, second tumors, infection, and cardiovascular disease. *Cancer J Sci Am* 1995;1:33.
90. Travis LB, Curtis RE, Glimelius B, et al. Second cancers among long-term survivors of non-Hodgkin's lymphoma. *J Natl Cancer Inst* 1993; 85:1932.
91. Cox DR. Regression models and life-tables. *J R Stat Soc B* 1972;334:187.
92. Breslow NE, Day NE. *Statistical methods in cancer research: the design and analysis of cohort studies, vol 2.* IARC Scientific Publications no. 82. Lyons, France: International Agency for Research on Cancer, 1987.
93. Kaldor JM, Day NE, Band P, et al. Second malignancies following testicular cancer, ovarian cancer and Hodgkin's disease: an international collaborative study among cancer registries. *Int J Cancer* 1987;39:571.
94. Boice JD Jr, Day NE, Andersen A, et al. Second cancers following radiation treatment for cervical cancer. An international collaboration among cancer registries. *J Natl Cancer Inst* 1985;74:955.
95. Storm HH, Prener A. Second cancer following lymphatic and hematopoietic cancers in Denmark, 1943–80. *Natl Cancer Inst Monogr* 1985;68:389.
96. Greene MH. Is cisplatin a human carcinogen? *J Natl Cancer Inst* 1992;84:306.
97. Dietrich PY, Henry-Amar M, Cosset JM, Bodis S, Bosq J, Hayat M. Second primary cancers in patients continuously disease-free from Hodgkin's disease: a protective role for the spleen? *Blood* 1994;84: 1209.
98. Valagussa P, Santoro A, Fossati-Bellani F, Banfi A, Bonadonna G. Second acute leukemia and other malignancies following treatment for Hodgkin's disease. *J Clin Oncol* 1986;4:830.
99. Ewertz M, Machado SG, Boice JD Jr, Jensen OM. Endometrial cancer following treatment for breast cancer: a case-control study in Denmark. *Br J Cancer* 1984;50:687.
100. Boice JD Jr, Harvey EB, Blettner M, Stovall M, Flannery JT. Cancer in the contralateral breast after radiotherapy for breast cancer [see comments]. *N Engl J Med* 1992;326:781.
101. Arseneau JC, Sponzo RW, Levin DL, et al. Nonlymphomatous malignant tumors complicating Hodgkin's disease. Possible association with intensive therapy. *N Engl J Med* 1972;287:1119.
102. Valagussa PA, Bonadonna G. Carcinogenic effects of cancer treatment. In: Peckham M, Pinedo H, Veronesi U, eds. *Oxford textbook of oncology.* Oxford: Oxford University Press, 1995:2348.
103. Abrahamsen JF, Andersen A, Hannisdal E, et al. Second malignancies after treatment of Hodgkin's disease: the influence of treatment, follow-up time, and age [see comments]. *J Clin Oncol* 1993;11:255.
104. Boivin JF, Hutchison GB, Zauber AG, et al. Incidence of second cancers in patients treated for Hodgkin's disease [see comments]. *J Natl Cancer Inst* 1995;87:732.
105. Henry-Amar M, Dietrich PY. Acute leukemia after the treatment of Hodgkin's disease. *Hematol Oncol Clin North Am* 1993;7:369.
106. Mauch PM, Kalish LA, Marcus KC, et al. Second malignancies after treatment for laparotomy staged IA–IIIB Hodgkin's disease: long-term analysis of risk factors and outcome. *Blood* 1996;87:3625.
107. Sankila R, Garwicz S, Olsen JH, et al. Risk of subsequent malignant neoplasms among 1,641 Hodgkin's disease patients diagnosed in childhood and adolescence: a population-based cohort study in the five Nordic countries. Association of the Nordic Cancer Registries and the Nordic Society of Pediatric Hematology and Oncology. *J Clin Oncol* 1996;14:1442.
108. Boivin JF, Hutchison GB, Lyden M, Godbold J, Chorosh J, Schottenfeld D. Second primary cancers following treatment of Hodgkin's disease. *J Natl Cancer Inst* 1984;72:233.
109. Cimino G, Papa G, Tura S, et al. Second primary cancer following Hodgkin's disease: updated results of an Italian multicentric study. *J Clin Oncol* 1991;9:432.
110. Devereux S, Selassie TG, Vaughan Hudson G, Vaughan Hudson B, Linch DC. Leukaemia complicating treatment for Hodgkin's disease: the experience of the British National Lymphoma Investigation. *Br Med J* 1990;301:1077.
111. Schellong G, Riepenhausen M, Creutzig U, et al. Low risk of secondary leukemias after chemotherapy without mechlorethamine in

childhood Hodgkin's disease. German-Austrian Pediatric Hodgkin's Disease Group. *J Clin Oncol* 1997;15:2247.

112. Canellos GP. Can MOPP be replaced in the treatment of advanced Hodgkin's disease? *Semin Oncol* 1990;17:2.
113. Viviani S, Bonadonna G, Santoro A, et al. Alternating versus hybrid MOPP-ABVD in Hodgkin's disease: the Milan experience. *Ann Oncol* 1991;2(Suppl 2):55.
114. Rosenberg SA. The management of Hodgkin's disease: half a century of change. The Kaplan Memorial Lecture. *Ann Oncol* 1996;7:555.
115. Tester WJ, Kinsella TJ, Waller B, et al. Second malignant neoplasms complicating Hodgkin's disease: the National Cancer Institute experience. *J Clin Oncol* 1984;2:762.
116. Mauch PM, Canellos GP, Rosenthal DS, Hellman S. Reduction of fatal complications from combined modality therapy in Hodgkin's disease. *J Clin Oncol* 1985;3:501.
117. Andrieu JM, Ifrah N, Payen C, Fermanian J, Coscas Y, Flandrin G. Increased risk of secondary acute nonlymphocytic leukemia after extended-field radiation therapy combined with MOPP chemotherapy for Hodgkin's disease [see comments]. *J Clin Oncol* 1990;8:1148.
118. Blayney DW, Longo DL, Young RC, et al. Decreasing risk of leukemia with prolonged follow-up after chemotherapy and radiotherapy for Hodgkin's disease. *N Engl J Med* 1987;316:710.
119. Tura S, Fiacchini M, Zinzani PL, Brusamolino E, Gobbi PG. Splenectomy and the increasing risk of secondary acute leukemia in Hodgkin's disease [see comments]. *J Clin Oncol* 1993;11:925.
120. van Leeuwen FE, Somers R, Hart AA. Splenectomy in Hodgkin's disease and second leukaemias (letter). *Lancet* 1987;2:210.
121. Meadows AT, Obringer AC, Marrero O, et al. Second malignant neoplasms following childhood Hodgkin's disease: treatment and splenectomy as risk factors. *Med Pediatr Oncol* 1989;17:477.
122. Swerdlow AJ, Douglas AJ, Vaughan Hudson G, Vaughan Hudson B, MacLennan KA. Risk of second primary cancer after Hodgkin's disease in patients in the British National Lymphoma Investigation: relationships to host factors, histology and stage of Hodgkin's disease, and splenectomy. *Br J Cancer* 1993;68:1006.
123. van der Velden JW, van Putten WL, Guinee VF, et al. Subsequent development of acute non-lymphocytic leukemia in patients treated for Hodgkin's disease. *Int J Cancer* 1988;42:252.
124. Burns CP, Stjernholm RL, Kellermeyer RW. Hodgkin's disease terminating in acute lymphosarcoma cell leukemia. A metabolic study. *Cancer* 1971;27:806.
125. Krikorian JG, Burke JS, Rosenberg SA, Kaplan HS. Occurrence of non-Hodgkin's lymphoma after therapy for Hodgkin's disease. *N Engl J Med* 1979;300:452.
126. Kim H, Zelman RJ, Fox MA, et al. Pathology Panel for Lymphoma Clinical Studies: a comprehensive analysis of cases accumulated since its inception. *J Natl Cancer Inst* 1982;68:43.
127. Bennett MH, MacLennan KA, Vaughan Hudson G, Vaughan Hudson B. Non-Hodgkin's lymphoma arising in patients treated for Hodgkin's disease in the BNLI: a 20-year experience. British National Lymphoma Investigation. *Ann Oncol* 1991;2(Suppl 2):83.
128. Penn I. Cancers complicating organ transplantation. *N Engl J Med* 1990;323:1767.
129. van Rijswijk RE, Verbeek J, Haanen C, Dekker AW, van Daal WA, van Peperzeel HA. Major complications and causes of death in patients treated for Hodgkin's disease. *J Clin Oncol* 1987;5:1624.
130. Zarate-Osorno A, Medeiros LJ, Longo DL, Jaffe ES. Non-Hodgkin's lymphomas arising in patients successfully treated for Hodgkin's disease. A clinical, histologic, and immunophenotypic study of 14 cases. *Am J Surg Pathol* 1992;16:885.
131. Boivin JF, O'Brien K. Solid cancer risk after treatment of Hodgkin's disease. *Cancer* 1988;61:2541.
132. Sont JK, van Stiphout WA, Noordijk EM, et al. Increased risk of second cancers in managing Hodgkins disease: the 20-year Leiden experience. *Ann Hematol* 1992;65:213.
133. Rodriguez MA, Fuller LM, Zimmerman SO, et al. Hodgkin's disease: study of treatment intensities and incidences of second malignancies. *Ann Oncol* 1993;4:125.
134. Biti G, Cellai E, Magrini SM, Papi MG, Ponticelli P, Boddi V. Second solid tumors and leukemia after treatment for Hodgkin's disease: an analysis of 1121 patients from a single institution. *Int J Radiat Oncol Biol Phys* 1994;29:25.
135. Bhatia S, Robison LL, Oberlin O. Late effects of treatment for childhood Hodgkin's disease. *N Engl J Med* 1996;335:353.
136. Tarbell NJ, Gelber RD, Weinstein HJ, Mauch P. Sex differences in risk of second malignant tumours after Hodgkin's disease in childhood. *Lancet* 1993;341:1428.
137. Tucker MA, Misfeldt D, Coleman CN, Clark WH Jr, Rosenberg SA. Cutaneous malignant melanoma after Hodgkin's disease. *Ann Intern Med* 1985;102:37.
138. Hancock SL, Cox RS, McDougall IR. Thyroid diseases after treatment of Hodgkin's disease. *N Engl J Med* 1991;325:599.
139. Birdwell SH, Hancock SL, Varghese A, Cox RS, Hoppe RT. Gastrointestinal cancer after treatment of Hodgkin's disease. *Int J Radiat Oncol Biol Phys* 1997;37:67.
140. Travis LB, Curtis RE, Boice JD Jr. Late effects of treatment for childhood Hodgkin's disease. *N Engl J Med* 1996;335:352.
141. Aisenberg AC, Finkelstein DM, Doppke KP, Koerner FC, Boivin JF, Willett CG. High risk of breast carcinoma after irradiation of young women with Hodgkin's disease. *Cancer* 1997;79:1203.
142. Hildreth NG, Shore RE, Dvoretsky PM. The risk of breast cancer after irradiation of the thymus in infancy. *N Engl J Med* 1989;321:1281.
143. Donaldson SS, Hancock SL. Second cancers after Hodgkin's disease in childhood [see comments]. *N Engl J Med* 1996;334:792.
144. Yahalom J, Petrek JA, Biddinger PW, et al. Breast cancer in patients irradiated for Hodgkin's disease: a clinical and pathologic analysis of 45 events in 37 patients [see comments]. *J Clin Oncol* 1992;10:1674.
145. Tucker MA. Solid second cancers following Hodgkin's disease. *Hematol Oncol Clin North Am* 1993;7:389.
146. Cadman EC, Capizzi RL, Bertino JR. Acute nonlymphocytic leukemia: a delayed complication of Hodgkin's disease therapy: analysis of 109 cases. *Cancer* 1977;40:1280.
147. De Witte T, Muus P, De Pauw B, Haanen C. Intensive antileukemic treatment of patients younger than 65 years with myelodysplastic syndromes and secondary acute myelogenous leukemia. *Cancer* 1990;66:831.
148. Hoyle CF, de Bastos M, Wheatley K, et al. AML associated with previous cytotoxic therapy, MDS or myeloproliferative disorders: results from the MRC's 9th AML trial. *Br J Haematol* 1989;72:45.

148a. Vaughan WP, Karp JE, Burke PJ. Effective chemotherapy of acute myelocytic leukemia occurring after alkylating agent or radiation therapy for prior malignancy. *J. Clin Oncol* 1983;1:204.

149. Preisler HD, Early AP, Raza A, et al. Therapy of secondary acute nonlymphocytic leukemia with cytarabine. *N Engl J Med* 1983;308:21.
150. Longmore G, Guinan EC, Weinstein HJ, Gelber RD, Rappeport JM, Antin JH. Bone marrow transplantation for myelodysplasia and secondary acute nonlymphoblastic leukemia. *J Clin Oncol* 1990;8:1707.
151. Jacquillat C, Khayat D, Desprez-Curely JP, et al. Non-Hodgkin's lymphoma occurring after Hodgkin's disease. Four new cases and a review of the literature. *Cancer* 1984;53:459.
152. Chung CT, Bogart JA, Adams JF, et al. Increased risk of breast cancer in splenectomized patients undergoing radiation therapy for Hodgkin's disease. *Int J Radiat Oncol Biol Phys* 1997;37:405.
153. Anonymous. Systemic treatment of early breast cancer by hormonal, cytotoxic, or immune therapy. 133 randomised trials involving 31,000 recurrences and 24,000 deaths among 75,000 women. Early Breast Cancer Trialists' Collaborative Group [see comments]. *Lancet* 1992;339:1.
154. Savitsky K, Bar-Shira A, Gilad S, et al. A single ataxia telangiectasia gene with a product similar to PI-3 kinase [see comments]. *Science* 1995;268:1749.
155. Easton DF. Cancer risks in A-T heterozygotes. *Int J Radiat Biol* 1994;66:S177.
156. Swift M, Morrell D, Massey RB, Chase CL. Incidence of cancer in 161 families affected by ataxia-telangiectasia [see comments]. *N Engl J Med* 1991;325:1831.
157. Boice JD Jr, Travis LB. Body wars: effect of friendly fire (cancer therapy) . *J Natl Cancer Inst* 1995;87:705.

Hodgkin's Disease, edited by P. M. Mauch,
J. O. Armitage, V. Diehl, R. T. Hoppe, and L. M. Weiss.
Lippincott Williams & Wilkins, Philadephia ©1999.

CHAPTER 34

Pulmonary Late Effects After Treatment of Hodgkin's Disease

Jean-Marc Cosset and Richard T. Hoppe

HISTORICAL ASPECTS

The pathology as well as the main clinical and radiologic features of lung injury resulting from therapeutic irradiation were described in detail in the 1960s and 1970s (1–4). Until recently, there was general agreement that there were two successive and distinct phases of lung damage secondary to irradiation and it was common to consider these two phases in defining the pulmonary problems observed after supradiaphragmatic radiotherapy for Hodgkin's disease (2).

The first phase of radiation injury is generally referred to as radiation pneumonitis. Because radiation pneumonitis usually occurs within the first 6 months after irradiation, it is often called the acute or early phase of radiation injury. It is characterized by local pulmonary edema with deposition of fibrin-like material in the alveolar spaces. These phenomena are responsible for both the clinical symptoms and radiologic changes of radiation pneumonitis.

The second phase, often referred to as the chronic or late phase, is characterized by the progressive development of a diffuse fibrosis of the septa in the irradiated lung. In some instances, this fibrosis can lead to a complete obliteration of the air spaces. Clinical and radiologic consequences clearly depend on the proportional volume of the lung irradiated and the severity of the fibrosis.

Clinicians felt there was no correlation between these two successive phases: patients experiencing severe acute radiation pneumonitis did not necessarily develop subsequent lung fibrosis, while other patients who experienced progressive severe pulmonary fibrosis did not show evidence of acute symptoms within the first 6 months after their irradiation. However, it was well known that the two phases of lung injury sometimes overlapped, and that the clinical and radiologic distinction between the so-called acute and chronic phases was not always easy to define. Recent studies, based in particular on molecular biology, shed new light on the question, and strongly suggest that the above-mentioned successive events could be viewed as a continuum, with no clear distinction between the temporal sequence of the different pulmonary reactions (5). Available data show an early (2 weeks) activation of an inflammatory reaction, involving in particular interleukin-1α (IL-1α) and transforming growth factor-β (TGF-β), leading to the expression and maintenance of a cytokine cascade, ultimately resulting in the overexpression of collagen genes (5,6). If confirmed, this concept could lead to possible countermeasures aimed at reducing the incidence and severity of postradiation pulmonary injury. Because so-called late pulmonary toxicity is no longer considered to be totally disconnected from the early phase, both early and late postradiation complications will be analyzed below.

In the late 1970s, ABVD [Adriamycin (doxorubicin), bleomycin, vinblastine, and dacarbazine] (7) combination chemotherapy was introduced and became rapidly successful. The potential pulmonary toxicity of the bleomycin component had been recognized (8), the most frequent observation being the development of an interstitial pneumonitis and subsequent fibrosis.

Recent data suggest that activation of interstitial macrophages to secrete an epidermal growth factor (EGF)-like growth factor (9), as well as an increase of tumor necrosis factor-α (TNF-α) (10), may contribute to this bleomycin-related pulmonary toxicity.

Therefore, two essential types of pulmonary toxicity that may occur after treatment of Hodgkin's disease are

J.-M. Cosset: Department of Radiation Oncology, Institut Curie, Paris, France.
R. T. Hoppe: Department of Radiation Oncology, Stanford University, Stanford, California.

analyzed in this chapter, the first one being linked to irradiation and the second to bleomycin. We also consider the combination of both irradiation and bleomycin, as well as the cofactors that modulate those toxicities.

TREATMENT-RELATED PULMONARY DAMAGES

Lung

Clinical Symptomatology

Clinical Symptoms After Irradiation

A dry hacking cough, otherwise unexplained, is the most common pulmonary symptom in the first months following standard mantle-field irradiation (2). It was reported to occur in as many as 66% of patients in the Stanford experience (11). Other papers confirmed this frequency (12). This cough usually lasts for 2 to 4 months and then gradually disappears, requiring only symptomatic treatment. Interestingly, a long-term analysis performed 10 to 18 years after mantle-field irradiation in a Dutch series (13) showed that patients reported a significantly higher rate of coughing (39.7%) than a control population of hospital visitors (21.1%). Early dyspnea on exertion (rarely at rest) is another frequent symptom after mantle-field irradiation. It was reported in 76% of the patients at Stanford (11) and in 47% in a French series (12). The evolution of this symptomatology usually parallels the one of coughing, with a progressive improvement after a few months. More recent data analyzed the long-term incidence of dyspnea. The above-mentioned Dutch study (13) found that 44.7% of patients treated 10 to 18 years before reported dyspnea (vs. 32.7% in the control group). In a smaller Swedish series, 20% of patients complained of dyspnea on exertion after a median follow-up of 15 years (14). A Norwegian study also reported dyspnea on exertion in 30% of patients, 5 to 13 years after supradiaphragmatic irradiation (15). These clinical symptoms (cough and dyspnea) are widely considered to be mild and transient after mantle-field irradiation. However, recent data seem to support the idea that a significant number of patients (about one-third) could still complain of some coughing and dyspnea more than 10 years after their treatment (Fig. 1).

Clinical Symptoms After Bleomycin

The most common clinical symptoms of bleomycin-induced interstitial fibrosis are dyspnea, nonproductive cough, and fever. The onset is usually subacute to insidious, although acute presentations or even fulminant courses have also been reported (8). Most often, symptoms develop 4 to 10 weeks posttreatment, but pulmonary toxicity can occur up to 6 months following discontinuation of chemotherapy.

Substernal and pleuritic chest pains have also been reported after bleomycin administration.

Only a few authors have reported in detail the degree of clinical impairment, most often after a combination of a bleomycin-containing regimen (ABVD) and radiotherapy. Six months to 3 years after three courses of ABVD and mediastinal irradiation, dyspnea was recorded in 15% of the patients in a French study (16).

Radiologic Changes

Radiologic Changes After Irradiation

The usual radiologic changes after conventional mantle-field irradiation were described in detail by Henry Kaplan (2). He reported that typically there was little or even no radiologic evidence of pulmonary reactions until 2 to 3 months posttherapy. The mediastinal silhouette could then show a somewhat shaggy appearance, with irregular stranding appearing in the paramediastinal pulmonary parenchyma. Modern techniques (computed tomographic [CT] scanning and nuclear magnetic resonance imaging) now confirm that these images can be closely linked to the size and shape of the mediastinal fields.

In the long term, a progressive fibrotic retraction is usually observed, sometimes leading to a near disappearance of the lesions on standard chest radiographs. However, residual lymph node masses (occasionally with calcifications) together with fibrosis, may persist for life, particularly after the treatment of bulky mediastinal disease. The severity of these changes is not systematically correlated with clinical symptoms or functional impairment (Figs. 1 to 3) (17–22). Splenic irradiation leads to limited radiation pneumonitis of the left lung base, followed by a local pleural thickening, often without any clinical symptoms.

Radiologic Manifestations of Bleomycin-Induced Toxicity

The classic radiographic pattern of bleomycin-induced interstitial fibrosis is marked by bibasilar reticular or fine nodular infiltrates (8,23,24). The earliest changes often occur as a triangular-shaped infiltrate in the costophrenic angles. Infiltrates may then progress to involve the middle and upper areas of the lungs. Various radiologic changes have been reported: reticular, reticulonodular, patchy alveolar or bandlike infiltrates, nodular shadows, and even lobar consolidation. Rarely, large nodules can even mimic metastatic lung disease.

The radiographic abnormalities associated with bleomycin toxicity are usually bilateral, but asymmetric or focal lesions have also been described. CT scans may show subtle changes that cannot be seen on chest radiographs. In a series of 100 patients receiving bleomycin,

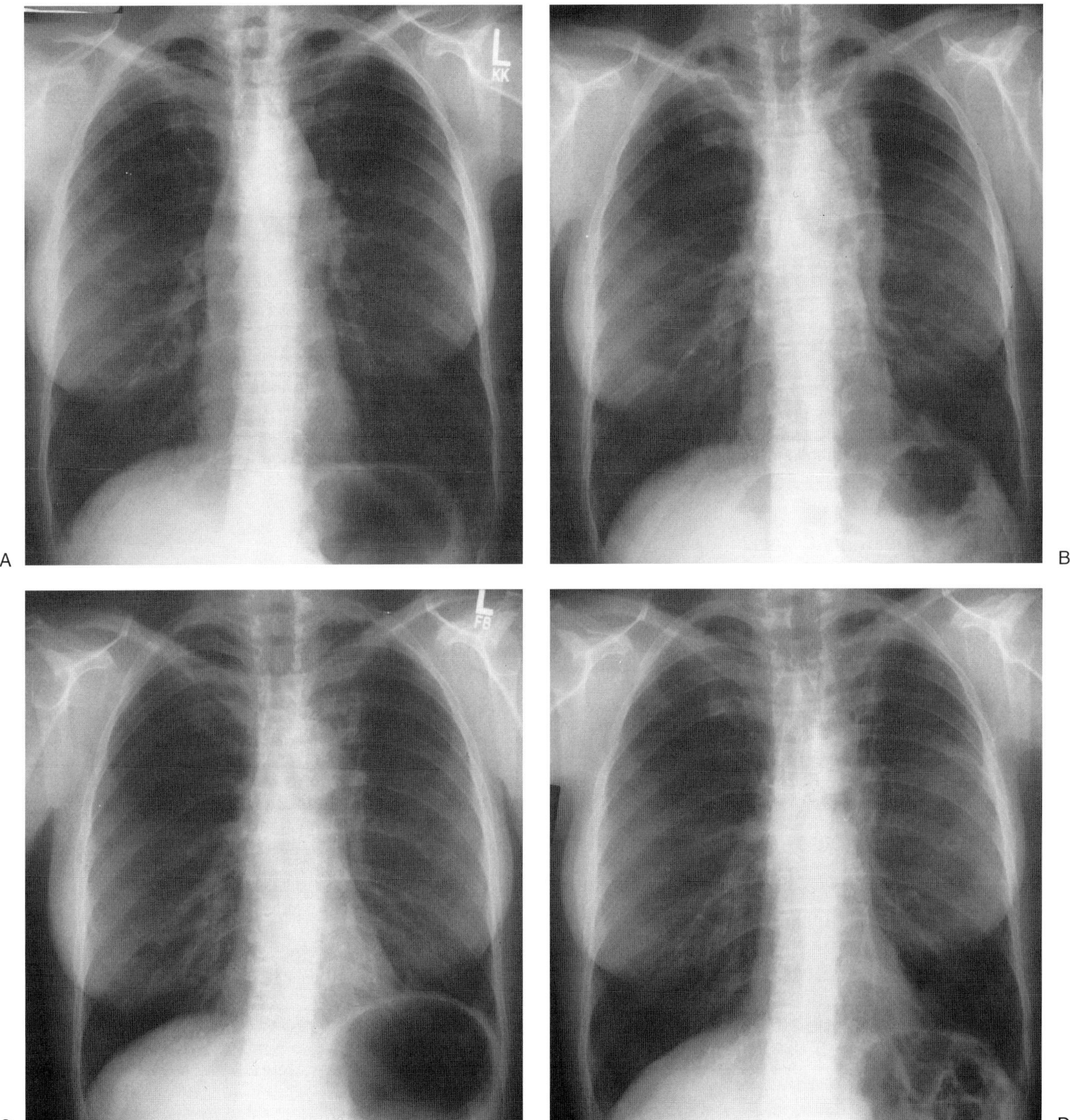

FIG. 1. Radiation fibrosis in a 49-year-old woman. **A:** Pretreatment chest radiograph showing mediastinal adenopathy in a woman with clinical stage (CS) IA nodular sclerosing Hodgkin's disease. **B:** Six weeks after the completion of mantle irradiation (43.8 Gy). Note acute radiation pneumonitis in the mantle-field distribution. This was an incidental finding; the patient was asymptomatic. **C:** Nine months after completion of therapy, radiation fibrosis has set in. **D:** Four and a half years after completion of irradiation, changes have stabilized on chest radiograph. The patient suffers from a chronic dry cough.

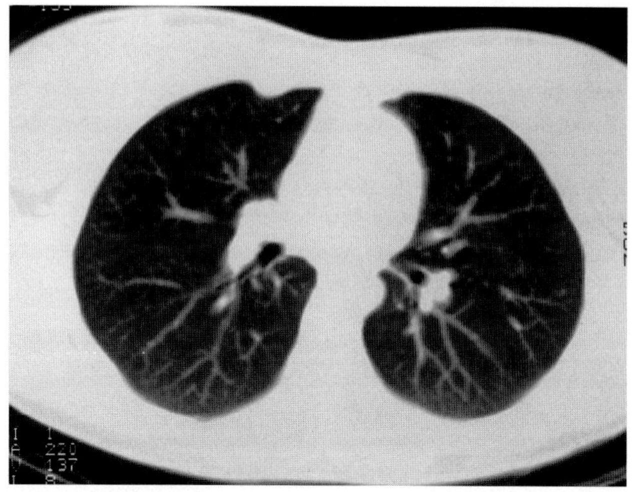

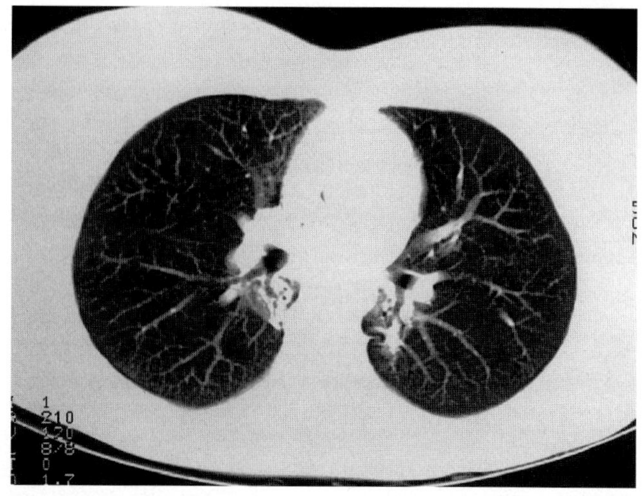

FIG. 2. Radiation pneumonitis in an 18-year-old woman. **A:** Pretreatment chest CT scan (lung window) through the region of the pulmonary hila. Note internal mammary adenopathy. **B:** Four months after completion of mantle irradiation (36 Gy). Note prominent pneumonitis posterior to the hila. The changes anterior to the right hilum are subtle. The patient was asymptomatic.

abnormalities visible on CT scans developed in 38 patients; only 15 of them had lesions on their plain radiographs (25). When associated with radiotherapy, bleomycin appears to amplify the radiation-induced changes described previously (Fig. 4).

Functional Impairment

Functional Impairment After Irradiation

Data going back to the 1970s have shown that pulmonary function tests (primarily vital capacity) usually

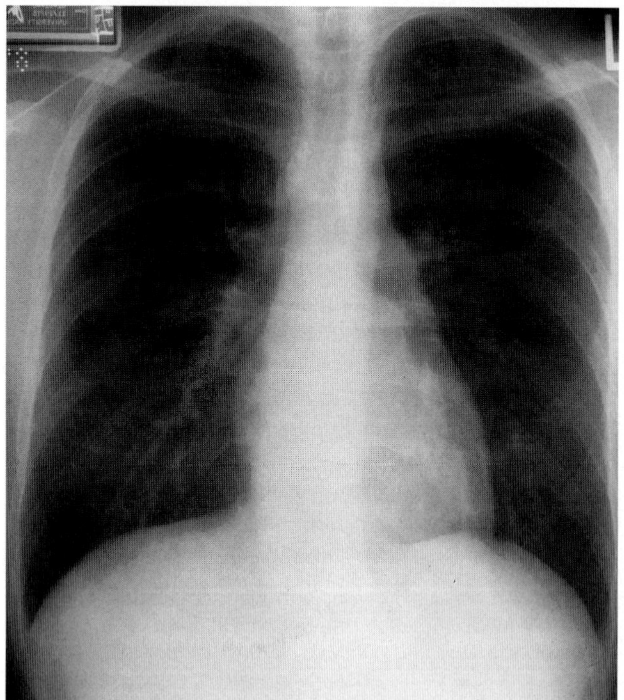

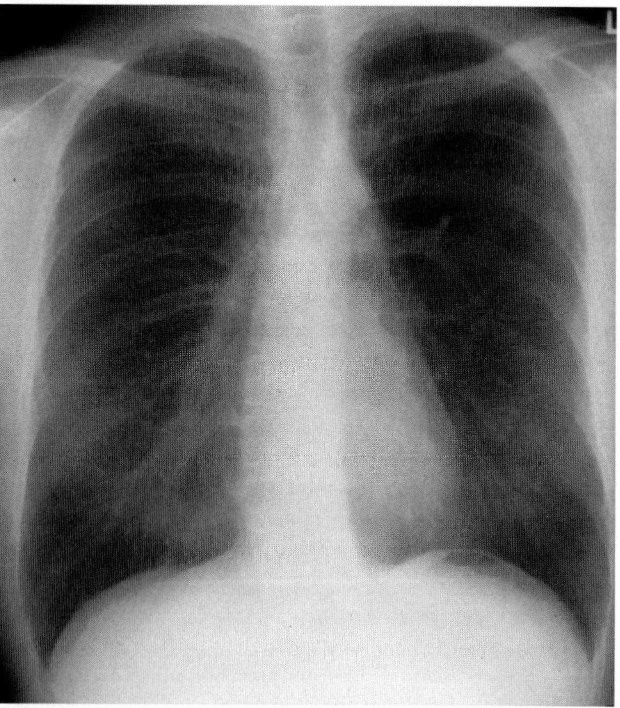

FIG. 3. Long-term changes after mantle irradiation. **A:** Chest radiograph in a 26-year-old man with pathologic stage (PS) IIIEB Hodgkin's disease immediately following MOPP [mechlorethamine, Oncovin (vincristine), procarbazine, and prednisone] chemotherapy and mantle irradiation (50 Gy to mediastinum and 15.6 Gy to left lung through partial transmission lung block). **B:** Chest radiograph 19 years later. Note apical changes, paramediastinal stranding, and upward retraction of hila. The patient never experienced any respiratory symptoms related to his radiation and at 19 years had normal screening stress echocardiography, baseline and stress electrocardiograms, and stress thallium studies.

drop to 70% to 80% of the normal theoretical value 6 to 12 months after completion of mantle therapy (26–30a). In a number of studies, a return to baseline has been noted for most patients after 1 to 2 years (26,27,31,32). However, other authors reported a persistent reduction in functional lung volumes (19,20,33,34). Recently, a number of (very) long-term analyses of pulmonary function appeared in the literature. Four to 13 years after mantle-field irradiation, Jensen et al. (35) detected some restrictive function impairment. Interestingly, they observed that static lung volumes were larger 8 to 13 years after treatment than at 4 to 8 years posttherapy, suggesting long-term recovery. With a median follow-up of 15 years, Gustausson et al. (14) reported minor restrictive ventilatory defects in 25 patients. Even when a significant decrease was detected, the impairment seemed small, with only four patients falling outside the normal range for vital capacity (VC) and total lung capacity (TLC). There was no evidence of airflow obstruction, and only minor abnormalities in gas exchanges. As would be expected, lung scintigrams showed perfusion and ventilation defects in 84% of the patients, located primarily in the apices. With a mean follow-up of 14 years, Hassink et al. (13) analyzed pulmonary morbidity in 78 patients. The mean value of all the function tests performed fell in a normal range.

At Stanford, pulmonary function was tested before treatment, early after treatment, and more than 3 years posttherapy. The decrease in forced vital capacity (FVC) and carbon monoxide diffusing capacity of the lungs (DLCO) observed in the first 15 months was followed by recovery in most patients. Overall, about 30% of patients had FVC values less than 80% of predicted, while only 7% of patients had a DLCO less than 80% of predicted. No patients experienced pulmonary toxicity severe enough to require hospitalization (36). In a series of patients tested 5 to 13 years after treatment, Lund et al. (15) detected a decrease in TLC, FVC, and DLCO in about one-third of their patients. However, the mean value of the total study group fell in the normal range.

A recent update at 5 years of the toxicity studies of the European Organization for the Research and Treatment of Cancer (EORTC) H_7 trial (M. Henry-Amar, personal communication) shows a mean vital capacity of 92% after subtotal nodal irradiation, and of 100% in the arms including MOPP [nitrogen mustard, Oncovin (vincristine), procarbazine, and prednisone]/ABV or EBVP [epirubicin, bleomycin, vinblastine, and prednisone] combined with irradiation. Boersma et al. (37) proposed calculating an overall response parameter, based on a three-dimensional dose distribution and average dose-effect relations for local perfusion or ventilation [calculated using single photon emission computed tomography (SPECT) and CT scanning]. This could be predictive of the radiation-induced change in pulmonary function.

This review of available data on long-term pulmonary function after mantle-field radiotherapy of Hodgkin's disease therefore seems to indicate that a large majority of patients can be cured without any clinically significant long-term functional pulmonary impairment. Severe acute functional impairment linked to acute pneumonitis usually dramatically improves after adequate treatment (see below), and resolves without long-term functional alterations.

Functional Impairment After Bleomycin

The large majority of the studies of functional pulmonary impairment after bleomycin administration report data for patients with solid tumors treated with bleomycin. A number of confounding factors in these patients (anemia, intercurrent surgery, pulmonary metastases, poor performance status) make it difficult to extrapolate the data to patients with Hodgkin's disease (8).

Most studies report a decrease of vital capacity and DLCO in patients showing bleomycin-induced interstitial fibrosis. A steep rate of fall of the vital capacity is considered by some authors as a warning of impending toxicity (38). However, the functional tests do not systematically parallel clinical symptoms and radiologic signs; there are reports of clinical toxicity and radiologic changes despite a normal DLCO (39). In contrast, a DLCO decrease may be detected in some patients in the absence of any clinical symptoms or radiologic signs of toxicity (8). Nevertheless, in clinical practice, the detection of abnormalities in pulmonary function tests usually lead to the discontinuation of bleomycin.

As with radiotherapy, long-term improvement in pulmonary function is possible after bleomycin administration. Experience of patients with germ-cell tumors show a potential for recovery, which may be better for vital capacity than for DLCO (8,40).

Pleura

Pleural Symptoms After Irradiation

Pleural problems were not even mentioned in the chapter devoted to complications of radiotherapy in Kaplan's 1980 book (2). When they are sought, minor pleural alterations (thickening, pleural effusions) are frequently found. Brice et al. (16) reported that CT scans showed small pleural effusions with pleural thickening after radiation in 19 out of 40 patients, and mediastinal and/or apical fibrosis in 15. However, clinically significant symptoms are rare, unless suboptimal irradiation has been delivered. Severe bilateral pleural effusions have been observed, for example, after irradiation delivered with large doses per fraction (41,42) (see below). Pneumothorax, probably due to irradiation of the pulmonary apex, has been reported in the absence of concurrent pul-

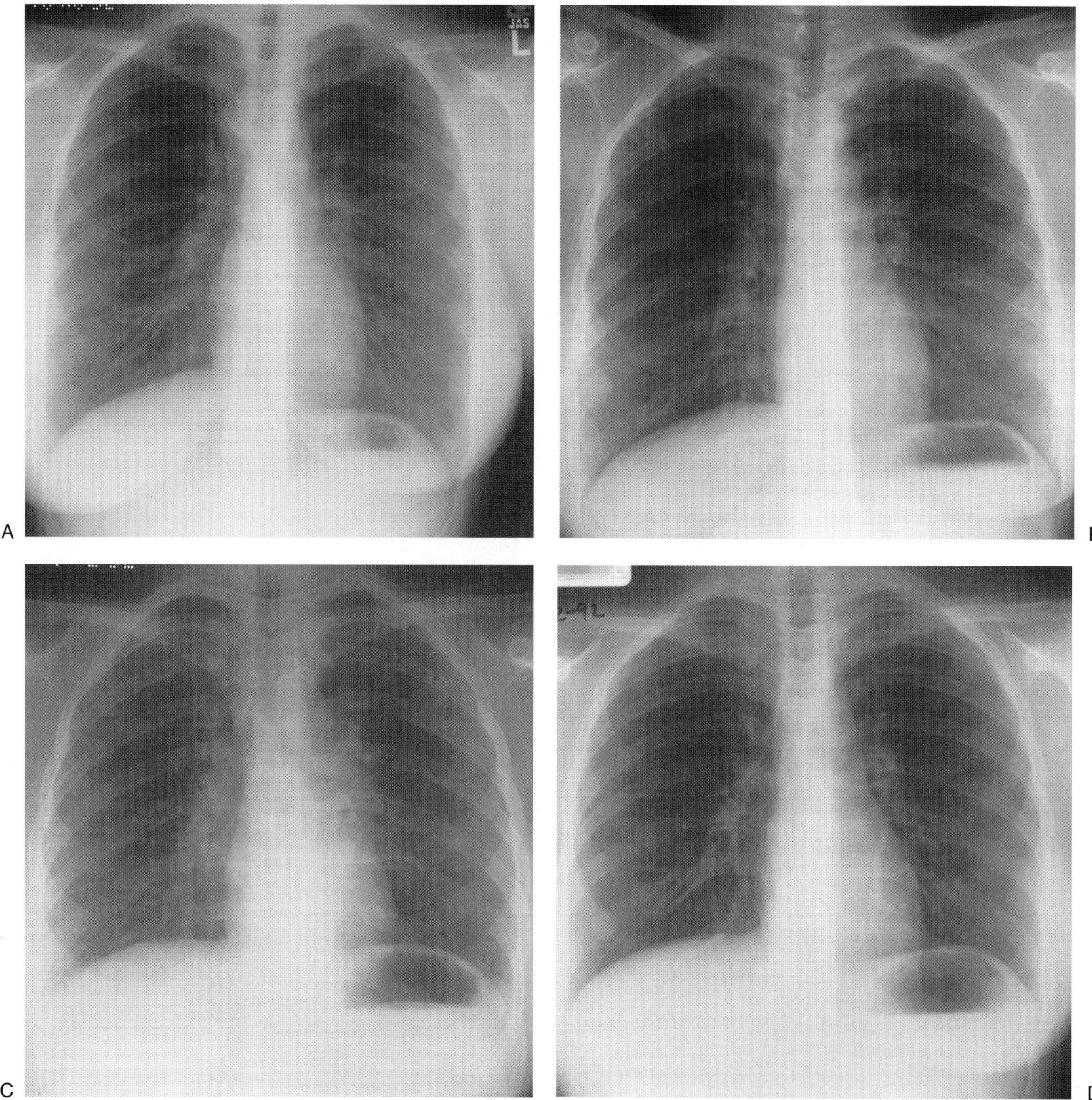

FIG. 4. Combined bleomycin/radiation pneumonitis. **A:** (3/30/92) Pretreatment chest radiograph from an 18-year-old woman with CS IIA Hodgkin's disease with a small superior mediastinal mass. **B:** (7/29/92) Four weeks after completion of two cycles of VBM (vinblastine, bleomycin, and methotrexate) chemotherapy (64 mg of bleomycin; 10 mg/m^2) and mantle irradiation (36 Gy). **C:** (8/1/92) Three days later, a diffuse interstitial infiltrate, with prominent paramediastinal and perihilar reaction. Patient was febrile, infectious-disease workup was negative. Corticosteroid treatment was initiated. **D:** (8/12/92) Eleven days later, the infiltrates have resolved completely. **E:** (8/17/98) Six-year follow-up evaluation. There are no residual abnormalities on chest radiograph.

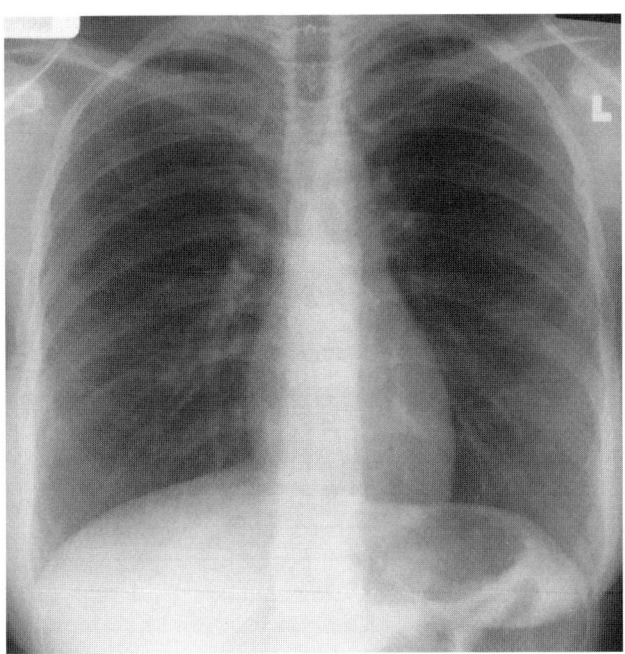

E

FIG 4. Continued.

monary disease (43,44). The frequency of this complication has been estimated to be about 2% (44). Late chylothorax, with recurring bilateral pleural effusions, has also been reported, but seems to be exceedingly rare and may be related to older techniques of therapy (45).

Pleural Symptoms After Bleomycin

A few pleural symptoms, mostly only radiologic—pleural thickening and even spontaneous pneumothorax or pneumomediastinum—have been reported after bleomycin administration. Pleural effusions are rarely seen (8).

TREATMENT PARAMETERS INVOLVED IN PULMONARY TOXICITY

Radiotherapy Parameters

Volume

Conventional mantle-field irradiation covers about 20% to 30% of the lung volume. This corresponds well to the 20% to 30% decrease in TLC observed when function tests are performed 6 to 12 months after completion of therapy (see above). The larger the lung volume to be irradiated, the greater the decrease in pulmonary function is likely to be, and probably the higher the risk of a long-term reduction in lung functional capacity. However, it is important to realize that the functional impact caused by irradiation varies according to the lung region. Studies in mice have shown that the response of lung is heterogeneous. The effect is always greater, for a similar volume irradiated, in the base compared to the apex (45a). Using SPECT and CT scanning, as proposed by some authors (37), it is possible to demonstrate lesser toxicity from irradiation when the lung volume is located in the apex. In addition to the conventional mantle field, it has been the practice in some situations to irradiate the entire lung (46). This has been shown to significantly increase the risk of radiation pneumonitis (13% vs. 3%, $p = .005$) (47). However, this risk is decreased by the use of partial transmission lung blocks, resulting in much smaller than conventional fraction size.

Dose

Limited data are available regarding the potential reduction in pulmonary complications that could be accomplished from a dose reduction in Hodgkin's disease. The reasons for this are as follows: (a) 40 Gy was considered thc gold standard of dose in Hodgkin's disease therapy for several decades; (b) even reduced to 30 to 35 Gy, the dose remains above the toxicity threshold for lung (usually set at 20 Gy); (c) follow-up is still too short to assess the long-term impact on pulmonary toxicity of the current dose de-escalation trials; and (d) even with a dose of 40 Gy, long-term pulmonary toxicity is relatively minor. Only one study (13) has been able to demonstrate that the radiation dose had a negative impact on VC and DLCO in the long term.

A careful conclusion could be that the current dose de-escalation trials (mainly aimed at limiting cardiac toxicity and second-cancer risk), are not likely to very significantly modify the long-term (modest) pulmonary toxicity in Hodgkin's disease.

Overall Treatment Time

There are some discrepancies in the literature about the impact of treatment time on late pulmonary toxicity. The animal data reviewed by Fowler (48) did not provide any evidence for an effect of treatment time. In contrast, the study of Van Dyk et al. (49), although questioned by others (50), suggests some impact of total treatment duration. Finally, the study by Dubray et al. (51) on 1,048 patients included in the first three EORTC Hodgkin's disease trials did not detect any influence of treatment time. This parameter therefore does not appear to have a significant impact on long-term pulmonary toxicity.

Fractionation

A large amount of experimental and clinical data has demonstrated clearly the high fractionation radiosensitivity of the lung. The α/β ratios derived from laboratory experiments or from clinical series have fallen consistently in the 2- to 4-Gy range, thereby confirming the major potential impact of the fraction size when irradiating the lung (52,53). In the H_1, H_2, and H_5 EORTC Hodgkin's disease trials, fraction size varied from 1.8 to 3.3 Gy, without changing the total dose. The derived α/β ratio was 3.07 Gy. Multivariate analysis confirms the increased risk of lung damage with increasing dose per fraction (51). The same pulmonary toxicity of large doses per fraction has also been reported for lung cancer, the use of a fraction greater than 2.67 Gy being the most significant factor associated with an increased risk of radiation pneumonitis (54). A last example of the fractionation sensitivity of the lung comes from the Stanford experience of whole-lung irradiation in Hodgkin's disease. After 16.2 Gy whole-lung irradiation using 2.2 to 2.75 Gy daily doses, the radiation pneumonitis rate was 35%. This percentage could be decreased to only 15% when using partial transmission blocks (thin lung blocks), allowing a fraction size of 0.81 Gy, without changing the total dose (46). This is consistent with the Boston experience, where the rate of pneumonitis was 13% after whole-lung irradiation delivered in 1.5 Gy fractions (47). It therefore seems clear that the fraction size should not exceed 1.8 to 2 Gy, to minimize the risk of pulmonary (and other) late complications.

Chemotherapy Parameters

Bleomycin Dose

The relationship between the cumulative dose of bleomycin and the incidence of pulmonary toxicity is complex, and the cumulative dose of bleomycin cannot be used reliably to predict toxicity in a given patient. The risk of bleomycin-induced interstitial fibrosis exists at all dose levels, and there are reports in the literature of patients who have developed interstitial fibrosis with cumulative doses of less than 50 mg. However, at cumulative doses above approximately 400 to 450 mg, the incidence of interstitial fibrosis appears to increase dramatically. Interstitial fibrosis should probably be considered sporadic below this threshold, occurring in particularly sensitive patients. On the other hand, the risk is about 13% at the 450- to 550-mg level, and appears to increase even more at higher doses (8).

Oxygen Therapy

The pulmonary toxicity of high inspired concentrations of oxygen in patients who received prior bleomycin therapy has been reported after treatment of testicular cancer (55). This toxicity has been confirmed in a large number of animal experiments (56,57). A study in rabbits showed that oxygen exposure as brief as 2 minutes was sufficient to increase the pulmonary toxicity of bleomycin (58). Anesthesiologists should be particularly concerned about this risk (59,60), and it seems prudent to avoid the use of any supplemental oxygen in patients who have received bleomycin (8).

Route of Administration

Bleomycin can be administrated by the subcutaneous, intramuscular, and intravenous routes. A few clinical studies (61,62), as well as an animal (mice) experiment (63), suggest that continuous infusion of bleomycin might have less toxicity than bolus injection. However, this has not been confirmed in other studies (8).

Renal Function

The presence of renal insufficiency at the time of bleomycin therapy has been reported to increase the risk of pulmonary toxicity. This could be explained by the prolongation of the half-life of bleomycin in case of severe renal impairment. Although the full relationship of renal function to the risk of developing bleomycin-induced pulmonary toxicity is unclear, it seems prudent to consider the possibility that the risk of toxicity may be increased in cases of a severe alteration of renal function (8).

Age

A number of studies suggested that older patients may be more susceptible to bleomycin toxicity. For example, Blum et al. reported that the incidence of bleomycin pulmonary toxicity was constant from age 20 to 70 years, but rose significantly in patients older than 70 years. Although this could not be confirmed in other studies (63a), the possibility that older patients may have a slight increase in risk cannot be ignored.

Combination with Other Chemotherapeutic Agents

Some authors report an unexpectedly high incidence of pulmonary toxicity (18–25%) after the administration of bleomycin together with doxorubicin, cyclophosphamide, and vincristine (64), or bleomycin in combination with doxorubicin, methotrexate, cyclophosphamide, vincristine, and dexamethasone (65). However, other authors using the same combination chemotherapy regimens did not observe an increase in pulmonary toxicity (8). The withdrawal of corticosteroids in some of these regimens has been linked to the development of toxicity for drugs such as methotrexate. However, there is no direct evidence to suggest that the tapering of corticosteroid dose, as used in many lymphoma protocols, could influence the development of bleomycin pulmonary toxicity.

In Hodgkin's disease, pulmonary toxicity related to the use of chemotherapy alone (as primary treatment) has rarely been reported. However, Canellos and colleagues (66) reported clinically significant severe pulmonary toxicity in 6% of 115 patients treated with ABVD chemotherapy, with death due to pulmonary toxicity in three patients (only one of whom had received mediastinal irradiation).

Combined Chemoradiotherapy

The bulk of the data that are available in the literature refer to pulmonary complications secondary to the use of combined chemotherapy and irradiation. It is reasonable to consider each chemotherapy combination independently.

A limited amount of data have been published on MOPP. Recall pneumonitis, resembling the recall pericarditis phenomenon (2), has been reported after the steroid withdrawal following cycles one and four of the classic MOPP regimen (which included prednisone only in those cycles). In the EORTC studies (31), the combination of MOPP radiotherapy did not appear to significantly alter the evolution of functional pulmonary tests when compared to irradiation alone. In the Canadian experience reported by Mah et al. (67), the combination of MOPP with radiation did not affect the risk for radiologic pneumonitis. In contrast, a number of studies have analyzed lung toxicity after the combination of ABVD with radiotherapy. Several studies report an increase in pulmonary toxicity when ABVD is combined with radiotherapy. In the EORTC H_6U trial, a significant difference in the decrement in vital capacity between ABVD (−19%) and MOPP (−13%) was reported. However, at 1 year, this difference was no longer significant (31). A more recent update of the trial shows that a significant vital capacity decrease persists in the ABVD arm, while there was a complete recovery in the MOPP arm.

In the previously mentioned Canadian series (67), it was concluded that the addition of ABVD "appeared to reduce the tolerance of lung to radiation." Santoro et al. (68), reporting on an Italian trial, observed radiographic evidence of pulmonary fibrosis in 59% of patients treated with ABVD and radiotherapy, compared to only 30% of patients treated with MOPP and radiotherapy. In the Norwegian experience (15), a multivariate analysis showed that chemotherapy with bleomycin and an anthracycline was the only significant predictor for lung function impairment. Hirsch et al. (69) recently reported the experience from the Memorial Sloan-Kettering Cancer Center. ABVD was found to induce acute pulmonary toxicity (requiring bleomycin dose modification) in a substantial number of patients. The addition of irradiation resulted in a further decrease in FVC. However, the long-term functional status did not seem to be altered.

In another Italian trial using an ABVD variant (EBVD) or MOPP/EBVD, 6 out of 95 patients suffered chronic lung toxicity (70). Finally, the Children's Cancer Study Group (71) reported a 9% incidence of acute pulmonary toxicity in 64 children with advanced-stage Hodgkin's disease treated with 12 cycles of ABVD followed by low-dose regional irradiation, with one fatality directly related to pulmonary toxicity.

However, in contrast, other authors did not detect any significant increase in lung toxicity with the addition of ABVD. Such is the case in the Stanford experience (36), although the authors note that the patient groups are small and that a possible effect could have been missed. Reporting on its experience with MOPP/ABVD (hybrid or alternating), the group from Milan concluded that no pulmonary toxicity due to bleomycin could be documented (72). In a recent study, Salloum et al. (73) reported that ABVD or MOPP/ABVD followed by low-dose mediastinal radiation did not result in a significant incidence of pulmonary toxicity, after a median follow-up of more than 6 years.

Few data are available concerning more recently introduced chemotherapy schedules. An exception is VBM (vinblastine, bleomycin, and methotrexate), with contradictory results. The Stanford group did not detect any increase in lung toxicity with VBM (36), while the British National Lymphoma Investigation (BNLI) reported a high rate of cough and dyspnea (14 out of 30 patients) after a split-course treatment with two cycles of VBM followed by involved-field irradiation and four more cycles of VBM. The British group concluded that the pulmonary toxicity of the schedule "makes the regimen unsuitable for routine use" (74). An Italian group, combining VBM with extended-field irradiation, reported eight cases of pulmonary toxicity, and one death, among 50 patients (75).

The comparison between the various chemoradiotherapy schedules is made difficult by the high intergroup variability in numerous parameters, both for radiotherapy and for chemotherapy. For radiotherapy, both the volumes and fractionation must be taken into account (see above). For chemotherapy, the cumulative dose of bleomycin must be considered. For example, while the cumulative dose of bleomycin is 120 mg/m^2 for six cycles of ABVD or VBM, it drops to 60 mg/m^2 for the same number of cycles of BEACOPP [bleomycin, etoposide, Adriamycin, cyclophosphamide, Oncovin (vincristine), procarbazine and prednisone] (76), MOPP/ABV (77), and EBVP II (78).

Apart from the potential long-term functional impairment due to combined chemotherapy and irradiation, it is important not to overlook the very severe unexpected toxicity of the combined modalities in a very small number of patients. Two pulmonary toxic deaths were reported in the ABVD arm of the EORTC H_6U trial (31), three in the report of Canellos (vide supra) (66), one (out of 60 patients) in the New York experience (69), and one in the previously noted Children's Cancer Study Group series (71).

The explanation for these undue severe complications is not clear. Is it simply hypersensitivity to bleomycin (79)? Does it correspond to the small proportion of hyperradiosensitive patients, well known to radiation oncologists? Or are some patients hypersensitive to both bleomycin and radiation? Ataxia-telangiectasia cells, well known to display increased radiation sensitivity, have been shown also to be hypersensitive to bleomycin (80). The recent report of a patient with a Nijmegen breakage syndrome showing both bleomycin and radiation hypersensitivity (81) and the indication of murine susceptibility to both radiation-induced and bleomycin-induced pulmonary fibrosis (82) would also support this hypothesis. The development of individual testing of normal tissue sensitivity to radiation and drugs could shed some light on this issue.

IMPORTANT RISK COFACTORS

Smoking

As could be reasonably expected, smoking has been found by several authors to have a negative impact on lung function in patients treated for Hodgkin's disease. A significant decrease with time in pulmonary function tests manifested by a progressive obstructive ventilatory defect, as observed in the series of Smith et al. (34), was confined to the subset of patients who smoked. In a Dutch study (13), smoking was found to have a detrimental influence on DLCO. Lund et al. (15) also reported that smokers had reduced diffusion capacity compared with nonsmokers (70% and 79% of predicted, $p = .002$), whereas ex-smokers (75% of predicted) did not significantly differ from either of the other two groups. The experience in patients with testicular cancer also showed that cigarette smoking is a risk factor for bleomycin-induced pulmonary toxicity (83).

Gender

In a recent survey (84), female gender was found to be linked to an increased risk of late pulmonary sequelae. Five to 13 years after mediastinal irradiation, gas transfer was found to be reduced in 41% of cases in females versus 22% in males ($p = .03$). This difference could not be explained by treatment-related differences. The possible negative impact of female gender on late pulmonary toxicity requires confirmation.

Surgery

Thoracic surgery may be considered after treatment of Hodgkin's disease for confirmation of relapse or diagnosis of other problems such as postradiation or bleomycin-induced fibrosis or infection. However, it seems reasonable to try to limit, as much as possible, the indications for such surgical procedures, especially in patients who previously received mediastinal irradiation and bleomycin. Apart from the risk of oxygen administration in patients previously treated with bleomycin (see above), surgery may add its own local fibrosis and alteration of chest compliance, to radiation and bleomycin-induced fibrotic processes, leading to more severe functional sequelae. With more sophisticated ways to detect relapse (magnetic resonance imaging and positron emission tomography scanning) and with the help of fibroscopy samplings, surgery should be reserved for a very small number of indications.

Systemic Symptoms

In an analysis of lung toxicity in the first three EORTC trials, a trend toward a higher incidence of pulmonary damage in patients with systemic symptoms was observed. In the three trials analyzed together, multivariate analyses confirmed the influence of the presence of systemic symptoms. One hypothesis to explain this finding could be that patients with systemic symptoms were more likely to present with larger mediastinal masses, thus leading to more extensive pulmonary irradiation and more aggressive chemoradiotherapy combinations, but this possible relationship could not be investigated in this series (51). Again, this potential detrimental factor requires confirmation in other series.

TREATMENT OF PULMONARY COMPLICATIONS

In the early phase, dry cough usually requires only symptomatic therapy. Only in rare cases of severe postirradiation acute symptoms, with dry hacking cough, dyspnea on rest, and infection, are antibiotics (often combined with steroids) indicated. Even in severe cases, this treatment may lead to a dramatic and rapid improvement of symptoms. Acute severe bleomycin-induced lung toxicity may also be reversible, if treated aggressively with high-dose corticosteroids (Fig. 4) (85). In both situations (postirradiation or postbleomycin pneumonitis) long-term taper of corticosteroids is required, in particular to avoid the recall syndrome (see above). However, corticosteroids increase the risk of superimposed infections, so that antibiotic prophylaxis (particularly against pneumocystis) is recommended.

In the long-term, symptomatology is linked mainly to fibrosis of lung parenchyma. Postradiation fibrosis generally has bccn considered to be nonreversible. At present, the new hypothesis on the role of the cytokine cascade in the genesis of such fibrosis (see above) leaves some hope of improving the functional impairment linked to fibrosis of the pulmonary septa, at least if this fibrosis is not too severe. Recent results obtained with superoxide dismutase (SOD) in postirradiation fibrosis, especially for the skin and mucosal tissues, would encourage the use of such therapy in patients with long-term reduced vital capacity and/or reduced gas transfer due to lung fibrosis (86). Several papers have also emphasized the potential efficacy of SOD on interstitial pneumonitis induced by bleomycin in animal models (87,88). Another recent study suggested that pretreatment of rats with alpha-tocopherol liposomes can provide significant protection against bleomycin-induced lung injury (89).

IMPACT ON LONG-TERM SURVIVAL

In contrast to cardiac complications, long-term pulmonary toxicity after treatment of Hodgkin's disease does not appear to show a significant impact on long-term survival when large cohorts of patients are analyzed. However, as previously noted, the functional impairment observed in some patients would likely affect their quality of life (90).

IMPACT ON CURRENT TREATMENT STRATEGY

The impact of late pulmonary toxicity on current treatment strategy has been relatively minor. However, the beneficial impact of reducing the irradiated lung volume after chemotherapy has been one of the reasons why combined chemotherapy-irradiation is clearly the standard treatment for stages I–II with bulky mediastinal involvement (47). In parallel, what has been learned about fractionation effects in the lung clearly mandates a fraction size of 2 Gy or less when irradiating part of the lung volume (52,53). In addition, when irradiating an entire lung, one should favor the use of partial lung transmission blocks (Fig. 3) (46). Finally, additional risk factors, especially smoking, should be avoided whenever possible.

RECOMMENDATIONS FOR ROUTINE PATIENT FOLLOW-UP

During Treatment

Close follow-up is necessary during chemotherapy, particularly if a bleomycin-containing regimen is used. Clinical examination at each cycle, together with a chest radiograph (often obtained to follow tumor regression), should detect minor changes that would lead to the performance of pulmonary function tests. Alterations of diffusion capacity should result in either a decrease in dosage or discontinuation of bleomycin. A number of groups agree that in the event of a large decrease in the diffusion capacity (to less than a third of the baseline), bleomycin should be dropped. During irradiation, as stated previously, very few clinical or radiologic symptoms are expected (see above).

After Completion of Treatment

In the absence of acute clinical or radiologic problems, routine chest radiographs, for example every 6 months during the first 5 years, seem sufficient to assess the type and severity of radiologic lesions and their evolution toward progressive fibrotic retraction. When necessary for further differential diagnosis, a CT scan can be performed. Functional evaluation may be performed in cases of significant dyspnea, at rest or on exertion. At times, these studies are proposed to patients in the context of prospective quality-of-life evaluations, especially in randomized trials.

CONCLUSIONS

Long-term pulmonary effects after treatment of Hodgkin's disease can be related to irradiation, to bleomycin, and, more and more often, to the combination of both. However, with recent improvements in radiotherapy administration (lower doses, adequate fractionation, and limited volumes) and chemotherapy delivery (with strict stopping rules as soon as bleomycin-induced toxicity is detected), long-term pulmonary effects are expected to be modest, and without any significant impact on survival. A few patients, hypersensitive to both radiation and bleomycin, are at risk of developing severe toxicity even with the usual doses of these agents, and efforts are ongoing to detect them in advance. Finally, for those few patients with significant long-term pulmonary fibrosis, new antifibrotic therapies, such as the ones based on superoxide dismutase, are being explored.

REFERENCES

1. Gross NJ. Pulmonary effects of radiation therapy. *Ann Intern Med* 1977;86(1):81–92.
2. Kaplan H. *Hodgkin's disease.* Cambridge, MA: Harvard University Press, 1980.
3. Phillips TL, Margolis LW. *Radiation pathology and the clinical response of lung and esophagus.* Basel: S. Karger, 1972.
4. Rubin P, Casarett G. *Clinical radiation pathology.* Philadelphia: WB Saunders, 1968.
5. Rubin P, Johnston C, Williams J, McDonald S, Finkelstein J. A perpetual cascade of cytokines postirradiation leads to pulmonary fibrosis. *Int J Radiat Oncol Biol Phys* 1995;33:99–109.
6. Morgan GW, Pharm B, Breit SN. Radiation and the lung: a reevaluation of the mechanisms mediating pulmonary injury. *Int J Radiat Oncol Biol Phys* 1995;31:361–369.
7. Santoro A, Bonfante V, Bonadonna G. Salvage chemotherapy with ABVD in MOPP-resistant Hodgkin's disease. *Ann Intern Med* 1982; 306(13):770–775.
8. Jules-Elysee K, White DA. Bleomycin-induced pulmonary toxicity. *Clin Chest Med* 1990;11:1–20.
9. Temelkovski J, Kumar RK, Maronese SE. Enhanced production of an EGF-like growth factor by parenchymal macrophages following bleomycin-induced pulmonary injury. *Exp Lung Res* 1997;23(5): 377–391.
10. Sleijfer S, Vujaskovic Z, Limburg PC, Schraffordt Koops H, Mulder NH. Induction of tumor necrosis factor-alpha as a cause of bleomycin-related toxicity. *Cancer* 1998;82(5):970–974.
11. Carmel R, Kaplan H. Mantle irradiation in Hodgkin's disease. An analysis of technique, tumor eradication, and complications. *Cancer* 1976;37:2813–2825.
12. Dixsaut G, Teillet F, Dana M, Miot C, Catherine N, Teillet-Thiebaud F. Conséquences de l'irradiation médiastinale et de la chimiothérapie sur la fonction respiratoire. *Nouv Presse Med* 1982;11:429–432.
13. Hassink E, Souren T, Boersma L, et al. Pulmonary morbidity 10–18 years after irradiation for Hodgkin's disease. *Eur J Cancer* 1993; 29A:343–347.
14. Gustavsson A, Eskilsson J, Landberg T, et al. Long-term effects on pulmonary function of mantle radiotherapy in patients with Hodgkin's disease. *Ann Oncol* 1992;3:455–461.

15. Lund M, Kongerud J, Nome O, et al. Lung function impairment in long-term survivors of Hodgkin's disease. *Ann Oncol* 1995;6:495–501.
16. Brice P, Tredaniel J, Monsuez J, et al. Cardiopulmonary toxicity after three courses of ABVD and mediastinal irradiation in favorable Hodgkin's disease. *Ann Oncol* 1991;2:73–76.
17. Jensen BV, Carlsen NLT, Peters K, Nissen NI, Sorensen PG, Walbom-Jorgensen S. Radiographic evaluation of pulmonary fibrosis following mantle field irradiation in Hodgkin's disease. *Acta Radiol Oncol* 1986;25:109–113.
18. Libshitz H, Brosof A, Southard M. Radiographic appearance of the chest following mantle field irradiation in Hodgkin's disease. *Cancer* 1973;32:206–215.
19. Morgan GW, Freeman A, McLean R, et al. Late cardiac, thyroid and pulmonary sequelae of mantle radiotherapy for Hodgkin's disease. *Int J Radiat Oncol Biol Phys* 1985;11:1925–1931.
20. Shapiro SJ, Shapiro SD, Mill W, Campbell E. Prospective study of long-term pulmonary manifestations of mantle irradiation. *Int J Radiat Oncol Biol Phys* 1990;19:707–714.
21. Slanina J, Musshof K, Rahner T, Stiasny R. Long-term side effects in irradiated patients with Hodgkin's disease. *Int J Radiat Oncol Biol Phys* 1977;2:1–19.
22. Svahn-Tapper G, Badetorp L, Landberg T. Mantle treatment of Hodgkin's disease. Results and side effects. *Acta Radiol Ther Phys Biol* 1976;15:369–386.
23. Balikian JP, Jochelson MS, Bauer KA, et al. Pulmonary complications of chemotherapy regimens containing bleomycin. *AJR* 1982;139: 455–496.
24. Bonadonna G, De Lena M, Monfardini S, et al. Clinical trials with bleomycin in lymphomas and in solid tumors. *Eur J Cancer* 1972;8: 205–215.
25. Bellamy EA, Husband JE, Blaquiere RM, Law MR. Bleomycin-related lung damage: CT Evidence. *Radiology* 1985;156:155–158.
26. Cionini L, Pacini P, de Paola E, et al. Respiratory function tests after mantle irradiation in patients with Hodgkin's disease. *Acta Radiol Oncol* 1984;23(6):401–409.
27. Do Pico G, Wiley A, Rao P, Dickie HA. Pulmonary reaction to upper mantle radiation therapy for Hodgkin's disease. *Chest* 1979;75(6): 688–692.
28. Evans R, Sagerman R, Ringrose T, Auchincloss J, Bowman J. Pulmonary function following mantle-field irradiation for Hodgkin's disease. *Radiology* 1974;111:729–731.
29. Host H, Vale J. Lung function after mantle field irradiation in Hodgkin's disease. *Cancer* 1973;32:328–332.
30. Landberg T, Svahn-Tapper G, Wintzell K. Preliminary report on side effects and early results. *Acta Radiol Ther Phys Biol* 1971;10: 174–186.
30a. Watchie J, Coleman C, Raffin T, et al. Minimal long-term cardiopulmonary dysfunction following treatment for Hodgkin's disease. *Int J Radiat Oncol Biol Phys* 1989;13:517–524.
31. Cosset JM, Henry-Amar M, Meerwaldt J. Long-term outcome of early stages of Hodgkin's disease therapy: the EORTC experience. *Ann Oncol* 1991;2(suppl 2):77–82.
32. Lokich J, Bass H, Eberly F, Rosenthal D, Moloney W. The pulmonary effect of mantle irradiation in patients with Hodgkin's disease. *Radiology* 1973;108:397–402.
33. Kadota R, Burget E, Driscoll D. Cardiopulmonary function in long-term survivors of childhood Hodgkin's lymphoma: a pilot study. *Mayo Clin Proc* 1988;63:362–367.
34. Smith L, Mendenhall N, Cigale M, Block E, Carter R, Million R. Results of a prospective study evaluating the effects of mantle irradiation on pulmonary function. *Int J Radiat Oncol Biol Phys* 1989;16: 79–84.
35. Jensen BV, Carlsen NL, Nissen NI. Influence of age and duration of follow-up on lung function after combined chemotherapy for Hodgkin's disease. *Eur Respir J* 1990;3:1140–1145.
36. Horning S, Adhikari A, Rizk N, Hoppe R, Olshen R. Effect of treatment for Hodgkin's disease on pulmonary function: results of a prospective study. *J Clin Oncol* 1994;12:297–305.
37. Boersma L, Damen E, de Boer R, et al. Estimation of overall pulmonary function after irradiation using dose-effect relations for local functional injury. *Radiother Oncol* 1995;36:15–23.
38. Samuels ML, Holoye PY, Johnson DE. Bleomycin combination chemotherapy in the management of testicular neoplasia. *Cancer* 1975;36:318–326.
39. Lewis BM, Izbicki R. Routine pulmonary function tests during bleomycin therapy. *JAMA* 1980;243:347–351.
40. Comis RL, Kuppinger MS, Ginsberg SJ, et al. The role of single-breath carbon monoxide diffusing capacity in monitoring the pulmonary effects of bleomycin in germ cell tumor patients. *Cancer Res* 1979;39:5076–5080.
41. Morrone N, Gama E, Silva Volpe V, Dourado A, et al. Bilateral pleural effusion due to mediastinal fibrosis induced by radiotherapy. *Chest* 1993;4:1276–1278.
42. Rodriguez-Garcia J, Fraile G, Moreno M, Sanchez-Corral JA, Penalver R. Recurrent massive pleural effusion as a late complication of radiotherapy in Hodgkin's disease. *Chest* 1991;100(4):1165–1166.
43. Penniment M, O'Brien P. Pneumothorax following thoracic radiation therapy for Hodgkin's disease. *Thorax* 1994;49:936–937.
44. Pezner R, Horak D, Sayegh H, Lipsett J. Spontaneous pneumothorax in patients irradiated for Hodgkin's disease and other malignant lymphomas. *Int J Radiat Oncol Biol Phys* 1989;18:193–198.
45. Promisloff R, Hogue D. Chylothorax: the result of previous radiation therapy? *J Am Osteopath Assoc* 1997;97:164–166.
45a. Liao Z, Travis E, Tucker S. Damage and morbidity from pneumonitis after irradiation of partial volumes of mouse lung. *Int J Radiat Oncol Biol Phys* 1995;32:1359–1370.
46. Hancock S, Hoppe R. Long-term complications of treatment and causes of mortality after Hodgkin's disease. *Semin Radiat Oncol* 1996;6:225–242.
47. Tarbell N, Thompson L, Mauch P. Thoracic irradiation in Hodgkin's disease: disease control and long-term complications. *Int J Radiat Oncol Biol Phys* 1990;18:275–281.
48. Fowler J. Radiation-induced lung damage: dose-time fractionation considerations. *Radiother Oncol* 1990;18:185–187.
49. Van Dyk J, Mah K, Keane T. Radiation-induced lung damage: dose-time fractionation considerations. *Radiother Oncol* 1989;14:55–69.
50. Bentzen S, Thames H. Incidence and latency of radiation reactions. *Radiother Oncol* 1989;14:261–262.
51. Dubray B, Henry-Amar M, Meerwaldt JH, et al. Radiation-induced lung damage after thoracic irradiation for Hodgkin's disease: the role of fractionation. *Radiother Oncol* 1995;36:211–217.
52. Cosset JM, Dubray B, Girinsky T, Maher M, Malaise E. Fractionation sensitivity of mammalian tissues. *Adv Radiat Biol* 1994;18:91–121.
53. Thames H, Hendry J. *Fractionation in radiotherapy.* Thames: Taylor and Francis, 1987.
54. Roach M, Gandara D, Yuo H, et al. Radiation pneumonitis following combined modality therapy for lung cancer: analysis of prognostic factors. *J Clin Oncol* 1995;13:2606–2612.
55. Goldiner PL, Carlon GC, Cvitkovic E, Schweizer O, Howland WS. Factors influencing postoperative morbidity and mortality in patients treated with bleomycin. *Br Med J* 1978;1(6128):1664–1667.
56. Sogal RN, Gottlieb AA, Bovtros AR. Effect of oxygen on bleomycin-induced lung damage. *Cleve Clin J Med* 1987;54:503–509.
57. Tryka AF, Skornik WA, Godleski JJ, Brain JD. Potentiation of bleomycin-induced lung injury by exposure to 70% oxygen. Morphologic assessment. *Am Rev Respir Dis* 1982;126:1074–1079.
58. Shen AS, Haslett C, Feldsien DC. Modulation of bleomycin lung injury by short exposure to hypoxia. *Chest* 1986;89:122S–123S.
59. Callery J, Brandl A. Oxygen toxicity in the bleomycin patient. *J Postanesth Nurs* 1988;3(3):139–143.
60. Waid-Jones MI, Coursin DB. Perioperative considerations for patients treated with bleomycin. *Chest* 1991;99(4):993–999.
61. Cooper KR, Hong WK. Prospective study of the pulmonary toxicity of continuously infused bleomycin. *Cancer Treat Rep* 1981;65:419–425.
62. Samuels ML, Johnson DE, Holoye PY, Lanzotti VJ. Large-dose bleomycin therapy and pulmonary toxicity. A possible role of prior radiotherapy. *JAMA* 1976;235:1117–1120.
63. Sikic BI, Collins JM, Mimnaugh EG, Gram TE. Improved therapeutic index of bleomycin when administered by continuous infusion in mice. *Cancer Treat Rep* 1978;62(12):2011–2017.
63a. Blum RH, Carter SK, Agre K. A clinical review of bleomycin. A new antineoplastic agent. *Cancer* 1973;31:903–914.
64. Schein PS, DeVita VT, Hubbard S, et al. Bleomycin, adriamycin, cyclophosphamide, vincristine, and prednisone (BACOP) combina-

tion chemotherapy in the treatment of advanced diffuse histiocytic lymphoma. *Ann Intern Med* 1976;85(4):417–422.
65. Bauer KA, Skarin AT, Balikian JP, Garnick MB, Rosenthal DS, Canellos GP. Pulmonary complications associated with combination chemotherapy programs containing bleomycin. *Am J Med* 1983;74: 557–563.
66. Canellos G, Anderson J, Propert K. Chemotherapy of advanced Hodgkin's disease with MOPP, ABVD or MOPP alternating with ABVD. *N Engl J Med* 1992;327:1478–1484.
67. Mah K, Keane T, Van Dyk J, Braban L, Poon P, Hao Y. Quantitative effect of combined chemotherapy and fractionated radiotherapy on the incidence of radiation-induced lung damage: a prospective clinical study. *Int J Radiat Oncol Biol Phys* 1994;28:563–574.
68. Santoro A, Bonadonna G, Valagussa P. Long-term results of combined chemotherapy-radiotherapy approach in Hodgkin's disease: superiority of ABVD plus radiotherapy versus MOPP plus radiotherapy. *J Clin Oncol* 1987;5:25–37.
69. Hirsch A, Vander EN, Straus DJ, et al. Effect of ABVD chemotherapy with and without mantle or mediastinal irradiation on pulmonary function and symptoms in early-stage Hodgkin's disease. *J Clin Oncol* 1996;14:1297–1305.
70. Pogliani E, Deliliers G, Baldini L, et al. EBVD and alternating MOPP/ EBVD with or without localized field radiotherapy in advanced or unfavorably presenting Hodgkin's disease. *Haematologica* 1996;8:8–14.
71. Fryer CJ, Hutchinson RJ, Krailo M, et al. Efficacy and toxicity of 12 courses of ABVD chemotherapy followed by low-dose regional radiation in advanced Hodgkin's disease in children: a report from the Children's Cancer Study Group. *J Clin Oncol* 1990;8:1971–1980.
72. Viviani S, Bonadonna G, Santoro A, et al. Alternating versus hybrid MOPP and ABVD combinations in advanced Hodgkin's disease: ten-year results. *J Clin Oncol* 1996;14:1421–1430.
73. Salloum E, Tanoue LT, Wackers FJT, Zelterman D, Cooper DL. Assessment of cardiac pulmonary function in adult patients treated with ABVD or MOPP/ABVD plus adjuvant low-dose mediastinal radiation for Hodgkin's disease. *Proc ASCO* 1997;(abstr.):9A.
74. Bates N, Williams M, Bessell E, Vaughan Hudson G, Vaughan Hudson B. Efficacy and toxicity of vinblastine, bleomycin and methotrexate with involved-field radiotherapy in clinical stage IA and IIA Hodgkin's disease: a British National Lymphoma Investigation pilot study. *J Clin Oncol* 1994;12:288–296.
75. Gobbi PG, Pieresca C, Frassoldati A, et al. Vinblastine, bleomycin, and methotrexate chemotherapy plus extended-field radiotherapy in early, favorably presenting, clinically staged Hodgkin's patients: the Gruppo Italiano per lo Studio dei Linfomi experience. *J Clin Oncol* 1996;14(2):527–533.
76. Diehl V, Sieber M, Ruffer U, et al. BEACOPP: an intensified chemotherapy regimen in advanced Hodgkin's disease. The German Hodgkin's Lymphoma Study Group. *Ann Oncol* 1997;8(2):143–148.
77. Klimo P, Connors JM. An update on the Vancouver experience in the management of advanced Hodgkin's disease treated with the MOPP/ ABV hybrid program. *Semin Hematol* 1988;25(2):34–40.
78. Hoerni B, Orgerie MB, Eghbali H, et al. Nouvelle association d'épirubicine, bléomycine, vinblastine et prednisone (EBVP II) avant radiothérapie dans les stades localisés de maladie de Hodgkin: Essai de phase II chez 50 malades. *Bull Cancer* 1988;8:789–794.
79. White DA, Stover DE. Severe bleomycin-induced pneumonitis. Clinical features and response to corticosteroids. *Chest* 1984;86:723–728.
80. Lavin MF. Radiosensitivity and oxidative signalling in ataxia telangiectasia: an update. *Radiother Oncol* 1998;47:113–123.
81. Perez-Vera P, Gonzales-del Angel A, Molina B, et al. Chromosome instability with bleomycin and X-ray hypersensitivity in a boy with Nijmegen breakage syndrome. *Am J Med Genet* 1997;70(1):24–27.
82. Haston CK, Travis EL. Murine susceptibility to radiation-induced pulmonary fibrosis is influenced by a genetic factor implicated in susceptibility to bleomycin-induced pulmonary fibrosis. *Cancer Res* 1997;57(23):2586–2591.
83. Senan S, Paul J, Thomson N, Kaye SB. Cigarette smoking is a risk factor for bleomycin-induced pulmonary toxicity. *Eur J Cancer* 1992; 28A(12):2084.
84. Lund M, Kongerud J, Nome B, Abrahamsen A, Ihlen H, Forfang K. Cardiopulmonary sequelae after treatment for Hodgkin's disease: increased risk in females? *Ann Oncol* 1996;7:257–264.
85. Maher J, Daly PA. Severe bleomycin lung toxicity: reversal with high dose corticosteroids. *Thorax* 1993;48(1):92–94.
86. Delanian S, Baillet F, Huart J, Lefaix J, Maulard C, Housset M. Successful treatment of radiation-induced fibrosis using liposomal Cu/Zn superoxide dismutase clinical trial. *Radiother Oncol* 1994;32: 12–20.
87. Ledwozyw A. Protective effect of liposome-entrapped superoxyde dismutase and catalase on bleomycin-induced lung injury in rats. I. Antioxydant enzyme activities and lipid peroxidation. *Acta Vet Hung* 1991;39(3–4):215–224.
88. Yamazaki C, Hoshino J, Hori Y, et al. Effect of lecithinized-superoxyde dismutase on the interstitial pneumonia model induced by bleomycin in mice. *Jpn J Pharmacol* 1997;75(1):97–100.
89. Suntres ZE, Shek PN. Protective effect of liposomal alpha-tocopherol against bleomycin-induced lung injury. *Biomed Environ Sci* 1997; 10(1):47–59.
90. Henry-Amar M, Joly F. Late complications after Hodgkin's disease. *Ann Oncol* 1996;7:S115–116.

Hodgkin's Disease, edited by P. M. Mauch,
J. O. Armitage, V. Diehl, R. T. Hoppe, and L. M. Weiss.
Lippincott Williams & Wilkins, Philadephia ©1999.

CHAPTER 35

Cardiovascular Late Effects After Treatment of Hodgkin's Disease

Steven L. Hancock

Cardiovascular diseases have been the most common nonmalignant sources of excess morbidity and mortality among survivors of Hodgkin's disease and provide some of the most difficult diagnostic and therapeutic dilemmas in the long-term care of patients after therapy. Clinical reactions in the cardiovascular system range from asymptomatic pericardial effusion or transient, acute pericarditis during or shortly after radiation therapy to fatal pancarditis, cardiomyopathy, myocardial infarction from premature coronary artery disease, or vascular stenosis and thrombosis. The magnitude of these problems is suggested by several series that feature prolonged follow-up. At Stanford, cardiovascular disease accounted for 16% of 754 deaths reported among 2,498 patients treated between 1960 and 1995 (1). Cardiovascular death (including cerebrovascular accident) accounted for 13.7% of the 124 deaths among 794 patients treated for Hodgkin's disease at the Joint Center for Radiation Therapy between 1969 and 1995 (2). Acute myocardial infarction was the second most common cause of intercurrent death among patients with early stages of Hodgkin's disease treated on the European Organization for the Research and Treatment of Cancer (EORTC) protocols and among patients cured of Hodgkin's disease after treatment before 30 years of age in British National Lymphoma Investigation (BNLI) trials. Myocardial infarction caused 7% of 240 deaths among 1,449 patients treated on EORTC studies between 1963 and 1986 (3), and 14% of 43 deaths among 1,043 BNLI patients (4). Although these risks are substantial, there is some evidence that they are decreasing with improvements in therapy. Among patients presenting with stage I or II Hodgkin's disease at Stanford, the incidence of cardiovascular death during the first 15 years of follow-up decreased from 5.4% among 812 patients treated between 1962 and 1980 to 0.8% among 628 patients treated from 1980 to 1996 (5). This chapter reviews the historical and clinical aspects of cardiovascular consequences of Hodgkin's disease treatment.

S. L. Hancock: Department of Radiation Oncology, Stanford University School of Medicine, Stanford, California.

HISTORICAL ASPECTS AND TREATMENT FACTORS AFFECTING RISK

During the era when supervoltage and megavoltage therapeutic radiation sources were first applied to the treatment of Hodgkin's disease, the heart was generally believed to be relatively resistant to radiation injury. Occasional case reports suggested potential risks of acute electrocardiographic changes, arrhythmia, fibrosis of the myocardium and/or pericardium, and acute myocardial infarction. In the late 1960s and early 1970s, systematic studies of patients who had been treated with mediastinal irradiation for Hodgkin's disease documented a more serious pattern of risk, as reviewed by Stewart and Fajardo (6). In 1967 Cohn et al. (7) reported a series of 21 cases of radiation-induced heart disease evaluated at Stanford, 11 of whom were treated for Hodgkin's disease using the mantle technique described by Kaplan (8). These cases presaged the findings of larger, population-based studies during the subsequent three decades, documenting episodes of acute pericarditis, chronic constrictive pericarditis, valvular heart disease, and premature coronary artery disease.

Most of the early studies focused on radiation carditis, a mixture of clinical entities that spanned the spectrum of acute pericarditis, postirradiation pericardial effusion, chronic pericarditis with constriction, and direct myocardial injury. Myocardial fibrosis was initially inferred from the observation that five of ten patients with severe late constrictive pericarditis did not derive clinical benefit from surgical pericardiectomy (6). Autopsies from such patients demonstrated diffuse pericardial, endocardial, and myocardial fibrosis. Observation of these clinical syndromes led to a series of pathologic and experimental studies characterizing the response of the parietal and visceral pericardium, myocardium, and endocardium to ionizing radiation (9–13). Direct valvular injury was sporadically reported in autopsy series of children (14) and young adults (15) but was not a feature of cardiac injury by irradiation in experimental systems. Similarly, premature coronary artery disease, although clinically suspected on the basis of sporadic case reports of acute myocardial infarction in younger patients, was not a common feature noted in early pathologic or experimental studies of radiation-induced heart disease. The role of radiation as an etiologic factor in valvular or coronary artery diseases was doubted by experts as late as 1984 (13).

Studies of patients treated for Hodgkin's disease with mantle-field irradiation at Stanford and the University of California provided the first indication of a dose-response for radiation pericarditis or myocardial injury (Table 1) (12). Most of the patients irradiated for Hodgkin's disease before 1971 had at least 60% of the cardiac volume included in the mediastinal portion of a mantle field. A dose of 40 Gy in 20 fractions over a treatment period of 4 weeks appeared to approximate the threshold for pericardial injury. No cases of pericarditis were observed after doses below 36 Gy. The risk was 2% with doses in the range of 36 to 40 Gy and 6% with doses of 40 to 48 Gy, which were the doses most often used for treatment of mediastinal Hodgkin's disease. Risks rose rapidly with the use of higher radiation doses—particularly among those patients who received more than one course of mediastinal irradiation for recurrent disease. Centers that had emphasized dose delivery through an anterior mediastinal field alone or had used anteriorly weighted ^{60}Co fields rather than equally weighted anterior and posterior fields generated by linear accelerators, soon reported a much higher incidence of constrictive pericarditis and myocardial injury (16,17). Based on these studies, it appeared that high dose per fraction was an important factor contributing to the risk of pericardial and myocardial injury. Therefore, daily treatment of both anterior and posterior fields and avoidance of excessive anterior field weighting became viewed as highly advisable to minimize high dose per fraction exposure of pericardium and myocardium.

TABLE 1. *Dose-response for the risk of radiation-induced pericarditis among 411 patients irradiated to the mediastinum at Stanford or University of California–San Francisco*

Approximate dose (cGy)	Patients at risk	Patients developing pericarditis	
		Number	%
<3600	23	0	0
3600–4000	87	2	2.3
4000–4400	156	7	4.5
4400–4800	75	6	8.0
4800–5000	63	6	9.5
>5000	7	3	43
Total	411	24	5.8

Adapted from data in ref. 12.

The use of subcarinal blocking was instituted at Stanford in 1971 and served to limit the radiation exposure of most of the myocardium to 30 to 35 Gy. This decreased the incidence of early pericardial injury to 2.5% from a 7% incidence observed with partial left ventricular shielding or a 20% incidence observed when radiation fields encompassed the entire heart (18). A study of cases of constrictive pericarditis that required surgery at Stanford suggested that such blocking techniques may have increased the latent interval between irradiation and the development of constriction without affecting the incidence of the problem (19). Patients who underwent pericardiectomy between 1970 and 1980 were usually irradiated before the routine use of subcarinal blocking and underwent surgery an average of 4.75 years after irradiation; those who underwent pericardiectomy between 1980 and 1985 usually had subcarinal blocking and underwent surgery an average of 11 years after irradiation. The authors of this study noted that no patients irradiated after 1980 at Stanford had required pericardiectomy. This complication has virtually vanished with modern treatment approaches.

The survival impact of limiting cardiac radiation dose was verified in a subsequent study from Stanford. The relative risk of death from cardiac diseases other than acute myocardial infarction decreased from 5.1 to 1.7 (not significantly increased) in association with the use of left ventricular and subcarinal blocking during mediastinal irradiation (20). The increased use of initial chemotherapy for patients who present with bulky mediastinal masses of Hodgkin's disease has also improved cardiac protection for many patients by reducing the volume of heart that is incidentally irradiated in order to encompass lymphadenopathy. These combined-modality programs also eliminated the need to use low-dose irradiation of the entire cardiac silhouette to treat cardiophrenic angle lymph nodes, which were relatively common sites for recurrence of mediastinal Hodgkin's disease when these nodal regions were initially untreated (21). The routine use of such strategies to limit the dose and volume of cardiac irradiation has virtually eliminated the complications of constrictive pericarditis and pancarditis from the management of patients treated for Hodgkin's disease. Whether or not the increased use of doxorubicin-based chemotherapy regimens will increase late myocardial injury in such combined-modality regimens remains to be established.

The first suggestions of an association between mediastinal irradiation for Hodgkin's disease and premature coronary artery disease were reports of acute myocardial infarction deaths in a 19-year-old man 4 years after mediastinal irradiation and a 15-year-old boy 16 months after mantle irradiation (7,22). Autopsy findings in the younger patient showed diffuse, severe intimal proliferation and atheromatous change in the proximal coronary arteries with no significant atherosclerosis apparent in other, unirradiated vessels. In the late 1970s Kopelson and Herwig (23) reported ten patients who developed angina pectoris, acute myocardial infarction, or sudden death from acute myocardial infarction before 40 years of age after receiving mediastinal irradiation for Hodgkin's disease. Pohjola-Sintonen et al. (24) reported severe coronary artery disease arising in two males at 12 and 31 years of age following treatment for Hodgkin's disease 7 and 10 years earlier. Both were treated with anterior radiation fields alone to estimated epicardial doses of 40 and 52 Gy.

In the first population-based study, Boivin and Hutchison (25) evaluated coronary heart disease mortality among 957 patients treated for Hodgkin's disease between 1942 and 1975 at either the Harvard Joint Center for Radiation Therapy or the Massachusetts General Hospital. They observed a higher annual probability of death from coronary disease among patients who had received mediastinal irradiation in comparison to those who received no cardiac irradiation. However, the relative risk for death from coronary artery disease in this population was 1.5, which was not significantly elevated. A subsequent analysis of 590 patients treated at the Joint Center for Radiation Therapy between 1969 and 1980 reported 13 deaths from acute myocardial infarction (only one of which occurred before 40 years of age) and a significantly elevated relative risk (RR) of myocardial infarction death of 6.7 [95% confidence interval (CI), 2.91–13.3] (26).

Among patients with early stages of Hodgkin's disease entered in EORTC trials, acute myocardial infarction was the second most common cause of intercurrent death. The standardized mortality ratio (SMR) for the risk of death from acute myocardial infarction was significantly increased for those treated either before or after 40 years of age [SMR, 14.9 (95% CI, 5.5–32.3) vs. SMR, 6.6 (95% CI, 3.3–11.9)], respectively (3). Cosset et al. (27) reported a 3.9% 10-year cumulative incidence rate of acute myocardial infarction after Hodgkin's disease treatment at Institut Gustave-Roussy; 13 acute myocardial infarctions occurred among 499 patients who received mediastinal irradiation for Hodgkin's disease. There were no myocardial infarctions in the 138 patients whose treatments did not include mediastinal irradiation.

In a case-cohort study that compiled records of 4,665 patients treated for Hodgkin's disease at 11 American and Canadian centers, Boivin (28) reported an age-adjusted relative risk of acute myocardial infarction death of 2.56 (95% CI, 1.11–5.93) after treatments that included mediastinal irradiation and 0.97 (95% CI, 0.53–1.77) after chemotherapy. The risk of death from myocardial infarction appeared to be higher among those irradiated after 60 years of age and lower among those treated before 40 years of age. The risk for death from myocardial infarction was significantly increased within 5 years of treatment and appeared to remain elevated with more prolonged follow-up.

Among 2,232 patients treated for Hodgkin's disease at Stanford between 1960 and 1991, 55 deaths were attributed to acute myocardial infarction, representing a relative risk or standardized mortality ratio of 3.2 (95% CI, 2.3–4.0) and an absolute risk of 17.8 excess deaths per 10,000 person-years of observation after therapy (20). The risk of myocardial infarction death tended to be higher among patients treated with radiation alone [RR, 4.1 (95% CI, 2.8–5.5)] than among those who received both chemotherapy and mediastinal irradiation [RR, 2.7 (95% CI, 1.5–3.8)]. The risk of death from myocardial infarction was not significantly increased for those who received no mediastinal irradiation [RR, 1.7 (95% CI, 0.7–3.5)] or who received mediastinal irradiation in doses less than 30 Gy [RR, 4.2 (95% CI, 0.7–13.8)]. The introduction of routine left ventricular and subcarinal blocking in 1971 had little impact upon the risk of death from acute myocardial infarction [RR before 1972: 3.7 (95% CI, 2.3–5.1) and RR after 1972: 3.4 (95% CI, 2.0–4.8)]. For most patients who received mediastinal irradiation, the proximal coronary arteries were likely to be located within the unblocked portion of the radiation field, adjacent to mediastinal lymphadenopathy.

In contrast to the study by Boivin et al., the study from Stanford showed that treatment at a young age conferred a higher relative risk of acute myocardial infarction death than treatment at an older age (Table 2). The risk of infarction death decreased significantly with advancing age at irradiation and was not significantly increased among patients irradiated at 50 years of age or older. The relative risk decreased from 44.7 for those irradiated at 10 to 19 years of age to 1.8 for those irradiated at 50 years of age or older. However, the annualized, absolute risk of death from myocardial infarction after exposure tended to increase with increasing age at irradiation from 12.4 excess cases per 10,000 person-years of observation for those treated between 10 and 19 years of age to 43.6 excess cases for those irradiated between 40 and 49 years of age.

In the Stanford experience, the risk of death from acute myocardial infarction was significantly increased within 5 years of irradiation with 12 events (twice the number expected) and an absolute risk of 6.4 excess events per 10,000 person-years of follow-up. Both the relative risk and the absolute risk after exposure increased significantly with more prolonged follow-up, reaching a relative risk of 5.6 and an absolute risk of 70.6 extra deaths per 10,000 person-years of observation among patients whose follow-up exceeded 20 years (Table 3). This trend to increased risk at more prolonged latency may have been confounded by variations in radiation technique, because patients treated in the earlier eras generally received less

TABLE 2. *Effect of age at irradiation on risk of death from acute myocardial infarction (AMI) after treatment of Hodgkin's disease*

Age at irradiation (years)	Observed/expected events	Relative risk (RR)[a]	95% confidence intervals	Absolute risk (AR)[a,b]
Less than 10	0/0.002	—	—	—
10 through 19	6/0.13	44.7	18.0–93.0	12.4
20 through 29	8/1.1	7.3	3.4–13.8	9.0
30 through 39	14/2.7	5.1	2.9–7.4	27.4
40 through 49	9/3.0	3.0	1.4–5.5	43.6
50 or more	12/6.8	1.8	1.0–3.0	—

[a]χ for trend in AMI-RR: $p < .0001$; χ for trend in AMI-AR: 2.6, $p = 0.01$.
[b]Absolute risk is expressed as excess cases per 10,000 person-years.
Adapted from ref. 20.

cardiac blocking, higher daily fraction size, higher total doses, and higher epicardial daily doses due to treatment of anterior and posterior fields on alternate days.

Acute myocardial infarction death tended to occur at a younger age than is common (Table 4). The relative risk was 52.4 for patients younger than 30 years of age; it declined progressively to 2.2 for those between 50 and 59 years of age, and was not significantly increased for those 60 years of age or older. There was no association between chemotherapy exposure and an increased risk of death due to premature coronary artery disease. Cardiac risk factors were not clearly documented among these patients, although the prevalence of cigarette smoking in the Stanford population appeared to be significantly lower than expected in the general population.

The association of increased myocardial infarction risk with high-dose mediastinal irradiation at a young age was underscored by another study that focused on 635 patients treated for Hodgkin's disease before 21 years of age at Stanford (29). Seven patients died of myocardial infarction, with a standardized mortality ratio of 41.5 (95% CI, 18.1–82.1). Three young patients sustained nonfatal myocardial infarctions, and three others required revascularization procedures for severe coronary artery disease. Among these younger patients, all coronary events arose from 6 to 20 years after mediastinal radiation doses that ranged from 42 to 45 Gy.

The effect of radiation dose in determining the subsequent risk for premature coronary disease is uncertain. Brierly et al. (30) summarized cardiac morbidity observed after treatment of Hodgkin's disease in 611 patients at Princess Margaret Hospital, where most patients received mediastinal radiation doses of 35 Gy in 20 fractions. The actuarial incidence of heart disease at 15 years was 10% for those whose mediastinum was irradiated and 12% for those who received no mediastinal irradiation. Mediastinal irradiation was not identified as a significant risk factor for cardiac disease. The relative risk of death from myocardial infarction was estimated at 1.55 (95% CI, 0.71–2.95)

Glanzmann et al. (31) reported a relative risk of acute myocardial infarction death of 4.2 (95% CI, 1.8–8.3) and a relative risk of either sudden death or myocardial infarction death of 6.7 (95% CI, 3.5–11.2) among 352 patients treated at University Hospital, Zurich, 93% of whom received 30 to 42 Gy with dose per fraction ranging from 1.3 to 2.1 Gy. Coronary mortality risk appeared to be confined to males and was higher after treatment with chemotherapy and irradiation [RR, 10 (95% CI, 4.3–19.7)] than with irradiation alone [RR, 5 (95% CI, 1.6–11.7)]. This analysis indicates that excess coronary artery disease mortality may occur despite lower mediastinal irradiation doses than were implicated in the Stanford experience. Unlike the experience reported from Stanford, the study from Zurich found that fatal or nonfatal coronary artery disease events were largely confined to individuals with known coronary risk factors of smoking, hypertension, obesity, or hypercholesterolemia. No adverse cardiac event

TABLE 3. *Latency of risk for death from acute myocardial infarction (AMI) after treatment of Hodgkin's disease*

Years after initial Hodgkin's disease Tx	Observed/expected events	Relative risk[a]	95% confidence intervals	Absolute risk[a,b]
0 through 4	12/6.0	2.0	1.1–3.3	6.4
5 through 9	17/4.7	3.6	2.2–4.5	20.1
10 through 14	11/3.7	3.0	1.6–5.2	20.5
15 through 19	11/2.2	5.0	2.6–8.7	54.2
Over 20	4/0.7	5.6	1.8–13.6	70.6

[a]χ for trend in relative risk of AMI death: 2.3, $p = .02$; χ for trend in absolute risk of AMI death: 3.8. $p = .0002$.
[b]Absolute risk is expressed as excess cases per 10,000 person-years.
Adapted from ref. 20.

TABLE 4. *Risk for death from acute myocardial infarction after treatment of Hodgkin's disease according to age at death*

Years of age at death from AMI	Observed/expected events	Relative risk	95% Confidence intervals	Absolute risk[a]
under 30	1/0.19	52.4	0.0–259	—
30 through 39	7/0.37	18.8	8.2–37.2	9.0
40 through 49	14/2.0	7.0	4.0–10.0	21.4
50 through 59	12/2.7	4.5	2.4–7.5	39.0
60 through 69	11/5.0	2.2	1.2–3.8	52.7
70 or more	10/6.2	1.6	0.8–2.9	—

[a]Absolute risk is expressed as excess cases per 10,000 person-years.
Adapted from ref. 20.

had occurred among the 74 patients who lacked identifiable risk factors and had received no chemotherapy. Nine of the 13 patients who had sudden death or a fatal myocardial infarction and two of three patients who sustained nonfatal myocardial infarctions had no antecedent angina pectoris or other cardiac symptoms in this series. This absence of prodromal symptoms was also common in the Stanford experience (20,29) and has led to assessment of strategies for screening populations at potential risk at both institutions, as discussed below.

Unusual valvular injury attributed to irradiation was reported in two necropsy studies of children and young adults treated with mediastinal irradiation (14,15), and mitral insufficiency was reported in early analyses from Stanford (6). Nonetheless, establishment of increased risks for valvular heart disease among Hodgkin's disease survivors has been a relatively recent finding. Most of the evidence for valvular disease derives from echocardiographic studies of Hodgkin's disease survivors. Mitral or aortic valve thickening was found in 27% of 41 Hodgkin's disease or mediastinal seminoma survivors studied in the early 1980s by Perrault et al. (32) and in 2 of 28 Hodgkin's disease patients studied by Pohjola-Sintonen et al. (24). Valvular insufficiency was the most common finding in echocardiographic studies of 25 young-adult Hodgkin's disease patients, with tricuspid regurgitation identified in 22, mitral regurgitation in nine, and aortic regurgitation in one. Studies of cardiopulmonary function in 116 Norwegians treated for Hodgkin's disease with mediastinal irradiation with or without chemotherapy identified cardiopulmonary dysfunction in 75% of females and 41% of males (33). On echocardiographic studies, 15% of these patients had aortic regurgitation, 7% had mitral regurgitation, and 2% had both aortic and mitral regurgitation that exceeded grade 1 severity (34). None of 40 control subjects had valvular regurgitation that exceeded grade 1 in severity. Valvular dysfunction affected 46% of the women and 16% of the men in this study, and female gender appeared to be an independent risk factor for valvular injury or symptomatic cardiopulmonary dysfunction in this population.

Female gender was not identified as a specific risk factor for cardiac dysfunction or valvular heart disease among 144 patients studied by Glanzmann (31) after mediastinal irradiation that generally ranged from 30 to 42 Gy for Hodgkin's disease. Only three patients had symptomatic valvular heart disease. However, the authors found abnormal valvular thickening in 29% of patients, with a cumulative incidence that rose from 8% after 10 years to 66% among patients treated more than 25 years before the study. Glanzmann et al. also found support for increased valvular abnormality with more prolonged follow-up through repeated echocardiography of 74 patients 1 to 6 years after an initial study that occurred more than 10 years after therapy; 8% of the subjects whose valves were normal developed signs of thickening, and 37% of the subjects with thickening had progression of valvular abnormality on subsequent study.

Although most of the valvular abnormalities identified by echocardiographic screening after mediastinal irradiation for Hodgkin's disease have not been associated with clinical symptoms, valvular heart disease has contributed to excess morbidity and mortality. Among 635 patients treated for Hodgkin's disease before 21 years of age at Stanford, three were reported to have died of complications related to valvular heart disease and three had undergone surgical replacement of damaged valves (29). Four of 1,597 patients treated at Stanford at 21 years of age or older died of valvular heart disease or complications related to valve replacement (20). Because age-specific rates for symptoms or death from valvular heart disease are not available in the general population, it has not been possible to quantitate the amount of additional risk that mediastinal irradiation for Hodgkin's disease has entailed.

RADIATION FACTORS ASSOCIATED WITH CARDIAC TOXICITY

The risks of acute radiation pericarditis and delayed constrictive pericarditis after irradiation for Hodgkin's disease have been clearly associated with the volume of the heart irradiated and the dose of radiation received. Stewart and Fajardo (12) and Stewart et al. (35) have estimated that the threshold for significant pericardial injury is 40 Gy if more than 60% of the heart is included in the radiation field and 55 to 60 Gy if less than 15% of the cardiac volume is irradiated. The risk of pericarditis rises steeply with doses above 40 Gy when subcarinal blocking is not employed (Table 1). Among patients treated with doses approximating 44 Gy, early pericarditis affected 20% of patients treated to 60% or more of the heart in the absence of blocking, 7% in whom blocks shielded the left ventricle, and 2.5% who had both left ventricular shielding and placement of a subcarinal block to limit ventricular exposure to 30 Gy (18). Late constrictive pericarditis has been exceedingly rare among patients treated with mediastinal doses of 44 Gy or less when exposure of the entire cardiac silhouette has been limited to 15 to 25 Gy and subcarinal blocking has been added between 25 and 35 Gy. Among patients treated at Stanford, the risk of death from cardiac diseases other than acute myocardial infarction has not been significantly increased among patients treated since the introduction of subcarinal blocking in 1971 or among cohorts who received mediastinal irradiation doses of 30 Gy or less (20).

Because the risk of premature coronary disease has varied with treatment technique, use of chemotherapy, age at treatment, and duration of observation, it is difficult to draw firm conclusions about the relationships between radiation dose, volume of the heart irradiated, and coronary-artery disease risk. Investigators at Princess Margaret Hospital have found no significant increase in the risk of acute myocardial infarction death among 611 patients with stage I or II Hodgkin's disease, 246 of whom received mantle irradiation to a usual dose of 35 Gy using a fraction size of 1.75 Gy (30). Among patients treated in Zurich Glanzmann et al. (31) observed a very high relative risk of acute myocardial infarction or sudden death of 8.6 (CI, 4.5–15.3) in men who received approximately 40 Gy in 1.5- to 1.8-Gy fractions but observed no excess risk among women who had received similar treatment [RR, 1.72 (CI, 0.04–9.6)]. They also found that the risk for fatal or nonfatal ischemic coronary events appeared to be confined to those who had known risk factors for coronary artery disease, including smoking, hypertension, diabetes, obesity, or hypercholesterolemia [RR, 2.36 (CI, 1.42–3.68) with risk factors vs. 0.96 (CI, 0.20–2.77) with no known risk factors]. The prevalence of known coronary risk factors was unknown in the population of patients irradiated at Stanford, where the usual mediastinal dose was 44 Gy administered in 1.8 to 2.2 Gy fractions (20). The relative risk of myocardial infarction death was significantly increased among women in this population [RR 2.6 (CI, 1.2–5.0)], suggesting some potential difference in risk associated with dose when compared with the Zurich experience. Dose effect remained unclear in the overall Stanford experience, because the relative risks were similar with or without subcarinal blocking [RR 3.4 (CI, 2.0–4.5) vs. RR 3.7 (CI, 2.3–5.1)] or with mediastinal doses above or below 30 Gy [RR, 3.5 (CI, 2.5–4.5) vs. 4.2 (CI, 0.7–13.8)]. Cosset et al. (27) were also unable to demonstrate a relationship between total dose or fraction size and the risk of acute myocardial infarction death in a comparison of 499 patients who had received mediastinal irradiation for Hodgkin's disease in comparison with 138 patients who were not irradiated.

The relationship between radiation dose, cardiac volume, and the subsequent development of valvular heart disease has also been difficult to discern due to the relatively small number of events, prolonged latency for the development of clinically apparent valvular disease, and evolving radiation techniques. Glanzmann et al. (31) demonstrated the latency of valvular abnormality after radiation by means of echocardiographic studies that were performed on 144 patients treated with mediastinal irradiation for Hodgkin's disease in Zurich between 1964 and 1994. Forty-two patients (29%) had aortic or mitral valvular thickening apparent on cardiac echogram, four of whom had grade 3 lesions. The cumulative incidence of valvular thickening 10 years after irradiation was 8% but rose to 45% at 20 years with grade 3 changes in 4.1%. Among patients who had repeat echocardiography from 1 to 6 years after an initial study, 8% of patients with normal heart valves at their initial study developed valvular thickening and 37% of those with abnormal valves showed progression of valvular abnormality.

IMPACT OF CHEMOTHERAPY

At present, studies in populations treated for Hodgkin's disease have shown variable associations between chemotherapy exposure in combined-modality regimens and subsequent risks for cardiac disease. The relative risk of death from acute myocardial infarction in the Stanford population was slightly lower among patients treated with mediastinal irradiation and MOPP [mechlorethamine, Oncovin (vincristine), procarbazine, and prednisone] than with irradiation alone [RR, 2.8 (CI, 1.6–4.0) vs. RR, 3.8 (CI, 2.0–5.1)] (20). Factors that contributed to this included the use of lower average mediastinal radiation doses and somewhat shorter follow-up duration with combined therapy. The mean mediastinal dose was 43.3 Gy for radiation alone versus 40.7 Gy for combined therapy, and the median follow-up was 9.1 years after radiation alone versus 8.1 years with combined treatment. Among patients treated in Zurich, the relative risk of acute myocardial infarction or sudden death was somewhat higher after combined therapy than after radiation alone [RR, 10 (CI, 4.3–19.7) vs. RR, 5 (CI, 1.6–11.7)] (31).

The increasing use of anthracycline-based chemotherapy regimens such as ABVD [Adriamycin (doxorubicin), bleomycin, vinblastine, and dacarbazine] raise new concerns about late cardiac toxicity after the treatment of Hodgkin's disease. Studies using clinical and morphologic end points have shown that mediastinal irradiation potentiates cardiac toxicity from anthracyclines. Using light and electron microscopic techniques Billingham et al. (36)

TABLE 5. *Pathologic grades of myocardial toxicity due to anthracyclines*

Grade	Definition
0	No changes from normal
1	Scanty cells with early change (early myofibrillar loss and/or distended sarcoplasmic reticulum)
2	Groups of cells with definite change (marked myofibrillar loss and/or cytoplasmic vacuolization)
3	Diffuse cell damage with marked change (total loss of contractile elements, loss of organelles, mitochondrial and nuclear degeneration)

From ref. 36.

developed a system for grading myofibrillary loss in endomyocardial biopsies obtained during cardiac catheterizations and found that histologic findings preceded and correlated with the risk of congestive cardiomyopathy (Table 5). Billingham et al. (37) found that patients who had received cardiac irradiation had greater myocyte degeneration and an increased incidence of congestive heart failure than patients who received comparable doses of Adriamycin without irradiation (Table 6). They also found evidence for Adriamycin recall of acute radiation injury, noting capillary endothelial cell damage typical of acute radiation injury in a patient who received Adriamycin 10.5 years after irradiation.

Late cardiac decompensation after anthracycline therapy has been better documented among individuals treated during childhood than among adults. Steinherz et al. (38) identified 15 patients among a screened population of 300 who developed abnormalities of cardiac conduction, dysrhythmias, or congestive failure between 6 and 19 years after exposure to daunorubicin or doxorubicin in doses ranging from 285 to 870 mg per square meter of body surface area. Some patients who had no early evidence of cardiac injury experienced cardiac decompensation more than 10 years after anthracycline exposure. Although stresses unique to adolescent development may have played a role in these occasional episodes of cardiac decompensation after anthracycline exposure, there is little published data regarding cardiac function beyond the first decade in individuals who received anthracycline therapy during early adulthood.

Several groups have used echocardiography and radionuclide imaging techniques to assess the contribution of doxorubicin to cardiac dysfunction in Hodgkin's disease survivors. LaMonte et al. (39) concluded that significant abnormalities were likely to be low, reporting normal resting and exercise function in 15 of 19 patients treated with the MOPP/ABVD regimen and varying doses of radiation to the mediastinum. Two patients had decreased left ventricular ejection fraction at rest, and two others had a diminished left ventricular response to exercise. Similarly, Allavena et al. (40) found signs of diminished left ventricular function in only 6% of Hodgkin's disease patients and could not differentiate between treatment with radiation alone or combined with MOPP or MOPP/ABVD. Among 40 patients screened with echocardiography after three cycles of ABVD and mediastinal irradiation to doses of 40 to 45 Gy, 38 had normal left ventricular ejection fraction and two had borderline low values of 50% (41). Functional impairment associated with combined irradiation and anthracycline-containing regimens for Hodgkin's disease may be greater when administered during childhood. Pihkala et al. (42) reported abnormally low left ventricular ejection fraction for 50% of children who had received both doxorubicin and mediastinal irradiation (to a median dose of 24 Gy with a range from 11 to 51 Gy) compared with 8% of children who had received mediastinal irradiation alone to a median dose of 40 Gy. Careful analyses of late intercurrent morbidity and mortality in large populations of

TABLE 6. *Effect of mediastinal radiation on the pathologic grade of doxorubicin-treated patients compared with unirradiated dose-matched controls*

	With radiation				Without radiation	
Patient no.	Dose (cGy)	Heart failure	Pathology grade	Dox. dose (mg/m^2)	Mean pathologic grade (±95% confidence limits)	Heart failure
6	3,500	No	0	90 ± 60	—	
10	4,900	No	1	216 ± 60	0.88 ± 0.54 (8 controls)	—
5	3,000	No	2	258 ± 60	0.89 ± 0.46 (9 controls)	No
8	4,510	No	1	262 ± 60	0.89 ± 0.46 (9 controls)	No
3	2,940	No	2	270 ± 60	1.11 ± 0.46 (9 controls)	No
7	4,000	No	1	270 ± 60	1.11 ± 0.46 (9 controls)	No
11	5,000	No	3	272 ± 60	1.11 ± 0.46 (9 controls)	No
12	5,700	Yes	3	330 ± 60	1.29 ± 0.70 (7 controls)	No
4	2,940	No	3	373 ± 60	1.5 ± 0.63 (8 controls)	No
1	<600	Yes	2	395 ± 60	1.38 ± 0.62 (8 controls)	No
2	<600	No	1	430 ± 60	1.38 ± 0.62 (8 controls)	Yes
9	4,800	Yes	3	445 ± 60	1.43 ± 0.73 (7 controls)	Yes
		Mean: 2.0 ± 0.89 (S.D.)			1.18 ± 0.23 (S.D.)	

Adapted from ref. 37.

Hodgkin's disease patients treated with anthracycline-based regimens such as ABVD with and without irradiation are clearly needed to confirm the lack of cardiac decompensation more than a decade beyond these therapies.

VASCULAR COMPLICATIONS

Elerding et al. (43) analyzed pooled retrospective data on 910 patients from M. D. Anderson Cancer Center who had received irradiation to the neck, including 247 patients treated for Hodgkin's disease, 119 patients treated for non-Hodgkin's lymphoma, and 537 patients with squamous cell carcinomas of the head and neck. The authors found a 6.9% incidence of cerebrovascular accidents over a 9-year period of observation. By their estimates the relative risk of stroke was nearly twice that expected in a general population, but this increase was not statistically significant (p = .39). These events occurred an average of 9 years after irradiation at an average of 64 years of age. The incidence of stroke among the patients treated for Hodgkin's disease was not specified. However, Elerding et al. also prospectively studied 77 patients more than 5 years after treatment radiation fields that included the neck for Hodgkin's disease with carotid phonoangiograms and ocular plethysmography. Seventeen patients (22%) had abnormal phonoangiogram studies, suggesting turbulent flow in the carotid system. Four others had audible bruits on auscultation and were excluded from the phonoangiogram study because turbulence may have originated in the innominate or subclavian system. Twelve of the patients studied (16%) had abnormal ocular plethysmography, suggesting significant impairment of blood flow through the carotid system due to stenosis. The Hodgkin's disease patients with apparent vascular stenosis averaged 38 years of age at the time of these studies. The impact of premature cerebrovascular disease has not been well quantified in other large populations of patients treated for Hodgkin's disease, although sporadic case reports have suggested that carotid artery disease and stroke may be potential late sources of morbidity or mortality (44–48).

Venous thrombotic disease that primarily involves the axillary-subclavian venous system has also been reported during chemotherapy or combined-modality therapy of Hodgkin's disease (49,50). The risk for these episodes has been primarily attributed to the desiccant action of some chemotherapy agents or the presence of indwelling infusion catheters, and appears to be unrelated to Hodgkin's disease activity .

CLINICAL PRESENTATIONS

The acute pericarditis that may develop during or after mediastinal irradiation for Hodgkin's disease has the same variety of clinical manifestations that occur with viral or idiopathic pericarditis or with the postcardiotomy syndrome and is usually transient and self-limited (18, 35). Patients report chest pains that are often pleuritic in character and may be affected by position. Auscultation may reveal a pericardial friction rub, and chest roentgenogram may or may not show an enlarged, globular cardiac silhouette. The electrocardiogram may show low voltage, when significant effusions are present, diffuse ST segment elevation across the precordium in the early phase, and diffuse T wave inversion during later stages. Acute pericarditis is generally treated with nonsteroidal antiinflammatory agents, unless symptoms are severe and persistent. Corticosteroids may be useful for refractory episodes, but are associated with risks for recurrent episodes of pericarditis during withdrawal and with a consequent risk of steroid dependency. Cardiac tamponade may develop during the course of acute pericarditis with effusion, and should be suspected when dyspnea is reported. Clinical signs include neck vein elevation and a paradoxical pulse. Echocardiography may be helpful in establishing the diagnosis. Therapy generally consists of pericardiocentesis, although thoracoscopic procedures or open pericardiectomy may be required when symptomatic pericardial effusion and constrictive pericarditis coexist. One episode of myocardial infarction without clinically significant coronary occlusion was reported to arise after irradiation for Hodgkin's disease due to vasospasm apparently induced by acute pericarditis (51).

Pericardial effusion may present as an increased heart size on routine follow-up chest radiograph in the absence of symptoms. Most such effusions resolve without intervention, although many patients are treated with nonsteroidal antiinflammatory agents. Tamponade is rare. Some small effusions may persist in an apparently benign form and have been observed as late findings on echocardiographic studies of asymptomatic patients.

Constrictive pericarditis may present insidiously with exertional dyspnea and pleural effusions or may present with signs of biventricular failure with exertional dyspnea, peripheral edema, hepatomegaly, and tamponade (Fig. 1) (6,20,27,29). Pericardial effusion may or may not be present on echocardiographic evaluation. Ventricular size and wall motion are usually normal on echogram. Echocardiography, computed tomography (CT), or magnetic resonance imaging (MRI) scans of the thorax may feature prominent pericardial thickening to support this diagnosis. Cardiac catheterization is usually necessary to document equalization of diastolic filling pressures in the left and right ventricles. Treatment requires surgical pericardiectomy, but this has been associated with increased morbidity and a 21% mortality rate in irradiated patients, presumably due to coexisting myocardial, pulmonary, and pleural fibrosis in many patients (19). The strategies used to decrease radiation dose and volume during mediastinal irradiation for Hodgkin's disease appear to have substantially reduced the incidence of constrictive pericarditis and should reduce surgical risks for the rare individual who may develop this complication.

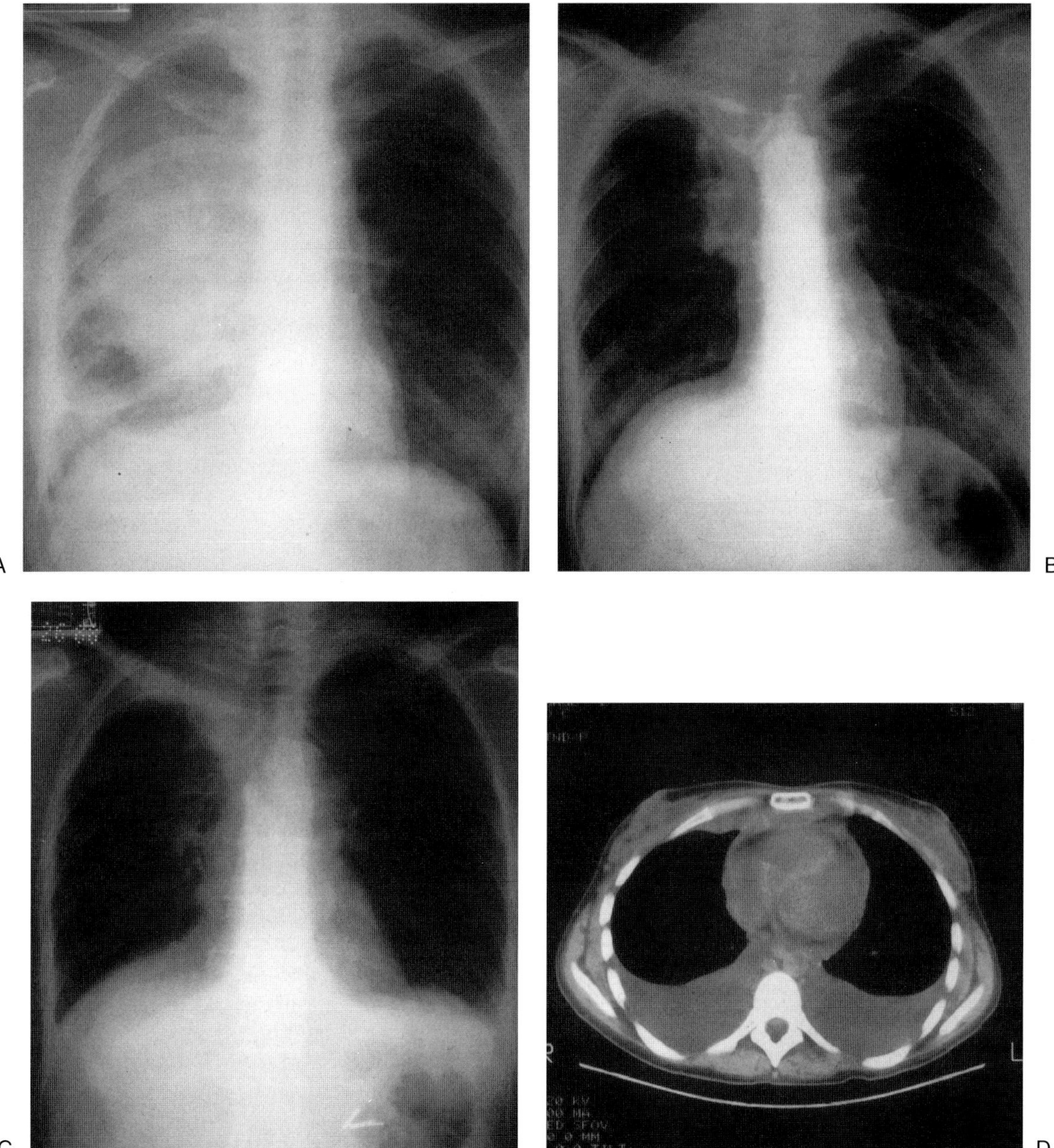

FIG. 1. Radiographs of a patient with delayed constrictive pericarditis. **A:** Chest radiograph at initial presentation with stage IIIeB nodular sclerosing Hodgkin's disease with massive mediastinal disease, bilateral hilar adenopathy, and extension of disease into the right lung. **B:** Routine follow-up chest radiograph obtained 4 years after therapy with procarbazine, Alkeran, and vinblastine (PAVe) chemotherapy alternating with Adriamycin (doxorubicin), bleomycin, vinblastine, and dacarbazine (ABVD) chemotherapy followed by mantle, paraaortic, and splenic pedicle irradiation. The residual mediastinal mass, fibrotic changes in the right lung apex and perimediastinal and hilar regions, and volume loss in the right lung had been stable on serial radiographs. **C:** Chest radiograph obtained 2 years after the film in B showing new, bilateral pleural effusions despite minimal change in the cardiac silhouette. **D:** Computerized tomographic scan of the chest obtained 2 days after the film in C showing massive bilateral pleural effusion but no significant pericardial effusion or thickening. Serial echocardiograms showed no signs of effusive or constrictive pericarditis. Subsequent cardiac catheterization documented equalization of ventricular filling pressures, indicating severe constrictive pericarditis. Effusions resolved after surgical pericardiectomy. Pathology revealed severe, diffuse pericardial fibrosis and pericardial aspergillosis.

Among the clinical sequelae of mediastinal irradiation, coronary artery disease has been particularly difficult to diagnose before cardiac injury from acute myocardial infarction or sudden death. In part, this may be attributable to cardiac symptoms that arise at an earlier age than is typical for coronary artery disease. However, many patients appear to have had no symptoms before a catastrophic event. Among 55 deaths attributed to myocardial infarction in Hodgkin's disease patients treated at Stanford, 38 patients had no prior history of heart disease or record of symptoms suggesting angina pectoris (20). Similarly, 9 of 13 acute myocardial infarction deaths or sudden deaths reported in Hodgkin's disease survivors from Zurich occurred in individuals who had no history of cardiac disease or angina pectoris (31). Two of these patients had normal electrocardiography, echocardiography, and myocardial perfusion scintigraphy within 6 months of death. Significant ischemia may be clinically silent, may produce unusual manifestations, such as exertional dyspnea, and may be associated with coronary ostial stenosis induced by radiation (52). Some have questioned whether a persistent sinus tachycardia that has been observed in occasional patients after mediastinal irradiation may represent functional denervation of the heart and a consequent inability to perceive chest pain. Similar phenomena have been documented among individuals after cardiac transplantation or associated with the autonomic dysfunction of severe diabetes mellitus (53,54).

Valvular heart disease that arises after irradiation should be identified by cardiac auscultation during routine follow-up of patients after treatment for Hodgkin's disease well before there are symptoms suggesting cardiac decompensation or the need for valve replacement. Cardiac murmurs indicating mitral or aortic regurgitation should be evaluated by echocardiography. Patients with more than minimal amounts of valvular insufficiency should have routine cardiologic follow-up with annual or biennial echocardiography to judge the need for and appropriate timing of valvular surgery.

Abnormalities of the cardiac conducting system may be manifestations of cardiac fibrosis and are well documented after mediastinal irradiation (11,15,24,55–57). Bundle branch block on electrocardiogram represents ventricular injury affecting the Purkinje branches and is the most common and earliest sign of conduction system abnormality (35). Bundle branch block may presage atrioventricular (AV) block, although this may also arise as a manifestation of direct AV nodal injury, which may be heralded by a prolonged PR interval on electrocardiography. AV block that causes symptoms or involves the His-Purkinje system requires implantation of a permanent pacemaker (35).

Chronic pleural effusions may be a late development after high-dose mediastinal irradiation for Hodgkin's disease and present a difficult diagnostic and therapeutic dilemma (35). Evaluation generally requires thoracentesis to evaluate potential malignant or infectious causes, assessment of thyroid and pulmonary function, thoracic CT scanning, and biopsy of pulmonary or pleural lesions that may be suspicious for malignancy. This often yields no adequate pulmonary or pleural pathology that is sufficient to explain persistent or recurrent effusion. Thorough cardiac evaluation should be performed including electrocardiography, echocardiography, and consideration of cardiac catheterization with coronary angiography to ensure the absence of pericardial constriction or potentially correctable left ventricular dysfunction, such as silent ischemia. Often, the etiology of such effusions remains obscure. These effusions may persist and vary in volume over many years and have generally been attributed to sclerosis of mediastinal lymphatics.

CARDIAC FUNCTIONAL EVALUATION AND SCREENING

Studies that have aimed to quantitate the extent of cardiopulmonary dysfunction in Hodgkin's disease survivors through various combinations of rest and exercise echocardiography and radionuclide scintigraphy scanning have reached variable conclusions. Watchie et al. (58) reported results of cardiac and pulmonary exercise testing for 57 patients an average of 5 years after treatment with extensive thoracic irradiation with or without chemotherapy at Stanford and concluded that symptomatic cardiopulmonary dysfunction was quite rare, with only one patient complaining of limitation. They identified conduction system abnormalities in seven patients, electrocardiogram (ECG) abnormalities of uncertain significance in 14 others, and diminished exercise tolerance in approximately one-third of patients. In contrast, Lund et al. (33) found a higher rate of cardiopulmonary dysfunction and disability among 116 patients treated for Hodgkin's disease in Norway and tested 5 to 14 years later. Signs of cardiac or pulmonary dysfunction affected 75% of women and 41% of the men who underwent echocardiography, exercise testing, and pulmonary function testing; 27% of those patients who had signs of diminished function on both cardiac and pulmonary testing reported disability, as did 4% of those with less impairment on testing. In a smaller series decreased left ventricular ejection fraction was found to correlate with irradiation techniques that encompassed the entire heart but was not observed in patients who had some portion of the heart shielded during Hodgkin's disease irradiation (59). None of the 16 patients studied in this series had symptomatic impairment. A high rate of cardiopulmonary dysfunction was also documented in a small series of patients treated with mantle-field irradiation during childhood (60).

There is growing interest in the use of exercise echocardiography and radionuclide perfusion imaging to screen for occult coronary artery disease or silent ischemia. In two early studies comparing resting and exercise thallium-201 single photon emission tomographic scans after irradiation for Hodgkin's disease, 61% and 84% of the patients had abnormal distribution of thallium uptake (61,62). Coronary angiography was not performed to confirm coronary obstruction. However, Maunoury et al. (62) reported that the patterns of the perfusion defects observed after irradiation were not typical for an obstruction in a single major coronary artery and attributed exercise-induced defects to small coronary vessel disease and fixed perfusion deficits to myocardial fibrosis. Functional testing has been reported for 144 patients treated for Hodgkin's disease in Zurich (31). Resting ECG was normal in 88%. During exercise testing ECG became abnormal in 8% of patients, with 4% having unequivocal signs of myocardial ischemia and 3% showing ascending ST segment depression suspicious for ischemia. One hundred of these patients underwent myocardial perfusion scintigraphy with technetium-99m–methoxy-isobutyl-isonitril (^{99m}Tc-MIBI): four patients had abnormalities suggesting ischemia, three were considered equivocal for ischemia, and 93 were normal. The report of this study did not specify whether these electrocardiographic or nuclear perfusion abnormalities suggesting ischemia were confirmed on subsequent angiography.

In an ongoing study of patients irradiated for Hodgkin's disease at Stanford, 5% of 274 patients have had stress-induced wall-motion abnormalities identified through comparison of resting and exercise echocardiograms and 11% have had stress-induced defects in myocardial perfusion imaging. Follow-up angiography in the 14% of patients who had abnormal screening studies showed that 55% of these had greater than 50% stenosis in at least one coronary artery. Four patients have undergone coronary artery bypass grafts and three have undergone percutaneous angioplasty for management of clinically occult coronary disease identified by screening. The role of cardiac screening in the routine follow-up of patients who have received mediastinal irradiation for Hodgkin's disease has not been clearly defined. Glanzmann et al. (31) have advocated exercise myocardial perfusion imaging at 5-year intervals after therapy.

MINIMIZING CARDIOVASCULAR RISKS

Several strategies have emerged to minimize late cardiovascular risks after treatment of Hodgkin's disease. Newer treatment approaches have attempted to limit the total radiation dose and radiation dose per fraction through treatment of involved fields, with chemotherapy regimens substituted for the prophylactic nodal irradiation previously used in extended-field, subtotal lymphoid, or total lymphoid irradiation regimens. It is likely that mediastinal irradiation can be avoided altogether in patients who have no evidence of intrathoracic involvement on CT imaging and have received chemotherapy regimens that have proven to be effective. The use of chemotherapy before irradiation causes regression of most mediastinal Hodgkin's disease and permits shielding a larger volume of heart from the radiation field. To minimize high epicardial radiation doses, mediastinal lymphadenopathy should be treated with equally weighted anterior and posterior radiation fields, with both fields irradiated each day instead of using anterior fields alone or anteriorly weighted fields.

Patients who have already received mediastinal irradiation should have periodic assessment of known cardiac risk factors and optimal medical management to minimize risk. This is underscored by the association of known cardiac risk factors with markedly increased risk for acute myocardial infarction death despite apparently conventional cardiac doses and dose rate in the University Hospital, Zurich study (31). Efforts should aim at cessation of cigarette smoking, and optimal management of lipids, glucose intolerance, and hypertension. Studies are under way to assess the value of follow-up cardiac screening tests in identifying clinically significant coronary artery disease, valvular degeneration, conduction deficits, and pericardial diseases. However, Glanzmann et al. (31) have reported that 2 of 112 patients that they screened with ECG, exercise testing, and perfusion scintigraphy died suddenly from acute myocardial infarction within 6 months of normal screening with no antecedent history of angina pectoris. This suggests a potentially important false-negative rate for noninvasive screening tests that remains to be quantified. At present, coronary angiography is considered the most accurate means for documenting the presence and severity of coronary artery disease. However, the costs and potential morbidity of angiography have precluded its use in validating noninvasive tests, such as stress echocardiography, electrocardiography, and radionuclide perfusion scintigraphy, in truly asymptomatic patients with no signs of potential ischemia on noninvasive testing. Whether developing techniques such as magnetic resonance or CT angiography will provide better vascular imaging with less risk remains to be determined.

Periodic patient assessment by careful history and physical examination are likely to contribute to decreased morbidity and mortality in survivors of Hodgkin's disease. Many physicians are hesitant to consider coronary artery disease as a cause of chest or arm pressure, epigastric distress, nausea or flu-like symptoms, or profound exertional fatigue in younger patients. Unusual symptoms such as these should prompt stress testing and careful cardiologic assessment. Auscultation of cardiac murmurs or carotid bruits should prompt ultrasound evaluation and a plan for periodic reevaluation when significant valvular stenosis, regurgitation, or vascular stenosis has been documented.

REFERENCES

1. Hoppe RT. Hodgkin's disease: complications of therapy and excess mortality. *Ann Oncol* 1997;8(suppl 1):115–118.
2. Mauch PM, Kalish LA, Marcus KC, et al. Long-term survival in Hodgkin's disease: relative impact of mortality, second tumors, infection, and cardiovascular disease. *Cancer J Sci Am* 1995;1:33–42.
3. Henry-Amar M, Hayat M, Meerwaldt JH, et al. Causes of death after therapy for early stage Hodgkin's disease entered on EORTC protocols. EORTC Lymphoma Cooperative Group. *Int J Radiat Oncol Biol Phys* 1990;19:1155–1157.
4. Vaughan Hudson B, Vaughan Hudson G, Linch C, Anderson L. Late mortality in young BNLI patients cured of Hodgkin's disease. *Ann Oncol* 1994;5:565–566.
5. Hancock SL, Hoppe RT. Long-term complications of treatment and causes of mortality after Hodgkin's disease. *Semin Radiat Oncol* 1996; 6:225–242.
6. Stewart JR, Fajardo LF. Radiation-induced heart disease. Clinical and experimental aspects. *Radiol Clin North Am* 1971;9:511–531.
7. Cohn KE, Stewart JR, Fajardo LF, Hancock EW. Heart disease following radiation. *Medicine (Baltimore)* 1967;46:281–298.
8. Kaplan HS. Role of intensive radiotherapy in the management of Hodgkin's disease. *Cancer* 1966;19:356.
9. Fajardo LF, Stewart JR. Experimental radiation-induced heart disease. I. Light microscopic studies. *Am J Pathol* 1970;59:299–316.
10. Fajardo LF, Stewart JR. Capillary injury preceding radiation-induced myocardial fibrosis. *Radiology* 1971;101:429–433.
11. Rubin E, Camara J, Grayzel DM, Zak FG. Radiation-induced cardiac fibrosis. *Am J Med* 1963;34:71–75.
12. Stewart JR, Fajardo LF. Dose response in human and experimental radiation-induced heart disease. Application of the nominal standard dose (NSD) concept. *Radiology* 1971;99:403–408.
13. Stewart JR, Fajardo LF. Radiation-induced heart disease: an update. *Prog Cardiovasc Dis* 1984;27:173–194.
14. Greenwood RD, Rosenthal A, Cassady R, Jaffe N, Nadas AS. Constrictive pericarditis in childhood due to mediastinal irradiation. *Circulation* 1974;50:1033–1039.
15. Broesius FC, Waller BF, Roberts WG. Radiation heart disease: analysis of 16 young (aged 15 to 33 years) necropsy patients who received over 3,500 rads to the heart. *Am J Med* 1981;70:519–530.
16. Byhardt R, Brace K. Dose and treatment factors in radiation-related pericardial effusion associated with the mantle technique for Hodgkin's disease. *Cancer* 1974;35:795–802.
17. Morton DL, Glancy DL, Joseph WL, et al. Management of patients with radiation-induced pericarditis with effusion: a note on the development of aortic regurgitation in two of them. *Chest* 1973;64:291–297.
18. Carmel RJ, Kaplan HS. Mantle irradiation in Hodgkin's disease: an analysis of technique, tumor eradication, and complications. *Cancer* 1976;37:2813–2825.
19. Cameron J, Oesterle SN, Baldwin JC, Hancock EW. The etiologic spectrum of constrictive pericarditis. *Am Heart J* 1987;113:354–360.
20. Hancock SL, Tucker MA, Hoppe RT. Factors affecting late mortality from heart disease after treatment of Hodgkin's disease. *JAMA* 1993; 270:1949–1955.
21. Blank N, Castellino RA. The intrathoracic manifestations of the malignant lymphomas and the leukemias. *Semin Roentgenol* 1980;15: 227–245.
22. Prentice RT. Myocardial infarction following radiation. *Lancet* 1965; 2:388.
23. Kopelson G, Herwig KJ. The etiologies of coronary artery disease in cancer patients. *Int J Radiat Oncol Biol Phys* 1978;4:895–906.
24. Pohjola-Sintonen S, Totterman KJ, Salmo M, Siltanen P. Late cardiac effects of mediastinal radiotherapy in patients with Hodgkin's disease. *Cancer* 1987;60:31–37.
25. Boivin JF, Hutchinson GB. Coronary heart disease mortality after irradiation for Hodgkin's disease. *Cancer* 1982;49:2470–2475.
26. Tarbell NJ, Thompson L, Mauch P. Thoracic irradiation in Hodgkin's disease: disease control and long-term complications. *Int J Radiat Oncol Biol Phys* 1990;18:275–281.
27. Cosset J-M, Henry-Amar M, Pellae-Cosset B, et al. Pericarditis and myocardial infarctions after Hodgkin's disease therapy. *Int J Radiat Oncol Biol Phys* 1991;21:447–449.
28. Boivin JF. Coronary artery disease mortality in patients treated for Hodgkin's disease. *Cancer* 1992;69:1241–1247.
29. Hancock SL, Donaldson SS, Hoppe RT. Cardiac disease following treatment of Hodgkin's disease in children and adolescents [see comments]. *J Clin Oncol* 1993;11:1208–1215.
30. Brierley JD, Rathmell AJ, Gospodarowicz MK, et al. Late effects of treatment for early-stage Hodgkin's disease. *Br J Cancer* 1998;77: 1300–1310.
31. Glanzmann C, Kaufmann P, Jenni R, Hess OM, Huguenin P. Cardiac risk after mediastinal irradiation for Hodgkin's disease. *Radiother Oncol* 1998;46:51–62.
32. Perrault DJ, Levy M, Herman JD, et al. Echocardiographic abnormalities following cardiac radiation. *J Clin Oncol* 1985;3:546–551.
33. Lund MB, Kongerud J, Boe J, et al. Cardiopulmonary sequelae after treatment for Hodgkin's disease: increased risk in females? *Ann Oncol* 1996;7:257–264.
34. Lund MB, Ihlen H, Voss BM, et al. Increased risk of heart valve regurgitation after mediastinal radiation for Hodgkin's disease: an echocardiographic study. *Heart* 1996;75:591–595.
35. Stewart JR, Hancock EW, Hancock SL. Radiation injury to the heart: risk factors, diagnosis, prevention and treatment. *Front Radiat Ther Oncol* 1998; in press.
36. Billingham ME, Mason JW, Bristow MR, Daniels JR. Anthracycline cardiomyopathy monitored by morphologic changes. *Cancer Treat Rep* 1978;62:865–872.
37. Billingham ME, Bristow MR, Glatstein E, Mason JW, Masek MA, Daniels JR. Adriamycin cardiotoxicity: endomyocardial biopsy evidence of enhancement by irradiation. *Am J Surg Pathol* 1977;1:17–23.
38. Steinherz LJ, Steinherz PG, Tan C. Cardiac failure and dysrhythmias 6–19 years after anthracycline therapy: a series of 15 patients. *Med Pediatr Oncol* 1995;24:352–361.
39. LaMonte CS, Yeh SDJ, Strauss DJ. Long-term follow-up of cardiac function in patients with Hodgkin's disease treated with mediastinal irradiation and combination chemotherapy including doxorubicin. *Cancer Treat Rep* 1986;70:439–444.
40. Allavena C, Conroy T, Aletti P, Bey P, Lederlin P. Late cardiopulmonary toxicity after treatment for Hodgkin's disease. *Br J Cancer* 1992;65: 908–912.
41. Brice P, Tredaniel J, Monsuez JJ, et al. Cardiopulmonary toxicity after three courses of ABVD and mediastinal irradiation in favorable Hodgkin's disease. *Ann Oncol* 1991;2(suppl 2):73–76.
42. Pihkala J, Saarinen UM, Lundstrom U, et al. Myocardial function in children and adolescents after therapy with anthracyclines and chest irradiation. *Eur J Cancer* 1996;32A:97–103.
43. Elerding SC, Fernandez RN, Grotta JC, Lindberg RD, Causay LC, McMurtrey MJ. Carotid artery disease following external cervical irradiation. *Ann Surg* 1981;194:609–615.
44. Atkinson JL, Sundt TM Jr, Dale AJ, Cascino TL, Nichols DA. Radiation-associated atheromatous disease of the cervical carotid artery: report of seven cases and review of the literature. *Neurosurgery* 1989; 24:171–178.
45. Eisenberg RL, Hedgcock MW, Wara WM, Jeffrey RB. Radiation-induced disease of the carotid artery. *West J Med* 1978;129:500–503.
46. Reed R, Sadiq S. Acute carotid artery thrombosis after neck irradiation. *J Ultrasound Med* 1994;13:641–644.
47. Rockman CB, Riles TS, Fisher FS, Adelman MA, Lamparello PJ. The surgical management of carotid artery stenosis in patients with previous neck irradiation. *Am J Surg* 1996;172:191–195.
48. Silverberg GD, Britt RH, Goffinet DR. Radiation-induced carotid artery disease. *Cancer* 1978;41:130–137.
49. Schreiber DP, Kapp DS. Axillary-subclavian vein thrombosis following combination chemotherapy and radiation therapy in lymphoma. *Int J Radiat Oncol Biol Phys* 1986;12:391–395.
50. Seifter EJ, Young RC, Longo DL. Deep venous thrombosis during therapy for Hodgkin's disease. *Cancer Treat Rep* 1985;69:1011–1013.
51. Yahalom J, Hasin Y, Fuks Z. Acute myocardial infarction with normal coronary arteriogram after mantle field radiation therapy for Hodgkin's disease. *Cancer* 1983;52:637–641.
52. Aronow H, Kim M, Rubenfire M. Silent ischemic cardiomyopathy and left coronary ostial stenosis secondary to radiation therapy. *Clin Cardiol* 1996;19:260–262.
53. O'Sullivan JJ, Conroy RM, MacDonald K, McKenna TJ, Maurer BJ. Silent ischemia in diabetic men with autonomic neuropathy. *Br Heart J* 1991;66:313–315.
54. Bertolet BD, Belardinelli L, Hill JA. Absence of adenosine-induced chest pain after total afferent denervation. *Am J Cardiol* 1993;72:483–484.

55. Cohen SI, Bharati S, Glass J, Lev M. Radiotherapy as a cause of complete atrioventricular block in Hodgkin's disease. *Arch Intern Med* 1981;141:676–679.
56. Totterman KJ, Pesonen E, Siltanen P. Radiation-related chronic heart disease. *Chest* 1983;83:875–878.
57. Slama MS, Le Guludec D, Sebag C, et al. Complete atrioventricular block following mediastinal irradiation: a report of six cases. *PACE* 1991;14:1112–1118.
58. Watchie J, Coleman CN, Raffin TA, et al. Minimal long-term cardiopulmonary dysfunction following treatment for Hodgkin's disease. *Int J Radiat Oncol Biol Phys* 1987;13:517–524.
59. Savage DE, Constine LS, Schwartz RG, Rubin P. Radiation effects on left ventricular function and myocardial perfusion in long term survivors of Hodgkin's disease. *Int J Radiat Oncol Biol Phys* 1990;19:721–727.
60. Kadota RP, Burgert EO Jr, Driscoll DJ, Evans RG, Gilchrist GS. Cardiopulmonary function in long-term survivors of childhood Hodgkin's lymphoma: a pilot study. *Mayo Clin Proc* 1988;63:362–367.
61. Gustavsson A, Eskilsson J, Landberg T, et al. Late cardiac effects after mantle radiotherapy in patients with Hodgkin's disease. *Ann Oncol* 1990;1:355–363.
62. Maunoury C, Pierga JY, Valette H, Tchernia G, Cosset J-M, Desgrez A. Myocardial perfusion damage after mediastinal irradiation for Hodgkin's disease: a thallium-201 single photon emission tomography study. *Eur J Nucl Med* 1992;19:871–873.

Hodgkin's Disease, edited by P. M. Mauch,
J. O. Armitage, V. Diehl, R. T. Hoppe, and L. M. Weiss.
Lippincott Williams & Wilkins, Philadephia ©1999.

CHAPTER 36

Other Complications of the Treatment of Hodgkin's Disease

Julie M. Vose, Louis S. Constine, and Simon B. Sutcliffe

Late complications of treatment are generally of two types: treatment-induced tissue or organ dysfunction, and mutagenic consequences of cytotoxic therapies. The differential diagnosis of symptomatology acquired after therapy must always include recurrent primary tumor (Hodgkin's disease), development of a new primary tumor (second malignancy), late effects of prior therapy, or other disease processes. Late complications can be a function of surgery, radiation, chemotherapy, the disease itself, or a combination of the etiologies. The damage that is caused by disease or its treatment includes vascular interruption, slowed tissue repair, altered metabolism or clearance of drugs, and genetic alterations. The long-term complications that may occur as a consequence of these therapies are outlined in this chapter.

ENDOCRINE

Thyroid

A spectrum of clinically significant thyroid abnormalities may occur in patients treated for Hodgkin's disease. Primary hypothyroidism is most frequent, but Graves' disease, autoimmune thyroiditis, euthyroid Graves' ophthalmopathy, benign cysts and nodules, and papillary or follicular thyroid cancers occur with a defined frequency (1,2). Among 1,787 patients treated for Hodgkin's disease at Stanford University, the 20-year actuarial risk for the development of any thyroid abnormality was 50% (2). Direct radiation exposure to the thyroid gland, incidental to cervical or mantle therapy, is the predominant therapeutic insult.

Hypothyroidism

Primary hypothyroidism is a frequent consequence of mantle or cervical irradiation. Subclinical hypothyroidism is defined as an elevation of the basal thyroid-stimulating hormone (TSH) level and an increased TSH response to thyrotropin-releasing hormone (TRH) provocation, but with normal serum triiodothyronine (T_3)/thyroxine (T_4) levels and no clinical symptoms of hypothyroidism. Clinical hypothyroidism is defined as the clinical symptoms of hypothyroidism associated with an elevation in basal TSH levels, increased TSH response to TRH, and depressed serum levels of T_4 or T_3. The legion of symptoms include cold intolerance, constipation, inordinate weight gain, dry skin, brittle hair, menorrhagia or spotting, muscle cramps or generalized muscle weakness, and slowed mentation. Signs include a round puffy face, slow speech, hoarseness, hypokinesia, delayed relaxation of deep tendon reflexes, periorbital or peripheral edema, and pleural or pericardial effusions (3). The incidence of hypothyroidism following therapeutic irradiation for Hodgkin's disease varies in different reports depending on radiation dose and technique, patient age, interval to and type of laboratory testing (e.g., T_4, T_3, free T_4, TSH, etc.), and the thoroughness of the history and physical examination. Consequently, if an elevated serum TSH concentration is the determinant, then 4% to 79% of patients become affected (4,5). A recent study by Hancock et al. (2) of 1,677 children and adults with Hodgkin's disease irradiated to the thyroid showed that the actuarial risk at 26 years for overt or subclinical hypothyroidism was 47%. Although the peak incidence occurred at 2 to 3 years, and half the risk was

J. M. Vose: Department of Internal Medicine, University of Nebraska Medical Center, Omaha, Nebraska.
L. S. Constine: Department of Radiation Oncology and Pediatrics, University of Rochester Medical Center, Rochester, New York.
S. B. Sutcliffe: Vancouver Cancer Center, Vancouver, British Columbia, Canada.

manifested within 5 years, some patients developed hypothyroidism as long as 20 years after therapy.

Radiation dose is the most relevant parameter in predicting the likelihood of hypothyroidism. Radiation technique determines dose deposition, including the use of differential anterior versus posterior field weighting and cervical or specific thyroid blocks (6). An increasing incidence of hypothyroidism above threshold doses of 20 to 30 Gy has been reported (4,5). Constine et al. (5) noted thyroid abnormalities in 4 of 24 children (17%) who received mantle irradiation of 26 Gy or less, and in 74 of 95 children (78%) who received greater than 26 Gy; the relationship of basal TSH to radiation dose was significant (p <.001). In a recent report by Bhatia et al. (4), the relative risk of hypothyroidism increased by 1.02/Gy, (p <.001) (Fig. 1). Other factors may affect risk for radiation-induced hypothyroidism. Prior to age 16 years, radiation therapy dose was the predominant determinant of risk, whereas female gender and chemotherapy were additional risk factors in older patients (2,4,5). The influence of chemotherapy on the development of thyroid dysfunction appears to be negligible (4,5).

Hyperthyroidism

Thyrotoxicosis may occur following mantle or cervical irradiation for Hodgkin's disease. Hancock et al. (2) report that approximately 2% of patients (n = 34) developed Graves' disease (2). Almost all had a diffuse goiter, high free thyroxine (FT_4), low TSH, and increased thyroid uptake of radioiodine. Half of these patients developed infiltrative ophthalmopathy, as did an additional four patients who did not have overt hyperthyroidism. The relative risk for Graves' disease was 7.2 to 20.4. Six patients developed silent thyroiditis characterized by transient mild symptoms of thyrotoxicosis, an increased serum FT_4 and low TSH, no thyroid enlargement or tenderness, and low thyroid uptake of radioiodine (7). All of these patients subsequently developed hypothyroidism. The mechanism of Graves' disease is an autoimmune dysregulation of unknown etiology.

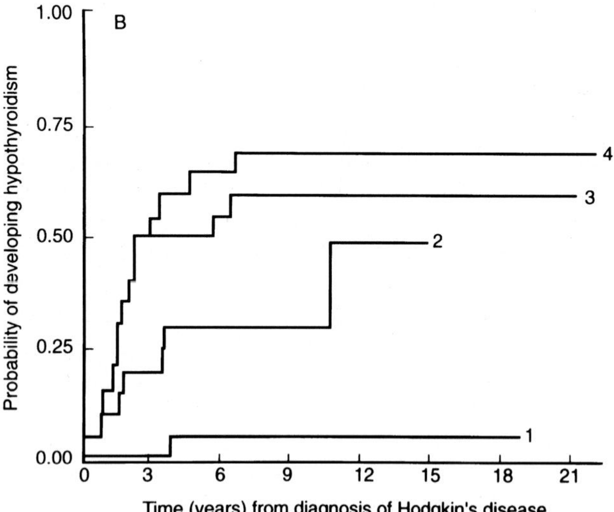

FIG. 1. Actuarial risk of hypothyroidism in 89 children treated for Hodgkin's disease. Curve 1 represents the risk in 13 children who did not undergo irradiation to the thyroid, curve 2 the risk in 10 children who received less than 30 Gy, curve 3 the risk in 26 children who received between 30 and 45 Gy, and curve 4 the risk in 40 children who received greater than 45 Gy (p =.002). (From ref. 4, with permission.)

Thyroid Enlargement, Benign and Malignant Nodules

An excess frequency of benign and malignant thyroid nodules occurs following radiation therapy for Hodgkin's disease. This risk appears to vary according to age at treatment, which may also reflect the known association of radiation dose and induced thyroid cancers. In a report by Boivin et al. (8) of 10,472 patients with Hodgkin's disease, the relative risk was 4.5 [95% confidence interval (CI) 2.4–7.7] overall, and 1.3 (95% CI 0.3–6.1) after radiation therapy. Children appear to be at greater risk. In a recent report on 1,380 children with Hodgkin's disease from the Late Effects Study Group, the relative risk was 32.7 (95% CI 15.3–55.3) (4).

Ovary

Radiation and chemotherapy for Hodgkin's disease can cause transient or permanent effects on reproductive capacity, endocrine integrity, and sexual function. The concerns of survivors range from their functional status to consequences on the health of their offspring. The complexity of defining these sequelae stems from the differential dose-dependent effects caused by different chemotherapy agents, radiation therapy, and their combination. Injury to the ovaries can cause both sterilization and suppressed hormone production because of the relationship of the latter to the presence of ova and maturation of the primary follicle (9).

Depending on the radiation dose, fertility may be transiently preserved due to survival of relatively radioresistant follicles in the late stages of development. Conversely, sterility may be transient due to survival of primordial follicles, although the duration of subsequent fertility may be shortened due to reduction of the total number of follicles or acceleration in the rate of follicular atresia. These observations may explain why girls treated prior to puberty, who have a greater complement of ova than do older women, are more likely to retain ovarian function after radiation therapy.

The dose of radiation that will ablate ovarian function depends on the patient's age and whether the dose is fractionated. Data from Ash (10) summarized the effect of fractionated radiation therapy on ovarian function in women of reproductive age (Table 1). Doses of 12 to 15

TABLE 1. *Effect of fractionated irradiation on ovarian function in women of reproductive age*

Minimum ovarian dose (Gy)[a]	Effect
0.6	No deleterious effect
1.5	No deleterious effect in most young women; some risk of sterilization especially in women age >40 years
2.5–5.0	Variable: age 15–40 years, 30–40% sterilized permanently; age >40 years, >90% sterilized permanently
5–8	Variable: age 15–40 years, 50–70% sterilized permanently, temporary amenorrhea in some of remainder; age >40 years, >90% sterilized permanently
>8	100% permanently sterilized

[a]No attempt has been made to allow for variation in mode of fractionation.
Modified from ref. 10, with permission.

TABLE 2. *Frequency of amenorrhea following treatment with combination chemotherapy*

Regimen	Patient age	Frequency of amenorrhea (patient numbers)
MVPP	All ages	63% (20/32)
	<30 years	52% (17/33)
	30–51 years	86% (31/36)
MOPP		
Full course	All ages	39% (17/44)
Full course	<30 years	11% (4/36)
Full course	30–45 years	56% (10/18)
3 cycles	16–30 years	3% (1/31)
3 cycles	31–45 years	61% (11/18)
ChlVPP	All ages	19% (6/32)
ChlVPP/EAV	All ages	80% (16/20)

M(O/V)PP, mechlorethamine, (vincristine/vinblastine), procarbazine, prednisone; ChlVPP, chlorambucil, vincristine, prednisone, procarbazine; EAV, etoposide, Adriamycin, vincristine.
Modified from ref. 15, with permission.

Gy in women 40 years of age or younger induced menopause, whereas women older than 40 years became menopausal after 4 to 7 Gy. Permanent sterility occurred in up to 60% of females 15 to 40 years of age who received 5 to 6 Gy. After single fractions, temporary sterility can occur with ovarian doses of 1.7 to 6.4 Gy, and permanent sterility after 3.2 to 10 Gy (11). Wallace et al. (12) reviewed data to estimate a median lethal dose (LD_{50}) of 6 Gy for the oocyte.

If pelvic irradiation is a potential component of therapy, the ovaries should be relocated in order to effectively shield them. An oophoropexy may be performed at the time of a staging laparotomy or as a separate procedure. Typically, the ovaries are moved to a midline position in front of or behind the uterus. Alternately, they may be moved laterally to the iliac wings or paracolic gutter, or even heterotopically autotransplanted into a remote location (e.g., the arm) (13).

Several chemotherapeutic agents used to treat Hodgkin's disease are capable of causing ovarian dysfunction, including cyclophosphamide and mechlorethamine (9, 14). The age of the patient, the dose of chemotherapy, and the combined use of irradiation are all relevant to the potential for ovarian injury. For example, prepubertal girls are apparently more resistant to large cumulative doses of cyclophosphamide than are adults. In Horning et al.'s (15) review of patients treated with MOP(P) [mechlorethamine, Oncovin (vincristine), procarbazine, and prednisone) or PAVe [procarbazine, Alkeran (L-phenylalanine mustard), and vinblastine] (15), 75% of women younger than 20 years maintained menses while only 30% of women 30 years or older continued to menstruate. In those patients who, in addition, received pelvic irradiation, 28% had irregular menses and 52% had amenorrhea (Table 2). Among the women treated with chemotherapy alone, ten pregnancies occurred in eight women, resulting in six normal births, one premature birth, and three therapeutic abortions. Among those receiving combined radiation and chemotherapy, seven pregnancies occurred among five women, resulting in six normal births, and one premature birth.

Strategies for protecting the ovary from chemotherapy-induced damage have been suggested. Administration of hormones to suppress ovarian function during chemotherapy might increase its resistance. Autotransplanting the ovary to a remote site, e.g., the arm, and then using a tourniquet to decrease the exposure to chemotherapy has also been suggested.

Testes

The testes can be exposed to radiation directly, by scatter, or by transmission through shielding blocks. Because the spermatogonia are exquisitely sensitive to radiation, even small doses can produce measurable damage. Depression of sperm counts is discernible at doses as low as 0.15 Gy. This decrease in sperm counts may evolve over 3 to 6 weeks following irradiation, and, depending on the dose, recovery may take 1 to 3 years. Complete sterilization may occur with fractionated irradiation to a dose of 1 to 2 Gy, though some patients will recover (16). Spermatocytes generally fail to complete maturation division at doses of 2 to 3 Gy and are visibly damaged after 4 to 6 Gy with resulting azoospermia. At the highest doses, permanent sterility is frequent. At lower doses this reduced sperm count is seen 60 to 80 days after exposure, which is the time that maturation would otherwise be complete (17). Multiple small fractions of radiation are more toxic to spermatogenesis than are large, single fractions. This reverse fractionation effect is due to the extreme radiosensitivity of the testicular germinal epithelium, the small number of stem cells, and rapid cell turnover (16,17). In contrast to the extreme radiosensitivity of the germinal epithelium, Leydig cell function is more resistant, and consequently testosterone production is generally normal below radiation doses of 10 to 20 Gy (18).

In a report from Stanford, 83% of men treated with pelvic irradiation utilizing testicular shielding were oligospermic or azoospermic when tested within 18 months of therapy, but only 12% remained azoospermic when tested more than 26 months after therapy (19). The testes of young children may be more difficult to protect from irradiation due to the smaller patient size. Stanford investigators assessed gonadal function in 20 boys treated for Hodgkin's disease, eight with radiation therapy alone (20). Four of the boys, irradiated at 13 to 15 years of age and receiving pelvic doses of 0, 40, 44, and 44 Gy, respectively, have fathered children 3 to 19 years after radiation therapy. Three had azoospermia 10 to 15 years after irradiation, and one other boy had testicular atrophy at biopsy 1 year after irradiation. Five additional boys had received chemotherapy and 20 to 44 Gy of pelvic irradiation at 8 to 15 years of age. Four were azoospermic 3 to 10 years later, and one had fathered a child.

The testicular germinal epithelium is susceptible to damage produced by several chemotherapeutic agents used in the treatment of Hodgkin's disease including cyclophosphamide, mechlorethamine, and procarbazine. The effects are almost certainly dose-related where data are available for this assessment (21). For example, azoospermia is consistently induced with a cumulative dose of 18 g of cyclophosphamide in men, and this effect is commonly permanent. When MOPP chemotherapy is used, six or more cycles will sterilize 90% of males, whereas three or fewer cycles will cause oligospermia in 25% (22,23). Reports are variable on the recovery of sperm numbers, with ranges from 0% to 50% (usually 10–25%), and latent intervals up to 10 years (usually 2–5 years) (22,24). ABVD (Adriamycin, bleomycin, vinblastine, and dacarbazine) appears to spare fertility, although transient azoospermia is reported in up to 50% of patients (25). A recent report from M. D. Anderson Cancer Center also documents rapid recovery (3–4 months) of spermatogenesis after three cycles of NOVP (Novantrone, Oncovin, vinblastine, and prednisone) chemotherapy (26).

Prepubertal patients may have a slightly decreased sensitivity to chemotherapy-induced gonadal toxicity compared with adults, but irreversible azoospermia can still occur after the use of alkylating agents. In a report by Sherins et al. (27), of 13 pubertal boys treated with MOPP, 9 (69%) demonstrated gynecomastia and had evidence of germinal aplasia on testicular biopsy.

Current efforts to protect patients from chemotherapy or radiation-induced damage to spermatogenesis involve eliminating those agents known to damage spermatogenesis, and optimizing testicular shielding from irradiation. Work in an animal model demonstrates that pretreatment with testosterone and estradiol, which reversibly inhibits the completion of spermatogenesis, protects spermatogonial stem cells from procarbazine and radiation (28). However, complete data are not yet available in clinical trials, with some trials demonstrating no protective effects.

BONE AND SOFT TISSUE

Detrimental effects of treatment for Hodgkin's disease on bone and soft tissue are most problematic in children (see Chapter 30), and predominantly result from radiation therapy. These effects are rarely seen in adults. The pathophysiology of radiation injury to growing bone is probably attributable to damage to the chondroblasts (29). Essentially the predominant effect on long bones is shortening, and on flat bones it is hypoplasia.

The crucial factors that determine outcome include the following: (a) the radiation total and fractional dose (as well as energy, beam type); (b) which bone(s), epiphyseal plate(s), and muscles are encompassed; (c) patient age and genetic constitution (including growth potential); and (d) other components of therapy (steroids, chemotherapeutic agents) (29,30). The greatest retardation of spinal growth occurred in children irradiated during the periods of most active growth (under 6 years of age and during puberty) and at doses greater than 35 Gy (31). Patients receiving less than 33 Gy demonstrated significant impairment in standing and sitting height for the prepubertal age group only (Fig. 2) (31).

Bone Damage

Although scoliosis and kyphosis may result from spinal or flank irradiation, children treated for Hodgkin's disease are uncommonly affected due to the relative symmetry of the radiation fields and the low doses currently used. Slipped femoral capital epiphysis is a clinically significant adverse effect observed in patients following irradiation of the femoral head (32). There is a threshold dose of 25 Gy for this complication. It occurred in about half the children irradiated at less than 4 years of age (7 of 15), as compared to only 1 of 21 children 5 to 15 years old. The mechanism of femoral capital epiphyseal plate slippage is postulated to be a radiation-induced delay in maturation of the epiphyseal plate with disruption of normal calcification and bone matrix deposition.

Avascular necrosis of the femoral or humeral heads can occur 2 to 3 years following irradiation, but most commonly occurs in the setting of combined-modality therapy (33). The etiology of this complication is unclear but may be related to the combined use of steroids and irradiation or corticosteroids alone. Libshitz and Edeikin (34) reported necrosis in 16 of 44 children receiving 30 to 60 Gy to the femoral heads; this was bilateral in four of five children treated to both hips. This debilitating injury is fortu-

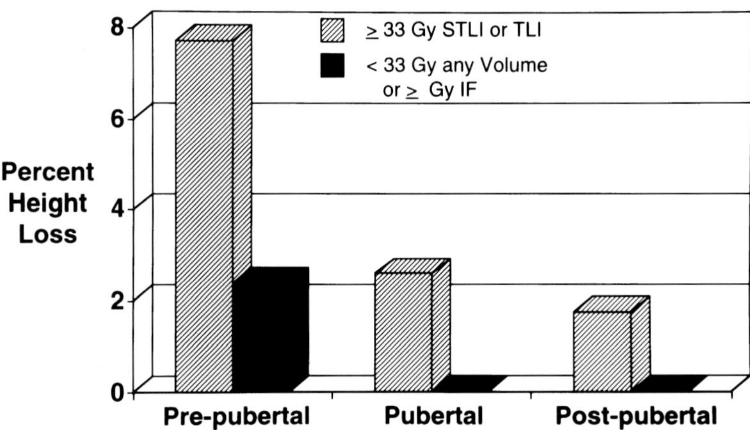

FIG. 2. Relative height impairment for six groups according to age at treatment and radiation dose/volume. (From ref. 31, with permission.)

nately rare when the femoral and humeral heads are shielded and/or when lower radiation doses are used (29).

A variety of other uncommon skeletal abnormalities can be seen after irradiation for Hodgkin's disease in young children, including sternal deformity (hypoplasia, asymmetry, pectus excavatum, pectus carinatum), clavicular shortening, hypoplasia of the iliac bones or lower ribs, cartilaginous exostoses, osteochondromata, and hypoplasia of the mandible (35). A common effect of chemotherapy is skeletal demineralization (osteoporosis) leading to fractures following use of corticosteroids.

The most common chronic radiation effect on muscle is hypoplasia. The muscles treated are smaller, although the effects on strength are not pronounced. Thus the effect is more cosmetic than functional. However, marked fibrosis can occur, which produces stiffness, a decrease in range of motion of a joint, and even pain. The frequency and severity of hypoplasia, as previously stated, essentially depends on the age, developmental status, sex, and growth potential of the patient. In young children, radiation doses of 15 to 25 Gy can cause varying degrees of hypoplasia. This is most evident in the neck and upper thorax (36). Certainly, doses of 35 to 45 Gy will impair muscle development in adolescent patients. Rare individuals who have been treated more than once with cumulative doses of greater than 50 Gy will demonstrate significant fibrosis (36).

Soft Tissue

In the growing breast, the most sensitive structure is the breast bud. Doses of as little as 10 Gy to the breast bud will cause the breast to be hypoplastic; doses above 20 Gy may ablate development altogether (37). Doses of 20 Gy or more to other areas of the breast will impair development in those areas. Even low doses of radiation during puberty may impair subsequent lactation (117).

Damage to developing teeth causes cosmetic and functional difficulties throughout life. The age of the child at the time of therapy, the radiation dose, and the use of chemotherapy determine the consequences. The defects that occur are most pronounced in children treated before age 6 and can include malocclusion, enamel hypoplasia, hypodontia, microdontia, enamel opacities, altered root development, shortening of premolar roots, and thinning of the roots with constriction (38). However, Hodgkin's disease is rare in patients younger than 6 years of age.

Salivary Glands

Radiation injury to the major salivary glands (parotid, submandibular, sublingual) primarily is associated with an increased risk for caries, alterations in taste, and discomfort due to mouth dryness. Salivary gland irradiation causes a qualitative and quantitative change in salivary flow. Chemotherapy may also independently diminish salivary function, though its effects are less severe and transient (39). However, anthracycline use may exacerbate radiation effects.

Salivary gland damage is evident after 20 Gy of fractionated irradiation. Salivary flow rate drops rapidly during a course of fractionated irradiation. Postradiotherapy xerostomia is irreversible if all major salivary glands are treated with doses of 50 to 60 Gy, which almost never occurs in the treatment of Hodgkin's disease. Excellent oral hygiene and attentive dental care are the keys to dealing with the effect of irradiation on teeth and salivation. Prior to radiation and chemotherapy, a dental evaluation is indicated. As possible foci of infection, loose exfoliating primary teeth and orthodontic appliances should be removed. The daily use of topical fluoride can dramatically reduce the frequency of radiation caries in the treated patient. Xerostomia is palliatively treated with saliva substitutes and sialagogues. Recent data support the efficacy of pilocarpine in improving saliva production and relieving symptoms of xerostomia, with minor risks that are predominantly limited to sweating.

Gastrointestinal Tract

The most systematic examination of late gastrointestinal tract complications following treatment for Hodgkin's disease is from the European Organization for the Research and Treatment of Cancer (EORTC) H_2 and H_5 trials conducted between 1972 and 1981 (40). These trials enrolled patients with clinical stage (CS) I and II Hodgkin's disease, registered all data including the type of complication prospectively, and comprised treatment groups with or without laparotomy, receiving radiation to mantle and paraaortic ± splenic fields according to three fractionation regimens. The report documented 36 late radiation injuries in 516 patients on the H_2 and H_5 protocols who received infradiaphragmatic irradiation—25 with ulcers of stomach or duodenum, two with severe gastritis, six with small-bowel obstruction or perforation, and three with both an ulcer and bowel obstruction. The complication rate was 2.7% in the nonlaparotomy cohort, and 11.5% in the laparotomy group. The highest risk of complications was in patients who had a laparotomy and subdiaphragmatic irradiation with large fractions. The median time to bowel injury from initiation of therapy was 14 months (3–92 months) for ulcers and gastritis, and 18 months (5–115 months) for small-bowel lesions.

In current practice, several factors would predict that gastrointestinal morbidity would be less prevalent than in the report from the EORTC (40). These include the abandonment of laparotomy as a staging technique, or its restriction to such favorably selected cases that extensive retroperitoneal dissection or mesenteric node biopsy can be omitted from the procedure; the established use of techniques to optimize dose, fractionation, and dosimetry; and the increasing use of combined-modality approaches that limit the necessity for abdominal irradiation encompassing structures other than limited axial nodal regions. Laparotomy without subsequent abdominal irradiation reduces the risks of gastrointestinal complications as compared to the use of both laparotomy and abdominal irradiation.

Irradiation of the liver beyond tolerance levels results in sclerosis and thrombosis of small hepatic veins; sinusoidal and hepatic congestion; centrilobular necrosis and subsequent fibrosis; and a resultant shrunken liver demonstrating severe vascular damage, liver cell atrophy, lobular collapse, and periportal vein and bile duct fibrosis. Clinically, early radiation injury may be manifest as abnormal liver function tests, hepatomegaly, radionuclide imaging abnormalities (absence of Kupffer cell uptake of radionuclide within the irradiated area), and ascites. In the absence of other predisposing factors, radiation tolerance of the whole liver is considered to be approximately 25 to 30 Gy using conventional fractionation techniques. Transient abnormalities of liver function and imaging tests have been reported in the majority of patients receiving 20 Gy to the whole liver plus 20 Gy to the left lobe for stage III Hodgkin's disease despite the absence of clinical symptomatology (41).

A wide variety of chemotherapeutic agents have applicability in Hodgkin's disease. Transient elevation of alkaline phosphatase and transaminases were reported in approximately 20% of patients treated with MOPP (42). Dimethyltriazeno imidazole carboxamide (dacarbazine or DTIC) commonly causes mild biochemical hepatic dysfunction at doses employed in the ABVD regimen (43), procarbazine has been associated with granulomatous hepatitis (44), and corticosteroids have a recognized association with acute pancreatitis and avascular necrosis of the femoral head (45). Despite these associations, clinically relevant chemotherapy-related hepatotoxicity is remarkably uncommon in the absence of other predisposing factors.

Late Treatment Injury to the Urinary Tract

The radiation tolerance of the kidney has been well established with a maximum tolerable dose limit of 20 Gy for whole kidney irradiation (46). In current practice, the configuration of abdominal radiation fields for the treatment of known or suspected Hodgkin's disease would comprise the midline upper abdominal nodes or an inverted Y with coverage of the splenic pedicle post-splenectomy, or the spleen in a clinically staged patient. Coverage of the spleen necessitates the irradiation of the upper third to half of the left kidney to full tumor dose (47). Such irradiation has not resulted in elevations of serum blood urea nitrogen or creatinine, or in hypertension. Appropriately executed therapy using accepted radiation techniques and established chemotherapy regimens usually do not result in clinically apparent long-term renal dysfunction.

Conventionally applied pelvic radiation fields for Hodgkin's disease do not necessitate inclusion of substantial portions of bladder within the tumor volume. In current practice, bulky pelvic disease that might otherwise require significant bladder irradiation to full tumor dose would be more appropriately managed using a combined-modality approach resulting in a more limited radiation volume. Partial bladder irradiation to 35 to 40 Gy and whole bladder scatter doses from inverted-Y fields do not result in clinical late bladder injury or dysfunction.

Bladder toxicity from cyclophosphamide is well recognized, both as fibrosis following cumulative long-term exposure (48) and as hemorrhagic cystitis following cyclophosphamide in various chemotherapy schedules or, more significantly in combination with radiation therapy (49). Appropriate hydration to prevent accumulation of toxic metabolites of cyclophosphamide within the bladder is the established procedure to avoid acute cystitis risk and subsequent progression to bladder fibrosis and the development of bladder carcinoma (50).

Late Treatment Injury to the Skin

The skin response to radiation is predictable, dose dependent, and characterized by an acute reaction during and shortly after the course of treatment. Chronic radiation injury may occur many months to years after radiation and may occur as a direct consequence of the acute reaction, or may develop without antecedent clinically apparent damage. Chronic injury is manifest as thin, atrophic, telangiectatic skin with variable pigmentation (both hyper- and hypopigmentation). Erosion and ulceration may occur, wound healing is poor and infection common, and the predisposition to the development of cutaneous malignancies of various histologic types is well recognized (51).

Chronic skin injury is usually seen in two circumstances. First is the use of radical irradiation where the full tumor dose is required either in the skin (cutaneous and/or subcutaneous tumor) or where the tumor volume of interest necessitates incorporation of the skin within the high-dose volume (subcutaneous lymph nodes, cutaneous lymphatic involvement, etc.). The other is the use of beam energies (orthovoltage or low-energy beam) or treatment techniques (e.g., inappropriate dosimetry, skin-applied bolus for missing tissue correction) that result in deposition of full dose in the skin and subcutaneous tissues and an inappropriate ratio of skin dose to tumor dose. In current practice, late skin injury should rarely, if ever, be seen, given appropriate consideration of tumor dose (35–40 Gy), fractionation (1.75–2 Gy per day), treatment of all fields daily, selection of appropriate beam energy to achieve skin sparing, and use of the technique to establish uniformity of dose within the volume of interest with remotely applied compensation or attenuation for missing tissue contour correction.

Alopecia within the radiation field is universal with fractionated doses to 35 to 40 Gy despite the use of skin-sparing techniques. Facial, scalp, and body hair epilates during radiation therapy and starts to regrow 3 months after completion of therapy. Similarly, radiation effects on sweat glands recover, although increased dryness of the skin may be a long-term effect. The use of combined-modality therapy with conventional radiation dose (35–40 Gy) and, more specifically, the ABVD regimen may result in enhanced acute skin reaction, and more variable recovery of body hair and sweat gland function.

Cutaneous hyperpigmentation commonly follows acute radiation reactions but usually resolves with natural desquamation over a period of weeks. Hyperpigmentation is frequently seen with bleomycin administration (52), often at sites of skin trauma, e.g., excoriations associated with pruritus, trauma, pressure, etc. Doxorubicin is also associated with hyperpigmentation, particularly of skin creases, palms and soles, face, oral mucosa, and tongue. Nail changes are not uncommon, consisting of darkening of the nail bed (bleomycin and doxorubicin), dystrophic change (bleomycin), and pigmented, hypopigmented, and/or transverse depressions of the nail occurring with successive courses of chemotherapy.

Radiation recall reactions are induced by administration of chemotherapy (certain drugs) or corticosteroids. They manifest themselves as a radiation effect (skin erythema or pneumonitis within the radiation field) and occur with or after the administration of the chemotherapy. These reactions may not have occurred previously or may have been seen with the radiation. Increased radiosensitivity of skin is associated with doxorubicin and bleomycin, and increased photosensitivity with dacarbazine and vinblastine. This may enhance the acute skin reaction during radiation therapy and delay recovery following radiation. Radiation recall reaction is also seen with doxorubicin and may occur when doxorubicin-based therapy is administered weeks to months following radiation and with each course of chemotherapy.

Late Treatment Effects on the Immune System

Even before any treatment is administered to patients diagnosed with Hodgkin's disease, an immunodeficiency state is often present. Patients with Hodgkin's disease often exhibit lymphocytopenia, which is mainly ascribed to a reduction of OKT4+ T cells. Blood lymphocytes of untreated Hodgkin's patients are poorly activated by mitogens and antigens, which preferentially stimulate T cells (53,54). Furthermore, the proliferative response of T lymphocytes cultured with autologous non–T lymphocytes is usually impaired or absent (55). Although lymphocytopenia is present in all clinical stages, it tends to be more pronounced in patients with advanced disease (53,56). Few studies have included patients who were tested both before and after treatment for Hodgkin's disease. In a relatively large study of patients retested 2 to 56 months following termination of radiotherapy for Hodgkin's disease, the responses to concanavalin A (ConA) and PPD, but not to pokeweed mitogen (PWM), were significantly reduced shortly after total nodal irradiation. The mitogen response did not increase with time after treatment; however, it did with PPD stimulation (57). Following cytotoxic chemotherapy, a moderate to severe T-cell depletion is also observed. In a prospective study by Van Rijswik et al. (58), 20 previously untreated patients with stage III and IV Hodgkin's disease were evaluated before modified MOPP therapy, after three courses, and within 3 months of the completion of six cycles. There was no change in the B cells; however, T lymphocytopenia was observed 2 years or more after cytotoxic drug therapy.

Deficiencies in the humoral immune system in untreated Hodgkin's disease patients are minimal. Antibody titers after immunization of untreated Hodgkin's patients with pneumococcal polysaccharide vaccine are normal (59). Radiotherapy and cytotoxic drug therapy may suppress a subsequent antibody response. Suppression was most pronounced following total-nodal irradiation plus cytotoxic drug therapy (59). The antibody response recovered with time after therapy and became normal in several patients after 3 years (60). Following curative radiotherapy and cytotoxic drug therapy, serum immunoglobulin IgG, IgA, and IgE concentrations are slightly decreased (61). The reduction of serum IgM in complete remission patients may be more pronounced. Splenectomy may partly contribute to the decline in serum IgM concentrations. Treated and potentially cured patients with Hodgkin's disease often have reduced serum IgM levels and a poor antibody response after immunization with microbial antigens.

Splenectomy was used in the past as a routine diagnostic and staging procedure in patients with Hodgkin's disease to assess the extent of abdominal disease. Splenectomy, however, may be associated with acute and late surgical complications and an increased risk of septicemia as a result of encapsulated bacteria, predominantly pneumococci (62). With splenectomy, 20% to 25% of the phagocytic cell mass of the body is removed, leading to a diminished capacity for clearing circulating bacteria (63). Removal of the spleen may also result in persistent blood-cell abnormalities. Neutrophilia, lymphocytosis, eosinophilia, and thrombocytosis are regular findings after splenectomy, but cell counts tend to return closer to normal over weeks to months (64). Splenectomy causes a relative increase in lymphocyte counts (both T and B cell), which can be observed in patients in long-term remission. However, reduced IgM levels, and possibly impaired B-cell response, contribute to the persistent lifelong threat of overwhelming postsplenectomy infections in splenectomized patients with Hodgkin's disease.

Due to the immunodeficiencies outlined above, patients with Hodgkin's disease are at increased risk for infections that depend on an intact cell-mediated immune capability for control. Infections seen with increased frequency in patients with Hodgkin's disease include varicella zoster, fungi, toxoplasmosis, listeriosis, and pneumocystis (65,66). Long-term survivors are also at increased risk for bacterial infections. Among identifiable factors predisposing patients to infection are advanced age, advanced disease, and prior extensive radiotherapy and cytotoxic drug therapy (67). *Streptococcus pneumoniae* is the most common and serious infection seen. Removal of the spleen predisposes patients to developing septicemia, which is caused predominantly by pneumococci, although *Haemophilus influenzae, Escherichia coli,* and *Staphylococcus aureus* may be isolated. Patients who are to have a splenectomy should be vaccinated for *S. pneumoniae* prior to the procedure to help to prevent infection with encapsulated organisms. In addition, all patients with Hodgkin's disease should be cautioned regarding their increased risk of bacterial sepsis and opportunistic infections.

Late Hematologic Complications

A number of chronic effects of Hodgkin's disease and its therapy on hematopoietic tissues can be demonstrated in long-term survivors of the disease. A decrease in the reserve of hematopoietic tissue can be evident in patients treated with chemotherapeutic agents such as alkylating agents and/or irradiation. This may be manifested only as slight cytopenias during times of normal health; however, under stress, such as a severe infection, an impaired response may be present due to the lack of a normal reserve capacity.

Although impaired immunocompetence is a feature present in most patients with Hodgkin's disease, evidence of immune activation is present as well. These alterations suggest that imbalances in cell populations, particularly of T cells, result in both compromised immunity and, at the same time, hyperreactivity. Autoantibodies directed against red blood cells, platelets, neutrophils, and lymphocytes are common in patients with Hodgkin's disease and can lead to immunohemolytic anemia, immune thrombocytopenic purpura, autoimmune neutropenia, and lymphopenia. These immune phenomena can predate the diagnosis of Hodgkin's disease and sometimes are a sign of relapse.

All chemotherapy agents used in the treatment of Hodgkin's disease affect hematopoietic cell proliferation. The inhibition of hematopoiesis is a reflection of a decline in DNA synthesis, most often by alkylation of nucleic acids, as well as mitotic inhibition. Because the stem cell population is predominantly noncycling, antimetabolites, generally cycle-specific, are less likely to result in stem cell depletion than alkylating agents. Chronic myelosuppressive effects of agents administered to patients with Hodgkin's disease appear more profound on occasion and may be demonstrated up to 2 years after the initial administration (68). There may also be effects on the marrow stromal elements, which could cause problems with bone marrow reserve for possible future autologous hematopoietic stem cell transplantation.

Radiation induces both stromal and stem cell compartment injury (69). Fibrosis in the bone marrow may be seen after radiation-induced injury and may effect long-term hematopoiesis (70,71). The combination of damage induced by chemotherapy and radiation therapy can be additive or synergistic, with resultant prolonged cytopenias that are never corrected to normal levels. These effects can also lead to reduced marrow reserve and problems with adequate collections for hematopoietic stem cell transplantation.

Patients have reduced marrow reserve after autologous bone marrow transplantation, which limits subsequent treatment with combination chemotherapy or large-field irradiation. This limit in marrow reserve is due to prior chemotherapy and transplantation of limited numbers of hematopoietic stem cells. Caution should be exercised in using myelosuppressive drugs after autologous bone marrow transplantation.

Numerous compounds have been recognized as lymphoma- or leukemia-inducing agents such as procarbazine, nitrosoureas, and alkylating agents (see Chapter

33) (72,73). Chemical carcinogenesis results from a multistep process of initiation and promotion. The development of secondary myelodysplasia may have a prolonged natural history with or without progression to acute leukemia, or alternatively the development of acute leukemia can appear to be very abrupt. Early in the course of dysmyelopoietic states, a blunted response to hematopoietic stress during infection may signal the appearance of the syndrome. As more severe changes progress, various degrees of pancytopenia my be present (74). Laboratory evaluation of dysmyelopoiesis also can identify abnormalities of red cell morphology, nucleated red blood cell forms, megaloblastoid cells, pseudo–Pleger-Huet neutrophils, immature white blood cells, monocytosis, dysmyelopoietic megakarocytic progenitors, and Auer rods.

Cytogenetic abnormalities are common, particularly involvement of chromosomes 5, 7, and 17 (75). Karyotypic evolution and the presence of complex cytogenetic abnormalities are indications of a leukemic evolution (75). Stanford University Medical Center analyzed the survival of 690 patients with Hodgkin's disease beginning 1 year after the initial diagnosis. The actuarial risks of developing acute leukemia at 5 and 7 years were 1.5% and 2%, respectively (76). These figures are similar to other studies with the cumulative risks of acute myelogenous leukemia development of 3% to 5.5% at 5 years and 8% to 10% at 10 years (77,78). The highest risk of development occurs at 6 to 7 years, with the critical window of 2 to 12 years. Chemotherapy and combined-modality therapy approaches appear to be the major risk factors for leukemia. The use of nitrosourea-containing combinations have been found to be a significant risk as compared to ABVD as front-line therapy (79). Treatment of secondary leukemias can often be difficult due to relative chemotherapy insensitivity and complex cytogenetic abnormalities. The goal of treatment of secondary leukemias in young patients otherwise cured of Hodgkin's disease should be eradication, and an aggressive approach with induction, consolidation, and high-dose therapy and transplantation when indicated should be planned.

Patients treated for Hodgkin's disease are also at increased risk for the development of non-Hodgkin's lymphoma (80). The etiology of lymphomas observed after treatment of Hodgkin's disease is not known, although several explanations are possible. The profound immunosuppression of Hodgkin's disease, both *de novo* and treatment related, may allow oncogenic viruses to proliferate and produce lymphomas. The appearance of non-Hodgkin's lymphomas may also represent a spectrum of the natural history of the disease. Patients who develop non-Hodgkin's lymphomas have an excellent chance of long-term survival and should be treated aggressively in hopes of eradicating the lymphoma. Chapter 33 has further details on this complication.

Late Neurologic Effects of Hodgkin's Therapy

Radiation therapy is associated with toxicity to normal tissue, which is unavoidably included in the port of treatment. This damage can result from either direct damage to the nerve tissue or indirect damage to supporting tissues, such as the arterial supply. Radiation disorders of the spinal cord are occasionally seen in patients with Hodgkin's disease because the spinal cord is unavoidably included in the radiation field of many patients. Two types of radiation-induced myelopathy have been reported. The first occurs within a few months of treatment and is manifested by the complaint of an electric shock–like sensation below the neck, precipitated by neck flexion (Lhermitte's sign) (81). The sensation is not accompanied by neurologic signs and is self-limiting. This syndrome probably represents reversible demyelination of sensory fibers in the cervical spinal cord. Chronic progressive radiation myelopathy is a disabling disorder usually presenting after mantle irradiation and paraaortic irradiation due to an overdose at the match line (82). The onset is insidious, with an initial slow progression and then often stabilization. Symptoms of chronic progressive radiation myelopathy include paresthesias, weakness, and bowel/bladder dysfunction. The signs are frequently of hemicord dysfunction (Brown-Séquard syndrome) or transverse myelopathy. The disorder may end in death or severe disability.

Peripheral nerves can also be affected adversely by radiation therapy. Areas adjacent to the spinal cord are most commonly affected. The brachial plexus is frequently in the portals of radiation for cervical, supraclavicular, and axillary lymph nodes as well as the apex of the lung. Brachial plexopathy usually begins with paresthesias or dysesthesias of the arm or hand, which is followed by weakness. Pain is usually not an early complaint and may not occur during the course of the disease. The onset is insidious and usually slowly progressive. In general, the dose of radiation to the brachial plexus that causes nerve injury is greater than 60 Gy (83). Because Hodgkin's patients usually receive 35 to 40 Gy, this complication is unusual except in cases of retreatment. The differential diagnosis of brachial plexopathy includes tumor as well as other benign causes, such as inflammatory plexopathy. A tumor often presents initially with pain, followed by neurologic disability and sometimes Horner's syndrome as well. Brachial plexus neuropathies can also occur with viral illnesses or related to a reaction to vaccination on rare occasions.

Several of the chemotherapeutic agents used to treat Hodgkin's disease can also cause neurotoxicity alone or in combination with radiation therapy. The most common agents used in Hodgkin's disease that have been associated with neurotoxicity are the *vinca* alkyloids such as vincristine and vinblastine. Neurotoxicity is caused by destruction of neurotubules and is the dose-limiting factor of these agents (84). Vincristine produces a peripheral neuropathy in patients treated with repeated doses (85). This neuropathy is usually manifested by paresthesias initially, depression of the ankle jerk reflex, and eventually areflexia (86). Sensation deficits are usually mild and typically partially or completely reversible once the treatment has been discontinued (87). Distal weakness may occur, usually after sensory complaints are prominent. The motor deficits may show little improvement and the patient may have chronic neuropathic disability. Vinblastine can cause similar neurotoxicity but it is often milder in nature than that of vincristine.

Paraneoplastic syndromes have also occasionally been associated with Hodgkin's disease (see Chapter 20). These disorders can either precede the diagnosis or occur when the tumor is quiescent. Occasional reports of syndromes such as the myasthenic syndrome as seen with small-cell cancer of the lung, the POEMS (polyneuropathy, organomegaly, endocrinopathy, M protein, skin changes) syndrome with osteosclerotic myeloma (88), and subacute cerebellar degeneration as seen in cancer of the ovary (89) have been reported. Most of these syndromes do not respond to treatment. Several of them are self-limited or respond to treatment of the primary tumor (90).

Corticocerebellar degeneration is a purely degenerative process largely confined to the cerebellar cortex. Patients with Hodgkin's disease who have this disorder, but have no inflammation, have also been described. This diagnosis has preceded the diagnosis of Hodgkin's disease in some patients by as much as 8 years. Most patients develop a pancerebellar deficit acutely or subacutely. Most patients are significantly disabled, having severe truncal and limb ataxia, and sometimes also having nystagmus, myoclonus, and mental symptoms. The pathologic hallmark is the loss of neurons in the Purkinje cell layer—the loss occurs evenly throughout the cerebellum.

REFERENCES

1. Hancock S, McDougall I, Constine L. Thyroid abnormalities after therapeutic external radiation. *Int J Radiat Oncol Biol Phys* 1995;31:1165.
2. Hancock S, Cox R, McDougall I. Thyroid diseases after treatment of Hodgkin's disease. *N Engl J Med* 1991;325:599.
3. McDougall IR. *Thyroid disease in clinical practice.* London: Chapman & Hall Medical, 1992:304.
4. Bhatia S, Ramsay N, Bantle J, Mertens A, Robson L. Thyroid abnormalities after therapy for Hodgkin's disease in childhood. *Oncologist* 1996;1:62.
5. Constine LS, Donaldson SS, McDougall IR, Cox RS, Link MP, Kaplan HS. Thyroid dysfunction after radiotherapy in children with Hodgkin's disease. *Cancer* 1984;53:878.
6. Marcial-Vega VA, Order SE, Lastner G, Cole PD, LaFrance N, O'Neill M. Prevention of hypothyroidism related to mantle irradiation for Hodgkin's disease: preoperative photon study. *Int J Radiat Oncol Biol Phys* 1990;18:613.
7. Petersen M, Keeling CA, McDougall IR. Hyperthyroidism with low radioiodine uptake after head and neck irradiation for Hodgkin's disease. *J Nucl Med* 1989;30:255.
8. Boivin J, Hutchison G, Zauber A, et al. Incidence of second cancers in patients treated for Hodgkin's disease. *J Natl Cancer Inst* 1995;87:732.
9. Green DM. Fertility and pregnancy outcome after treatment for cancer in childhood or adolescence. *Oncologist* 1997;2:171.
10. Ash P. The influence of radiation on fertility in man. *Br J Radiol* 1980;53:271.
11. Lushbaugh CC, Casarett GW. The effects of gonadal irradiation in clinical radiation therapy: a review. *Cancer* 1976;37:1111.
12. Wallace WHB, Shalet SM, Hendry JH, Morris-Jones PH, Gattameneni HR. Ovarian failure following abdominal irradiation in childhood: the radiosensitivity of the human oocyte. *Br J Radiol* 1989;62:995.
13. Leporrier M, vonTheobald P, Roffe J, Muller G. A new technique to protect ovarian function before pelvic irradiation: heterotopic ovarian autotransplantation. *Cancer* 1987;60:2201.
14. Mackie E, Radford M, Shalet S. Gonadal function following chemotherapy for childhood Hodgkin's disease. *Med Pediatr Oncol* 1996;27:24.
15. Horning WJ, Hoppe RT, Kaplan HS, Rosenberg SA. Female reproductive potential after treatment for Hodgkin's disease. *N Engl J Med* 1981; 304:1377.
16. Griffin JE, Wilson JD. Disorders of the testes and the male reproductive tract. In: Wilson JD, Foster DW, eds. *Williams' textbook of endocrinology.* Philadelphia: WB Saunders, 1992:799.
17. Heller GC. Effects on the germinal epithelium of radiobiological factors in manned space flight. In: Langham WH, ed. *NRC publication 1487.* Washington, DC: National Academy of Sciences, National Research Council, 1967:124.
18. Izard M. Leydig cell function and radiation: a review of the literature. *Radiother Oncol* 1995;34:1.
19. Pedrick TJ, Hoppe RT. Recovery of spermatogenesis following pelvic irradiation for Hodgkin's disease. *Int J Radiat Oncol Biol Phys* 1986; 12:117.
20. Sy Ortin TT, Shastak CA, Donaldson SS. Gonadal status and reproductive function following treatment for Hodgkin's disease in childhood: the Stanford experience. *Int J Rad Oncol Biol Phys* 1990;19:873.
21. Sanders JE. Effects of bone marrow transplantation on reproductive function. In: Green DM, D'Angio GJ, eds. *Late effects of treatment for childhood cancer.* New York: Wiley-Liss, 1992:95.
22. da Cunha M, Meistrich M, Fuller L, et al. Recovery of spermatogenesis after treatment for Hodgkin's disease: limiting dose of MOPP chemotherapy. *J Clin Oncol* 1984;2:571.
23. Braumswig J, Heimes U, Heiermann E, et al. The effects of different cumulative doses of chemotherapy on testicular function. Results in 75 patients treated for Hodgkin's disease during childhood or adolescence. *Cancer* 1990;65:1298.
24. Heikens J, Behrendt H, Adriaanse R, Berghout A. Irreversible gonadal damage in male survivors of pediatric Hodgkin's disease. *Cancer* 1996; 78:2020.
25. Kulkarni S, Sastry P, Saikia T, Parikh P, Gopal R, Advani S. Gonadal function following ABVD therapy for Hodgkin's disease. *Am J Clin Oncol* 1997;20:354.
26. Meistrich M, Wilson G, Mathur K, et al. Rapid recovery of spermatogenesis after mitoxantrone, vincristine, vinblastine, and prednisone chemotherapy for Hodgkin's disease. *J Clin Oncol* 1997;15:3488.
27. Sherins RJ, Olweny CLM, Ziegler JL. Gynecomastia and gonadal dysfunction in adolescent boys treated with combination chemotherapy for Hodgkin's disease. *N Engl J Med* 1978;299:12.
28. Kurdoglu B, Wilson G, Parchuri N, Ye W, Meistrick M. Protection from radiation-induced damage to spermatogenesis by hormone treatment. *Radiat Res* 1994;139:97.
29. Dawson WB. Growth impairment following radiotherapy in childhood. *Clin Radiol* 1968;19:241.
30. Eifel P, Donaldson S, Thomas P. Response of growing bone to irradiation: a proposed late effects scoring system. *Int J Radiat Oncol Biol Phys* 1995;31:1301.
31. Willman K, Cox R, Donaldson S. Radiation induced height impairment in pediatric Hodgkin's disease. *Int J Radiat Oncol Biol Phys* 1994;28:85.
32. Chapman JA, Deakin DP, Green JH. Slipped upper femoral epiphysis after radiotherapy. *J Bone Joint Surg* 1980;62B:337.
33. Prosnitz LR, Lawson JP, Friedlaender GE, Farber LR, Pezzimenti JF. Avascular necrosis of bone in Hodgkin's disease patients with combined modality therapy. *Cancer* 1981;47:2793.
34. Libshitz A, Edeikin BS. Radiotherapy changes of the pediatric hip. *AJR* 1981;137:585.
35. Rutherford H, Dodd GD. Complications of radiation therapy; growing bone. *Semin Roentgenol* 1974;9:15.
36. Gillette E, Mahler P, Powers B, Gillette S, Vujaskovic Z. Late radiation

injury to muscle and peripheral nerve. *Int J Radiat Oncol Biol Phys* 1995;31:1309.
37. Rosenfield N, Haller J, Berdon W. Failure of development of the growing breast after radiation therapy. *Pediatr Radiol* 1989;19:124.
38. Maguire A, Craft A, Evans R, et al. The long-term effects of treatment on the dental condition of children surviving malignant disease. *Cancer* 1987;60:2570.
39. Schubert M, Izutsu K. Iatrogenic causes of salivary gland dysfunction. *J Dent Res* 1987;66:680.
40. Cosset J-M, Henry-Amar M, Burgers JMV, et al. Late radiation injuries of the gastrointestinal tract in the H2 and H5 EORTC Hodgkin's disease trials: emphasis on the role of exploratory laparotomy and fractionation. *Radiother Oncol* 1988;13:61.
41. Poussin-Rosillo H, Nisee LZ, D Angio GJ. Hepatic radiation tolerance in Hodgkin's disease patients. *Radiology* 1976;121:461.
42. DeVita VT, Serpick AA, Carbone PP. Combination chemotherapy in the treatment of advanced Hodgkin's disease. *Ann Intern Med* 1970;73:881.
43. Johnson RO, Metter G, Wilson W et al. Phase I evaluation of DTIC (NSC-45388) and other studies in malignant melanoma in the Central Oncology Group. *Cancer Treat Rep* 1976;60:183.
44. Stolinsky DC, Solomon J, Pugh RP, et al. Clinical experience with procarbazine in Hodgkin's disease, reticulum cell sarcoma, and lymphosarcoma. *Cancer* 1979;26:984.
45. Nakashima Y, Howard JM. Drug induced acute pancreatitis. *Surg Obstet Gynecol* 1977;145:105.
46. Kunkler PB, Farr FR, Luxton RW. The limit of renal tolerance to x-rays. *Br J Radiol* 1952;25:190.
47. Koster A, Kimmig B, Müller-Schmipfle et al. MR tomographie und MR angiographic-eine neue methode zur bestrahlungs-planung abdomineller gross felder. *Strahlenther Onkol* 1992;168:230.
48. Johnson WW, Meadows DC. Urinary-bladder fibrosis and telangiectasia associated with long term cyclophosphamide therapy. *N Engl J Med* 1977;284:290.
49. Jayalkshamma B, Pinkel D. Urinary bladder toxicity following pelvic irradiation and simultaneous cyclophosphamide therapy. *Cancer* 1976; 28:701.
50. Pathak AB, Advani SH, Gopal R, Nadkarni KS, Saikia TK. Urinary bladder cancer following cyclophosphamide therapy for Hodgkin's disease. *Leuk Lymphoma* 1992;8:503.
51. Tranenkle HL. Late radiation injury and cutaneous neoplasms. In: Helm F, ed. *Cancer dermatology.* Philadelphia: Lea & Febiger, 1979:99.
52. Yagoda A, Mukherji B, Young C, et al. Bleomycin, an antitumour antibiotic. Clinical experience in 274 patients. *Ann Intern Med* 1972; 77:861.
53. Holm G, Mellstedt H, Bjorkholm M, et al. Lymphocyte abnormalities in untreated patients with Hodgkin's disease. *Cancer* 1976;37:751.
54. Case DC, Hansen JA, Corrales E, et al. Comparison of multiple in vivo and in vitro parameters in untreated patients with Hodgkin's disease. *Cancer* 1976;38:1807.
55. Begemann M, Claas G, Falke H. Impaired autologous mixed lymphocyte reactivity in Hodgkin's disease. *Klin Wochenschr* 1982;60:19.
56. Wedelin C, Bjorkholm M, Johansson B, et al. Clinical and laboratory findings in untreated patients with Hodgkin's disease with special reference to age. *Med Oncol Tumor Pharmacother* 1984;1:33.
57. Bjorkholm M, Wedelin C, Holm G, Johansson B, Mellstedt H. Longitudinal studies of blood lymphocyte capacity in Hodgkin's disease. *Cancer* 1981;48:2010.
58. Van Rijswijk REN, Sybesm JPHB, Kater L. A prospective study of the changes in the immune status before, during, and after multiple-agent chemotherapy for Hodgkin's disease. *Cancer* 1983;51:637.
59. Levine AM, Overturf GD, Field RF, Holdorf D, Paganini-Hill A, Feinstein DI. Use and efficacy of pneumococcal vaccine in patients with Hodgkin's disease. Blood 1979;54:1171.
60. Minor DR, Schiffman G, McIntosh LS. Response of patients with Hodgkin's disease to pneumococcal vaccine. *Ann Intern Med* 1979; 90:887.
61. Amlot PL, Green L. Serum immunoglobulins G, A, M, D, and E concentration in lymphomas. *Cancer* 1979;40:371.
62. Singer DB. Postsplenectomy sepsis. In: Rosenberg HS, Bolands RP, eds. *Perspectives on pediatric pathology.* Chicago: Year Book Medical, 1973:185.
63. Schulkind ML, Ellis EF, Smith RT. Effect of antibody upon clearance of I-125-labelled pneumococci by the spleen and liver. *Pediatr Res* 1967;1:178.
64. Lipson RL, Bayrd ED, Watkins CH. The postsplenectomy blood picture. *Am J Clin Pathol* 1959;32:526.
65. Goffinet DR, Glatstein EJ, Merigan TC. Herpes zoster-varicella infections and lymphoma. *Ann Intern Med* 1972;76:235.
66. Ruskin J, Remington JS. *Pneumocystis carinii* infection in the immunosuppressed host. *Antimicrob Agents Chemother* 1967;7:70.
67. Notter D, Grossman P, Rosenberg SA, et al. Infections in patients with Hodgkin's disease: a clinical study of 300 consecutive adult patients. *Rev Infect Dis* 1980;2:761.
68. Botnick LE, Hannon EC, Hellman S. Multisystem stem cell failure after apparent recovery from alkylating agents. *Cancer Res* 1978;38:1942.
69. Nelson DF, Chaffey JT, Hellman S. Late effects of x-irradiation on the ability of mouse bone marrow to support hematopoiesis. *Int J Radiat Oncol Biol Phys* 1977;2:39.
70. Knospe WA, Blom J, Crosby WH. Regeneration of locally irradiated bone marrow—I. Dose dependent long term changes in the rat, with particular emphasis upon vascular and stromal reaction. *Blood* 1966; 28:398.
71. Slanina J, Musshoff K, Rahner T, Stiasny R. Long-term side effects in irradiated patients with Hodgkin's disease. *Int J Radiat Oncol Biol Phys* 1977;2:1.
72. Dexter TM, Schofield R, Lajtha LG, Moore M. Studies on the mechanism of chemical leukaemogenesis. *Br J Cancer* 1974;30:325.
73. O'Gara RW, Adamson RH, Kelly MG, Dalgaard DW. Neoplasms of the hematopoietic system in nonhuman primates: report of one spontaneous tumor and two leukemias induced by procarbazine. *J Natl Cancer Inst* 1971;46:1121.
74. Weiden PL, Lerner KG, Gerdes A, et al. Pancytopenia and leukemia in Hodgkin's disease: report of three cases. *Blood* 1973;42:571.
75. Anderson RL, Bagby GC, Richert-Boe K, et al. Therapy-related preleukemic syndrome. *Cancer* 1981;47:1867.
76. Coleman CN, Williams CJ, Flint A, et al. Hematologic neoplasia in patients treated for Hodgkin's disease. *N Engl J Med* 1977;297:1249.
77. Pedersen-Bjergaard J, Larsen SO. Incidence of acute nonlymphocytic leukemia, preleukemia, and acute myeloproliferative syndrome up to 10 years after treatment of Hodgkin's disease. *N Engl J Med* 1982;307:965.
78. Blayney DW, Longo DL,Young RC, et al. Decreasing risk of leukemia with prolonged follow-up after chemotherapy and radiotherapy for Hodgkin's disease. *N Engl J Med* 1987;316:710.
79. Yahalom J, Voss R, Leizerowitz R, et al. Secondary leukemia following treatment of Hodgkin's disease: ultra structural and cytogenetic data in two cases with a review of the literature. *Am J Clin Pathol* 80:1983;231.
80. Razis DV, Diamond HD, Craver LF. Hodgkin's disease associated with other malignant tumors and certain non-neoplastic diseases. *Am J Med Sci* 1959;238:327.
81. Carmel RJ, Kaplan HS. Mantle irradiation in Hodgkin's disease. *Cancer* 1976;37:2813.
82. Reagan TJ, Thomas JE, Colby MY Jr. Chronic progressive radiation myelopathy: its clinical aspects and differential diagnosis. *JAMA* 1968;203:128.
83. Kori SH, Foley KM, Posner JB. Brachial plexus lesions in patients with cancer: 100 cases. *Neurology* 1981;31:45.
84. Jellinger K. Pathologic effects of chemotherapy. In: Walker MD, ed. *Oncology of the nervous system.* Martinus Nijhoff, 1983:416.
85. Young DF, Posner JB. Nervous system toxicity of chemotherapy agents. In: Vinken PJ, Bruyn GW, eds. *Handbook of clinical neurology,* vol 39. Amsterdam: North-Holland, 1980:126.
86. Casey EB, Jellife AM, LeQuesne PM, et al. Vincristine neuropathy: clinical and electrophysiological observations. *Brain* 1973;96:69.
87. Sandler SG, Tobin W, Henderson ES. Vincristine-induced neuropathy: a clinical study of fifty leukemic patients. *Neurology* 1969;19:367.
88. Kelly JJ, Kyle RA, Miles JM, et al. Osteosclerotic myeloma and peripheral neuropathy. *Neurology* 1983;33:202.
89. Greenlee JE, Brashear HR. Antibodies to cerebellar Purkinje cells in patients with paraneoplastic cerebellar degeneration and ovarian carcinoma. *Ann Neurol* 1983;14:609.
90. Carr I. The Ophelia syndrome: memory loss in Hodgkin's disease. *Lancet* 1982;1:844.

Hodgkin's Disease, edited by P. M. Mauch,
J. O. Armitage, V. Diehl, R. T. Hoppe, and L. M. Weiss.
Lippincott Williams & Wilkins, Philadephia ©1999.

CHAPTER 37

Assessing Quality of Life in Patients with Hodgkin's Disease: Instruments and Clinical Trials

Michel Henry-Amar, Henning Flechtner, Patricia Fobair, Florence Joly, and S. Jens-Ulrich Rüffer

HISTORY AND BACKGROUND

What are the effects of cancer on quality of life? Despite improvements in cancer survival rates and in the control of the side effects of treatment, there is little formal documentation on patients' quality of life after treatment for Hodgkin's disease.

How do the symptoms and treatment of cancer affect the emotional, social, and spiritual dimensions of patients' lives? The desire of health care providers and patients to predict the impact of different medical interventions on patients' lives has led to the concept of quality of life and the means to measure it (1).

Historical Aspects

A number of events contributed to the development of measurements of quality of life since the end of World War II. In 1948, the World Health Organization (WHO) offered a redefinition of health as a state of complete physical, mental, and social well-being and not merely the absence of disease or infirmity (2). In the same year, Karnofsky and Burchenal (3) proposed a rating scale designed to help physicians assess the effects of treatment by comparing patients' performance before and after therapeutic intervention. In 1960, the term *quality of life* was used by the United States Presidential Commission on National Goals. In 1964, these goals were used to stimulate programs that would examine the quality and needs of individual lives, and develop programs to improve quality of life (4). By 1977, "quality of life" became a key word for the retrieval of journal articles in the United States National Library of Medicine. Since 1987, there have been more than 400 articles per year referring to quality of life (5). In 1989, the United States Congress passed the Outcomes Assessment Research Act to create the Agency for Health Care Policy and Research, whose task it is to measure functional status, well-being, and satisfaction with care along with other end points to evaluate policies that affect patient outcomes (2). Numerous conferences have been held during the 1990s on the aspects of quality of life. Each of these landmark events has been important in further developing the concept of quality of life for health care providers. Today, quality-of-life assessment tools are frequently used as part of prospective and randomized trials (6).

Background

Quality of life can be seen as a metaphor for the physical, psychological, and social health of patients after treatment for cancer. Health-related quality of life can be defined as the value assigned for the duration of life as modified by social opportunities, perceptions, functional

M. Henry-Amar: Department of Clinical Research, Centre François Baclesse, Caen, France.

F. Joly: Department of Medicine, Centre François Baclesse, Caen, France.

H. Flechtner: Department of Child and Adolescent Psychiatry, Universität zu Köln and Clinic of Child and Adolescent Psychiatry, University Hospital, Köln, Germany.

P. Fobair: Department of Radiation Oncology, Stanford University Medical School, Stanford, California.

S. J.-U. Rüffer: Department of Hematology/Oncology, Klinik I für Innere Medizin, der Universität zu Köln, Köln, Germany.

states, and impairments that are influenced by disease or treatment (7). Quality of life includes psychological and social functioning as well as physical functioning, and incorporates positive as well as negative aspects of disease or infirmity (8).

Qualitative and Quantitative Measurements

Qualitative aspects of quality of life include the subjective expression or evaluation of an individual's physical, mental, and social status, that is, the patient's sense of well-being (6,9). The patient's perspective or subjective view, defined as how a patient perceives his current level of functioning compared to his sense of the ideal, is a major component of the quality-of-life concept (10). Quality of life is also a quantifiable, multidimensional concept, encompassing perceptions of both positive and negative aspects of somatic discomfort and other symptoms produced by a disease or its treatment (11). It is the multidimensionality of life that provides the various domains or dimensions to be evaluated using quantitative methods. These domains include physical, functional, emotional or psychological, social (12–14), and spiritual well-being (15).

Psychosocial Aspects of Quality of Life

The aspects of physical well-being include symptoms of the disease, side effects of treatment, and acute or chronic limitations in physical activity, self-care, mobility, sleep, body image, and energy (fatigue) (7,12,13,15). These may occur acutely as a result of the disease or treatment, and long-term as part of the recovery process.

A review of the literature on late effects and psychosocial recovery after cancer suggests that physical adjustment after treatment is associated with the stage of the disease and the extent of treatment required. In a cross-sectional Stanford University study that highlighted problems with fatigue, 37% of 403 survivors of Hodgkin's disease (mean survival, 9 years) reported that their energy had not returned to normal and that they continued to experience fatigue following normal activities (16). Many patients (43%) also noticed reduced activity levels affecting work and leisure activities following treatment. Patients whose energy was normal were compared to those who had persistent fatigue. Four factors predicted for persistent fatigue—advanced disease, greater treatment, younger age, and higher depression scores—and these factors accounted for the difference between the two subgroups. Subsequent analysis demonstrated a close association between patients' scores of body image, treatment, and return of energy.

Functional well-being includes the ability to perform both work and leisure activities (12,15). A Stanford University study comparing activity and work patterns of men with Hodgkin's disease found that the men with more sedentary activity patterns experienced greater fatigue scores on the Profile of Mood States (POMS), whereas those with more active patterns enjoyed higher POMS vigor scores, and higher self-reports of energy and health status (17). An earlier analysis found that Hodgkin's disease survivors had more difficulties in completing work tasks than a comparison group of patients treated for testicular cancer. Using a measure of physical performance at work and at leisure, it was found that compromised physical performance was more likely to be observed in leisure activities than in work-related activities (18).

Psychological or emotional well-being includes both positive and negative aspects (distress) (12,13,15). It is estimated that some degree of emotional distress may occur in more than 40% of patients during the course of their illness (1). In three studies of survivors of Hodgkin's disease at Stanford University, the overall scores for depression and emotional distress were within the range of normal. The percentage of patients with scores above the norm for depression was 29% within the first year of treatment compared to 18% for patients treated an average of 9 years earlier. Similarly, 31% of the newly diagnosed patients had high emotional distress scores, and 21% continued to report similar distress patterns an average of 9 years later (16).

Social well-being includes perceived social support, functional family support, ability to engage in leisure activities and work, and financial success (12,13,15). Cella (12) also suggests that measures of intimacy and sexuality be added to the assessment of social well-being. Patients with poor support systems have been found to be more depressed, vulnerable, angry, and unsettled, and more likely to reject overtures from others (19). Examining social support among the Stanford series of Hodgkin's disease survivors, Bloom et al. (20) found positive associations between the emotional support patients received and their social well-being. They also found that successful social integration led to lower levels of depression.

Hannah et al. (21) found that survivors of Hodgkin's disease often reported difficulties in communication in the marital relationship; these difficulties in part were founded on a fear of recurrence or death and the avoidance of talking about problems. In their study, 41% of men with Hodgkin's disease reported problems with sexual frequency 3 years after treatment; 21% of patients in the Stanford series reported similar problems (16).

Spiritual well-being includes the sense of purpose and meaning in life, and emphasis on religious issues and values (15,22). This important domain has been noted but not frequently studied. Among the long-term survivors of Hodgkin's disease at Stanford University, 44% of patients reported that they changed their view of life, 23% found that their self-esteem increased, 22% found that the importance of relationships increased, and 11% found that there were no benefits (16). Coping with the disease and its treatment were the toughest problem for 60% of survivors of Hodgkin's disease, while 40% reported that family and career problems provided greater challenges to them than the cancer. The greatest source of social support came from family and friends (56%), and faith in religion, self-belief, and treatment (44%).

Why Should the Quality of Life of Cancer Patients be Assessed?

Despite the fact that patients with cancer are surviving in greater numbers today (23), there continues to be little data on the effects of the cancer and its treatment on the quality of life of those affected (6). Concern about the late effects of the disease and treatment (including quality of life) for survivors of cancer provides the impetus to more formally study these issues. Health practitioners and providers will increasingly seek qualitative and quantitative data to support their choices in treatment based on differing concerns for mortality, morbidity, and quality of life. For example, patients with Hodgkin's disease now enjoy increased survival due to improvements in treatment (24), and many are young and have potentially productive years after completion of treatment. Clinical trials that may not demonstrate differences in survival or event-free survival may allow recommendations for less toxic treatment based on quality-of-life measurements, which might allow increased productivity at work and improved functioning outside of work. Thus, studies that lead to reducing late effects and psychosocial burdens among survivors of Hodgkin's disease will continue to provide benefit to patients as survival and freedom from recurrence continue to improve.

QUALITY-OF-LIFE ASSESSMENT IN HODGKIN'S DISEASE

Historically, from the 1950s to the early 1980s, the focus among health professionals was in improving treatment and reducing mortality among patients with Hodgkin's disease (24a). As the major efforts have been directed toward increasing cure and minimizing late effects, it is understandable that quality-of-life assessment has had less effect on the treatment of Hodgkin's disease than on the treatment of other malignancies such as lung or breast cancer (25,26). Major developments in quality-of-life assessment have been accomplished in palliative treatment, where there has been concern about the value of treatment to patients (27,28). To date, most studies on quality of life have been conducted in patients with lung and breast cancer, two of the most common cancers (29,30).

The majority of the quality-of-life instruments developed in the early 1980s were directed at assessing the short-term effects of the disease and treatment, including the acute effects of chemotherapy and radiotherapy (nausea and vomiting, hair loss). Most of the quality-of-life assessments measured the general and physical condition of the patient. Measurements included assessment of pain, gastrointestinal problems (diarrhea, constipation), and sleep disturbance among other more psychological issues (31,32). Patients were usually older, typically in their 50s or 60s or older, and thus, the studies provided an assessment of quality of life for an aging individual having to cope with a life-threatening illness. There were few studies that focused on younger patients and their quality of life after returning to their jobs, new marriages, and families (10).

Large differences exist between pediatric and adult oncology in the development of quality-of-life instruments (33). Assessment of quality of life in pediatric and young-adult oncology patients has focused on cure and the psychosocial consequences after inducing complete remission (34,35). An increasing number of studies have also assessed quality of life in children and adolescents long after cure (36,37). These quality-of-life assessments have included interactions with family and peers, status of leisure activities, school and academic performance, child and adolescence development, and psychosexual development. Many of the assessment tools were derived from existing research tools taken from the fields of child psychology and psychiatry, and family and developmental psychology (38). There are instruments to measure family interaction, emotional relations, and psychopathologic phenomena such as anxiety and depression. Cross-sectional studies (studies conducted at one period in time) were employed rather than longitudinal trials due to limitations in resources and measurements (39). These early measurements were lengthy, time-consuming, and unsuitable for longitudinal follow-up studies. Since the focus has been on curing the patient, quality-of-life research for patients treated for Hodgkin's disease has not been connected to clinical trials (40,41).

Studies investigating the late effects and sequelae in Hodgkin's disease were often conducted with a cross-sectional design and utilized instruments from a variety of research fields including data on socioeconomic and occupational status (16,42–46), while disease-specific instruments were developed for many of the more common adults cancers. As a consequence, there are no quality-of-life instruments ready to use for Hodgkin's disease. There are also no internationally field-tested instruments in different language versions, and no quality-of-life assessments in children and adolescents in pediatric oncology (47).

In contrast there are a number of well-established, internationally investigated instruments for quality-of-life assessment that focus on acute effects of treatment and shorter periods of follow-up in the palliative treatment of patients (48,49). From the beginning, these instruments were developed for longitudinal studies, using repeated measurements in clinical trials (50,51). There still is a need for quality-of-life instruments that inquire about the needs of surviving patients after active treatment and recovery have taken place (52).

To further enhance the effectiveness of treatment and reduce as much as possible the acute and late side effects, more information is needed about how patients cope with the illness and late effects of treatment and whether they are able to return to normal life. This makes a prospective longitudinal approaches desirable, i.e., data taken on quality of life during and following treatment. To obtain information from the patient's point of view, instruments are needed to address the relevant issues from the beginning of therapy to 10 and 15 years later (53,54). This task is made more difficult as instruments can become outdated, treatments change, our ideas of what are the most important areas for assessment change, and patients with a chronic illness need to be seen in health care settings for many years.

METHODS AND INSTRUMENTS

The main constructs of assessing the quality of life of a patient do not aim at fixed definitions of quality of life but consider the important influences on a patient's quality of life (31,55,56). The two major sources that influence quality of life are the disease itself and the treatment administered. This has led to a change over the years from the notion of quality of life as a broader concept to the more restricted notion of health-related quality of life (48). Three broad domains of quality of life—physical, psychoemotional, and social—are defined by the WHO. Although these domains are widely accepted internationally, major problems remain as to how to arrive at valid, reliable, and meaningful data reflecting the influence of illness and treatment (57–59).

Two approaches are available. The first has an expert rater do the assessment, such as the physician or health professional; examples are the Karnofsky performance scale, used in the assessment of the physical effects of the disease and treatment (3,26), and the Spitzer Index, which assesses five dimensions of quality of life (60). The second approach has patients rating their own experience and quality of life; this subjective information can be collected through interviews, questionnaires, or a combination of the two (61).

Interviews

The interview approach is useful in informing the research team about important issues with which patients cope. Interviews can improve the reliability of data when patients are disadvantaged by age, language, or disease process. However, the interview method can be time-consuming and expensive, as it requires personnel skilled in interviewing. Interview methods vary from face-to-face, psychologically oriented interviews lasting a couple of hours, to structured telephone interviews lasting a few minutes (62). One format involves a highly structured interview that holds the interviewer tightly to the questionnaire. Bloom (63) benefited from this approach in a recent study of breast cancer patients in a multiethnic population. At the other extreme are open, exploratory interviews that refrain from restricting the patient's answer. Trained interviewers are used and a method of analyzing the thematically based qualitative information is needed (64). Telephone interviews are sometimes used to supplement data not collected, or to complete partial answers on forms (62).

Since health-related quality of life of patients is largely dependent on the current status of the disease and treatment, we believe that it would be helpful to physicians and patients if repeated quality-of-life measurements were made over time. Developing studies using repeated measures over many points of time would create a database that could help health care professionals gain insight into the physical and emotional changes patients experience as a result of the disease and treatment.

Questionnaires

The most established method of assessing quality of life is the use of self-administered questionnaires. Over the last two decades, a number of questionnaires have been developed for assessment of quality of life or the more specific health-related quality of life. In general, most instruments measure either generic health quality of life or cancer-specific quality of life. Basic principles have been established internationally on how to construct quality-of-life instruments and how to validate them. Most instruments approach quality of life as a multidimensional construct by employing multiitem scales and single items for the different domains of quality of life (65). For the generic health quality-of-life instrument, there is wide agreement that at least the domains of physical, emotional, and social functioning as well as global assessments of health and well-being should be assessed. This is also true for the more specific cancer-oriented instruments where these domains constitute the core of what is assessed and are complemented by other domains more specifically pertaining to cancer (assessment of the side effects of treatment and symptoms of the disease). Recent developments make use of a modular approach by which the main domains are covered by a core instrument, and other domains, dealing with tumor or treatment-specific phenomena, are available as add-on modules (31,66).

A time frame has to be given to the patient for which an assessment is requested. Apart from the diary-type instruments, where patients are asked to assess their quality of life daily or weekly on different items, the time frames most often given are 1 and 2 weeks. Usually four- to seven-point scales are used to obtain severity ratings. Widely used áre Liekert-type scales (a numerical seven-point scale from worst to best or highest to lowest) and the scaling technique of summated scales. Each item has equal weight within the scale and the grading of the item uses equal intervals. Equal weighting is, in principle, questionable, but sufficient data from many sources are available to show that this kind of scaling exhibits the necessary robustness. Although other scoring techniques have been scientifically explored, the standard procedure for the scoring of scales uses unweighted summed scores of the contributing items. Other instruments use the visual or linear analog type of scales where only the ends of the poles are defined and the distance between them (usually 10 cm) is held constant. The patient marks a cross on the line where appropriate or at given linear intervals (28). Most questionnaires do not produce an overall sum score but generate scale scores and single-item scores, usually transformed uniformly on a 0 to 100 (worst to best) scale like the European Organization for the Research and Treatment of Cancer (EORTC) Quality of Life Core Questionnaire (QLQ-C30) (51). The psychometric (ability to correctly and reliably measure) properties of the instrument are of utmost importance. Validity, reliability, and responsiveness to change over time are anchor points and have to be investigated and proven.

Aspects of *validity* usually referred to in the context of quality-of-life research are face validity, content validity, criterion-related validity, construct validity, and discriminant and predictive validity. Discriminant and predictive validity are of particular clinical relevance and importance because they refer to the properties of an instrument that can distinguish between groups of patients and predict outcome, which is the main interest of quality-of-life research in the clinical trials.

Such aspects of *reliability* as test-retest reliability and interrater reliability are not very important for quality-of-life assessment because interrater reliability is not applicable to self-report (exceptions are instruments such as the Spitzer Index, which use rater assessments), and test-retest is in many situations difficult to perform because of the natural changes that occur in the treatment and disease process. Since quality-of-life measures do not address trait variables, stability over time should only be expected for shorter periods of time (days). As a third measure, the internal consistency (Cronbach's alpha) of scales is often used, and values above 0.7 are regarded as sufficient for conducting group comparisons (67).

Responsiveness over time refers to sensitivity and specificity and to the clinical significance of observed changes in health status or quality of life over time (68). Investigation of responsiveness will become more important because for most quality-of-life questionnaires there are no normative reference data, and an increasing amount of reported data need interpretation frames for controls for determining the clinical value of the observed changes (69). Due to increasing international collaboration, the psychometric properties also need cross-cultural validation. Most of the major questionnaires have either gone from national development to international field testing procedures or from the start have undergone international testing. Guidelines for translation (forward-backward procedures) and adaptation to language (e.g., in some languages male, female, and mixed gender forms of the questionnaires are necessary) have been developed and are standardized.

The general disadvantage of all available standard instruments is the lack of a Hodgkin's disease–specific module. The wide range of key interval times (treatment period, follow-up, long-term surveillance) is not adequately covered by existing instruments. Most published trials in Hodgkin's disease that address late effects and quality of life use different instruments (mainly questionnaires but often mixed questionnaire-interview approaches) that focus on psychological outcome including mood (POMS), depression [Center for Epidemiologic Studies Depression Scale (CES-D)], psychosocial adaptation [Psychosocial Adjustment to Illness Scale (PAIS)], and psychiatric symptoms [90-item symptoms checklist (SCL 90)] (70–75). Besides this complex of psychological outcomes, the socioeconomic impact of the disease is also evaluated, for example, living circumstances, occupational situation, leisure activities, family life, and drinking and smoking habits (52,76,77). Infertility and sexual problems as a consequence of treatment have received particular attention. As outlined above, these assessment instruments were derived from the general assessment of late effects from a variety of research fields and illnesses. They are not derived from quality-of-life assessment in clinical trials that may have the goal of developing more successful treatment with fewer consequences. Only recently have explicit quality-of-life measures, such as the EORTC QLQ-C30, been included in cross-sectional studies (46,76,77). These measures have not been specific for Hodgkin's disease quality of life.

Few published reports have addressed both late effects and longitudinal quality-of-life assessment. For quality-of-life assessment, a variety of instruments have been tested (validated) that can distinguish between generic health outcome measures. They include the Nottingham Health Profile (NHP) (78), Sickness Impact Profile (SIP) (79), Medical Outcome Study Short Form 36 (MOS SF-36) (80), EuroQoL (81), World Health Organization Quality of Life WHOQOL (82), Dartmouth COOP Function Charts (83), and cancer-specific questionnaires such as the EORTC QLQ-C30/36 (51), Functional Assessment of Cancer Therapy (FACT) (84), Functional Living Index: Cancer (FLIC) (85), Spitzer Index (60), Cancer Rehabilitation Evaluation System (CARES) (86,87), and the Rotterdam Symptom Checklist (88). Apart from the Spitzer Index, which is rater assessment oriented, all newer instruments use patient self-assessment of the perceived quality of life. Apart from the broader and general domains of quality of life, there is agreement about the necessity of assessing specific disease- and treatment-related problems (e.g., body image, sexuality, fatigue, spirituality, and gender issues, as well as issues pertaining to very old or very young patients). To accomplish this, a number of groups follow the modular approach in the development of questionnaires (FACT-G and the QLQ-C30 represent core instruments) and supplement the core instrument by specific modules (50,89). As an example, the structure and the dimensions of the EORTC QLQ-C30 are given in Table 1, together with the available phase III and IV modules (Table 2).

One of the difficulties in designing Hodgkin's disease–specific modules is that, unlike other cancers, the particular problems are not easily identified. Apart from problems of sexuality and fertility, many side effects of radiation therapy (xerostomia) and chemotherapy (alopecia and peripheral neuropathy) are only temporary. One frequently reported problem after treatment for Hodgkin's disease is fatigue (90). Although certainly not restricted to or in any way pathognomonic of Hodgkin's disease, fatigue seems to occur in a high proportion of patients successfully treated for Hodgkin's disease.

Over the last 5 years, there has been increased research on assessment of fatigue, and instruments are now available to measure the different aspects of this symptom (90). As with quality of life in general, current opinion perceives fatigue as a combined construct with a number of dimensions. One dimension refers to physical and mental fatigue in accordance with what would be seen after intensive exercise or work. Other aspects include motivation, activity, and cognition, and the connection with mood states such as depression. Interestingly, the available data suggest that a great proportion of the fatigue reported by patients is not due primarily to physical condition. Particularly in surviving patients after Hodgkin's disease or breast cancer, high levels of fatigue occur with normal levels of physical functioning.

TABLE 1. *EORTC QLQ-C30—core questionnaire*

Scale	Number of items
Functional scales	
Physical functioning	5
Role functioning	2
Emotional functioning	4
Cognitive functioning	2
Social functioning	2
Global quality of life	2
Symptom scales	
Fatigue	3
Nausea and vomiting	2
Pain	2
Single questions	
Dyspnea	1
Sleep disturbance	1
Appetite loss	1
Constipation	1
Diarrhea	1
Financial impact	1
Total number of items	30

EORTC, European Organization for the Research and Treatment of Cancer.

TABLE 2. *EORTC QLQ-C30—phase III and IV modules*

Module		Number of items
Lung cancer module	QLQ-LC13	13
Breast cancer module	QLQ-BR23	23
Head and neck cancer module	QLQ-H&N37	37
Esophageal cancer module	QLQ OES24	24
Colorectal cancer module	QLQ-CR38	38

An example of an instrument that assesses fatigue is the Multiple Fatigue Index (MFI), which uses 20 items on five subscales (91). To date no Hodgkin's- or lymphoma-specific module has been published. Therefore, the EORTC Lymphoma Cooperative Group devised an alternative way to measure fatigue in patients with Hodgkin's disease (52). Rather than using a separate module as the core, the main elements of the core were supplemented by already-existing instruments or modules addressing, in particular, the dimensions of fatigue, sexuality, and fear of childlessness, and, as single questions, the special side effects of chemotherapy and radiotherapy.

The first results of the EORTC H_8 Quality of Life (QL) questionnaire, developed for repeated measurement and extensively tested within two large trial cooperative groups [EORTC and German Hodgkin's Study Group (GHSG)], have yielded promising results concerning psychometrics, applicability, and appropriateness of content. Complementing the H_8-QL questionnaire is the Life Situation Questionnaire (LSQ) developed in Caen, France, to systematically investigate the quality of life of patients at the end of treatment and at several points thereafter. The questionnaire is available in French, German, and English and is being prepared for further international evaluation. It addresses the following areas: general living circumstances (housing), work history and current occupational status, marital status and family relationships, health records, family medical history, current health status, leisure activities, and economic and insurance problems related to Hodgkin's disease (76). Due to the development of international collaborations in Hodgkin's disease over the last decade, internationally tested instruments for quality-of-life assessment in Hodgkin's disease are needed. The most applicable instruments are the EORTC QLQ-C30 and the FACT; both are available in many languages and are brief and easy to administer (51,84). The EORTC and the GHSG are carrying out standardized module development internationally, including the forward-backward method of translation.

Children and Adolescents

Only very recently has there been progress in the development of instruments to measure quality of life and late effects in pediatric oncology (92). Quality-of-life assessment in children must address normal developmental issues in such areas as peer relations, school, family, and play, which differ from the topics addressed in adult instruments. Questionnaires must also be suitably administered. In children under the age of 10 or 11, self-reporting is neither reliable nor feasible; proxy ratings by the parents or caregivers are necessary. A number of proxy and self-rating tools are already available from the disciplines of child psychology and psychiatry; no established and tested instruments exist for quality-of-life research in children and, in particular, in children with Hodgkin's disease (27,38).

Quality-Adjusted Life Years

The concept of quality-adjusted life years (QALY) (93,94) adjusts survival time (months/years) by a factor derived from quality-of-life measures, integrating quantity and quality of survival into one measurement. The use of QALY allows integrating quality-of-life data into standard survival data (curves) to facilitate clinical decision making. Despite the attractiveness of this concept, a number of problems have arisen. One problem concerns calculated comparisons, since by this method 1 year with a 100% quality of life equals 10 years with a 10% quality of life. Obviously, a number of assumptions have to be made in comparing time and the quality of life. A second problem is related to the generation of adjustment factors and the time interval to which they are assigned. One of the assumptions is that time intervals with constant quality of life can be identified and that the corresponding adjustment factor (ranging from 0 to 1) can be measured accurately. Even if time intervals can be identified with a sufficient reliability to obtain quality-of-life indicators, it is still uncertain which quality-of-life domains are the most relevant for generating adjustment factors. In attempting to address some of these problems, different approaches have been taken to define time intervals and to generate quality-of-life adjustment factors for them.

One of the more advanced methods is known as Time Without Symptoms and Toxicity (TWiST) or more recently Q-TWiST, which applies a patient-derived qualifying component to the adjustment process (95,96). Evaluations of TWiST/Q-TWiST have been carried out in two populations of breast cancer patients: those receiving palliative treatment (patients with a limited survival) and those on adjuvant trials. TWiST evaluates the different components of time on treatment with or without side effects, and time of remission with or without symptoms or side effects and without other restrictions or limitations to the patients' quality of life in order to assess the overall outcome of treatment (97). The patients who have been studied with TWiST have had cancers with different outcomes and side effects than patients with Hodgkin's disease (in which there is an emphasis on a high probability of late survival, and late complications of treatment are extremely important). However, the impact of long-term effects and late sequelae from these other cancers could be used for generating adjustment factors for Hodgkin's disease as well. Since most patients with Hodgkin's disease will be successfully treated (and cured), it may be hard to distinguish between treatment or disease-related issues and the influence of normal life events on perceived quality of life. Years after treatment, normal life events can be as influential as the prior life-threatening illness. To make valid judgments, normal populations must be included to control for these variables. Thus, QALY concepts rarely have been employed in Hodgkin's disease, but there are studies that have applied the methodology to cost-effectiveness analyses (98). However, unless prospective longitudinal long-term trials are available to provide insight into the course of disease and clarify the important changes in quality of life over long periods of time, it is questionable whether QALY will influence clinical decisions in patients with Hodgkin's disease (99–101).

USE OF QUALITY-OF-LIFE DATA

Quality-of-life data are utilized in both psychosocial and medical research (102). There are three general uses for quality-of-life measures to assist professionals in predicting patient outcomes and in planning patient care programs: (a) to evaluate the extent of change in the quality of life of an individual or group across time or as an end point in evaluating treatment outcome (3,6,9,10); (b) to predict outcome, prognosis, patient survival, or response to future treatment (9,10,103,104); and (c) to assess rehabilitation needs, and determine problem areas and coping patterns among various patient subgroups (10,16).

Quality of Life as an Independent Variable

Quality-of-life measures can be used as either independent or dependent variables in research (6). In effectiveness of treatment studies, quality of life is used as an independent variable. In Example 1, quality of life after an intervention in patients versus controls is the independent variable, while survival time, or time to recurrence, is the dependent variable. Spiegel et al. (104a) used quality-of-life measures among breast cancer patients randomized to treatment or controls. In an analysis of survival time (the dependent measure), they found that those patients in the group with intervention enjoyed a survival benefit of 18 months compared to patients in the control group.

Example 1: Effectiveness of Treatment Studies

$$= \frac{\textit{QL + Treatment vs. Controls}}{\textit{Survival Time, Time to Recurrence}}$$

Rehabilitation studies provide a second example of quality of life used as an independent variable. In Example 2, quality-of-life measures are combined with medical variables to form the independent variable, with the dependent variable being a predictor such as depression or anxiety. Rehabilitation studies provide an example of data from quality-of-life measures that might be grouped as both independent and dependent variables.

Example 2: Rehabilitation Studies

$$= \frac{\textit{Quality of Life + Medical Variables}}{\textit{Patient Depression/QL Measures}}$$

Using data from a cross-sectional group of Hodgkin's patients, Fobair et al. (16) examined how return of energy and severity of treatment were predicted by depression scores at follow-up. Although the intent of the study was to describe the patients' problems, there was interest in using the results to inform the support services of the patient care problems. In this analysis of data from 403 patients treated for Hodgkin's disease, the independent variables were energy loss, physical functioning, medical condition, stage of disease and type of treatment, and age at treatment. The dependent variable was the depression score on the CES-D. When the results indicated that overall energy loss after treatment was a problem for 37% of the patients, a program was developed for a posttreatment group session, and the development of the "Surviving!" newsletter.

Quality of Life as a Dependent Variable

Quality-of-life scores are used as the dependent or outcome measure in clinical trials (Example 3) comparing two treatments of similar biologic effectiveness, to determine which treatment had the least emotional, social, or physical dysfunctioning.

Example 3: Comparison of Treatment Studies

$$= \frac{\textit{Treatment 1 vs. Treatment 2}}{\textit{Quality of Life Scores}}$$

In psychosocial studies, quality-of-life scores are used as dependent measures when data on the effectiveness of one or more interventions versus controls is analyzed for outcome. In medical outcome studies, quality of life can be viewed as being "as important as the conventional outcomes of survival and toxicity of therapy" (105). Coates and Gebski (104) found that quality-of-life scores provided an independent predictor of survival duration for cancer patients when assessing the impact of the disease and its treatment.

The clinical applications of quality-of-life data benefit both the analysis of clinical trials and of clinical practice. When used as an independent or predictive variable, quality-of-life data guide clinical decisions based on the effectiveness of treatment and assist in the early detection of morbidity. Used as a dependent measure, in the comparison of different treatments, quality of life helps to determine patient preferences among treatment choices in a systematic and quantifiable manner (6), and has prognostic value in predicting survival among patients treated for advanced disease "as patients perceive disease progression before it is clinically evident" (103).

APPLYING QUALITY-OF-LIFE INSTRUMENTS TO PATIENTS

There are three main reasons why investigators might measure quality of life: (a) to assess need for rehabilitation resources, (b) to use information as a predictor of outcome or prognosis, and (c) to have an end point in evaluating treatment outcome (27). The main characteristics and instruments used in the most recent published studies are listed in Table 3.

To Address the Need for Rehabilitation

Cancer and its treatment affect many aspects of quality of life in long-term survivors of malignancy (including physical, psychological, social, and spiritual well-being) (111). Information from several different questionnaires can help better understand the needs of patients and improve support after treatment. Most validated questionnaires only consider overall quality of life (80,112, 113) or contain a limited number of aspects of quality of life such as depression or anxiety (114). Although assessment of sexuality is present in 34% of studies on quality of life of cancer survivors, spiritual (10.4%) and economic (12.3%) patient-specific outcomes are infrequently addressed (115). Aspects of quality of life, including difficulties in family, professional, and social settings, in using medical resources, and in financial security (one recent population-based study found that patients had difficulties in borrowing from banks), must be correlated with standard quality-of-life scales (76,116). Several of the above questions have been included in a few validated questionnaires such as the CARES (117). To cover all aspects of quality of life, multiple questionnaires should be used during each assessment, although this will entail some duplication.

Predictors of Outcome or Prognosis

Performance status has been shown to significantly predict survival for a number of tumors. Patients with good scores on quality-of-life measures have longer survival times (118,119). One explanation for this is that patients with fewer effects of the tumor have either an earlier stage of disease and thus a better prognosis or are more likely to tolerate and benefit from effective treatment (120). Quality-of-life measures performed prior to treatment are used as variables for stratification in randomized clinical trials (103,121). Although this represents progress, such stratification usually is based on a single measure, while quality of life can be highly depen-

TABLE 3. *Quality of life studies in Hodgkin's disease*

Author	Study type and study population	Survey modality	Instruments used	Follow-up (yrs)	Participation rate (%)	Areas explored
Cella and Tross 1986 (106) (*n* = 60)	Cross-sectional study Adults with HD compared with 20 healthy men	SAD Interview	BSI Subscales of Derogatis sexual functioning IES RSES DAQ GAS	0.5–10	—	Psychosocial adaptation Emotion Sexuality Body image
Fobair et al. 1986 (16) (*n* = 403)	Cross-sectional study Adults with HD	SAD Interview	CES-D POMS	9 (1–21)	95	Psychosocial adaptation Sense of well-being Family relationship Employment
Wasserman 1987 (107) (*n* = 40)	Cross-sectional study Children with HD	Interview	No validated questionnaires	7–19	—	Physical sequelae Social difficulties Experience of having a cancer
Devlen et al. 1987 (108) (*n* = 120)	Prospective study Adults with HD and lymphoma	Interview at diagnosis, and 2, 6, and 12 months posttreatment	Toxicity of treatment (not validated) Wechsler memory test	—	95	Toxicity of treatment Psychiatric morbidity Social morbidity
Bloom et al. 1989 (18) (*n* = 85)	Cross-sectional study Adults with HD compared with adults with testicular cancer	SAD Interview	POMS Social Support Scale SAS	3	—	Social morbidity Employment
Carpenter et al. 1989 (109) (*n* = 43)	Cross-sectional study Adults with HD	Interview	PAIS BDS Subscales of Derogatis sexual functioning State-Trait Anxiety Scale	4.7 (0.5–13)	—	Psychosocial status Anxiety Sexuality
Hannah et al. 1992 (21) (*n* = 24)	Cross-sectional study Adults with HD and their spouses compared with 34 adults with testicular cancer and their spouses	Interview	FES	—	—	Marital functioning Sexual functioning
Kornblith et al. 1992 (110) (*n* = 93)	Cross-sectional study Adults with HD	Interview	PAIS BSI POMS IES	2.2 (1–5)	76	Psychological, sexual, familial and vocational functioning
Kornblith et al. 1992 (74) (*n* = 273)	Cross-sectional study Adults with HD	Interview	PAIS BSI POMS IES Subscales of Derogatis sexual functioning	6.3 (1–20)	91	Psychosocial adaptation Sexuality Employment
Bloom et al. 1993 (42) (*n* = 85)	Cross-sectional study Adults with HD compared with 88 adults with testicular cancer	Interview	POMS CES-D SCL-90 SAS	1–7.5	88	Physical functioning Psychological distress Social outcome
van Tulder et al. 1994 (77) (*n* = 81)	Cross-sectional study Adults with HD compared with 160 hospital visitors	SAD	SF36 No validated questionnaire (insurance, sexuality)	14 (10–18)	92	Psychosocial adaptation Sexuality Insurance
Ferrell et al. 1995 (43) (*n* = 687)	Cross-sectional study Long-term adult survivors: 43% breast cancer 17% lymphoma and HD 8% ovarian cancer	SAD	QOL-CS FACT-G	—	57	Physical, psychological adaptation Social outcome Spiritual well-being
Joly et al. 1996 (76) (*n* = 93)	Cross-sectional study Adults with HD compared with 186 healthy men	SAD	QLQ-C30 No validated questionnaire (insurance, work situation, medical consumption)	10 (4–17)	91	Physical, psychological adaptation Social outcome Insurance
Norum and Wist 1996 (46) (*n* = 42)	Cross-sectional study HD	SAD	QLQ-C30	5 (1–12)	95	Physical, psychological adaptation Social outcome Insurance

SAD, self-administered questionnaire; HD, Hodgkin's disease; BSI, Brief Symptoms Inventory; IES, Impact of Events Scales; RSES, Rosenberg Self-Esteem Scales; DAQ, Death Anxiety Questionnaire; GAS, Global Assessment Scale; CES-D, Center for Epidemiologic Studies—depression scale; POMS, Profile of Mood States; SAS, Social Activities Scale; PAIS, Psychosocial Adjustment to Illness Scale; BDS, Beck Depression Scale; FES, Family Environment Scale; SCL-90, 90-item symptoms checklist; SF36, Mos 36-item short-form healthy survey; QOL-CS, Quality of life cancer survivors; FACT-G, Functional Assessment of Cancer Therapy—general; QLQ-C30, EORTC Quality of Life Core Questionnaire.

dent on the time of assessment. Also, the use of only one score, which may have been arbitrarily selected for stratification or as a predictor, may be less than optimal as multiple scores are provided that correspond to well-defined quality-of-life dimensions that cannot be used separately. Also there are concerns that "the use of quality-of-life data as part of the characterization of patients raises the possibility that such data might also be used as a basis for discrimination" (9). Quality-of-life measurements have never been applied to the design of studies of patients with Hodgkin's disease. Validated quality-of-life questionnaires have not been used as indicators for response to therapy, clinical outcome, or survival.

End Points in Evaluating Treatment Outcome

In evaluating treatment outcome, the purpose is not to identify problems for rehabilitation but to compare the quality of life across competing (alternative) treatments. Repeated quality-of-life data might be used as an end point or outcomes measure in clinical trials in addition to more conventional end points such as survival and time to relapse. Disease specific measures are clinically sensible in that patients and clinicians intuitively find the items directly relevant. This increases the potential for compliance and is particularly compelling in the clinical trial setting. The disadvantages of this approach are the multiple comparisons and the lack of a unified scoring system that may lead to difficulties in interpretation (122). In clinical trials that have equivalent disease-free and overall survival results, quality-of-life assessment may help in selecting the best treatment arm. However, quality-of-life assessment should not be considered as a surrogate end point (123,124).

Single Versus Multiple Modality of Evaluation

There is no single standard quality-of-life instrument available. The use of psychometric instruments (health profiles) provide the most common approach. These can be replaced by and/or utilized with utility measures such as Q-TWiST (125).

Generic Versus Specific Questionnaires

Generic questionnaires cover a broad range of quality-of-life dimensions in a single instrument. Their use facilitates comparisons among various individuals or diseases (126). This approach is particularly important for studies aimed at evaluating rehabilitation and long-term sequelae of treatment. Generic questionnaires can be applied to both normal volunteers and to patients. The use of both generic and specific questionnaires can improve quality-of-life assessment because items included in specific questionnaires relate more to a particular disease than do generic questionnaires. For example, the EORTC core questionnaire is a generic, validated questionnaire for oncology; it can be used together with specific modules adapted to a given cancer (e.g., breast cancer) or aspect of cancer treatment (e.g., palliative care, patient satisfaction) (107). Therefore, the type of questionnaire used (generic, specific, or both) depends on the objectives of the study; during the time of therapy, disease-specific measures might be of greatest interest, whereas generic measures, because they permit comparisons across conditions and populations, are of greatest interest in post-treatment longitudinal studies or in cross-sectional studies in long-term survivors (122). The use of multiple questionnaires can be difficult because of the large number of questions and the long time needed to complete them, which can adversely affect patient compliance.

Psychometric Versus Utility Measures

Utility measures of quality of life, another type of generic instrument, are derived from economic and decision theory. Their use is particularly appropriate when choices exist between length of life or length of remission and quality of life. In this approach (Q-TWiST), the survival time is weighed by disease progression and adverse events of treatment. Q-TWiST can add complementary data to the standard evaluation of survival as was recently demonstrated in postmenopausal patients with breast cancer (127). In clinical trials where the major focus is patient benefit, the Q-TWiST can be integrated with a psychometric scale (59,122). The association of two such complementary approaches can be of great interest in trials comparing two treatment modalities with similar efficacy but different toxicity. This is particularly the case in clinical trials aiming at scaling down treatment modalities such as in early-stage Hodgkin's disease. Because the methodology in assessing quality of life is not yet perfected, the results of quality-of-life studies should be regarded as a process to facilitate discussion, and not merely a process of measurement (128).

When Should Quality-of-Life Instruments Be Administered?

The timing of quality-of-life assessment and its frequency depend on the study aim, the expected sensitivity of the survey, and constraints from both patients and medical staff. In the absence of previous experience with longitudinal studies, it is difficult to suggest a schedule. The use of infrequent evaluations may miss transient effects that are likely to appear during and after therapy. On the other hand, repeated inquiries may increase patient stress or decrease compliance (129). Patient compliance may also vary according to the way the study aims are explained (130). The more frequent the evaluation, the more explanation needed. In randomized clinical trials, a baseline quality-of-life assessment before initiation of treatment is necessary. Subsequent quality-of-life assessments, during or after treatment, may need to take into account any preexisting intragroup differences in baseline quality-of-life characteristics. This may help to assess whether or not observed changes can be attributed to treatment.

The timing of quality-of-life evaluation depends on the questions asked. The impact of cumulative toxicity can be measured at two or more points during treatment, whereas disease-related impact on quality of life should be measured after acute toxicity has subsided, generally months or years following the end of therapy (131). This quality-of-life assessment could be coupled with routine follow-up visits. Later quality-of-life assessment in long-term survivors would help in distinguishing the respective impacts of the treatment and the cancer. The number and the timing of follow-up quality-of-life assessments depend on whether it is desirable to measure long-term treatment and disease-related toxicity as well as the entire duration of the beneficial effects of therapy. Development of specific questionnaires on rehabilitation needs is particularly appropriate in long-term quality-of-life assessment. Short questionnaires should improve long-term compliance. Ideally long-term quality-of-life assessments should be prospective and continuous. If these are not possible, cross-sectional studies with comparison to a healthy population can facilitate understanding of patients' long-term difficulties (18,76).

USE OF QUALITY-OF-LIFE INSTRUMENTS IN CLINICAL TRIALS

In a review of the literature in pediatric oncology, Bradlyn et al. (132) demonstrated that only 3% of all reports of randomized clinical trials ($n = 70$) included quality-of-life data. A review of the most important randomized clinical trials in Hodgkin's disease also reveals that quality of life is disregarded as a primary or even as a secondary outcome measure. However, retrospective analyses of long-term survivors of Hodgkin's disease have demonstrated that a substantial subgroup of patients has demonstrable effects of the disease and its treatment even years after the end of treatment (46,74,76,77). In one study, men earning less than $15,000 a year, and persons currently unemployed, single, less educated, or experiencing serious illness since treatment, were found to be at high risk, years after treatment, for poor adaptation. Furthermore, in one study 22% of patients met the criteria suggested for a psychiatric diagnosis (74). It remains unclear when in the course of the disease one can distinguish patients with good coping mechanisms from those without. To more precisely characterize the difficulties in adjustment after treatment, quality-of-life assessment has to be included in prospective randomized clinical trials.

Most randomized clinical trials are conducted by cooperative groups because of the low incidence of Hodgkin's disease. A major challenge to prospective multicenter trials using longitudinal data on quality of life is the completeness of data sets as missing data limits the value of the results. A high standard of data collection is essential for the trial to be successful (133). To obtain completeness of data, quality-of-life assessments have to be a mandatory component of the clinical trial design and part of the inclusion criteria (134). However, assurance of a complete data set will only be guaranteed by convincing the patient and the participating physicians and nurses of the importance of, and the future therapeutic impact of, quality-of-life assessment in randomized clinical trials (135).

The prognosis of Hodgkin's disease has dramatically improved over the last three decades (136). Today, almost 80% of all Hodgkin's disease patients are cured (24). The clinical stage at presentation remains the strongest predictor of outcome of treatment. Prognosis is based on stage: early, intermediate, or advanced. With a cure rate of 85% to 90% and a 5-year rate of freedom from treatment failure of 80% to 85% for patients with early- and intermediate-stage Hodgkin's disease, improvement of treatment results is an improbable goal (137). In patients with early- and intermediate-stage Hodgkin's disease, future therapeutic efforts should aim at reducing early and late toxicity. In recent years, several advances in reducing treatment-related toxicity in early and intermediate stages have been achieved. For example, in the H_6 twin study, the EORTC Lymphoma Cooperative Group demonstrated that diagnostic staging laparotomy is no longer routinely recommended in the workup of patients with early-stage Hodgkin's disease since overall survival was similar in patients with or without laparotomy (137). The advantage of more extensive staging was counterbalanced by the morbidity and mortality of the procedure.

A metaanalysis conducted by Specht et al. (138) demonstrated that combined-modality treatment consisting of chemotherapy and irradiation results in lower recurrence rates than radiation alone in early-stage Hodgkin's disease. Thus, modern treatment strategies should consider the combination of chemotherapy and involved-field irradiation as a standard treatment option for patients with early- and intermediate-stage Hodgkin's disease. This strategy, however, may have a substantial impact on early and late toxicity as well as on quality of life. Because late toxicities, such as cardiopulmonary toxicities or secondary neoplasia (139,140; see Chapters 32,33, and 34), occur years after treatment, long-term follow-up has to be performed. Quality-of-life assessments can help in demonstrating an advantage of a new treatment strategy (141); thus, quality-of-life assessment has to be included in studies aiming at reducing the treatment-related toxicity, especially if a known less aggressive treatment is not proposed in the study design.

Until recently, treatment results were not satisfactory for patients with advanced Hodgkin's disease (142). Present studies, however, suggest that dose-intensive chemotherapy regimens might induce cure rates comparable to that observed in patients with early- and intermediate-stage disease. With the escalated BEACOPP [bleomycin, etoposide, Adriamycin (doxorubicin), cyclophosphamide, Oncovin (vincristine), procarbazine, and prednisone] regimen, a freedom-from-treatment failure rate of 90% and a survival rate of 95% were achieved by the GHSG after a median observation time of 27 months (142a). This improvement is accompanied by a considerable increase in acute toxicity such as myelosuppression and infections. Whether or not late toxicity will also increase remains to be seen. Future efforts should concentrate on the search for the most effective regimen with the lowest toxicity. In early-stage Hodgkin's disease, quality-of-life assessment can help in defining the toxicity profile of the therapeutic regimens tested.

Quality of Life as Primary or Secondary Outcome

Before starting a new randomized clinical trial, one should decide what significant adverse side effects would require interrupting the study. Quality-of-life assessment in patients with Hodgkin's disease is not established yet as a standard part of clinical trials and it remains unclear whether quality-of-life scores are able to detect differences between treatment arms. Furthermore, the evaluation of potential differences in quality-of-life assessment is still under debate. Considering that it is unknown what amount of time is required before long-term disadvantages in quality of life become obvious, the length of time during which patients should be evaluated cannot be anticipated. The EORTC Lymphoma Cooperative Group and the GHSG are presently performing longitudinal assessment of quality of life (Table 4). It is hoped these ongoing trials will contribute answers to the questions posed.

In general, quality-of-life assessment is regarded as a secondary outcomes measure. Before it can be regarded as a primary outcomes measure, quality-of-life assessment must fulfill various requirements. The method of assessment must be shown to be applicable in a multicenter setting. In a study aiming at reducing treatment-related toxicities, assessment of quality of life is mandatory.

Does QALY Add to the Final Treatment Decision?

Recently, there have been attempts to evaluate treatment outcome using surrogate parameters of overall survival or freedom from treatment failure. Efforts have been made to set up a correlation between life years gained and the patients' self-reported quality of life (97,98,133). However, there is still a substantial debate on how to measure health-related quality of life (143,144).

Norum et al. (98) have shown that the cost-benefit correlation for patients with Hodgkin's disease is very favorable in the Norwegian setting. The cost per gained life year was estimated at 1,651 English pounds. Compared with other cancer entities, the cost appears to be very low. However, this should not be surprising as there is a positive relationship between cost-benefit and outcomes in Hodgkin's disease because of its very favorable prognosis.

The QALY approach is used to include patients' self-reported quality of life in the evaluation or comparison of treatment strategies. In a palliative setting, QALY can help in decision making and counseling. In patients with curable disease, one can argue that curing the patient is more important than the consequences of treatment, especially when there is not much difference from one strategy to another. However, early data are available on loss of quality of life years after treatment. Should longitudinal assessment of quality of life demonstrate that a significant loss in quality of life is dependent on the type of treatment administered and that it varies with treatment modality, an evaluation using the QALY approach might help identify which treatment is associated with the optimal cost-benefit. Nevertheless, to compare several Hodgkin's disease treatment strategies, methods of measuring health-related quality of life remain to be standardized (144).

To prove small differences in therapy-related toxicity or in improvement of treatment results, large numbers of

TABLE 4. *Instruments used in quality-of-life assessment in GHSG and EORTC/GELA ongoing prospective trials*

Time	GHSG-HD8 trial	EORTC-H_8 trial
Before treatment start	EORTC QLQ-C30 Additional scales Life situation questionnaire	No evaluation
At the end of initial treatment	EORTC QLQ-C30 Additional scales	EORTC QLQ-C30 Additional scales
Follow-up, first year	EORTC QLQ-C30 Additional scales (every 3 months)	EORTC QLQ-C30 Additional scales (every 2 months for 6 months, every 3 months thereafter)
Follow-up, second year	EORTC QLQ-C30 Additional scales (every 3 months)	EORTC QLQ-C30 Additional scales (every 4 months)
Follow-up, third to fifth year	EORTC QLQ-C30 Additional scales (every 6 months)	EORTC QLQ-C30 Additional scales (every 6 months)

GHSG, German Hodgkin's Study Group; GELA, Groupe d'Etude des Lymphomes de l'Adulte.

patients are needed (145). Because of the disease's low incidence rate, randomized clinical trials must be conducted in a multicenter setting. In 1998, the GHSG included 312 participating centers, of which 15 are located outside of Germany; the EORTC Lymphoma Cooperative Group and the Groupe d'Etude des Lymphomes de l'Adulte (GELA) in France together included 125 participating centers in eight European countries. Therefore, the instrument used in the assessment of quality of life in Hodgkin's disease has to meet several requirements (134). It should be validated and highly independent of the local environment. This is most likely to occur by the use of prevalidated quality-of-life self-administered questionnaires. These questionnaires must focus on the disease-specific needs. Also, the questionnaires should consider not only toxicity, acute or late, but also rehabilitation and changes in quality of life.

GENERAL POPULATION COMPARISON

The Importance of Control Comparison

The aim of randomized clinical trials is usually to compare the efficacy of two or more treatments. When the compared treatments are expected to differ, quality of life can be considered as an additional end point; when the treatments are expected to be equivalent, quality of life can be considered as the main end point (123,146,147). Because in randomized clinical trials patient characteristics are similar in both treatment arms, it is not necessary to use a healthy control population. In contrast, the use of a control group is particularly important in epidemiologic studies where the objectives are to evaluate the incidence and the impact of the disease and/or its treatment on the patients' quality of life (148). In long-term cancer survivors, the use of a healthy population as control is fundamental to evaluate the respective impact of cancer and its treatment compared to baseline socioeconomic quality of life. This approach contains two difficult aspects: the choice of a questionnaire that can be administered to both cancer patients and controls, and the selection of a reference population (146).

Quality-of-Life Reference Data

When many patients or controls are enrolled in quality-of-life studies, conducting interviews becomes costly. Under these circumstances, self-administered questionnaires are used instead. A number of questionnaires were developed for and validated on the healthy population. All of them are generic, for example, the NHP questionnaire (112), the SIP questionnaire (149), and the MOS SF-36 questionnaire (80). The advantages and disadvantages of using such questionnaires are listed in Table 5. Questionnaires that explore various aspects of a specific disease and treatment are constructed for patients and therefore are not suitable for general population comparison.

TABLE 5. *Advantages and disadvantages of population quality-of-life questionnaires*

Advantages	Disadvantages
Can be applied to healthy and patient populations	Limited exploration of quality of life in healthy population
Quick to administer and easy to complete	Socioprofessional parameters in long-term survivors not explored
Reference scores from healthy population are known	Specific aspects of disease and treatment not evaluated

Validated generic quality-of-life questionnaires have been used in various healthy population studies and the results published (150–153). These studies provide data on quality of life for use as a comparison with questionnaires issued to patients with cancer. However, these control data have some limitations. First, comparison is effective only at the time of the study since socioeconomic conditions are likely to influence the quality of life of healthy subjects as well as that of cancer survivors. Second, even for a particular group of individuals, it might not be possible to extrapolate the available data from one country to another, or from one area of a given country to another, because of potential cross-cultural biases. Third, information obtained is restricted to that explored by the generic questionnaire(s) used.

Case-Control Studies

Case-control studies can be used to avoid the potential biases of quality-of-life reference data. Their advantages are that controls can be matched to patients at the time of the study, and that other questionnaires can be added to the generic one to assess marital and familial issues, socioprofessional status, medical care, etc. (as in the LSQ). This information might be particularly relevant in long-term cancer survivor studies.

Patients to be Enrolled

The selection of cases (i.e., patients) is important; it can greatly affect the results of the study. In general population studies, patients obtained from cancer registry databases, where available, represent unbiased cases. This approach controls for the characteristics and the specificity of medical practice in a given area. In contrast, cases from hospital series are only representative of the recruitment and the clinical practice of the specific hospital.

Selection of Controls

The designation of the type of control group is the most difficult task in planning a case-control study (154). The selection of the controls depends on the study-specific aims and circumstances. If the aim of the study is to evaluate the quality of life of long-term cancer survivors in comparison with that of a healthy population, a population-based series is the best choice because such controls are especially comparable with the cases. When a hospital-based series of cases is assembled, the use of population controls is also recommended because multiple biases can occur in the selection of hospital controls. There are two main disadvantages associated with the use of the general population based controls. First, the individuals selected are often not cooperative, and response tends to be worse than that from other types of controls and that from cases (76,155,156). Second, a substantial proportion of controls might present with a cancer history. These controls will be excluded and replaced. However, in order not to influence the participation rate of controls and the quality of their response, the cover letter sent with the questionnaires or given at the time of interview should not mention that their questionnaires are to be matched to those of patients who have suffered from cancer. For example, in the Rieker et al. (157) study, cases from hospital series were matched to general population controls on sociodemographic characteristics, while in the Joly et al. (76) study, both cases and controls issued from the general population. An alternative to the selection of a general population control group is that of controls from among cases' neighbors (158), hospital visitors (77), or cases' siblings (159). This alternative, however, should be considered with caution because of multiple potential biases.

When the objective of the study is to explore the impact of site-specific outcomes, because of disease-specific treatment, controls should be selected among patients treated for another type of cancer with a similar clinical outcome. This approach was used by Bloom et al. (42), who compared the psychosocial outcomes of patients treated for testicular cancer and patients treated for Hodgkin's disease (42).

Short Review on Ongoing and Completed Research

Case-controls studies performed in Hodgkin's disease survivors are listed in Table 6. Only one study concerned cases derived from a population cancer registry. Two studies involved healthy controls (one population based), and one compared quality of life in Hodgkin's disease

TABLE 6. *Case-control studies in long-term survivors of Hodgkin's disease*

Study	Cases (patients)	Controls	Instruments	Follow-up time in years	Main results
Cella and Tross 1986 (106)	60 male survivors	20 healthy males matched on age	Interview	0.5–12	Significant lower intimacy motivation, increasing avoidant thinking about illness, prolonged difficulty in returning to premorbid work status and illness-related concerns Cancer patients were significantly more appreciative of life than controls
Kornblith et al. 1992 (110)	33 patients treated with ABVD	Patients treated with MOPP (n = 31) or MOPP-ABVD (n = 29) within a clinical trial	Interview SAD	1–5	No significant long-term advantage in psychological adaptation or psychosexual function for survivors of HD treated with the less gonadally toxic ABVD regimen
Bloom et al. 1993 (42)	85 males treated in three university hospitals	88 men with testicular cancer	Interview	1–7.5	More focused symptoms among controls (decrease in sexual enjoyment, poor health habits) More generalized symptoms among cases (fatigue, energy loss, work impairment) Similar levels of infertility and erectile dysfunction Most of these differences were site-related
van Tulder et al. 1994 (77)	81 patients treated at a single institution	116 hospital visitors	SAD	10–18	More physical, role, sexuality impairment, and low perception of overall health among cases
Joly et al. 1996 (76)	93 patients derived from a cancer registry	186 population-based controls matched on age and sex	SAD	4–17	More physical, role, and cognitive impairment among cases Major limitation in borrowing from banks remained the major problem in cases

MOPP, mechlorethamine, Oncovin (vincristine), procarbazine, prednisone; ABVD, Adriamycin, bleomycin, vinblastine, dacarbazine; SAD, self-administered questionnaire.

survivors to that of testicular-cancer survivors. Half of the studies used an interview alone or in combination with self-administrated questionnaires. Results mainly depend on the choice of controls. When controls are healthy individuals, similar results are observed.

CONCLUSIONS

The assessment of quality of life has become important, especially in the evaluation of treatment given to patients with a chronic illness such as cancer. Although overall survival and survival without disease have long been used as the end points in clinical trials, evaluation of these end points alone is no longer accepted today because other characteristics are now considered as important as survival by both patients and physicians. Among these, treatment burden, treatment-related toxicity, as well as their psychological and social impacts are of great importance.

This change stems from the dramatic improvement in the efficacy of cancer treatments, particular those for Hodgkin's disease. Effective therapies, however, have several drawbacks that might limit their use. Chemotherapy as well as radiation therapy can induce severe acute and late toxicities that may lead to death long before what would be expected in patients (see Chapter 32). Because most Hodgkin's disease patients have a very long life expectancy after diagnosis and treatment, one should always keep in mind the distinction that exists between curing the disease and curing the patient. Several studies have highlighted the difficulties that survivors may experience long after treatment ends, such as general fatigue, health fragility, and social and financial problems. These findings have been demonstrated in studies where a quality-of-life approach has been used.

In this chapter, we have attempted to illustrate how difficult it is to properly study the quality of life of patients both in the clinical trial setting and in epidemiologic studies. Instruments (questionnaires) have been developed specifically for the general population or for patients, although there are no instruments specific to Hodgkin's disease. Most of these instruments are validated, but they are not always available in other languages, which limits their use. Also, they generally do not include items on family and social issues, professional limitations, and medical care. Thus, several research teams have begun developing a so-called life situation questionnaire, but its reliability remains to be demonstrated.

Like happiness, quality of life is an ambiguous concept, with various definitions. Therefore, it is difficult for a questionnaire to adequately summarize all aspects of patient quality of life even though cured patients might have contributed to its production. Interviews are less impersonal than questionnaires. Their reliability, however, depends on the experience the interviewer has gained and on his fairness in analyzing the patient's responses. In Hodgkin's disease, there has been no analysis of the results of interviews and of generic or specific questionnaires administered to the same patients. Such a study would potentially help interpret the results of studies limited to the use of self-administered questionnaires.

Before starting a quality-of-life assessment, one should always consider the following questions: What is the question being asked? Will quality-of-life assessment help answer the question? What is the population to be studied? How many patients should be enrolled? What should the study design be (e.g., cross sectional or longitudinal)? Do validated instruments exist that can be used to assess quality of life? Can they be used in a longitudinal study, i.e., can they be repeated over time? What would an interview add to questionnaires? Is the study feasible? Are its time demands reasonable? These questions are not very different from the questions researchers have to answer before undertaking a clinical study. Quality-of-life assessment should not be considered an end in itself, but rather a way to help physicians evaluate the efficacy and toxicity of treatment and help in making medical decisions among treatment strategies with similar efficacy but different toxicity. Quality-of-life assessment should also benefit patients by defining issues that are important to them, even long after they have been cured.

REFERENCES

1. Iscoe N, Williams JI, Szalai JP, Osoba D. Prediction of psychosocial distress in patients with cancer. In: Osoba D, ed. *Effect of cancer on quality of life.* Boca Raton, FL: CRC Press, 1991:42.
2. Ware JE. Measuring functioning, well-being, and other generic health concepts. In: Osoba D, ed. *Effect of cancer on quality of life.* Boca Raton, FL: CRC Press, 1991:9.
3. Karnosfky DA, Burchenal JH. The clinical evaluation of chemotherapeutic agents in cancer. In: MacLeod CM, ed. *Evaluation of chemotherapeutic agents.* New York: Columbia University Press, 1949:191.
4. Strain JJ. The evolution of quality of life evaluations in cancer therapy. *Oncology* 1990;4:22.
5. Gough IR. Quality of life as an outcome variable in oncology and surgery. *N Z J Surg* 1994;64:227.
6. Osoba D. Measuring the effect of cancer on quality of life. In: Osoba D, ed. *Effect of cancer on quality of life.* Boca Raton, FL: CRC Press, 1991:29.
7. Patrick DL. Assessing health-related quality of life outcomes. In: Heithoff KA, Lohr KN, eds. *Effectiveness and outcomes in health care.* Washington, DC: National Academy Press, 1990:139.
8. Till JE, McNeil BJ, Bush RS. Measurement of multiple components of quality of life. *Cancer Treat Symp* 1984;1:177.
9. Till JE. Use (and some possible abuses) of quality-of life measures. In: Osoba D, ed. *Effect of cancer on quality of life.* Boca Raton, FL: CRC Press, 1991:137.
10. Cella DF. Quality of life: the concept. *J Palliat Care* 1992;8:8.
11. Osoba D. Lessons learned from measuring health-related quality of life in oncology. *J Clin Oncol* 1994;12:608.
12. Cella DF. Quality of life: concepts and definition. *J Pain Symptom Manage* 1994;9:186.
13. Ganz PA. Quality of life and the patient with cancer: individual and policy implications. *Cancer* 1994;74(suppl):1445.
14. Gotay CC. Trial-related quality of life: using quality-of-life assessment to distinguish among cancer therapies. *J Natl Cancer Inst Monogr* 1996;20:1.
15. Hollen PJ, Gralla RJ. Comparison of instruments for measuring quality of life in patients with lung cancer. *Semin Oncol* 1996;23(suppl):31.

16. Fobair P, Hoppe RT, Bloom J, Cox R, Varghese A, Spiegel D. Psychosocial problems among survivors of Hodgkin's disease. *J Clin Oncol* 1986;4:805.
17. Bloom JR, Gorsky RD, Fobair P, et al. Physical performance at work and at leisure: validation of a measure of biological energy in survivors of Hodgkin's disease. *J Psychosoc Oncol* 1990;8:49.
18. Bloom JR, Hoppe RT, Fobair P, et al. Effects of treatment on the work experiences of long-term survivors of Hodgkin's disease. *J Psychosoc Oncol* 1989;6:65.
19. Fobair P, Mages NL. Psychosocial morbidity among cancer patients survivors. In: Ahmed P, ed. *Coping with cancer.* New York: Elsevier, 1981:285.
20. Bloom JR, Fobair P, Spiegel D, et al. Social supports and the social well-being of cancer survivors. In: Algrecht G, ed. *Advances in medical sociology,* vol 2. New York: JAI Press, 1991:95.
21. Hannah MT, Gritz ER, Wellisch DK, et al. Changes in marital and sexual functioning in long- term survivors and their spouses: testicular cancer versus Hodgkin's disease. *Psychooncology* 1992;1:89.
22. Donovan K, Sanson-Fisher RW, Redman S. Measuring quality of life in cancer patients. *J Clin Oncol* 1989;7:959.
23. Cole P, Rodu B. Declining cancer mortality in the United States. *Cancer* 1996;78:2045.
24. Rosenberg SA. The management of Hodgkin's disease: half a century of change. *Ann Oncol* 1996;7:555.
24a. Frei E. The National Cancer Chemotherapy Program. *Science* 1982; 217:600.
25. Bernhard J, Ganz PA. Psychosocial issues in lung cancer patients. *Cancer Treat Res* 1995;72:363.
26. Ganz PA, Haskell CM, Figlin RA, La-Soto N, Siau J. Estimating the quality of life in a clinical trial of patients with metastatic lung cancer using the Karnofsky performance status and the Functional Living Index-Cancer. *Cancer* 1988;61:849.
27. Cella DF, Tulsky DS. Quality of life in cancer: definition, purpose, and method of measurement. *Cancer Invest* 1993;11:327.
28. Coates A, Dillenbeck CF, McNeil DR. On the receiving end. II. Linear analogue self-assessment (LASA) in evaluation of aspects of the quality of life of cancer patients receiving therapy. *Eur J Cancer Clin Oncol* 1983;19:1633.
29. Coates A, Gebski V, Bishop JF. Improving the quality of life during chemotherapy for advanced breast cancer. A comparison of intermittent and continuous treatment strategies. *N Engl J Med* 1987;317:1490.
30. Bernhard J, Hürny C, Bacchi M, et al. Initial prognostic factors in small-cell lung cancer patients predicting quality of life during chemotherapy. *Br J Cancer* 1996;74:1660.
31. Aaronson NK, Bullinger M, Ahmedzai S. A modular approach to quality-of-life assessment in cancer clinical trials. *Recent Results Cancer Res* 1988;111:231.
32. Ahles TA, Blanchard EB, Ruckdeschel JC. The multidimensional nature of cancer-related pain. *Pain* 1983;17:277.
33. Copeland DR, Worchel FF. Psychosocial aspects of childhood cancer. *Tex Med* 1986;82:46.
34. Eiser C. Psychological effects of chronic disease. *J Child Psychol Psychiatry* 1990;31:85.
35. Holmes HA, Holmes FF. After ten years, what are the handicaps and life styles of children treated for cancer. *Clin Pediatr* 1975;14:819.
36. van Dongen-Melman JEWM, Sanders-Woudstra JAR. Psychosocial aspects of childhood cancer: A review of the literature. *J Child Psychol Psychiatry* 1986;27:145.
37. O'Malley JE, Koocher G, Foster D, Slavin L. Psychiatric sequelae of surviving childhood cancer. *Am J Orthopsychiatry* 1979;49:608.
38. Achenbach T, Edelbrock C. *Manual for child behavior checklist and revised child behavior profile.* Burlington, VT: University of Vermont, 1983.
39. Derogatis LR. *The SCL-90R.* Baltimore, MD: Clinical Psychometric Research, 1977.
40. Herr HW. Quality of life measurement in testicular cancer patients. *Cancer* 1987;60:1412.
41. Ferrell BR, Hassey-Dow K, Grant M. Measurement of the quality of life in cancer survivors. *Qual Life Res* 1995;4:523.
42. Bloom JR, Fobair P, Gritz E, et al. Psychosocial outcomes of cancer: a comparative analysis of Hodgkin's disease and testicular cancer. *J Clin Oncol* 1993;11:979.
43. Ferrell BR, Hassey-Dow K, Leigh S, Ly J, Gulasekaram P. Quality of life in long-term cancer survivors. *Oncol Nurs Forum* 1995;22:915.
44. Flechtner H, Rüffer U, Eisenbarth M, et al. Quality of life and life situation after cure from Hodgkin's disease. *Psychooncology* 1996;5:10.
45. Kornblith AB, Anderson J, Cella DF. et al. Quality of life assessment of Hodgkin's disease survivors: a model for cooperative clinical trials. *Oncology* 1990;4:93.
46. Norum J, Wist EA. Quality of life in survivors of Hodgkin's disease. *Qual Life Res* 1996;5:367.
47. Flechtner H. Quality of life research in somatic medicine and psychiatry. *Pharmacopsychiatry* 1997;30:239.
48. Anderson RT, Aaronson NK, Wilkin D. Critical review of the international assessments of health-related quality of life. *Qual Life Res* 1993; 2:369.
49. Cella DF, Bonomi AE. Measuring quality of life: 1995 update. *Oncology* 1995;9:47.
50. Sprangers MA, Cull A, Bjordal K, Groenvold M, Aaronson NK. The European Organization for Research and Treatment of Cancer approach to quality of life assessment: guidelines for developing questionnaire modules. *Qual Life Res* 1993;2:287.
51. Aaronson NK, Ahmedzai S, Bergman B, et al. The European Organization for Research and Treatment of Cancer QLQ-C30: a quality-of-life instrument for use in international clinical trials in oncology. *J Natl Cancer Inst* 1993;85:365.
52. Flechtner H, Rüffer U, Eisenbarth M, et al. Quality of life and life situation in survivors of Hodgkin's disease. *Psychooncology* 1996;5:158.
53. Greer S. Improving quality of life: adjuvant psychological therapy for patients with cancer. *Support Care Cancer* 1995;3:248.
54. Fawzy IF, Fawzy NW, Arndt LA, Pasnau RO. Critical review of psychosocial interventions in cancer care. *Arch Gen Psychiatry* 1995;52:100.
55. Aaronson NK. Methodologic issues in assessing the quality of life of cancer patients. *Cancer* 1991;67:844.
56. Ware JE. Methodology in behavioral and psychosocial cancer research. Conceptualizing disease impact and treatment outcomes. *Cancer* 1984;53:2316.
57. van Knippenberg FC, de Haes JC. Measuring the quality of life of cancer patients: psychometric properties of instruments. *J Clin Epidemiol* 1988;41:1043.
58. de Haes JC, van Knippenberg FC. The quality of life of cancer patients: a review of the literature. *Soc Sci Med* 1985;20:809.
59. Cella DF. Methods and problems in measuring quality of life. *Support Care Cancer* 1995;3:11.
60. Spitzer WO, Dobson AJ, Hall J, et al. Measuring the quality of life of cancer patients. *J Chron Dis* 1981;34:585.
61. Cella DF, Tulsky DS. Measuring quality of life today: methodological aspects. *Oncology (Williston Park)* 1990;4:29.
62. Kornblith AB, Holland JC. Model for quality of life research from the Cancer and Leukemia Group B: the telephone interview, conceptual approach to measurement, and theoretical framework. *NCI Monogr* 1996;20:55.
63. Bloom JR, Stewart SL, Johnston M, Banks P. Intrusiveness of illness and quality of life in young women with breast cancer. *Psychooncology* 1998;7:89.
64. Mages N, Castro J, Fobair P, et al. Patterns of psychosocial response to cancer: can effective adaptation be predicted? *Int J Radiat Oncol Biol Phys* 1981;7:385.
65. Anderson LF. Enthusiasm for quality-of-life research rises (news). *J Natl Cancer Inst* 1995;87:712.
66. de Haes JC, Stiggelbout AM. Assessment of values, utilities and preferences in cancer patients. *Cancer Treat Rev* 1996;22(suppl A):13.
67. Cronbach LJ. Coefficient alpha and the internal structure of tests. *Psychometrika* 1951;16:297.
68. Osoba D, Rodrigues G, Myles J, Zee B, Pater J. Interpreting the significance of changes in health-related quality-of-life scores. *J Clin Oncol* 1998;16:139.
69. Ganz PA. Impact of quality of life outcomes on clinical practice. *Oncology* 1995;9:61.
70. Arai Y, Kawakita M, Hida S, et al. Psychosocial aspects in long-term survivors of testicular cancer. *J Urol* 1996;155:574.
71. Harrer ME, Mosheim R, Richter R, Walter MH, Kemmler G. Coping and life satisfaction in patients with Hodgkin's disease in remission. A contribution to the question of adaptive aspects of coping processes. *Psychother Psychosom Med Psychol* 1993;43:121.
72. Hoerni B, Eghbali H. Quality of life during and after treatment of Hodgkin's disease. *Recent Results Cancer Res* 1989;117:257.
73. Hoerni B, Hoerni-Simon G, Eghbali H, Richaud P. Quality of life dur-

ing and following radiochemotherapy for Hodgkin's disease. Evaluation of 60 patients. *Bull Cancer* 1983;70:284.
74. Kornblith AB, Anderson J, Cella DF, et al. Hodgkin's disease survivors at increased risk for problems in psychosocial adaptation. *Cancer* 1992;70:2214.
75. Yellen SB, Cella DF, Bonomi A. Quality of life in people with Hodgkin's disease. *Oncology* 1993;7:41.
76. Joly F, Henry-Amar M, Arveux P, et al. Late psychosocial sequelae in Hodgkin's disease survivors: a French population-based case-control study. *J Clin Oncol* 1996;14:2444.
77. van Tulder MW, Aaronson NK, Bruning PF. The quality of life of long-term survivors of Hodgkin's disease. *Ann Oncol* 1994;5:153.
78. Hunt SM, McEwen J, McKenna SP. The Nottingham Health Profile user's manual, 1981.
79. Bergner M, Bobbitt RA, Kressel S, et al. The sickness impact profile: conceptual foundation and methodology for the development of a health status measure. *Int J Health Serv* 1976;6:393.
80. Ware JE, Sherbourne CD. The MOS 36-item short form health survey (SF-36) I. Conceptual framework and item selection. *Med Care* 1992;30:473.
81. The EuroQol Group. EuroQol—a new facility for the measurement of health-related quality of life. *Health Policy* 1990;16:199.
82. WHOQOL Group. Study protocol for the World Health Organization project to develop a quality of life assessment instrument (WHOQOL). *Qual Life Res* 1993;2:153.
83. Nelson E, Wasson J, Kirk J, et al. Assessment of function in routine clinical practice: description of the COOP chart method and preliminary findings. *J Chron Dis* 1987;40:55s.
84. Cella DF, Tulsky DS, Gray G, et al. The Functional Assessment of Cancer Therapy scale: development and validation of the general measure. *J Clin Oncol* 1993;11:570.
85. Schipper H, Clinch J, McMurray A, et al. Measuring the quality of life of cancer patients. The functional living index-cancer: development and validation. *J Clin Oncol* 1984;2:472.
86. Coscarelli-Shag CA, Heinrich RL. Development of a comprehensive quality of life measurement tool: CARES. *Oncology* 1990;4:135.
87. Schag CA, Ganz PA, Heinrich RL. CAncer Rehabilitation Evaluation System–short form (CARES-SF). A cancer specific rehabilitation and quality of life instrument. *Cancer* 1991;68:1406.
88. de Haes JC, van Knippenberg FC, Neijt JP. Measuring psychological and physical distress in cancer patients: structure and application of the Rotterdam Symptom Checklist. *Br J Cancer* 1990;62:1034.
89. Cella DF, Bonomi AE, Lloyd SR, Tulsky DS, Kaplan E, Bonomi P. Reliability and validity of the Functional Assessment of Cancer Therapy-Lung (FACT-L) quality of life instrument. *Lung Cancer* 1995;12:199.
90. Smets EMA, Garssen B, Schuster-Uitterhoeve, ALJ, de Haes JCJM. Fatigue in cancer patients. *Br J Cancer* 1993;68:220.
91. Smets EMA, Garsson B, Bonke B, de Haes JCJM. The Multidimensional Fatigue Inventory (MFI); Psychometric qualities of an instrument to assess fatigue. *J Psychosom Res* 1995;39:315.
92. Schuler D, Bakos M, Zsambor A, et al. Psychological late effects of leukemia in children and their prevention. *Med Pediatr Oncol* 1981; 9:191.
93. Fryback DG. QALYs, HYEs, and the loss of innocence. *Med Decis Making* 1993;13:271.
94. Coast J. Reprocessing data to form QALYs. *Br Med J* 1992;305:87.
95. Gelber RD, Goldhirsch A. A new endpoint for the assessment of adjuvant therapy in postmenopausal women with operable breast cancer. *J Clin Oncol* 1986;4:1772.
96. Goldhirsch A, Gelber RD, Simes RJ, Glasziou P, Coates AS. Costs and benefits of adjuvant therapy in breast cancer: A quality-adjusted survival analysis. *J Clin Oncol* 1989;7:36.
97. Kaplan RM. Quality of life assessment for cost/utility studies in cancer. *Cancer Treat Rev* 1993;19(suppl A):85.
98. Norum J, Angelsen V, Wist E, Olsen JA. Treatment costs in Hodgkin's disease: A cost-utility analysis. *Eur J Cancer* 1996;32A:1510.
99. Singer PA, Tasch ES, Stocking C, Rubin S, Siegler M, Weichselbaum R. Sex or survival: trade-offs between quality and quantity of life. *J Clin Oncol* 1991;9:328.
100. Turner S, Maher EJ, Young T, Young J, Vaughan Hudson G. What are the information priorities for cancer patients involved in treatment decisions? An experienced surrogate study in Hodgkin's disease. *Br J Cancer* 1996;73:22.
101. Vaughan Hudson B, Vaughan Hudson G, Linch DC, Anderson L. Late mortality in young BNLI patients cured of Hodgkin's disease. *Ann Oncol* 1994;5(suppl):65.
102. Kaasa S. The dimensions of quality of life. In: Zittoun R, ed. *Quality of life of cancer patients:* a review. *Proceedings of the International Congress of Psychosocial Oncology.* Beaune, France: 1992(December 10):19.
103. Coates AS, Gebski V, Signorini D, et al. Prognostic value of quality-of-life scores during chemotherapy for advanced breast cancer. *J Clin Oncol* 1992;10:1833.
104. Coates A, Gebski V. On the receiving end. VI. Which dimensions of quality-of-life scores carry prognostic information? *Cancer Treat Rev* 1996;22(suppl A):63.
104a. Spiegel D, Bloom JR, Kraemer HC, Gottheil E. Effect of psychosocial treatment on survival of patients with metastatic breast cancer. *Lancet* 1989;2:888.
105. Osoba D. Rationale for the timing of health-related quality-of life assessments in oncological palliative therapy. *Cancer Treat Rev* 1996; 22(suppl A):69.
106. Cella DF, Tross S. Psychological adjustment to survival from Hodgkin's disease. *J Consult Clin Psychol* 1986;54:616.
107. Wasserman AL, Thompson EI, Wilimas JA, et al. The psychological status of survivors of childhood/adolescent Hodgkin's disease. *Am J Dis Child* 1987;141:626.
108. Devlen J, Maguire P, Phillips P, et al. Psychological problems associated with diagnosis and treatment of lymphomas: prospective study. *Br Med J* 1987;295:955.
109. Carpenter PJ, Morrow GR, Schmale AH. The psychosocial status of cancer patients after cessation of treatment. *J Psychosoc Oncol* 1989; 7:95.
110. Kornblith AB, Anderson J, Cella DF, et al. Comparison of psychosocial adaptation and sexual function of survivors of advanced Hodgkin disease treated by MOPP, ABVD, or MOPP alternating with ABVD. *Cancer* 1992;70:2508.
111. Ferrell BR, Hassey Dow K. Quality of life among long-term survivors. *Oncology* 1997;11:565.
112. Bucquet D, Condon S, Ritchie K. The French version of the Nottingham Health profile. A comparison of items weights with those of the source version. *Soc Sci Med* 1990;30:829.
113. Aaronson NK, Culi A, Kaasa S, Sprangers MAG. The EORTC modular approach to quality of life. Assessment in oncology. *Int J Mental Health* 1994;23:75.
114. Hamilton M. The assessment of anxiety states. *Br J Psychol* 1959; 32:50.
115. Curbow B. Quality of life among long-term survivors (Comments). *Oncology* 1997;11:572.
116. Siegel K, Christ GH. Hodgkin's disease survivorship: psychosocial consequences. In: Lacher MD, Mortimer J, Redman JR, eds. *Hodgkin's disease: the consequences of survival.* Philadelphia: Lea & Febiger, 1989:383.
117. Schag CC, Heinrich RL, Ganz PA. Cancer inventory of problem situations: An instrument for assessing cancer patients' rehabilitation needs. *J Psychosoc Oncol* 1983;1:11.
118. Ruckdeschel JC, Piantadosi S. Quality of life assessment in lung surgery for brochogenic carcinoma. *J Thorac Surg* 1991;6:201.
119. Ganz PA, Lee JJ, Siau J. Quality of life assessment. An independent prognostic variable for survival in lung cancer. *Cancer* 1991;67:3131.
120. Selby P. Measurement of quality of life in cancer patients. *J Pharm Pharmacol* 1993;45:384.
121. Kaasa S, Mastekaasa A, Lund E. Prognosis factors for patients with inoperable non-small cell lung cancer, limited disease: the importance of patient's subjective experience of disease and psychosocial well-being. *Radiother Oncol* 1989;15:235.
122. Guyatt GH, Feeny DH, Patrick DL. Measuring health-related quality of life. *Ann Intern Med* 1993;118:622.
123. McMillen Moinpour C, Feigl P, Metch B, Hayden KA, Meyskens FL, Crowley J. Quality of life end points in cancer clinical trials: review and recommendations. *J Natl Cancer Inst* 1989;81:485.
124. Hunt SM. The problem of quality of life. *Qual Life Res* 1997;6:205.
125. Guyatt GH, Veldhuyzen van Zanten SJO, Feeny DH, Patrick DL, Measuring quality of life in clinical trials: a taxonomy and review. *Can Med Assoc J* 1989;140:1441.
126. Fletcher A, Gore S, Jones D, et al. Quality of life measures in health care. II: Design, analysis, and interpretation. *Br Med J* 1992;305: 1145.

127. Gelber RD, Cole BF, Goldhirsch A, Rose C, et al. Adjuvant chemotherapy plus tamoxifen compared with tamoxifen alone for postmenopausal breast cancer: meta-analysis of quality-adjusted survival. *Lancet* 1996;347:1066.
128. Turnbull HR, Brunk GL. Quality of life and public philosophy. In: Schalok RL, ed. *Quality of life: perspectives and issues.* Washington, DC: American Association on Mental Retardation, 1990:193.
129. Uyl de Groot CA. *Economic evaluation of cancer treatments.* Den Haag, The Netherlands: CIP-Gegevens Koninklijke Bibliotheek, 1995:51.
130. Fayers PM, Jones DR. Measuring and analysing quality of life in cancer clinical trials: a review. *Stat Med* 1983;2:429.
131. Obosa D. Rationale for the timing of health-related quality-of-life assessments in oncology palliative therapy. *Cancer Treat Rev* 1996; 22:69.
132. Bradlyn A, Harris C, Spieth L. Quality of life assessment in pediatric oncology: a retrospective review of phase III reports. *Soc Sci Med* 1995;41:1463.
133. Morris J, Goddard M. Economic evaluation and quality of life assessment in cancer clinical trials: the CHART trial. *Eur J Cancer* 1993; 5:766.
134. Aaronson NK. Assessing the quality of life of patients in cancer clinical trials: common problems and common sense solution. *Eur J Cancer* 1992;8:1304.
135. Taylor KM, Macdonald K, Bezjak A, Ng P, DePetrillo AD. Physicians' perspectives on quality of life: An exploratory study of oncologists' attitudes. *Qual Life Res* 1996;5:5.
136. Diehl V, Engert A. An overview of the Second International Symposium on Hodgkin's Disease. *Ann Oncol* 1992;3(suppl 4):1.
137. Carde P, Hagenbeek A, Hayat M, et al. Clinical staging versus laparotomy and combined modality with MOPP versus ABVD in early-stage Hodgkin's disease: the H6 twin randomized trials from the European Organization for Research and Treatment of Cancer Lymphoma Cooperative Group. *J Clin Oncol* 1993;11:2258.
138. Specht L, Gray RG, Clark MJ, Peto R. Influence of more extensive radiotherapy and adjuvant chemotherapy on long-term outcome of early-stage Hodgkin's disease: a meta-analysis of 23 randomized trials involving 3888 patients. *J Clin Oncol* 1998;16:830.
139. Henry-Amar M. Second cancer after the treatment for Hodgkin's disease: a report from the International Database on Hodgkin's Disease. *Ann Oncol* 1992;3(suppl 4):117.
140. Henry-Amar M. Treatment sequelae and quality of life. *Baillieres Clin Haematol* 1996;9:595.
141. van Holten-Verzantvoort ATM, Zwinderman AH, Aaronson NK, et al. The effect of supportive pamidronate treatment on aspects of quality of life of patients with advanced breast cancer. *Eur J Cancer* 1991;27:544.
142. Canellos GP, Anderson JR, Propert KJ, et al. Chemotherapy of advanced Hodgkin's disease with MOPP, ABVD, or MOPP alternating with ABVD. *N Engl J Med* 1992;327:1478.
142a. Diehl V, Franklin J, Hasenclever, et al. BEACOPP: A new regimen for advanced Hodgkin's disease. *Ann Oncol* 1998;9:67.
143. Bonsel GJ, Rutten FFH, Uyl de Groot CA. Economic evaluation alongside cancer trials: methodological and practical aspects. *Eur J Cancer* 1993;29A(suppl 7):10.
144. Fryback DG, Lawrence WF. Dollars may not buy as many QALYs as we think: a problem with defining quality-of-life adjustments. *Med Decis Making* 1997;17:276.
145. Pfreundschuh M, Lathan B, Löffler M, Rüffer U, Hasenclever D, Diehl V. Workshop III: Recommendations for future clinical trials. *Ann Oncol* 1992;3(suppl 4):101.
146. Yabroff KR, Linas BP, Schulman K. Evaluation of quality of life for diverse patient populations. *Breast Cancer Res Treat* 1996;40:87.
147. Ganz PA. Quality of life measures in cancer chemotherapy: methodology and implications. *Pharmacoeconomics* 1994;5:376.
148. Bloom JR. Quality of life after cancer: a policy perspective. *Cancer* 1991;67(suppl):855.
149. Selby PJ, Chapman JAW, Etazadi-Amoli J. The development of a method for assessing the quality of life of cancer patients. *Br J Cancer* 1984;50:13.
150. Klee M, Groenvold M, Machin D. Quality of life of Danish women: population-based norms for the EORTC QLQC30.*Qual Life Res* 1997;6: 27.
151. Briançon S, Guillemin F, Presiozi P, et al. Determinants of quality of life in general population. *Qual Life Res* 1997;6:626(abst).
152. Rumpold G, Söllner W. Quality of life in a healthy population. An epidemiologic research. *Qual Life Res* 1997;6:711(abst).
153. Hjermstad MJ, Fayers P, Bjordal K, Kaasa S. Health-related quality of life in the general Norwegian population assessed by the European Organization for Research and Treatment of Cancer Core Quality-of-Life questionnaire: the QLQ-C30 (-3). *J Clin Oncol* 1998;16: 1188.
154. Breslow NE, Day NE. *Statistical methods in cancer research. I: The analysis of case-control studies.* IARC Scientific publication no. 32. Lyon, France: International Agency for Research on Cancer, 1980: 14.
155. Ware JE, Brook RH, Davies AR, et al. Choosing measures of healthy status for individuals in general population. *Am J Public Health* 1981; 71:620.
156. Dorval M, Maunsell E, Deschênes L, et al. Long-term quality of life after breast cancer: comparison of 8-year survivors with population controls. *J Clin Oncol* 1998;16:487.
157. Rieker P, Fitzgerald E, Kalish L, et al. Psychosocial factors, curative therapies, and behavioral outcomes. *Cancer* 1989;64:2399.
158. Olweny C, Juttner C, Rofe P, et al. Long-term effects of cancer treatment and consequences of cures: cancer survivors enjoy quality of life similar to their neighbours. *Eur J Cancer* 1993;29A:826.
159. Byrne J, Fears T, Steinhorn S, Mulvihill J, et al. Marriage and divorce after childhood and adolescent cancer. *JAMA* 1989;262:2693.

SECTION VIII

Special Topics

Hodgkin's Disease, edited by P. M. Mauch,
J. O. Armitage, V. Diehl, R. T. Hoppe, and L. M. Weiss.
Lippincott Williams & Wilkins, Philadephia ©1999.

CHAPTER 38

The Management of Hodgkin's Disease during Pregnancy

Carol S. Portlock and Joachim Yahalom

Since 1911, when the first case of Hodgkin's disease complicated by pregnancy was reported (1), the management of Hodgkin's disease during pregnancy has presented difficult choices that are not always supported by a solid body of data. Pregnancy is more common in patients with Hodgkin's disease than in those with non-Hodgkin's lymphoma because the period of peak incidence of Hodgkin's disease coincides with the female reproductive years. Nevertheless, this association remains sufficiently rare (3.2% of all cases of Hodgkin's disease at the M. D. Anderson Cancer Center) (2) that only a few large series have examined the many aspects of patient presentation, management, the interaction of malignancy and pregnancy, and the effects of treatment on the developing fetus and delivered infant (3).

Ultimately, the collection of limited data from pregnant women with a variety of malignancies must form the basis for individual management decisions made in the care of a pregnant patient with Hodgkin's disease. The incidence of pregnancy associated with Hodgkin's disease is difficult to estimate accurately. Stewart and Monto (4) reported three cases within a period of 10 years at the Henry Ford Hospital, where about 18,000 deliveries were handled during the same period. Palacios Costa et al. reported five cases of Hodgkin's disease associated with 30,000 pregnancies, a similar incidence of one case in 6,000 pregnancies (5).

In the past, the influence of pregnancy on the course of Hodgkin's disease was controversial (4,6). However, later studies suggested no significant effect of pregnancy on the course of Hodgkin's disease (6,7). Barry et al. (8) reviewed all cases of Hodgkin's disease diagnosed at Memorial Sloan-Kettering Cancer Center from 1910 until 1960. Female patients between the ages of 18 and 40 were chosen for the study, resulting in the selection of 347 patients of childbearing age with Hodgkin's disease. One age-corrected control group was established from the cases in which no pregnancy occurred. Of the 347 patients, 84 became pregnant and yielded a total of 112 pregnancies associated with Hodgkin's disease. The survival curve and median survival time of 90 months were similar in both groups. Survival statistics were similar for patients whose pregnancy was aborted and for patients whose pregnancy was allowed to continue. Hennessy and Rottino (7) reviewed 35 patients whose Hodgkin's disease was associated with pregnancy and reached the same conclusions. Stewart and Monto (4) were able to show that Hodgkin's disease did not affect the obstetric course of pregnancy and that women affected with Hodgkin's disease did well during pregnancy, parturition, and puerperium. Only a single case report (9) suggesting a possible "transmission" from a mother with Hodgkin's disease to her newborn, who died at the age of 5 months with disseminated Hodgkin's disease.

PRESENTATION

Lishner et al. (10) have reported the largest recent series, comprising 48 women with 50 pregnancies occurring during active Hodgkin's disease; they utilized the Princess Margaret Hospital (Toronto, Canada) database for 1958–1984. Each pregnant patient was matched with three non-pregnant controls. The analysis revealed a median age of 26 (range, 18–38 years). A similar age distribution was reported in a literature review by Yahalom (3). In the 50 pregnancies in the Toronto series, the diagnosis of Hodgkin's disease was made in 12 patients before conception, in 27 patients within 9 months after delivery

C. S. Portlock: Department of Medical Oncology, Memorial Sloan-Kettering Cancer Center, New York, New York.

J. Yahalom: Department of Medicine, Cornell University Medical College and Department of Radiation Oncology, Memorial Sloan-Kettering Cancer Center, New York, New York.

or termination of pregnancy, and in only 10 patients (20%) during pregnancy. Hodgkin's disease was treated during pregnancy in 22 patients. The stage of disease at diagnosis did not appear to differ significantly from that of nonpregnant controls in the Lishner series: stage I, 25%; stage II, 45.8%; stage III, 16.7%; and stage IV, 12.5%.

Several American series appear to reflect similar age and stage distributions (2,3,11,12). An exception to these data in regard to stage was reported by Aviles of the Mexican National Medical Center (13); of 14 pregnant patients, five had stage II, three stage III, and six stage IV disease. Eight of the 14 patients had Hodgkin's disease of the mixed-cellularity subtype, and the other six had nodular sclerosing Hodgkin's disease. These distributions most likely reflect the background of these women, residents of a developing country, in contrast to the distributions of their North American counterparts.

The most carefully evaluated pathology analysis of pregnancy-associated Hodgkin's disease was reported by Gelb et al. (12). The Stanford investigators reviewed 17 cases, classifying 13 of them as nodular sclerosis Hodgkin's disease and three as mixed cellularity Hodgkin's disease; one case was unclassified. Nodal tissue was obtained from peripheral sites in 14 patients, the mediastinum in one, and lung in one (unknown site in one). In an earlier Stanford series, Jacobs et al. (11) found 14 of 15 patients with nodular sclerosis Hodgkin's disease; similarly, the investigators from M. D. Anderson (2) reported that 16 of 16 patients had nodular sclerosis Hodgkin's disease.

FETAL GROWTH AND DEVELOPMENT

Treatments for Hodgkin's disease, whether radiation therapy or chemotherapy, are potentially teratogenic. The risk for fetal malformation or death depends on the stage of fetal development, fetal susceptibility, the agent utilized, and the fetal dose of that agent (14–16).

The first trimester is the most critical period for agent exposure, as implantation (the first 2 weeks) and embryogenesis (weeks 3–8) proceed. Spontaneous abortion is the most likely consequence of treatment exposure during implantation, whereas major morphologic abnormalities can be a consequence during weeks 3 to 8 of embryogenesis. Some structures, such as the limbs and palate, are vulnerable during limited periods of embryogenesis, whereas the central nervous system may be affected throughout all phases of embryogenesis and fetal development.

With radiation therapy, another consideration related to possible fetal toxicity is the increasing uterine fundal height, as it influences total dose exposure from internal radiation scatter (2). The closer the fetus is to the diaphragm, the greater the possible whole-body fetal dose when the mother receives radiation above the diaphragm.

With chemotherapy, the placenta plays a pivotal role in drug transfer (15). It is of interest that the placenta has a multidrug-resistant phenotype (16), which may help to prevent or reduce the transfer of such natural products as doxorubicin, vinblastine, and vincristine to the fetus. However, case reports regarding the efficiency of placental transfer of doxorubicin are inconclusive.

A consideration of fetal drug metabolism and excretion must also take into account the recirculation of amniotic fluid (15). This feature helps to explain the marked teratogenicity of the folate antagonists aminopterin and methotrexate when fetal doses are within the therapeutic range.

Finally, during the second and third trimesters, effects on the fetus may be more subtle (3,14). Low birth weight, intrauterine growth retardation, premature birth, stillborn fetus, impaired functional development, mental retardation, and diminished learning capability are all possible effects of therapy for Hodgkin's disease.

STAGING DURING PREGNANCY

Hodgkin's disease presenting during pregnancy is a rare event. Most patients in North American series present without B symptoms (2,3,11,12), whereas the Aviles series (13) from Mexico reveals a predominance of B symptoms in 10 of 14 patients. A peripheral lymph node is usually the site of biopsy (12).

Recommended staging studies have evolved with changing technology and therapeutic options (Table 1). A single posteroanterior chest roentgenogram with adequate abdominal shielding, blood work (complete blood count, tests of hepatic and renal function, sedimentation rate, and alkaline phosphatase and lactic dehydrogenase levels), and bone marrow biopsy continue to be indicated. In 1981, the Stanford group (11) recommended a single-view lymphogram to evaluate intraabdominal disease. Lymphangiography exposes the fetus to radiation and has become less available during the last

TABLE 1. *Staging studies in the pregnant patient with Hodgkin's disease*

History and physical examination
Routine blood work
Chest assessment
Single-view chest roentgenogram with adequate abdominal shielding (see text)
Magnetic resonance imaging (as indicated)
Computed tomography (as indicated)
Abdominal assessment (see text)
Ultrasound (as indicated)
Magnetic resonance imaging (as indicated)
Computed tomography (as indicated)
Bone marrow biopsy
Not indicated:
Gallium scanning
PET scan
Bone scan

PET, positron emission tomography.

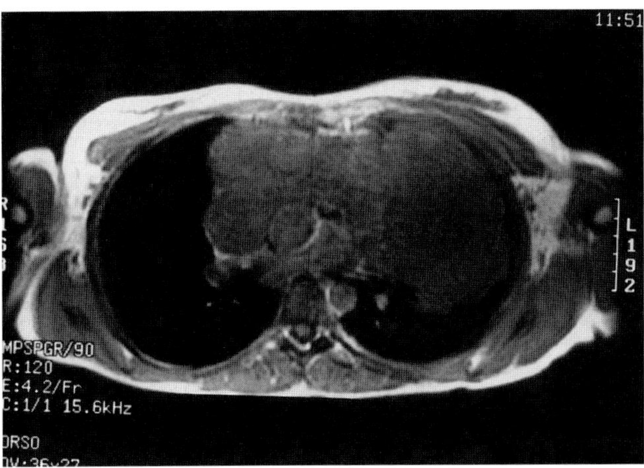

FIG. 1. Chest magnetic resonance image in a pregnant patient reveals a large mediastinal mass.

decade. Without multiple viewing angles and expert interpretation, its accuracy may be limited. More recently, magnetic resonance imaging (MRI) has been utilized, with the advantage that it can be used to evaluate nodes, liver, and spleen with good accuracy (Fig. 1). Although it is thought that MRI is probably safe in pregnant patients, no data are yet available to support this assumption. Abdominal ultrasonography is much less sensitive than MRI but may be adequate to screen for involvement with bulky disease, and it does permit serial examinations when needed in follow-up (Fig. 2). Gallium scanning and positron emission tomography (PET) are contraindicated. Computed axial tomography (CT) is rarely indicated if abdominal ultrasonography and MRI are available.

As precise pathologic staging in Hodgkin's disease (with laparotomy) has been supplanted by clinical staging and therapy, the need for more careful definition in the pregnant patient has diminished. Moreover, it is acknowledged that Hodgkin's disease in most patients is a rather indolent neoplasm that may often be monitored safely during pregnancy until fetal development and growth are adequate to permit a safe delivery.

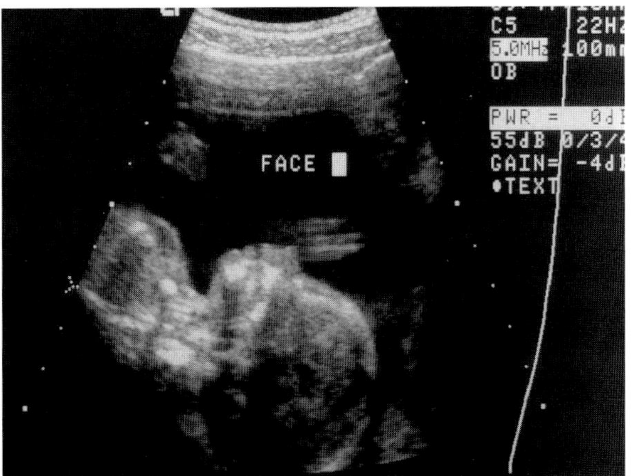

FIG. 2. Abdominal ultrasonogram of a pregnant patient reveals a healthy fetus and no abdominal adenopathy.

TREATMENT

Radiation Therapy

Many series have documented the effectiveness of radiation therapy for the treatment of Hodgkin's disease during pregnancy (1,3,10,11). Several principles are conducive to a successful outcome: delay irradiation until the second or third trimester, limit the whole-body fetal dose to 10 cGy or less, and realistically consider radiotherapy during pregnancy to be a holding or partial therapy rather than a definitive therapy.

The details of radiotherapy are limited in some reports. Radiotherapy experience since 1960 is available [reviewed in (2)], and estimations of radiation dose from several sources are summarized in Table 2. Woo et al. (2) have provided a complete analysis of 16 pregnant patients with clinical stage (CS) I or IIA treated at the M. D. Anderson Cancer Center. Involved-field irradiation was administered to the neck (3,500 cGy) in two cases, extended-field to the neck and mediastinum (4,000 cGy) in three cases, and full-mantle irradiation to the remaining 11 patients (4,000 cGy).

Uterine shielding was maximized by utilizing four to five half-value layers of lead. The dose to the fetus was estimated in nine patients and was 1.4 to 5.5 cGy with 6-MV photons and 10 to 13.6 cGy with cobalt 60. After delivery, 10 patients underwent lymphangiography and five underwent staging laparotomy (two with positive findings). Eight patients subsequently had additional radiation therapy and/or chemotherapy. All offspring were reported to be physically and mentally normal, and the 10-year survival of the patients was 83%.

In a review of 47 patients with Hodgkin's disease during pregnancy from several series, 23 patients received supradiaphragmatic radiation therapy (five in the first trimester), with no apparent harm to the fetus. Seventy-four percent of the patients remained without evidence of Hodgkin's disease at the time of the report (3).

The Stanford group (11) reported the details of radiation therapy in nine patients. Involved or mantle fields were used and doses were generally low (≤3,300 cGy in six, full dose only in three who became pregnant during preplanned radiotherapy). Full staging and therapy were completed after delivery. These investigators recommended treatment delay whenever possible if Hodgkin's disease is detected during the last half of the second or during the third trimester. If radiation therapy is recommended, limited fields and dose should be considered.

Fetal outcome following radiotherapy depends on gestational age at radiation therapy, whole-body fetal dose, and maternal health. Although one would expect a higher frequency of spontaneous abortions and congenital

TABLE 2. *Estimated radiation dose to the fetus as percentage of the total mantle[a] dose in different studies (phantom measurements)*

Study (ref.)	Energy	Trimester 1	Trimester 2	Trimester 3
Zucali et al. (17)[a]	Co 60	0.21	0.45	3.0
Zucali et al. (17)[a]	6 MV	0.15	0.34	2.0
Covington and Baker (18)	6 MV	0.19–0.4	0.9–1.4	3.7–7.1
Sharma et al. (20)	10 MV	0.4[c]–0.8[d]	0.6[c]–1.1[d]	1.2[c]–2.2[d]
Wong et al. (19)	10 MV	1.3[c]–1.4[d]	1.9[c]–2.0[d]	4.3[c]–5.0[d]
Woo et al. (2)	6 MV		0.2–0.5	0.32–0.42
Woo et al. (2)	Co 60		0.48–0.82	
Yahalom (3)	6 MV	0.23	0.1–0.83	3.2

MV, megavolt; Co 60, cobalt isotope.
[a]Supraclavicular field 11 × 11 cm and opposed mediastinal fields 13 × 13 cm.
[b]Distances from the lower border of the field are slightly smaller than in Sharma et al.
[c]With shielding LMR-13 Toshiba accelerator.
[d]Without shielding Clinac 18.

anomalies, this has not been clearly evident from the literature. The M. D. Anderson series (2) had 16 full-term infants; the Stanford series (11) had one spontaneous abortion in a patient irradiated during the first trimester and six normal infants (three therapeutic abortions). The Princess Margaret Hospital case-control study (10) of 50 pregnancies associated with Hodgkin's disease included 13 patients treated with radiation therapy (six during and seven after the first trimester). Interestingly, for the entire cohort of 50 pregnancies, there were no significant differences in gestational age, number of preterm births, birth weight, malformations, or number of stillbirths in comparison with matched controls. Unfortunately, the analysis did not assess the impact of radiation therapy alone in these cases.

In all reported series, it is obviously impossible to assess the confounding factor of therapeutic abortion in improving pregnancy outcome in the data. The general recommendation has been to terminate pregnancy in patients requiring radiotherapy during the first trimester, although this has not been consistently applied (3).

Chemotherapy

Like radiation therapy, combination chemotherapy offers potentially curative treatment of Hodgkin's disease. However, because of concern regarding possible immediate and delayed side effects to the offspring, conventional combination chemotherapy has seldom been administered to pregnant patients.

In a comprehensive review of antineoplastic agents and pregnancy by Doll et al. (15), the incidence of fetal malformations was approximately 15% with exposure during the first trimester. Alkylating agents and antimetabolites had the most consistent risk. Vinblastine was associated with the least risk in Doll's review, with only one abnormality among 14 patients treated in the first trimester. Similar data were reported elsewhere (3). No data were available for vincristine alone.

During the second and third trimesters, chemotherapy is associated with a low risk for fetal malformation (1.3% of 150 exposed patients), probably not significantly different from that in the normal population (3.1%) (24). However, as emphasized by Doll et al. (15), the relative lack of anomalies should not be interpreted as fetal safety, as delayed effects remain a significant concern.

Both MOPP [Mustargen (mechlorethamine), Oncovin (vincristine), procarbazine, prednisone] and ABVD [Adriamycin (doxorubicin), bleomycin, vinblastine, dacarbazine] have been administered to pregnant patients with Hodgkin's disease. The largest series is that of Aviles et al. (13), in which 14 patients were treated, five during the first trimester and nine during the second and third trimesters. All patients completed successful pregnancies (at 34–40 weeks), with no congenital anomalies noted. Eleven patients remain in complete remission 3 to more than 17 years after treatment. These authors have also reported their experience with CHOP [cyclophosphamide, hydroxydaunomycin, Oncovin (vincristine), prednisone] or its variants in 18 pregnant patients with non-Hodgkin's lymphomas, with nine treated during the first trimester and nine during the second and third trimesters. Similarly, no congenital malformations were noted, and all fetuses were successfully delivered at 35 to 40 weeks.

In other reports (15), procarbazine appears to be the most teratogenic agent in these drug combinations. During the first trimester, one congenital malformation occurred with single-agent procarbazine therapy, and four of seven cases exposed to MOPP had malformations.

The timing of chemotherapy may also be important before delivery. The ability of a neonate to metabolize and excrete drugs is diminished (14). Reynoso et al. (21) reported that 5 of 15 infants born to leukemic mothers who received chemotherapy within 30 days of delivery were cytopenic. Aviles et al. (13) noted no cytopenia in the infants of mothers treated for Hodgkin's disease, whereas 3 of 18 infants whose mothers were treated for non-Hodgkin's lymphoma experienced transient cytopenia.

MONITORING DURING PREGNANCY

Because of concern regarding the possible teratogenic effects of therapy, many authors have recommended no active treatment of Hodgkin's disease during pregnancy. The eligibility criteria for this strategy are poorly defined but would include the following:

- "Limited" CS IA or IIA presenting during the late second and third trimester
- Stable, "nonurgent" presentations of disease diagnosed after 20 weeks of gestation

Few data are available to assess the application of these criteria. The Stanford group (11,12,27) has reported five cases of delayed therapy: three with CS IIA Hodgkin's disease, all in continuous complete remission following successful therapy after delivery, and two with infradiaphragmatic Hodgkin's disease, both of whom died of disease despite therapy after delivery. As emphasized by Jacobs et al. (11), the decision to treat or monitor the pregnant patient must be individualized. Clearly, it is important that the site(s) of disease can be easily assessed if this strategy is to be undertaken.

DELIVERY

The timing of delivery must be a joint decision between the obstetrician and oncologist. Whenever possible, the fetus should be carried to term without compromising the health of mother or infant. Cesarean section is not necessary unless obstetrically indicated. Staging laparotomy performed in conjunction with delivery is not warranted and is to be discouraged.

If the pregnant patient has received therapy for Hodgkin's disease before delivery, it is important to keep in mind that the blood counts of both mother and infant may be adversely affected. Ideally, no potentially myelosuppressive therapy should be administered within 3 weeks of delivery.

MANAGEMENT AFTER DELIVERY

Staging assessment after delivery may proceed as in the nonpregnant patient. It is recommended that breastfeeding be discontinued once staging and therapy have begun. There is a risk that agents used for contrast and nuclear imaging, chemotherapeutic drugs, and ancillary, supportive medications may concentrate in breast milk. Lactating breasts show intense uptake on gallium scan, again suggesting possible concentration in breast milk (although data are unavailable on this point).

During and after gallium scanning, it is advisable not to hold the infant for 1 week. For PET, a 1-day wait is advisable.

PROGNOSIS OF PREGNANT PATIENTS WITH HODGKIN'S DISEASE

The outcomes of patients with Hodgkin's disease presenting during pregnancy appear to be similar to those of their nonpregnant counterparts (3,7,8). The largest modern experience is that of Lishner et al. (10), in which the cause-specific survival of 33 pregnant patients was compared with that of 67 case-matched controls. Approximately 70% of both groups were alive at 25 years, with no significant effect of age or stage at diagnosis on outcome.

Among 17 patients managed at Stanford (11), only one died of disease after delivery, with more than 90% alive at 5 years. Similarly, among 16 patients with CS IA and IIA disease treated with radiotherapy at M. D. Anderson (2), the cause-specific survival was 83% at 10 years. The National Medical Center of Mexico series (13) of 14 patients treated with combination chemotherapy (MOPP in four patients, ABVD in seven, and MOPP/ABVD in three) for stages II (five patients), III (three patients), and IV (six patients) revealed 11 patients in complete remission 3 to more than 17 years after treatment and two disease-related deaths; one patient was lost to follow-up.

OUTCOME OF OFFSPRING OF PREGNANCIES ASSOCIATED WITH HODGKIN'S DISEASE

As discussed in detail by Garber (22), the late manifestations of *in utero* exposure to antineoplastic agents may include impaired growth, diminished neurologic and/or intellectual function, decreased gonadal and reproductive function, mutagenesis of germline tissue, and carcinogenesis. Unfortunately, very few data are available regarding these critical questions.

Aviles et al. (13) reported the status of 43 Mexican children exposed to chemotherapy during pregnancy (14 mothers and children had MOPP and/or ABVD). Their ages ranged from 3 to 19 years. All were examined, blood work was obtained, and intelligence testing was performed. A case-control group of 25 children was also evaluated. In this comprehensive evaluation, all children were normal in regard to routine blood work, lymphocyte function, immunoglobulins, cytogenetics, bone marrow aspirate and biopsy, school performance, neurologic testing, and medical histories. Sexual development appeared normal.

Reynoso et al. (21) reported the long-term follow-up of eight children, ages 1 to 17 years, who were exposed *in utero* to antileukemic therapy. All but one child appeared normal. A male fraternal twin in whom neuroblastoma and thyroid cancer developed in childhood had congenital malformations and a low intelligence quotient. Of interest, his female fraternal twin was normal. Both had been exposed to cyclophosphamide and prednisone throughout gestation.

RECOMMENDATIONS FOR MANAGEMENT DURING PREGNANCY

How should the above data affect routine recommendations for the therapy of pregnant patients with Hodgkin's disease?

1. Risks to the fetus are greatest during the first trimester, and so it is reasonable to delay therapy during the first trimester whenever possible.
2. Based on the available data, it appears unreasonable to delay appropriate therapy for patients with symptomatic, bulky, subdiaphragmatic, or progressive Hodgkin's disease after the first trimester.
3. Treatment options include supradiaphragmatic radiotherapy (involved field or mantle field) for early-stage disease and single-agent vinblastine or combination chemotherapy with ABVD for bulky or subdiaphragmatic disease, as well as for symptomatic or advanced-stage presentations.
4. Radiation fields should be designed to decrease the fetal dose by allowing for the maximal distance between the inferior border of the field and the uterus. The uterus should be protected during radiotherapy with 10 half-value layer shielding. The maximal dose to the fetus should be calculated before treatment, and the dose to the fetus should be monitored during treatment.
5. One should not be reluctant to use combination chemotherapy when it is clearly indicated during the second or third trimester.
6. All pregnant patients with Hodgkin's disease should be managed as high-risk cases by an obstetrician. Early delivery may not be required if the patient has received, or is receiving, adequate therapy.
7. Termination of pregnancy is rarely medically indicated in cases of newly diagnosed Hodgkin's disease; combination chemotherapy has been successfully administered during the first trimester, and vinblastine is even safer during embryogenesis.
8. Termination of pregnancy is often medically indicated in cases of relapsed Hodgkin's disease following combination chemotherapy, as high-dose chemoradiotherapy with stem cell support is then usually indicated. If relapse occurs after radiotherapy alone, the pregnant patient may be satisfactorily managed with chemotherapy (as discussed above), and termination of the pregnancy is not required.
9. All women of childbearing age receiving therapy for Hodgkin's disease should undergo pregnancy testing before treatment and should be counseled regarding birth control measures during therapy.

PREGNANCY AFTER TREATMENT

Ovarian function is usually maintained in women of childbearing age successfully treated for Hodgkin's disease. Pelvic shielding with primary irradiation, oophoropexy for those requiring pelvic radiotherapy, and utilization of combination chemotherapy regimens not containing MOPP have all contributed to the preservation of fertility. Reports of pregnancy outcome among patients previously treated for Hodgkin's disease are also generally favorable (Table 3). In 1993, Aisner et al. (28) found that 35 of 43 premenopausal women (81%) who desired children had successful pregnancies. The median treatment-free interval to the birth of a child after treatment was 5.5 years (range, 0.6–14 years), and the median age at delivery was 30 years (range, 16–35 years). In this group of 35 women, 54 pregnancies resulted in delivery of 42 children, one spontaneous and nine elective abortions, and two stillbirths. No major birth defects were reported in the 42 children, whose median birth weight was 6 lb 4 oz and whose 5-minute Apgar score (9) was within normal range.

The pregnancy rate among premenopausal survivors of Hodgkin's disease now appears similar to that of the normal female population (85%). The probability of a successful pregnancy, as reported by Horning et al. (30), is related to menopausal status and age at Hodgkin's disease therapy. This study, published in 1981, reported a 50% probability of pregnancy for Hodgkin's disease survivors who were treated as teen agers, in contrast to a probability approaching zero for those survivors treated at age 30. Total-lymphoid irradiation with or without MOPP-containing combination chemotherapy most likely accounts for this low probability of fertility.

Guidelines for planning subsequent pregnancy are empirically derived but based on the following observations:

TABLE 3. *Female survivors of Hodgkin's disease: outcome of pregnancies begun after therapy*

Prior therapy	Pregnancies	Live births/ stillborn	Spontaneous/ therapeutic abortions	Congenital anomalies	Reference
Radiation	36[a]	34/0	2[a]/0	1	26
	11	9/0	0/2	0	30
	22	16/3	0/3	1	29
Totals	**69[a]**	**59/3**	**2[a]/5**	**2**	
Chemotherapy					
with/without	16	14/0	0/1	2	26
irradiation	17[a]	15[a]/0	0/3	0	30
	11	8/1	2/0	1	29
Totals	**44[a]**	**37[a]/1**	**2/4**	**3**	

[a]One pregnancy with twins.

1. Most relapses of Hodgkin's disease occur within 2 to 3 years of definitive therapy (see Chapters 25–27).

2. Follow-up imaging is performed less frequently after years 2 to 3 and can safely be delayed in the pregnant patient (see Chapter 16).

3. Chemotherapy-induced menstrual irregularity is often transient and resolves within 1 to 2 years after therapy (see Chapter 36).

4. The risk for congenital abnormalities in children conceived after treatment for Hodgkin's disease (and also other malignancies) does not appear to be greater than that in the general population. The largest study reported to date of children born to survivors of prior cancer treatment is that of Byrne et al. (24). Among 2,198 offspring of survivors of pediatric and adolescent cancer treated before 1976, genetic disease was not significantly increased (3.4% in offspring of cancer survivors vs. 3.1% in 4,544 control children). Moreover, the kinds of genetic abnormalities noted (simple malformations, single-gene defects, and cytogenetic syndromes) were not significantly different from those of controls. A similar population-based study has examined the incidence of cancer among offspring of 14,652 survivors of childhood and adolescent cancer. Utilizing data from patients in Scandinavian countries in whom disease was diagnosed after 1940, Sankila et al. (25) report no evidence of a significantly increased risk for nonhereditary cancers based on offspring follow-up of 86,780 person-years (standardized incidence ratio of 1:3).

RECOMMENDATIONS FOR MANAGEMENT OF PREGNANCY CONCEIVED AFTER TREATMENT

Based on these observations, it is generally recommended that women delay pregnancy for 2 years after all treatment. Practical precautions that may be considered include the following:

1. Follow-up imaging should be performed before the patient attempts to conceive.

2. Thyroid function should be assessed and closely monitored among patients at risk for hypothyroidism (e.g., prior mantle irradiation). Hypothyroidism during pregnancy can result in hypertension, preterm delivery, and prematurity (23). Moreover, thyroid replacement needs may increase during pregnancy.

3. A Hodgkin's disease-related physical examination should be performed at least once during pregnancy.

4. The patient should receive high-risk obstetric care.

5. Infertility should be evaluated promptly if conception is not achieved within 6 to 12 months.

6. No imaging is necessary while the patient is pregnant unless it is indicated by physical findings or symptoms.

REFERENCES

1. Davis AB. Report of a case of Hodgkin's disease complicated by pregnancy. *Bull Lying-in Hosp N Y* 1911;7:151–158.
2. Woo SY, Fuller LM, Cundiff JH, et al. Radiotherapy during pregnancy for clinical stages IA–IIA Hodgkin's disease. *Int J Radiat Oncol Biol Phys* 1992;23:407–412.
3. Yahalom J. Treatment options for Hodgkin's disease during pregnancy. *Leuk Lymphoma* 1990;2:151–161.
4. Stewart HL, Monto RW. Hodgkin's disease and pregnancy. *Am J Obstet Gynecol* 1952;63:570–578.
5. Palacios Costa N, Chavanne FC, Zebel Fernancdez D. *An de ateneo.* Buenos Aires: , 1945:127.
6. Bichel J. Hodgkin's disease and pregnancy. *Acta Radiol* 1950;33: 427–434.
7. Hennessy JP, Rottino A. Hodgkin's disease in pregnancy. *Am J Obstet Gynecol* 1963;87:851–853.
8. Barry RM, Diamond HD, Carver LF. Influence of pregnancy on the course of Hodgkin's disease. *Am J Obstet Gynecol* 1962;84:445–454.
9. Priesel A, Winkelbauer A. Placetnare ubertagung des lymphogranulomas. *Virchows Arch* 1926;262:749–796.
10. Lishner M, Zemlickis D, Degendorfer P, Panzarella T, Sutcliffe SB, Koren G. Maternal and foetal outcome following Hodgkin's disease in pregnancy. *Br J Cancer* 1992;65:114–117.
11. Jacobs C, Donaldson SS, Rosenberg SA, Kaplan HS. Management of the pregnant patient with Hodgkin's disease. *Ann Intern Med* 1981;95: 669–675.
12. Gelb AB, Van de Rijn M, Warnke RA, Kamel OW. Pregnancy-associated lymphomas. A clinicopathologic study. *Cancer* 1996;78:204–210 (*see comments*).
13. Aviles A, Diaz-Maqueo JC, Talavera A, Guzman R, Garcia EL. Growth and development of children of mothers treated with chemotherapy during pregnancy: current status of 43 children. *Am J Hematol* 1991; 36:243–248.
14. Barnicle MM. Chemotherapy and pregnancy. *Semin Oncol Nurs* 1992; 8:124–132.
15. Doll DC, Ringenberg QS, Yarbro JW. Antineoplastic agents and pregnancy. *Semin Oncol* 1989;16:337–346.
16. Cordon-Cardo C, O'Brien JP, Casals D, et al. Multidrug-resistance gene (P-glycoprotein) is expressed by endothelial cells at blood-brain barrier sites. *Proc Natl Acad Sci U S A* 1989;86:695–698.
17. Zucali R, Marchesini, R, DePalo O. Abdominal dosimetry for supradiaphragmatic irradiation of Hodgkin's disease in pregnancy. Experimental data and clinical considerations. *Tumori* 1981;67:203–208.
18. Covington EE, Baker AS. Dosimetry of scattered radiation to the fetus. *JAMA* 1969;209:414–415.
19. Wong PS, Rosemark PJ, Exler MC, Greenberg SH, Thompson RW. Doses to organs at risk from mantle field radiation therapy using 10 MV x-rays. *Mt Sinai J Med* 1985;52:216–220.
20. Sharma SC, Williamson JF, Khan FM, Lee CK. Measurement and calculation of ovary and fetus dose in extended field radiotherapy for 10 MV x-rays. *Int J Radiat Oncol Biol Phys* 1981;7:843–846.
21. Reynoso EE, Shepherd FA, Messner HA, Farquharson HA, Garvey MB, Baker MA. Acute leukemia during pregnancy: the Toronto Leukemia Study Group experience with long-term follow-up of children exposed *in utero* to chemotherapeutic agents. *J Clin Oncol* 1987;5:1098–1106.
22. Garber JE. Long-term follow-up of children exposed *in utero* to antineoplastic agents. *Semin Oncol* 1989;16:437–444.
23. Montoro MN. Management of hypothyroidism during pregnancy. *Clin Obstet Gynecol* 1997;40:65–80.
24. Byrne J, Rasmussen SA, Steinhorn SC, et al: Genetic disease in offspring of long-term survivors of childhood and adolescent cancer. *Am J Hum Genet* 1998;62:45–52.
25. Sankila R, Olsen JH, Anderson H, et al. Risk of cancer among offspring of childhood cancer survivors. *N Engl J Med* 1998;338:1339–1344.
26. Holmes GE, Holmes FF. Pregnancy outcome of patients treated for Hodgkin's disease: a controlled study. *Cancer* 1978;41:1317–1322.
27. Ortin TT, Shostak CA, Donaldson SS. Gonadal status and reproductive function following treatment for Hodgkin's disease in childhood: the Stanford experience. *Int J Radiat Oncol Biol Phys* 1990;19:873–880.
28. Aisner J, Wiernik PH, Pearl P. Pregnancy outcome in patients treated for Hodgkin's disease. *J Clin Oncol* 1993;11:507–512.
29. Green DM, Hall B. Pregnancy outcome following treatment during childhood or adolescence for Hodgkin's disease. *Pediatr Hematol Oncol* 1988;54:269–277.
30. Horning SJ, Hoppe RT, Kaplan HS, Rosenberg SA. Female reproductive potential after treatment for Hodgkin's disease. *N Eng J Med* 1981;304:1377–1382.

Hodgkin's Disease, edited by P. M. Mauch,
J. O. Armitage, V. Diehl, R. T. Hoppe, and L. M. Weiss.
Lippincott Williams & Wilkins, Philadephia ©1999.

CHAPTER 39

HIV-related Hodgkin's Disease

Umberto Tirelli, Antonino Carbone, and David J. Straus

Hodgkin's disease is the most common non–AIDS-defining tumor that occurs in the HIV population. More than 300 cases of Hodgkin's disease in HIV-infected persons have been reported, mainly from the European countries (i.e., Italy, Spain, and France) and to a lesser extent from the United States (1–8). All series have documented unusually aggressive tumor behavior, including a higher frequency of unfavorable histologic subtypes, advanced stages, and poorer therapeutic outcomes, in comparison with Hodgkin's disease outside the HIV setting.

EPIDEMIOLOGY

Is Hodgkin's disease more frequent in patients with HIV infection? Are there differences in the incidence of Hodgkin's disease among the various HIV risk groups?

Male Homosexuals

In the early 1980s, analysis of data from the Surveillance, Epidemiology and End Results (SEER) program detected a marked increase in the incidence of Kaposi's sarcoma and non-Hodgkin's lymphoma among never-married young men, a surrogate group for the male homosexual population, but no similar increase in Hodgkin's disease was observed (9,10). The analysis was confounded by the fact that unlike non-Hodgkin's lymphoma and Kaposi's sarcoma, which occur in older persons in the general population who are not infected with HIV, Hodgkin's disease occurs in similar young-adult and middle-aged populations with and without HIV infection. However, subsequent analyses indicated a slightly increased incidence of Hodgkin's disease among men in the male homosexual risk group. Among never-married young men from San Francisco, Biggar et al. (11) found a small but nonsignificant increase in the occurrence of Hodgkin's disease. Rabkin and Yellin (12) observed a slight overall increase that actually started before the AIDS epidemic, although the incidence of the mixed cellularity subtype was further increased 2.2 to 3.4 times more than expected. Analyses of data from a cancer registry in New York State, not part of the SEER data, revealed a marked increase in Hodgkin's disease among never-married men in 1985 (13).

Medeiros and Greiner (14) used data from the SEER program to study trends in Hodgkin's disease during three time periods (1973–77, 1978–82, and 1983–87). In San Francisco County, where young men are known to have a high prevalence of HIV infection, the age-specific incidence rates for mixed cellularity Hodgkin's disease increased for men, and the mixed cellularity subtype was the most common subtype by the age of 50. This was in contrast to an unchanged age-adjusted rate in the mixed cellularity subtype among men in the entire SEER database.

In another study based on SEER data, the risk for development of another primary cancer after a diagnosis of Kaposi's sarcoma was evaluated. Because of the more than 40,000-fold increase in risk for Kaposi's sarcoma among never-married men since the beginning of the HIV epidemic, this tumor was used as a surrogate for HIV-positivity. No indication of an increased risk for Hodgkin's disease was found among never-married men with Kaposi's sarcoma (15).

Reynolds et al. (16) linked data from AIDS and cancer registries in San Francisco between 1980 and 1987. Compared with concurrent rates for the population in the same geographic area, the standardized incidence rate for Hodgkin's disease in men with AIDS increased from 1.9 in 1980–81 to 18.3 in 1986–87. This observation was

U. Tirelli: Department of Oncology, University of Udine, Udine, Italy and Division of Medical Oncology and AIDS, Instituto Nazionale Tumori, Aviano (PN), Italy.

A. Carbone: Department of Pathology, University of Padua, Padua, Italy and Department of Pathology, Centro di Riferimento Oncologico, Instituto Nazionale Tumori, Aviano, Italy.

D. J. Straus: Department of Medicine, Weill Medical College of Cornell University and Department of Medicine, Lymphoma Service, Memorial Sloan-Kettering Cancer Center, New York, New York.

based on only 16 cases, and the standardized intervals overlapped for each of the four periods studied.

Hessol et al. (17) compared the risk for Hodgkin's disease in a cohort of 6,704 homosexual men included in the San Francisco City Clinic Cohort Study from 1978 to 1989 with population-based rates from the SEER database. Information on cancer events in the cohort was obtained by computer-matched identification of participants with the records of the Northern California Cancer Registry. Among HIV-infected men, the age-adjusted standardized relative risk for Hodgkin's disease was 5.0 (95% CI, 2.0–10.3), a significant increase. A subsequent analysis of the San Francisco City Clinic cohort combined with a similar cohort of homosexual men from New York City, which was not restricted to HIV-positive men, also found a statistically significant, slightly increased SIR that was 2.5 times greater than expected (18).

Lyter et al. (19) studied cancer events occurring in 1984–93 in a cohort of 769 HIV-seronegative and 430 HIV-seropositive homosexual men in the Pittsburgh component of the Multicenter AIDS Cohort Study (MACS). Cancer information was collected through semiannual visits, medical records, and death certificates. There was no difference in the rate of Hodgkin's disease between the seronegative homosexual men and the general population of Pennsylvania, whereas the two cases observed in the HIV-seropositive group were more than expected (SIR, 19.8; 95% CI, 2.4–71.5). More recently, the same authors analyzed the data from the entire MACS cohort (5,579 homosexual men) and confirmed a significant increase in the rate of Hodgkin's disease in the group of patients with HIV infection (20).

Serraino et al. (21) compared the incidence rates of Hodgkin's disease among seroconverters for HIV infection with the rates in the general population of Italy. The study was part of an ongoing cohort investigation conducted by the HIV Italian Seroconversion Study Group, in which 1,255 persons between the ages of 20 and 49 years were enrolled. Hodgkin's disease was observed in three men (two homosexuals and one intravenous drug user), which was 38 times more often in the cohort of HIV seroconverters (95% CI, 8–111) than in the general population.

Intravenous Drug Users

In 1988, the Italian Cooperative Group on AIDS and Tumors (GICAT) reported on 35 HIV-infected patients with Hodgkin's disease, noting an unusually high frequency among infected intravenous drug users and suggesting that this particular group was at higher risk (22). An increased incidence of Hodgkin's disease had also been reported among intravenous drug users in New York prisons (23). Rubio (2) in Spain observed a significantly higher ratio of Hodgkin's disease to non-Hodgkin's lymphoma in intravenous drug users than in homosexual men (0.81 vs. 0.24; p <.01). A significantly higher ratio in intravenous drug users compared with homosexual men has also been reported in France (24) and Italy (25). The higher frequency of Hodgkin's disease in Spain and Italy occurs in a similar epidemiologic context, the predominant high-risk group in both countries being intravenous drug users. In Italy, the percentage of intravenous drug users among all AIDS cases is lower than the percentage of intravenous drug users among cases of HIV-related Hodgkin's disease as observed by GICAT.

Other Risk Groups

In a study of women ages 20 to 49 from New York and New Jersey, whose age was based on cancer registry and AIDS surveillance data, an increased incidence of Hodgkin's disease during 1976–88 was not detected, although the incidences of Kaposi's sarcoma, non-Hodgkin's lymphoma, and AIDS were increased during the same period (26).

Ragni et al. (27) found no increased incidence of Hodgkin's disease among 3,041 hemophiliac patients from the United States between 1978 and 1989. In fact, no case of Hodgkin's disease was reported among the 1,295 HIV-positive patients.

In the National Cancer Institute Multicenter Hemophilia Cohort Study, there were two cases of Hodgkin's disease among 1,065 HIV-seropositive subjects and one case among 636 HIV-seronegative subjects (28), representing frequences of 6.6 and 8.2 times those expected in HIV-seropositive and HIV-seronegative subjects, respectively, although neither excess was statistically significant.

Conclusions

In summary, the majority of recent studies demonstrate a slight increase in the incidence of Hodgkin's disease in the young-adult and middle-aged male homosexual population; however, an increased incidence among women in a specific age group and location associated with an increased risk for AIDS and among hemophiliacs has not been convincingly demonstrated.

Available data support the finding that Hodgkin's disease associated with HIV infection occurs preferentially in intravenous drug users. This could be explained by the lower age of intravenous drug users relative to homosexual men and other groups at risk for AIDS, as Hodgkin's disease affects mainly young persons. Moreover, some other, unknown epidemiologic factor favoring the higher incidence of Hodgkin's disease might be associated with intravenous transmission of HIV infection. The area where infected patients live as well as the route of HIV infection must be carefully examined to obtain an accurate evaluation of the incidence of Hodgkin's disease in the HIV-positive population. Although the majority of evidence suggests that Hodgkin's disease may be more common in HIV-infected intravenous drug users than in other groups at risk for HIV infection, the disease does not appear to be restricted to this group alone (17,19, 21,28). The question of whether this evidence is sufficient for Hodgkin's disease to be considered an AIDS-defining illness remains open to debate.

PATHOLOGIC FEATURES

Distribution of Histologic Subtypes among HIV-infected Persons

The diagnosis of Hodgkin's disease in HIV-infected persons is primarily based on the histopathologic criteria proposed by Lukes et al. in 1965 (Fig. 1A) (29). However, it is important to remember that the pathologic features of Hodgkin's disease in HIV-infected persons are different from those in the general population (29–31). First of all, recent studies have documented a significant difference between the distribution of Hodgkin's disease subtypes in HIV-infected persons and the distribution in the HIV-uninfected population. Hodgkin's disease in HIV-infected persons is characterized by a predominance of unfavorable histologic subtypes (1–3,7,32). In several series reported from Europe and the United States (Table 1), mixed cellularity was the most frequent histologic subtype among HIV-infected persons (41–100%), and nodular sclerosis was less frequent (0–40%) than in HIV-uninfected persons. In the HIV-infected group, the incidence of the lymphocyte predominance subtype was notably low (0–4%), whereas more than 20% of cases were classified as being of the lymphocyte-depletion subtype. These histologic data were confirmed by a recent multicentric study including a large number of Italian patients with Hodgkin's disease (1). The study documented a frequency of mixed cellularity plus lymphocyte depletion in an HIV setting of 66%, compared with a frequency of 29% in HIV-uninfected patients (p <.001). On the other hand, lymphocyte predominance plus nodular sclerosis subtypes were more frequent in the HIV-uninfected group (34% vs. 71%; p <.001) (1).

Special Morphologic Features in HIV-infected Persons

The Lukes et al. classification of Hodgkin's disease was based on the quantitative relationship between lymphocytes and diagnostic Reed-Sternberg cells (lymphocyte predominance vs. lymphocyte depletion) and the different types of connective tissue proliferation (nodular sclerosis vs. lymphocyte depletion, diffuse fibrosis) (30). In this context, it is important to note that Hodgkin's disease in HIV-infected persons exhibits special features related to the cellular background and the abundance of neoplastic cells. Notably, these special features, which include a proliferation of fibrohistiocytoid stromal cells and an abundance of Reed-Sternberg cells and their morphologic atypia, may pose difficulties in diagnosing and classifying the disease.

Regarding the cellular background, some studies have shown that the pathologic spectrum of HIV-associated

A 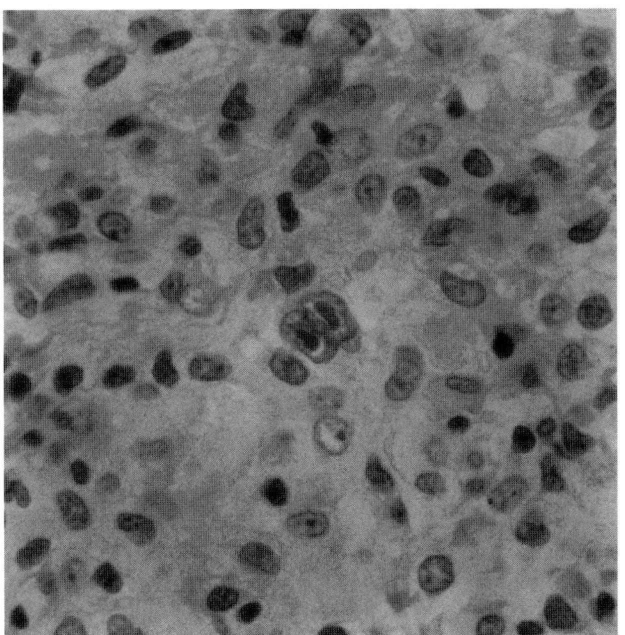

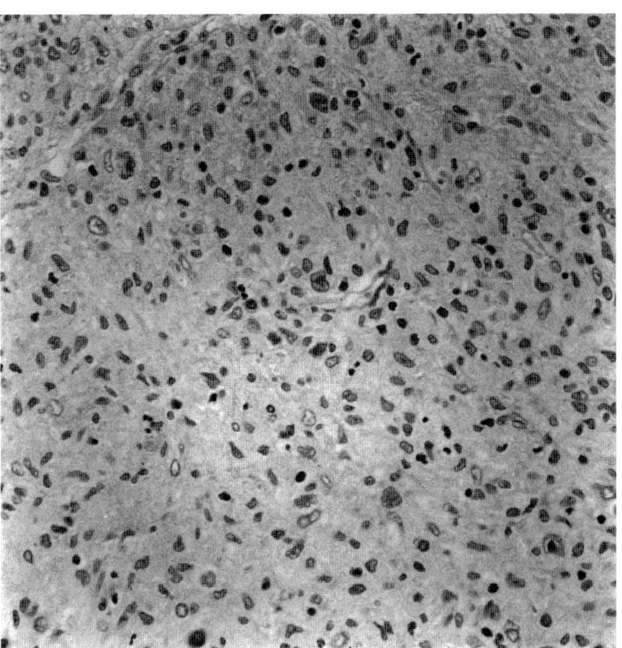 B

FIG. 1. Histologic section of a lymph node involved by mixed cellularity Hodgkin's disease from an HIV-infected person. **A:** The microphotograph demonstrates a Reed-Sternberg cell of classic type (*center*). The background consists of histiocytes and lymphocytes. (Hematoxylin and eosin, x400.) **B:** Same node as in A, showing a background rich in fibrohistiocytoid stromal cells. Lymphocytes are reduced in number. (Hematoxylin and eosin, x180.)

TABLE 1. *Histopathologic characteristics of Hodgkin's disease in HIV-infected persons (studies with more than 20 patients)*

Study (ref.)	Period	No. cases	Median age (range)	No. male patients	No. female patients	Histopathology (%) Mixed cellularity	Lymphocyte depletion	Nodular sclerosis	Lymphocyte predominance
Ree at al., 1991, U.S. (7)	1983–90	24	34 (24–51)	23	1	100	0	0	0
Andrieu et al., 1993, France (3)	1987–89	45[a]	30 (NR)	39	6	49	4	40	0
Rubio, 1994, Spain (2)	1984–91	46	27 (mean) (18–55)	43	3	41	22	22	4
Tirelli et al., 1995, Italy (1)	1986–94	114[b]	29 (19–57)	103	11	45	21	30	4
Bellas et al., 1996, Spain (32)	NR	24[c]	NR (18–41)	22	2	42	21	33	0

NR, not reported.
[a]Three cases had undetermined histologic subtype.
[b]Seven cases were not classified histopathologically.
[c]One case was not classified histopathologically.

Hodgkin's disease characteristically includes fibrohistiocytoid stromal cell proliferation (Fig. 1B) (7,32). The fibrohistiocytoid stromal cells are usually arranged in bundles surrounding nodular areas, thus mimicking the classic pattern of the nodular sclerosis subtype. The fibrohistiocytoid pattern was initially considered as part of the mixed cellularity spectrum because of the absence of a polarizable sclerosing reaction (7). On the other hand, a recent report has documented that cases of Hodgkin's disease with fibrohistiocytoid cell proliferation also show distinct nodules surrounded by polarizable collagen bands (32). For this reason, the fibrohistiocytoid pattern may be considered as part of the nodular sclerosis spectrum when it is associated with the histopathologic findings fulfilling the criteria for the nodular sclerosis subtype.

Another morphologic characteristic of Hodgkin's disease in HIV-infected persons is the predominance of cases rich in Reed-Sternberg cells (32,33). This finding contrasts with the rather low population of neoplastic cells usually found in HIV-unrelated Hodgkin's disease.

Differential Diagnosis and Immunophenotyping

The high frequency of cases rich in Reed-Sternberg cells poses special diagnostic problems (33). In an HIV setting, the admixture of scarce amounts of the reactive components with high numbers of neoplastic cells may result in histopathologic patterns that encompass obvious cases of Hodgkin's disease and cases of non-Hodgkin's lymphoma displaying anaplastic large-cell populations (33).

Major problems may occur in distinguishing between Hodgkin's disease and the so-called CD30+ anaplastic large-cell lymphomas (34,35), because both entities also share several phenotypic features, including the consistent expression of the CD30 molecule and the frequent expression of B cell-associated lymphoid antigens (32,34–37). However, although these phenotypic features exaggerate the diagnostic difficulties entailed in separating cases of Hodgkin's disease from cases of CD30+ anaplastic large-cell lymphoma in the HIV setting, a combination of several markers, including activation antigens and leukocyte common antigen (LCA, or CD45), can be applied to obtain a reliable immunodiagnosis of Hodgkin's disease. In fact, the CD30+, CD45-, CD15+, and epithelial membrane antigen-negative phenotypic profile is consistently expressed by Reed-Sternberg cells (36,38) and is very helpful for the diagnosis of Hodgkin's disease (31). Conversely, the neoplastic cells of anaplastic large-cell lymphoma usually express a CD30+, CD45+, CD15- profile. This is the most frequent phenotype of anaplastic large-cell lymphomas in HIV-infected persons (34,35).

Relationship with Epstein-Barr Virus

The frequency of Epstein-Barr viral (EBV) infection in AIDS-related non-Hodgkin's lymphoma has been a matter of controversy (39). Discrepancies may depend on the different methods used for viral detection and on the different histologic types or sites of disease investigated. A high frequency of association with EBV (80–100%) has been demonstrated in Hodgkin's disease tissues from HIV-infected persons (1,40–42), which is in contrast to the findings in tissues from persons with systemic non-Hodgkin's lymphoma. The EBV genomes in such cases have been reported to be episomal and clonal (33), even when detected in multiple lesions (43). On the other hand, the association of EBV with Hodgkin's disease in HIV-uninfected persons has been shown globally to be about 50%, although a higher association of EBV (around 60%) has been found with the mixed cellularity subtype (1, 32,38).

The elevated frequency of EBV in association with Hodgkin's disease indicates that unlike human herpes virus 6 (HHV-6) (36,44,45) and HHV-8 (46,47), EBV probably does represent a relevant factor involved in the pathogenesis of HIV-associated Hodgkin's disease.

Hodgkin's Disease in HIV-infected Persons as an EBV-related Lymphoma Expressing Latent Membrane Protein 1

A pathogenetic role of EBV is further supported by data showing that at least some EBV-transforming proteins, namely EBV-encoded latent membrane protein 1 (LMP1), are expressed in EBV+ cases of Hodgkin's disease. In fact, in cases of EBV+ Hodgkin's disease, the virus adopts a latency type 2 pattern—namely, positive for LMP1 and negative for Epstein-Barr nuclear antigen 2 (EBNA2) (Fig. 2) (33,36). Notably, the fact that LMP1 is expressed in virtually all HIV-associated Hodgkin's disease cases suggests that EBV plays an etiologic role in the pathogenesis of HIV-associated Hodgkin's disease (32). For these reasons, Hodgkin's disease in HIV-infected persons appears to be an EBV-related lymphoma expressing LMP1 (37,48,49).

The grouping of the different pathologic subtypes of AIDS-related lymphoproliferative disorders based on EBV association and EBV latent gene expression (40) is shown in Table 2. The frequent association between EBV infection and some lymphomas in HIV-infected persons (50), including those arising primarily in the brain and body cavities (46,51–53), as well as anaplastic large-cell lymphomas (35,37) and Hodgkin's disease (1,32), suggests that EBV is an important cofactor in the pathogenesis of these conditions. Furthermore, the presence of EBV in these lymphoma cells appears to be important for the expression of certain morphologic and immunophenotypic features in the context of HIV infection.

TABLE 2. *Grouping of pathologic types of AIDS-related lymphomas based on EBV latent gene expression*

Lymphomas not associated with expression of EBV-encoded LMP1
- Large noncleaved cell
- Small noncleaved cell

Lymphomas that may be associated with expression of EBV-encoded LMP1
- Immunoblastic (either systemic or arising in the brain as a primary site)
- Occasional cases of small noncleaved cell
- Body cavity-based lymphoma (associated with HHV-8 infection), also called primary effusion lymphoma

Lymphomas associated with monoclonal EBV infection and expression of LMP1
- Anaplastic large-cell (CD30/Ki-1$^+$) lymphoma
- Hodgkin's lymphoma (mixed cellularity and lymphocyte depletion)

EBV, Epstein-Barr virus; LMP1, latent membrane protein 1. Updated and adapted from ref. 40.

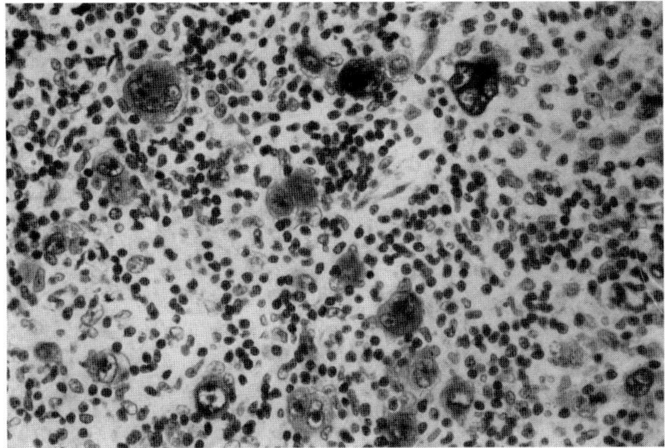

FIG. 2. Latent membrane protein 1 (LMP1) staining in a fixed, paraffin-embedded section of a lymph node involved by mixed cellularity Hodgkin's disease from an HIV-infected person. The microphotograph shows strong LMP1 staining within the cytoplasm of some Reed-Sternberg cells. (Alkalene phosphatase, antialkaline phosphatase method, hematoxylin counterstain, x400.)

CLINICAL ASPECTS

Clinical Presentation

One of the most peculiar features of HIV-related Hodgkin's disease is the widespread extent of the disease at presentation and the frequency of systemic "B" symptoms, including fever, night sweats, and/or weight loss of more than 10% of the normal body weight. At the time of diagnosis, 70% to 96% of the patients have B symptoms, and 74% to 92% have advanced disease (stage III–IV according to the Ann Arbor staging classification) with frequent involvement of extranodal sites, the most common being bone marrow, liver, and spleen.

In HIV-uninfected patients, Hodgkin's disease typically involves contiguous lymph node groups, and dissemination and infiltration of extranodal sites are late occurrences. In HIV-infected patients, noncontiguous spread of tumor may be observed, such as liver involvement without splenic disease or lung involvement without mediastinal adenopathy (Fig. 3), and extranodal disease has been described in approximately 60% of cases at presentation. Bone marrow involvement is common, occurring in 40% to 50% of patients, and it may be the first indication of the presence of Hodgkin's disease in approximately 20% of cases (1–7,54). The liver becomes

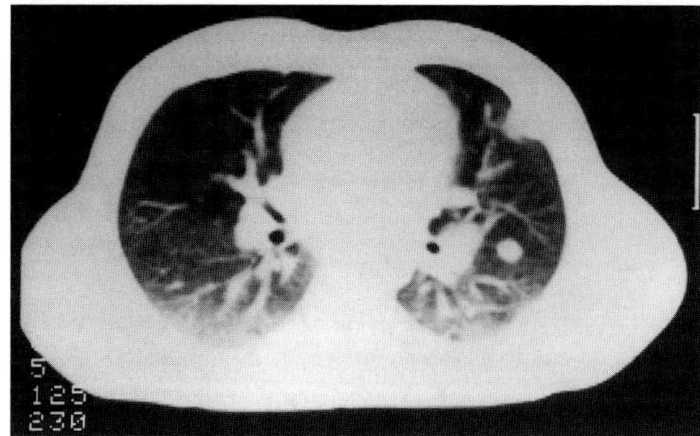

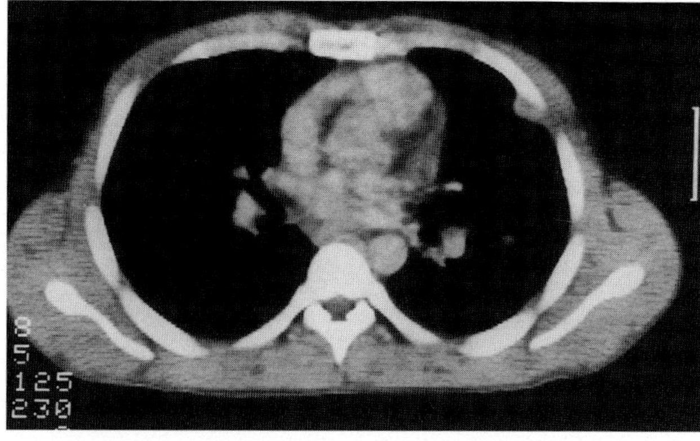

FIG. 3. Computed tomogram (CT) of the chest showing involvement of the left lung and parietal pleura (*arrows*) in a patient with Hodgkin's disease and HIV infection. No mediastinal adenopathy was observed in the upper slices (*not shown*). **A:** Parenchymal window. **B:** Mediastinal window.

involved in 15% to 40% of the patients, and the spleen in approximately 20% (1–7). In contrast to HIV-related non-Hodgkin's lymphoma, HIV-related Hodgkin's disease uncommonly involves unusual sites, but case reports of central nervous system, skin, rectum, tongue, and lung involvement have been reported (6,55,56).

Hodgkin's disease, like Burkitt's non-Hodgkin's lymphoma, tends to develop as an earlier manifestation of HIV infection, with a higher median count of CD4+ cells (range, 275–306/μL), than does diffuse large-cell lymphoma (1–7).

At the time of diagnosis, the majority of patients with Hodgkin's disease (65% of cases in the Italian series) have persistent generalized lymphadenopathy, and in approximately 50% of cases the lymphoma may be concurrently present with persistent generalized lymphadenopathy in the same lymph node group (57,58). Hodgkin's disease may be clinically confused with persistent generalized lymphadenopathy; therefore, an increase in size of preexisting adenopathy in patients with persistent generalized lymphadenopathy should be evaluated with a biopsy. The initial diagnostic workup may also require, in particular cases, lymph node biopsies at multiple sites. On the other hand, clinicians should recognize the possibility that HIV-positive patients will be overstaged with computed tomography (CT) of the abdomen as well as lymphangiography, owing to the presence of persistent generalized lymphadenopathy in retroperitoneal lymph nodes (Fig. 4). Hilar and mediastinal lymphadenopathy are not part of HIV-related persistent generalized lymphadenopathy (59).

Systemic symptoms are frequently associated with both advanced HIV infection and opportunistic infections. Thus, these symptoms mandate a careful evaluation to exclude other causes, including tuberculosis, cryptococcosis, or cytomegalovirus infection.

All case reports and case series describe a particular natural history and histologic distribution of Hodgkin's disease in HIV-infected persons that are different from those of Hodgkin's disease in HIV-uninfected persons.

In the Italian series (the largest published so far), 77% and 81% of HIV-infected patients had systemic symptoms and stage III–IV disease, respectively, in comparison with 35% and 44% of a group of 104 patients with "primary" Hodgkin's disease diagnosed at the same institution (1). Another distinctive feature of HIV-related Hodgkin's dis-

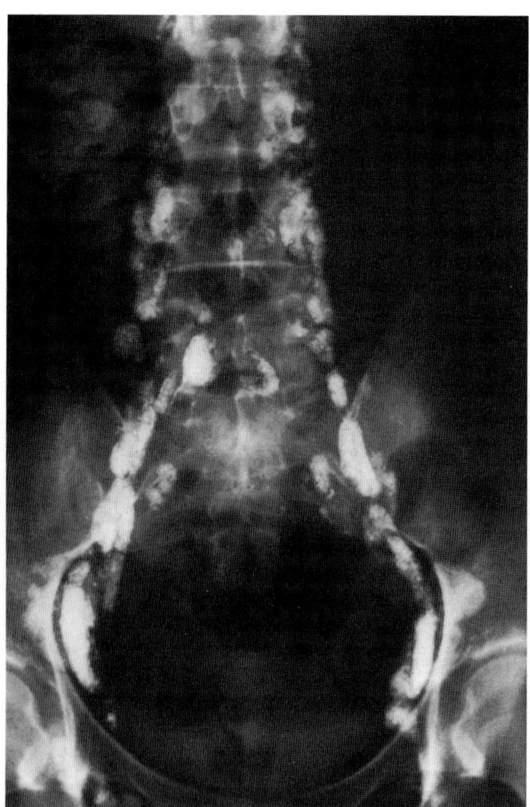

FIG. 4. Generalized increase in the size of abdominal and pelvic lymph nodes with a small filling defect (persistent generalized lymphadenopathy). The lymphangiography films of this patient, referred to the Aviano Cancer Center with an erroneous histologic diagnosis of HIV-related Hodgkin's disease, were previously read as consistent with involvement by lymphoma.

ease is the lower frequency of mediastinal adenopathy in comparison with "primary" Hodgkin's disease. Overall, mediastinal disease is absent in between 77% and 87% of HIV-infected patients, versus only 29% to 42% of HIV-negative control cases (1–7). It is noteworthy that in the Italian series, this difference was also significant in patients with the nodular sclerosis subtype (27% in HIV-positive vs. 80% in HIV-negative patients; $p < .001$) (1).

Andrieu et al. (3) compared all 45 cases of Hodgkin's disease collected by the French registry of HIV-associated tumors between 1987 and 1989 with a cohort of 407 HIV-negative patients having Hodgkin's disease for whom similar diagnostic criteria had been used. The groups had a similar median age (30–31 years) but differed significantly with respect to advanced clinical stage (75% vs. 33%), proportion of mixed cellularity (49% vs. 20%), and absence of mediastinal disease (87% vs. 29%). Errante et al. (60) studied treatment response and survival in 84 HIV-negative and 92 HIV-positive patients. Complete remission was achieved in 51% of HIV-infected patients and in more than 90% of the HIV-negative patients. When HIV-infected patients were compared with only the older HIV-negative patients, in whom the mixed cellularity type of Hodgkin's disease was primarily diagnosed, similar differences were observed. The estimated 4-year survival was 33% in HIV-positive patients, compared with 88% to 100% in HIV-negative patients, depending on the age group.

Infections described in patients with Hodgkin's disease without HIV infection are mostly caused by gram-positive cocci and bacilli and gram-negative bacilli (84% of microbiologically documented infections) (61). Opportunistic infections are infrequent in these patients (61,62). In contrast, in patients with Hodgkin's disease and HIV infection, opportunistic infections diagnostic of AIDS develop, many of them concomitantly with administration of combination chemotherapy (1–8).

Ames et al. (6) described the development of opportunistic infections in 27 of 50 such patients, including *Pneumocystis carinii* pneumonia, cytomegalovirus infection, extrapulmonary tuberculosis, disseminated or esophageal candidiasis, cryptococcal meningitis, cryptosporidiosis, and cerebral toxoplasmosis. Most of these episodes were fatal. In the Italian series (1), the causes of death of patients included tumor progression in 33%, opportunistic infections in 35%, tumor progression with infection in 12%, and nonopportunistic infections in 7%.

The classic prognostic criteria for the general population (i.e., advanced stage, bulky disease, bone marrow involvement, inguinal node involvement, age of more than 40 years, high lactate dehydrogenase level, high erythrocyte sedimentation rate, and anemia) (63) must be supplemented by host prognostic criteria in the HIV setting—namely, a low number of CD4+ cells and prior AIDS diagnosis, both of which reflect the underlying immunodeficiency. In the Italian series, statistically significant predictors for survival included achievement of a complete response, absence of a prior AIDS diagnosis, and presence of more than 250 CD4+ cells per microliter. The median survival of patients achieving a complete response was 58 months, whereas the median survival of the remaining patients was 11 months ($p < .001$). The median survivals of patients without or with a diagnosis of AIDS were 20 and 7 months, respectively ($p < .001$). Patients with more than 250 CD4+ cells per microliter had a median survival of 38 months, whereas patients with fewer than 250 CD4+ cells per microliter had a median survival of 11 months ($p < .002$) (1). The importance to survival of the same prognostic factors was also demonstrated in other studies (2,3).

Treatment

The optimal therapy for HIV-related Hodgkin's disease has not been defined. Because most patients have advanced Hodgkin's disease, they have been treated with combination chemotherapy regimens such as MOPP [mechlorethamine, Oncovin (vincristine), procarbazine, and prednisone], and more recently with ABVD [Adriamycin (doxorubicin), bleomycin, vinblastine, and dacarbazine], but their response rate remains poorer than that of patients with "primary" Hodgkin's disease. Moreover, the therapy of HIV-related Hodgkin's disease, as well as that of other HIV-related tumors, presents many problems. The main one is that of immunosuppression induced by antineoplastic treatment, which can further compromise the immunocellular deficit of HIV-infected patients and facilitate the onset of opportunistic infections and/or the evolution of the HIV infection itself. A complex qualitative immunologic deficiency is also known to be associated with "primary" Hodgkin's disease. Furthermore, although the numbers of CD4+ cells in these patients are usually normal or slightly decreased at diagnosis, they may become severely depressed during and after treatment, and these patients are known for their higher susceptibility to opportunistic infections. Finally, leukopenia, frequently present in patients with HIV-related Hodgkin's disease because of previous therapy with nucleoside analogs and/or HIV-related myelodysplasia, often makes conventional dosages of chemotherapy difficult to administer.

In the retrospective evaluations reported in the literature (2–7,57), the complete response rate was far below that usually observed in HIV-uninfected patients with Hodgkin's disease, tolerance to chemotherapy was poor, and reduction of doses or delay of chemotherapy was often necessary (at least when bone marrow growth factors were not available); the overall median survival time was approximately 1.5 years (Table 3).

In a retrospective evaluation conducted within the GICAT of 41 patients with HIV-related Hodgkin's disease who received chemotherapy, the 22 who received MOPP appeared to have a worse outcome than those who received MOPP alternating with or followed by ABVD (25). The rate of complete response was 65% in MOPP/ABVD-

TABLE 3. *Characteristics, treatments, and outcome of 232 patients with HIV-associated Hodgkin's disease (retrospective series from Europe and U.S.)*

	Italy (57)	France (3)	Spain (2)	U.S. (7)	U.S. (6)	U.S. (5)	U.S. (4)
No. patients	71	45	46	24	23	13	10
Median age (y)	28	30	27	34	34	38	38
Advanced stages (%)	80	75	89	92	74	92	90
B symptoms (%)	82	80	83	96	70	85	80
Prior AIDS (%)	16	11	7	0	22	46	30
No treatment	12	1	3	0	3	0	0
Treatments							
MOPP ± RT	22	13	6	11	10	0	2
ABVD ± RT	5	14	4	3	1	0	0
MOPP/ABVD ± RT	19	14	21	5	2	12	8
RT alone	7	3	3	0	6	1	0
Others CT regimens	6	0	9	5	1	0	0
Complete response (%)	55	79	44	63	53	54	57
Median survival (mo)	14	20	15	15	8	14	NR

MOPP: mechlorethamine, vincristine, procarbazine, and prednisone; ABVD: doxorubicin, bleomycin, vinblastine, and dacarbazine; RT, radiotherapy; CT, chemotherapy; NR, not reported.

treated patients, versus 46% in those who received MOPP alone. Furthermore, a lower rate of opportunistic infections was observed in the MOPP/ABVD-treated group.

In a prospective trial conducted within the GICAT between March 1989 and March 1992, 17 previously untreated patients with HIV-related Hodgkin's disease were enrolled in a study in which a regimen of epirubicin, vinblastine, and bleomycin (EBV) was used (64). EBV is a modification of the EBVP (epirubicin, vinblastine, bleomycin, and prednisone) regimen, which is an ABVD-like regimen with low bone marrow toxicity developed by Zittoun et al. (65) for patients with "primary" Hodgkin's disease. The patients were stratified into two groups: those with an Eastern Cooperative Oncology Group (ECOG) performance status of less than 3 and without a history of opportunistic infection (group A), and those with an ECOG performance status of 3 or more or a previous opportunistic infection (group B). The latter group received half-doses of epirubicin and vinblastine and full-dose bleomycin, and zidovudine (the only anti-HIV drug available at that time) was also administered from the outset of chemotherapy to this group. Patients in group A received full-dose chemotherapy, with zidovudine started after the third cycle. Courses were repeated every 21 days for 6 cycles. Overall, complete response was achieved in 53% of the whole group, which lasted a median of 20 months. Sixty-seven percent of group A patients had a complete response, whereas only one of five patients in group B (20%) had a complete response, which lasted for a median of 5 months. The median survival for the group as a whole was 11 months, and the 2-year disease-free survival rate was 55% (64). This study also showed that a combination of tailored chemotherapy regimens and zidovudine in patients with HIV-related Hodgkin's disease may result in a substantial decrease in opportunistic infections in comparison with conventional chemotherapy such as MOPP or ABVD without zidovudine.

In an attempt to improve upon these results, a second prospective trial (1993–1996) of full-dose EBV plus prednisone (EBVP regimen), concomitant antiretroviral therapy (zidovudine or didanosine), primary use of granulocyte colony-stimulating factor (G-CSF), and *Pneumocystis carinii* pneumonia prophylaxis was conducted. Preliminary results of this trial, in which 29 patients were enrolled, showed a complete response rate of 69% and an opportunistic infection rate during or after chemotherapy of 28% (median follow-up, 14 months). Toxicity was moderate, with grade 3–4 leukopenia and thrombocytopenia in 34% and 10% of patients, respectively. Thirty percent of the patients who achieved complete response relapsed. Overall, Hodgkin's disease progression alone or in association with opportunistic infections was the cause of death in 50% and 5% of patients, respectively. The 2-year survival rate and the 2-year disease-free survival were 35% and 58%, respectively (66).

The AIDS Clinical Trials Group (ACTG) reported the preliminary results of a phase II study of 15 patients treated with ABVD chemotherapy for 4 to 6 cycles and primary use of G-CSF. Antiretroviral therapy was administered after the second cycle of ABVD. New HIV-related illness developed in 80% of patients during the study. Complete response was obtained in nine (60%), partial remission in three (20%), and stable disease in three patients. The median survival for all patients was 18 months (67). The available data from the literature on prospective treatment studies are summarized in Table 4 (64,66–68).

Because Hodgkin's disease is an earlier manifestation of HIV infection than is non-Hodgkin's lymphoma (i.e., higher numbers of CD4+ cells, significantly lower percentage of cases with previous AIDS) and because patients with non-Hodgkin's lymphoma are generally much sicker, the treatment approaches may be different. In fact, although it is possible that chemotherapy in less

TABLE 4. *Prospective treatment clinical trials in patients with HIV-associated Hodgkin's disease*

Regimen	Evaluable patients	Median age (range)	Stages III and IV (%)	B symptoms (%)	Median CD4+ count (cells/μL)	Prior AIDS (%)	Response OR (%)	Response CR (%)	Median survival (mos)	Reference
EBV	17	30 (24–58)	88	82	184	24	82	53	11	64
EBVP	29	34 (21–49)	80	90	219	24	90	69	14	66
ABVD	15	34 (24–52)	62[a]	86	128	33	80	60	18	67
BOSE	5	33 (NR)	100	NR	278	0	100	80	NR	68

OR, objective response; CR, complete response; EBV, epirubicin, vinblastine, bleomycin; EBVP, epirubicin, vinblastine, bleomycin, prednisone; ABVD, doxorubicin, bleomycin, vinblastine, dacarbazine; BOSE, bleomycin, vincristine, streptozocin, etoposide; NR not reported.

[a]Stage IV only.

than conventional doses may be an effective alternative to conventional chemotherapy for the treatment of patients with non-Hodgkin's lymphoma, in patients with Hodgkin's disease, for whom there is a real probability of cure, the same therapeutic strategy should be employed as for the general population.

The outcome of patients with HIV-related Hodgkin's disease should be improved with better combinations of antineoplastic and antiretroviral therapies. The availability of efficacious new antiretroviral drugs (i.e., protease inhibitors) to be used in conjunction with nucleoside analogs might improve the control of underlying HIV infection during treatment with chemotherapy. In fact, being able to reduce the viral load to undetectable levels and increase the numbers of CD4+ cells reduces the risk for opportunistic infections during antineoplastic treatment.

The inclusion of hematopoietic growth factors in the treatment of patients with HIV-related Hodgkin's disease might allow for the administration of chemotherapy at a higher dose intensity and the prolonged use of antiretroviral drugs, with the aim of improving the survival times of these patients. Finally, more effective antineoplastic regimens, as the aggressive nature of HIV-related Hodgkin's disease would warrant, should be used to improve the response rate and disease-free survival of patients with HIV-related Hodgkin's disease.

SUMMARY

In summary, the above studies indicate that Hodgkin's disease in the presence of HIV infection is more likely to have mixed cellularity or lymphocyte depletion histology and to be clinically more aggressive. The absolute incidence of Hodgkin's disease may also be increased in HIV-infected persons, particularly intravenous drug users, but the association is not proven because the observed increases are of modest magnitude. The EBV genome may be involved in the pathogenesis of the disease. It is also apparent from treatment and outcome data that if significant improvements in long-term survival are to be attained, future investigations must deal with the underlying HIV-induced immunodeficiency in patients with HIV-related Hodgkin's disease.

REFERENCES

1. Tirelli U, Errante D, Dolcetti R, et al. Hodgkin's disease and human immmunodeficiency virus infection: clinicopathologic and virologic features of 114 patients from the Italian Cooperative Group on AIDS and Tumors. *J Clin Oncol* 1995;13:1758.
2. Rubio R. Hodgkin's disease associated with human immunodeficiency virus infection. A clinical study of 46 cases. *Cancer* 1994;73:2400.
3. Andrieu JM, Roithmann S, Tourani JM, et al. Hodgkin's disease during HIV-1 infection: the French registry experience. *Ann Oncol* 1993;4:635.
4. Lowenthal DA, Straus DJ, Campbell SW, Gold JWM, Clarkson BD, Koziner B. AIDS-related lymphoid neoplasia. The Memorial Hospital experience. *Cancer* 1988;61:2325.
5. Knowles DM, Chamulak GA, Subar M, et al. Lymphoid neoplasia associated with the acquired immunodeficiency syndrome (AIDS). *Ann Intern Med* 1988;108:744.
6. Ames ED, Conjalka MS, Goldberg AF, et al. Hodgkin's disease and AIDS. Twenty-three new cases and a review of the literature. *Hematol Oncol Clin North Am* 1991;5:343.
7. Ree HJ, Strauchen JA, Khan AA, et al. Human immunodeficiency virus-associated Hodgkin's disease. Clinicopathologic studies of 24 cases and preponderance of mixed cellularity type characterized by the occurrence of fibrohistiocytoid stromal cells. *Cancer* 1991;67:1614.
8. Newcom SR, Ward M, Napoli VM, Kutner M. Treatment of human immunodeficiency virus-associated Hodgkin's disease. Is there a clue regarding the cause of Hodgkin's disease? *Cancer* 1993;71:3138.
9. Biggar RJ, Horm J, Lubin JH, Goedert JJ, Greene MH, Fraumeni JF. Cancer trends in a population at risk of acquired immunodeficiency syndrome. *J Natl Cancer Inst* 1985;74:793.
10. Bernstein L, Levin D, Menck H, Ross RK. AIDS-related secular trends in cancer in Los Angeles County men: a comparison by marital status. *Cancer Res* 1989;49:466.
11. Biggar RJ, Horm J, Goedert JJ, Melbye M. Cancer in a group at risk of acquired immunodeficiency syndrome (AIDS) through 1984. *Am J Epidemiol* 1987;126:578.
12. Rabkin CS, Yellin F. Cancer incidence in a population with a high prevalence of infection with human immunodeficiency virus type 1. *J Natl Cancer Inst* 1994;86:1711.
13. Biggar RJ, Burnett W, Mikl J, Nasca P. Cancer among New York men at risk of acquired immunodeficiency syndrome. *Int J Cancer* 1989;43:979.
14. Medeiros LJ, Greiner TC. Hodgkin's disease. *Cancer* 1995;75:357.
15. Biggar RJ, Curtis RE, Coté TR, Rabkin CS, Melbye M. Risk of other cancers following Kaposi's sarcoma: relation to acquired immunodeficiency syndrome. *Am J Epidemiol* 1994;139:362.
16. Reynolds P, Saunders LD, Layefsky ME, Lemp GF. The spectrum of acquired immunodeficiency syndrome (AIDS)-associated malignancies in San Francisco, 1980–1987. *Am J Epidemiol* 1993;137:19.
17. Hessol NA, Katz MH, Liu JY, Buchbinder SP, Rubino CJ, Holmberg SD. Increased incidence of Hodgkin's disease in homosexual men with HIV infection. *Ann Intern Med* 1992;117:309.
18. Koblin PA, Hessol NA, Zauber AG, et al. Increased incidence of cancer

among homosexual men, New York City and San Francisco, 1978–1990. *Am J Epidemiol* 1996;144:916.
19. Lyter DW, Bryant J, Thackeray R, Rinaldo CR, Kingsley LA. Incidence of human immunodeficiency virus-related and nonrelated malignancies in a large cohort of homosexual men. *J Clin Oncol* 1995;13:2540.
20. Lyter DW, Kingsley LA, Rinaldo CR, Bryant J. Malignancies in the Multicenter AIDS Cohort Study (MACS), 1984–1994. *Proceedings of the American Society of Clinical Oncology* 1996;15:305(abst).
21. Serraino D, Pezzotti P, Dorrucci M, Alliegro MB, Sinicco A, Rezza G, for the HIV Italian Seroconversion Study Group. Cancer incidence in a cohort of human immunodeficiency virus seroconverters. *Cancer* 1997; 79:1004.
22. Monfardini S, Tirelli U, Vaccher E, et al. Malignant lymphomas in patients with or at risk for AIDS. *J Natl Cancer Inst* 1988;80:855.
23. Ahmed T, Wormser GP, Stahl RE, et al. Malignant lymphomas in a population at risk for acquired immunodeficiency syndrome. *Cancer* 1987; 60:719.
24. Roithmann S, Tourani JM, Andrieu JM. Hodgkin's disease in HIV-infected intravenous drug abusers. *N Engl J Med* 1990;323:275.
25. Tirelli U, Vaccher E, Rezza G, et al. Hodgkin's disease and infection with the human immunodeficiency virus (HIV) in Italy. *Ann Intern Med* 1988;108:309.
26. Rabkin CS, Biggar RJ, Baptiste MS, Abe T, Kohler BA, Nasca PC. Cancer incidence trends in women at high risk of human immunodeficiency virus (HIV) infection. *Int J Cancer* 1993;55:208.
27. Ragni MV, Belle SH, Jaffe RA, et al. Acquired immunodeficiency syndrome-associated non-Hodgkin's lymphomas and other malignancies in patients with hemophilia. *Blood* 1993;81:1889.
28. Rabkin CS, Hilgartner MW, Hedberg KW, et al. Incidence of lymphomas and other cancers in HIV-infected and HIV-uninfected patients with hemophilia. *JAMA* 1992;267:1090.
29. Lukes RJ, Craver LF, Hall TC, Rappaport H, Ruben P. Report of the Nomenclature Committee. *Cancer Res* 1966;26:1311.
30. Lukes RJ, Butler JJ, Hicks EB. Natural history of Hodgkin's disease as related to its pathological picture. *Cancer* 1966;19:317.
31. Harris NL, Jaffe ES, Stein H, et al. A revised European-American classification of lymphoid neoplasms: a proposal from the International Lymphoma Study Group. *Blood* 1994;84:1361.
32. Bellas C, Santón A, Manzanal A, et al. Pathological, immunological, and molecular features of Hodgkin's disease associated with HIV infection. Comparison with ordinary Hodgkin's disease. *Am J Surg Pathol* 1996;20:1520.
33. Boiocchi M, De Re V, Gloghini A, et al. High incidence of monoclonal EBV episomes in Hodgkin's disease and anaplastic large-cell Ki-1-positive lymphomas in HIV-1-positive patients. *Int J Cancer* 1993;54:53.
34. Tirelli U, Vaccher E, Zagonel V, et al. CD30 (Ki-1)-positive anaplastic large-cell lymphomas in 13 patients with and 27 patients without human immmunodeficiency virus infection: the first comparative clinicopathologic study from a single institution that also includes 80 patients with other human immunodeficiency virus-related systemic lymphomas. *J Clin Oncol* 1995;13:373.
35. Carbone A, Gloghini A, Zanette I, Canal B, Volpe R. Demonstration of Epstein-Barr viral genomes by *in situ* hybridization in acquired immune deficiency syndrome-related high grade and anaplastic large cell CD30+ lymphomas. *Am J Clin Pathol* 1993;99:289.
36. Carbone A, Dolcetti R, Gloghini A, et al. Immunophenotypic and molecular analyses of acquired immune deficiency syndrome-related and Epstein-Barr virus-associated lymphomas: a comparative study. *Hum Pathol* 1996;27:133.
37. Carbone A, Gloghini A, Volpe R, Boiocchi M, Tirelli U, and the Italian Cooperative Group on AIDS and Tumors. High frequency of Epstein-Barr virus latent membrane protein-1 expression in acquired immunodeficiency syndrome-related Ki-1 (CD30)-positive anaplastic large cell lymphomas. *Am J Clin Pathol* 1994;101:768.
38. Carbone A, Weiss LM, Gloghini A, Ferlito A. Hodgkin's disease: old and recent clinical concepts. *Ann Otol Rhinol Laryngol* 1996;105:751.
39. Gaidano G, Pastore C, Lanza C, Mazza U, Saglio G. Molecular pathology of AIDS-related lymphomas. Biologic aspects and clinicopathologic heterogeneity. *Ann Hematol* 1994;69:281.
40. Carbone A, Tirelli U, Gloghini A, Volpe R, Boiocchi M. Human immunodeficiency virus-associated systemic lymphomas may be subdivided into two main groups according to Epstein-Barr viral latent gene expression. *J Clin Oncol* 1993;11:1674.
41. Hamilton-Dutoit SJ, Pallesen G, Karkov J, Skinh JP, Franzmann MB, Pedersen C. Identification of EBV-DNA in tumour cells of AIDS-related lymphomas by *in situ* hybridization. *Lancet* 1989;1:554.
42. Herndier BG, Sanchez HC, Chang KL, Chen YY, Weiss LM. High prevalence of Epstein-Barr virus in the Reed-Sternberg cells of HIV-associated Hodgkin's disease. *Am J Pathol* 1993;142:1073.
43. Boiocchi M, Dolcetti R, De Re V, Gloghini A, Carbone A. Demonstration of a unique Epstein-Barr virus-positive cellular clone in metachronous multiple localizations of Hodgkin's disease. *Am J Pathol* 1993;142:33.
44. Di Luca D, Dolcetti R, Mirandola P, et al. Human herpesvirus 6: a survey of presence and variant distribution in normal and peripheral lymphocytes and lymphoproliferative disorders. *J Infect Dis* 1994;170:211.
45. Dolcetti R, Di Luca D, Carbone A, et al. Human herpesvirus 6 in human immunodeficiency virus-infected individuals: association with early histologic phases of lymphadenopathy syndrome but not with malignant lymphoproliferative disorders. *J Med Virol* 1996;48:344.
46. Cesarman E, Chang Y, Moore PS, Said JW, Knowles DM. Kaposi's sarcoma-associated herpesvirus-like DNA sequences in AIDS-related body-cavity-based lymphomas. *N Engl J Med* 1995;332:1186.
47. Gaidano G, Pastore C, Gloghini A, et al. Distribution of human herpesvirus-8 sequences throughout the spectrum of AIDS-related neoplasia. *AIDS* 1996;10:941.
48. Gaidano G, Carbone A. AIDS-related lymphomas: from pathogenesis to pathology. *Br J Haematol* 1995;90:235.
49. Carbone A, Gloghini A, Vaccher E, et al. Kaposi's sarcoma-associated herpesvirus DNA sequences in AIDS-related and AIDS-unrelated lymphomatous effusions. *Br J Haematol* 1996;94:533.
50. Carbone A, Tirelli U, Gloghini A, Vaccher E, Gaidano G. Herpesvirus-like DNA sequences selectively cluster with body-cavity-based lymphomas throughout the spectrum of AIDS-related lymphomatous effusions. *Eur J Cancer* 1996;32A:555.
51. Horenstein MG, Nador RG, Chadburn A, et al. Epstein-Barr virus latent gene expression in primary effusion lymphomas containing Kaposi's sarcoma-associated herpesvirus/human herpesvirus-8. *Blood* 1997;90:1186.
52. Audouin J, Diebold J, Pallesen G. Frequent expression of Epstein-Barr virus latent membrane protein-1 in tumour cells of Hodgkin's disease in HIV-positive patients. *J Pathol* 1992;167:381.
53. Siebert JD, Ambinder RF, Napoli VM, Quintanilla-Martinez L, Banks PM, Gulley ML. Human immunodeficiency virus-associated Hodgkin's disease contains latent, not replicative, Epstein-Barr virus. *Hum Pathol* 1995;26:1191.
54. Karcher DS. Clinically unsuspected Hodgkin disease presenting initially in the bone marrow of patients infected with the human immunodeficiency virus. *Cancer* 1993;71:1235.
55. Hair LS, Rogers JD, Chadburn A, Sisti MBJ, Knowles DM, Powers JM. Intracerebral Hodgkin's disease in a human immunodeficiency virus-seropositive patient. *Cancer* 1991;67:2931.
56. Shaw MT, Jacobs SR. Cutaneous Hodgkin's disease in a patient with human immunodeficiency virus infection. *Cancer* 1989;64:2585.
57. Tirelli U, Errante D, Vaccher E, et al. Hodgkin's disease in 92 patients with HIV infection: the Italian experience. *Ann Oncol* 1992;3:S69.
58. Monfardini S, Tirelli U, Vaccher E, Foà R, Gavosto F, for the Gruppo Italiano Cooperativo AIDS e Tumori (GICAT). Hodgkin's disease in 63 intravenous drug users infected with human immunodeficiency virus. *Ann Oncol* 1991;2(Suppl 2):201.
59. Tirelli U, Vaccher E, Serraino D, et al. Comparison of presenting clinical and laboratory findings of patients with persistent generalized lymphadenopathy (PGL) syndrome and malignant lymphoma (ML). *Haematologica* 1987;72:563.
60. Errante D, Zagonel V, Vaccher E, et al. Hodgkin's disease in patients with HIV infection and in the general population: comparison of clinicopathological features and survival. *Ann Oncol* 1994;5(Suppl 2):S37.
61. Coker DD, Morris DM, Coleman JJ, Schimpff SC, Wiernik PH, Elias EG. Infections among 210 patients with surgically staged Hodgkin's disease. *Am J Med* 1983;75:97.
62. Notter DT, Grossman PL, Rosenberg SA, Remington JS. Infections in patients with Hodgkin's disease: a clinical study of 300 consecutive adult patients. *Rev Infect Dis* 1980;2:761.
63. Coiffier B. Prognostic factors in Hodgkin's disease and non-Hodgkin's lymphomas. *Curr Opin Oncol* 1991;3:843.
64. Errante D, Tirelli U, Gastaldi R, et al. Combined antineoplastic and antiretroviral therapy for patients with Hodgkin's disease and human immunodeficiency virus infection. A prospective study of 17 patients. *Cancer* 1994;73:437.

65. Zittoun R, Eghbali H, Audebert A, et al. Association d'épirubicine, bléomycine, vinblastine et prednisone (EBVP) avant radiothérapie dans les stades localisés de la maladie de Hodgkin. *Bull Cancer* 1987;74:151.
66. Tirelli U, Errante D, Gisselbrecht C, et al. Epirubicin, bleomycin, vinblastine and prednisone (EBVP) chemotherapy (CT) in combination with antiretroviral therapy and primary use of G-CSF for patients with Hodgkin's disease and HIV infection (HD-HIV). *Proceedings of the American Society of Clinical Oncology* 1996:15:304(abst).
67. Levine AM, Cheung T, Tulpule A, Huang J, Testa M. Preliminary results of AIDS Clinical Trials Group (ACTG) Study No. 149: phase II trial of ABVD chemotherapy with G-CSF in HIV-infected patients with Hodgkin's disease (HD). *AIDS* 1997;14:A12(abst).
68. Kaplan L, Kahn J, Northfelt D, Abrams D, Volberding P. Novel combination chemotherapy for Hodgkin's disease in HIV-infected individuals. *Proceedings of the American Society of Clinical Oncology* 1991; 10:33(abst).

SUGGESTED READINGS

Audouin J, Diebold J, Pallesen G. Frequent expression of Epstein-Barr virus latent membrane protein-1 in tumour cells of Hodgkin's disease in HIV-positive patients. *J Pathol* 1992;167:381.

Bellas C, Santón A, Manzanal A, et al. Pathological, immunological, and molecular features of Hodgkin's disease associated with HIV infection. Comparison with ordinary Hodgkin's disease. *Am J Surg Pathol* 1996; 20:1520.

Biggar RJ, Horm J, Goedert JJ, Melbye M. Cancer in a group at risk of acquired immunodeficiency syndrome (AIDS) through 1984. *Am J Epidemiol* 1987;126:578.

Boiocchi M, De Re V, Gloghini A, et al. High incidence of monoclonal EBV episomes in Hodgkin's disease and anaplastic large-cell Ki-1-positive lymphomas in HIV-1-positive patients. *Int J Cancer* 1993;54:53.

Boiocchi M, Dolcetti R, De Re V, Gloghini A, Carbone A. Demonstration of a unique Epstein-Barr virus-positive cellular clone in metachronous multiple localizations of Hodgkin's disease. *Am J Pathol* 1993;142:33.

Carbone A, Tirelli U, Gloghini A, Volpe R, Boiocchi M. Human immunodeficiency virus-associated systemic lymphomas may be subdivided into two main groups according to Epstein-Barr viral latent gene expression. *J Clin Oncol* 1993;11:1674.

Carbone A, Dolcetti R, Gloghini A, et al. Immunophenotypic and molecular analyses of acquired immune deficiency syndrome-related and Epstein-Barr virus-associated lymphomas: a comparative study. *Hum Pathol* 1996;27:133.

Carbone A, Weiss LM, Gloghini A, Ferlito A. Hodgkin's disease: old and recent clinical concepts. *Ann Otol Rhinol Laryngol* 1996;105:751.

Errante D, Zagonel V, Vaccher E, et al. Hodgkin's disease in patients with HIV infection and in the general population: comparison of clinicopathological features and survival. *Ann Oncol* 1994;5(Suppl 2):S37.

Levine AM. HIV-associated Hodgkin's disease. Biologic and clinical aspects. *Hematol Oncol Clin North'20Am* 1996;10:1135.

Lyter DW, Bryant J, Thackeray R, Rinaldo CR, Kingsley LA. Incidence of human immunodeficiency virus-related and nonrelated malignancies in a large cohort of homosexual men. *J Clin Oncol* 1995;13:2540.

Rabkin CS, Yellin F. Cancer incidence in a population with a high prevalence of infection with human immunodeficiency virus type 1. *J Natl Cancer Inst* 1994;86:1711.

Ree HJ, Strauchen JA, Khan AA, et al. Human immunodeficiency virus-associated Hodgkin's disease. Clinicopathologic studies of 24 cases and preponderance of mixed cellularity type characterized by the occurrence of fibrohistiocytoid stromal cells. *Cancer* 1991;67:1614.

Reynolds P, Saunders LD, Layefsky ME, Lemp GF. The spectrum of acquired immunodeficiency syndrome (AIDS)-associated malignancies in San Francisco, 1980–1987. *Am J Epidemiol* 1993;137:19.

Tirelli U, Errante D, Dolcetti R, et al. Hodgkin's disease and human immunodeficiency virus infection: clinicopathologic and virologic features of 114 patients from the Italian Cooperative Group on AIDS and Tumors. *J Clin Oncol* 1995;13:1758.

Hodgkin's Disease, edited by P. M. Mauch, J. O. Armitage, V. Diehl, R. T. Hoppe, and L. M. Weiss. Lippincott Williams & Wilkins, Philadephia ©1999.

CHAPTER 40

Hodgkin's Disease in the Elderly

Vincent F. Guinee, Johan Magnus Björkholm, and Silvio Monfardini

THE ELDER EFFECT

Hodgkin's disease in older adults, "the elderly," has been considered an enigma. The "elder effect" is not a defined entity or condition. It is measured by a decreasing responsiveness to treatment with increasing age at diagnosis. It is reflected in rates of complete remission (CR), relapse, and survival. Several factors have made it difficult to determine when this phenomenon actually occurs.

First, the numbers of patients available to study have been small. Of the published studies specifically concerned with older patients during the past decade, four reports had fewer than 50 patients (1–4), three reports had about 65 patients (5–7), and only six reports had 99 or more patients (8–13). Three of these 13 studies chose a "cutoff" of 50 years of age, and the others used age 60 or 65. Second, studies have often chosen a single age as the cutoff and have compared the clinical course of patients above and below that age. As might be expected, whatever age is chosen can be supported by poor results in the older group, with patients in their 80s, and good results in the younger group, with patients in their 20s. It should also be noted that in studies in which the apparently same cutoff of 60 years or more is used, the age distributions above 60 can be completely different.

To address these problems, a large international study (8) of the International Cancer Patient Data Exchange System intentionally limited its age groups to the four decades from 40 to 79 years. This allowed for the comparison of a continuum and also eliminated cases representing extreme values. When the survival curves for patients with Hodgkin's disease in each decade were examined, patients in the groups comprising 40 to 49 and 50 to 59 years had essentially overlapping curves. The change in prognosis appeared in the cohort of patients who were 60 to 69 years old. This was seen in survival based on all causes of death (Fig. 1) as well as in disease-specific survival based only on deaths resulting from Hodgkin's disease (Fig. 2).

When another set of parameters was used, a somewhat different picture emerged (Table 1). The percentage of patients with CR was the same for patients 50 to 79 years old (85%), but it was somewhat better for patients in the 40- to 49-year cohort (91%). The percentage of patients who relapsed by 2 years was the same for patients 40 to 69 years old (12–19%), but it was dramatically different for patients in the oldest decade (41%).

The Swedish National Cancer Programme, a population-based study (1985–89), also reported results by age in the four decades comprising 40 to 79 years (12) (Table 2). Among the patients treated with a curative intent, a steady decline in survival was seen based on total deaths and disease-specific deaths. The largest difference in percentages of deaths and deaths resulting from Hodgkin's disease was at the decade of 60 to 69 years. The CR rate was best in the youngest decade, intermediate in the two middle decades, and definitely decreased in the 70- to 79-year age group. The percentages for "freedom from progression" were comparable for the three younger decades but lower for the 70- to 79-year group.

Based on an analysis of 1,197 patients with Hodgkin's disease treated at Stanford (1981–96), Rosenberg (5) reported essentially identical disease-specific survival curves for 933 patients ages 10 to 39 years and 174 patients ages 40 to 59 years. Patients 60 years and older had a decreased survival (64).

In a study of patients with Hodgkin's disease diagnosed between 1979 and 1988 in three Swedish counties, Enblad (6) found cause-specific survival was very similar for patients less than 40 years old and those from 40 to 60 years old. However, the 61 patients above the age of 60 years had poor survival.

V. F. Guinee: Department of Internal Medicine, University of Texas—Houston Medical School, Houston, Texas.

M. Björkholm: Department of Medicine, Karolinska Institute and Hospital, Stockholm, Sweden.

S. Monfardini: Division of Medical Oncology, Azienda University Hospital, Padova, Italy.

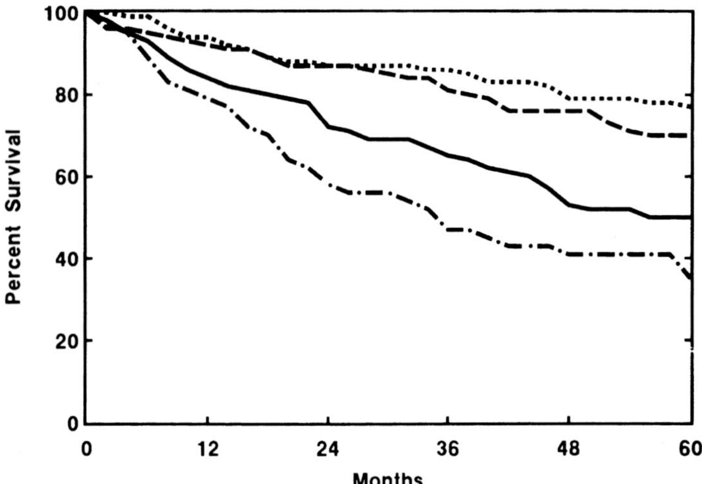

FIG. 1. Survival of patients with Hodgkin's disease by age. Patients (...) 40–49 years (n = 116), (– –) 50–59 years (n = 107), (——) 60–69 years (n = 88), (–·–) 70–79 years (n = 48). (From ref. 8, with permission.)

It would be expected that a biologic response measured by different parameters, in different populations, would vary somewhat in presentation. If one were to seek a strict age demarcation for the onset of the "elder effect," it would be the 60- to 69-year decade. However, these large studies with defined age groups would support the view that the "elder effect" is not an all-or-none phenomenon at any age. It affects an increasing proportion of patients with each successive decade of age. It would appear to affect some patients in the 50-year age group, is evident in the 60-year age group, and is a prominent factor in the poor prognosis of the 70- to 79-year age group.

Components of the Elder Effect

In reality, what is known and not known about this older patient population has become better defined. Although cure rates comparable with those in younger patients have not yet been achieved, progress has been made. A number of clinical concerns linked to poor prognosis have been addressed and clarified in an international study involving eight cancer centers in five countries (8).

Delay in diagnosis has been offered as an explanation for the poor prognosis of elderly patients. In this study, there was no major difference in the time span between initial symptoms and registration in the four decades from 40 to 79 years of age. In fact, in the 70- to 79-year-old group, the median time lapse of 18 weeks was less than that seen in the three younger decades (21 to 24 weeks). In addition, for the total study population, survival was the same for patients with intervals between first symptom to registration of 0 to 6 weeks, 7 to 20 weeks, and 21 or more weeks. Of interest, the median interval between the first symptom and registration was the same for patients with and without B symptoms (22 weeks).

Advanced stage at presentation has also been thought to contribute to the poor prognosis of older adults with Hodgkin's disease. This was not apparent in this study population. Whereas 24% of the 223 patients ages 40 to 59 had stage I, 36% of the 136 patients ages 60 to 79 pre-

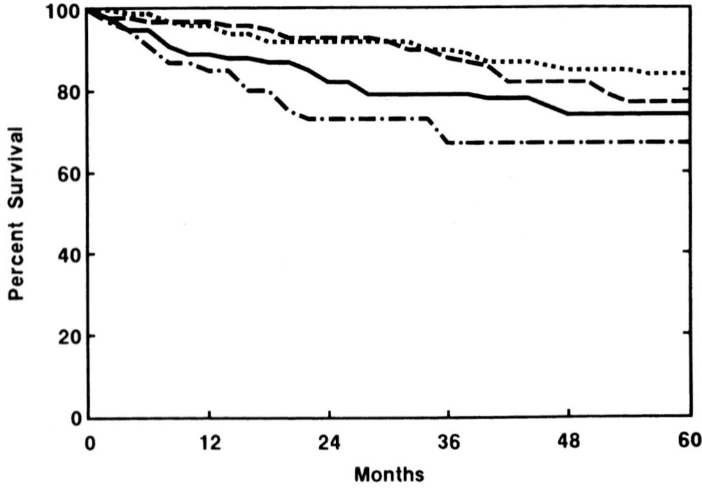

FIG. 2. Disease-specific survival of patients with Hodgkin's disease by age. Patients (...) 40–49 years (n = 116), (– –) 50–59 years (n = 107), (——) 60–69 years (n = 88), (–·–) 70–79 years (n = 48). (From ref. 8, with permission.)

TABLE 1. *Complete remission and relapse among 356 patients with Hodgkin's disease by age*

Age (y)	No. patients	CR (%)	Relapse (%)
40–49	115	91	12
50–59	105	85	16
60–69	88	83	19
70–79	48	85	41

CR, complete remission.
From ref. 8.

sented with stage I. The two age groups had essentially the same percentages of stage IV, 19% for the younger and 18% for the older patients.

Histology has also been linked to poor prognosis, primarily because mixed cellularity is more common in older adults, who have a poor prognosis. In this study, the survival of patients with nodular sclerosis and mixed cellularity histologic subtypes was found to be the same within the younger and older patient cohorts. In the 40- to 59-year-old age group, the 5-year survival was 82% for nodular sclerosis and 79% for patients with mixed cellularity disease. In the 60- to 79-year age cohort, 5-year survival showed a similar decline for both histologic subtypes, to 71% for nodular sclerosis and 70% for mixed cellularity.

The prognosis of elderly patients with Hodgkin's disease was obscured in older studies by the inclusion of deaths from other causes in survival calculations. A visual comparison between the survival curves by age based on all causes (Fig. 1) and curves based solely on deaths from Hodgkin's disease (Fig. 2) shows the dramatic difference achieved by removing deaths from other causes from survival calculations. In this international study, a series of Cox proportional hazards models was used to delineate factors that predicted the risk for death. It was found that the risk for death from Hodgkin's disease among the 60- 79-year age group was 2.17 times that of the 40- to 59-year-old group (CI, 1.37–3.43). However, of particular interest, the older patient group had a risk for death from "other causes" that was four times that of the younger group. It is now obvious that in earlier studies, deaths from other causes were sufficiently frequent to suppress the calculated survival rates of older patients with Hodgkin's disease to a significant degree.

Of note, the "elder effect" should be distinguished from the clinical course of patients in whom disease was diagnosed and treated when they were in their 40s and in whom second tumors then developed when they were in their 60s (14). For these patients, the therapeutic approach is to reduce the extent of initial treatment.

The above-mentioned factors have not been found to play a major role in the prognosis of older patients with Hodgkin's disease. However, in subsequent discussions dealing with the poor prognosis of the elderly, two basic problems do emerge as a recurrent theme—toxicity early in treatment and relapse early in recovery.

TABLE 2. *Treatment results in 193 patients with advanced Hodgkin's disease according to age at diagnosis*

Age (y)	No. patients[a]	CR (%)	FFP (%)	Deaths (%)	Deaths from Hodgkin's disease (%)
40–49	48	88	54	29	19
50–59	39	79	67	36	26
60–69	56	73	55	52	41
70–79	50	50	42	68	52

CR, complete remission; FFP, freedom from progression.
[a]Only patients for whom the treatment intention was curative are included.
From ref. 12.

TREATMENT EXPERIENCE

A few reports have stated that elderly patients may do as well as younger patients provided "adequate" therapy is given. One major factor explaining the discrepancy in treatment results of elderly patients between different series is patient selection. When interpreting therapeutic studies of Hodgkin's disease in the elderly, one should be aware of the fact that differences in patient selection may be very pronounced. This may be related to type of hospital or health care system, or to geographic and many other factors. In addition, it is well-known that in a rather large proportion of elderly patients (10–20%), Hodgkin's disease is diagnosed postmortem (15,16). Some of these patients might have benefited from a correct diagnosis and a potentially curative treatment.

In many early reports, before the introduction of modern principles of therapy, survival in elderly patients was shorter than in the young (17,18). The development of effective, wide-field, megavoltage radiation techniques and the introduction of combination chemotherapy have dramatically improved the prognosis in Hodgkin's disease. However, this has mainly been achieved in series with young patients, whereas the outcome in elderly patients remains uncertain. In most large series, a decline in response to treatment starts around the age of 40, and with increasing age the survival becomes progressively shorter (18,19). Older age (above 50–60 years) has been reported as an adverse prognostic factor for survival in many studies of patients treated according to modern principles, both with primary Hodgkin's disease (12,15, 20–23) and in relapse (24). This seems to be true also for localized (25) and infradiaphragmatic (26) disease. In contrast, the significance of age as a factor predicting freedom from first and second relapse is less certain (10,20,21). The causes of these less favorable survival rates of older patients compared with younger patients remain in part undetermined. Increased risks for intercurrent death, death from complications of treatment, or death from Hodgkin's disease are all possibilities (23).

The German Hodgkin Study Group compared the toxicity and efficacy of standard regimens in adult patients with Hodgkin's disease who were older and younger than 60 years. Older patients experienced more World Health Organization grade 3–4 hematologic and nonhematologic toxicity and had more and longer delays in chemotherapy and more dose reduction than did younger patients. Freedom from treatment failure and overall survival were significantly worse for patients older than 60 years. The authors stated that the twofold to fourfold higher toxicity and death rates of the older age group could not be explained by preexisting impairment of lung, liver, heart, and kidney function, as the presence of such impairment was a criterion for exclusion from these trials (27).

No specific chemotherapy regimens are recommended for elderly patients with Hodgkin's disease. Most investigators have used the same multiagent schedules as in the younger population, with necessary modifications to avoid unacceptable toxicity. The use of well-tolerated low-aggressivity chemotherapy programs such as CVP/CEB (chlorambucil, vinblastine, procarbazine/cyclophosphamide, etopside, bleomycin) has been unsuccessful with regard to event-free and overall survival (9). In the Swedish National Care Program (1985–88), elderly patients who received conventional MOPP or MOPP/ABVD [mechlorethamine, Oncovin (vincristine), procarbazine, prednisone/Adriamycin (doxorubicin), bleomycin, vinblastine, dacarbazine] treatment with a curative intent had a disease-specific 5-year survival of just over 40% (12). The overall toxicity was significant. To decrease treatment-related morbidity and mortality, patients were given LVPP/OEPA (leukeran, vinblastine, procarbazine, prednisone/Oncovin, etoposide, prednisone, Adriamycin), with initial doses reduced by 10% to 50% of those recommended for younger patients (1989–92). Chemotherapy doses were to be increased according to patient tolerance. Unfortunately, no differences in toxicity or outcome were seen in comparison with the previous cohort (12; Enblad et al., *personal communication).* In addition, a response-adapted strategy (MOPP/ABVD to CR, with a minimum of 2 full courses) did not prove superior in elderly (or younger) patients to 4 courses of MOPP/ABVD (28; *unpublished findings*).

Another highly relevant issue is whether the association between age and outcome in Hodgkin's disease differs from that seen in other potentially curable hematologic malignancies. In a comparison with other systemic hematologic neoplasms, such as acute leukemia and non-Hodgkin's lymphoma, this does not appear to be the case (29). In non-Hodgkin's lymphoma, there seems to be no clear difference between elderly and younger patients with regard to the proportion of patients with advanced stage, B symptoms, number and sites of extranodal disease, presence of anemia, or levels of lactate dehydrogenase (30). However, as in Hodgkin's disease, a higher percentage of patients present with concomitant disease and a low probability of being included in prospective clinical trials. In almost all studies, the survival of elderly patients with non-Hodgkin's lymphoma is reported to be inferior to that of younger patients. This difference persists when cause-specific survival is analyzed and causes of death not related to the lymphoma or its treatment are excluded. Older age as an adverse prognostic factor was also confirmed in the International Non-Hodgkin's Lymphoma Prognostic Factors Project (31). In that analysis, the complete remission rates of older patients (above 60 years) were only slightly lower than those of younger patients. However, both relapse-free and overall survival rates were much lower in the elderly population. Slightly longer survival of elderly patients with aggressive lymphoma has been observed for patients treated with an anthracycline-containing regimen (32).

Factors such as inadequate therapy, decreased tolerance to treatment, presence of intercurrent diseases, and accumulation of certain clinical, "biologic," and other risk factors, such as immunologic impairment and short familial life span, may all to a varying degree contribute to poor outcome in elderly patients with Hodgkin's disease. However, based on the results of various patient series, there seems to exist a subpopulation of elderly patients who can undergo adequate diagnostic procedures and also tolerate intensive treatment. These patients appear to have an outcome (complete remission rate and relapse-free and overall survival) as good as that seen in younger patients (8,10,33). The discrepancy in reported treatment results in the elderly is probably mainly the consequence of a broad variation of selection mechanisms. For the whole group of elderly patients, the paradox remains: elderly patients need more effective antitumor treatment but at the same time less toxic therapy.

Given this background, what should be the optimal treatment strategy for the individual elderly patient with Hodgkin's disease? Certain factors need to be considered. These include the patient's physical and mental condition, disease history, presence of concurrent disorders, and the patient's attitude to the disease and its treatment. The elderly person with a preserved good physical and mental capacity should undergo the same diagnostic and staging procedure as the younger patient. However, exploratory laparotomy should be avoided. In biologically "young" patients with clinical stage (CS) IA disease, mantle and inverted-Y fields can be irradiated, just as in younger patients. However, the majority of elderly patients will receive radiotherapy with reduced volumes according to biologic age. In patients with disease presentation in the upper neck, the axillae and lower part of the mediastinum may be excluded. Radiotherapy should be given at least to the involved and adjacent lymph node regions. Possibly, treatment to somewhat larger volumes (24–33 Gy) can be given, followed by involved-field treatment to 33 to 38 Gy. For intermediate stages (IB, IIA), 2 cycles of chemotherapy may be administered before radiotherapy. For stage IIA disease, radiotherapy alone may be given to patients who are adequately staged and expected to tolerate relatively large volumes and whose involvement is limited to two lymph node regions.

In advanced stages, treatment should also be given with a curative intent, and the same treatment strategy should be followed as in the younger patient population. However, recently developed chemotherapy programs (not proven to be more efficacious in either young or old patients) associated with known severe hematologic toxicity should be avoided. The well-established ABVD combination or variants thereof may be considered as a first-line combination for patients judged to be in need of chemotherapy. Radiotherapy to initially bulky disease should be considered. Support with hematopoietic growth factors should be given liberally. Close monitoring of toxicity and response to treatment are important to adjust treatment at an early point. Granulocyte colony-stimulating factor (G-CSF) should be given to patients who experience the infectious complications of neutropenia. In addition, G-CSF is indicated in patients when the recommended time interval between courses is exceeded and when major dose reductions (>50% on one or >75% on two occasions) are required. However, there are no studies to support a better outcome with G-CSF when it is used to maintain the relative dose intensity.

Very old patients with Hodgkin's disease and disabled patients with concurrent disorders that preclude any curative treatment should be given good palliative care, which may include symptomatic involved-field radiotherapy and oral combination chemotherapy; CEP (CCNU, etoposide, and prednimustine) or similar combinations may be a useful alternative (34).

In the remaining categories of elderly patients with Hodgkin's disease, it is more difficult to recommend a uniform treatment strategy. Less intensive staging procedures may be considered, and extensive radiotherapy should probably be avoided. Lower-aggressivity chemotherapy programs, such as the combination of vinblastine, bleomycin, and methotrexate, may be given as primary treatment (35,36). Patients showing a good tolerance and response to this kind of chemotherapy may be switched to conventional ABVD-like chemotherapy.

SELECTION OF PATIENTS

Only a small fraction of patients with cancer receive treatment in clinical trials. Martin and colleagues (37) reported a survey of potential study subjects in 13 Veterans Administration hospitals that identified 2,687 patients with one of several tumor sites. Of these, only 437 (16%) actually participated in the protocol. Similarly, a cross-sectional survey by Begg and colleagues (38) of 2,487 patients being treated in hospitals affiliated with a cooperative oncology group showed just 16% enrolled in any protocol.

To determine the representation of elderly patients in clinical trial protocols sponsored by the National Cancer Institute (NCI), Trimble and colleagues (39) used incidence data from the Surveillance, Epidemiology, and End Results (SEER) program to compare accrual of both men and women for studies of five major cancer sites. With respect to incidence, older patients were significantly ($p < .001$) underrepresented in cancer treatment trials, with the exception of treatment for prostate cancer. This is particularly interesting because age *per se* was not a valid eligibility criterion for these trials. In all 10 sex-site combinations, the mean ages of patients in the NCI trials were less than the mean ages of patients in the SEER groups.

The authors proposed several factors to explain this situation. They felt that older patients would be more likely to have a prior malignancy or a comorbid condition. They noted that there appeared to be perceptions among clinicians, patients, and family members that older patients are less likely to benefit from aggressive therapy and are less likely to tolerate it.

Benson (40) investigated the reasons why physicians do not place patients in clinical trials in a survey of 437 physician members of the Illinois Cancer Center. Responses were received from 244 practicing oncologists. Ninety-three physicians (38%) were community-based, and 144 (59%) were hospital-based. Nearly three-fourths of the physicians (73%) stated that excessive time is required in trials for patient follow-up. Ninety-one percent indicated that trials are inconvenient for patients, and 79% felt that participation in trials imposes a financial burden on patients. Each of these factors was cited by about 25% of respondents as reasons why they had not entered patients into trials. One of the most significant findings was that more than 50% of physicians in this survey had excluded patients from clinical trials on the basis of age.

These documented reasons for reluctance to refer patients into trials were in addition to the most frequently cited reason for not enrolling patients—the rigid design of protocols. On this point, the authors stated that rigid protocol exclusion criteria not only decreased accrual but also limited the applicability of results to the total spectrum of patients. What is particularly interesting is that this survey involved physicians closely associated with an urban cancer center, physicians who would be considered to view clinical trials most favorably.

Specifically in regard to the topic of exclusion criteria, the Toronto Leukemia Study Group examined the effect of exclusions on the analysis of chemotherapy regimens for adults with acute myelogenous leukemia (41). All patients with this diagnosis admitted consecutively to 14 general hospitals in the Toronto region were included. The complete remission rate for a group of 142 patients was 52% if no exclusions were applied, but it was 91%

for the 68 patients who were evaluated after five exclusion criteria were applied based on such factors as previous disease, completion of treatment, and age.

Concerning exclusion criteria for protocols, an editorial by Kennedy (42) stated that patients older than 70 years have been excluded from almost all clinical trials, resulting in a real lack of information on therapeutic management in this age group. Further, the sparsity of pharmacokinetic and phase I or II studies of older persons makes it impossible to select the best regimens in older persons. Fentiman et al. (43) stated the problem succinctly: "The elderly, disenfranchised as they are from entry to clinical trials, receive either untested treatments, inadequate treatment, or even none at all."

Thus, we have the obvious exclusionary practices associated with protocol research documented in writing, while the more subtle influences on patterns of referral to cancer centers and other teaching hospitals remain unexpressed in writing. With this in mind, we can better assess the variations in clinical research reports.

IS HODGKIN'S DISEASE IN OLDER PATIENTS A DIFFERENT DISEASE?

The constant biomodality of the age-specific incidence and mortality rate curves led MacMahon in 1966 (44) to propose the hypothesis that Hodgkin's disease in younger and older adults comprised different entities with probably distinct etiologies. The younger group, with a peak risk at about 25 to 30 years, included most patients between 15 and 34 years old. The older subgroup included most patients over 50 years of age. In the data available at that time, the younger group had a male-to-female ratio of 1:1, in contrast to a 2:1 ratio in the group 50 years old and over. Subsequent data were not as clear-cut.

MacMahon also noted a confirmatory international variation in mortality rates, with two modes of approximately equal prominence in Denmark, a second mode of greater prominence in the United States, and a striking absence of the first mode in Japan. He felt that the epidemiologic subdivision of Hodgkin's disease based on age was particularly meaningful in terms of survival. Persons over 50 years of age had a 5-year survival percentage less than half that of younger patients. At this time, he felt that the disease in young adults was probably infectious and in the "elderly" most likely a neoplasm.

In a subsequent analysis in 1971 (45), MacMahon quoted recently published data from the Royal Marsden Hospital showing the nodular sclerosis histology to be predominant in young adults and MC in the older group. It is indicative of the literature of the time that MacMahon wrote, "One can search in vain for the ages of patients that were the source of material for many reported studies of potential causal factors in Hodgkin's disease." To put these observations in perspective, MacMahon did comment that even if patients with Hodgkin's disease encompassed persons with diseases of different etiologies, they might still constitute a group that could usefully be considered as a single disease category for diagnostic and therapeutic purposes.

Medeiros and Greiner (46) reported that incidence data from the SEER program suggest that Hodgkin's disease, "as it is currently defined," is a heterogeneous entity composed of at least two different diseases—nodular sclerosis and MC, which represent the early and late modes of the bimodal curve, respectively. This analysis dealt with 9,418 microscopically confirmed cases of Hodgkin's disease collected between 1973 and 1987.

Nodular sclerosis was essentially unimodal, with a peak in young adults ages 20 to 24 years. In this age group,

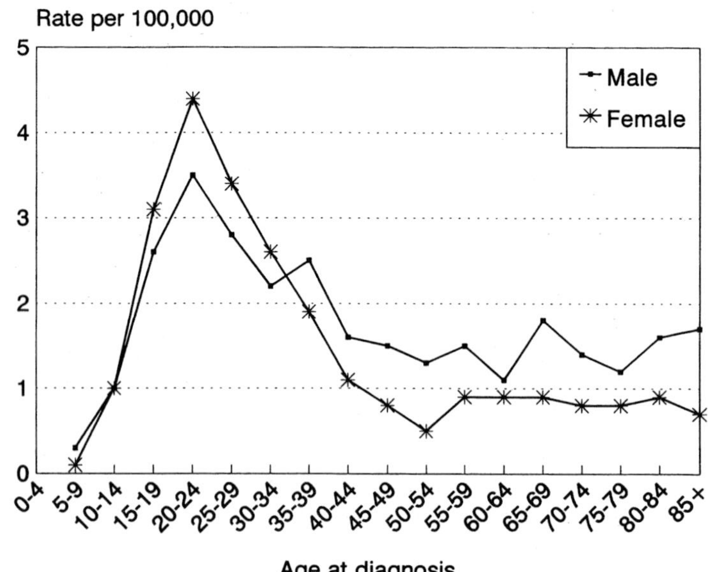

FIG. 3. Nodular sclerosis Hodgkin's disease: age-specific incidence rates by sex, all races. Surveillance, Epidemiology, and End Results (SEER), 1983–1987. (From ref. 46, with permission.)

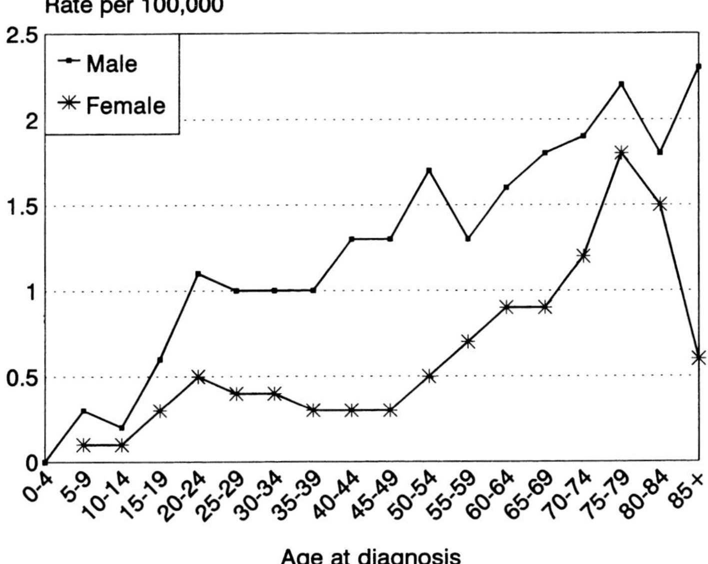

FIG. 4. Mixed-cellularity Hodgkin's disease: age-specific incidence rates by sex, all races. Surveillance, Epidemiology, and End Results (SEER), 1983–1987. (From ref. 46, with permission.)

about 75% of all cases of Hodgkin's disease were of the nodular sclerosis subtype (Fig. 3). Mixed cellularity also presented in a unimodal distribution and gradually increased with age, with a peak age-specific incidence rate in the elderly (Fig. 4). In men older than 70 years, the proportion of mixed cellularity cases approached 50%. These authors quoted studies showing the Epstein-Barr virus (EBV) to be present in most cases of mixed cellularity but in only a small subset of cases of nodular sclerosis. But the situation was not that clear-cut. They also pointed out that studies of DNA content and molecular genetics showed Hodgkin's disease subtypes also to be heterogeneous.

In an international study by Glaser et al. (47), the tumor EBV status was assessed in 1,546 patients with Hodgkin's disease collected from 14 investigator groups. A total of 618 study subjects (40%) were EBV-positive. The highest percentages of EBV-positive cases occurred in children younger than 10 and in adults older than 80. EBV gene products were present in approximately 75% of mixed cellularity tumors but in only 25% of nodular sclerosis cases. The authors concluded that the epidemiologic characteristics considered in their study did not discriminate "neatly" between the two virus-defined subtypes of Hodgkin's disease.

Histologic and viral data aside, one of the main arguments in favor of the hypothesis that Hodgkin's disease in the elderly is a different disease was the poor prognosis observed in patients more than 50 years of age. In some respects, this is circular reasoning, as follows: (a) it must be a different disease because the prognosis is poor, and (b) the prognosis is poor because it is a different disease. Changes in therapy since the 1970s have improved survival for all age groups, including the elderly. In addition, the observed survival rates have better reflected the response to treatment of Hodgkin's disease in older patients, as actuarial presentations have been replaced by disease-specific survival calculations. The latter survival estimates do not include deaths from other causes, a significant factor in the older patient group.

In an overview of this topic, Gustavsson (48) pointed out that several consequences of normal aging may contribute to a different course of Hodgkin's disease in the elderly. Normal tissues show a decreasing regenerative capacity. Because of a decline in bone marrow proliferative capacity, sensitivity to drugs increases. Reduction in the total amount of body water leads to increased blood levels of water-soluble drugs. And finally, many older patients have coexisting diseases being treated with medicines that can interact adversely with antineoplastic chemotherapy. She concluded that the specific features of Hodgkin's disease in the elderly should not be a reason for it to be interpreted as a different disease; rather, these differences should be ascribed to the fact that the hosts are different.

ROLE OF IMMUNOCOMPETENCE

Parker et al. (49) and Steiner (50) were the first to postulate that the susceptibility to tuberculosis of persons with Hodgkin's disease might reflect an immunologic derangement. Since then, numerous studies have confirmed the depression of delayed skin hypersensitivity, not only to tuberculin but also to other recall antigens and neoantigens, in a high proportion of untreated patients with Hodgkin's disease (51). Other organisms, control of which also depends in large part on an intact cell-mediated immune capability, have been frequently encountered in patients with Hodgkin's disease. They include varicella-zoster virus, various fungi, *Toxoplasma, Listeria,* and other unusual infectious agents. Indeed, patients with Hodgkin's disease show severe abnormalities in variables related to cellular immune responses, including lymphocytopenia, total (CD3+, CD4+, CD8+) and relative (CD3+, CD4+) T lymphocytopenia, decreased mitogen- and antigen-induced blood lymphocyte DNA synthesis, impaired response in the mixed lymphocyte reaction, and increased number of lymphocytes (mainly T cells) activated *in vivo* (51). It is generally agreed that B-lymphocyte functions (including serum immunoglobulin levels) are well preserved in untreated patients except in far-advanced disease. The exact nature of the mechanisms of the cellular immune defect in Hodgkin's disease is not known. However, it seems likely that T-cell activation and accumulation in the tumor tissue (lymphocyte maldistribution), resulting in an intense but ineffective immune response, may contribute (52,53).

Today, infectious complications in the untreated patient with Hodgkin's disease are a limited clinical problem. The large majority of serious infections are encountered during treatment and more often in the elderly population. These infections are commonly caused by bacterial pathogens and related to the myelosuppressive effects of cytotoxic drug therapy and radiotherapy (54). In addition, an increased incidence of bacterial infections is observed in patients likely to be cured of their disease. Among identifiable factors predisposing patients to infection are older age and advanced disease at diagnosis and prior extensive treatment. Splenectomy and irradiation to the spleen predispose patients to the development of septicemia, which is caused predominantly by pneumococci, although other pathogens, such as *Haemophilus influenzae, Escherichia coli,* and *Staphylococcus aureus*, may be isolated. The risk for infection does not seem to decrease with time following splenectomy or with increasing age (55,56).

Normal aging is also accompanied by a decline in immune reactivity, which to a major extent can be attributed to changes in the level of regulatory CD4+ T cells. Blood lymphocyte blastogenesis and DNA synthesis induced by T-cell mitogens decline in adults older than 30 years and are severely impaired in healthy persons older than 70 years (Fig. 5) (57). However, in centenarians (who are a good example of successful aging), several immune variables are well conserved (58). Thus, longitudinal studies will tell whether the number, type, and function of T cells (partly related to the genetic background) are associated with longevity, morbidity, and mortality in free-living elderly humans.

In larger series of patients, certain facets of the immunodeficiency, such as lymphocytopenia, a high spontaneous blood lymphocyte DNA synthesis and decreased mitogen-induced blood lymphocyte DNA synthesis, were strongly associated with a poor prognosis (survival). Despite the fact that functional lymphocyte abnormalities were more frequent in patients with an advanced clinical stage, older age, and the presence of B symptoms, lymphocyte DNA synthesis was besides age the strongest

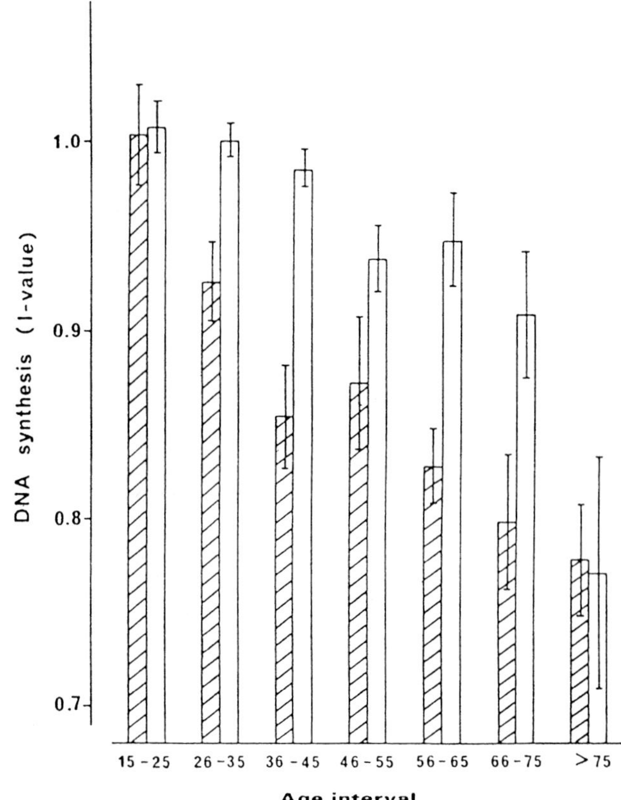

FIG. 5. Age dependency of lymphocyte DNA synthesis induced by 20 μg/mL of concanavalin A in patients ▨ and controls □. (From ref. 57, with permission.)

prognostic indicator in a multivariate analysis of 262 patients (59). Thus, as in the aging normal population, there is a conspicuous premature age-dependent decrease in the blood lymphocyte response to mitogen stimulation in patients with Hodgkin's disease (Fig. 5). Does the immunodeficiency affect response to treatment? One cannot exclude the possibility that the recorded immune impairment may be just a good surrogate marker for the severity/aggressiveness of the host-tumor interaction. Although there is a clear association between certain facets of cell-mediated immunity and outcome, there is no direct evidence to support any causal relationship. Moreover, from a clinical standpoint, the effects of immunopotentiating therapy have had no influence on the long-term course.

T lymphocytopenia and impairment of T-cell functions have also been observed in long-term survivors with Hodgkin's disease, which is in contrast to the normalization of these variables in patients with non-Hodgkin's lymphoma following successful therapy (60,61). To elucidate whether a persistent (and possibly preexisting) immune impairment (in part unrelated to tumor-associated immunosuppressive factors and treatment) is characteristic of a subpopulation of patients with Hodgkin's disease, studies of immune function were performed in the

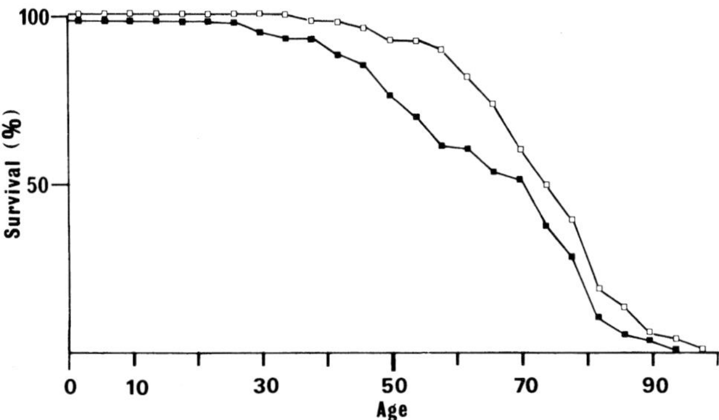

FIG. 6. Survival of parents and grandparents of living patients >50 years (n = 90; □–□) and of deceased patients >50 years (n = 79; ■–■). (From ref. 66, with permission.)

relatives of patients with Hodgkin's disease. In summary, the results of these studies show that otherwise healthy persons (including twin partners of patients who have died of progressive disease) who have a first-degree relative with Hodgkin's disease display a significantly increased frequency of T-cell impairment (62–65).

In an attempt to explore other potential factors related to prognosis in Hodgkin's disease, we studied the influence of familial longevity on outcome in a well-studied cohort of patients with Hodgkin's disease followed for a long time (66). The survival of parents and grandparents of patients more than 50 years old who died of progressive Hodgkin's disease was significantly shorter than that of ancestors of survivors in the same age group (Fig. 6). The excess death rate among relatives (less than 70 years old) of the deceased patients was caused mainly by tuberculosis, which suggests a T-cell defect. The prognostic information obtained by analyzing the life span of ancestors was superior to that derived from the clinical stage. No association between familial longevity and prognosis was observed in younger patients (50 years old or less) (Fig. 7). These findings may have important implications

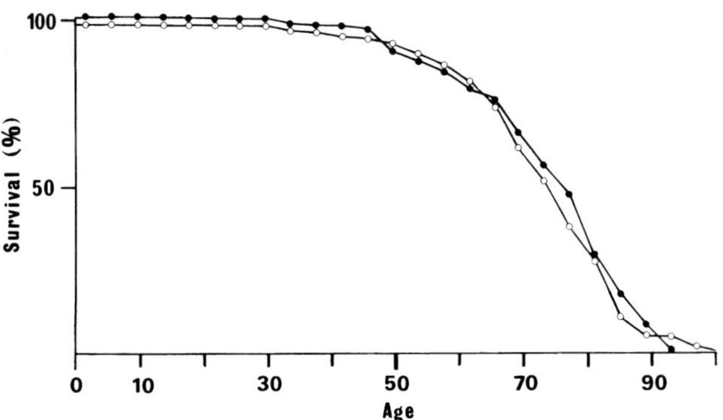

FIG. 7. Survival of parents and grandparents of living patients ≤50 years (n = 89; ○–○) and of deceased patients ≤50 years (n = 91; ●–●). (From ref. 66, with permission.)

regarding the understanding and treatment of Hodgkin's disease in the elderly.

Does immunodeficiency predispose to Hodgkin's disease? The weight of evidence suggests that close relatives of patients with Hodgkin's disease in the young adult form have a significantly increased risk for development of the disease in comparison with persons in the general population (67). Studies in identical twins suggest a genetic susceptibility (68). However, if certain defects in cell-mediated immunity are related to the pathogenesis of Hodgkin's disease or merely mirror the patient's ability to cope with Hodgkin's disease and/or its treatment, they remain to be clarified.

EVALUATION OF THE OLDER PATIENT

It is well-known that there is a wide variability in number and degree of age-associated disabilities and pathologic conditions among the elderly. The widely used performance-status test does not allow for a comprehensive evaluation of various age-related factors in the elderly. A methodic and systematic analysis of these variables has been developed and used by geriatric specialists to set up the best therapeutic plan for each patient, but this methodology is not yet well-known by clinical oncologists. In essence, the multidimensional geriatric assessment takes into consideration the presence and degree of comorbidity, physical functioning, cognitive status, and the presence and degree of depressive symptoms. Among several evaluation tools that have been validated in the elderly population, the Folstein's Mini Mental State Examination (FMMSE) can be used to evaluate cognitive status (69), information on depressive symptoms can be collected with the short form of the Geriatric Depression Scale (GDS) (70), and "self-reported" disability can be measured through the Lawton's Instrumental Activities of Daily Living (IADL) scale (71).

It should also be determined whether family and/or social support is present. Medical oncologists and hematologists are accustomed to performing a careful evaluation of cardiac, respiratory, renal, and hepatic function, but the complete spectrum of comorbid conditions present after 65 years should be considered. Preliminary observations on elderly cancer patients also confirm the coexistence of other associated diseases. For example, chronic backache, arthritis, aural and visual defects, and diabetes may not seem to be major problems, but they should not be underestimated. Chronic arthritis and backache may make it difficult for a patient to maintain a fixed position during radiotherapy. Pain medications before treatment may solve this problem. Physical disability does not seem to interfere in a strict sense with the administration of chemotherapy, but it certainly influences its continuation and regular follow-up. A patient's capability to travel to the cancer center, self-administer drugs, and call the physician or nurse by phone in case of need is important for treatment and can easily be measured with the Instrumental Activities of Daily Living (IADL) scores. There is no need to stress that mental deterioration in the elderly may lead to real problems in administration of treatment, especially if family and social support are insufficient or totally lacking. The degree of mental depression, especially in elderly women, needs to be assessed to determine whether it will be an obstacle to treatment, so that if necessary measures can be taken to overcome it.

Oncologists who have experience in the management of elderly patients with Hodgkin's disease may think that the above-described scenario is too broad and dark, but this is probably because older patients with malignant lymphomas and obvious mental or physical deterioration are not even referred to them (i.e., cancer specialists) for active treatment. This is also true for other types of neoplasia, which are treated empirically, generally not as part of a clinical trial and therefore without reports on the results of treatment. The utilization of comprehensive geriatric assessment in elderly patients with Hodgkin's disease could be useful in the context of both clinical trials and clinical practice (72). First, it could help to identify different subgroups of patients with a different natural history and survival expectancy that are not necessarily related to the underlying neoplastic condition. Second, responsible physicians would be obliged to take into account all age-associated conditions that might possibly interfere with administration of treatment and determine whether and how these could be overcome, instead of being dissuaded from recommending active and appropriate treatment because of their own or the family's ageism. With the aging of the population, elderly patients will become more aware of ageism, and more "frail" elderly patients with Hodgkin's disease will be treated appropriately. Management will be better designed based on the "host factors" (described above) present and the results of multidimensional geriatric evaluation.

The way in which the complications of Hodgkin's disease are anticipated and managed in the elderly is really no different than in other adult patients, but the severity of treatment-related complications may be more pronounced in elderly patients because of decreased organ function or comorbidity.

The consensus of opinion, based on results of a wide number of studies, is that elderly patients display a somewhat higher degree of hematologic toxicity, a more prolonged and severe neutropenia, and a higher rate of infection-related deaths secondary to chemotherapy than do younger patients. It has been shown that the hematologic response to G-CSF and GM-CSF (granulocyte-macrophage colony-stimulating factor) is well maintained in patients and normal volunteers ages 65 years and over (73,74). The possibility of preventing or overcoming bone marrow toxicity by the administration of GM-CSF might be hampered by the expression of specific receptors on tumor cells (75). G-CSF, and not GM-CSF, should then be used to treat or prevent infection-related neutropenia. Because older patients may be particularly prone to the development of infection-related fatal complications, the prompt addition of G-CSF to combination chemotherapy appears to be justified and cost-effective.

Retrospective analysis indicates that the probability of development of congestive heart failure increases from 0 to 3% at total cumulative doses of doxorubicin of 400 mg/m_2 to 18% to 31% at doses greater than 600 mg/m_2. Doses larger than 400 mg/m_2 are rarely reached with the ABVD combination, which is usually delivered in up to 6 cycles of treatment. However, reported risk factors for the development of doxorubicin cardiotoxicity include increasing age and a history of heart disease. Therefore, elderly patients with Hodgkin's disease who might potentially benefit from treatment with ABVD or other doxorubicin combinations are categorized as being at high risk for development of cardiotoxicity and may be excluded from treatment. As an alternative, doxorubicin can be started, with administration continued until a 10% reduction of the ejection fraction is noted. Another possible alternative is the addition of dexrazoxane, whose cardioprotective action was definitely demonstrated in doxorubicin-based combination chemotherapy in breast cancer (76). Determination of oxygen tension before treatment and tests of lung function to check for lung disease can guide the administration of combinations including bleomycin (e.g., ABVD).

Concurrent illnesses such as diabetes may be an obstacle to administration of treatment. Prednisone, which is included in MOPP and other combinations, can be omitted in patients with insulin-treated diabetes but can usually be given to patients being treated with oral antidiabetic agents if their blood glucose levels can be periodically checked during administration.

Hypnotics are frequently prescribed for the elderly. Procarbazine, one of the drugs of the MOPP combination, may induce drowsiness or depression. These changes in mental status may be related to the inhibition of monoamine oxidase. Other monoamine oxidase inhibitors, as well as the tricyclic antidepressants often prescribed for elderly patients, should be discontinued while MOPP is administered.

In a review, Vestal (77) outlined several important physiologic factors that may influence drug distribution in older patients. The proportion of body fat is increased, which may result in an increase in volume distribution of lipid-soluble drugs. Total body water is decreased, which can lead to higher peak concentrations of hydrophilic drugs in plasma. Liver mass is decreased, with a corresponding decrease in hepatic flow and diminished liver perfusion. Finally, renal mass is decreased, with a corresponding reduction of renal blood flow, tubular function, and glomerular filtration.

Vestal observed that few studies have dealt with aging and cancer chemotherapy. He concluded that this relative dearth of information presents many opportunities for clinical research. The same sentiments were expressed 8 years earlier by Balducci et al. (78), who cited Hodgkin's lymphoma as a likely model for the investigation of age-related alterations in drug pharmacodynamics.

FUTURE APPROACHES TO TREATMENT

We do currently lack apt biologic or clinical predictors of tolerance and outcome that could guide us in choosing treatment. However, a patient's advanced chronologic age should not deter the treating physician from maintaining a curative attitude toward treatment. It is well established that a considerable fraction of older patients may tolerate as aggressive an approach as younger patients and may have the same chance of achieving remission and relapse-free survival.

With the use of treatment programs developed for younger patients in elderly patients, the overall outlook for these patients as a group has improved. However, although the poorer survival of older patients with Hodgkin's disease has long been recognized, clinical studies exploring the potential reasons for it have been infrequent.

In addition, few studies have adequately addressed important treatment issues in the elderly population. It may be concluded that elderly patients with Hodgkin's disease constitute a heterogeneous patient population with regard to tolerance of staging and treatment as well as to outcome. Elderly patients are also more heterogeneous than younger patients in regard to comorbidity, organ function, and general functional status. This is also true for a number of other malignancies, including non-Hodgkin's lymphoma (79).

If there is an intention to treat all patients, the multidimensional geriatric evaluation can be of help in understanding whether the patient is self-sufficient or will need family and/or social support for the entire duration of treatment, treatment-related complications, and follow-up. Even depression and physical disabilities can be overcome with a proper plan. All the possible comorbidities, in addition to those that classically induce decreased organ function and interfere with the administration of chemotherapy (heart, lung, liver, kidney), should be evaluated.

The concept of sequential, moderate-dose, single-agent chemotherapy may be considered as well as immunopotentiating therapy. Low-aggressivity chemotherapy, with the option to increase doses according to patient tolerance, and a response-adapted strategy have so far not been successful.

Because the more frequent early relapse of the elderly compared with younger adults is probably often the consequence of a decreased dose intensity, the prophylactic or therapeutic use of G-CSF should be considered to accelerate bone marrow recovery after combination chemotherapy. In the case of patients at higher risk for heart toxicity who are to be treated with doxorubicin (including combinations), the administration of cardioprotective agents can be considered.

Whereas hematopoietic growth factors are a well-established modality for bone marrow protection, a prospect for the future is amifostine (ULR-2721, Ethyol), an agent developed to protect tissues from hematologic, cardiac, renal, and peripheral nervous system toxicity (80). Amifostine is well tolerated and might be quite useful to prevention toxic reactions in older patients induced by the drugs included in the most common schedules of combination chemotherapy for Hodgkin's disease (MOPP, ABVD). Specific studies are not yet available in elderly patients.

Owing to recent developments indicating that CD30 and CD40 antigens or cytokine receptors on Reed-Sternberg cells represent critical molecules regulating tumor cell growth in Hodgkin's disease, the possibility of targeting tumor cells through these specific surface structures provides an appealing future prospect. The use of toxic conjugated ligands (CD30L/CD40L) to target CD30+/CD40+ tumor cells in the treatment of Hodgkin's disease in elderly patients should be actively investigated, because of the predicted low toxicity and high biologic activity (79,81).

To establish treatment approaches specifically designed for "elderly" patients, we need the results of large series with "unselected" patients who are uniformly staged and treated. We also need to delineate and quantify the effects of decreased liver and kidney function on pharmacokinetics. In elderly patients with several risk factors, conventional treatment should be compared with best palliative treatment in regard to end points other than remission rate and relapse-free survival (e.g., functional status and quality of life). With such studies, our efforts to improve the outcome for elderly patients with Hodgkin's disease will, it is hoped, prove rewarding.

A final cautionary note—this chapter has used the term "elderly" as it commonly appears in the medical literature. "Elderly" is more of a literary word than a scientific term. It can have a negative or pessimistic connotation. It is important that our choice of words not influence our choice of treatment. A more appropriate designation for this group of patients might be "older adults."

REFERENCES

1. Zietman AL, Linggood RM, Brookes AB, Convery K, Piro A. Radiation therapy in the management of early stage Hodgkin's disease. *Cancer* 1991;68:1869.
2. Bennett JM, Andersen JW, Begg CB, Glick JH. Age and Hodgkin's disease: the impact of competing risks and possible salvage therapy on long-term survival. An E.C.O.G. study. *Leuk Res* 1993;17:10:825.
3. Erdkamp FL, Breed WP, Bosch LJ, Wijnen JT, Blijham GB. Hodgkin disease in the elderly. *Cancer* 1992;70:830.
4. Diaz-Pavon JR, Cabanillas F, Majlis A, Hagemeister FB. Outcome of Hodgkin's disease in elderly patients. *Hematol Oncol* 1995;13:19.

5. Rosenberg SA. The management of Hodgkin's disease: half a century of change. *Ann Oncol* 1996;7:555.
6. Enblad G. Hodgkin's disease in young and elderly patients, clinical and pathological studies. *Ups J Med Sci* 1994;99:1.
7. Norberg B, Dige U, Roos G, Johansson H, Lenner P. Hodgkin's disease in northern Sweden 1971–1981. *Acta Oncol* 1991;30:597.
8. Guinee VF, Giacco GG, Durand M, et al. The prognosis of Hodgkin's disease in older adults. *J Clin Oncol* 1991;9:947.
9. Levis A, Depaoli L, Bertini M, et al. Results of a low aggressivity chemotherapy regimen (CVP/CEB) in elderly Hodgkin's disease patients. *Haematologica* 1996;81:450.
10. Specht L, Nissen NI. Hodgkin's disease and age. *Eur J Haematol* 1989; 43:127.
11. Bosi A, Ponticelli P, Casini C, et al. Clinical data and therapeutic approach in elderly patients with Hodgkin's disease. *Haematologica* 1989;74:463.
12. Glimelius B. Enblad G, Kalkner M, et al. Treatment of Hodgkin's disease: the Swedish National Care Programme experience. *Leuk Lymphoma* 1996;21:71.
13. Kennedy BJ, Loeb V Jr, Peterson V, Donegan W, Natarajan N, Mettlin C. Survival in Hodgkin's disease by stage and age. *Med Pediatr Oncology* 1992;20:100.
14. Mauch PM, Kalish LA, Marcus K, et al. Long-term survival in Hodgkin's disease: relative impact of mortality, infection, second tumors, and cardiovascular disease. *Cancer* J Sci Am 1995;1:33.
15. Wedelin C, Björkholm M, Biberfeld P, Holm G, Johansson B, Mellstedt H. Prognostic factors in Hodgkin's disease with special reference to age. *Cancer* 1984;53:1202.
16. Hasle H, Mellemgaard A. Hodgkin's disease diagnosed post mortem: a population-based study. *Br J Cancer* 1993;67:185.
17. Uddströmer M. On the occurrence of lymphogranulomatosis (Sternberg) in Sweden 1915–1931 and some considerations as to its relation to tuberculosis. *Acta Tubercul Scand* 1934;1(Suppl):1.
18. Westling P. Studies of the prognosis in Hodgkin's disease. *Acta Radiol* 1965;245(Suppl):5.
19. Nordentoft AM, Pedersen-Bjergaard J, Brincker H, et al. Hodgkin's disease in Denmark. A national clinical study by the Danish Hodgkin Study Group. LYGRA. *Scand J Haematol* 1980;24:321.
20. Peterson BA, Pajak TF, Cooper MR, et al. Effect of age on therapeutic response and survival in advanced Hodgkin's disease. *Cancer Treat Rep* 1982;66:889.
21. Vaughan Hudson B, MacLennan KA, Easterling MJ, Jelliffe AM, Haybittle JL, Vaughan Hudson G. The prognostic significance of age in Hodgkin's disease: examination of 1500 patients (BNLI report no 23). *Clin Radiol* 1983;34:503.
22. Walker A, Schoenfeld ER, Lowman JT, Mettlin CJ, MacMillan J, Grufferman S. Survival of the older patient compared with the younger patient with Hodgkin's disease. *Cancer* 1990;65:1635.
23. Enblad G, Glimelius B, Sundström C. Treatment outcome in Hodgkin's disease in patients above the age of 60: a population-based study. *Ann Oncol* 1991;2:297.
24. Healey EA, Tarbell NJ, Kalish LA, et al. Prognostic factors for patients with Hodgkin's disease in first relapse. *Cancer* 1993;71:2613.
25. Tubiana M, Henry-Amar M, van der Werf-Messing B. A multivariate analysis of prognostic factors in early stage Hodgkin's disease. *Int J Radiat Oncol Biol Phys* 1985;11:23.
26. Källner KM, Enblad G, Gustavsson G, et al. Infradiaphragmatic Hodgkin's disease: the Swedish National Care Programme experience. *Eur J Haematol* 1997;59:31.
27. Sextro M. Differences in clinical presentation and course between adult patients with Hodgkin's disease older and younger than 60 years. American Society of Hematology, December 1996. *Blood* 1997;88(Suppl 1): 227A (abst).
28. Björkholm M, Axdorph U, Grimfors G, et al. Fixed versus response-adapted MOPP/ABVD chemotherapy in Hodgkin's disease. *Ann Oncol* 1995;6:895.
29. Walsh SJ, Begg CB, Carbone PP. Cancer chemotherapy in the elderly. *Semin Oncol* 1989;16:66.
30. Coiffier B. What treatment for elderly patients with aggressive lymphoma? [Editorial]. *Ann Oncol* 1994;5:873.
31. Shipp MA, Harrington DP, Anderson JR, The International Non-Hodgkin's Lymphoma Prognostic Factors Project. A predictive model for aggressive non-Hodgkin's lymphoma. *N Engl J Med* 1993; 329:987.
32. Bastion Y, Blay JY, Divine M, et al. Elderly patients with aggressive non-Hodgkin's lymphoma: disease presentation, response to treatment, and survival—a Groupe d'Etude des Lymphomes de l'Adulte study on 453 patients older than 69 years. *Clin Oncol* 1997;15:2945.
33. Austin-Seymour MM, Hoppe RT, Cox RS, Rosenberg SA, Kaplan HS. Hodgkin's disease in patients over sixty years old. *Ann Intern Med* 1984;100:13.
34. Santoro A, Viviani S, Valagussa P, Bonafante V, Bonadonna G. CCNU, etoposide and prednimustine (CEP) in refractory Hodgkin's disease. *Semin Oncol* 1986;13:23.
35. Horning SJ, Hoppe RT, Hancock SL, Rosenberg SA. Vinblastine, bleomycin, and methotrexate: an effective adjuvant in favorable Hodgkin's disease. *J Clin Oncol* 1988;6:1822.
36. Gherlinzoni F, Zinzani PL, Magagnoli M, et al. VMB regimen for Hodgkin's disease in the elderly. Presented at the Fourth International Symposium on Hodgkin's Lymphoma, March 28–April 1, 1998. *Leuk Lymphoma* 1998;29(Suppl 1):71(abst).
37. Martin JF, Henderson WG, Zacharski LR. Accrual of patients into a multihospital cancer clinical trial and its implications on planning future studies. *J Clin Oncol* 1984;7:173.
38. Begg CB, Zelen M, Carbone PP, et al. Cooperative groups and community hospitals: measurement of impact in the community hospitals. *Cancer* 1983;52:1760.
39. Trimble EL, Carter CL, Cain D, et al. Representation of older patients in cancer treatment trials. *Cancer* 1994;7:2208.
40. Benson AB. Oncologists' reluctance to accrue patients onto clinical trials: an Illinois Cancer Center study. *J Clin Oncol* 1991;9:2067.
41. The Toronto Leukemia Study Group. Results of chemotherapy for unselected patients with acute myeloblastic leukemia: effect of exclusions on interpretation of results. *Lancet* 1986;1:786.
42. Kennedy BJ. Needed: clinical trials for older patients [Editorial]. *J Clin Oncol* 1991;9:718.
43. Fentiman I, Tirelli U, Monfardini S, et al. Cancer in the elderly: why so badly treated? *Lancet* 1990;335:1020.
44. MacMahon B. Epidemiology of Hodgkin's disease. *Cancer Res* 1966; 26:1189.
45. MacMahon B. Epidemiological considerations in staging of Hodgkin's disease. *Cancer Res* 1971;31:1854.
46. Medeiros LJ, Greiner TC. Hodgkin's disease. *Cancer* 1995;75:357.
47. Glaser SL, Ruby JL, Stewart SL, et al. Epstein-Barr virus-associated Hodgkin's disease: epidemiologic characteristics in international data. *Int J Cancer* 1997;70:375.
48. Gustavsson A. Hodgkin's disease of the elderly. A different disease? *Hematol Oncol* 1993;11:73.
49. Parker F Jr, Jackson H Jr, FitzHugh G, et al. Studies of diseases of the lymphoid and myeloid tissues IV. Skin reactions to human and avian tuberculin. *J Immunol* 1932;22:277.
50. Steiner PE. Etiology of Hodgkin's disease. II. Skin reaction to avian and human tuberculin proteins in Hodgkin's disease. *Arch Intern Med* 1934;54:11.
51. Björkholm M. Immunodeficiency in Hodgkin's disease and its relation to prognosis [Academic Thesis]. *Scand J Haematol* 1978;20 (Suppl 3):3.
52. Grimfors G, Holm G, Mellstedt H, Schnell PO, Tullgren O, Björkholm M. Increased blood clearance rate of indium-111 oxine-labeled autologous CD4+ blood cells in untreated patients with Hodgkin's disease. *Blood* 1990;76:583.
53. Gruss H-J, Pinto A, Duyster J, Poppema S, Herrman F. Hodgkin's disease: a tumor with disturbed immunological pathways. *Immunol Today* 1997;18:156.
54. Notter D, Grossman P, Rosenberg SA, et al. Infections in patients with Hodgkin's disease: a clinical study of 300 consecutive adult patients. *Rev Infect Dis* 1980;2:761.
55. Askergren J, Björkholm M. Post-splenectomy septicemia in Hodgkin's disease and other disorders. *Acta Chir Scand* 1980;146:569.
56. Shimm DS, Linggood RM, Weitzman SA. Overwhelming post-splenectomy infection in Hodgkin's disease: pathogenesis and prevention. *Clin Radiol* 1983;34:95.
57. Björkholm M, Wedelin C, Holm G, Ogenstad S, Johansson B, Mellstedt H. Immune status of untreated patients with Hodgkin's disease and prognosis. *Cancer Treat Rep* 1982;66:701.
58. Franceschi C, Monti D, Sansoni P, Cossarizza A. The immunology of exceptional individuals: the lesson of centenarians. *Immunol Today* 1995;16:12.

59. Tullgren O, Grimfors G, Holm G, et al. Lymphocyte abnormalities predicting a poor prognosis in Hodgkin's disease. *Cancer* 1991;68:768.
60. Lindemalm C, Biberfeld P, Björkholm M, et al. Longitudinal studies of blood lymphocyte functions in non-Hodgkin's lymphoma. *Eur J Cancer Clin Oncol* 1983;19:499.
61. Björkholm M, Wedelin C, Holm G, Johansson B, Mellstedt H. Longitudinal studies of blood lymphocyte capacity in Hodgkin's disease. *Cancer* 1981;48:2010.
62. McBride A, Fennelly JJ. Immunological depletion contributing to familial Hodgkin's disease. *Eur J Cancer* 1977;13:549.
63. Björkholm M, Holm G, de Faire U, Mellstedt H. Immunological defects in healthy twin siblings to patients with Hodgkin's disease. *Scand J Haematol* 1977;19:396.
64. Björkholm M, Holm G, Mellstedt H. Immunological family studies in Hodgkin's disease. Is the immunodeficiency horizontally transmitted? *Scand J Haematol* 1978;20:297.
65. Dworsky R, Baptista J, Parker J, et al. Immune function in healthy relatives of patients with malignant disease. *J Natl Cancer Inst* 1978;60:27.
66. Björkholm M, Wedelin C, Holm G, Essy-Ehsing B. Familial longevity and prognosis in Hodgkin's disease. *Cancer* 1984;54:1088.
67. Ferraris AM, Racchi O, Rapezzi D, Gaetani GF, Boffetta P. Familial Hodgkin's disease: a disease of young adulthood? *Ann Hematol* 1997; 74:131.
68. Mack TM, Cozen W, Shibata DK, et al. Concordance for Hodgkin's disease in identical twins suggesting genetic susceptibility to the young-adult form of the disease. *N Engl J Med* 1995;332:413.
69. Folstein MF, Folstein SE, McHugh PR. Mini Mental State. A practical method for grading the cognitive state of patients for the clinicians. *J Psychiatr Res* 1975;12:189.
70. Brink TL, Yesavage JA, Lum O, Hevesuma PH, Adey M, Rose TL. Screening test for geriatric depression. *Clin Gerontol* 1982;1:37.
71. Lawton MP, Bordy EM. Assessment of older people: self-maintaining and instrumental activities of daily living. *Gerontologist* 1969;9:179.
72. Monfardini S, Ferrucci L, Fratino L, Del Lungo I, Serraino D, Zagonel V. Validation of a multidimensional evaluation scale for use in elderly cancer patients. *Cancer* 1996;77:395.
73. Vose JM. Cytochine use in older patients. *Semin Oncol* 1995;22 (Suppl 1):6.
74. Chatta GS, Proce TH, Stratton JR, Dale DC. Aging and marrow neutrophil reserves. *J Am Geriatr Soc* 1994;42:77.
75. Gruss H-J, Dower SK. Tumor necrosis factor ligand superfamily: involvement in the pathology of malignant lymphomas. *Blood* 1995;85: 3378.
76. Swain SM, Whaley FS, Gerber MC, et al. Cardioprotection with dexrazoxane for doxorubicin-containing therapy in advanced breast cancer. *J Clin Oncol* 1997;15:1318.
77. Vestal RE. Aging and pharmacology. *Cancer* 1997;80:1302.
78. Balducci L, Parker M, Sexton W, Tantranond P. Pharmacology of antineoplastic agents in the elderly patient. *Semin Oncol* 1989;16:76.
79. Pinto A, Gioghini A, Gattei V, et al. Expression of the c-kit receptor in human lymphomas is restricted to Hodgkin's disease and C-30 positive anaplastic large cell lymphomas. *Blood* 1994;83:785.
80. Capizzi RL. Protection of normal tissues from the cytotoxic effects of chemotherapy by amifostine (Ethyol): clinical experiences. *Semin Oncol* 1994;21(Suppl 11):8.
81. Carbone A, Gioghini A, Gattei V, et al. Expression of functional CD40 antigen on Reed Sternberg cells and Hodgkin's disease cell lines. *Blood* 1995;85:780.

Hodgkin's Disease, edited by P. M. Mauch, J. O. Armitage, V. Diehl, R. T. Hoppe, and L. M. Weiss. Lippincott Williams & Wilkins, Philadephia ©1999.

CHAPTER 41

Hodgkin's Disease Presenting Below the Diaphragm

Michael Barton and Peter O'Brien

This chapter describes the specific features of stage I–II infradiaphragmatic Hodgkin's disease. Whenever a detailed review appears elsewhere in the text pertaining to general aspects of the treatment of early-stage Hodgkin's disease, the reader is referred to the appropriate section. Hodgkin's disease occurring below the diaphragm has always been regarded with interest because of the relative infrequency of infradiaphragmatic in comparison with supradiaphragmatic presentations of stage I–II disease. Collation of 13 published series (1–15) in which the numbers of all patients with stage I–II disease have been reported shows that infradiaphragmatic cases account for 7% of all such presentations (range, 4–13%). The reason for the disparity in presentations above and below the diaphragm is unknown; however, it is generally accepted that the histopathologic features of infradiaphragmatic presentations are identical (although, as discussed later, there are differences in the proportions of histologic subgroups) and that there is no inherent difference in response to treatment. Any attempt to make definitive statements regarding the features of infradiaphragmatic Hodgkin's disease in regard to patient demographics, clinical presentations, pathologic subtypes, and treatment outcomes is handicapped by the small numbers of patients reported in the literature. Further confounding the analysis of the available data are the variations in treatment and staging procedures in the individual studies, which often extend over significant time periods. The veracity of pathologic review, techniques of radiology and radiotherapy, and regimens of combination chemotherapy have all evolved as knowledge of the biologic behavior of Hodgkin's disease has increased during these periods. The published series have been collated by a combination of computer and manual searches. Many series have reported individual patient data, and these have been summated when possible. However, several patients have been included in multiple series, and when these have been identifiable, the multiple references have been removed (1,2,8,9,15–17).

M. Barton: Department of Medicine, University of New South Wales Roadwick, New South Wales, Australia and Collaboration for Cancer Outcomes, Research and Evaluation, Liverpool Hospital, New South Wales, Australia.

P. O'Brien: Department of Radiation Oncology, Newcastle Mater Hospital, Waratah, New South Wales, Australia.

PRESENTING FEATURES

Clinical Features

There appear to be demographic differences between patients presenting with early-stage infradiaphragmatic disease and their counterparts with supradiaphragmatic disease (Table 1). The data in Table 1 have been drawn from 20 published series involving a total of more than 600 patients. The patients with infradiaphragmatic disease are slightly older than those with supradiaphragmatic disease, and the male-to-female ratio is much higher. The proportion of patients presenting with stage I disease is, however, similar for both groups. The comparative data for supradiaphragmatic Hodgkin's disease have been taken from the International Database (18). There is no definitive explanation for the difference in clinical features—in particular, the striking increase in the male-to-female ratio. As discussed later, the increased proportion of cases with the lymphocyte-predominance histologic subtype may in part explain the excess of male cases (19).

Mode of Presentation

The most common presenting feature in patients with stage I or II Hodgkin's disease confined to infradiaphragmatic sites is a peripheral nodal mass, classically in the

TABLE 1. *Clinical features of infradiaphragmatic Hodgkin's disease*

	Infradiaphragmatic (1–15, 17, 23, 24, 64)	Supradiaphragmatic (18)
Mean age[a] (y)	40 (range, 30–50)	33
Male: female ratio	3.0:1	1.5:1
Stage I (%)	31	34

[a]Represents a mean derived from reported medians and range of medians.

inguinofemoral region (Table 2). An inguinal mass accounts for more than 90% of all stage I presentations and for slightly more than 70% of stage II presentations. Less commonly, patients present with an abdominal mass, and laparotomy may be required for histologic diagnosis. More recently, laparoscopically guided biopsy or localized biopsy performed with a needle has been increasingly used (20). In addition to the lymph nodes of the inguinofemoral region, the iliac and paraaortic nodes are less frequently involved, and uncommon but well-recognized involvement occurs in the nodes of the porta hepatis and/or mesentery. Splenic involvement is particularly common in patients with paraaortic nodal disease (*see below*) and may be equated with a greater potential for hepatic infiltration (8,21). Gastrointestinal tract involvement presenting as obstruction has been described, as has involvement of the gonads and other pelvic and abdominal organs. These rarer sites of involvement tend to occur only in patients with disease resistant to treatment and/or very advanced disease (16,21). Some degree of circumspection is needed in assessing older reports of extranodal sites, as some of these cases may have been non-Hodgkin's lymphoma. There are well-documented cases of patients presenting with jaundice, hepatomegaly, long-tract signs caused by extradural compression, and even pancreatic masses (9,15,22,23). The original lymph node regions defined by Kaplan included the popliteal fossa, but this is an extremely rare site of involvement. Systemic symptoms at the time of presentation are rare in patients with stage I disease but occur in more than 25% of stage II cases. Pyrexia of unknown origin has been the presenting complaint in a number of patients with abdominal disease (15). Such patients represent a very small proportion of all cases of pyrexia of unknown origin, which remains a diagnostic challenge even in the modern era of medicine.

TABLE 2. *Sites at presentation, pathology, and systemic symptoms*

	Stage I (%)	Stage II[a] (%)
Site		
Inguinal	93	74
Pelvic or abdominal	6	54
Other	1	11
Pathology		
Lymphocyte predominance	49	25
Nodular sclerosis	31	41
Mixed cellularity	15	31
Lymphocyte depletion	5	3
B symptoms	1	28

[a]Sites for Stage II patients add up to more than 100%, as some presented with disease at more than one site.

PATHOLOGIC FEATURES

There is no difference in pathologic classification between patients with infradiaphragmatic and supradiaphragmatic Hodgkin's disease, but many authors have commented on the differences in the relative proportions of subtypes. The data in Table 3 represent 501 patients from 17 series from which it was possible to extract information on pathologic subtypes (1–10,12–15,17,23,24). The most striking difference between the proportions of pathologic subtypes for infradiaphragmatic and supradiaphragmatic presentations is the decrease in nodular sclerosis histology. In comparing these data with the International Database, representing 9,091 patients with supradiaphragmatic disease, it can be seen that nodular sclerosis histology occurs only half as frequently in the patients with infradiaphragmatic disease. The decrease in nodular sclerosis subtype is counterbalanced by an increase in lymphocyte predominance histology and, to a lesser extent, mixed cellularity. The increase in lymphocyte predominance histologic subtype is consistent with the high proportion of cases presenting with peripheral (i.e., inguinofemoral) adenopathy (*see below*). Although the decrease in the proportion of patients with nodular sclerosis histology is consistent across many series, there is quite a wide variation, ranging from 11% to 62% of all cases (1–5,14,17,24). This serves to emphasize the comment made in the opening paragraph that the small numbers of patients, reported over lengthy time periods with

TABLE 3. *Frequency of pathologic subtypes of Hodgkin's disease*

	Infradiaphragmatic (%) (1–10, 12–15, 17, 23, 24)	Supradiaphragmatic (%) (18)
Lymphocyte predominance	27	8
Nodular sclerosis	32	64
Mixed cellularity	32	24
Lymphocyte depletion	5	2
Unspecified or unclassified	4	2

undoubtedly varying pathologic interpretation, may confound the interpretation of these grouped data.

STAGING

The staging of Hodgkin's disease is reviewed in detail elsewhere in this book (Chapters 15–18). The Ann Arbor staging system as modified at the Cotswolds meeting (25) is used for both supradiaphragmatic and infradiaphragmatic Hodgkin's disease. The investigations that are indicated for supradiaphragmatic Hodgkin's disease [i.e., complete blood cell count; erythrocyte sedimentation rate; biochemical tests of liver, bone, and renal function; computed tomography (CT) of the chest and abdomen] are also appropriate for infradiaphragmatic Hodgkin's disease. Lymphangiography has been widely used. Gallium scanning is of limited use for assessing infradiaphragmatic disease because of normal uptake in the liver, spleen, and intestine (26,27). Accordingly, the false-positive rate is higher than in assessment of the mediastinum, although the sensitivity in assessment of suspected abdominal relapse was high in one reported series (28), which can partly be explained by the use of delayed images when bowel activity was high. Similarly, SPECT (single-photon emission computed tomography) may further improve the sensitivity and specificity of gallium scanning in the assessment of infradiaphragmatic disease. The role of magnetic resonance imaging (MRI) is still under investigation, but preliminary reports suggest that it is of limited value in assessing the spleen (26). The major diagnostic question is the role, if any, of staging laparotomy.

Lymphangiography

Lymphangiography has been extensively reported in the published series of infradiaphragmatic Hodgkin's disease (1,3,6,7,9–11,14–17,23,24). Of a total of 670 patients, 373 were documented to have had a lymphangiogram. Results were reported in 203 cases, with a positivity rate of 65%. However, there are several biases in these reports. Patients with large masses often did not receive lymphangiography, and pathologic correlation is infrequently reported. The specificity and sensitivity for supradiaphragmatic presentations have been reported to be high, but the information for infradiaphragmatic presentations is limited. Lymphangiography does not assess the spleen and is highly dependent on the skills and experience of the radiologist. Nevertheless, lymphangiography provides several advantages over other imaging modalities in the assessment of infradiaphragmatic Hodgkin's disease. It accurately determines the location of lymph node chains, and this information can be utilized in designing radiotherapy fields to help minimize the radiation exposure of normal tissue, such as bowel and kidney. Lymphangiography is also the only method of assessing nodes of normal size that may contain Hodgkin's disease. In such cases, the abnormalities appear as filling defects. In comparison with the positivity rate in supradiaphragmatic disease, that in infradiaphragmatic disease is considerably higher. Unfortunately, lymphangiography has been performed less frequently in recent years and, given its dependence on the skills and experience of the radiologist, is now rarely performed outside of select centers (26).

Laparotomy

Staging laparotomy is discussed in detail in Chapter 18. In this chapter, we deal only with those issues pertinent to infradiaphragmatic presentations.

Diagnostic Laparotomy

One-fifth of laparotomies are performed to establish a histologic diagnosis, usually to resolve the cause of pelvic or abdominal lymphadenopathy (Table 4). The lymph nodes are usually bulky enough to be symptomatic, which may explain the worse prognosis of this group in some series (3,10,17). A diagnostic laparotomy is rarely performed with staging in mind and therefore does not provide a reliable sample of abnormal nodes identified on lymphangiogram, nor is the spleen routinely removed for pathologic examination. Laparoscopic biopsy in many instances may avoid the need for laparotomy, and there are a number of reports of laparoscopic splenectomy (20,29). Only occasionally can Hodgkin's disease be diagnosed by fine-needle cytology, although it may be useful in the setting of recurrent disease (30).

Staging Laparotomy

Staging laparotomy has been used to make individual treatment decisions and to acquire knowledge of the natural history and routes of spread of infradiaphragmatic Hodgkin's disease. In the past, it was one of the few reliable ways to assess tumor bulk. That role has been taken over by high-quality CT, which is now widely available. Staging laparotomy remains the only way to assess splenic involvement. Its continued use can be justified only if it alters treatment decisions and patient outcomes. The accumulated data from collected series now provide a clear picture of risk factors from which rational treatment policies can be derived. Table 4 shows that stage is altered in about 14% of cases. Some individual series quote higher rates of upstaging (8). They refer to the detection of splenic involvement or of a greater number of sites of disease. Such findings would now rarely alter treatment regimens. Overall, the rates for alteration of

TABLE 4. *Staging laparotomy*

Author (ref.)	No. patients	Laparotomy			Change in stage	
		Total	Diagnostic	Staging	Up	Down
Barton et al. (17)	106	59	9	50	1	3
Cionini et al. (3)	41	31	3	28	0	2
Dorreen et al. (4)	23	17	1	16		
Frassica et al. (14)	26	20	10	10	1	1
Givens et al. (24)	60	22	12	10		
Krikorian et al. (16)	23	23	7	16	6	1
Lanzillo et al. (7)	17	7	0	7	0	4
Leibenhaut et al. (8)	49	49	5	44	6	0
Liew et al. (9)	16	8	5	3	0	0
Mai et al. (23)	19	19			0	0
Mason et al. (2)	53	21	0	21	0	0
Mauch et al. (10)	36	25	11	14	1	0
Roos et al. (15)	15	8			0	0
Specht and Nissen (12)	35	11	0	11	1	
Total	**519**	**320**	**63**	**230**	**16**	**11**
Percentage		62%	20%	72%	8%	6%

stage following laparotomy for infradiaphragmatic presentations are lower than those reported for supradiaphragmatic presentations (26). Another reason for formerly advocating staging laparotomy was the difficulty of diagnosing splenic involvement with noninvasive investigations. However, splenic involvement can be predicted from the clinical stage (CS) (Table 5) and site of involvement. The rate of splenic involvement was 7% in CS IA, 15% in CS IIA, and 52% in CS IIB. Analysis of pooled data from the published reports (2,3,8,10,14,17) shows that CS IA affecting only the inguinal region was rarely associated with splenic involvement but that CS IA with abdominal involvement was frequently associated with splenic involvement at laparotomy (4% vs. 45%). Even when the series of Leibenhaut et al. (8), in which the incidence of splenic involvement is highest, is removed from consideration, the rate of splenic involvement in abdominal CS IA is still high (35%). Given the morbidity, potential mortality (26), and lack of a survival benefit (31), laparotomy can rarely be justified for staging alone.

SITE, STAGE, AND PATHOLOGY

A potential relationship between the site of presentation and pathologic subtype has been postulated by Mauch et al. (19), in which certain sites of involvement are correlated with a higher probability of disease at other individual sites. In particular, this analysis found that the lymphocyte predominance subtype is more common in

TABLE 5. *Splenic involvement at laparotomy*

Author (ref.)	CS I spleen-positive	Total no. laparotomies	CS IIA spleen-positive	Total no. laparotomies	CS IIB spleen-positive	Total no. laparotomies
Barton et al. (17)	1	59	0	47		
Cionini et al. (3)	0	3	0	7	2	4
Dorreen et al. (4)	1	7	8	9		
Enrici et al. (5)	4	22				
Frassica et al. (14)	0	8	1	8	2	2
Krikorian et al. (16)	1	3	1	11	3	6
Lanzillo et al. (7)	0	5	0	12		
Leibenhaut et al. (8)	0	6	8	32	8	9
Liew et al. (9)	1	3	0	5	0	8
Mai et al. (23)	0	4	0	10	2	3
Mason et al. (2)	0	5	5	9	3	6
Mauch et al. (10)	1	8	1	9	4	8
Roos et al. (15)	0	0	1	6	4	8
Total	**9**	**133**	**25**	**165**	**28**	**54**
Percentage	7%		15%		52%	

CS, clinical stage.

inguinal presentations and less common in central nodal sites, including the upper abdomen and spleen; these findings are consistent with other data concerning presentations and behavior of supradiaphragmatic lymphocyte predominance Hodgkin's disease (32). These authors also suggested that certain sites are associated with a higher probability of stage I disease, including the inguinal regions. As might be expected, there was a correlation between the lymphocyte predominance histologic subtype and presentation with stage I disease.

The most common presentation for patients with infradiaphragmatic Hodgkin's disease is that of a mass in the inguinofemoral region. Nine series present a sufficiently detailed breakdown of patient characteristics to determine the site of involvement and correlate it with histology (1,3,7,9,10,14–16,23), and further details have been extracted from the Australasian Radiation Oncology Lymphoma Group database (17). The data in Table 2 confirm that more than 90% of patients who have stage I disease present with disease in the inguinal nodes, and, as Mauch et al. found, stage I patients show a striking excess of lymphocyte predominance histologic subtype. In comparison with patients who have supradiaphragmatic Hodgkin's disease, in which lymphocyte predominance histology accounts for 8% of all presentations, almost 50% of patients with stage I infradiaphragmatic disease have the lymphocyte predominance subtype. B symptoms and bulky disease are also extremely uncommon. At least two other series with summary data on sites of involvement confirm the very high proportion of stage I cases presenting as an inguinal mass (8,24). In stage II disease, the relationship between sites of involvement and histology is more difficult to ascertain, but for 160 patients in 10 series, some patterns do emerge (1,3,7,9,10,14–17,23). The incidence of lymphocyte predominance is less common than in stage I, affecting 25% of patients, and there is a corresponding rise in nodular sclerosis and mixed cellularity histology. Just over one-fourth of all stage II patients presented with B symptoms. Very few series documented the incidence of bulky disease; as might be expected, however, this is more common in patients presenting with primarily abdominal involvement. Even with stage II disease, the most common site of involvement remains the inguinal region. The incidence of splenic involvement and its relationship to other sites has been discussed (*vide supra*).

TREATMENT

Radiotherapy

The classic radiotherapy fields described in Chapter 21 are also used to treat infradiaphragmatic Hodgkin's disease. Briefly, involved-field radiotherapy encompasses the known involved nodal site as defined by the Ann Arbor staging system (33), with a suitable margin of 3 to 5 cm around macroscopic disease. An inverted-Y field covers both groins and the iliac, femoral, and paraaortic lymph nodes. A splenic field may be added. Total-nodal irradiation is defined as the combination of an inverted-Y field and a mantle field covering supradiaphragmatic lymph node regions. All field arrangements should be administered by opposed anterior and posterior beams with use of customized shielding. To reduce the incidence of late sequelae, both fields should be treated daily.

An inverted-Y field extends from the lower border of T-10 cranially to include the femoral nodes caudally. Lymphangiography is useful in delineating the anatomic extent of the inguinal, external, common iliac, and paraaortic lymph nodes. The paraaortic portion of the field is generally 8 to 10 cm wide, depending on individual patient size and the position of the kidneys, which are best delineated by use of intravenous contrast at simulation. The anatomic position of the inguinal nodes, in particular the femoral group, can vary, so the placement of the inferior border should not be less than 3 cm inferior to the ischial tuberosity (34). It is unusual for these nodes to be less than 3 cm from the midline. This should be considered in the design of the midline block, which will affect the gonadal dose in both male and female patients. An increase in shielding thickness to 6 to 10 half-value layers will reduce the contribution to the gonadal dose from the primary beam; however, internal scatter remains a problem. When oophoropexy has been performed, every effort should be made to achieve a distance of 2 cm between the ovaries (as marked by metal clips) and shielding blocks (35). In male patients, a secondary shield around the scrotum is desirable to reduce the scattered dose to the testes. However, in individual cases, there may be a risk for underdosing the tumor because of the proximity of involved inguinal lymph nodes (Fig. 1).

Total doses of radiation should be identical with those used for supradiaphragmatic disease—namely, 30 to 35 Gy and a dose per fraction of not greater than 2 Gy. There is little evidence to support total doses greater than 30 Gy when given in combination with chemotherapy. A small daily fraction (about 1.5 Gy daily) may improve acute tolerance by reducing the incidence of nausea and vomiting.

Chemotherapy

The introduction of combination chemotherapy for Hodgkin's disease has made a dramatic difference in the numbers of patients cured. The inherent rarity of infradiaphragmatic Hodgkin's disease has resulted in a very small number of patients being treated with chemotherapy, most commonly with MOPP (mechlorethamine, vincristine, prednisone, and procarbazine) or MOPP-like regimens such as ChlVPP, in which chlorambucil is

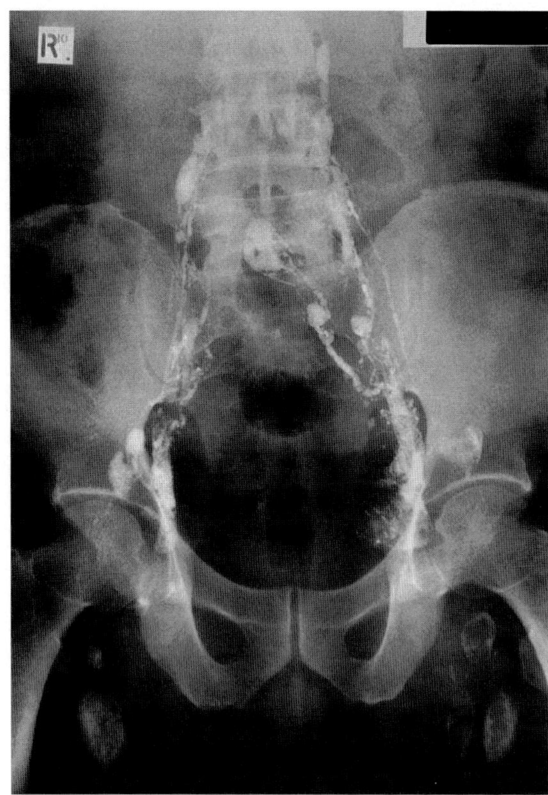

FIG. 1. Pelvic component of an inverted-Y field showing the proximity of the involved right inguinal nodes to the scrotal shadow.

substituted for mechlorethamine. With the advent of doxorubicin and regimens based on it, such as ABVD (doxorubicin, bleomycin, vinblastine, and dacarbazine), fewer patients are being treated with MOPP, including the small number of patients with infradiaphragmatic disease. The increasing use of ABVD is probably based more on the leukemogenic potential of MOPP rather than a clear therapeutic advantage of ABVD, and there is no clear evidence that ChlVPP avoids this problem. The principles of adequate dose intensity for a minimum of 6 cycles are the same as for other presentations of Hodgkin's disease in which chemotherapy alone is appropriate treatment. For a fuller discussion of drug doses and the importance of dose intensity, the reader is referred to Chapter 22. There is no evidence that infradiaphragmatic differs in any way from supradiaphragmatic disease in terms of inherent response to chemotherapy. Lymphocyte predominance histology accounts for significant proportion of patients with disease confined to infradiaphragmatic sites. It is not clear which combination regimens are likely to be effective for cases with lymphocyte predominance histology, and given that most patients present with stage I disease, radiotherapy may be the preferred modality. In assessing the results of chemotherapy in patients with infradiaphragmatic disease, it should be remembered that selection criteria may have been applied that are not apparent in the published reports. The most obvious of these is bulky disease, but the decision to use a doxorubicin-based regimen (with or without involved-field radiotherapy) may be based equally on a wish to maximize the chances of preserving fertility in a given patient. Similar considerations apply to combined-modality therapy, for which the selection criteria also are not necessarily clear from the reported data. In terms of the number of cycles of chemotherapy used in combined-modality therapy, again there is no difference between infradiaphragmatic and supradiaphragmatic disease. Commonly, this has varied from 3 to 6 cycles before radiotherapy, based more on institutional preference than guidance from randomized studies. Similarly, the volumes irradiated are not always presented, particularly when involved-field radiotherapy is used in combined-modality therapy.

TREATMENT ISSUES AND RESULTS

The major treatment questions concern the appropriate use of radiotherapy as a single modality, the extent of fields, and the role of combined-modality therapy. There are few reports on the use of chemotherapy alone. Surprisingly, the results of chemotherapy alone for other than stage I patients are poor, but again selection criteria are a likely influence. Results of all the published series are given in Tables 6, 7, and 8. The control rates quoted are all crude rates owing to the difficulties of producing more sophisticated analyses from the published data. It is often unclear why one treatment is given instead of another, and one must suspect that unreported tumor bulk or other prognostic factors have been considered in individual treatment decisions. Nevertheless, the summation of the published reports provides considerable insight into the management of infradiaphragmatic Hodgkin's disease.

Stage IA

In the vast majority of cases, stage IA disease is confined to the inguinal region. As is shown in Table 6, an inverted-Y field achieves a high absolute rate of freedom from relapse (82%) and is superior to an involved field (59%). A high rate of freedom from relapse is also seen with combined-modality therapy (94%), but the small improvement in freedom from relapse is not statistically significant and hardly justifies the extra morbidity. Total-nodal irradiation was given to only 12 patients, and the reasons for choosing a more aggressive approach are unclear. The lower rate of disease control (67%) suggests that this regimen was used with more advanced cases (e.g., abdominal or bulky presentations).

TABLE 6. *Treatment results stage 1A*

Author (ref.)	No. patients	IF		IY/PA		TNI		MOPP		CMT	
		No.	NED	No.	NED	No.	NED	No.	NED	No.	NED
Barrett et al. (1)	5			5	5						
Barton et al. (17)	59	12	7	43	37	4	3				
Cionini et al. (3)	5	2	1	1	1	2	1				
Enrici et al. (5)	10										
Frassica et al. (14)	13			9	7	3	2			1	1
Ifrah et al. (6)	7									7	7
Krikorian et al. (22)	2									2	1
Lanzillo et al. (7)	9			8	8	1	1				
Leibenhaut et al. (8)	8			3	2	2	1			3	3
Liew et al. (9)	3	2	2	1	1						
Mai et al. (23)	4			4	3						
Mason et al. (2)	11	1	1	10	7						
Mauch et al. (10)	7			7	7						
Pene et al. (64)	4			4	1						
Roos et al. (15)	1			1	0						
Specht and Nissen (12)	8			2	1			1	1	5	5
Total	**156**	**17**	**11**	**98**	**80**	**12**	**8**	**1**	**1**	**18**	**17**
Total NED	**117**										
Percentage	75%		65%		82%		67%		100%		94%

IF, involved-field; IY/PA, inverted-Y/paraaortic; TNI, total-nodal irradiation; MOPP, mechlorethamine, vincristine, prednisone, procarbazine; CMT, combined-modality therapy; NED, no evidence of disease.

Chemotherapy either alone or combined with radiotherapy has been used so infrequently that its role, if any, remains uncertain.

For patients with inguinal presentations of stage IA disease, treatment of the spleen is not required because of the low risk for involvement. Elective treatment of the spleen is justified in stage IA cases with abdominal involvement, for which pooled data suggest a risk for splenic involvement of 45%. Stage IA abdominal disease may present later and therefore may be bulkier. In addition, the adjacent lymph node groups include those of the spleen, neck, and mediastinum. For that reason, a

TABLE 7. *Treatment results stage IIA*

Author (ref.)	No. patients	IF		IY/PA		TNI		MOPP		CMT	
		No.	NED	No.	NED	No.	NED	No.	NED	No.	NED
Barrett et al. (1)	6			4						2	4
Barton et al. (17)	47	4	2	41	27	2	0				
Cionini et al. (3)	10	0	0	5	1	5	3				
Frassica et al. (14)	9			5	0	3	1			1	1
Ifrah et al. (6)	10									10	8
Krikorian et al. (22)	12	1	1	2	1	5	5			4	4
Lanzillo et al. (7)	6	1	1	2	2	2	2			1	1
Leibenhaut et al. (8)	29			4	0	13	11			11	8
Liew et al. (9)	5			4	2			1	0		
Mai et al. (23)	12			4	3	6	4			2	1
Mason et al. (2)	26			21	12			8	2	13	10
Mauch et al. (10)	15			5	3	6	4			4	3
Pene et al. (64)	12			12	2						
Roos et al. (15)	6	1	0	1	1			3	2	1	0
Specht and Nissen (12)	26			7	2			3	1	16	11
Total	**231**	**7**	**4**	**117**	**56**	**42**	**30**	**15**	**5**	**65**	**51**
Total NED	**146**										
Percentage	63%		57%		48%		71%		33%		78%

IF, involved-field; IY/PA, inverted-Y/paraaortic; TNI, total-nodal irradiation; MOPP, mechlorethamine, vincristine, prednisone, procarbazine; CMT, combined-modality therapy; NED, no evidence of disease.

TABLE 8. *Treatment results stage IIB*

Author (ref.)	No. patients	IY/PA		TNI		MOPP		CMT	
		No.	NED	No.	NED	No.	NED	No.	NED
Barrett et al. (1)	6	1	1			1	0	4	4
Cionini et al. (3)	5	2	0	1	0			2	2
Frassica et al. (14)	4			1	0	1	1	2	2
Ifrah et al. (6)	11							11	9
Krikorian et al. (22)	5			1	1			4	3
Lanzillo et al. (7)	2							2	2
Leibenhaut et al. (8)	8			2	1			6	6
Liew et al. (9)	8	4	1			4	2		
Mai et al. (23)	3							3	2
Mauch et al. (10)	11	1	0			2	0	8	6
Roos et al. (15)	8	1	0			4	0	3	3
Total	**71**	**9**	**2**	**5**	**2**	**12**	**3**	**45**	**39**
Total NED	**46**								
Percentage	65%		22%		40%		25%		87%

IY/PA, inverted-Y/paraaortic; TNI, total-nodal irradiation; MOPP, mechlorethamine, vincristine, prednisone, procarbazine; CMT, combined-modality therapy; NED, no evidence of disease.

more aggressive treatment approach with either total-nodal irradiation or combined-modality therapy is warranted in a stage IA abdominal presentation, with combined-modality therapy potentially producing less gonadal toxicity through avoidance of pelvic and inguinal irradiation.

Stage IIA

Better initial control of tumor is seen with total-nodal irradiation (71%) or combined-modality therapy (78%) than with either inverted-Y-field (48%) or involved-field (57%) irradiation (Table 7). Chemotherapy alone has been reported in only a very small number of cases, and again it is difficult to disentangle the effects of selection in the treatment of stage IIA patients. When an inverted-Y field alone was used, failure frequently occurred in lymph node areas that would have been covered by a mantle field (17). Combined-modality therapy may be preferable to total-nodal irradiation, especially when gonadal toxicity is an issue. As in stage I disease, the radiation dose to the testes or ovaries will be less if irradiation of one or both inguinal regions is avoided.

Krikorian et al. in 1986 (22) raised the question of whether optimal management of patients with disease confined to the pelvis should include staging laparotomy to rule out abdominal involvement, with a view to treating with an inverted-Y field. There are six series comprising a total of 25 patients with disease confined to the pelvis (9,10,14–17). Of the 11 pathologically staged patients, eight relapsed following treatment with an inverted-Y field, and the relapse was supradiaphragmatic in the majority of cases. Of 14 clinically staged patients, five relapsed. These data show that there is no good case for advocating pathologic staging in this subgroup of patients, as inverted-Y radiotherapy is still associated with an unacceptably high rate of relapse.

Splenic involvement in the laparotomy series was 17%, and the rate is higher when paraaortic lymph nodes are involved (8). Splenic irradiation should be given for stage IIA with pelvic or paraaortic involvement and should be considered in other cases.

Stage IIB

Combined-modality therapy consistently provides the best tumor control in stage IIB (87%); radiation or chemotherapy alone yields much lower rates of control (Table 8), although again the reported numbers are small (of 26 patients, seven with no evidence of disease). The only randomized study evaluating the extent of radiotherapy fields in combined-modality therapy showed no advantage for wide-field over involved-field radiation, and the toxicity of the former is greater (36). However, the high rate of splenic involvement in stage IIB reported in the laparotomy series and the difficulty of diagnosing splenic involvement clinically suggest that the spleen should be included in radiotherapy fields in combined-modality therapy.

Treatment of the Spleen

Indications

Splenic involvement may be predicted from the CS and site of presentation. The risk in stage IA inguinal presentation is 4%, and splenic radiotherapy is therefore not indicated. However, elective treatment of the spleen is clearly justified in stage IA with abdominal involvement, in which the pooled reports suggest a risk for splenic involvement of 45%. In stage IIA, the laparotomy series suggest that the risk for splenic involvement is 15%, so the spleen should be treated. The high rates of splenic involvement in stage IIB and the insensitivity of nonsurgical methods of splenic assessment suggest that the spleen should be routinely irradiated as part of the combined-modality approach to stage IIB, regardless of whether the spleen is clinically involved at diagnosis.

Planning

The spleen lies immediately below the left hemidiaphragm, adjacent to the left kidney. It is not easily identifiable on a plain film, but the medial border may be localized by use of an intravenous pyelogram to outline the kidney. A line drawn horizontally through the space between the second and third lumbar vertebrae is a useful mark of the lower extent of the spleen. Gas in the splenic flexure of the colon may also point to the lower extent of the spleen. Laterally, the spleen extends to the chest wall and underlies ribs 9, 10, and 11.

Such indirect localizers are rarely necessary for planning with the widespread availability of CT. Care must still be taken, however, because the overlying diaphragm is associated with a large range of respiratory movement of the spleen (Fig. 2). CT should be performed in quiet respiration. A margin of at least 2 cm should be given to the splenic volume determined by CT. The treatment field should be checked by image intensification to ensure adequate coverage of the diaphragm.

Bulky Disease

Bulky disease, defined as a tumor diameter of 7 cm or larger, has been reported in two series (9,24). Givens et al. (24) achieved high rates of cure with either total-nodal irradiation (13 of 15 with no evidence of disease) or combined-modality therapy (8 of 9 with no evidence of disease). In contrast, Liew et al. (9) had no survivors among eight patients who had bulky disease treated with either an inverted-Y field or chemotherapy alone. In other series, abdominal presentations are recorded but bulk is not specifically described. Abdominal presentation may be a surrogate for tumor bulk, as it is most likely that only large lymph node masses will be symptomatic. This may account for the poorer results seen with abdominal presentations.

TOXICITY OF TREATMENT FOR INFRADIAPHRAGMATIC DISEASE

Radiotherapy

Acute gastrointestinal toxicity from irradiation to volumes such as inverted-Y fields is usually mild but occurs in a significant proportion of patients (37). Emesis is rarely severe, and if so, it can be well controlled with serotonin antagonists (38). Metoclopramide or dexamethasone is often sufficient for milder emesis. Diarrhea may also occur and responds to agents such as loperamide. Significant myelosuppression will not develop in most patients during and immediately after a course of infradiaphragmatic irradiation, but complete blood cell counts should be performed weekly, particularly during radiotherapy given as part of combined-modality therapy or during total-nodal irradiation.

The effect of therapeutic irradiation on fertility has been studied in patients undergoing infradiaphragmatic irradiation for Hodgkin's disease and testicular tumors (39–44). The dose to the testis is often higher for patients with infradiaphragmatic Hodgkin's disease as a consequence of irradiating the femoral group of nodes (Fig. 2). In a detailed study of male patients undergoing pelvic irradiation for Hodgkin's disease, there appeared to be a time-dependent recovery of spermatogenesis, with 88% of patients being fertile more than 26 months after completion of treatment, compared with one-sixth at less than

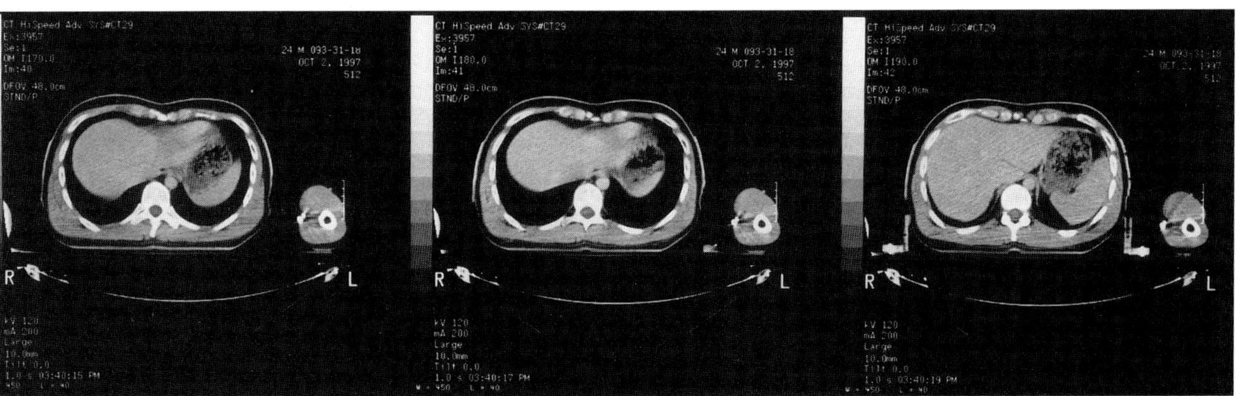

FIG. 2. Movement of the spleen in quiet respiration as demonstrated on three sequential CT slices taken at one cm intervals.

18 months (44). Patients in this study almost certainly benefited from efforts to reduce the gonadal dose, which ranged from 0.28 to 1.35 Gy. A 10-cm-thick midline pelvic block reduced the dose contribution from the primary beam to 0.5% of the incident dose. However, the major contribution to testicular dose is from internal scatter. Testicular shielding will reduce the dose to 3% of the incident dose, but care must be taken to avoid shielding tumor (Fig. 1). The proportion of patients becoming azoospermic or oligospermic and the duration of the decrease in sperm counts shows a significant dose dependence over a range of 1 to 3.5 Gy (39,45,46). It should be remembered that fertility may be impaired in patients with Hodgkin's disease before treatment (47). Storage of semen is advisable if fertility is likely to be an issue for the patient.

A literature review of reproductive outcomes following various treatments for Hodgkin's disease failed to show any increased risk for congenital malformations, low birth weight, stillbirths, or cancer in offspring, or an altered sex ratio (41). The rate of successful reproductive outcomes was found to be highest in the group that underwent radiotherapy alone. Similar findings were made in patients having infradiaphragmatic radiotherapy for testicular cancer (40), with 65% of men who wished to do so fathering at least one child. Irradiation for Hodgkin's disease in female patients has been associated with decreasing fertility with older age at treatment (41,42). Horning et al. in 1981 (42) reported on 19 women who underwent midline oophoropexy before pelvic irradiation (as part of total-lymphoid irradiation). A 10-cm-thick midline block was used to shield the ovaries. Of 10 women in whom menses resumed and pregnancy was a desired outcome, seven became pregnant at a median interval of 48 months following treatment. Interestingly, temporary amenorrhea developed in five of these. Hadar et al. in 1994 (43) radiologically assessed the position of transposed ovaries in relation to radiation fields in patients receiving pelvic radiotherapy for Hodgkin's disease and carcinoma of the cervix. They suggested that medial transposition of the ovaries is less likely to result in successful protection of ovarian function than is lateral transposition, although the midline pelvic block used was narrower than that reported by the Stanford group (42). One series has suggested a potential role for laparoscopic transposition of the ovaries to the medial position (48).

That splenectomy predisposes patients to potentially fatal septicemia is a well-recognized danger. Patients with asplenia induced by irradiation may also be at increased risk for septicemia (49). The immunosuppression occurring in Hodgkin's disease *per se* increases the risk for overwhelming sepsis resulting from splenectomy. *Streptococcus pneumoniae*, *Haemophilus influenzae*, and *Neisseria meningitidis* are the organisms most commonly associated with severe infection following splenectomy or splenic irradiation. For patients scheduled for elective splenectomy or splenic irradiation, it is recommended that vaccination against pneumococci, meningococci, and *Haemophilus influenzae* B be performed at least 72 hours before the procedure (50). In practice, the patients should be immunized as soon as possible following the diagnosis of Hodgkin's disease and before splenectomy or splenic irradiation (51). The role of prophylactic antibiotics is still debated, but patients and their families should be advised that in the presence of fever, urgent medical attention is required and antibiotics should be used if there is any suspicion of bacterial infection (51).

An analysis of patterns of care data from the United States indicates that the most frequent late complication of infradiaphragmatic irradiation is gastrointestinal injury, including peptic ulceration, hemorrhage, chronic diarrhea, and intestinal obstruction (52). Bowel complications increased as dose increased, with only 1% of patients who received less than 35 Gy having a major complication. The European Organization for the Research and Treatment of Cancer (EORTC) encountered similar complications but emphasized the influence of staging laparotomy and the dose per fraction of radiotherapy (53,54). In patients who underwent both a staging laparotomy and infradiaphragmatic radiation with fractional doses greater than 2 Gy, there was an increase in late gastrointestinal complications that was maximal (cumulative incidence at 5 years of 28%) for those who received 3.3 Gy.

Possibly the major concern after therapeutic irradiation for Hodgkin's disease in any site, including infradiaphragmatic sites, is the induction of second malignancies. Cancers of the stomach, colon, rectum, pancreas, cervix, ovary, vulva, prostate, testes, kidney, and bladder have all been described following irradiation (55–61). Often, these are grouped according to whether they affect gastrointestinal or genitourinary/gynecologic sites for the purposes of statistical evaluation. It has been postulated that splenectomy and splenic irradiation may increase the risk for second malignancies (58). A full discussion of the problem of second malignancies can be found in Chapter 33. Because infradiaphragmatic presentations are relatively rare, no specific data are available pertaining to second malignancies in these cases, but it is unlikely that they differ essentially from those associated with other presentations.

Chemotherapy and Combined-Modality Therapy

The acute toxicities encountered with chemotherapy for infradiaphragmatic Hodgkin's disease are no different from those for other sites and stages. The majority of patients reported in the literature and treated with chemotherapy or combined-modality therapy have received MOPP or MOPP-like regimens (most commonly ChlVPP) and, less commonly, ABVD or other doxorubicin-based regimens. The excess of patients treated with MOPP reflects the long period of time encompassed by most reports of treatment for infradiaphragmatic Hodgkin's disease rather than any therapeutic advantage. The major disadvantage with MOPP is the detrimental effect on fertility occurring in both male and female patients, largely caused by mechlorethamine and with a likely contribution from procarbazine. Vincristine neuropathy can also be troublesome for patients. Both MOPP and ABVD are emetogenic, although in the era of 5HT3 antagonists, severe nausea and vomiting are unusual. The substitution of chlorambucil for mechlorethamine in the ChlVPP regimen probably reduces acute toxicity, but the disadvantages of impairment of fertility and leukemogenesis remain. ABVD or similar regimens have the significant advantage of not impairing fertility in most patients and of being associated with a minimal risk for leukemogenesis. The well-recognized pulmonary complications of bleomycin and the capacity of anthracycline to induce cardiomyopathy still remain, but elimination of the need for supradiaphragmatic irradiation lessens the additive effects seen with combined-modality therapy. When its reduced leukemogenic potential and likely therapeutic advantages are taken into account, there is little doubt that ABVD should be used in combined-modality regimens when appropriate for infradiaphragmatic disease (55,62, 63). Combined-modality therapy based around ABVD may be optimal when it is possible to minimize pelvic and/or inguinal irradiation and improve the chances of preserving fertility. This is particularly so when irradiation of one or both inguinal regions can be avoided in male patients and bilateral pelvic irradiation can be avoided in female patients. Under these circumstances, the use of 3 cycles of ABVD and involved-field irradiation not only minimizes acute morbidity but also results in a dose of doxorubicin that is very unlikely to produce cardiomyopathy. Furthermore, a radiation dose can be used that is associated with minimal risk for late gastrointestinal morbidity. For a complete review of the potential toxicities of chemotherapy and combined-modality therapy, the reader is referred to Chapters 22 and 23.

CONCLUSION

Infradiaphragmatic Hodgkin's disease accounts for only 7% of all early-stage presentations. The patients are older, with a higher male-to-female ratio. The majority (90%) of stage I presentations are inguinal, and half of these patients have lymphocyte predominance histopathology. Nodular sclerosis histopathology is less common than in supradiaphragmatic Hodgkin's disease. Laparotomy may be necessary for diagnosis, but formal staging laparotomy has no established role in the management of infradiaphragmatic Hodgkin's disease.

CS IA disease of the inguinal region should be treated with inverted-Y-field radiation therapy. The incidence of splenic involvement in such cases is 4% and therefore does not justify splenic irradiation. In selected cases in which preservation of fertility is an important issue, combined-modality therapy based around ABVD with involved-field irradiation may be preferable. Cases of lymphocyte predominance histology, for which there is a paucity of data to support the use of chemotherapy, are the exception. CS IA disease of the abdomen or pelvis and CS IIA nonbulky disease requires either total-nodal irradiation or combined-modality therapy. Combined-modality therapy is preferable from the viewpoint of toxicity. The presence of bulky disease and/or B symptoms indicates the need for combined-modality therapy. In stage IA disease with abdominal involvement or stage IIA or IIB disease, the spleen should be irradiated as part of combined-modality therapy. There are very few data to support a role for chemotherapy alone.

REFERENCES

1. Barrett A, Gregor A, McElwain TJ, Peckham MJ. Infra-diaphragmatic presentation of Hodgkin's disease. *Clin Radiol* 1981;32:221.
2. Mason MD, Law M, Ashley S, et al. Infradiaphragmatic Hodgkin's disease. *Eur J Cancer* 1992;28A:1851.
3. Cionini L, Magrini S, Mungai V, Biti GP, Ponticelli P. Stage I and II Hodgkin's disease present in infradiaphragmatic nodes. *Tumori* 1982; 68:519.
4. Dorreen MS, Wrigley PMF, Jones AE, Shand WS, Stansfeld AG, Lister TA. The management of localized, infradiaphragmatic Hodgkin's disease: experience of a rare clinical presentation at St. Bartholomew's Hospital. *Hematol Oncol* 1984;2:349.
5. Enrici RM, Osti MF, Anselmo AP, et al. Hodgkin's disease stage I and II with exclusive subdiaphragmatic presentation. The experience of the Departments of Radiation Oncology and Hematology, University "La Sapienza" of Rome. *Tumori* 1996;82:48.
6. Ifrah N, Hunault M, Jais J-P, et al. Infradiaphragmatic Hodgkin's disease: long-term results of combined-modality therapy. *Leuk Lymphoma* 1996;21:79.
7. Lanzillo JH, Moylan DJ, Mohiuddin M, Kramer S. Radiotherapy of stage I and II Hodgkin disease with inguinal presentation. *Ther Radiol* 1985;154:213.
8. Leibenhaut MH, Hoppe RT, Varghese A, Rosenberg SA. Subdiaphragmatic Hodgkin's disease: laparotomy and treatment results in 49 patients. *J Clin Oncol* 1987;5:1050.
9. Liew KH, Ding JC, Cruickshank D, Quong GG, Wolf MM, Cooper IA. Infradiaphragmatic Hodgkin's disease: long-term follow-up of a rare presentation. *Aust N Z J Med* 1991;21:16.
10. Mauch P, Greenberg H, Lewin A, Cassady JR, Weichselbaum R. Prognostic factors in patients with subdiaphragmatic Hodgkin's disease. *Hematol Oncol* 1983;1:205.
11. Sutcliffe SB, Gospodarowicz MK, Bergsagel DE, et al. Prognostic groups for management of localized Hodgkin's disease. *J Clin Oncol* 1985;3:393.
12. Specht L, Nissen NI. Hodgkin's disease stages I and II with infradiaphragmatic presentation: a rare and prognostically unfavourable combination. *Eur J Haematol* 1988;40:396.
13. Villamor N, Reverter JC, Marti JM, Montserrat E, Rozman C. Clinical

features and response to treatment of infradiaphragmatic Hodgkin's disease. *Eur J Haematol* 1991;46:38.

14. Frassica DA, Schomberg PJ, Banks PM, Colgan JP, Ilstrup DM, Earle JD. Management of subdiaphragmatic early-stage Hodgkin's disease. *Int J Radiat Oncol Biol Phys* 1989;16:1459.
15. Roos DE, O'Brien PC, Wright J, Willson K. Treatment of sub-diaphragmatic Hodgkin's disease: is radiotherapy alone appropriate only for inguino-femoral presentations? *Int J Radiat Oncol Biol Phys* 1994;28: 683.
16. Krikorian JG, Portlock CS, Rosenberg SA, Kaplan HS. Hodgkin's disease, stages I and II occurring below the diaphragm. *Cancer* 1979;43: 1866.
17. Barton M, Boyages J, Crennan E, et al. Radiotherapy for early infradiaphragmatic Hodgkin's disease: the Australasian experience. *Radiother Oncol* 1996;39:1.
18. Henry-Amar M, Aeppli DM, Anderson J, et al. Workshop statistical report. In: Somers R, Henry-Amar M, Meerwaldt JK, Carde P, eds. *Treatment strategy in Hodgkin's disease*. London: John Libbey Eurotext, 1990:169.
19. Mauch PM, Kalish LA, Kadin M, Coleman CN, Osteen R, Hellman S. Patterns of presentation of Hodgkin disease: implications for etiology and pathogenesis. *Cancer* 1993;71:2062.
20. Green FL, Brown PA. Laparoscopic approaches to abdominal malignancy. *Semin Surg Oncol* 1994;10:386.
21. Kaplan HS. *Hodgkin's disease*, 2nd ed. Cambridge, MA: Harvard University Press, 1980.
22. Krikorian JG, Portlock CS, Mauch PM. Hodgkin's disease presenting below the diaphragm: a review. *J Clin Oncol* 1986;4:1551.
23. Mai DH-W, Peschel RE, Portlock C, Knowlton A, Farber L. Clinical trials: stage I and II subdiaphragmatic Hodgkin's disease. *Cancer* 1991; 68:1476.
24. Givens SS, Fuller LM, Hagemeister FB, Gehan EA. Treatment of lower torso stages I and II Hodgkin's disease with radiation with or without adjuvant mechlorethamine, vincristine, procarbazine, and prednisone. *Cancer* 1990;66:69.
25. Lister TA, Crowther D, Sutcliffe SB, et al. Report of a committee convened to discuss the evaluation and staging of patients with Hodgkin's disease: Cotswolds meeting. *J Clin Oncol* 1989;7:1630.
26. Mendenhall NP. Diagnostic procedures and guidelines for the evaluation and follow-up of Hodgkin's disease. *Semin Radiat Oncol* 1996; 6:131.
27. King SC, Reiman RJ, Prosnitz LR. Prognostic importance of restaging gallium scans following induction chemotherapy for advanced Hodgkin's disease. *J Clin Oncol* 1994;12:306.
28. Hagemeister FB, Fesus SM, Lamki LM, Haynie TP. Role of the gallium scan in Hodgkin's disease. *Cancer* 1990;65:1090.
29. Ferzli G, Fiorillo MA, Solis R, et al. Laparoscopic staging of Hodgkin's disease. *J Laparoendosc Adv Surg Tech A* 1997;7:353.
30. Dmitrovsky E, Martin SE, Krudy AG, et al. Lymph node aspiration in the management of Hodgkin's disease. *J Clin Oncol* 1986;4:306.
31. Carde P, Hagenbeek A, Hayat M, et al. Clinical staging versus laparotomy and combined modality with MOPP versus ABVD in early stage Hodgkin's disease: the 146 twin randomised trials from the European Organisation for Research and Treatment of Cancer Lymphoma Cooperative Group. *J Clin Oncol* 1993;11:2258.
32. Russell KJ, Hoppe RT, Colby TV, et al. Lymphocyte predominant Hodgkin's disease: clinical presentation and results of treatment. *Radiother Oncol* 1984;1:199.
33. Carbone PP, Kaplan HS, Mushoff K, Smithers DW, Tubiana M. Report of the Committee on Hodgkin's Disease Staging Classification. *Cancer Res* 1971;31:1860.
34. Wang CJ, Chin YY, Leung SW, Chen HC, Sun LM, Fang FM. Topographic distribution of inguinal lymph nodes metastasis: significant in determination of treatment margin for elective inguinal lymph nodes irradiation of low pelvic tumors. *Int J Radiat Oncol Biol Phys* 1996; 35:133.
35. LeFloch O, Donaldson SS, Kaplan HS. Pregnancy following oophoropexy and total nodal irradiation in women with Hodgkin's disease. *Cancer* 1976;38:2263.
36. Zittoun R, Hoerni AB, Bernadou A, et al. Extended versus involved fields irradiation combined with MOPP chemotherapy in early clinical stages of Hodgkin's disease. *J Clin Oncol* 1985;3:207.
37. Aass N, Fossa S, Host H. Acute and subacute side effects due to infradiaphragmatic radiotherapy for testicular cancer: a prospective study. *Int J Radiat Oncol Biol Phys* 1992;22:1057.
38. Aass N, Hatun DE, Thoreson M, Fossa SD. Prophylactic use of tropisetron of metoclopramide during adjuvant abdominal radiotherapy of seminoma stage I: a randomised, open trial in 23 patients. *Radiother Oncol* 1997;45:125.
39. Hansen PV, Trykker H, Svennekjaer IL, Hvolby J. Long-term recovery of spermatogenesis after radiotherapy in patients with testicular cancer. *Radiother Oncol* 1990;18:117.
40. Fossa S, Aass N, Kaalhus O. Long-term morbidity after infradiaphragmatic radiotherapy in young men with testicular cancer. *Cancer* 1989; 64:404.
41. Swerdlow AJ, Jacobs PA, Marks A, et al. Fertility, reproductive outcomes, and health of offspring of patients treated for Hodgkin's disease: an investigation including chromosome examinations. *Br J Cancer* 1996;74:291.
42. Horning SJ, Hoppe RT, Kaplan HS, Rosenberg SA. Female reproductive potential after treatment for Hodgkin's disease. *N Engl J Med* 1981; 304:1377.
43. Hadar H, Loven D, Herskovitz P, Bairey O, Yagoda A, Levavi H. An evaluation of lateral and medial transposition of the ovaries out of radiation fields. *Cancer* 1994;74:774.
44. Pedrick TJ, Hoppe RT. Recovery of spermatogenesis following pelvic irradiation for Hodgkin's disease. *Int J Radiat Oncol Biol Phys* 1986; 12:117.
45. Clifton DK, Bremner WJ. The effect of testicular X-irradiation on spermatogenesis in man. *J Androl* 1983;4:387.
46. Rowley MJ, Leach DR, Warner GA, Heller CG. Effect of graded doses of ionizing radiation on the human testis. *Radiat Res* 1974;59:901.
47. Shekarriz M, Tolentino MVJr, Ayzman I, Lee J-C, Thomas AJ, Agarwal A. Cryopreservation and semen quality in patients with Hodgkin's disease. *Cancer* 1995;75:2732.
48. De Wilde RL, Hesseling M. No more radiogenic castration in women with Hodgkin's disease? *Am J Obstet Gynecol* 1995;173:1639.
49. Coleman CN, McDougall IR, Dailey MO, Ager P, Bush S, Kaplan HS. Functional hyposplenia after splenic irradiation for Hodgkin's disease. *Ann Intern Med* 1982;96:44.
50. Shurin SB. Disorders of the spleen. In: Handin RH, Lux SE, Stossel TP, eds. *Blood: principles and practice of hematology*. Philadelphia: JB Lippincott Co, 1995:1359.
51. Siber GR, Gorham C, Martin P, Corkery JC, Schiffman G. Antibody response to pre-treatment immunization and post-treatment boosting with bacterial polysaccharide vaccines in patients with Hodgkin's disease. *Ann Intern Med* 1986;104:467.
52. Coia LR, Hanks GE. Complications from large field intermediate dose infradiaphragmatic radiation: an analysis of the Patterns Of Care outcome studies for Hodgkin's disease and seminoma. *Int J Radiat Oncol Biol Phys* 1988;15:29.
53. Cosset J-M, Henry-Amar M, Meerwaldt JH. Long-term toxicity of early stages Hodgkin's disease therapy: the EORTC experience. *Ann Oncol* 1991;2:77.
54. Cosset J-M, Henry-Amar M, Burgers JMV, et al. Late injuries of the gastro-intestinal tract in the H_2 and H_5 EORTC Hodgkin's disease trials: emphasis on the role of exploratory laparotomy and fractionation. *Radiother Oncol* 1988;13:61.
55. Boivin J-F, Hutchison GB, Zauber AG, et al. Incidence of second cancers in patients treated for Hodgkin's disease. *J Natl Cancer Inst* 1995; 87:732.
56. Mauch PM, Kalish LA, Marcus KC, et al. Second malignancies after treatment for laparotomy staged IA–IIIB Hodgkin's disease: long-term analysis of risk factors and outcome. *Blood* 1996;87:3625.
57. Swerdlow AJ, Barber JA, Horwich A, Cunningham D, Milan S, Ozmar RZ. Second malignancy in patients with Hodgkin's disease treated at the Royal Marsden Hospital. *Br J Cancer* 1997;75:116.
58. Dietrich P-Y, Michel H-A, Cosset J-M, Bodis S, Bosq J, Hayat M. Second primary cancers in patients continuously disease-free from Hodgkin's disease: a protective role for the spleen. *Blood* 1994;84:1209.
59. Hancock SL, Hoppe RT. Long-term complications of treatment and causes of mortality after Hodgkin's disease. *Semin Radiat Oncol* 1996; 6:225.
60. Tucker MA, Coleman CN, Cox RS, Varghese A, Rosenberg SA. Risk of second cancers after treatment for Hodgkin's disease. *N Engl J Med* 1988;318:76.

61. Birdwell SH, Hancock SL, Varghese A, Cox RS, Hoppe RT. Gastrointestinal cancer after treating of Hodgkin's disease. *Int J Radiat Oncol Biol Phys* 1997;37:67.
62. Viviani S, Santoro A, Regni G, et al. Gonadal toxicity after combination chemotherapy for Hodgkin's disease: comparative results of MOPP vs ABVD. *Eur J Cancer* 1985;21:601.
63. Canellos GP, Anderson JR, Propert KJ, et al. Chemotherapy of advanced Hodgkin's disease with MOPP, ABVD, or MOPP alternating with ABVD. *N Engl J Med* 1992;327:1478.
64. Pene F, Henry-Amar M, Le Bourgeois JP, et al. A study of relapse and course of 153 cases of Hodgkin's disease (clinical stages I and II) treated at the Institut Gustave-Roussy from 1963 to 1970 with radiotherapy alone or with adjuvant monochemotherapy. *Cancer* 1980; 46:2131.

Hodgkin's Disease, edited by P. M. Mauch, J. O. Armitage, V. Diehl, R. T. Hoppe, and L. M. Weiss. Lippincott Williams & Wilkins, Philadephia ©1999.

CHAPTER 42

Contributions of the International Database on Hodgkin's Disease

Markus Loeffler, Michel Henry-Amar, and Reinier Somers

Throughout this textbook several authors repeatedly refer to the International Database on Hodgkin's Disease (IDHD) and analyses performed in this context. The IDHD initiative has been a milestone in the history of international collaboration in the field. This chapter serves as a description of what has been done by the IDHD, what results have been obtained, and the impact it has had on further research.

The idea for the IDHD originated at the First International Symposium on Hodgkin's Disease held 1987 in Cologne, Germany. Several prognostic-factor analyses had been performed by various groups by that time. However, there was no consensus about which prognostic factors should be taken into account, what their relative importance was, and how this depends on the endpoints considered. Available analyses differed remarkably in the spectrum of patients included, parameters considered, and statistical methodology. A second controversy at the Cologne Symposium centered around the long-term sequelae experienced by Hodgkin's disease patients, particularly those who had achieved a complete remission. Reports were available indicating increased risks of secondary neoplasms and other health hazards. However, the data sets reported by various groups were small and potentially biased. Several investigators therefore agreed at the Cologne meeting to plan a systematic metaanalysis on these issues.

The initiative was then taken over by the colleagues of the European Organization for Research and Treatment of Cancer (EORTC), who coordinated the project, aiming to present a first analysis on the occasion of an international symposium planned to be held in Paris in 1989 to commemorate the retirement of Professor Maurice Tubiana. Drs. Michel Henry-Amar and Reiner Somers deserve the credit for having pursued this tremendous effort.

Most of the larger institutions and cooperative groups in the Western World with extensive experience in the management of Hodgkin's disease were approached in 1988 for potential interest in contributing to the development of such a large database. A steering committee was formed to promote the IDHD, to regulate access to the data, and to stimulate new studies using the data collected. Twenty institutions/cooperative groups (see Appendix) agreed to participate by sending data in a standardized coding format to be analyzed by a common statistical design specified in a written protocol. In a sequence of meetings held in London, Paris, and Toronto, study protocols and regulations for data submission, publication, and data access were agreed on. During these meetings, adjustments of the study protocol and of the biostatistical evaluation strategies were discussed.

Data were obtained from patients randomized on prospective trials and from patients treated by standardized observational protocols. Requested data were restricted to factors previously reported to be of prognostic importance. Initial clinical presentation, extent of staging, type of treatment, treatment outcome, site and time to relapse, length of survival, cause of death, and development of second cancers were requested. Data were often simplified to facilitate statistical analysis. For example, radiation therapy was categorized into three groups: localized or involved-field, regional, or extended-field radiation therapy. Data were analyzed by one of us

M. Loeffler: Institute of Medical Statistics and Epidemiology, University of Leipzig, Leipzig, Germany.

M. Henry-Amar: Department of Clinical Research, Centre François Baclesse, Caen, France.

R. Somers: Valeriusstraat 42 II, 1071 MK Amsterdam, The Netherlands.

(M. H.-A.) with the use of a specific database management program developed at the Institut Gustave Roussy Department of Biostatistics and Epidemiology in Paris. The data were first presented at the Paris International Workshop and Symposium held on June 28–30, 1989. The proceedings were published in 1990 (1,2). The collaborative group subsequently had several plenary meetings on the occasion of international meetings related to lymphomas in Lugano 1990, Cologne 1991, Lugano 1993, and Cologne 1995 and 1998. A summary of the important results is presented subsequently.

After 1990, several additional studies were initiated, which are also discussed below: (a) salvage of relapse of early Hodgkin's disease initially treated with radiotherapy; (b) direct estimate at diagnosis of the prognosis of Hodgkin's disease patients; (c) risk of intercurrent death after Hodgkin's disease; and (d) treatment-related acute leukemia risk after Hodgkin's disease.

General meetings of all contributors were organized at the Second and Third International Symposia on Hodgkin's Lymphoma held in Cologne, Germany, in 1991 and 1994, during which updated information was presented (3–5).

THE INTERNATIONAL DATABASE ON HODGKIN'S DISEASE DATA SET

Overall data on 14,308 adult patients diagnosed from the early 1960s to 1984 were collected. Table 1 describes the contributions of the cancer centers and study groups. Table 2 provides a description of the study cohort. Most of the patients were treated in the 1970s, and only a few in the 1960s. Radiotherapy alone was the most frequent therapy, but combined-modality treatment has become more popular in the last decade. It should be noted that most of the patients registered were treated with MOPP or MOPP-like regimens if chemotherapy was applied. Adriamycin-containing modalities are rare in this data set. Although complete data were submitted for most parameters, there were some with a great deal of missing data, such as hemoglobin, ESR, albumin, and the extent of massive mediastinal tumor. Futhermore, several data items were not collected, such as date of primary treatment evaluation, treatment duration, dose of chemotherapy or radiotherapy, relapse treatment, and outcome.

In several respects the data submitted had varying degrees of accuracy. Some but not all trial groups coded histopathologic diagnosis reviewed by an expert panel. Coding of causes of death also varied with regard to completeness and accuracy. Biological parameters often could not be provided in relation to the normal values used in the respective laboratories. It therefore became obvious that the dataset and any analyses based on it would have limitations related to data completeness, accuracy, and consistency. On the other hand, the data set comprised the vast majority of all data collected in prospective trials available at that time. It can therefore be considered as representative of the status achieved in diagnosis and treatment in Western Europe, North America, and other countries meeting these standards.

TABLE 1. *Distribution of patients included by center and clinical stage*

Center	Clinical Stage				Total
	I	II	III	IV	
B.N.L.I. (UK)	623	837	615	463	2,538
EORTC Lymphoma Group	593	987	110	111	1,801
Stanford Univ Med Center (USA)	186	886	481	110	1,663
Princess Margaret Hospital (Canada)	228	430	229	160	1,047
Southwest Oncology Group (USA)	72	274	334	255	935
M. D. Anderson Cancer Center (USA)	190	422	157	101	870
Royal Marsden Hosp., London (UK)	214	357	159	0	730
St. Bartholomew's Hosp., London (UK)	129	231	146	104	610
G.A.T.L.A. (Argentina)	64	163	250	114	591
Universita di Pavia (Italy)	41	180	222	86	529
Joint Center for Radiation Therapy (USA)	133	303	83	3	522
Finsen Institute (Denmark)	122	182	88	86	478
Fondation Bergonié Bordeaux (France)	117	179	116	29	441
German Hodgkin Study Group (FRG)	29	140	144	87	400
Groupe Pierre et Marie Curie (France)	105	204	26	0	335
Christie Hospital, Manchester (UK)	38	76	58	127	299
The Institute of Oncology, Lubljana (Yugoslavia)	47	64	71	18	200
University of Minnesota Health Sciences Center (USA)	39	135	7	0	181
University of Nebraska (USA)	10	32	28	8	78
Yale University (USA)	6	23	23	8	60
Total	2,986	6,105	3,347	1,870	14,308

BNLI, British National Lymphoma Investigation; EORTC, European Organization for the Research and Development of Cancer; GATLA, Grupo Argentina de Tratamiento de la Leucemia Agoda.

TABLE 2. *Description of the IDHD cohort*

Initial Patient characteristics	
Sex	
Male	59.8%
Age (mean, in years)	33.5
15–19	12.4%
20–29	36.3%
30–39	23.6%
40–49	12.8%
50–59	8.2%
60–69	4.9%
70–79	1.4%
80+	0.4%
Clinical stage	
I	23.5%
II	45.1%
III	22.1%
IV	9.3%
Histologic type	
Lymphocytic predominance (LP)	7.7%
Nodulor sclerosing (NS)	62.0%
Mixed cellularity (MC)	25.9%
Lymphocytic depletion (LD)	2.1%
Unclassified	2.3%
Date of diagnosis	
1960–1969	8.2%
1970–1979	57.4%
1980–1984	34.4%
Treatment characteristics	
Splenectomy	45.0%
Irradiation alone	46.9%
Localized	6.5%
Regional	17.8%
Extended	22.6%
Chemotherapy alone	18.4%
MOPP-like	16.0%
Other types	2.4%
Combined modalities	34.7%
Localized RT and MOPP-like	9.2%
Localized RT and CT other types	2.1%
Regional RT and MOPP-like	8.4%
Regional RT and CT other types	2.7%
Extended RT and MOPP-like	11.9%
Extended RT and CT other types	0.4%

RT, radiotherapy; CT, chemotherapy; localized RT, involved-field RT; regional RT, mantle-field or inverted-Y RT; extended RT, (sub)total nodal RT; MOPP-like chemotherapy, combination of mechlorethamine, vincristine, procarbazine, and prednisone (MOPP) or alternatives with minor variations; CT other types, mostly Adriamycin-containing regimens.

TRENDS

The IDHD dataset shows several systematic trends in diagnostic and treatment policies over the years. It is remarkable that the relative frequency of nodular sclerosis subtype was steadily increasing while those of the mixed-cellular and lymphocyte predominant subtypes were diminishing from the 1960s to the 1980s. The reasons are unclear but are likely related to a shift in diagnostic techniques than to epidemiologic changes.

Laparotomy frequency changed. For example, it was performed in fewer than 20% of the CS III patients in the 1960s and 1980s, but over half of the patients underwent this procedure in the 1970s. This was accompanied by a gradual shift from radiotherapy alone to combined modality and chemotherapy alone over the years.

An important result of the IDHD was the insight that a remarkable gain in disease control and a reduction of mortality were obtained in the 1970s compared with the 1960s. However, surprisingly little further improvement was evident in the cohort diagnosed in the 1980s. Figure 1 illustrates this finding for overall survival and relapse-free survival. It is noteworthy that the trials conducted in the 1960s frequently were unicenter trials with a standardized strategy whereas data of the later periods stem from cooperative multicenter trials. Hence, one can speculate about a certain regression-to-the-mean effect in Figure 1. However this effect is unlikely to change the general judgment of only very limited improvement of treatment outcomes between the 1970s and the 1980s.

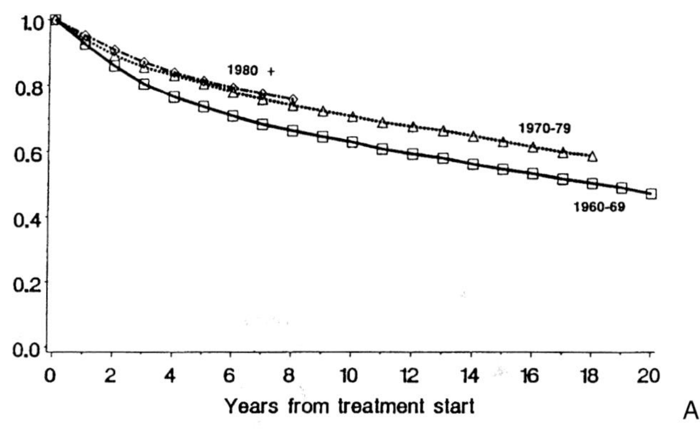

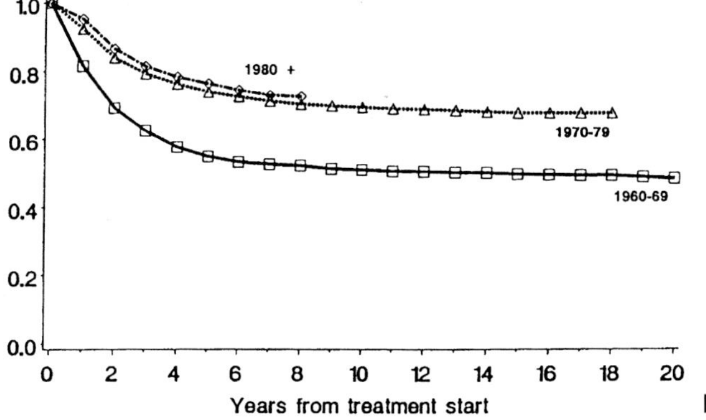

FIG. 1. Trends in treatment efficacy over the decades. **A:** Overall survival of all stages by treatment period (1960–1969, 1,115 patients; 1970–1979, 8,104 patients; 1980–, 5,096 patients). **B:** Relapse-free survival for all stages by treatment period (1960–1969, 1,008 patients; 1970–1979, 6,970 patients; 1980–, 4,338 patients). (Modified from ref. 1.)

TABLE 3. *Prognostic factors for positive laparotomy findings in patients staged clinically*

	CS IA	CS IIA	CS IB, CS IIB
Adverse factors			
Male gender	+	+	+
MC, LD histology	+	+	
Age over 50	+		
No mediastinal involvement		+	+
Many lymph node areas involved		+	+
Extranodal disease			+
High ESR		(+)	
Observed proportion of positive laparotomy			
No risk factor	0.11	0.19	0.11
All risk factors	0.38	0.69	0.51

CS, clinical stage; MC, mixed cellularity; LD, lymphocyte depletion, ESR, erythrocyte sedimentation rate.

PROGNOSTIC FACTORS FOR LAPAROTOMY FINDINGS

An important question addressed by the IDHD was whether the outcome of a staging laparotomy could be reliably predicted on the basis of the clinical stage and additional noninvasive measurements, that is, serum parameters.

Data on 4,049 laparotomized patients in CS I and II were analyzed using logistic regression methodology. Table 3 summarizes the results. In stage CS IA, only male gender, mixed cellularity and lymphocyte depletion histology, and age over 50 were associated with a higher probability of a positive laparotomy. In CS IIA, male gender, mixed cellularity and lymphocyte depletion histology, absence of mediastinal involvement, involvement of many lymph node areas, and high ESR were associated with positive laparotomy. In CS IB and IIB, male gender, absence of mediastinal involvement, and extranodal disease were predictive for infradiaphragmatic involvement.

It is, however, remarkable that in over 10% of the patients having none of these adverse factors, abdominal disease was detected by laparotomy. On the other hand, patients with many or all factors present frequently had no infradiaphragmatic disease. Depending on the clinical stage, this proportion varied between 30% and 60%. A more detailed description of these issues is presented in this volume in Chapter 18.

Thus, although a variety of noninvasive factors could be shown to be of prognostic value for laparotomy findings, the overall sensitivity and specificity obtained by the best prediction models were generally not sufficient to base rigorous treatment decisions (e.g., radiation alone to involved fields based on clinical staging) on them.

PROGNOSTIC FACTORS FOR ACHIEVING COMPLETE REMISSION

Table 4 summarizes the prognostic factors for achieving complete remission after primary treatment. They were analyzed separately for each clinical stage, and two different multivariate logistic regression models were used. In the first model (A) serum parameters were ignored. In this case, age, histology (lymphocyte depletion or mixed cellularity) and B symptoms were prognostic, with relative risks between 1.2 and 1.5. In the alternative model (B) systemic symptoms were deliberately ignored to assess the role of serum parameters. In this case, ESR and serum albumin took over the role of B symptoms. This is understandable because a strong correlation between serum parameters and B symptoms was revealed. However, taken together, only a few factors appeared to be prognostic for achievement of a complete response. Ann Arbor stage and B symptoms were confirmed to be the most reliable predictors, and other parameters were of minor importance.

TABLE 4. *Prognostic factors for CR (nonlaparotomized patients)*[a]

Models	CS I (*n* = 1,509)	CS II (*n* = 2,880)	CS III (*n* = 1,856)	CS IV (*n* = 1,512)
Model A B symptoms included Serum parameters excluded	Age Histology	Age B symptoms	Age B symptoms	Age Infradiaphragmatic
Model B B symptoms excluded Serum parameters included	ESR	Age ESR/albumin	Age ESR/albumin	Age Albumin Infradiaphragmatic

[a]Relative risks between 1.2 and 1.5.
CR, complete remission; CS, clinical stage; ESR, erythrocyte sedimentation rate.

TABLE 5. *Prognostic factors for relapse*[a]

CS I (n = 2,783)	CS II (n = 5,414)	CS III (n = 2,568)	CS IV (n = 819)
Age	Age	Age	Age
Gender	Gender	Gender	
Histology[b]	Histology[b]	Histology	Histology
Laparotomy	Laparotomy	Laparotomy	
B symptoms[b]	B symptoms	B symptoms	
Infradiaphragmatic[b]	No. LN areas	No. LN areas	
ESR, Hb[b]	ESR, Hb, Alb[b]	MT	

CS, clinical stage; LN, lymph node; MT, mediastinal disease; ESR, erythrocyte sedimentation rate; Hb, hemoglobin; ALB, albumin.
[a]Relative risks between 1.2 and 1.8.
[b]RR > 1.5.

PROGNOSTIC FACTORS FOR RELAPSE-FREE SURVIVAL

In contrast to complete response, more factors were found to contribute to the prediction of the quality of a complete response once it was achieved. Table 5 summarizes the result of a multivariate analysis based on the proportional hazard model, which was stratified for treatment period and type of treatment. These models were constructed under the simplifying assumptions that prognostic factors are effective over the entire time of the observation and that there are no interactions with treatment modalities. Because data were pooled from various risk-adapted treatment protocols, it was evident that expectations of detecting many new prognostic factors had to be moderate. It was therefore remarkable to find evidence that several factors beyond the Ann Arbor factors had independent contributions to the prediction of relapse-free survival. Old age and male gender were already well known to be unfavorable; lymphocyte depletion and mixed cellularity histology had an adverse role in all stages but most prominently in CS I and CS II, where the relative risks exceeded 1.5. B symptoms and infradiaphragmatic disease appeared to be associated with unfavorable prognosis in stage I. It was particularly noteworthy that clinical stages II and III proved to be heterogeneous. The extent of the disease, as measured by the number of lymph node areas involved, plays a role in stages II and III. This finding suggests a considerable heterogeneity of these stages, which could be taken into account in the treatment allocation. Furthermore, serum parameters such as ESR, hemoglobin, and serum albumin appeared to play a role in stages I and II if added as single factors to the above models. However, because of the missing-value problem, their role had to be interpreted with some caution. No relevant prognostic factors could be identified for stage IV. As a conclusion of the IDHD analysis, it was not considered justified to identify a very high-risk group that might be submitted to very aggressive forms of primary treatments such as high-dose chemotherapy.

A few years later an improved prognostic metaanalysis for advanced-stage disease was undertaken by Hasenclever et al. (6). In their analysis a more complete and better standardized data set was submitted, and the endpoints considered were time to treatment failure and disease-specific survival. The analysis showed seven independent factors to be relevant, the first five of which were similar to findings in the IDHD: stage, old age, male gender, low hemoglobin, low serum albumin, leukocytosis, and lymphocytopenia (for details see Chapter 19).

PROGNOSTIC FACTORS FOR DISEASE-SPECIFIC SURVIVAL

Disease-specific survival was also analyzed using proportional hazard models as mentioned above. In contrast to relapse-free survival, the prognostic factors for survival remained few (Table 6). The role of age and gender is not surprising. The lymphocyte-depleted subtype, and to a smaller degree the mixed-cellularity subtype were unfavorable indicators. This was not new. A new factor was the number of lymph node areas involved in stages I, IIB, and

TABLE 6. *Prognostic factors for death from Hodgkin's disease*

CS I and IIA	CS I and IIB	CS IIIA	CS IIIB	CS IV
Age[a]	Age[a]	Age[a]	Age[a]	Age[a]
Histology[a]	Gender	Histology[a]	Histology	Gender
	Histology[a]	No. LN areas		Histology
	No. LN areas			

CS, clinical stage; LN, lymph node; MT, mediastinal disease; ESR, erythrocyte sedimentation rate; Hb, hemoglobin; ALB, albumin.
[a]RR > 2.0.

IIIA. This parameter quantifying the extent of the disease added to the information of the stage. No contribution could be detected for serum parameters or for bulky disease, but this may have been because of the missing-value problem.

The three preceding analyses about prognostic factors for complete remission, relapse free survival, and disease-specific survival were all conducted in the first round of analyses published in 1990 (1). The key lessons were that the Ann Arbor staging system and the histopathologic classification were confirmed to be major prognostic factors for the disease with respect to all endpoints. However, there was evidence that this list could and should be amended by additional parameters related to more details on the spread of disease and tumor burden (e.g., infradiaphragmatic disease, number of lymph node areas), to biological activity (e.g., hemoglobin, ESR, serum albumin), and to constitutive parameters such as age and gender.

SURVIVAL AFTER RELAPSE

The data gathered in the IDHD permitted some insight into survival after relapse. When occurrence of a relapse was included as a time-dependent covariate into proporional hazard models, it was by far the most prominent adverse prognostic factor with respect to overall survival. Relative risks increased by more than fivefold. Figure 2 illustrates that relapses after initial stage I and II disease had a somewhat better prognosis than after an initial advanced stage. Only 30% of advanced-stage patients experiencing a relapse survived more than 10 years.

Recently a more detailed reanalysis of the IDHD data was undertaken to investigate survival in patients with limited disease who were initially treated with radiotherapy alone. In patients who relapsed after a laparotomy staged PS I or PS II disease treated with radiation alone, over 30% died within 10 years of Hodgkin's disease (7). It was irrelevant in this context whether the relapse occurred within the first year after the initial treatment or many years later. Disease-specific survival after relapse was shown to be worse if the patient was over 40 years of age or had MC histology or extranodal involvement. Almost identical results were found when the analysis was repeated for patients in clinical stages I and II who underwent radiotherapy alone (8).

PROGNOSTICATING OVERALL SURVIVAL

An analysis of prognostic factors for long-term outcomes usually has the objective of investigating heterogeneity in a population with respect to specific endpoints. For this purpose, proportional hazard models are widely used. They belong to a family of semiparametric models that specify relative risks under restrictive assumptions about the proportionality of hazard functions. However, these models do not require quantitative specifications of the shape of these hazard functions or the related survival functions.

If the objective of modeling is not to analyze population heterogeneity but to predict the survival of individual patients, it is advantageous to have a quantitative specification of the survival function. In a reanalysis of IDHD data, Gobbi and co-workers (9) investigated a variety of different parametric survival functions. They found that a log-normal model would fit the observed overall survival data best. This model was then fitted to the data on 12,647 patients treated from 1970 to 1984, adjusting for several prognostic factors.

As a result, the authors derived an equation for the median expected survival time. In this equation the following seven factors were taken into account: stage, B symptoms, age, gender, histopathology, serum albumin, and number of lymph node areas involved. Thus, this model also illustrated the role of several prognostic factors besides Ann Arbor stage with respect to survival.

CAUSES OF DEATH

The IDHD data set permitted an analysis of the causes of death. Figure 3 illustrates that the mortality after diagnosis of Hodgkin's disease is increased over the mortality

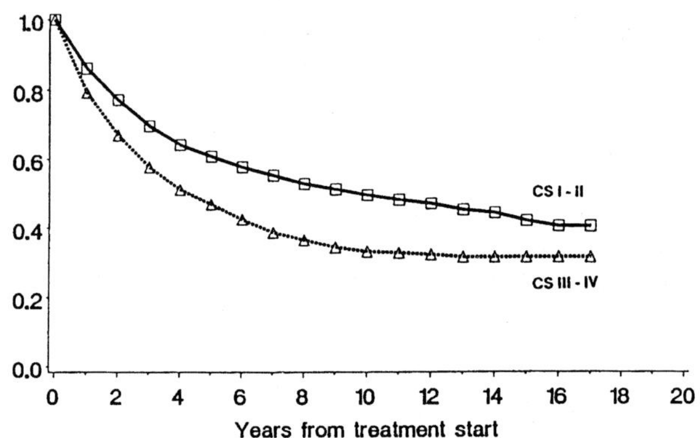

FIG. 2. Survival after relapse in patients treated between 1970 and 1984 by clinical stage at first presentation (CS I–II, 1,878 patients; CS III–IV, 1,257 patients). (Modified from ref. 1.)

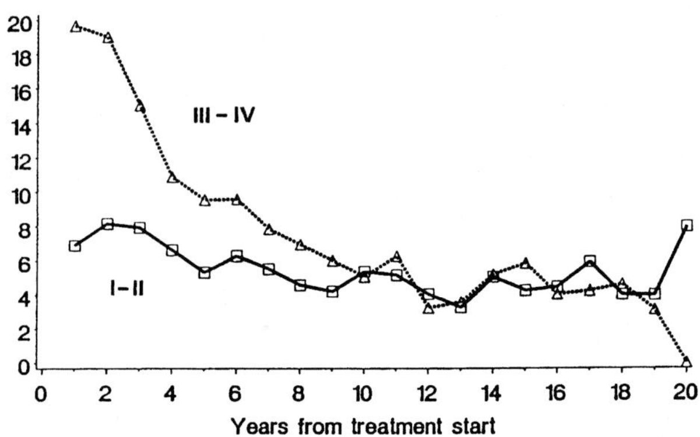

FIG. 3. Standardized mortality ratio (SMR) for all stages as a function of time by clinical stage including all causes of death (CS I–II, 9,041 patients; CS III–IV, 5,184 patients). (Modified from ref. 1.)

in the normal reference population not only in the first years after diagnosis but for at least 20 years thereafter. The high mortality in CS III and IV is certainly expected, and the elevation for several years reflects to some degree the high risk for relapse. However, there remains a four- to sixfold increase in risk of death compared with a comparable general population. With regard to clinical stages I and II, it is even more remarkable that the initial risk of death is only slightly higher than the risk in subsequent years.

Figure 4 provides some more detailed insight. It describes the cumulative incidence in the IDHD cohort, separating death from Hodgkin's disease from that of other causes. It is evident that death from disease was the overwhelming process in advanced stages. After a steep increase in the first 6 to 8 years, the disease continued to cause death virtually over 20 years at a low rate. In limited stages, the cumulative incidence of death from disease had a strikingly different pattern. Death from disease and other causes of death were of the same order of magnitude over the entire time course and finally the disease contributed less than other causes.

A more detailed analysis was undertaken to discriminate causes of death not related to the disease (1,2). Figure 4C shows that treatment-related mortality had a prominent contribution with a cumulative incidence of almost 3% after 20 years. Another important cause of death was the occurrence of secondary neoplasms. A total of 413 deaths were reported to be caused by either acute leukemias, non-Hodgkin's lymphomas, or solid tumors. The cumulative incidence of this cause of death rose continuously over the observation period and reached about 10% after 20 years. Taken together, treatment-related deaths and secondary neoplasms accounted for about half of the deaths not caused by the disease. Because, however, the standard mortality ratio was increased about four- to sixfold (see Fig. 3), a large proportion of the deaths coded as "intercurrent death" or "cause unspecified" must be assumed to be associated with the disease and/or treatment as well. This issue is discussed in greater depth in Chapters 32, 34, and 35 of this volume.

SECONDARY NEOPLASMS

An important contribution of the IDHD was an insight into the epidemiology of secondary neoplasms following Hodgkin's disease. When the analysis was restricted to those 12,411 patients who had survived at least 1 year after diagnosis, overall, 631 secondary neoplasms were observed. Of these, 158 were acute leukemias or myelodysplastic syndromes (AL), 106 were non-Hodgkin's lymphomas (NHL), and 367 solid tumors (ST, male 229, female 138). The most frequent solid tumors in men were long carcinomas (68), basal cell carcinoma of the skin (31), and carcinomas of the digestive tract (53). In women, long carcinomas (27), breast cancer (39), basal cell carcinoma of the skin (14), and *in situ* cervical carcinomas (9) were most frequent.

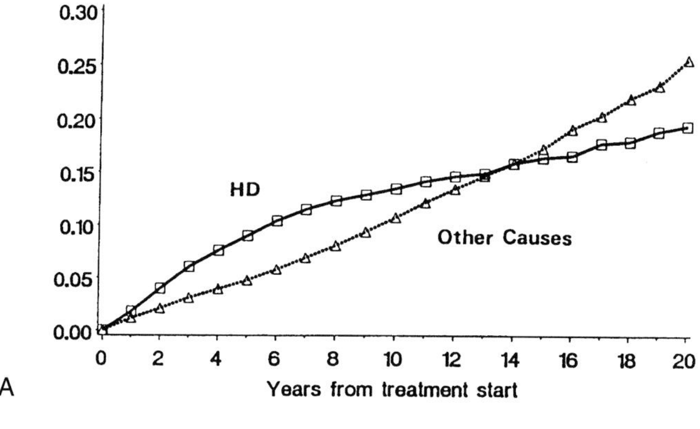

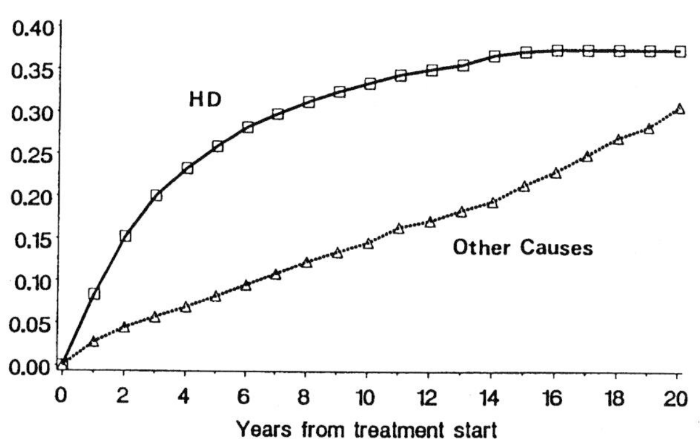

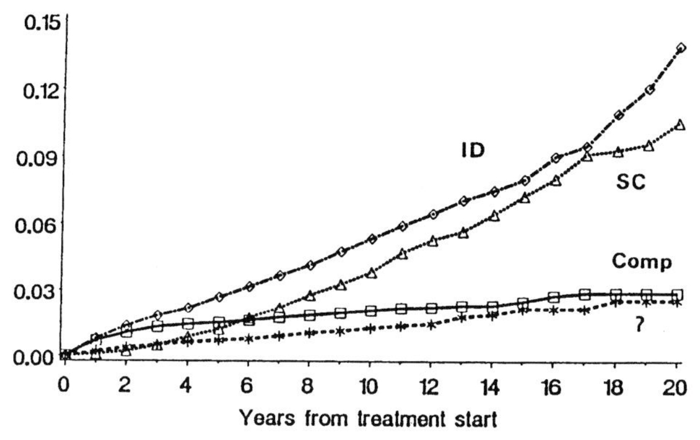

FIG. 4. Cumulative incidence of death by stage and cause of death. **A:** Early stages (9,041 patients; deaths from disease, 1,242; other causes, 715). **B:** Advanced stages (5,184 patients; death from disease, 1,768; other causes, 414). **C:** Causes of death other than disease (ID, intercurrent death, 577 patients; SC, secondary cancers, 413 patients; TRD, treatment-related death, 233 patients; ?, cause unspecified, 139 patients). (Modified from ref. 1.)

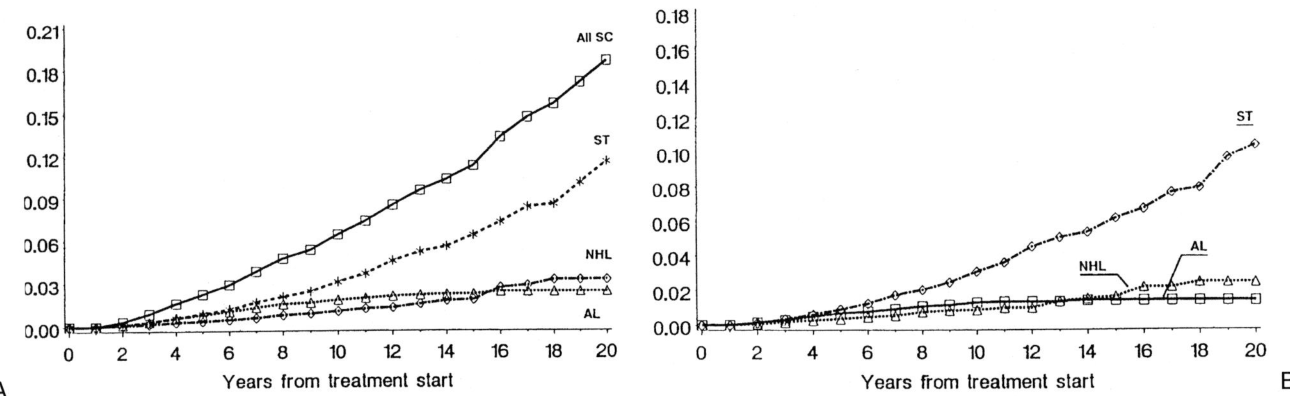

FIG. 5. Cumulative incidence of secondary neoplasms. **A:** All patients who survived primary treatment at least 1 year (12,411 patients; acute leukemia, 158; NHL, 106; solid tumors, 367). **B:** All patients in continuous complete remission who survived primary treatment at least 1 year (11,241 patients; acute leukemia, 87; NHL, 68; solid tumors, 231). (Modified from ref. 1.)

TABLE 7. *Time-dependent proportional hazards model on selected second cancer risk (relative risk) for 12,411 patients who survived at least 1 year after Hodgkin's disease diagnosis*

	AL (204–208)	NHL (200)	ST (140–194)
Sex ratio (male/female)	1.1	1.9	1.2
Age			
15–19 years	1.0	1.0	1.0
20–29 years	1.3	1.4	0.8
30–39 years	1.4	3.7[d]	1.3
40–49 years	2.5[d]	6.0[e]	3.1[e]
50–59 years	4.0[e]	10.5[e]	8.4[e]
≥60 years	4.5[e]	21.6[e]	12.0[e]
Histology			
LP	1.5	1.8[e]	0.9
NS	1.0	1.0	1.0
MC	0.9	1.0	0.9
LD	0.6	0.4	1.2
Unclassified	0.9	2.1	1.6
Response to initial treatment			
No complete remission/CR	2.1[d]	0.9	1.0
Initial treatment			
Splenectomy (yes/no)	1.3[b]	1.4[b]	1.0
Localized RT	1.0	1.0	1.0
Regional RT	1.2	0.9	1.2
Extended RT	1.3	1.2	1.7[e]
MOPP-like CT	3.5[d]	2.0[b]	1.2
Other CT	4.3[c]	2.4	1.0
RT (any type) and MOPP-like CT	5.3[e]	1.8	—
Localized/regional RT and MOPP-like CT	—	—	0.8
Extended RT and MOPP-like CT	—	—	1.8[b]
RT (any type) and CT other types	3.0	4.5[d]	0.7
Clinical outcome (time-dependent covariate)			
No relapse	1.0	1.0	1.0
First relapse treated with RT	1.7	3.7[d]	1.1
First relapse treated with CT	5.3[e]	2.3[d]	1.2
First relapse treated with RT + CT	2.8[e]	2.2[d]	1.3[b]
Global chi-square	168	159	411
p value (df)	<.001 (22)	<.001 (22)	<.001 (23)

[a]AL, acute leukemia; NHL, non-Hodgkin's lymphoma; ST, solid tumor. IC D0-9 codes shown in parentheses. ICD0-9 173 and 180 excluded from ST. Relative risk for a model allowing all the variables to be considered together.

[b]$p < .10$; [c]$p < .05$; [d]$p < .01$; [e]$p < .001$; two-sided test.

LP, lymphocyte predominance; NS, nodular sclerosis; MC, mixed cellularity; LD, lymphocyte depletion; RT, radiation therapy.

When compared to the general population, the ratio of observed (O) to expected (E) cases was 1.7 in both male and female patients for solid tumors. This risk increase appears moderate but accounted for about 170 excess tumors. In contrast the O/E-risk was found to be elevated for about 10 years by a factor of 30, accounting for about 150 excess cases.

Figure 5A illustrates the cumulative incidence measures for all secondary neoplasms and the various subtypes for the entire cohort. The cumulative incidence for ST increased from 6% after 10 years to 11% after 15 years and to 19% after 20 years. For acute leukemia the respective rates were 1.8%, 2.2%, and 2.4%. For non-Hodgkin's lymphoma they were 1.0%, 1.8% and 3.2%, respectively. Figure 5B describes the same analysis restricted to patients who were in continuous complete remission. The difference between the two figures illustrates the contribution treatment for relapse makes with repect to the occurrence of secondary neoplasms.

A more thorough analysis of prognostic factors for incidence of secondary tumors was performed (1,5). Variables included in the model were gender, age, histology, response to initial treatment, initial treatment type (involved-field or extended-field irradiation, total nodal irradiation, MOPP-like chemotherapy, combined-modality therapy), relapse, and type of treatment at relapse. Results are summarized in Table 7. Factors significantly correlated with an increased risk of acute leukemia were age above 40 and MOPP-like chemotherapy given alone or in combination with radiation therapy. In addition, chemotherapy-treated relapses were associated with a higher risk for acute leukemia. This was considered an indication that chemotherapy played a role in leukemia induction. However, it was not clear whether Hodgkin's disease itself is associated with an intrinsic risk for leukemia.

Factors associated with increased risk of secondary non-Hodgkin's lymphoma were age above 30, male gender, combination chemotherapy other than MOPP and radiation therapy, as treatment for relapse.

Only age above 40 and extended-field radiation given alone or in combination with chemotherapy were associated with an increased incidence of solid tumor.

To further highlight the remarkable contribution of relapse treatment to this phenomenon, Figure 3B illustrates the cumulative incidence of these malignancies if restricted to those patients who are in continuous complete remission. For acute leukemia the incidence was 1.3% and 1.5% after 10 and 15 years, respectively. A separate prognostic analysis was performed for these patients. Combined-modality treatments including MOPP-like chemotherapies were associated with the higher risk of secondary acute leukemia. In contrast, MOPP-like chemotherapy alone had only slightly increased risks. Furthermore, there was a small but significant relationship between acute leukemia and splenectomy.

SPECIFIC ASPECTS OF LEUKEMIA INDUCTION

Some further insight into the induction of AL was recently obtained by a sophisticated reanalysis of IDHD data using a novel biometric technique (10,11). The approach was based on a parametric model of latent carcinogenesis, which had been shown to be an effective method in analyzing time to tumor occurence. The basic model assumptions can be summarized as follows. It is assumed that there is an induction step that causes preleukemic lesions (e.g., microscopic clones). The number of such lesions indicates the strength of the induction process and may be related to dose and timing of the hazardous process. Such lesions are assumed to follow a Poisson distribution. The development of such lesions to a manifest leukemia usually depends on a complex sequence of events. For simplicity, it is assumed that this time, called progression time, has a distribution that, in particular, considers that some lesions never develop into a leukemia. If several lesions are induced, the time for the first to develop a manifest leukemia is called latency time. Clearly, such latency times are also distributed over a population.

When this model was fit to the IDHD data, it was considered that leukemia induction could occur during initial treatment and during relapse treatment. Relapse treatment implied that lesions could be induced at later times in addition to the lesions left from initial treatment. Two groups of patients in the IDHD were considered. One group received radiotherapy alone as primary treatment (5,403 cases) and MOPP-like treatment in case of relapse (1,777 such relapses). A second group received MOPP-like chemotherapy as primary treatment (6,113 cases) and some other kind of chemotherapy in case of relapse (1,223 such relapses).

The major findings are summarized in Figure 6. Of the treatment regimens considered, radiotherapy alone had the lowest leukemia induction potency. MOPP-like chemotherapy, in contrast, had a much higher potency (about sevenfold) to lead to leukemia than radiation alone. An even higher leukemia induction was revealed by relapse treatments with chemotherapy other than the primary MOPP-like schemes. Unfortunately, the IDHD did not provide more detailed data on the type of these relapse treatments, but it can be assumed to have incorporated a wide variety of schemes including high-dose chemotherapy and subsequent bone marrow transplantation. The most remarkable finding, however, is that the hazard curves in fact had very similar shapes, with peaks at about 4 years, medians at about 8 years, and steep declines after 10 years. This was true following primary and relapse treatment. This finding can hence be interpreted as strong evidence for treatment-related effects.

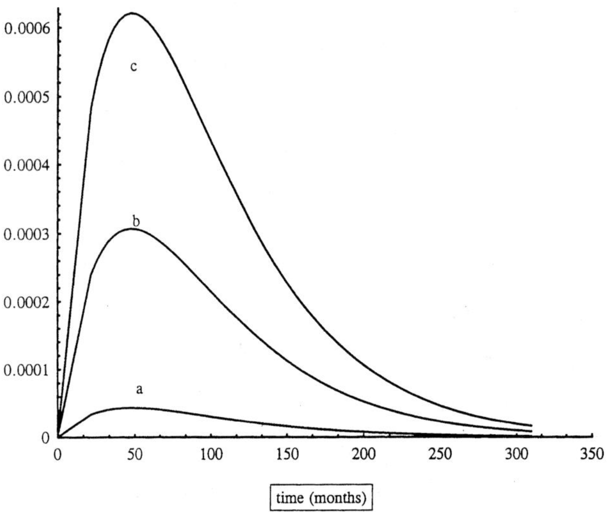

FIG. 6. Hazard functions and latency times for acute leukemia. Estimates based on parametric modeling: *lower curve,* radiotherapy alone; *middle curve,* MOPP-like chemotherapy; *upper curve,* relapse chemotherapy other than MOPP-like.

DISCUSSION

The IDHD is a historic milestone in the research on Hodgkin's disease, as it represented for the first time a collaborative effort among many of the leading cancer centers and cooperative trial groups to answer burning questions in the management of the disease. This type of metaanalysis, pooling individual patient data into one comprehensive database and analyzing them according to a jointly designed study protocol, turned out to be feasible and subsequently encouraged a couple of successor metaanalyses in this field. In particular, it encouraged the project that led to the international index for high-grade non-Hodgkin lymphomas (11), the international prognostic factor project for Hodgkin's disease (6), and a meta-analysis on chemotherapy versus combined-modality treatment in advanced-stage Hodgkin's disease (12).

The IDHD analyses have certainly influenced the scientific community remarkably. They made clear that the Ann Arbor staging system needed amendments if one were to use them to decide on treatment strategies. The analyses provided a sound platform to establish a series of such factors. They showed that prediction of laparotomy outcomes on the basis of noninvasive parameters is limited. They showed a variety of prognostic factors other than stage and their dependency on the choice of the endpoint. They revealed important insights into the mortality patterns in relation to the corresponding population but also with repect to the causes of death. In particular, they focused attention on the issue of secondary neoplasms and their relation to treatment. The data also highlighted the necessity to investigate in greater detail the so-called intercurrent deaths and treatment-related mortality.

Despite these remarkable aspects, the IDHD suffered from several limitations. One limitation was the quality of the data submitted. There were many missing values for biological parameters (e.g., size of mediastinal tumors, reviewed histology, serum parameters). There were defects in the data abstraction process (e.g., no date of primary treatment outcome, no coding of outcomes other than CR, no distinction between treatment intended and treatment given, limited attempts to quantify treatment intensity). The major limitation, however, was that any treatment comparisons were strictly excluded. It was decided that all data would be blinded with respect to the centers and treatment protocols from which they stemmed. Hence, it was impossible to compare arms of randomized trials. Therefore, it was also impossible to investigate whether prognostic factors depend on treatment strategies. Another limitation is that data on children were hardly included.

Now, 10 years after the IDHD was inaugurated, perhaps the most important limitation is that it only contains data on patients diagnosed before 1984. In particular, the contribution of Adriamycin-containing regimens was small in the database, but these regimens are now widely used. We, however, do not know to what extent the results discussed above for prognostic factors are different under these regimens. There is some evidence that leukemia induction from primary treatment might have decreased, but we do not know whether more aggressive relapse treatments outweigh this effect.

In summary, the International Database on Hodgkin's Disease collected data on over 14,000 individual patients treated in different cancer centers and trial groups according to standardized observational or randomized trial protocols. The data were collected to be submitted to a joint statistical analysis on prognostic factors for various endpoints and investigations on mortality patterns and on late sequelae. The IDHD was a milestone in the international cooperation of many trial groups, and many successor projects have directly or indirectly originated from this highly successful effort.

APPENDIX

IDHD steering committee members: D. E. Bergsagel (Toronto, Canada); M. Henry-Amar, Scientific Secretary (Villejuif, France); R. T. Hoppe (Stanford, USA); A. Horwich (London, UK); M. Loeffler (Cologne, Germany); K. A. MacLennan (London, UK); P. Mauch, present Chairman (Boston, USA); R. Somers, first Chairman (Amsterdam, The Netherlands); L. Specht (Copenhagen, Denmark); B. Vaughan Hudson (London, UK).

IDHD cooperating centers and cooperating groups: British National Lymphoma Investigation (BNLI), London, UK (M. H. Bennett, B. W. Hancock, K. A. MacLennan, B. Vaughan Hudson, G. Vaughan Hudson); EORTC Lymphoma Cooperative Group (M. Henry-Amar,

J. H. Meerwaldt, R. Somers, J. Thomas); Stanford University Medical Center, Stanford, USA (R. S. Cox, R. T. Hoppe); Princess Margaret Hospital, Toronto, Canada (D. E. Bergsagel, M. Gospodarowicz, S. Sutcliffe); Southwest Oncology Group (SWOG), USA (C. A. Coltman, S. J. Dahlberg); University of Texas M. D. Anderson Cancer Center, Houston, USA (D. O. Dixon, L. M. Fuller, F. B. Hagemeister); Royal Marsden Hospital, London, UK (S. Ashley, A. Horwich); St. Bartholomew's Hospital, London, UK (W. Gregory, T. A. Lister); Grupo Argentina de Tratamiento de la Leucemia Agoda (GATLA), Argentina (S. Pavlovsky, M. T. Santarelli); Universita di Pavia, Italy (M. Comelli, P. G. Gobbi); Joint Center for Radiation Therapy, Boston, USA (C. N. Coleman, P. Mauch); Finsen Institute, Copenhagen, Denmark (N. I. Nissen, L. Specht); Fondation Bergonié, Bordeaux, France (F. Bonichon, H. Eghbali, B. Hoerni); German Hodgkin Study Group, Germany (V. Diehl, D. Hasenclever, M. Loeffler, M. Pfreundschuh); Groupe Pierre et Marie Curie, France (H. Eghbali, A. Najman, R. Zittoun); Christie Hospital and Holt Radium Institute, Manchester, UK (D. Crowther, R. Swindell); The Institute of Oncology, Ljubljana, Slovenia (V. Pompe Kirn, M. Vovk); University of Minnesota Health Science Center, Minneapolis, USA (D. M. Aeppli, C. K. K. Lee, S. H. Levitt); University of Nebraska, Omaha, USA (J. Anderson, J. O. Armitage); and Yale University, New Haven, USA (S. Dowling, C. S. Portlock).

REFERENCES

1. Somers R, Henry-Amar M, Meerwaldt IH, et al, eds. *Treatment strategy in Hodgkin's disease. Colloque Inserm Vol 196.* Paris: Les Editions INSERM; London: John Libbey Eurotext 1990.
2. Henry-Amar M, Somers R. Survival outcome after Hodgkin's disease: A report from the IDHD. *Semin Oncol* 1990;17:758–768.
3. Mauch P, Henry-Amar M, International database on Hodgkin's disease: A cooperatiave effort to determine treatment outcome. *Ann Oncol* 1992;3(Suppl 4):9–61.
4. Loeffler M, Mauch P, MacLennon K, Specht L, Henry-Amar M. Review on prognostic factors. *Ann Oncol* 1992;3(Suppl 4):63–66.
5. Henry-Amar M. Second cancer after the treatment for Hodgkin's disease: A report from the IDHD. *Ann Oncol* 1992;3(Suppl 4):117–128.
6. Hasenclever D, Diehl V. A numerical index to predict tumor control in advanced Hodgkin's disease. *Blood* 1996;88:673a.
7. Specht L, Horwich A, Ashley S. Salvage of relapse of patients with Hodgkin's disease in clinical stages I or II who were staged with laparotomy and initially treated with radiotherapy alone. A report from the IDHD. *Int J Radiat Oncol Biol Phys* 1994;30:S805–S811.
8. Horwich A, Specht L, Ashley S. Survival analysis of patients with clinical stages I or II Hodgkin's disease who have relapsed after initial treatment with radiotherapy alone. *Eur J Cancer* 1997;33:848–853.
9. Gobbi P, Comelli M, Grignani GE, Pieresca C, Bertoloni D, Asconi E. Estimate of expected survival at diagnosis in Hodgkin's disease: A means of weighting prognostic factors and a tool for treatment choice and clinical research. A report of the IDHD. *Haematologica* 1994;79:241–255.
10. Tsodikov AD, Loeffler M, Yakovlev AY. Assessing the risk of secondary leukemia in patients treated for Hodgkin's disease. A report from the IDHD. *J Biol Systems* (in press).
11. Tsodikov A, Loeffler M, Yakovlev A. A cure model with time changing risk factors: An application to the analysis of secondary leukemia. A report from the IDHD. *Stat Med* (in press).
12. Loeffler M, Brosteanu O, Hasenclever D, et al. Meta-analysis of chemotherapy versus combined modality treatment trials in Hodgkin's disease. International Database on Hodgkin's Disease Overview Study Group. *J Clin Oncol* 1998;16:818–829.

Hodgkin's Disease, edited by P. M. Mauch,
J. O. Armitage, V. Diehl, R.T. Hoppe, and L. M. Weiss.
Lippincott Williams & Wilkins, Philadephia ©1999.

CHAPTER 43

Hodgkin's Disease in Africa

Peter Jacobs, Werner Bezwoda, Geoffrey Falkson, and Dalila Sellami

Data from Africa regarding Hodgkin's disease is generally sketchy. This is, in part, a reflection of the priorities in underdeveloped countries, where imperatives are usually basic survival rather than the nuances of exacting disease classification. Data gathering by registries and attempts to treat lymphoma in a consistent and acceptable manner are often hampered by a shortage of resources. These range from a lack of trained staff to inadequate facilities for investigation and are aggravated by limited supplies of cytotoxic drugs or poor access to radiotherapeutic equipment.

There are vast population and cultural variations on the continent. It is thus impossible to give a comprehensive picture of differences in natural history and response to treatment of Hodgkin's disease in Africa. This is particularly true when the diverse populations, that include black, white, and those of mixed ancestry, together with others of Mediterranean stock, are considered. The available data are derived from relatively few centers, making generalization difficult.

Despite these daunting limitations, it has been possible to assemble an overview of this entity as reported during the last three decades and as presently seen by practitioners in those countries where there is access to medical records. With such observations in mind, five aspects are sufficiently circumscribed to allow more detailed analysis. Included are the issues of epidemiologic difference, if any, by race or geographic region; patterns of disease at presentation; childhood Hodgkin's disease; the association with retroviral or other infectious disease; and prevailing management programs. From this some global comments emerge.

First, there are significant differences in the pattern of Hodgkin's disease in the various populations. It appears to be less common in blacks, particularly in central Africa as well as those living in the northern and southern extremities of the continent. In addition, the mean age at diagnosis is highest in whites and lowest in blacks, with those of mixed ancestry occupying an intermediate position. Similarly, histologic subtypes vary: nodular sclerosis predominates in the Caucasian patients, whereas mixed-cellularity and lymphocyte-depleted disease are more frequent in blacks. Second, late presentation is more common among lower socioeconomic and less educated groups. This may, however, be caused more by perceptions and lack of access to medical care than by any unique or disparate disease biology. Finally, the coexistence of tuberculosis with Hodgkin's disease and the acquired immunodeficiency syndrome is widespread, thus distorting natural history and survival in this lymphoma.

Conclusions about Hodgkin's disease in Africa inevitably attract comparisons with findings in other economically underdeveloped populations, including black Americans. Such contrasts provide a chance to examine common genetic influences based on the slave routes of yesteryear and to explore those differences that may have an environmental basis. We have also had the opportunity to review experiences in the northern and southern parts of the continent and briefly to compare our findings with what is reported from other Third World countries. The conclusions are that, stage for stage, there are no fundamental disparities in regard to presentation or response to treatment. The constellation of environmentally determined adverse prognostic features that culminate in advanced stage when first seen, seem to be the major factors that impact negatively on outcome, rather than any genetically determined or ethnic differences in host or host response to the neoplasm.

P. Jacobs: Department of Hematology and Bone Marrow Transplant Unit, Constantiaberg Medi-Clinic, Plumstead, South Africa.

W. Bezwoda: Department of Medicine, University of Witatersrand, Parktown, South Africa.

G. Falkson: Department of Medical Oncology, University of Pretoria, Pretoria, South Africa.

D. Sellami: Radiotherapie, Institut Salah Azaiz, Tunis, Tunisia.

The way in which these variables exert their influence leads to a perspective of poorly nourished patients who delay seeking medical attention for prolonged periods of time and, consequently, present with extensive disease. Superimposed on this is significant infectious comorbidity. Additionally, there is a lack of disciplined protocol treatment, except in a few centers where First World standards prevail. These circumstances combine to result in an outcome for this lymphoma in Africa that ranges from appallingly poor remission figures to those comparable with developed countries.

BACKGROUND

During the past three decades research in Hodgkin's disease on the African continent has concentrated largely on epidemiology, with descriptions of clinical patterns of disease as reported in the different population groups. Pioneering studies, such as those of H. Falkson (1), focused on what was seen predominantly in white South Africans during the era before effective chemotherapy was available. Only more recently has information become available on black and other ethnic groups.

Over the last decade there has been a worldwide paradigm shift in understanding the spectrum of lymphoproliferative disorders. This was occasioned, in part, by emerging consensus in revised classification systems (2) that now include immunophenotyping and data from molecular genetics. This improved knowledge extends to Hodgkin's disease and has led to better understanding of the entity. Wherever feasible, given the limited resources available in Africa, the newer concepts have been incorporated into classification (3,4), investigation, and treatment of these patients.

The most significant change, however, came from the introduction of effective drugs, rapidly culminating in the development of combination chemotherapy with resultant high complete remission rates. Consequently, cure is now possible in many, if not most, cases, given only that they are correctly staged and treated early. This, however, seldom happens in Africa, where a major determinant of prognosis remains high-bulk lymphadenopathy and organ involvement when patients are first seen. This phenomenon appears to be explicable by environmental factors rather than there being some unique or continent-specific difference in tumor biology. Additional adverse factors include rampant undernutrition and associated infectious disease, with human immunodeficiency virus and tuberculosis holding pride of place. To try to gain perspective on what the current situation is in Africa, five topics have been singled out for examination. In each of these a brief commentary is appended to highlight differences between data from more affluent Western patients and their counterparts from this continent. Furthermore, where possible, findings have been compared to those in blacks from other parts of the world because it is here that we have the opportunity to contrast populations with a common genetic pool but living under vastly different environmental conditions and variable levels of medical care.

EPIDEMIOLOGY WITH GEOGRAPHY AND RACE AS INDEPENDENT VARIABLES

Westernized Societies

Extensive publications, mostly from the developed or First World, show little variation in incidence when geographic areas are compared. There is a well-defined bimodal pattern of incidence and mortality with two distinct peaks evident, the first at 25 and the other at 70 years (5). These findings, which occur typically in North America, have parallels in Denmark and The Netherlands, but they are distinctly different from Japanese, Singaporean, and Indian reports.

One hypothesis advanced to explain this distribution is that the pathogenesis may differ with age. In young adults the disease has similarities to a chronic granulomatous or inflammatory process, with an extensive host reaction but paucity of malignant cells. By contrast, in the elderly, truly neoplastic behavior is more evident. This concept has precedent in the model for paralytic poliomyelitis. Here, infection with a virus of low virulence at an early age confers life-long immunity, but without such exposure, the subsequent manifestations are much more severe (6). This paradigm, however, fails to deal adequately with this lymphoma in childhood, which has a higher frequency in Africa than elsewhere, and where the predominant histologic subtype appears to be mixed cellularity with a relatively high proportion of neoplastic Reed-Sternberg cells.

An alternative hypothesis to explain these two peaks, based on Colombian studies, suggests that there is a common cause but that different presentations reflect different host and environmental factors.

African Experience

Whatever the explanation ultimately turns out to be, there are regional and socioeconomically based variations in incidence, age at presentation, distribution of histologic subtype, and therapeutic outcome when Hodgkin's disease in different parts of the continent are compared (7–15).

Considerable geographic variation in the incidence of this lymphoma is evident in Africa, with the frequency increasing from the equator to more temperate zones. Age-standardized rates for men and women recorded in the Kampala (Uganda) Cancer Registry from 1964 to 1968 (16) were far below those from Europe and North America. Accounts from other African countries within the tropical zone are based largely on single-institution findings from academic centers or large regional hospitals. In most of these, the prevalence of Hodgkin's disease is low, except in childhood, when compared with other malignancies. Uniquely, a much higher incidence rate, approaching that seen in the Northern Hemisphere, was reported from the Ibadan Province of Western Nigeria (17). This may reflect intraregional variation related to undefined local factors. Relatively low frequencies are reported from Zambia (18), Kenya (19), and Zimbabwe (20). Similar data sourced from other sub-Saharan countries with cancer registries, such as Mali, Uganda, and Gambia, show figures less than 0.8 per 100,000 population (21,22).

From Algeria, based on the regional register at Sétif, rates are 2.4/100,000 in adults and 0.7/100,000 in male and 0.4/100,000 in female children, respectively (21). Tunisia has epidemiologic data from the Institut Pasteur going back to 1950 (23–25) as well as classification, clinical staging, and outcome data from 1969, when the Institut Salah Azaiz (ISA) was founded as a national cancer center (26) (Tables 1 and 2). There do not seem to be significant differences in the pattern of Hodgkin's disease in Algeria and Tunisia, but incidence is difficult to evaluate precisely because there is no national cancer registry. The ISA figures show the disease to comprise 4% of all cancers in adults and 11% of those in children (26). In Tunisia, this lymphoma accounts for 7.43% of all cancers in both sexes (26). In Morocco the corresponding rate was 6.6% of all malignancies (27).

The pattern in the Maghreb thus appears to be that the disease affects children and young adults. Children under the age of 15 account for approximately one-third of the cases (23–27). In childhood the male-to-female ratio is approximately 3:1, whereas in adults it is greater than 2:1. Among adults, nodular sclerosing Hodgkin's disease appears to be the most common variant. Stage distribution between stage I and II and stages III and IV is about equal. Delayed diagnosis seems relatively common, with 40% of people being seen more than 6 months after the onset of symptoms, thereby perhaps explaining the extensive disease at presentation. In children from this region, most have nodular sclerosing or mixed cellularity, with stages III and IV predominating.

TABLE 1. *Hodgkin's disease in Tunisia and Algeria: Demographic data*

	Tunisia		Algeria	
	No. patients	%	No. patients	%
Total	113	100	262	100
Age				
0–15	34	30	80	31
16–25	18	16	62	23.5
26–40	37	33	83	31.5
>40	24	21	35	13.5
Histology[a]				
LP	7	6	30	11.5
NS	55	49	105	40
MC	45	40	66	25
LD	4	4	7	3
Unclassified	2	1	56	21.5
Sex				
Male	70	62	180	68
Female	43	38	84	32
Median age (y)	28.5		—	
M/F ratio	1.6:1		2:1	

[a]LP, lymphocyte predominant; NS, nodular sclerosis; MC, mixed cellularity; LD, lymphocyte depleted.

TABLE 2. *Hodgkin's disease in Tunisia and Algeria: Clinical characteristics*

	Tunisia		Algeria	
	No. patients	%	No. patients	%
Stage				
I–II	58	51.5	139	53
III–IV	55	48.5	123	47
B symptoms	77	68	—	—
Mediastinal Involvement				
No	80	71	—	—
Bulky	25	22	—	—
ESR (mm/L)				
<40	34	30	—	—
>40	79	70	—	—

ESR, erythrocyte sedimentation rate.

In Egypt, epidemiologic data are based on studies conducted in ten different cancer centers that are attached to various universities. The major repositories for data are the Egyptian National Cancer Institute (ENCI) and the Cairo University Hospital Oncology Center, or NEMROCK. As a generalization, lymphoreticular tumors and leukemias in Egypt constitute between 7% and 15.9% of all malignancies. In a survey of 557 cases, high-grade lymphoma (previously designated as reticulum cell sarcoma) occurred most frequently, followed by Hodgkin's disease. For Hodgkin's disease, the highest incidence rate was in the second decade, and a male-to-female ratio of 3 to 1 was noted. Mixed cellularity was the most common subtype of Hodgkin's disease, and nodular sclerosis was rare (28). In another report, differences were found comparing Egypt and the Gaza strip. In Egyptian men, lymphoma occurred more frequently than in men in the Gaza strip, whereas the inverse situation was found among women. The authors noted that this kind of comparison may provide improved approaches for discerning risk factors for cancer and advocate increased cooperation among participating countries (29).

Additional data from ENCI, analyzing a series of 4,382 newly diagnosed cancer patients, all reviewed by a single pathologist, yielded 526 cases of malignant lymphoma (7%) but only 193 cases of Hodgkin's disease (2.57%) (30). Mixed cellularity accounted for 50.71%, lymphocyte predominant 23.78%, nodular sclerosis 17%, and lymphocyte depleted 8.29% of the patients with Hodgkin's disease. Unfortunately, age and sex distribution within the histologic variants was not recorded. In addition, at NEMROCK, 7,325 adults with cancer were reviewed between 1992 and 1995. There were 420 cases of non-Hodgkin's lymphoma (5.7%) and 107 with Hodgkin's disease (1.5%), giving a ratio of 3.8:1 (31). These data showed similar trends to the ENCI series, with 42% of patients having mixed-cellularity Hodgkin's disease. Here the male-to-female ratio was equal. Lymphocyte predominant Hodgkin's disease accounted for only 5.6% of cases with a male predominance in this subtype, and lymphocyte-depleted occurred in 7.4%, again with male predominance. Nodular sclerosis Hodgkin's disease accounted for 48 of the 107 patients over the age of 15 years, and within this subtype the male-to-female ratio was approximately 2 to 1.

Clinical staging in the Cairo University Hospital series (31) showed that 12% were in stage I, most of these without constitutional symptoms; 43% were in stage II, with half showing weight loss or other evidence of systemic involvement; 35% had stage III disease, and 10% stage IV disease: in both of the latter two categories, two-thirds to three-quarters were accompanied by systemic symptoms. Supradiaphragmatic presentation occurred in 73%, the mediastinum was involved in 20%, the liver in 30%, and only sporadic cases had disease demonstrable in bone marrow, skin, or nasopharynx (31).

The investigation of cancer patterns in migrant populations has been used as an epidemiologic tool. Migrants from North Africa to France provide useful insights into the changing pattern of lymphoreticular malignancy following relocation. When Egyptian-born settlers were compared to local-born French, with appropriate adjustment for confounding factors such as social status and areas of residence, there was a trend for higher risk of lymphoma among the migrants, although specific data on Hodgkin's disease are not available (32).

South of the equator, Hodgkin's disease in Zimbabwe shows a pattern similar to that found in North Africa, although the age split is slightly different. Approximately one-third of cases are seen before 20 years, with a male-to-female ratio of 1.8:1. A striking predominance of the lymphocyte-depleted variant was noted (Table 3).

South African data are available for the Gauteng (33) area (previously known as Pretoria and Johannesburg) and the Western Cape, and they show regional trends. Conversely, countrywide patterns are documented in the National Cancer Registry (34), which reflect a consistent pattern since the time of its establishment in 1989, with an age-adjusted rate of 0.81 for black women as compared to 1.42 for their white counterparts, and 0.95 and 3.27 for black and white men, respectively (Fig. 1). The apparently lower frequency of Hodgkin's disease in the black population may, in part, be related to underreporting because this is a pathology database. Nevertheless, these figures are consistent with that previously declared for this region (33).

TABLE 3. *Hodgkin's disease in Zimbabwe: Demographic and stage characteristics*

	Number	Percent
Total	170	100
Age by decile		
0–9	4	2.4
10–19	48	28.2
20–29	40	23.5
30–39	37	21.8
40–49	21	12.3
50–59	8	4.7
60–69	9	5.3
70–79	3	1.8
Histology[a]		
LP	7	4.1
NS	30	17.7
MC	92	54.1
LD	41	24.1
Sex		
Male	109	64
Female	61	36
Stage		
I–II	35	20.6
III–IV	135	79.4
Median age 28 years		
M/F ratio 1.8		

[a]LP, lymphocyte predominant; NS, nodular sclerosis; MC, mixed cellularity; LD, lymphocyte depleted. Data from L. Levy (unpublished).

There is also a marked difference between the histologic subtypes found in blacks and whites in South Africa. In the former, mixed cellularity or lymphocyte depletion predominates, whereas in the latter, nodular sclerosing is most frequently encountered. This pattern, illustrated by the Gauteng data (Table 4), also occurs in Natal and in the Freestate. The Western Cape, however, has a different population mix. In the past the population in the Cape was predominantly white or of mixed ancestry. More recently there has been a large black population influx. These population differences appear to be responsible for changes in Hodgkin's disease subtypes seen in the Cape, the pattern previously conforming to northern European data but with a significant trend toward the more frequent African pattern becoming evident since 1994.

Points of Contrast

Prominent differences are seen in the epidemiologic patterns between Africa and Europe or North America. In the terminology recommended by the International Union Against Cancer (35), Hodgkin's disease epidemiology is seen to fall into one of four categories. Type I Hodgkin's disease occurs primarily in children and is associated with less favorable histologic subtypes. Type III Hodgkin's disease predominates in developed countries and prevails in young adults, where a better outcome is associated with more frequent occurrence of lympho-

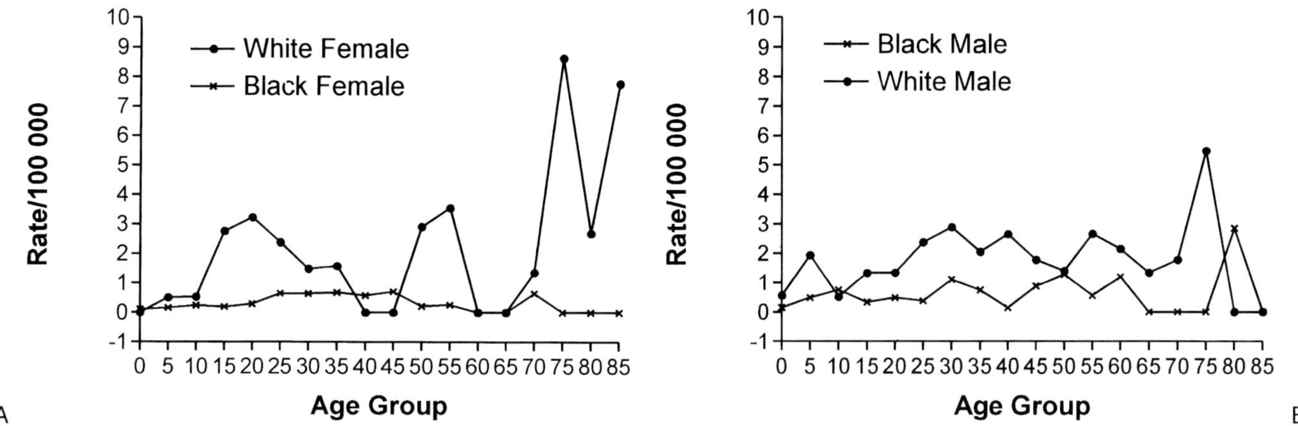

FIG. 1. Distribution by age at diagnosis of Hodgkin's disease in black and white female (**A**) and male (**B**) South Africans. (Data from ref. 34.)

cyte predominant and nodular sclerosing subtypes. Type II is intermediate between type I and type III. The type IV epidemiologic pattern is largely limited to Asia and is not discussed further here.

Viewed in this way, the type I pattern appears to be predominant in the central part of Africa (16–20). A few additional studies do deserve mention here, although in general the data were considered too sparse to be included in our main analysis of geographic pathology. A report from Zambia showed that Hodgkin's disease accounted for 18.6% of malignant lymphomas, with 44% of the cases occurring the first two decades of life. The patients were predominantly of more advanced stage and had either mixed-cellularity or lymphocyte-depleted subtypes (18). Similar clinical presentations are reported from Nigeria (17,36–39), Kenya (19,40–42), Uganda (43,44), Gabon (45), and Zimbabwe (46–48). One set of Ugandan (44) data that may represent intraregional variation, however, describes a bimodal age-specific incidence curve approximating the type III pattern.

The pattern of Hodgkin's disease in North African littoral and South Africa is mostly intermediate or type II (49). This epidemiologic pattern approximates that seen in North America during the 1950s and 1960s (50–52), where this lymphoma occurred less frequently in blacks than whites. Hodgkin's disease in the former group had aggressive histology and was of advanced stage. These features were attributed to socioeconomic rather than genetic factors. In this regard, indications are that there has been a shift during the last 25 to 30 years among the North American black population (51) to a pattern more closely approximating type III. Based on similar inferential reasoning, one may conclude that the intermediate pattern seen in South Africa represents a transitional phase in epidemiology. However, this postulate needs to be confirmed by direct investigation to establish whether HLA or immune response–linked gene frequencies, or other genetic factors, might still play a significant role in the incidence and/or subtype distribution.

It might also be debated whether a drift in epidemiologic pattern from a lower overall frequency to a higher incidence, albeit to one with better prognostic features, represents a step forward in cancer control. It may rather be argued that available studies have not, as yet, provided any real clues to suggest a strategy of prevention of Hodgkin's disease in any population group.

TABLE 4. *Distribution of Hodgkin's disease by age group and histologic subtype in South Africa: Crude rates based on pathologic diagnosis*

	Ethnic Group: Black Age range							Ethnic Group: White Age range						
Histologic subtype[a]	10–14	15–24	25–34	35–44	45–54	>55	Total	10–14	15–24	25–34	35–44	45–54	>55	Total
LP	1	0	1	1	4	0	7	0	2	2	2	0	0	6
NS	2	4	7	6	2	7	28	2	6	5	3	0	5	21
MC	5	4	1	4	2	2	18	3	1	1	1	4	3	13
LD	1	5	4	2	1	4	17	0	1	0	1	1	4	7
NOS	9	15	20	17	6	15	82	3	8	16	10	9	18	64
Total	18	28	33	30	15	28	152	8	18	24	17	14	30	111

[a]LP, lymphocyte predominant; NS, nodular sclerosis; MC, mixed cellularity; LD, lymphocyte depleted; NOS, not otherwise specified.

Data from National Cancer Registry of South Africa (62).

CLINICAL PRESENTATION, STAGING, AND PROGNOSTIC FACTORS

Westernized Societies

The clinical features reported in North American adults and children (50–53) provide a convenient orientation against which to examine intercontinental differences. Although, predictably, attention is drawn to this entity by the finding of enlarged glands, with diagnosis dependent on node biopsy, in both developed and emerging societies there are, nevertheless, contrasting features.

TABLE 5. *International Study of Prognostic Factors in Hodgkin's Disease: Factors identified as leading to a significant reduction in failure-free survival*

Age ≤ 45 years
Male sex
Stage IV disease
Albumin < 40 g/L
Hemoglobin < 10.5 g/dL
Total WCC ≤ 1.5 × 10^9/L
Lymphocyte count < 0.6 × 10^9/L

WCC, white cell count.
Adapted from ref. 56.

African Experience

Throughout the length of this continent, the four-stage Ann Arbor classification (54–56) with modifications, as proposed at follow-up meetings in the Cotswolds (57,58), is recommended and is in general use. The problems of applying this approach to individual patients are organizational rather than methodologic. A large rural population with a limited number of centers that offer sophisticated investigations, such as computerized axial tomography, lymphangiography, and nuclear medicine techniques, have made accurate staging difficult. However, because this is a potentially curable disease, it is felt that all patients should be referred to available specialist establishments, where full and adequate investigations can be carried out. Imaging facilities are accessible along the North African littoral; in southern Africa, including Zimbabwe and South Africa; and in Kenya in East Africa, Nigeria, Ghana, and the Francophone countries.

The significant frequency of chronic bacillary and parasitic infections throughout Africa that are capable of giving rise to granulomatous or other inflammatory processes that may coexist with the lymphoma needs to be taken into account when evaluating lesions detected either clinically or radiologically (59). Such complications include, in our experience, tuberculosis, with its associated lymphadenopathy; human immunodeficiency virus infections; amebic abscesses; lymphogranuloma inguinale; hydatid cyst; syphilitic gummas; and schistosomiasis. Delay in diagnosis and empiric treatment for tuberculous lymphadenopathy, particularly among patients from rural areas, has, in our experience, been a significant cause of delay in diagnosis of Hodgkin's disease. Although these disorders usually demonstrate features that are sufficiently distinctive for separation from Hodgkin's disease, this does require experience and awareness of the condition.

The absence of pulmonary involvement by typical tuberculous changes should alert the clinician to the possibility that lymphadenopathy may have a cause other than this common infection. Ultimately, however, the diagnostic problem can only be resolved by adequate investigation. Access to and provision of laboratories that can make diagnoses on microbiologic and histologic grounds, rather than reliance on empiric treatment, are urgent needs in many African countries.

Enlarged spleens from endemic malarial infestation give rise to the tropical splenomegaly syndrome. Here the question of staging laparotomy and splenectomy requires judgment. The risk of malaria and other infectious diseases, on the one hand, and the fact that the majority of patients have stage IIB or more advanced illness on the other, make removal of this organ inappropriate in most of our cases. Not surprisingly, splenectomy has virtually not been used for staging in southern Africa since 1985.

Stage at presentation and prognostic features have been examined in some detail in northern and southern Africa. Data from Tunisia and Algeria (Table 2) show striking similarity, with approximately half of the patients presenting with advanced disease, B symptoms, elevated erythrocyte sedimentation rate, and a significant delay in time to diagnosis. In addition, the experience of ISA, unfortunately repeated throughout the rest of the continent, is that as many as 20% of the patients are lost to follow-up or receive inadequate treatment. The experience

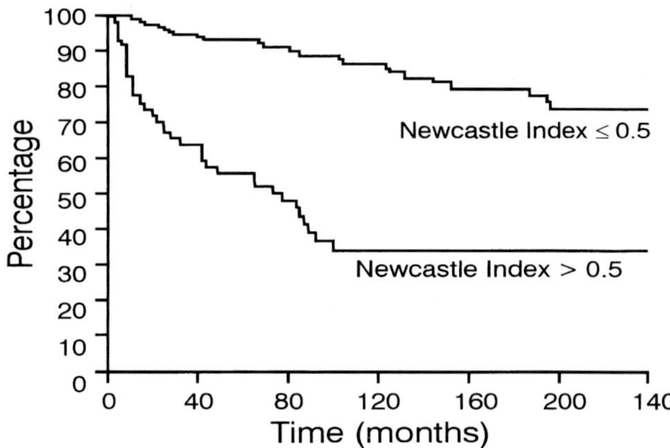

FIG. 2. Disease-free survival of chemotherapy-treated (MOPP/ABVD) white patients with Hodgkin's disease, stratified according to the Newcastle Prognostic Index (p = .001). (Data from ref. 62.)

TABLE 6. *Distribution of histologic subtype among 494 adult black and white patients with Hodgkin's disease*

	Lymphocyte predominant		Nodular sclerosis		Mixed cellularity		Lymphocyte depleted		
Age (decile)	Black	White	Black	White	Black	White	Black	White	*p* Value
10–19	2	6	12	24	12	10	5	0	NS
20–29	2	13	13	51	26	12	15	5	$\chi^2 = 16.8$
30–39	0	9	18	24	27	22	12	2	$\chi^2 = 19.2$
40–49	2	2	12	20	10	10	3	3	NS
50–59	1	4	3	33	4	13	3	1	$<.3$, $\chi^2 = 15.5$
60–69	—	—	0	9	4	8	1	1	NS
>70	—	12	—	10	—	10	—	3	NS
Totals	7	36	58	171	83	85	39	15	

Adapted from ref. 63. Overall $\chi^2 = 60.52$; $p < .001$. NS, not significant.

from Zimbabwe shows an even more striking predominance of advanced disease (Table 3). Little is known about the specific clinical presentation of these lymphomas in equatorial Africa, where data reporting is sparse (41).

Egyptian data are not distinctive and essentially appear to overlap those reported from other areas in North Africa, particularly Algeria, Morocco, and Tunisia. However, when migrant populations are reviewed, differences appear to exist but are limited by small numbers (32).

In South Africa, as elsewhere, the prognosis is influenced by a number of factors, not all of which are included in the anatomically based staging systems (57,58). Although the impact of histologic subtype as an independent variable remains controversial, there is general agreement that mixed-cellularity and lymphocyte-depleted variants are usually associated with more advanced stage and the presence of B symptoms at presentation (Table 4). Proctor and co-workers developed a numerical index (60) that included disease extent, age, hemoglobin level, lymphocyte count, and tumor bulk and was able to discriminate between patients with a good prognosis, with a failure-free survival over 80% at 10 years, and those with less satisfactory outcome, for whom the corresponding figure was less than 59% at 10 years. The predictive effect of some of these elements has been confirmed in another international analysis, where seven factors (Table 5) were identified, each of which reduced tumor control by 7% to 8% at 5 years (61).

There are few corresponding studies from Africa, although data from Johannesburg (62) confirmed the ability of the Newcastle Prognostic Index (60) to discriminate between good and poor outcome in Caucasian patients (Fig. 2). The frequency distribution of histologic subtypes and other features in this population group were similar to those reported from elsewhere in the world (Table 6). This index, however, failed to discriminate between prognostic groups in black patients (Fig. 3).

Points of Contrast

Striking confirmation of these differences comes from an updated study (Table 7) that showed significant differences to persist in the relative frequency distribution of components of the prognostic index, particularly histologic subtype and age, between the two populations. Despite the black patients being younger (age was a significant factor with substantial weighting toward good prognosis in the Newcastle Index), the overall outcome in these patients remained similar to that of the poor prognostic group among Caucasians. One consideration, which may be a major one in assessing the relative impact of prognostic factors on outcome of Hodgkin's disease between blacks and whites, is that economic and educational level may be more predictive than race. However, these socioeconomic factors are correlated with race. Patient education and better socioeconomic support networks will, it is hoped, improve this situation in the future.

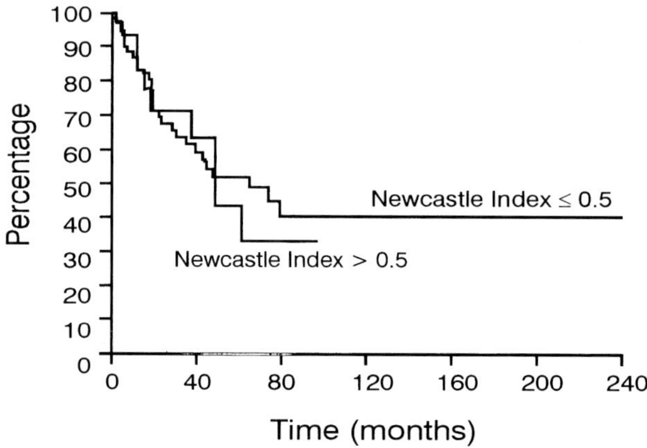

FIG. 3. Disease-free survival of chemotherapy-treated (MOPP or MOPP/ABVD) black patients with Hodgkin's disease stratified according to the Newcastle Prognostic Index ($p = .1$). (Data from ref. 62.)

TABLE 7. *Relative distribution of factors considered to be important in predicting outcome of Hodgkin's disease among adult black and white patients treated with combination therapy*

	Black		White		
	Number	%	Number	%	p Value
Stage					
I and II	32	17	171	56	0.001
III and IV	155	83	136	44	
Symptoms					
A	29	11	95	31	<0.001
B	158	89	212	69	
Age					
<50	171	91	203	66	0.001
≥50	16	9	104	34	
Hemoglobin					
≥10	129	69	280	91	0.001
<10	58	31	27	9	
Disease bulk					
Bulky (≥10cm)	90	48	98	32	0.02
Nonbulky (<10cm)	97	52	209	68	
Lymphocyte count					
$<1.0 \times 10^9$/L	87	47	85	28	0.01
$>1.0 \times 10^9$/L	100	53	222	72	
Newcastle index					
≤0.5	109	76	212	76	NS
>0.5	35	24	67	24	

Updated from Ref. 62.

SPECIFIC ASPECTS IN CHILDREN

Westernized Societies

Childhood Hodgkin's disease is rare in developed countries (63–66).

African Experience

Pediatric Hodgkin's disease occurring in Egypt has been analyzed in a consecutive group of 242 children treated at the National Cancer Institute in Cairo between 1975 and 1980. There was a male predominance of 3:1. The most common histopathologic type was mixed cellularity (accounting for 60.74%). Late stages (defined as III and IV) comprised 63.2%, usually with bulky disease. Not unexpectedly, staging laparotomy (which was done in 154 cases) revealed more infradiaphragmatic disease than was clinically evident. Although an association between infradiaphragmatic Hodgkin's disease and schistosomal hepatic fibrosis was described, this is probably no more than coincidental (67).

Currently available data from South Africa suggest that, although there may be a peak incidence between the ages of 15 and 19 in black children (34), the overall frequency is lower in blacks of all ages, including the childhood years, relative to whites (Fig. 1).

In a study from the Western Cape, including 39 children under 15 years of age, there were seven black, 12

TABLE 8. *Childhood Hodgkin's disease in the Western Cape: Distribution of histology by ethnic group*

	Black		Mixed		White	
Histology[a]	No. of patients	%	No. of patients	%	No. of patients	%
MC	0	0	8	40	4	33
NS	2	29	7	35	7	59
LD	3	43	4	20	1	8
LP	1	14	0	0	0	0
Other	1	14	1	5	0	0
Total	7		20		12	

[a]MC, mixed cellularity; NS, nodular sclerosis; LD, lymphocyte depleted; LP, lymphocyte predominant.

Data from ref. 71. Nodular sclerosing was present in 59% of white patients, whereas mixed cellularity dominated in those of mixed ancestry at 40%, and lymphocyte depletion in blacks at 43%. Mixed cellularity was present in 37% of the children under 11 and 25% of the older group, while lymphocyte depletion occurred in 30% of the older group and only 12% of the younger cases. The incidence of nodular sclerosing histopathology in whites and those of mixed ancestry did not achieve significant differences, again probably because of small numbers.

TABLE 9. *Childhood Hodgkin's disease in the Western Cape: Distribution of stage by ethnic group*

	Whole group		Black		Mixed		White	
Stage	No.	%	No.	%	No.	%	No.	%
I	2	5	0	0	1	5	1	9
II	16	41	2	29	8	40	6	50
III	11	28	2	29	4	20	5	41
IV	10	26	3	42	7	35	0	0
Total	39		7		20		12	

Data from ref. 71.

white and 20 children of mixed ancestry (68–70) (Tables 8 and 9). The male-to-female ratio was 2.9:1, and the median ages were 147, 124, and 119 months in children of white, mixed, and black ancestry, respectively. The latter two groups came mainly from a poor socioeconomic background. Systemic symptoms were present in 51% of cases. Histologic subtypes included nodular sclerosis in 59% of white patients, mixed-cellularity in 40% of mixed ancestry patients, and lymphocyte-depleted in 43% of black patients. Five percent of the entire group had clinical stage I; 41% stage II; 28% stage III; and 26% stage IV disease. By contrast, the majority of white children presented with stages I and II.

Points of Contrast

A recent study in children (<13 years old) from Johannesburg (62) emphasizes the Capetown data (Table 10). Notably, in this group of 91 patients, of whom 61 were black and 30 were white, there was a clear demonstration of a difference in distribution of prognostic factors, with late-stage disease and lower hemoglobin levels among black children as compared to their white counterparts.

Similar observations were noted in Namibia (71). Significantly, here, the increased risk of developing tuberculosis was sufficient to lead to the suggestion that

TABLE 10. *Clinical and pathologic features among 91 children with Hodgkin's disease from Johannesburg (Gauteng)*

	Black		White		
	Number	%	Number	%	*p* Value
Sex					
Male	47	52	22	24	
Female	14	15	8	9	
Histologic subtype[a]					
LP	1	1	3	3	
NS	20	22	12	13	
MC	39	43	14	16	
LD	1	1	1	1	
Stage					
I and II	18	20	19	21	
III and IV	43	47	11	12	.001
Symptoms					
A	25	27	20	21	
B	36	40	10	12	<.03
Hemoglobin					
≤ 10	24	26	18	20	
< 10	37	41	12	13	.06
Lymphocyte count × 10^9L					
≤1.0	50	55	18	19	
< 1.0	11	12	12	12	<.03
Disease bulk					
Bulky	31	34	5	5	<.03
Nonbulky	30	33	25	27	
Age					
Mean ± SD	8.2 ± 3.1		9.4 ± 4.1		

[a]LP, lymphocyte predominant; NS, nodular sclerosis; MC, mixed cellularity; LD, lymphocyte depleted. Percents reflect proportion of the population as a whole.

Data from ref. 63.

prophylactic anti-TB therapy is appropriate in all children with malignancy being treated in the developing countries of Africa (72).

VIRAL INFECTION AND HODGKIN'S DISEASE

Epstein-Barr Virus

Westernized Societies

Numerous studies have examined the role of Epstein-Barr virus (EBV) (73,74) in Hodgkin's disease. Although initial serologic studies were unable to show any clear clinical relationship between this lymphoma and the virus, the advent of *in situ* hybridization studies revealed an integrated genome in the Reed-Sternberg cells in 35% of cases (75). Furthermore, at least one gene product, the latent membrane protein (LMP-1), can be found on the surface of the multinucleate tumor cells. The LMP may function as a target for cytotoxic T lymphocytes and thereby facilitate host control over the neoplasm. Conversely, if this surveillance mechanism is lost, the same molecule appears to have the capacity to enhance proliferation of the infected cells, leading to the emergence of a histologically aggressive tumor (73–75). These apparently opposing effects might underlie differences in the course of this lymphoid malignancy and raise the interesting possibility that prevention may be achieved by means of vaccination.

African Experience

The role of Epstein-Barr in Hodgkin's disease occurring in different geographic areas has been investigated in a number of studies (76,77). Differences in the frequency of expression of EBV in neoplastic cells of Hodgkin's disease have been noted when cases from Kenya and Italy were compared (78). In another study biopsy material from cases of childhood Hodgkin's disease occurring in ten different countries were compared: LMP-1 was found in 50% to 100% of cases, with the highest rates of expression tending to occur in cases from underdeveloped countries. By a sensitive polymerase chain reaction–based EBV strain–typing procedure (76), EBV strain type I was shown to be predominant in childhood Hodgkin's disease from the United Kingdom, South Africa, Australia, and Greece; EBV strain type II was predominant in Egypt. Both EBV strain types I and II were detected in some cases of childhood Hodgkin's disease from the United Kingdom, Costa Rica, and Kenya, with the frequency of dual infection being highest in cases from developing countries. The authors speculated that the high incidence of EBV and the presence, especially in developing countries, of dual infections with both type I and type II may reflect socioeconomic conditions leading to malnutrition-induced immunologic impairment (76).

The Human Immunodeficiency Virus

Westernized Societies

The possible role of the human immunodeficiency virus (HIV) in Hodgkin's disease is attracting increasing attention. A number of recent publications from Europe and the United States have suggested an association between the two (79–85). In this setting, at-risk individuals are homosexual men with HIV disease and/or intravenous drug abusers with low CD4 counts and with significant evidence of impaired immunologic integrity.

African Experience

High rates of immunodeficiency viral infection and clinical AIDS occur throughout Africa. A causal relationship could be expected to have a major impact on Hodgkin's disease incidence. HIV seropositivity rates of approximately 7% to 10% have been recorded among antenatal clinic attendees in South Africa (86). Even higher figures have been reported from Central Africa.

However, no increased incidence of Hodgkin's disease has emerged in cancer registry data. In a recent case-control study involving 913 blacks with malignant disease (87) conducted in Johannesburg, a notable correlation between HIV infection and neoplasia was observed only for Kaposi's sarcoma, with 27 of 35 patients being seropositive (odds ratio 61.8, 95% C.I. 19.7 to 194.2), and for non-Hodgkin's lymphoma (27 of 40 individuals seropositive for HIV, with an odds ratio of 4.8, 95% C.I. 1.5 to 14.8). This association is similar to that noted in several other sub-Saharan African communities (88–90), where HIV viral prevalence is high. The odds ratio for the association of HIV and non-Hodgkin's lymphoma was, however, lower than that reported in developed countries. The reasons for these findings are not clear but may include early mortality from tuberculosis in African HIV cases. This infectious complication occurs at higher CD4 counts (about 300 to 400/μL) counts than those associated with the development of non-Hodgkin's lymphoma. No other cancer observed, including Hodgkin's disease, as well as those arising from liver, vagina, penis, esophagus, cervix, or the oropharynx (all of which may have an infectious etiology), showed a significant relationship to infection with HIV. The Johannesburg study showed an HIV seropositivity rate of 10.8% in patients with Hodgkin's disease, giving an odds ratio of 2.0 (95% C.I. 0.6 to 6.6).

Although there was no notable correlation between HIV and Hodgkin's disease, the coincidental occurrence of the two entities does exist, particularly because both occur in younger patients. Of the 37 patients with Hodgkin's disease who were HIV positive, clinical data were available for 28. The identification of these individuals allowed some observations to be made regarding the clinical aspects of Hodgkin's disease with HIV in black

TABLE 11. *Presenting clinical and laboratory features in 28 black HIV-positive patients with Hodgkin's disease*

	Number	%
Histologic subtype[a]		
NS	8	29
MC	13	46
LD	7	25
Stage		
IIB	4	14
IIIA	1	4
IIIB	19	68
IVB	4	14
Male	18	64
Female	10	36
Bulky disease (> 10 cm)	11	39
Nonbulky disease (<10 cm)	17	61
Hemoglobin (g/dL)	10.3 ± 1.2[b]	
Lymphocytes (× 10^9/L)	0.849 ± 0.102[b]	
Age (years)	20.9 ± 4.2[b]	

[a]NS, nodular sclerosis; MC, mixed cellularity; LD, Lymphocyte depleted.
[b]Mean ± SD.
Data from ref. 80.

patients (Table 11). Of note was the finding that the median CD34 count (488 ± 195 × 10^9/L) was not significantly different from that found in HIV-negative black patients with Hodgkin's disease (80) (Table 11). There seem, therefore, to be no specific features that identify HIV patients with Hodgkin's disease, and no reason not to treat them with standard therapeutic approaches, provided they are not, in addition, suffering from advanced acquired immunodeficiency disease.

Data from Zimbabwe collected between 1988 and 1996 (Table 12) for 105 new patients with Hodgkin's disease showed that of 89 tested, 37% were HIV positive. These figures need to be seen in the context of an even higher frequency of HIV positivity in that country than in South Africa. Again, clinical features were similar, irrespective of retroviral status.

TREATMENT OUTCOMES

Westernized Societies

Evidence from an expanding literature clearly demonstrates that Hodgkin's disease is curable. Cardinal determinants are reliable diagnosis, accurate staging, and management with appropriate and well-tested multimodality programs that comprise combination chemotherapy alone or combined with irradiation (91–93).

There has been a major shift from the early days when clinical assessment was converted to pathologic staging by surgery (94,95). Currently favored are less invasive methods that center on technological advances, including high-resolution imaging procedures (96,97).

Despite the favorable outcome for most patients treated with conventional approaches, there are still a number of problems. The first is refractory, slowly responding, or relapsed disease, which does better with high-dose chemotherapy and myeloprotection using peripheral blood hematopoietic stem and progenitor cells (98–100). Equally important is the ever-increasing appreciation that, although conventional treatment has curative capacity in sensitive patients, late complications arise and adversely affect outcome. Safer but equally effective regimens are needed (101–102).

African Experience

Treatment has been modified to keep abreast of new advances. In summarizing contemporary practice, radia-

TABLE 12. *Hodgkin's disease and HIV in Zimbabwe: 89 patients of known HIV status*

	HIV positive		HIV negative	
	Number	%	Number	%
Histologic subtype[a]				
LP	0	0	5	8.9
NS	3	9.1	13	23.3
MC	24	72.7	25	44.6
LD	6	18.2	13	23.2
Age				
Median	34		25	
Range	17–70		9–70	
Stage				
I–II	3		16	
III–IV	30		40	
Sex				
M/F ratio	3.7:1		1.3:1	

[a]LP, lymphocyte predominant; NS, nodular sclerosis; MC, mixed cellularity; LD, lymphocyte depleted; M, male; F, female.
Data from L. M. Levy (*unpublished data*).

tion and chemotherapy have been somewhat artificially isolated, and children are considered separately.

Adults: Radiation Therapy

In a report from Johannesburg (62), the outcome after laparotomy, for stage I to IIIA Hodgkin's disease treated between 1976 and 1986 with total nodal irradiation, was much poorer for black patients than for whites. However, in this retrospective analysis, when patients with stage I disease and those with nonbulky stage II disease with normal hemoglobin levels were considered, the outcome in blacks did not differ from that in whites with corresponding early stage similarly managed. These results suggest that radiation treatment can play a significant role on this continent, as elsewhere, provided diagnosis is prompt and referral appropriate. One problem is, however, access to radiation therapy centers. To this end, the World Health Organization, in association with the International Atomic Energy Commission, has embarked on a project of installing the necessary equipment and providing oncology training.

Adults: Chemotherapy

Systemic treatment is based on the traditional MOPP combinations. With few exceptions, the response rates in blacks emerge as significantly poorer than those observed with similar treatment regimens in other parts of the world (103–106).

From the evidence available, patients with unfavorable histology and advanced disease have a better outcome following six or even eight cycles of multidrug therapy combining MOPP, or its variant, with one or another form of ABVD than following MOPP alone (107–111). A significant factor may be the higher dose intensity achieved with the hybrid regimens (112–114). There have, however, been no randomized studies to determine whether this observation applies equally to all population groups. Our own experience, based on a retrospective analysis, is that there may be a trend toward improvement in blacks when the MOPP-ABVD era (1985 to 1995) is compared to earlier experience (1970 to 1985), when MOPP alone was used (Figs. 2 and 3). However, despite some improvements, the discrepancy between black and white individuals with Hodgkin's disease, equivalently treated, remains evident (Fig. 4). Costs are also significantly higher for regimens containing anthracycline, such as ABVD.

Data from the Cairo University Center are instructive. The overall and disease-free survival is shown in Figure 5. Survival appears, in general, to be inferior by 10% to 15% to that reported for Western series except for those cases with stage I disease, treated with mantle or inverted-Y radiation therapy, where survival exceeds 88% at 5 years. The corresponding figures are 48% for stage II, 39% for stage III, and 33% for stage IV. As elsewhere, the explanation may be related to irregular treatment courses, with 47% being delayed more than 2 weeks because of social circumstances (31).

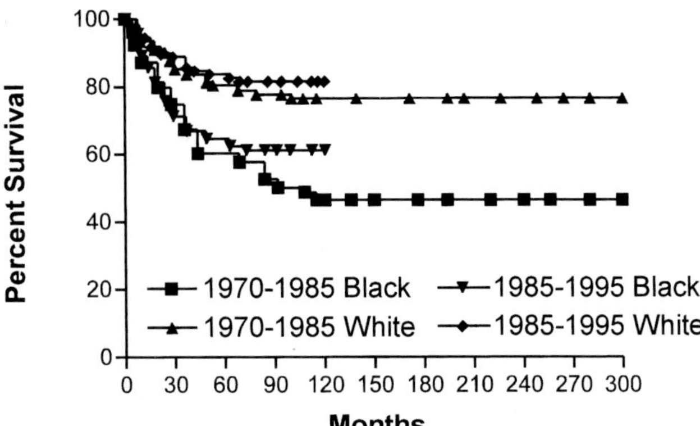

FIG. 4. Overall survival of patients with Hodgkin's disease treated during 1970 to 1985 (MOPP alone) and during 1985 to 1995 (MOPP/ABVD). The difference between the survival curves for black and white patients was statistically significant ($p < .01$) for both time periods.

A significant dose–response relationship has been shown for Hodgkin's disease with favorable results for high-dose chemotherapy linked to autologous bone marrow transplantation for patients with recurrent disease (115–116).

Because both dose intensification and better treatment compliance might be achieved using high-dose chemotherapy with autologous bone marrow support for advanced poor prognosis disease, a trial was initiated in Johannesburg using this as the initial approach. Twenty-six patients are currently evaluable. The regimen consists

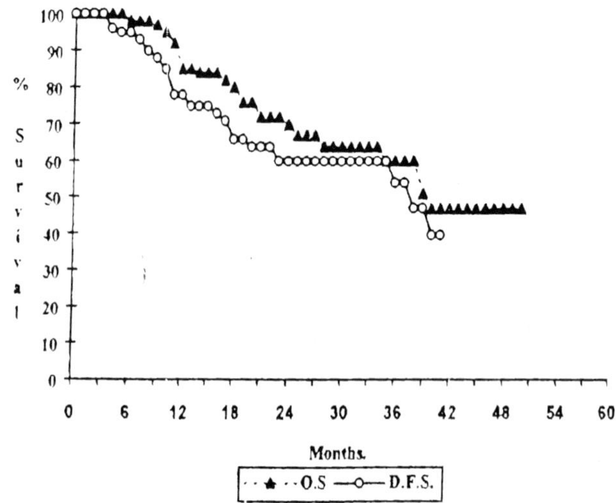

FIG. 5. Actual 5-year survival for 107 patients with adult Hodgkin's disease. (Data from ref. 31.) O.S., overall survival; D.F.S., disease-free survival.

of melphalan (140 mg/m^2 IV) combined with etoposide (VP16, 2.5 g/m^2). Hematologic rescue is effected using noncryopreserved autologous marrow (four patients) or G-CSF-stimulated peripheral blood stem and progenitor cells (22 patients). Not having to freeze and store the rescue products has made the whole procedure technically simpler and cheaper. All patients have reconstituted (to $>1.0 \times 10^9$/L neutrophils and $>40 \times 10^9$/L platelets, without transfusion dependency) with median recovery time of 17 days. Median hospitalization time was 19 days. Twenty-four of the 26 patients achieved complete remission following one cycle of treatment. Only one patient had a partial response, and one failed, giving an overall complete response rate (24 of 26) of 92%. The first six patients in this study underwent only a single course of high-dose chemotherapy. There were three recurrences (at 18, 22, and 25 months, respectively) (117). All subsequent patients had the induction cycle repeated and were autografted (as outlined above) with the second cycle, administered 4 to 6 weeks after the first procedure. Time to hematologic recovery was not significantly different following the second course of therapy in comparison to the first. Among the 20 patients given double high-dose chemotherapy with peripheral blood stem-cell rescue, the complete remission rate was 100%. At a median follow-up of 30 months, there have been no recurrences among the patients who were treated twice (118). The disease-free survival for all 26 patients is shown in Figure 6.

Although this is not a randomized study, it is of interest to note that the single cycle of chemotherapy has an inadequate cure rate, even though the disease is chemotherapy sensitive. The efficacy of a double induction cycle remains to be established on further follow-up. However, if successful, this approach is likely to provide an acceptable method because it is additionally associated with a reduction in total treatment time for patients with poor prognostic Hodgkin's disease in Africa.

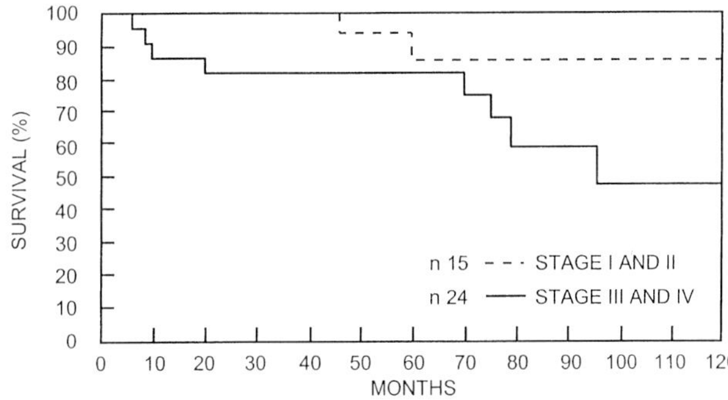

FIG. 7. Disease-free survival of children (<15 years) with Hodgkin's disease treated at Tygerberg Hospital (Western Cape). (Data from ref. 70.)

Children

Although reported series are small, results suggest an outcome superior to that achieved in adults (119,120). Exceptionally good results have been reported with MOPP for childhood disease in Africa with initial complete response rates of 85% to 100% (67,68,121,122). This outcome is noticeably better than that achieved in adults using the same therapeutic regimen. In a series reported from the Tygerberg Academic Hospital, those under 15 years of age (Tables 8 and 9) treated with MOPP, or its equivalent, ChlVPP, or the MOPP/ABVD hybrid together with 20 to 30 Gy involved-field radiotherapy to bulky mediastinal disease (70) had a projected survival at 10 years of 85% for stage I and II disease and 82% and 48% at 5 and 10 years, respectively, for stage III and IV disease (Fig. 7). Survival in children was identical, irrespective of chemotherapy used (Fig. 8). Disease- and treatment-related complications were, however, frequent. Of the infections, tuberculosis was common in the Western Cape and caused significant morbidity; one-third of the patients required antituberculosis treatment

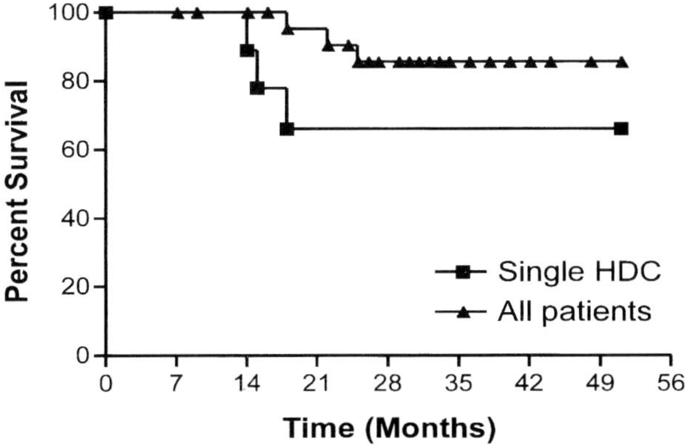

FIG. 6. Disease-free survival of patients with Hodgkin's disease treated with primary high-dose chemotherapy (melphalan—VP16) and autologous hematopoietic rescue.

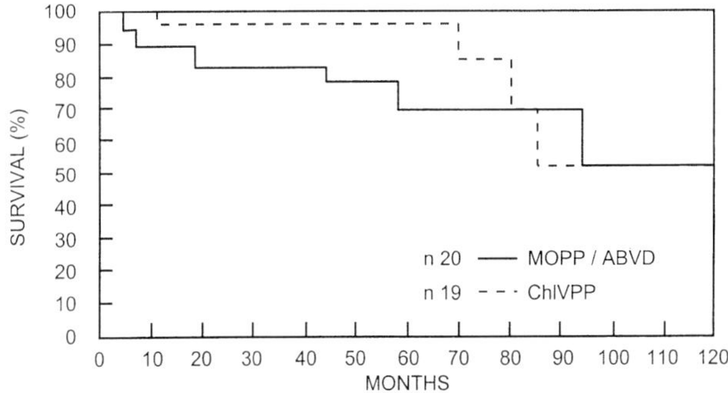

FIG. 8. Disease-free survival of children with Hodgkin's disease analyzed by type of chemotherapy. (Data from ref. 70.)

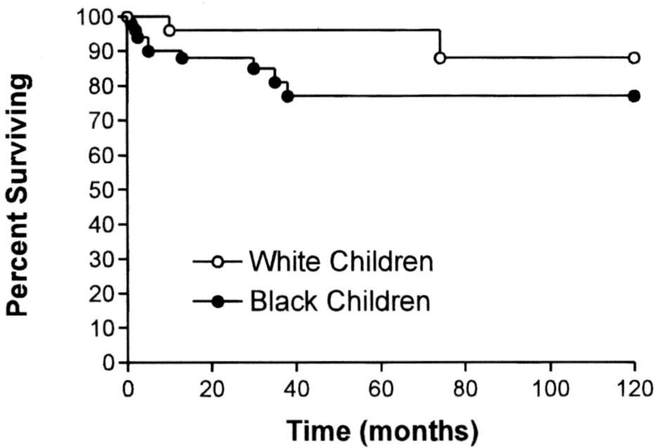

FIG. 9. Disease-free survival of children with Hodgkin's disease in Gauteng. (Data from ref. 62.) (p = .03).

(72). Varicella was encountered in six cases. It is probably noteworthy that two patients who had undergone staging splenectomy developed overwhelming sepsis and died (at 7 months and 8 years, respectively). Three children died of therapy-related complications, including marrow failure, tuberculous bronchiectasis and osteitis, and a second malignancy.

The survival experience of children with Hodgkin's disease seen in the Gauteng area more closely approximated that seen in Western countries (Fig. 9), with an observed 10-year disease-free survival in excess of 80%. This latter group came from a fully urbanized population, attended a clinic with intensive support services, and were all treated with chemotherapy (MOPP or MOPP/ABVD) alone. Compliance was excellent (over 85% received optimal dose as scheduled). The incidence and range of infectious complications were significantly less, with only one recorded case of TB. The results emphasize the importance of socioeconomic elements, and adequacy of treatment is the major factor influencing prognosis of Hodgkin's disease. Although the results in black children appeared significantly better than those in black adults, there was, nevertheless, still a significant difference as compared to white children (62).

CONCLUSION

Hodgkin's disease, as seen among children and adults throughout Africa, creates a sense of *déjà vu* among investigators working in First World centers. Our understanding of the available evidence is that there is a single causative pathophysiologic process, but the impact of environmental factors is much more profound than in the more uniform societies generally evolved in the Western World. Of these, the presentation and clinical course are profoundly and adversely influenced by malnutrition and by rampant and escalating human immunodeficiency disease positivity, with its linked epidemic of tuberculosis. Logic would dictate that, if these compounding factors could be corrected, little difference would be seen either between blacks and whites on the continent or in comparison with more affluent societies in other parts of the world. On currently available evidence, these appear to be unobtainable and even receding goals. Perhaps the most frightening reality to be faced is a continent-wide deterioration in medical standards, with reduction and restriction of available resources that range from unavailability of chemotherapy drugs to the nondelivery of radiation and radiation therapy equipment. If this is the truth, as seems to be the case, Africa will continue to provide a model for the study of differences between affluent and poor. This is a chilling scenario and the antithesis of what all dedicated doctors strive toward. The goal must be improvement in the investigation and management of these individuals. Only in this way can the outcome be elevated to levels that in the future will differ in no significant way from the standard-setting academic centers in the First World.

ACKNOWLEDGMENTS

The authors wish to thank many colleagues in Africa who provided data for this chapter. Included are Lorraine Levy, Associate Professor, Department of Medicine, at the University of Zimbabwe and the Zimbabwean Cancer Registry; Dr. Hamdy Azim, of the Cairo Oncology Center; Peter Hesseling, Professor and Head of the Department of Paediatrics and Child Health, University of Stellenbosch, who was particularly helpful in providing additional data from his own experience and records; Gary Culligan, Professor, Medical University of Southern Africa; Coenrad F. Slabber from the Department of Medical Oncology, University of Pretoria; Sedick Isaacs from the University of Cape Town, Groote Schuur Hospital; and Pauline Close, Department of Anatomical Pathology, University of Cape Town and Groote Schuur Hospital. We would also like to thank Christine Dölling for providing invaluable bibliographic assistance; and Deirdre Collins and Gillian Ganz, who prepared and typed drafts and the final manuscript.

REFERENCES

1. Falkson HC. *The value of N-isopropyl-alpha-(2-methyl-hydrazino)-p-toluamide hydrochloride relative to ionizing radiations in the treatment of Hodgkin's disease.* Dissertation, University of Pretoria, 1965.
2. The Non-Hodgkin's Lymphoma Classification Project. A clinical evaluation of the International Lymphoma Study Group classification of non-Hodgkin's lymphoma. *Blood* 1997;89:3909–3918.
3. Jacobs P. The malignant lymphomas in Africa. *Hematol Oncol Clin North Am* 1991;5:953–982.
4. Jacobs P. Hodgkin's disease and the malignant lymphomas. *Disease-a-Month* 1993;39:215–297.
5. MacMahon B. Epidemiology of Hodgkin's disease. *Cancer Res* 1966;26(Pt 1):1189–1200.
6. Newell GR, Mills PK, Johnson DE. Epidemiologic comparison of cancer of the testis and Hodgkin's disease among young males. *Cancer* 1984;54:1117–1123.

7. Anderson RE, Ishida K, Li Y, Ishimaru T, Nishiyama H. Geographic aspects of malignant lymphoma and multiple myeloma: select comparisons involving Japan, England and the United States. *Am J Pathol* 1970;61:85–97.
8. Burn C, Davies JNP, Dodge OG, Nias BC. Hodgkin's disease in English and African children. *J Natl Cancer Inst* 1971;46:37–41.
9. Cook PJ, Burkitt DP. Cancer in Africa. *Br Med Bull* 1971;27:14–20.
10. Correa P, O'Conor GT. Epidemiologic patterns of Hodgkin's disease. *Int J Cancer* 1971;8:192–201.
11. Burkitt DP. Distribution of cancer in Africa. *Proc R Soc Med* 1973;66: 312–314.
12. Stewart A, Davies JNP, Dalldorf G, Barnhart FE. Malignant lymphomas of African children. *Proc Natl Acad Sci USA* 1973;70:15–17.
13. Olweny CLM. Lymphomas and leukaemias. Part 1: Tropical Africa. *Clin hematol* 1981;10:873–893.
14. Fleming AF. The epidemiology of lymphomas and leukaemias in Africa: an overview. *Leuk Res* 1985;9:735–740.
15. Colonna P, Belhadj-Merzoug K, Henni T, Andrieu JM. Changes in patterns of Hodgkin's disease in Algeria, 1966–1985: influence of health care delivery system. *Acta Hematol* 1988;80:227–228.
16. Wright DH. Epidemiology and histology of Hodgkin's disease in Uganda. *Natl Cancer Inst Monogr* 1973;36:25–30.
17. Edington GM, Osankoya BO, Hendrickse M. Histological classification of Hodgkin's disease in the Western State of Nigeria. *J Natl Cancer Inst* 1973;50:1633–1637.
18. Naik KG, Bhagwandeen SB. Hodgkin's disease in Zambia. *East Afr Med J* 1976;53:459–467.
19. Kung'u A. Hodgkin's disease in Kenya: a histopathological and epidemiological study. *East Afr Med J* 1983;60:416–427.
20. Emanuel DJ, Gelfand M. A survey into the clinical presentation of Hodgkin's disease at Harare Hospital, Salisbury, Rhodesia. *J Trop Med Hyg* 1975;78:44–46.
21. Hamdi Cherif M, Sekfali N, Benlatrech K. Algeria. In: Parkin DM, Muir CS, Whelan SL, Gao YT, Ferlay J, Powell J, eds. *Cancer incidence in five continents,* Vol 6. *IARC Scientific Publication No. 120.* Lyons: IARC, 1992:182–185.
22. Parkin DM, Muir CS, Whelan SL, Gao YT, Ferlay J, Powell J. *Cancer incidence in five continents,* Vol 6. *IARC Scientific Publication No. 120.* Lyon: IARC, 1992:186–193.
23. Chadli A, Philippe E. La physionomie du cancer en Tunisie. *Arch Inst Pasteur* 1960;37:391–392.
24. Chadli A, Rethers L, Landreat A, Habanec B. La physionomie du cancer en Tunisie (II): etude de 7.959 cancers primitifs. *Arch Inst Pasteur* 1976;53:318–423.
25. Cosset J-M. *Etude anatomo-pathologique et clinique de 112 cas de maladies de Hodgkin vus à l'Institut Salah Azaiz de Tunis du 01.01.1969 au 31.12.1972.* These de medecine, Universite de Paris XI, 1975.
26. Ben Abdallah M. *Epidemiologie des cancers en Tunisie: registre de l'Institut Salah Azaiz.* Tunis, 1997.
27. Chaouki N, El Gueddari B. Epidemiological descriptive approach of cancer in Morocco through the activity of the National Institute of Oncology, 1986–7. *Bull Cancer (Paris)* 1991;78:603–609.
28. Nasr ALA, Tawfik HN, El-Einen MA. Lymphoreticular tumors and leukemias in Egypt. *J Natl Cancer Inst* 1973;50:1619–1621.
29. Kahan E, Ibrahim AS, El Najjar K, et al. Cancer patterns in the Middle East: special report from the Middle East Cancer Society. *Acta Oncol* 1997;36:631–636.
30. El-Boulkainy MN. *General pathology of cancer.* Cairo: Al-Asdekaa Graphics Center; 1991.
31. Azim HA, Moussa M, Hamada E, Kamel YM. *Adult Hodgkin's disease: clinical presentation and results of treatment in NEMROCK (1992–1995).* Dissertation, Cairo University; 1998.
32. Bouchardy C, Parkin DM, Wanner P, Khlat M. Cancer mortality among north African migrants in France. *Int J Epidemiol* 1996;25: 5–13.
33. Cohen C, Hamilton DG. Epidemiologic and histologic patterns of Hodgkin's disease: comparison of the black and white populations of Johannesburg, South Africa. *Cancer* 1980;46:186–189.
34. Sitas F, Blaauw D, Terblanche M, Madhoo J, Carrara H. *Cancer in South Africa 1988. National Cancer Registry of South Africa: incidence of histologically diagnosed cancer in South Africa, 1992.* Johannesburg: South African Institute for Medical Research, 1997: 46–51.
35. Correa P, O'Conor GT. Geographic pathology of lymphoreticular tumors: summary of survey from the Geographic Pathology Committee of the International Union Against Cancer. *J Natl Cancer Inst* 1973;50:1609–1617.
36. Edington GM, Hendrickse M. Incidence and frequency of lymphoreticular tumors in Ibadan and the Western State of Nigeria. *J Natl Cancer Inst* 1973;50:1623–1631.
37. Williams CKO. Influence of life-style on the pattern of leukaemia and lymphoma subtypes among Nigerians. *Leuk Res* 1985;9:741–745.
38. Adedeji MO. The malignant lymphomas in Benin City, Nigeria. *East Afr Med J* 1989;66:134–140.
39. Okpala IE, Akang EE, Okpala UJ. Lymphomas in University College Hospital, Ibadan, Nigeria. *Cancer* 1991;68:1356–1360.
40. Kasili EG. Leukaemia and lymphoma in Kenya. *Leuk Res* 1985;9: 747–752.
41. Kinuthia DM, Kasili EG. Hodgkin's disease in Kenya children: a six-year report on management. *East Afr Med J* 1980;57:769–780.
42. Riyat MS. Hodgkin's disease in Kenya. *Cancer* 1992;69:1047–1051.
43. Dhru R, Templeton AC. Post-mortem findings in Ugandans with Hodgkin's disease. *Br J Cancer* 1972;26:331–334.
44. Amsel S, Nabembezi JS. Two-year survey of hematologic malignancies in Uganda. *J Natl Cancer Inst* 1974;52:1397–1401.
45. Walter PR, Klotz F, Alfy-Gattas T, Minko-Mi-Etoua D, Nguembi-Mbina C. Malignant lymphomas in Gabon (Equatorial Africa): a morphologic study of 72 cases. *Hum Pathol* 1991;22:1040–1043.
46. French TJ, Ross M. Hodgkin's disease at Harare Hospital. *Cent Afr J Med* 1976;22:237–241.
47. Levy LM. Hodgkin's disease in black Zimbabweans: a study of epidemiologic, histologic, and clinical features. *Cancer* 1988;61: 189–194.
48. Levy LM. The pattern of hematological and lymphoreticular malignancy in Zimbabwe. *Trop Geogr Med* 1988;40:109–114.
49. Vianna NJ, Thind IS, Louria DB, Polan A, Kirmss V, Davies JNP. Epidemiologic and histologic patterns of Hodgkin's disease in blacks. *Cancer* 1977;40:3133–3139.
50. Glaser SL. Hodgkin's disease in black populations: a review of the epidemiologic literature. *Semin Oncol* 1990;17:643–659.
51. Glaser SL. Black–white differences in Hodgkin's disease incidence in the United States by age, sex, histology subtype and time. *Int J Epidemiol* 1991;20:68–75.
52. Hooper WC, Holman RC, Strine TW, Chorba TL. Hodgkin's disease mortality in the United States: 1979–1988. *Cancer* 1992;70: 1166–1171.
53. Zaki A, Natarajan N, Mettlin CJ. Early and late survival in Hodgkin disease among whites and blacks living in the United States. *Cancer* 1993;72:602–606.
54. Lukes RJ, Craver LF, Hall TC, Rappaport H, Ruben P. Report of the Nomenclature Committee. *Cancer Res* 1966;26(Pt 1):1311.
55. Rosenberg SA. Report of the Committee on the Staging of Hodgkin's Disease. *Cancer Res* 1966;26(Pt 1):1310.
56. Carbone PP, Kaplan HS, Musshoff K, Smithers DW, Tubiana M. Report of the Committee on Hodgkin's Disease Staging. *Cancer Res* 1971;31:1860–1861.
57. Lister TA, Crowther D, Sutcliffe SB, et al. Report of a committee convened to discuss the evaluation and staging of patients with Hodgkin's disease: Cotswolds meeting. *J Clin Oncol* 1989;7:1630–1636.
58. Crowther D, Lister TA. The Cotswolds report on the investigation and staging of Hodgkin's disease. *Br J Cancer* 1990;62:551–552.
59. Stanford JL, Grange JM, Pozniak A. Is Africa lost? *Lancet* 1991;338: 557–558.
60. Proctor SJ, Taylor P, Mackie MJ, et al. A numerical prognostic index for clinical use in identification of poor-risk patients with Hodgkin's disease at diagnosis. The Scotland and Newcastle Lymphoma Group (SNLG) Therapy Working Party. *Leuk Lymphoma* 1992;7(Suppl):17–20.
61. Hasenclever D, Diehl V, for the International Prognostic Factors Project on Advanced Hodgkin's Disease. A numerical index to predict tumor control in advanced Hodgkin's disease (abstract). *Blood* 1996; 88(Suppl 1):673a.
62. Bezwoda WR, MacPhail AP, Dawey R, et al. Hodgkin's disease in sub-Saharan Africa. Cambridge Medical Reviews. In: Armitage J, Newland A, Keating A, Burnett A, eds. *Hematological oncology,* Vol 4. Cambridge: Cambridge University Press, 1995:21–40.
63. Donaldson SS. Hodgkin's disease in children. *Semin Oncol* 1990;17: 736–748.

64. Donaldson SS. Making choices in the staging of children with Hodgkin's disease. *Med Pediatr Oncol* 1991;19:211–213.
65. Donaldson SS, Link MP. Hodgkin's disease: treatment of the young child. *Pediatr Clin North Am* 1991;38:457–473.
66. Cleary SF, Link MP, Donaldson SS. Hodgkin's disease in the very young. *Int J Radiat Oncol Biol Phys* 1993;28:77–83.
67. Gad-el-Mawla N, Hussein MH, Abdel-Hadi S, el-Taneer O, Adde M, Magrath I. Childhood non-Hodgkin's lymphoma in Egypt: preliminary results of treatment with a new ifosfamide-containing regimen. *Cancer Chemother Pharmacol* 1989;24(Suppl 1):S20–S23.
68. Hesseling PB, Wessels G, van Riet FA. The Tygerberg Hospital Children's Tumor Registry 1983–1993. *Eur J Cancer* 1995;31A: 1471–1475.
69. Jacobson RJ, Klappenbach RS, Clinton C, de Moor NG, Wong O. Hodgkin's disease in South African children. *S Afr Med J* 1981;59: 133–137.
70. Hesseling PB, Wessels G, van Jaarsveld D, van Riet FA. Hodgkin's disease in children in southern Africa: epidemiological characteristics, morbidity and long-term outcome. *Ann Trop Paediatr* 1997;17: 367–373.
71. Wessels G. *Paediatric cancer in Namibia (1983–1990).* Dissertation, University of Stellenbosch, 1994.
72. Wessels G, Hesseling PB, Gie RP, Nel E. The increased risk of developing tuberculosis in children with malignancy. *Ann Trop Paediatr* 1992;12:277–281.
73. Pallesen G, Hamilton-Dutoit SJ, Rowe M, Young LS. Expression of Epstein-Barr virus latent gene products in tumor cells of Hodgkin's disease. *Lancet* 1991;337:320–322.
74. Pallesen G, Sandvej K, Hamilton-Dutoit SJ, Rowe M, Young LS. Activation of Epstein-Barr virus replication in Hodgkin and Reed-Sternberg cells. *Blood* 1991;78:1162–1165.
75. Knecht H, Odermatt BF, Bachmann E, et al. Frequent detection of Epstein-Barr virus DNA by the polymerase chain reaction in lymph node biopsies from patients with Hodgkin's disease without genomic evidence of B- or T-cell clonality. *Blood* 1991;78:760–767.
76. Weinreb M, Day PJR, Niggli F, et al. The role of Epstein-Barr virus in Hodgkin's disease from different geographical areas. *Arch Dis Child* 1996;74:27–31.
77. Geser A, de Thé G, Lenoir G, Day NE, Williams EH. Final case reporting from the Ugandan prospective study of the relationship between EBV and Burkitt's lymphoma. *Int J Cancer* 1982;29: 397–400.
78. Leoncini L, Spina D, Nyong'o A, et al. Neoplastic cells of Hodgkin's disease show differences in EBV expression between Kenya and Italy. *Int J Cancer* 1996;65:781–784.
79. Tirelli U, Vaccher E, Rezza G, et al. Hodgkin disease and infection with the human immunodeficiency virus (HIV) in Italy. *Ann Intern Med* 1988;108:309–310.
80. Beral V. The epidemiology of cancer in AIDS patients. *AIDS* 1991; 5(Suppl 2):S99–S103.
81. Pelstring RJ, Zellmer RB, Sulak LE, Banks PM, Clare N. Hodgkin's disease in association with human immunodeficiency virus infection: pathologic and immunologic features. *Cancer* 1991;67:1865–1873.
82. Rabkin CS, Blattner WA. HIV infection and cancers other than non-Hodgkin lymphoma and Kaposi's sarcoma. *Cancer Surv* 1991;10: 151–160.
83. Rabkin CS, Biggar RJ, Horm JW. Increasing incidence of cancers associated with the human immunodeficiency virus epidemic. *Int J Cancer* 1991;47:692–696.
84. Hessol NA, Katz MH, Liu JY, Buchbinder SP, Rubino CJ, Holmberg SD. Increased incidence of Hodgkin disease in homosexual men with HIV infection. *Ann Intern Med* 1992;117:309–311.
85. Tirelli U, Serraino D, Carbone A. Hodgkin disease and HIV. *Ann Intern Med* 1993;118:313.
86. *Fifth national HIV survey attending antenatal clinics of the public health services in South Africa 1995.* Pretoria: Department of Health, 1996.
87. Sitas F, Bezwoda WR, Levin V, et al. Association between human immunodeficiency virus type 1 infection and cancer in the black population of Johannesburg and Soweto, South Africa. *Br J Cancer* 1997;75:1704–1707.
88. Wabinga HR, Parkin DM, Wabwire-Mangen F, Mugerwa JW. Cancer in Kampala, Uganda, in 1989–91: changes in incidence in the era of AIDS. *Int J Cancer* 1993;54:26–36.
89. Bassett MT, Chokunonga E, Mauchaza B, Levy L, Ferlay J, Parkin DM. Cancer in the African population of Harare, Zimbabwe, 1990–1992. *Int J Cancer* 1995;63:29–36.
90. Newton R, Grulich A, Beral V, et al. Cancer and HIV infection in Rwanda. *Lancet* 1995;345:1378–1379.
91. DeVita VT Jr, Serpick AA, Carbone PP. Combination chemotherapy in the treatment of advanced Hodgkin's disease. *Ann Intern Med* 1970; 73:881–895.
92. Henry-Amar M, Somers R. Survival outcome after Hodgkin's disease: a report from the International Data Base on Hodgkin's Disease. *Semin Oncol* 1990;17:758–768.
93. van Spronsen DJ, Dijkema IM, Vrints LW, et al. Improved survival of Hodgkin's disease patients in south-east Netherlands since 1972. *Eur J Cancer* 1997;33:436–441.
94. Høst H, Abrahamsen AF, Jørgensen OG, Normann T. Laparotomy and splenectomy in the management of Hodgkin's disease. *Scand J Hematol* 1973;10:327–336.
95. Green DM, Ghoorah J, Douglass HO Jr, et al. Staging laparotomy with splenectomy in children and adolescents with Hodgkin's disease. *Cancer Treat Rev* 1983;10:23–38.
96. Munker R, Stengel A, Stäbler A, Hiller E, Brehm G. Diagnostic accuracy of ultrasound and computed tomography in the staging of Hodgkin's disease. *Cancer* 1995;76:1460–1466.
97. Hoh CK, Glaspy J, Rosen P, et al. Whole-body FDG-PET imaging for staging of Hodgkin's disease and lymphoma. *J Nucl Med* 1997;38: 343–348.
98. Nademanee A, O'Donnell MR, Snyder DS, et al. High-dose chemotherapy with or without total body irradiation followed by autologous bone marrow and/or peripheral blood stem cell transplantation for patients with relapsed and refractory Hodgkin's disease: results in 85 patients with analysis of prognostic factors. *Blood* 1995;85: 1381–1390.
99. O'Brien MER, Milan S, Cunningham D, et al. High-dose chemotherapy and autologous bone marrow transplant in relapsed Hodgkin's disease: a pragmatic prognostic index. *Br J Cancer* 1996;73:1272–1277.
100. Horning SJ, Chao NJ, Negrin RS, et al. High-dose therapy and autologous hematopoietic progenitor cell transplantation for recurrent or refractory Hodgkin's disease: analysis of the Stanford University results and prognostic indices. *Blood* 1997;89:801–813.
101. Goffman TE, Raubitschek A, Glatstein E. Survivors of Hodgkin's disease: prevention of sequelae. *South Med J* 1991;84:1108–1110.
102. DeVita VT Jr. Late sequelae of treatment of Hodgkin's disease. *Curr Opin Oncol* 1997;9:428–431.
103. Olweny CLM, Ziegler JL, Berard CW, Templeton AC. Adult Hodgkin's disease in Uganda. *Cancer* 1971;27:1295–1301.
104. Oluboyede OA, Esan GJF. The therapy of Hodgkin's disease in Nigeria: a five year study. *Afr J Med Sci* 1976;5:201–207.
105. Olweny CLM, Katongole-Mbidde E, Kiire C, Lwanga SK, Magrath I, Ziegler JL. Childhood Hodgkin's disease in Uganda: a ten year experience. *Cancer* 1978;42:787–792.
106. Williams CKO. Prospective studies on Hodgkin's disease in Ibadan: a preliminary report. *Afr J Med Sci* 1985;14:37–43.
107. Canellos GP, Anderson JR, Propert KJ, et al. Chemotherapy of advanced Hodgkin's disease with MOPP, ABVD or MOPP alternating with ABVD. *N Engl J Med* 1992;327:1478–1484.
108. Longo DL, Duffey PL, DeVita VT Jr, et al. Treatment of advanced-stage Hodgkin's disease: alternating noncrossresistant MOPP/CABS is not superior to MOPP. *J Clin Oncol* 1991;9:1409–1420.
109. Somers R, Carde P, Henry-Amar M, et al. A randomized study in stage IIIB and IV Hodgkin's disease comparing eight courses of MOPP versus an alternation of MOPP with ABVD: A European Organization for Research and Treatment of Cancer Lymphoma Cooperative Group and Groupe Pierre-et-Marie-Curie Controlled Clinical Trial. *J Clin Oncol* 1994;12:279–287.
110. Radford JA, Crowther D, Rohatiner AZS, et al. Results of a randomized trial comparing MVPP chemotherapy with a hybrid regimen, ChlVPP/EVA, in the initial treatment of Hodgkin's disease. *J Clin Oncol* 1995;13:2379–2385.
111. Viviani S, Bonadonna G, Santoro A, et al. Alternating versus hybrid MOPP and ABVD combinations in advanced Hodgkin's disease: ten-year results. *J Clin Oncol* 1996;14:1421–1430.
112. Carde P, MacKintosh FR, Rosenberg SA. A dose and time response analysis of the treatment of Hodgkin's disease with MOPP chemotherapy. *J Clin Oncol* 1983;1:146–153.

113. Longo DL, Young RC, Wesley M, et al. Twenty years of MOPP therapy for Hodgkin's disease. *J Clin Oncol* 1986;4:1295–1306.
114. Bezwoda WR, Dansey R, Bezwoda MA. Treatment of Hodgkin's disease with MOPP chemotherapy: effect of dose and schedule modification on treatment outcome. *Oncology* 1990;47:29–36.
115. Jagannath S, Armitage JO, Dicke KA, et al. Prognostic factors for response and survival after high-dose cyclophosphamide, carmustine, and etoposide with autologous bone marrow transplantation for relapsed Hodgkin's disease. *J Clin Oncol* 1989;7:179–185.
116. Kessinger A, Nademanee A, Forman SJ, Armitage JO. Autologous bone marrow transplantation for Hodgkin's and non-Hodgkin's lymphoma. *Hematol Oncol Clin North Am* 1990;4:577–587.
117. Seymour LK, Dansey RD, Bezwoda WR. Single high-dose etoposide and melphalan with non-cryopreserved autologous marrow rescue as primary therapy for relapsed, refractory and poor-prognosis Hodgkin's disease. *Br J Cancer* 1994;70:526–530.
118. Bezwoda WR, Dansey R. High dose chemotherapy with bone marrow rescue for treatment of relapsed and refractory Hodgkin's disease. *Leuk Lymphoma* 1989;1:71–76.
119. Martin J, Radford M. Current practice in Hodgkin's disease. The United Kingdom Children's Cancer Study Group. In: Kamps WA, Humphrey GB, Poppema S, eds. *Hodgkin's disease in children: controversies and current practice.* Boston: Kluwer, 1989:263–275.
120. Hunger SP, Link MP, Donaldson SS. ABVD/MOPP and low-dose involved-field radiotherapy in pediatric Hodgkin's disease: the Stanford experience. *J Clin Oncol* 1994;12:2160–2166.
121. Oberlin O, Leverger G, Pacquement H, et al. Low-dose radiation therapy and reduced chemotherapy in childhood Hodgkin's disease: the experience of the French Society of Pediatric Oncology. *J Clin Oncol* 1992;10:1602–1608.
122. Sankila R, Garwicz S, Olsen JH, et al. Risk of subsequent malignant neoplasms among 1,641 Hodgkin's disease patients diagnosed in childhood and adolescence: a population-based cohort study in the five Nordic countries. *J Clin Oncol* 1996;14:1442–1446.

Hodgkin's Disease, edited by P. M. Mauch,
J. O. Armitage, V. Diehl, R. T. Hoppe, and L. M. Weiss.
Lippincott Williams & Wilkins, Philadephia ©1999.

CHAPTER 44

Hodgkin's Disease in Asia

Raymond H. S. Liang, C. C. Yau, Mary Ann Muckaden,
Ketayun A. Dinshaw, and David Todd

A great variation in the incidence rates of Hodgkin's disease has been observed in different ethnic populations (1). In Western populations, the incidence rates of Hodgkin's disease range from 1.5 to 4.5/100,000 for men and between 0.9 and 3.0/100,000 for women (2). In Asian countries, the corresponding figures are in general very much lower (1). There is at the present no satisfactory explanation for the discrepancy. Genetic susceptibility may be important. Infective or other environmental factors, however, may also contribute. Furthermore, very little information is currently available on how the disease may present, behave, and respond to treatment differently in Asian patients as compared with those in the West.

EPIDEMIOLOGY

In Western populations, the crude incidence of Hodgkin's disease is estimated to be about three per 100,000 population (1,2). On the other hand, the figure is considerably lower in most Asian countries (2). The pattern has been consistent in most places and cannot be accounted for by occasional cases being misdiagnosed, for example, as peripheral T-cell lymphoma.

Extensive data on the cancer incidence of different geographic locations have been collected systematically by the International Agency for Research on Cancer (2). Figures were obtained from local cancer registries of countries around the world. Hodgkin's disease has been highlighted as a separate entity in their report, and data can be easily retrieved. Based on the information reported in 1992 covering the period of 1983 to 1987, a summary of the crude incidences of Hodgkin's disease in Asia has been compiled (2) (Table 1).

Table 1 shows the crude incidence of Hodgkin's disease in various places in Asia (2). In men, low incidence rates of less than 1.0 per 100,000 are observed consistently in China, Japan, Philippines, and Thailand (2). The pattern appears to vary very little in different areas within each of these countries. Figures of around 2.0 to 4.0 per 100,000 are found in the Jewish population of Israel and are similar to those of the Western populations. Intermediate rates between 1.0 and 2.0 per 100,000 are observed in other places, such as India, Kuwait, and Kyrazstan. Singaporean Chinese have an incidence rate of Hodgkin's disease that is similar to those observed in China, Japan, Philippines, and Thailand but is much lower than those of the Indians and Malays in Singapore (2).

The overall incidence of Hodgkin's disease in Asian women is lower than that of men, but the overall pattern is still very similar (2) (Table 1). Low incidence rates of around 0.5 per 100,000 or less are observed in China, Japan, Philippines, and Thailand. Again, the pattern varies very little in different cities within these countries. Similarly, a relatively higher incidence rate of more than 2.0 per 100,000 is seen in the Jewish population of Israel and is similar to those of the Western populations. Intermediate rates between 0.5 and 2.0 per 100,000 are observed in other places, such as India, Kuwait, and Kyrgyzstan. In Singapore, the overall incidence rate of Hodgkin's disease in women is low and is less than 0.5 per 100,000. However, unlike the men, the difference between Chinese and the Indians/Malay is less obvious.

The incidence rates of Hodgkin's disease are also available for Asian immigrants in the United States (2) (Table 2). In Los Angeles and Hawaii, the rates for Asian immi-

R. H. S. Liang: Department of Medicine, University of Hong Kong and Division of Hematology/Oncology, Queen Mary Hospital, Hong Kong.

C. C. Yau: Department of Radiotherapy and Oncology, Queen Mary Hospital, Hong Kong.

M. A. Muckaden and K. A. Dinshaw: Department of Radiation Oncology, Tata Memorial Center, Mumbai, India.

D. Todd: Department of Medicine, University of Hong Kong, Queen Mary Hospital, Hong Kong.

TABLE 1. *The annual crude incidence rates of Hodgkin's disease in different parts of Asia (per 100,000)*

	Male	Female
China		
Hong Kong	0.6	0.4
Qidong	0.1	0.0
Shanghai	0.4	0.3
Tianjin	0.4	0.3
India		
Ahmedabad	1.4	0.5
Bangalore	1.2	0.5
Mumbai	1.0	0.4
Chennai	1.5	0.6
Israel		
Jews	2.9	2.3
Jews (Africa)	3.0	2.0
Jews (Europe)	3.9	2.7
Jews (Israel)	2.5	2.7
Non-Jews	2.0	1.0
Japan		
Hiroshima City	0.4	0.1
Miyagi	0.5	0.3
Nagasaki City	0.6	0.3
Osaka	0.5	0.3
Saga	0.6	0.3
Yamagata	0.1	0.0
Kuwait		
Kuwaitis	1.4	0.5
Non-Kuwaitis	1.8	1.3
Kyrgyzstan	1.2	1.1
Philippines		
Manila	0.4	0.3
Rizal	0.4	0.3
Singapore		
Chinese	0.5	0.3
Indian	1.1	0.3
Malay	1.0	0.5
Thailand		
Chiang Mai	0.7	0.6
Khon Kaen	0.8	0.2

Adapted from ref. 2.

TABLE 2. *The annual crude incidence rates of Hodgkin's disease in Asian immigrants of the United States (per 100,000)*

	Male	Female
Los Angeles		
Black	2.8	2.0
Chinese	0.6	1.1
Filipino	0.2	0.5
Japanese	0.7	0.4
Korean	1.1	0.0
Spanish	2.0	1.5
White	3.9	2.8
Hawaii		
Chinese	0.9	3.7[a]
Filipino	1.4	0.7
Hawaiian	0.6	1.2
Japanese	0.7	0.8
White	2.5	3.6

[a]Very few cases only.
Adapted from ref. 2.

grants from China, Japan, Korea, and Philippines are consistently below 1.0 per 100,000. The figures are very similar to those observed in their native countries. The incidence rate for Native Hawaiian is comparable to that of the Asian immigrants. On the other hand, the blacks and Hispanics in Los Angeles have rates between 1.0 and 2.0 per 100,000, which are intermediate between Asian immigrants and whites.

Interestingly, reports from United Kingdom suggest that children of Asian ethnic origin, mainly from the Indian subcontinent, have been observed to have a twofold increased risk of developing Hodgkin's disease, especially men (3–6). A nonsignificant excess for Hodgkin's disease has also been noted in the British ethnic population born in India. It is postulated that the migrants of both Indian and British ethnicities may have an opportunity for early-life infectious exposure in India and for later exposure to new infections at migration (7).

Tables 3 and 4 summarize the average annual incidence rates of Hodgkin's disease by age groups in Asian men and women, respectively (2). A bimodal age distribution for Hodgkin's disease has been observed in Western populations. There is an early peak at the second or third decade and a late one at sixth or seventh. The early age peak appears to be absent in Japanese. For the other Asian countries with a low incidence of Hodgkin's disease, the early peak is also not obvious. The data from Asian immigrants in the United States are more difficult to interpret, as the number of cases in each age subgroup is relatively small.

Table 5 summarizes the proportion of Hodgkin's disease among all lymphomas in Asia as reported in the literature (8–26). In Western populations, Hodgkin's disease commonly comprises up to one-third of all lymphomas. Only about a tenth of all patients with lymphoma have Hodgkin's disease in most parts of Asia, except in the Middle East. In Japan, there appears to be a trend that the proportion decreased further in the last decade. This observation is probably the result of the relatively low incidence rates of Hodgkin's disease in most of these places. On the other hand, the overall incidence rates of non-Hodgkin's lymphoma are quite similar in different populations around the world, although the rates for some histologic subtypes may be markedly different.

The incidence rates of various histologic subtypes of Hodgkin's disease may also vary in different ethnic populations (27–29). Table 6 summarizes the results obtained in California as reported by Perkin et al. (29). The racial difference is most prominent for the nodular sclerosing subtype of Hodgkin's disease. Because the nodular sclerosing subtype accounts for a great majority of the cases of Hodgkin's disease at the early age peak, this may explain the lack of this peak in many Asian populations. The incidence rate of the nodular sclerosing type is only 0.5 per 100,000 in Asians, in contrast to a much higher rate of 1.9 for whites. The differences were less obvious for the mixed-cellularity subtype (0.2 for Asian versus 0.5 for

TABLE 3. *The average annual incidence rates of Hodgkin's disease according to age groups in Asian men (per 100,000)*

	0–	1–	5–	10–	15–	20–	25–	30–	35–	40–	45–	50–	55–	60–	65–	70–	75–	80–	85+
China																			
Hong Kong	0.2	—	0.8	0.5	0.5	0.3	0.6	0.7	0.3	0.4	1.1	0.5	0.6	1.1	1.3	1.1	3.9	—	4.3
Qidong	—	—	—	—	—	—	—	—	—	—	—	—	—	1.1	1.5	—	—	—	—
Shanghai	0.3	—	0.7	0.2	0.3	0.4	0.2	0.1	0.2	—	0.4	0.5	0.3	0.1	1.4	0.8	0.5	1.1	3.7
Tianjin	—	—	0.3	0.2	0.5	0.2	0.2	0.4	0.5	1.2	0.9	1.0	1.1	0.3	—	0.6	—	—	—
India																			
Ahmedabad	0.6	—	1.4	1.3	1.0	1.2	1.4	1.3	1.4	2.1	1.8	1.5	3.4	2.0	3.6	3.1	—	—	—
Bangalore	—	—	1.9	1.2	0.7	0.2	1.0	0.7	1.3	1.9	1.3	3.1	3.7	3.8	2.0	3.7	2.4	—	—
Bombay	0.3	—	1.4	0.5	0.6	0.5	0.9	1.4	1.0	0.9	1.1	1.4	2.0	3.2	4.1	3.9	2.1	—	—
Madras	0.2	—	1.6	2.0	1.1	0.9	1.5	1.7	1.6	1.3	3.1	2.3	1.5	2.4	3.4	1.1	2.6	—	—
Israel																			
Jews	—	0.1	1.2	1.9	4.3	3.4	3.8	3.6	3.2	3.2	4.6	4.6	1.8	2.8	4.4	3.2	5.8	—	—
Jews (Africa)	—	—	—	—	—	3.0	3.7	2.4	2.9	2.3	4.3	2.6	1.6	3.9	2.8	3.4	5.9	—	—
Jews (Europe)	—	—	—	4.1	7.0	2.8	3.5	2.7	4.2	6.7	1.8	5.9	2.5	2.5	4.8	2.7	6.1	—	—
Jews (Israel)	—	0.1	1.3	1.8	4.2	3.5	3.9	4.4	2.6	1.7	8.3	6.9	—	—	10.4	11.0	—	—	—
Non-Jews	—	0.9	0.7	2.0	1.4	1.7	3.0	3.9	1.2	2.9	1.8	9.3	6.3	—	—	12.4	8.6	—	—
Japan																			
Hiroshima City	—	—	—	—	1.1	—	—	—	—	0.5	—	—	0.9	2.6	5.1	2.2	—	—	—
Miyagi	—	—	—	—	0.2	0.5	0.3	0.2	0.4	—	0.6	0.6	0.9	1.7	1.8	0.8	1.1	6.8	5.1
Nagasaki City	—	—	—	—	—	—	—	1.1	2.2	—	—	—	1.6	—	2.9	3.7	—	—	—
Osaka	—	0.1	0.2	0.1	0.2	0.5	0.1	0.3	0.2	0.4	0.6	0.6	1.2	0.7	2.8	3.5	2.1	3.5	—
Saga	—	—	—	—	—	—	—	—	2.0	—	—	—	—	3.3	—	5.3	3.5	—	12.8
Yamagata	—	—	—	—	—	—	—	0.5	0.5	—	—	—	—	—	—	—	—	—	—
Kuwait																			
Kuwaitis	1.5	1.1	1.4	1.3	0.5	2.7	—	—	4.3	1.6	—	2.5	—	—	6.3	—	16.9	—	—
Non-Kuwaitis	—	—	1.3	2.9	1.0	2.1	2.3	1.3	2.0	2.8	2.1	1.7	1.7	8.1	—	—	—	—	—
Kyragzstan	0.8	—	1.2	1.1	0.7	0.3	1.1	0.7	1.0	1.9	4.3	2.0	3.4	2.3	2.3	2.9	—	—	—
Philippines																			
Manila	—	0.2	—	—	0.2	0.1	0.4	0.6	0.8	0.2	0.9	1.5	1.0	3.6	2.0	1.5	3.4	—	—
Rizal	—	—	0.1	—	—	0.3	0.5	0.3	0.4	0.8	1.8	2.9	2.9	—	2.8	2.1	2.2	—	—
Singapore																			
Chinese	—	—	0.2	0.2	0.8	0.4	0.2	—	0.5	—	0.9	1.5	2.6	1.6	1.0	1.4	—	—	—
Indian	—	—	—	—	—	2.2	—	—	—	—	—	3.9	—	9.2	7.3	—	—	—	—
Malay	1.1	—	—	1.2	2.0	—	1.0	1.3	—	—	—	—	—	—	12.7	10.6	—	—	—
Thailand																			
Chiang Mai	0.3	—	—	—	0.3	0.6	0.3	—	1.1	—	1.6	0.9	3.2	2.9	2.2	6.5	10.8	—	—
Khon Kaen	—	—	—	—	—	—	—	2.6	2.0	2.4	2.9	3.7	—	3.0	—	14.0	—	—	—

Adapted from ref. 2.

TABLE 4. *The average annual incidence rates of Hodgkin's disease according to age groups in Asian women (per 100,000)*

	0–	1–	5–	10–	15–	20–	25–	30–	35–	40–	45–	50–	55–	60–	65–	70–	75–	80–	85+
China																			
Hong Kong	—	—	0.1	0.2	0.4	0.3	0.5	0.8	0.2	0.4	0.2	1.1	0.7	0.2	0.5	1.8	0.5	0.8	1.1
Qidong	—	—	—	—	—	—	—	—	—	—	—	—	—	—	—	—	—	—	—
Shanghai	0.1	—	—	0.5	0.4	0.4	0.3	0.3	0.1	0.3	0.1	0.2	0.4	0.5	0.6	0.2	—	—	—
Tianjin	—	—	0.5	—	0.4	0.2	0.1	0.2	—	0.2	0.4	0.4	0.7	1.5	0.9	0.6	—	3.9	4.2
India																			
Ahmedabad	0.1	—	0.6	0.4	0.5	0.1	0.4	0.4	0.5	—	0.7	1.8	1.3	2.2	1.3	—	3.8	—	—
Bangalore	—	—	0.2	0.3	0.5	0.7	0.8	0.5	0.2	0.6	0.7	0.8	0.6	0.6	2.1	2.5	—	—	—
Bombay	0.1	—	0.2	0.2	0.2	0.2	0.2	0.4	0.5	0.4	1.2	1.1	1.7	0.8	2.7	2.5	1.1	—	—
Madras	0.1	—	0.4	0.6	1.0	0.8	0.9	0.3	0.4	0.7	1.1	1.3	0.5	—	—	1.1	3.5	—	—
Israel																			
Jews	—	0.1	0.4	0.9	3.4	3.9	4.3	3.8	2.2	1.8	1.3	2.9	2.6	2.2	3.1	3.4	4.2	—	—
Jews (Israel)	—	0.1	0.4	1.0	3.5	3.5	4.2	4.5	0.5	2.6	1.0	4.9	2.3	—	8.9	9.2	17.1	—	—
Jews (Europe)	—	—	—	—	1.8	5.6	4.1	3.2	4.0	2.0	0.8	2.5	2.9	1.3	2.0	4.3	3.3	—	—
Jews (Africa)	—	—	—	—	3.8	4.6	4.6	2.4	2.4	1.1	1.7	2.4	2.2	4.5	4.9	—	5.3	—	—
Non-Jews	—	—	0.4	1.2	1.0	1.1	3.7	1.0	—	1.5	—	6.5	—	—	—	—	—	—	—
Japan																			
Hiroshima City	—	—	—	—	—	—	—	—	—	—	—	0.7	—	—	1.3	1.6	—	—	—
Miyagi	—	—	—	—	0.5	0.3	0.8	0.2	—	—	—	0.3	0.3	—	0.5	1.7	0.8	—	—
Nagasaki City	—	—	—	—	—	—	—	1.1	—	—	—	—	—	—	4.3	—	—	—	—
Osaka	—	0.1	—	0.1	0.3	0.4	—	0.1	0.0	0.2	0.3	0.3	0.5	0.7	0.4	1.0	0.5	2.0	2.3
Saga	—	—	—	—	1.1	—	—	—	—	—	—	1.1	—	—	1.6	1.7	—	—	—
Yamagata	—	—	—	—	—	—	—	—	—	—	—	—	—	—	—	—	—	—	—
Kuwait																			
Kuwaitis	—	0.4	0.4	—	1.0	0.6	0.7	1.0	1.2	1.6	—	—	—	—	—	—	—	—	—
Non-Kuwaitis	—	0.4	2.2	0.5	0.6	2.1	1.3	1.5	2.6	1.9	—	—	—	—	—	—	—	—	—
Kyragzstan	—	0.4	0.2	0.2	1.9	0.8	1.8	1.4	1.4	2.8	—	0.6	1.7	0.7	1.2	6.5	3.5	—	—
Philippines																			
Manila	—	0.1	—	—	0.3	0.2	0.5	0.4	—	1.1	0.3	1.7	1.4	1.2	2.4	—	—	—	—
Rizal	—	—	0.1	0.1	0.1	0.2	0.3	0.6	0.4	—	1.5	0.5	1.3	1.7	—	—	1.7	—	—
Singapore																			
Chinese	—	—	—	0.5	—	—	0.2	—	0.3	0.6	—	0.5	0.6	0.7	—	2.2	1.6	—	—
Indian	—	—	—	—	—	—	2.4	—	—	—	—	—	—	—	—	—	—	—	—
Malay	—	—	1.2	—	—	1.0	1.1	—	1.9	—	—	—	—	—	—	—	—	—	—
Thailand																			
Chiang Mai	—	—	0.3	—	—	—	1.8	0.4	—	1.5	0.8	1.7	4.1	—	1.9	2.8	—	—	—
Khon Kaen	—	—	—	—	—	—	—	—	—	—	1.6	1.8	—	—	4.3	—	—	—	—

Adapted from ref. 2.

TABLE 5. *Hodgkin's disease as a percentage of the total number of lymphoma patients in Asia*

	Percentage
China	9%
Hong Kong	9%
Iran	33%
Japan	10%
Kuwait	35%
Malaysia	14%
Oman	35%
Papua New Guinea	8%
Saudi Arabia	44%
Singapore	20%

white). Both the lymphocyte predominant and lymphocyte-depleted are uncommon entities in all ethnic populations, and there appear to be no ethnic differences for these two subtypes.

GENETIC AND VIRAL FACTORS

The variation in incidence rates of Hodgkin's disease in different ethnic populations strongly suggests that inherited susceptibility plays an important role in its pathogenesis (1). There may be interaction between genetic and other environmental factors (30). It has been shown that the association of Hodgkin's disease and Epstein-Barr virus is strongest in the group of patients with evidence of genetic susceptibility and familial clustering (31). Reports of familial aggregation and human leukocyte antigen (HLA) association further support the importance of genetic influence.

Familial aggregation for Hodgkin's disease has been reported frequently (32–38). A twin study has nicely demonstrated a very good concordance for Hodgkin's disease in identical twins. Monozygotic twins of young adults with Hodgkin's disease are estimated to have a 99-fold increased risk of the disease (39). The result suggested that genetic predisposition accounts for at least a subgroup of patients with Hodgkin's disease.

The association of HLA with Hodgkin's disease has been studied (40–47). It is postulated that HLA-linked recessive susceptibility may be responsible for about 60% of the familial cases of Hodgkin's disease (40). It is possible that there are candidate genes that lie within various histocompatibility gene loci. An international collaborative study has recently shown that the frequency of HLA-DPB1*0301 allele was significantly higher in white patients with Hodgkin's disease, as compared with the ethnically matched controls (43). At the same time, the HLA-DPB1*0301 allele is associated significantly with a 1.95-fold increased risk of developing Hodgkin's disease. On the other hand, there is also a significant reduction in the frequency of HLA-DPB1*0401 allele in patients from Japan and Taiwan. Furthermore, clinical analysis in the study demonstrates a significantly inferior remission duration in Hodgkin's disease patients with the HLA-DPB1*0901 allele, which is most prevalent in Asian populations. The significance of these findings is uncertain, and further investigations are warranted (43).

A strong association between Epstein-Barr virus (EBV) and Hodgkin's disease has been demonstrated by molecular techniques (48–52). However, the significance of EBV in the pathogenesis of Hodgkin's disease remains uncertain. The presence of EBV DNA, RNA, and LMP-1 protein in practically all neoplastic cells in the positive samples of Hodgkin's disease and the demonstration of EBV in a clonal episomal form in tissues provide strong evidence for a possible causative role of EBV. Table 7 shows the positive rates for EBV as reported in different ethnic populations (53–68). A relatively lower rate of 20% to 30% is seen in non-Hispanic populations in the United States. On the other hand, EBV is almost invariably positive in all cases of Hodgkin's disease in Latin America. An intermediate pattern is seen in Asia. It appears that there is a stronger association of EBV with Hodgkin's disease at the extremes of life. In Japan, the bimodal age distribution for Hodgkin's disease is not seen, and there is only a single age peak in elderly patients (57,58); EBV is found mainly in specimens from Japanese patients above the age of 40 years. The frequency of EBV detection in Hodgkin's disease also varies with histologic subtype: EBV positivity correlates with the mixed-cellularity histology and is rarely seen in lymphocyte predominant type (53). As discussed earlier, Asian populations have a much lower incidence rate for nodular sclerosing type. This may account for a higher proportion of EBV-positive cases. It has been suggested that other factors such as nutrition may also be important in contributing to a high positive rate for EBV in developing countries (68).

TABLE 6. *The incidence rates of various histologic subtypes of Hodgkin's disease in different ethnic population in California (per 100,000)*

	Nodular sclerosing	Lymphocyte predominant	Mixed cellularity	Lymphocyte depleted
White	1.9	0.2	0.5	0.1
Black	1.2	0.3	0.5	0.1
Hispanic	0.9	0.1	0.6	0.1
Asian	0.5	0.1	0.2	0.1

TABLE 7. *Positive rates for Epstein-Barr virus for Hodgkin's disease*

Asia	
China	65–82%
India	70%
Japan	26–64%
Korea	76%
Philippines	43%
Latin America	~100%
United States	
Hispanic	53%
Non-Hispanic	23%

CLINICAL PRESENTATIONS AND MANAGEMENT

Other than having a lower overall incidence rate, there are suggestions that Hodgkin's disease may present, behave, and respond to treatment differently in Asian patients (69–75). Similar to the Western populations, Hodgkin's disease affects men more commonly than women in Asia. The bimodal age distribution, however, is not as obvious, and there is a relatively higher proportion of more elderly patients with Hodgkin's disease in Asian countries. There is also apparently a higher proportion of the mixed-cellularity rather than nodular sclerosing subtype, as discussed earlier.

Hodgkin's disease may also present differently in Asian patients (69–75). There are reports of more advanced disease being seen at presentation, such as the involvement of liver, spleen, and marrow involvement (69,70). The incidence rate of B symptoms also appears to be higher. Furthermore, there has been a report of a high proportion of subdiaphragmatic disease (71). These findings can be partly explained by the late presentation of patients to doctors as a result of low awareness of the disease and/or difficulty in access to medical care facilities in some parts of Asia. There are also some concerns about diagnostic accuracy in some of the cases. Peripheral T-cell lymphoma is known to be more commonly seen many places in Asia and can be mistaken for Hodgkin's disease histologically (76,77). Similar to Hodgkin's disease, EBV association has also been reported for some cases of T-cell lymphoma. Without immunophenotyping, it is possible that some of them may have been misdiagnosed as Hodgkin's disease. It is known that most cases of peripheral T-cell lymphoma affect the more elderly, and the tumor often presents as advanced disease with the presence of B symptoms.

There is an impression that Asian patients with Hodgkin's disease do not respond as well to treatment. This may be a consequence of the aggressiveness of the disease or of late presentation of patients for therapy. As discussed earlier, it is possible that occasional cases of peripheral T-cell lymphoma may be treated as for Hodgkin's disease. It is also known that advanced age of patient is an important prognostic factor and is often associated with poorer tolerance to therapy (78). A higher median age of Asian patients with Hodgkin's disease may also contribute to the inferior treatment results being observed. In some areas of Asia, adequate treatment facilities are not always available or accessible to patients. However, if optimal therapy is available, satisfactory treatment results for Asian patients with Hodgkin's disease can still be observed (72–75).

TABLE 8. *The treatment results of 92 Hong Kong Chinese patients (Pts) with Hodgkin's disease*

	Complete response (CR)	Relapses following CR	Disease-free survival of CR patients at 5 years	Overall survival of all patients at 5 years
Staging of disease				
Ia	13/16 (81%)	3/13 (23%)	73%	100%
Ib	1/2 (50%)	0/1 (0%)	—[a]	—
IIa	13/14 (93%)	1/13 (8%)	92%	100%
IIb	8/10 (80%)	5/8 (63%)	31%	37%
IIIa	7/10 (70%)	4/7 (57%)	43%	58%
IIIb	6/8 (75%)	3/6 (50%)	—[a]	0%
IVa	7/10 (70%)	3/7 (43%)	50%	50%
IVb	8/22 (36%)	5/8 (63%)	45%	48%
p-Value	<0.02	NS	NS	<0.0075
Rye classification				
LP	9/9 (100%)	1/9 (11%)	86%	100%
NS	24/34 (70%)	8/24 (24%)	63%	66%
MC	21/29 (73%)	11/21 (52%)	28%	65%
LD	5/9 (56%)	3/5 (60%)	0%	30%
UC	4/11 (36%)	1/4 (25%)	100%	48%
p-Value	NS	NS	NS	0.0045
Age				
>60 years	6/10 (60%)	3/6 (50%)	—[a]	19%
<60 years	57/82 (70%)	21/57 (37%)	54%	78%
p-Value	NS	NS	NS	<0.02

[a]Not reached.
From ref. 75, with permission.

THE HONG KONG EXPERIENCE

The experience of managing 92 Hong Kong Chinese patients with Hodgkin's disease seen at Queen Mary Hospital, Hong Kong, was reported previously (75). There were 54 male and 38 female patients in the series. Their median age was 34 years (range 5 to 79 years). A bimodal age distribution with peaks at 16 to 20 and 51 to 55 years of age was observed. Their histologic subtypes were: lymphocyte predominant (10%), nodular sclerosing (37%), mixed-cellularity (31%), lymphocyte-depleted (10%), and unclassifiable (12%). Their clinical stages were: IA (17%), IB (2%), IIA (15%), IIB (11%), IIIA (11%), IIIB (9%), IVA (11%), and IVB (24%). Thirteen percent of them had bulky mediastinal disease. Twenty-five stage I and II patients were staged by laparotomy, and six of them were found to have more advanced disease after operation.

A variety of treatments were given to the 92 patients. Patients with stage I or II disease received radiotherapy alone except for those with B symptoms, bulky disease, or lymphocyte-depleted histology, who were given combination chemotherapy with or without radiotherapy. All patients with stage III or IV disease received combination chemotherapy with or without additional radiotherapy, except two patients with stage IIIA disease who had total nodal irradiation. A variety of chemotherapeutic regimens were used, including MOPP, COPP, ChlVPP, ABVD, and MOPP/ABVD.

The treatment results of these 92 Hong Kong Chinese patients are summarized in Table 8. On multivariate analysis, significant independent prognostic factors predicting survival included Ann Arbor staging and age of patients at diagnosis.

THE INDIAN EXPERIENCE

The clinical experience at Tata Memorial Hospital of India was reviewed (73,74). Similar to the pattern seen in many developing countries but in contrast to the observation in Western populations, Hodgkin's disease in India appeared to behave more aggressively at presentation. They were more likely to have advanced-stage disease at presentation. A total of 657 patients were seen at Tata Memorial Hospital, India, during a 10-year period between 1983 and 1992. This included 229 pediatric patients (35%) under 15 years of age. Table 9 shows their age at presentation. The typical bimodal age distribution was not seen. Table 10 shows the clinical stage of the disease. Almost half of the patients had advanced-stage disease, and they were more likely to have B symptoms.

Their histologic subtypes were lymphocyte-rich classical (11.8%), nodular lymphocyte predominant (5.3%), diffuse lymphocyte predominant (11.2%), mixed-cellularity (30.2%), lymphocyte-depleted (3%), and nodular sclerosing (37.9%). In contrast to the other reports from India, the nodular sclerosing subtype was the most common in this series. A relatively high proportion of the lymphocyte predominant subtype was also observed. The discrepancy may be related to the difference in the criteria being used by different pathologists. Table 11 shows the relationship of the different histologic subtypes and the clinical Ann Arbor stage. Patients with lymphocyte predominant Hodgkin's disease were more likely to present with early-stage disease. In contrast, the lymphocyte-depleted subtype was more likely to have advanced-stage disease.

Table 12 shows the EBV positivity rates according to different histologic subtypes. Similar to other experience, EBV positivity was found more commonly in the mixed-cellularity subtype and less frequently in lymphocyte predominant Hodgkin's disease. Table 13 shows the EBV positivity rates in different age groups. It was highest in the youngest age group (1 to 10 years) and declined with age.

Figure 1 shows the treatment strategy adopted at Tata Memorial Hospital. The treatment results were similar to those reported in the literature. Only a small proportion of the patients seen had clinically early-stage disease (I_A or II_A), and staging laparotomy was performed for these patients. Table 14 shows the results of staging laparotomy. Forty-one percent of the patients were found to have more advanced disease after laparotomy.

TABLE 9. *Hodgkin's disease in India: age at presentation (n = 657)*

Age (years)	No. of patients (%)
1–10	158 (24%)
11–20	142 (22%)
21–30	135 (21%)
31–40	99 (15%)
41–50	68 (10%)
51–60	43 (7%)
61–70	9 (1%)
71†	3 (0.5%)

TABLE 10. *Hodgkin's disease in India: Ann Arbor stage at presentation (n = 657)*

Stage	A	B
I	20.2%	6.3%
II	16.6%	15.4%
III	15.4%	16%
IV	1.4%	9.7%

TABLE 11. *Hodgkin's disease in India: Histological subtypes and Ann Arbor stage*

Histologic subtypes	Ann Arbor stage: cases (%) I	II	III	IV
Lymphocyte-rich classical	10 (50.0%)	6 (30.0%)	3 (15.0%)	1 (5.0%)
Nodular lymphocyte predominant	3 (33.3%)	1 (11.1%)	3 (33.3%)	2 (22.2%)
Diffuse lymphocyte predominant	12 (63.2%)	2 (10.5%)	5 (26.3%)	
Mixed cellularity	10 (19.6%)	13 (25.5%)	23 (45.1%)	5 (9.8%)
Lymphocyte depleted	1 (20.0%)	—	2 (40.0%)	2 (40.0%)
Nodular sclerosis	10 (15.9%)	19 (30.2%)	23 (36.5%)	11 (17.5%)
Total	45 (27.5%)	41 (24.6%)	59 (35.3%)	21 (12.65)

TABLE 12. *Hodgkin's disease in India: EBV positivity in different subtypes of Hodgkin's disease*

	Lymphocyte-rich classical	Nodular lymphocyte predominant	Diffuse lymphocyte predominant	Mixed cellularity	Lymphocyte depleted	Nodular sclerosis	Total
Proportion of (%) positive cases	12/16 (75.0%)	2/8 (25.0%)	4/13 (30.8%)	43/50 (86.0%)	1/2 (50.0%)	36/52 (69.2%)	98/141 (69.5%)

TABLE 13. *Hodgkin's disease in India: EBV positivity in different age groups*

Age (years)	EBV positive Cases	% pos.
1–10	36/38	94.7%
11–20	26/26	72.2%
>20	36/68	52.9%
Total	98/142	69.0%

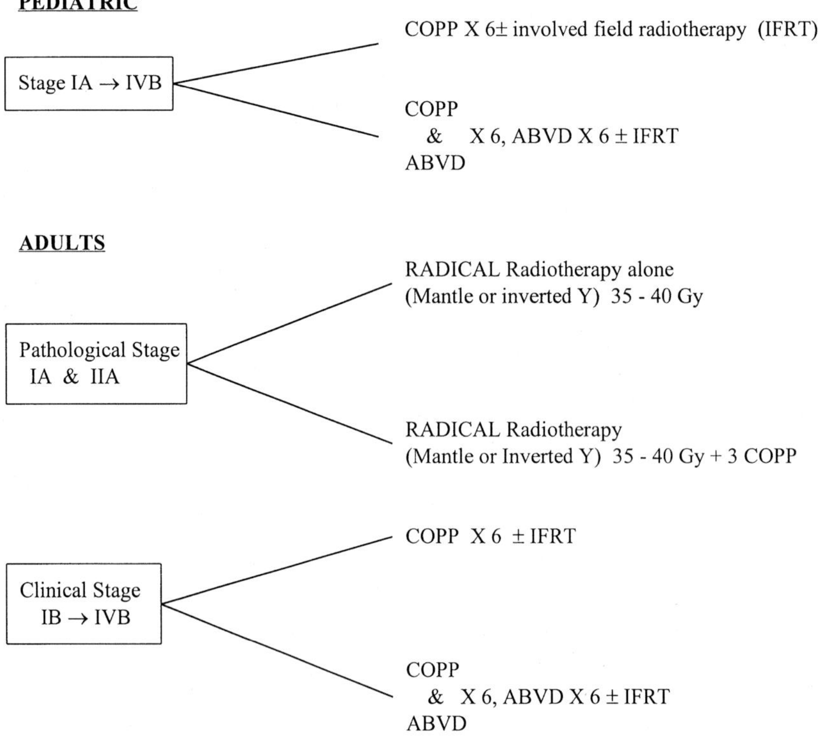

FIG. 1. Treatment strategy adopted at Tata Memorial Hospital.

TABLE 14. *Hodgkin's disease in India: staging laparotomy (n = 134)*

Clinical stage	Result of pathologic staging	*n*
IA and IIA		110
	IA	45
	IIA	19
	IIIA	45
	IVA	1
IB and IIB		55
	IB	3
	IIB	12
	IIIB	7
	IVB	2

REFERENCES

1. Glaser SL, Jarrett RF. The epidemiology of Hodgkin's disease. *Bailliere's Clin Haematol* 1996;9:401–416.
2. Parkin DM, Muir CS, Whelan A. *Cancer incidence in five continents,* Vol VI, *IARC Scientific Publication No. 120.* Lyons: International Agency for Research on Cancer, 1992.
3. Varghese C, Barrett JH, Johnston C, Shires M, Rider L, Forman D. High risk of lymphomas in children of Asian origin, ethnicity or confounding by socioeconomic status. *Br J Cancer* 1996;74:1503–1505.
4. Powell JE, Parkes SE, Cameron AH, Mann JR. Is the risk of cancer increased in Asians living in the UK? *Arch Dis Child* 1994;71:398–403.
5. Stiller CA, Mckinney PA, Bunch KJ, Bailey CC, Lewis IJ. Childhood Cancer and Ethnic Group in Britain: A United Kingdom children s cancer study group (UKCCSG) study. *Br J Cancer* 1991;64:543–548.
6. Stiller CA, Parkin DM. International variations in the incidence of childhood lymphomas. *Paediatr Perinatol Epidemiol* 1990;4:303–324.
7. Swerdlow AJ, Marmot MG, Grulich AE, Head J. Cancer mortality in Indian and British ethnic immigrants from the Indian subcontinent to England and Wales. *Br J Cancer* 1995;72:1312–1319.
8. Mancer KL. The spectrum of lymphoma in Malaysia, a histopathological study utilizing immunophenotyping. *Malaysia J Pathol* 1990;12: 77–88.
9. Tajima K, Suchi T, Oyama A. Changes in clinico-pathological features of Hodgkin's disease and follicular lymphoma in Nagoya, Japan, over a 21-year period (1965–1985). *Acta Pathol Jpn* 1990;40:713–721.
10. MacFaarlane GJ, Evstifeevs T, Boyle P, Grufferman S. International patterns in the occurrence of Hodgkin's disease in children and young males. *Int J Cancer* 1995;61:165–169.
11. Aozasa K, Ueda T, Tamai M, Tsujimura T. Hodgkin's disease in Osaka, Japan (1964–1985). *Eur J Cancer Clin Oncol* 1986;22:1117–1119.
12. Albebouyeh M, Vossough P. Hodgkin's disease in Iranian children. *Eur J Pediatr* 1993;152:21–23.
13. Tabrizchi H, Gupta RK, Rafii MR. A study of malignant lymphomas in Iran, based on the updated Kiel classification. *Virchows Arch A Pathol Anat Histopathol* 1991;419:451–454.
14. Miller RW. The US–Japan Cooperative Cancer Research Program, some highlights of seminars and interdisciplinary program area, 1981–1996. *Jpn J Cancer Res* 1996;87:221–226.
15. Park SH, Shin SS, Kim CW, Chi JG. Malignant lymphomas in children. Kor J Pathol 1990;24:137–147.
16. Chi JG, Kim CW, Cho KJ, Lee SK. Malignant lymphoma in Korea. *J Kor Med Sci* 1987;2:231–237.
17. Ali M, Akhtar M, Amaer M. Morphological and immunologic spectrum of malignant lymphomas, a review of 211 cases. *Ann Saudi Med* 1989;9:344–348.
18. Revesz T, Mpofu C, Oyejide C. Ethnic differences in the lymphoid malignancies of children in the United Arab Emirates, a clue to etiology. *Leukemia* 1995;9:189–193.
19. Motawy MS, Omar YT. Hodgkin's disease in Kuwait. *Cancer* 1986; 57:2255–2259.
20. Bamanikar S, Thunold S, Devi KRL, Bamanikar A. The pattern of malignant lymphoma in Oman. *J Trop Med Hyg* 1995;98:351–354.
21. Al-Bahar S, Pandita R, Al-Bahar E, Al-Muhana A, Al-Yassseen N. Recent trends in the incidence of lymphoma in Kuwait. *Neoplasma* 1996;43:253–257.
22. SenGupta SK, Ades CJ, Cooke RA. Malignant lymphoma in Papua New Guinea, an immunohistological study of 125 cases. *Pathology* 1996;28:36–38.
23. Paulino AFG, Paulino-Cabrera E, Weiss LM, Medeiros LJ. Hodgkin's disease in Philippines. *Mod Pathol* 1996;9:115–119.
24. Ho FCS, Todd D, Loke SL, Ng RP, Khoo RKK. Clinico-pathological features of malignant lymphomas in 294 Hong Kong Chinese patients-retrospective study covering an eight-year period. *Int J Cancer* 1984; 34:143–148.
25. Xiaolong J, Weihua L. Malignant lymphoma in Beijing. *J Environ Pathol Toxicol Oncol* 1992;11:327–329.
26. Tan KK, Kshanmugaratnam K. Incidence and histologic classification of malignant lymphoma in Singapore. *J Natl Cancer Inst* 1973;50: 1681–1683.
27. Cozen W, Katz J, Mack TM. Risk patterns of Hodgkin's disease in Los Angeles by cell type. *Cancer Epidemiol Biomark Prev* 1992;1: 261–268.
28. Wakasa H. Hodgkin's disease in Asia, particularly in Japan. *Natl Cancer Inst Monogr* 1973;36:15–22.
29. Perkin CI, Morris CR, Wright WE, Young JL Jr. *Cancer incidence and mortality in California by detailed race and ethnicity, 1988–1992.* Sacramento: California Department of Health Services Surveillance Section, 1995.
30. Cozen W, Katz J, Mack TM. Risk patterns of Hodgkin's disease in Los Angeles vary by cell type. *Cancer Epidemiol Biomark Prev* 1992;1: 261–268.
31. Diehl V, Tesch H. Hodgkin's disease, environmental or genetic? *Lancet* 1995;332:461–462.
32. Creagan ET, Fraumeni JF Jr. Familial Hodgkin's disease. *Lancet* 1972; 1:547.
33. Buehler SK, Fodor G, Marshall WH, Firme F, Fraser GR, Vaze P. Common variable immunodeficiency, Hodgkin's disease and other malignancies in a Newfoundland family. *Lancet* 1975;1:195–197.
34. Bjerrum OW, Hasselbalch HC, Drivsholm A, Nissen NI. Non-Hodgkin's malignant lymphoma and Hodgkin's disease in first-degree relatives. Evidence for a mutual genetic predisposition. *Scand J Haematol* 1986;36:398–401.
35. Donhuijsen-Ant R, Abken H, Bornkamm G, et al. Fatal Hodgkin's and non-Hodgkin's lymphoma associated with persistent Epstein-Barr virus in four brothers. *Ann Intern Med* 1988;109:946–952.
36. Fraumeni JF Jr. Family studies in Hodgkin's disease. *Cancer Res* 1974; 34:1164–1165.
37. Bohunicky L, Poliakova L, Krizan Z, Cerny V, Halko J. The incidence of lymphogranulomatosis in single-ovum twins. *Neoplasma* 1971;18: 283–288.
38. Cimo G, Lo Cocco F, Cartoni C, et al. Immuno-deficiency in Hodgkin's disease, a study of patients and healthy relatives in families with multiple cases. *Eur J Cancer Clin Oncol* 1988;24:1595–1601.
39. Mack TM, Cozen W, Shibata DK, et al. Concordance for Hodgkin's disease in identical twins suggesting genetic susceptibility to the young adult form of the disease. *N Engl J Med* 1995;332:413–418.
40. Chakreavarti AM, Halloran SL, Bale SJ, Tucker MA. Etiological heterogeneity in Hodgkin's disease, HLA linked and unlinked determinants of susceptibility independent of histological concordance. *Genet Epidemiol* 1989;3:407–415.
41. Maldonado JE, Taswell HF, Kiely JM. Familial Hodgkin's disease. *Lancet* 1972;2:1259.
42. Poppema S, Visser L. Epstein-Barr virus positivity in Hodgkin's disease does not correlate with an HLA A2 negative phenotype. *Cancer* 1994;73:3059–3063.
43. Oza AM, Tonks S, Lim J, Fleetwood MA, Lister TA, Bodmer JG. A clinical and epidemiological study of human leukocyte antigen-DPB alleles in Hodgkin's disease. *Cancer Res* 1994;54:5101–5105.
44. Klitz W, Aldrich CL, Fildes N, Horning SJ, Begovich AB. Localization of predisposition to Hodgkin's disease in the HLA class II region. *Am J Hum Genet* 1994;54:497–505.
45. Tonks S, Oza AM, Lister TA, Bodmer JG. Association of HLA-DPB with Hodgkin's disease. *Lancet* 1992;340:968–969.
46. Taylor GM, Gokhale DA, Crowther D, et al. Increased frequency of HLAA-DPB10301 in Hodgkin's disease suggests that susceptibility is HVR-sequence and subtype-associated. *Leukemia* 1996;10:854–859.

47. Dorak MT, Mills KI, Poynton CH, Burnett AK. HLA and Hodgkin's disease (letter). *Leukemia* 1996;10:1671–1672.
48. Masih A, Weisenburger DD, Duggan M. Epstein-Barr viral genome in lymph nodes from patients with Hodgkin disease may be not specific to Reed-Sternberg cells. *Am J Pathol* 1991;139:37–43.
49. Morris JDH, Eddleston ALWF, Crook T. Viral infection and cancer. *Lancet* 1995;346:754–758.
50. Preciado MV, De Matteo E, Diez B, Menarguez J, Grinstein S. Presence of Epstein-Barr virus and strain type assignment in Argentine childhood Hodgkin's disease. *Blood* 1995;86:3922–3929.
51. Aarate-Osorno A, Roman LN, Kingma DW, Meneses-Garcia A, Jaffe ES. Hodgkin's disease in Mexico, prevalence of Epstein-Barr virus sequences and correlation with histologic subtypes. *Cancer* 1995;75:1360–1366.
52. O'Grady J, Stewart S, Elton RA, Krajewski AS. Epstein-Barr virus in Hodgkin's disease and site of origin of tumor. *Lancet* 1994;343:265–266.
53. Chan JKC, Yip TTC, Tsang WYW, Lau WH, Wong CSc, Ma VWS. Detection of Epstein-Barr virus in Hodgkin's disease occurring in an Oriental population. *Hum Pathol* 1995;26:314–318.
54. Ko DWT, Loke SSL, Srivastava G, Ho FCS. *Epstein-Barr virus in Hodgkin's disease can be both clonal or nonclonal.* Paper presented at the seventh congress of the Asian Pacific division of the International Society of Hematology, November 1991, Hong Kong.
55. Jarrett RF, Gallagher A, Jones DB. Detection of Epstein-Barr virus genomes in Hodgkin's disease, relation to age. *J Clin Pathol* 1991;44:844–848.
56. Gulley ML, Eagan PA, Quintanilla-Martinez L. Epstein-Barr virus DNA is abundant and monoclonal in Reed-Sternberg cells of Hodgkin's disease, association with mixed cellularity subtype and Hispanic American ethnicity. *Blood* 1994;83:1595–1602.
57. Chang KL, Albujar PF, Chen YY. High incidence of Epstein-Barr virus in reed-Sternberg cells of Hodgkin's disease occurring in Peru. *Blood* 1993;81:496–501.
58. Ambinder RF, Browning PJ, Lorenzana I. Epstein-Barr virus status and childhood Hodgkin's disease in Honduras and the United States. *Blood* 1993;81:462–467.
59. Ohshima K, Kikuchi M, Eguchi F. Analysis of Epstein-Barr viral genomes in lymphoid malignancy using Southern blotting, polymerase chain reaction and *in-situ* hybridization. *Virchows Arch B* 1990;59:383–390.
60. Uhara H, Sata Y, Mukai K. Detection of Epstein-Barr virus DNA in Reed-Sternberg cells of Hodgkin's disease using polymerase chain reaction and *in-situ* hybridization. *Jpn J Cancer Res* 1990;81:272–278.
61. Tomita Y, Ohsawa M, Kanno H, et al. Epstein-Barr virus in Hodgkin's disease patients in Japan. *Cancer* 1996;77:186–192.
62. Zhou XG, Hamilton-Dutoit SJ, Yan QH. The association between Epstein-Barr virus and Chinese Hodgkin's disease. *Int J Cancer* 1993;55:359–365.
63. Park CS, Juhng SW, Brigati DJ, Montone KT. Analysis of Epstein-Barr virus in Hodgkin's disease: experience of a single university hospital in Korea. *J Clin Lab Anal* 1994;8:412–417.
64. Li PJ, Zhou XG, Liu SR. The association of Epstein-Barr virus with Hodgkin's lymphoma in childhood. *Chin J Pathol* 1994;23:224–226.
65. Huh J, Park CS, Juhng A, Kim CE, Poppema S, Kim C. A pathological study of Hodgkin's disease in Korea and its association with the Epstein-Barr virus infection. *Cancer* 1996;77:949–955.
66. Tomita Y, Ohsawa M, Kanno H, et al. Epstein-Barr virus in Hodgkin's disease patients in Japan. *Cancer* 1996;77:186–192.
67. Mikata Am Li D, Oda K, Kuroshu K, Yumoto N, Furukawa R, Takenouchi T. EBV genome in Hodgkin's disease in Japan (abstract). *J Pathol* 1994;1759(Suppl 8):153A.
68. Weinreb PS, Day PJR, Niggli F, et al. The role of Epstein-Barr virus in Hodgkin's disese from different geographical areas. *Arch Dis Child* 1996;74:27–31.
69. Rana R, Chopra R, Masih K, Zzchariah A, Prabhakar BR, Mahajan MK. Hodgkin's disease, a clinicopathological study. *Indian J Pathol Microbiol* 1995;38:245–249.
70. Gupta R, Parikh PM, Advani SH, et al. Hodgkin's disease with bone marrow involvement. *Indian J Cancer* 1989;26:58–66.
71. Ramadas K, Sankaranarayanan R, Nair MK, Nair B, Padmanabhan TK. Adult Hodgkin's disease in Kerala. *Cancer* 1994;73:2213–2217.
72. Dinshaw KA, Pande SC, Shrivastava SK, et al. The relevance of a staging laparotomy for Hodgkin's disease in India. *J Surg Oncol* 1992;49:39–44.
73. Muckaden MA, Dinshaw KA, Shrivastava SK, et al. *Early stage Hodgkin's disease, Tata Memorial Centre experience.* Paper presented at Radiotherapy and Oncology 1995: Association of Radiation Oncologists of India, Sixteenth Annual Meeting and Roentgen Centenary Celebration, February 2–4, 1995, Kerala, India, pp 232–233.
74. Kapoor G, Advani SH, Dinshaw KA, et al. Treatment results of Hodgkin's disease in Indian children. *Pediatr Hematol Oncol* 1995;12:559–569.
75. Liang R, Choi P, Todd D, Chan TK, Choy D, Ho F. Hodgkin's disease in Hong Kong Chinese. *Hematol Oncol* 1989;7:395–403.
76. Liang R, Todd, Chan TK, Wong KL, Ho F, Loke SL. Peripheral T-cell lymphoma. *J Clin Oncol* 1987;5:759–765.
77. The Non-Hodgkin's Lymphoma Classification Project. A clinical evaluation of the International Lymphoma Study Group Classification of non-Hodgkin's lymphoma. *Blood* 1997;89:3909–3918.
78. Levi F, La Vecchia, Lucchini F, Negri E. Worldwide trends in cancer mortality in the elderly. *Eur J Cancer* 1996;32A:652–672.

Subject Index

D

Q

R